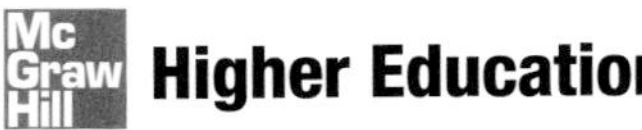

CLINICAL PROCEDURES FOR MEDICAL ASSISTING, SECOND EDITION

Published by McGraw-Hill, a business unit of The McGraw-Hill Companies, Inc., 1221 Avenue of the Americas, New York, NY 10020.

This book is printed on acid-free paper.

1 2 3 4 5 6 7 8 9 0 QPD/QPD 0 9 8 7 6 5

ISBN 0-07-321394-2

Publisher: *David Culverwell*
Senior Sponsoring Editor: *Roxan Kinsey*
Developmental Editor: *Patricia Forrest*
Editorial Coordinator: *Connie Kuhl*
Outside Developmental Services: *Julie Scardiglia*
Senior Marketing Manager: *James F. Connely*
Senior Project Manager: *Sheila M. Frank*
Senior Production Supervisor: *Laura Fuller*
Media Project Manager: *Sandra M. Schnee*
Media Technology Producer: *Janna Martin*
Designer: *Laurie B. Janssen*
Cover Designer: *Studio Montage*
Lead Photo Research Coordinator: *Carrie K. Burger*
Supplement Producer: *Tracy Konrardy*
Compositor: *Interactive Composition Corporation*
Typeface: *10/12 Slimbach*
Printer: *Quebecor World Dubuque Inc.*

Cover photo credits: Front (left to right); Photodisc: Medicine & Health Care, © Jose Luis Pelaez, Inc./CORBIS, Medical Still Life Brand X Pictures, Medical Perspectives Photodisc, Medical Still Life Brand X Pictures, Medical Still Life Brand X Pictures, Total Care Programming, Inc. Back (left to right); Photodisc: V40 Health & Medicine 2, Total Care Programming, Inc., © JFPI Studies, Inc./CORBIS, Photodisc: V18 Health & Medicine, Total Care Programming, Inc., Medical Still Life Brand X Pictures, Total Care Programming, Inc.

Library of Congress Cataloging-in-Publication Data

Clinical procedures for medical assisting/Barbara Ramutkowski . . . [et al.]. — 2nd ed. update.
p. cm.
Includes index.
ISBN 0-07-321394-2 (hard copy : alk. paper)
1. Physicians' assistants. 2. Clinical medicine.
[DNLM: 1. Physician Assistants. W 21.5 C641 2005b]. I. Ramutkowski, Barbara.

R697.P45C557 2005
610.73'7069—dc22 2005007145
CIP

WARNING NOTICE: The clinical procedures, medicines, dosages, and other matters described in this publication are based upon research of current literature and consultation with knowledgeable persons in the field. The procedures and matters described in this text reflect currently accepted clinical practice. However, this information cannot and should not be relied upon as necessarily applicable to a given individual's case. Accordingly, each person must be separately diagnosed to discern the patient's unique circumstances. Likewise, the manufacturer's package insert for current drug product information should be consulted before dministering any drug. Publisher disclaims all liability for any inaccuracies, omissions, misuse, or misunderstanding of the ormation contained in this publication. Publisher cautions that this publication is not intended as a substitute for the essional judgment of trained medical personnel.

hhe.com

Brief Contents

Clinical Medical Assisting 2

SECTION 7

Externship 768

APPENDIXES

Contents

Procedures

Preface

Clinical Procedures for Medical Assisting, 2nd Edition, is a complete clinical textbook for the medical assisting student at the postsecondary level. It acquaints the student with all the clinical knowledge, skills, and duties expected of a medical assistant, from the general to the specific. The book speaks directly to the student, with chapter introductions, case studies, procedures, and chapter summaries written to engage the student's attention and build a sense of positive anticipation about joining the profession of medical assisting.

When referring to patients in the third person, we have alternated between passages that describe a male patient and passages that describe a female patient. Thus, the patient will be referred to as "he" half the time and as "she" half the time. The same convention is used to refer to the physician. The medical assistant is consistently addressed as "you."

Patient Education

Throughout the book we provide the medical assistant with the information needed to educate patients so that patients can participate fully in their health care. Whenever tasks involving interaction with patients are described, the focus is on the patient's needs and on the role of the medical assistant in making the patient an active participant in her own care. Several chapters are primarily or exclusively devoted to interaction with patients—such as Chapter 18, on interviewing the patient.

There is a particular focus on patient education. It is always desirable for patients to be as knowledgeable as possible about their health. Patients who do not understand what is expected of them may become confused, frightened, angry, and uncooperative; educated patients are better able to understand why compliance is important.

We have also made a consistent effort to discuss patients with special needs. A number of chapters in the book contain special sections of text devoted to the particular concerns of certain patient groups. These groups include the following:

- **Pregnant women.** Pregnancy has profound effects on every aspect of health, all of which must be taken into account when working with pregnant patients. Where appropriate, we have addressed special concerns for pregnant patients, such as positioning them for an examination, recommending changes in diet, and taking care to avoid harming the fetus with drugs or procedures that would ordinarily pose little or no risk to the patient. Chapter 38, on the general physical examination, includes a separate procedure for meeting the needs of the pregnant patient during an examination.
- **Elderly patients.** Special care is often required with elderly patients. The body undergoes many changes with age, and patients may have difficulty adjusting to their changing physical needs. Several chapters deal with the special needs of elderly patients, such as Chapter 21, which includes an Educating the Patient feature on preventing falls of the elderly.
- **Children.** The special needs of children are complex, because not only their bodies but also their minds and social situations are very different from those of adults. Dealing with children usually means dealing with their parents as well, and medical assistants must hone their communication skills to meet the needs of both patient and parent when working with children. One chapter that focuses on children is Chapter 22, which discusses the medical specialty of pediatrics.
- **Patients with disabilities.** Many different diseases and disabilities require extra effort or consideration on the part of the medical assistant. Patients in wheelchairs and patients with diabetes, hemophilia, or visual or hearing impairments all require specific accommodations. For example, Chapter 4 addresses the needs of such patients; it includes a section that discusses the Americans With Disabilities Act and a procedure for making the examination room safe for patients with visual impairments.
- **Patients from other cultures.** Communicating with patients from other cultures, especially when language barriers are involved, poses a special challenge for the medical assistant. In addition, patients from other cultures may have attitudes about medicine or about social interaction that differ sharply from those of the medical assistant's culture. Chapter 20 is one chapter that deals in depth with patients from other cultur It contains a text section and a Caution: Handl Care feature about different cultures' attitu medicine.

Because safety is a primary concern tient and the medical assistant, we have aspect of medical assisting work. Every procedure includes appropriate icons, discussed in Chapter 1, for safety precautions required by the Occupational Safety and Health Administration (OSHA) guidelines. These icons for the OSHA guidelines appear in order of use within each procedure. If hand washing is necessary more than once, the hand washing icon appears twice. If biohazardous waste is generated during the procedure, the biohazardous waste container icon will appear, and so on.

Areas of Competence

A key feature of *Clinical Procedures* that will enhance its usefulness to both students and instructors is its reference to the areas of competence defined in the 2003 AAMA (American Association of Medical Assistants) Role Delineation Study. The study, which replaces the 1990 DACUM (*D*eveloping *A* Curricul*UM*) analysis, provides a comprehensive list of duties and skills that medical assistants must master at the entry level. The Committee on Accreditation of Allied Health Education Personnel (CAAHEP) requires that all medical assistants be proficient in the 71 entry-level areas of competence when they begin medical assisting work. The opening page of each chapter provides a list of the areas of competence that the chapter covers, and the complete Medical Assistant Role Delineation Chart is provided as an appendix. (A correlation chart also appears in the *Instructor's Resource Binder.*) The chapter-by-chapter listing of areas of competence allows instructors to identify skills that have been covered in the course and helps students find the chapters that cover specific skills and duties.

We have been careful to ensure that the text provides ample coverage of topics used to construct the AMT (Association of Medical Technologists) Registered Medical Assistant (RMA) Exam. A correlation chart appears in the *Instructor's Resource Binder.*

Organization of the Text

Clinical Procedures for Medical Assisting, 2nd Edition, is divided into seven sections, each of which relates to a broad topic or area of skills. Each section is set apart, and the general areas of competence covered, with the exception of the chapters in the section on anatomy and physiology, are included within each chapter. The ordering of sections, and of chapters within each section, allows the student and the instructor to build a knowledge base starting with the fundamentals and working toward an understanding of highly specialized tasks.

Section 1 begins with a grounding in principles of asepsis, a concept that is crucial to all clinical procedures, before delving into the details of infection control and blood-borne pathogens. Section 2 provides the student with information on anatomy and physiology, beginning with a chapter on the organization of the body; each chapter that follows addresses a particular body system. The chapters in this section also include information on the most common disease and disorders of each body system. Section 3 leads the student into details of the general physical examination; Section 4 builds on that knowledge as it explores highly specialized physical examinations. Section 5 explores the technical details of laboratory testing, and Section 6 involves the most complex and challenging aspects of clinical medical assisting, including drug administration, electrocardiography, and radiology. Section 7 provides the student with information about the medical assisting externship and preparing to find a position as a medical assistant.

Each chapter opens with a page of material that includes the chapter outline and objectives, a list of key terms, and the areas of competence covered in the chapter. The main text of each chapter begins with an overview of chapter content and includes a case study for students to consider as they read the chapter. The main text of each chapter is organized into topics that move from the general to the specific. Color photographs, anatomic and technical drawings, tables, charts, and text features help educate the student about various aspects of medical assisting. The text features, set off in boxes within the text, include the following:

- **Case Studies** are provided at the beginning of all chapters. They represent situations similar to those that the medical assistant may encounter in daily practice. Students are encouraged to consider the case study as they read each chapter. Case Study Questions in the end-of-chapter review check students' understanding and application of chapter content.
- **Procedures** give step-by-step instructions on how to perform the specific administrative tasks a medical assistant will be required to perform. A list of the procedures, which follows the Table of Contents, details the procedures found in each chapter, the AAMA competency number associated with each specific procedure, and if information related to that procedure is included on the student CD.
- **"Tips for the Office"** features provide guidelines on keeping the administration of the medical office running smoothly and efficiently.
- **"Educating the Patient"** focuses on ways to instruct patients about caring for themselves outside of the medical office.
- **"Diseases and Disorders"** features give detailed information on specific medical conditions, including how to recognize, prevent, and treat them.
- **"Pathophysiology"** features within the chapters on anatomy and physiology provide a description about the most common diseases and disorders, including information on the causes, signs and symptoms, and treatment options.
- **"Caution: Handle With Care"** boxes cover the precautions to be taken in certain situations or when performing certain tasks.
- **"Career Opportunities"** provide the student with information on various specialized medical professions

or duties related to the medical assistant's role within the healthcare team.

Each chapter closes with a summary of the chapter material, focusing on the role of the medical assistant. The summary is followed by an end-of-chapter review that consists of the following elements:

- Case Study Questions
- Discussion Questions
- Critical Thinking Questions
- Application Activities
- Internet Activities

These questions and activities allow students to practice specific skills.

The book also includes a glossary and several appendices for use as reference tools. The Glossary lists all the words presented as key terms in each chapter, along with a pronunciation guide and the definitions of each term. The appendices include the Medical Assistant Role Delineation Chart, commonly used prefixes and suffixes, Latin and Greek terms, abbreviations and symbols used in medical terminology, and a comprehensive list of professional organizations and agencies.

The Student CD-ROM provides a comprehensive learning program that is correlated to each chapter of the text and reinforces competencies required to become a medical assistant. Short video clips and pictures introduce skills and case studies for application. In addition, numerous interactive exercises and applications are provided for every chapter in the text. The Student CD, included with each student textbook, provides the following menu choices:

- Administrative Practice
- Clinical Practice
- Anatomy and Physiology Review
- Games
    - Spin the Wheel
    - Key Term Concentration
- Interactive Review
- Audio Glossary
- Progress Report
- Online Learning Center

The Online Learning Center is a text-specific website that offers an extensive array of learning and teaching tools, including chapter quizzes with immediate feedback, newsfeeds, links to relevant websites, and many more study resources. Log on at www.mhhe.com/medicalassisting

Ancillaries

The *Student Workbook* provides an opportunity for the student to review the material and skills presented in the textbook. On a chapter-by-chapter basis, it provides:

- Vocabulary review exercises, which test knowledge of key terms in the chapter
- Content review exercises, which test the student's knowledge of key concepts in the chapter
- Critical thinking exercises, which test the student's understanding of key concepts in the chapter
- Application exercises, which test mastery of specific skills
- Case studies, which apply the chapter material to real-life situations or problems
- Competency checklists for the procedures in the text

The *Instructor's Resource Binder* provides the instructor with materials to help organize lessons and classroom interactions. It includes:

- A complete lesson plan for each chapter, including an introduction to the lesson, teaching strategies, alternate teaching strategies, case studies, assessment, chapter close, resources, and an answer key to the student textbook
- Procedure competency checklists, reproduced from the *Student Workbook*
- An answer key to the *Student Workbook*
- Charts that show the location in the student textbook, the *Student Workbook*, and the *Instructor's Resource Binder*, of material that correlates with the 2003 AAMA Role Delineation Study Areas of Competence, the SCANS Competencies, the National Health Care Skill Standards, and the AMT Registered Medical Assistant (RMA) Certification Exam Topics
- Power Point Presentations on the IPC CD-ROM

Computer software for the student and instructor is also available. The Student CD-ROM is packaged with each student textbook. The Instructor Resource CD-ROM provides easy-to-use resources for class preparation. The Instructor Resource CD-ROM includes the following:

- Exam*View*® Pro Test Generator with answer rationales and correlations to AAMA competencies
- PowerPoint® Presentations
- Correlations to AAMA and AMT Standards
- Course syllabi

Together, the Student Edition, the *Student Workbook*, and the *Instructor's Resource Binder* form a complete teaching and learning package. The *Medical Assisting* course will prepare students to enter the medical assisting field with all the knowledge and skills needed to be a useful resource to patients, a valued asset to employers, and a credit to the medical assisting profession.

Acknowledgments

The publisher and authors would like to
viewers and contributors for their assist
this revision. We appreciate their sugg

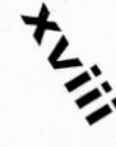

Case studies represent situations similar to those that the medical assistant may encounter in daily practice

CHAPTER 26

Medical Emergencies and First Aid

AREAS OF COMPETENCE

2003 Role Delineation Study

CLINICAL

Patient Care

- Adhere to established patient screening procedures
- Obtain patient history and vital signs
- Recognize and respond to emergencies

GENERAL

Professionalism

- Prioritize and perform multiple tasks

Instruction

- Locate community resources and disseminate information

CHAPTER OUTLINE

- Understanding Medical Emergencies
- Preparing for Medical Emergencies
- Accidental Injuries
- Common Illnesses
- Less Common Illnesses
- Common Psychosocial Emergencies
- The Patient Under Stress
- Educating the Patient
- Disasters
- Bioterrorism

OBJECTIVES

After completing Chapter 26, you will be able to:

26.1 Discuss the importance of first aid during a medical emergency.
26.2 Describe the purpose of the emergency medical services (EMS) system and explain how to contact it.
26.3 List items found on a crash cart or first-aid tray.
26.4 List general guidelines to follow in emergencies.
26.5 Compare various degrees of burns and their treatments.
26.6 Demonstrate how to help a choking victim.
26.7 Demonstrate cardiopulmonary resuscitation (CPR).
26.8 Demonstrate four ways to control bleeding.

KEY TERMS

automated external defibrillator (AED)
bioterrorism
cast
chain of custody
concussion
contusion
crash cart
dehydration
dislocation
epistaxis
hematemesis
hematoma
hyperglycemia
hypoglycemia
hypovolemic shock
palpitations
recovery position
septic shock
splint
sprain
strain
stroke
tachycardia
ventricular fibrillation
xiphoid process

Chapter openers include chapter outlines, objectives, key terms, and the competencies covered in each chapter.

Introduction

Medical assisting is one of the fastest-growing occupations in allied health care today. Health care is changing at a rapid rate, from advanced technology to implementing cost-effective medicine while maintaining quality patient care. The medical assistant is the perfect complement to this changing industry. Employers are looking for health care professionals who are "generalists." A generalist is someone who is trained in all departments in the facility in which they are employed. Medical assistants who graduate from an accredited institution will gain the skills that enable them to multitask. A multitasking professional is someone who is able to work in the administrative areas, the clinical areas, and the financial areas. Employers are seeking credentialed health care professionals who are dedicated to the profession and the patient.

This chapter will introduce the professional standards that are required in medical assisting.

CASE STUDY

Medical assistants are considered generalists in most medical environments. The following scenarios describe how the medical assistant functions as a generalist or multiskilled professional. As you review the scenarios, make note of the many duties the medical assistant performs.

Scenario 1 Kim is 28 years old. She has been working as a medical assistant for 6 years. She is currently working in a family practice office with two doctors, two other medical assistants, and a medical records clerk. Her role is primarily administrative; she is mainly responsible for phone reception and patient check-in and check-out.

A 29-year-old female patient calls complaining of lower back pain. As Kim listens ... scribe her condition, she determines the severity of the patient's discomfo... appointment. When the patient arrives at the office, Kim greets he... and insurance information, and escorts her to an exam ... patient is instructed to see Kim on the way ou... diagnostic test and laboratory work ... and gives the patient a ... ment and files ...

Subcutaneous. Orally referred to as sub Q by most health-care professionals, a subcutaneous injection provides a slow, sustained release of a drug and a relatively long duration of action. Generally, 1 mL or less of a drug can be delivered by SC injection (Procedure 33-5). Various drugs, such as insulin and heparin, are commonly administered by SC injection.

Common subcutaneous injection sites include an area on the back between the shoulder blades, the outer sides of the upper arms and thighs, and the abdomen (except for a 2-inch area around the umbilicus). To prepare for an SC injection, select a site away from bones and blood vessels. Do not use an area that is edematous (swollen), scarred, or hardened or one that has a large amount of fat, because

PROCEDURE 33.5

Giving a Subcutaneous Injection

Objective: To administer a subcutaneous injection safely and effectively, using sterile technique

OSHA Guidelines

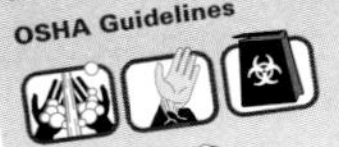

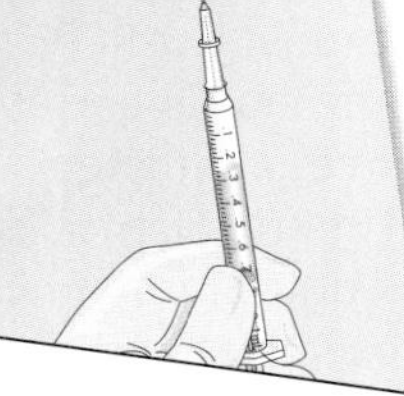

...chart), alcohol

Specific administrative or clinical tasks are illustrated in a step-by-step format in the Procedures boxes.

Educating the Patient

Teaching Patients About Sexually Transmitted Diseases

You must provide complete and detailed information with a nonjudgmental and supportive attitude when you teach patients about sexually transmitted diseases. Begin with the principle that all STDs are preventable. The key to prevention is avoiding sexual activities in which blood, semen, or vaginal secretions pass from one person to another.

There are various levels of protection in connection with STDs. The only absolute methods of "safe sex" are abstinence (no sex) and masturbation (self-stimulation). The next level is mutual monogamy, in which partners have sex only with each other. Emphasize that monogamy provides protection from STDs only if neither partner has an STD when the relationship begins. A final level of prevention applies to people who do not practice abstinence or mutual monogamy but wish to protect themselves and others from STDs. The following measures provide some protection.

- Use a latex condom and spermicide for every act of intercourse. (Use a latex condom during oral sex.)
- Know all your sexual partners, and discuss STD prevention with them.
- Have a physician regularly screen you for STDs because many people, especially men, have no signs when they are infected.
- Consult a physician if any signs of STDs develop, such as a blister, sore, discharge, rash, or abdominal pain.

Encourage patients to ask questions and discuss any concerns they have. Explain the need to make follow-up appointments with a physician if appropriate.

Teaching a patient who has been diagnosed with an STD how to treat or manage the disease is especially important. Make sure the patient understands all directions and the necessity for treatment. Bacterial infections such as chlamydia, gonorrhea, and syphilis can be cured with antibiotics as long as the patient takes all the medication in the prescribed manner. Viral infections such as AIDS, genital herpes, and genital warts cannot be cured, although they can be treated and managed to differing degrees.

Emphasize to patients with an STD that they should avoid all sexual contact until the infection has been treated completely. Many STDs can be spread through any type of genital contact, including vaginal intercourse, anal sex, and oral sex. Herpes can be spread through kissing if there are herpes sores in the mouth. Encourage patients to inform each person with whom they had sexual contact that they have contracted an STD. Explain that unless all sexual partners are treated successfully, the disease will pass back and forth indefinitely.

You can reinforce your education efforts by providing patients with materials on the prevention and treatment of STDs. Keep a variety of pamphlets, books, and other resources in your office to help patients cope with and manage STDs.

drug to kill the organism, and the organism will build up a tolerance to the antibiotic.

Sexually Transmitted Diseases. Sexually transmitted diseases (STDs)—diseases acquired through sexual contact with an infected person—are also infectious diseases. The number and severity of these diseases, their high incidence, and the great amount of misinformation about them warrant a discussion apart from other infectious diseases. (AIDS is discussed in Chapter 3.) Internists, infectious disease specialists, pediatricians, urologists, and gynecologists are all involved in the diagnosis and treatment of STDs.

Patient Education About STDs. Your role as an educator is vital in dealing with patients who have STDs. Some patients may be hesitant to ask for information. Providing educational materials in the examination room will help answer their questions and put them at ease. These materials deal with sensitive or embarrassing topics, and the patient's privacy must be maintained. Printed materials are available from several medical agencies and should be provided to your patients. In addition, you must educate patients about prevention and treatment of STDs. The Educating the Patient section provides more information on this topic.

Common Types of STDs. Your role in assisting the doctor in the treatment of STDs will involve emphasizing to the patient the importance of completing the course of therapy and avoiding sexual contact while the infection is still active. Sexual partners must also be treated to avoid reinfection. Several types of STDs are fairly common.

Candidiasis is a yeast infection. It is not a true STD but is included with the STDs because the infection can be transmitted between sexual partners. Symptoms include severe genital itching, redness and swelling of the vaginal or vulval tissue, light yellow or white patches (usually cheesy

Assisting With Examinations in the Basic Specialties 357

Patient instruction on self care outside the medical office is the focus in the Educating the Patient boxes.

Handle With Care boxes cover precautions to be taken when performing certain tasks.

CAUTION Handle With Care

Preventing Transmission of Viruses in the Health-Care Setting

Certain procedures are thought to cause the transmission of infection from a medical worker to a patient, and other procedures may also carry that risk. For example, skin-puncture injuries in medical workers are not uncommon. Therefore, many procedures involving needles are considered exposure-prone. If the worker's skin is cut or punctured, the patient could be exposed to the worker's blood.

The risk that a health-care worker will transmit an infection to a patient is small, if proper precautions are taken. Workers participating in high-risk procedures, however, should take extra precautions. Workers with skin conditions characterized by sores that secrete fluid should forgo direct patient care and the handling of equipment used for exposure-prone procedures until the condition has healed. Workers performing high-risk procedures should know their HIV and HBV status. (HIV refers to the virus that causes AIDS; HBV refers to the hepatitis B virus.) HBV vaccination is strongly recommended.

A health-care worker who is infected with HIV or HBV should not perform procedures that might result in exposure without the advice of an expert review panel. This panel might include the health-care worker's own physician, someone with expert knowledge about the transmission of infectious disease, a medical professional with expert knowledge about the procedures in question, public health officials, and a member of the infection control committee of the institution.

The panel will advise the worker about when she will be allowed to perform certain procedures. The panel will require her to inform potential patients of the infection before the procedure. The panel must, however, otherwise protect the health-care worker's confidentiality.

Although there has been great controversy on the subject, there are no recommendations in place for required testing of all health-care workers for HIV or HBV because the risk of transmission from ... patient is not considered great ... expense. Educational ... reinforce the ... ers sh...

- Hepatitis D (delta agent he... in people infected ... make th...

Career Opportunities boxes provide information on professions and duties related to medical assisting.

Career Opportunities

HIV/AIDS Instructor *(continued)*

- The Workplace HIV/AIDS Program, which is tailored for each specific work site and covers topics such as rights and responsibilities, disability laws, local resources, and other issues of interest to employers and employees.
- Act SMART, developed by the Red Cross and the Boys & Girls Clubs of America to provide prevention knowledge and skills through age-appropriate activities for people ages 6 through 17.

Workplace Settings

HIV/AIDS instructors work in a variety of settings. They may run programs in schools, universities, offices, places of worship, community meeting rooms, clinics, hospitals, and people's homes.

Education

To become an HIV/AIDS instructor, you must be trained and ...fied by your local American Red Cross chapter. There are no specific educational requirements to be eligible for the training. This is often an unpaid volunteer position.

More than 26,000 instructors were teaching one or more of the Red Cross HIV/AIDS programs in 1995. To date, instructors trained by the Red Cross have reached more than 12 million people through HIV/AIDS education sessions. With the increasing awareness of AIDS and other sexually transmitted diseases, this field is expected to grow.

Where to Go for More Information

The American Red Cross
HIV/AIDS Education, Health and Safety Services
8111 Gatehouse Road, 6th Floor
Falls Church, VA 22042
703-206-7180

diseases to perform your job effectively. This knowledge ...ut diseases is useful to you for several reasons. ...ify symptoms that may indicate patients ...d-borne disease ...ation they can use

Diseases and Disorders boxes detail medical conditions and how torecognize, prevent, and treat them.

Diseases and Disorders

Preventing Nosocomial Infections

Patients in hospital settings are at risk not only from the disease or injury that caused the hospitalization but also from nosocomial, or hospital-related, infection. The Centers for Disease Control and Prevention (CDC) publishes a seven-part series discussing techniques for control of nosocomial infections. The guidelines cover the following topics:

- Catheter-associated urinary tract infections
- Hand washing and environmental control
- Infection control in hospital personnel
- Intravascular device-related infections
- Isolation precautions in hospitals (discussed later in this chapter)
- Nosocomial pneumonia
- Surgical wound infections

Researchers at the CDC have found that if hospital personnel pay careful attention to the care of instruments and devices used to deliver care to patients, significant improvements can be made regarding patients' chances for avoiding infection. In addition, new, less-invasive techniques for delivering medications are promising an even greater reduction in patient risk.

To obtain a copy of these guidelines, contact:

National Technical Information Service (NTIS)
5285 Port Royal Road
Springfield, VA 22161
703-487-4650

The CDC can also be found on the World Wide Web at http://www.cdc.gov.

The patient must be isolated from others and undergo antibiotic therapy until tissue cells taken from the nose and the throat show negative results. Once a leading cause of death among young children, diphtheria is now rare in the United States because of widespread immunization. Cases of diphtheria must be reported to the state or county health department.

Haemophilus Influenzae Type B

Haemophilus influenzae type B (Hib) is a frequent cause of bacterial infections—including blood infections, epiglottitis, and pneumonia—in infants and young children in the United States. It is spread through direct, indirect, and droplet transmission. The incubation period is approximately 3 days. The patient may experience upper respiratory symptoms, fever, drowsiness, body aches, and diminished appetite. The infection can also cause bacterial meningitis (a swelling or inflammation of the tissue covering the spinal cord and brain) and should be carefully monitored.

Influenza (Flu)

Nearly everyone has experienced symptoms of influenza, or the flu: fever, chills, headaches, body aches, and upper respiratory congestion. Isolation and other commonsense precautions can greatly reduce transmission of this viral infection.

Measles (Rubeola)

Measles, also called rubeola, is an infectious viral disease spread through droplets or direct transmission. Normally, the disease requires 8 to 13 days for the initial symptom of fever to appear. The characteristic itchy rash appears 14 days after exposure. Patients should follow isolation procedures for 7 days after the rash first appears. Children under the age of 3 are especially at risk for contagion and should be kept apart from family members who have contracted the disease. The CDC requires reporting measles to the state or county health department.

Meningitis

Meningitis is an inflammation and infection of the protective coverings of the brain and spinal cord, and the fluid that surrounds these tissues. Meningitis is usually caused by an infection with a virus or bacteria. Viral meningitis is usually relatively mild. It clears up in a week or two without specific treatment. Viral meningitis is also called aseptic meningitis.

Bacterial meningitis is a serious, life-threatening condition that requires immediate medical treatment. Severe bacterial meningitis can result in brain damage and even death. It affects more men than women. At highest risk are the elderly, children under age 5, and people with chronic illnesses. Risk groups include children in daycare, schools, and college students living in dorms or other close environments.

Between 5% and 20% of the population normally carry the bacteria that cause meningitis. These bacteria are commonly found in the nose and throat. Occasionally, a person who carries these bacteria develops meningitis. A person with an ear or sinus infection is at greater risk for meningitis. In addition, persons who have certain types of skull fractures also have a higher risk for developing meningitis.

For patients over the age of 2, symptoms may include a red, blotchy rash; confusion and delirium (delusions or

40 CHAPTER 2

A summary of the chapter material and an end-of-chapter review close out each chapter.

REVIEW

CHAPTER 14

CASE STUDY QUESTIONS

Now that you have completed this chapter, review the case study at the beginning of the chapter and answer the following questions:

1. Where is the pituitary gland located?
2. What structures are likely to be compressed by a tumor of the pituitary gland?
3. What hormones are normally produced by the pituitary gland?
4. What signs and symptoms would this patient have if she did not take supplemental hormones following the removal of her pituitary gland?

Discussion Questions

1. Explain the difference between an endocrine gland and an exocrine gland.
2. Name the major endocrine organs of the body and give their locations.
3. Explain how the body responds to stress.
4. Explain why the testes and ovaries are described as both endocrine organs and reproductive organs.

Critical Thinking Questions

1. If a patient had his pituitary gland removed, what hormone supplements would he need?
2. What is the danger of a diabetic injecting too much insulin?
3. Why is hyposecretion (insufficient secretion) of thyroid hormone in newborns more serious than hyposecretion in adults?

Application Activities

1. Tell which endocrine gland secretes the following hormones:
   a. Insulin
   b. ADH
   c. Testosterone
   d. Prolactin
   e. Growth hormone
2. Describe the effects the following hormones produce:
   a. Oxytocin
   b. Cortisol
   c. LH and FSH
   d. Glucagon
   e. Estrogen
3. For each of the following diseases, name the hormone that is involved:
   a. Acromegaly
   b. Myxedema
   c. Dwarfism
   d. Diabetes
   e. Cushing's disease
4. Define what a stressor is and give an example.

Internet Activity

Find a Web site that discusses endocrinology. Research t... roles of an endocrinologist and how weight managemen... and endocrinology are related.

228 CHAPTER 14

and commitment to providing information that is relevant and valuable to medical assisting students.

In addition, many people and organizations provided invaluable assistance in the process of illustrating the highly technical and detailed topics covered in the text. Their contributions helped ensure the accuracy, timeliness, and authenticity of the illustrations in the book.

We would like to thank the following organizations for providing source materials and technical advice: the American Association of Medical Assistants, Chicago, Illinois; Becton Dickinson Microbiology Systems, Sparks, Maryland; Becton Dickinson VACUTAINER Systems, Franklin Lakes, New Jersey; Bibbero Systems, Petaluma, California; Burdick, Schaumberg, Illinois; the Corel Corporation, Ottawa, Ontario, Canada; Hamilton Media, Hamilton, New Jersey; Nassau Ear, Nose, and Throat, Princeton, New Jersey; Princeton Allergy and Asthma Associates, Princeton, New Jersey; Richmond International, Boca Raton, Florida; Winfield Medical, San Diego, California.

We would like to express our appreciation to the following New Jersey physicians and medical facilities for allowing us to photograph a variety of procedures and procedural settings at their facilities: the Eric B. Chandler Medical Center, New Brunswick; Helene Fuld School of Nursing of New Jersey, Trenton; Mercer Medical Center, Trenton; Mercer County Vocational-Technical Health Occupations Center, Trenton; Plainfield Health Center, Plainfield; Princeton Allergy and Asthma Associates, Princeton; the Princeton Medical Group, Princeton; Robert Wood Johnson University Hospital, New Brunswick; Robert Wood Johnson University Hospital at Hamilton, Hamilton; St. Francis Medical Center, Trenton; St. Peter's Medical Center, New Brunswick; Dr. Edward von der Schmidt, neurosurgeon, Princeton; Wound Care Center/Curative Network, New Brunswick.

We would also like to thank the following facilities and educational institutions for graciously allowing us to photograph procedures and other technical aspects related to the profession of medical assisting: Total Care Programming, Henrico, North Carolina; Wildwood Medical Clinic, Henrico, North Carolina; Central Piedmont Community College, Charlotte, North Carolina; and Roanoke Rapids Clinic, Roanoke Rapids, Virginia.

Reviewers

Every area of the text was reviewed by practitioners and educators in the field. Their insights helped shape the direction of the book.

Kaye Acton, CMA
Alamance Community College
Graham, NC

Jannie R. Adams, PhD, RN, MS-HSA, BSN
Clayton College and State University,
School of Technology
orrow, GA

Cathy Kelley Arney, CMA, MLT (ASCP), AS
National College of Business and Technology
Bluefield, VA

Joseph Balatbat, MD
Dean of Academics
Sanford Brown Institute

Marsha Benedict, CMA-A, MS, CPC
Baker College of Flint
Flint, MI

Michelle Buchman
Springfield College
Springfield, MO

Patricia Celani, CMA
ICM School of Business and Medical Careers
Pittsburgh, PA

Theresa Cyr, RN, BN, MS
Heald Business College
Honolulu, HI

Barbara Desch
San Joaquin Valley College
Visalia, CA

Herbert J. Feitelberg, BA, DPM
King's College
Charlotte, NC

Geri L. Finn
Remington College, Dallas Campus
Garland, TX

Kimberly L. Gibson, RN, DOE
Sanford Brown Institute
Middleburg Heights, OH

Barbara G. Gillespie, MS
San Diego & Grossmont Community College Districts
El Cajon, CA

Cindy Gordon, MBA, CMA
Baker College
Muskegon, MI

Mary Harmon
MedTech College
Indianapolis, IN

Glenda H. Hatcher, BSN
Southwest Georgia Technical College
Thomasville, GA

Helen J. Hauser, RN, MSHA, RMA
Phoenix College
Phoenix, AZ

Christine E. Hetrick
Cittone Institute
Mt. Laurel, NJ

Beulah A. Hofmann, RN, MSN, CMA
Ivy Tech State College
Terre Haute, IN

Karen Jackson
Remington College
Dallas Campus, Dallas, TX

Latashia Y. D. Jones, LPN
CAPPS College, Montgomery Campus
Montgomery, AL

Donna D. Kyle-Brown, PhD, RMA
CAPPS College, Mobile Campus
Mobile, AL

Sharon McCaughrin
Ross Learning
Southfield, MI

Tanya Mercer, BS, RMA
Kaplan Higher Education Corporation
Roswell, GA

T. Michelle Moore-Roberts
CAPPS College, Montgomery Campus
Montgomery, AL

Linda Oprean
Applied Career Training
Manassas, VA

Julie Orloff, RMA, CMA, CPT, CPC
Ultrasound Diagnostic School
Miami, FL

Delores W. Orum, RMA
CAPPS College
Montgomery, AL

Katrina L. Poston, MA, RHE
Applied Career Training
Arlington, VA

Manuel Ramirez, MD
Texas School of Business
Friendswood, TX

Beatrice Salada, BAS, CMA
Davenport University
Lansing, MI

Melanie G. Sheffield, LPN
Capps Medical Institute
Pensacola, FL

Kristi Sopp, RMA
MTI College
Sacramento, CA

Carmen Stevens
Remington College, Fort Worth Campus
Fort Worth, TX

Deborah Sulkowski, BS, CMA
Pittsburgh Technical Institute
Oakdale, PA

Fred Valdes, MD
City College
Ft. Lauderdale, FL

Janice Vermiglio-Smith, RN, MS, PhD
Central Arizona College
Apache Junction, AZ

Erich M. Weldon, MICP, NREMT-P
Apollo College
Portland, Oregon

Terri D. Wyman, CMRS, CMS
Ultrasound Diagnostic School
Springfield, MA

Contributors

Kaye Acton, CMA
Alamance Community College
Graham, North Carolina

Jannie R. Adams, PhD, RN, MS-HSA, BSN
Clayton College and State University, School of Technology
Morrow, Georgia

Cathy Kelley Arney, CMA, MLT (ASCP), AS
National College of Business and Technology
Bluefield, Virginia

Russell E. Battiata
National School of Technology
Miami, Florida

Marti A. Burton, RN, BS
Canadian Valley Technology Center
El Reno, Oklahoma

Ann Coleman
Society of Nuclear Medicine
Reston, Virginia

Barbara G. Gillespie, MS
San Diego and Grossmont Community College Districts
El Cajon, California

Regina Hoffman, PhD
Midlands Technical College
Columbia, South Carolina

Donna D. Kyle-Brown, PhD, RMA
CAPPS College, Mobile Campus
Mobile, Alabama

Cynthia Newby, CPC
Chestnut Hill Enterprises

Melanie G. Sheffield, LPN
Capps Medical Institute
Pensacola, Florida

Cynthia T. Vincent, MMS, PA-C
Wildwood Medical Clinic
Henrico, North Carolina

Terri D. Wyman, CMRS, CMS
Sanford Brown Institute

Previous Edition Reviewers

Janet Aaberg, MS
San Diego Community Colleges
San Diego, CA

Jeri Adler, BA, AA, CMA, CMT
Lane Community College
Eugene, OR

Sr. Patricia Carter, BSN, MS
Stautzenberger College
Findlay, OH

Gwendolyn J. Coleman, RN
Weakley County Vocatonal Center
Dresden, TN

Lisa Cook, RMA, CMA
Eton Technical Institute
Port Orchard, WA

Barbara Dahl, CMA
Whatcom Community College
Bellingham, WA

Joyce Deutsch, RN, CPC-H, CMA
Indiana Business College
Evansville, IN

Suzanne Ezzo, RN, AST, BS, LVT
Sawyer School
Pittsburgh, PA

Tracie Fuqua, AAS, CMA
Wallace State College
Hanceville, AL

Jeanette Girkin, EdD, CMA
Tulsa Junior College
Tulsa, OK

Glenn Grady, MEd, BSMT (ASCP), CMA
Miller-Motte Business College
Wilmington, NC

Christine E. Hollander, CMA, BS
Denver Institute of Technology
Denver, CO

Sue A. Hunt, MA, RN, CMA
Middlesex Community College
Bedford/Lowell, MA

Gwynne Mangiore
Missouri College For Doctors' Assistants
St. Louis, MO

Diane Morlock, CMA
Stautzenberger College
Toledo, OH

Deborah Newton, BS, MA, EMT-I, CMA
Montana State University, College of Technology
Great Falls, MT

Virginia Opitz, RN, BSN, MS, CRRN
North Western Business College
Chicago, IL

Tom Palko, MEd, MCS, MT (ASCP)
Arkansas Tech University
Russellville, AR

Hilda Palko, BS, MT (ASCP), CMA
Russellville, AR

Savatore M. Passanese, AS, BA, MS, PhD
Niagara County Community College
Sanborn, NY

Debra Rosch, CMA
Minnesota School of Business
Brooklyn Center, MN

Jay Shahed, BS, PhD
Robert Morris College
Chicago, IL

Connie W. Stack, BSAH, MLT (ASCP), CMA
Anson Community College
Polkton, NC

Patricia A. Stang, CMA, CPT
Medix School
Baltimore, MD

Geraldine M. Todaro, CMA, CLPLb
Stark State College of Technology
Canton, OH

Kimberly C. Wilson, MT (AMT), CMA
Spencerian College
Louisville, KY

Chris Kientzle, CMA-C, RMA
Sanford Brown College
Hazelwood, MO

Clare Lewandowski, BS, MA, PhD
Columbus State Community College
Columbus, OH

Joan Winters, BS, MS, DLM (ASCP), MT (ASCP)
Wayne Community College
Goldsboro, NC

CLINICAL PROCEDURES

for Medical Assisting

2

Clinical Medical Assisting

"One of the most important things you must remember when assisting with patients is to put yourself in the patient's place. How would you feel if you were told to do something you didn't know how to do? Wouldn't you want to know ahead of time what will be expected of you?

"As a medical assistant, it is your job to anticipate the physician's every need during a physical exam. Compare the process with that of surgery, where the doctor is handed an instrument even before he asks for it. You should try to make as smooth a transition as possible from one step to the next; everyone benefits."

Diane Morlock
Medical Assisting Instructor
Stautzenberger College
Toledo, Ohio

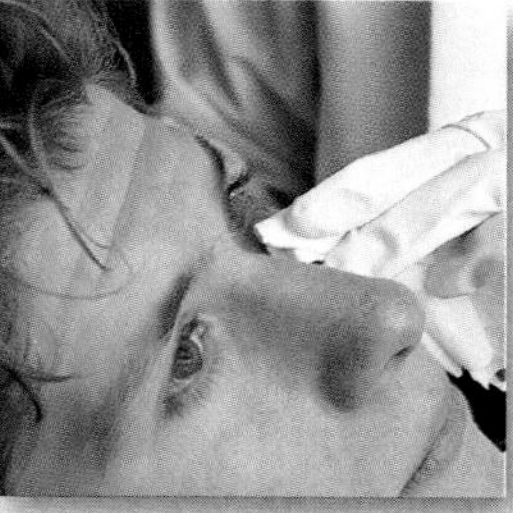

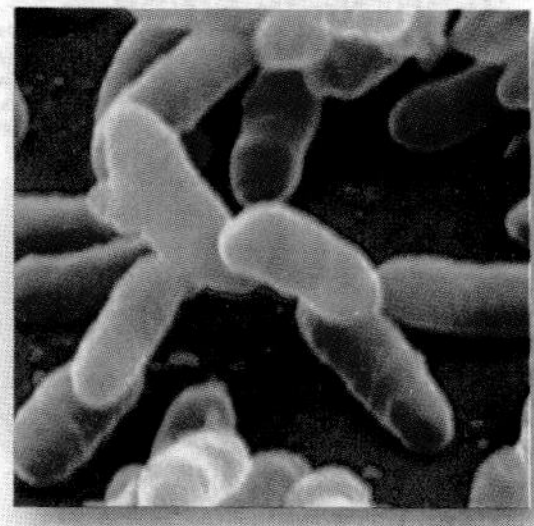

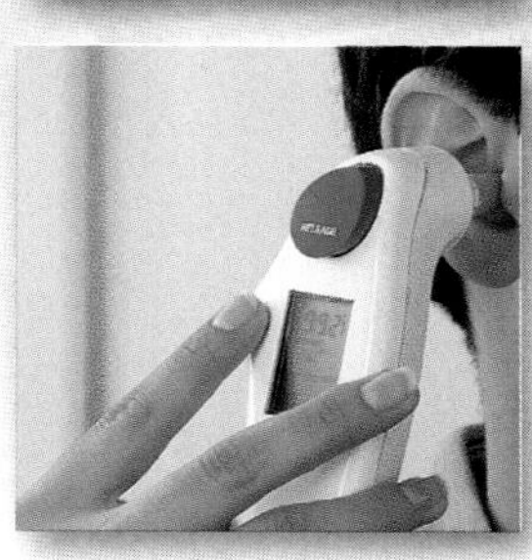

SECTION 1

THE MEDICAL OFFICE ENVIRONMENT

CHAPTER 1

Principles of Asepsis

AREAS OF COMPETENCE

2003 Role Delineation Study

CLINICAL

Fundamental Principles

- Apply principles of aseptic technique and infection control

Patient Care

- Prepare and maintain examination and treatment areas

GENERAL

Instruction

- Teach methods of health promotion and disease prevention

CHAPTER OUTLINE

- History of Infectious Disease Prevention
- Microorganisms and Disease
- The Disease Process
- The Body's Defenses
- The Cycle of Infection
- Breaking the Cycle
- Medical and Surgical Asepsis
- OSHA Blood-borne Pathogens Standard and Universal Precautions
- Educating Patients About Preventing Disease Transmission

OBJECTIVES

After completing Chapter 1, you will be able to:

1.1 Explain the historical background of infectious disease prevention.
1.2 Identify the types of microorganisms that cause disease.
1.3 Explain the disease process.
1.4 Explain how the body's defenses protect against infection.
1.5 Describe the cycle of infection.
1.6 Identify and describe the various methods of disease transmission.
1.7 Explain how you can help break the cycle of infection.
1.8 Compare and contrast medical and surgical asepsis.
1.9 Describe how to perform aseptic hand washing.
1.10 Define the Blood-borne Pathogens Standard and Universal Precautions as described in the rules and regulations of the Occupational Safety and Health Administration (OSHA).
1.11 Explain the role of Universal Precautions in the duties of a medical assistant.
1.12 List the procedures and legal requirements for disposing of hazardous waste.
1.13 Explain how to educate patients in preventing disease transmission.

KEY TERMS

antibodies
antigen
asepsis
bacterial spore
biohazardous materials
biohazardous waste container
carrier
disinfection
endogenous infection
exogenous infection
fomite
immunity
macrophage
microorganism
normal flora
opportunistic infection
pathogen
phagocyte
reservoir host
sanitization
Standard Precautions
sterilization
subclinical case
susceptible host
Universal Precautions
vector
virulence

Introduction

Our bodies are amazing structures that defend us against infections under normal circumstances. As you read this chapter you will learn about disease-causing microorganisms, how the body defends itself against infections, and ways that infections might occur. You also learn how, as a medical assistant, you can be instrumental in helping to break the cycle of infection by practicing asepsis in the office setting as well as by educating patients in the prevention of disease transmission. The chapter concentrates on OSHA's role in the health-care setting and introduces the Blood-borne Pathogens Standard; it also explains how these regulations apply to you.

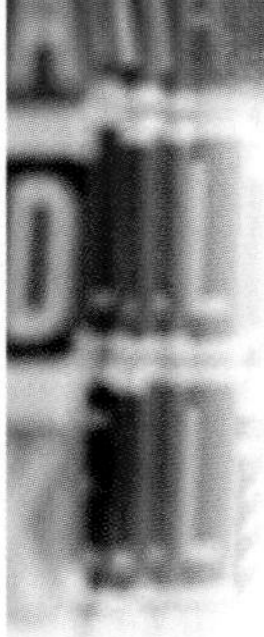

CASE STUDY

The medical assistant employed at the doctor's office was scratched on the hand last week by her kitten, and the scratch subsequently became infected. The office was very busy this week with patients, and the medical assistant did not observe Standard Precautions when assisting with a Category I minor surgical procedure. Two days later, the patient returned to the office with an infected surgical site.

While reading this chapter, consider the following questions:

1. What part of the cycle of infection caused the problem for the medical assistant?
2. How did the patient become infected?
3. How does the Blood-borne Pathogens Standard apply to the medical assistant?
4. Because the medical assistant did not observe the regulation, what penalties, if any, could be imposed by OSHA?

History of Infectious Disease Prevention

Throughout history, doctors have tried to solve the problem of infection: what causes it, how it spreads, how to prevent it, and how to treat it. Some infections, such as the plague in the Middle Ages, have changed the course of history.

During the past century, remarkable advances have taken place in knowledge regarding the causes, prevention, and treatment of infectious disease. The threat of infection, however, is as great as it has ever been. Medical science still wrestles with relatively new infectious diseases, such as acquired immunodeficiency syndrome (AIDS) and Ebola virus disease. In addition, some older diseases (such as methicillin-resistant *Staphylococcus aureus,* or MRSA, and tuberculosis) continue to challenge researchers because they have become resistant to established medications.

As a medical assistant, you need to understand how to perform specific tasks to control infection and prevent disease transmission. Prior to this, you need an understanding of the disease process and spread of infection.

Hippocrates

The Greek physician Hippocrates (circa 460 to 377 B.C.) made the first recorded attempt to control infection. Although Hippocrates is usually associated with the Hippocratic oath, the code of ethics for physicians, his scientific beliefs were as influential as his ethical beliefs. Instead of basing his practice of medicine on religion, he used logic. He believed that environmental and natural forces, such as diet, exercise, climate, and occupation, play the greatest role in disease and health. He taught his students to study disease by observing with the senses and by keeping careful records of patients' symptoms.

Hippocrates believed in simple and natural treatments, using strong drugs and surgery only as a last resort. He often prescribed a diet of basic foods. Some of his treatments—for example, honey in vinegar or boiled water—alleviated the symptoms of infection by causing the body to expel phlegm and urine. One of his innovations, the treatment of wounds with coal tar, was effective in controlling infection. Centuries after Hippocrates' time, scientists discovered that coal tar contains carbolic acid, a natural germ-killing chemical. Carbolic acid, also known as phenol, is a common chemical ingredient in today's antiseptics and disinfectants. It is now used in low concentrations (1.0% to 1.5%) because it is readily absorbed by the body; however, it is carcinogenic at higher levels.

Joseph Lister

Joseph Lister was a British surgeon, scientist, and researcher who lived from 1827 to 1912 (Figure 1-1). He discovered how to use chemical antiseptics to control surgery-related infections caused by invisible organisms known as microorganisms. **Microorganisms** are simple forms of life commonly made up of a single cell. These

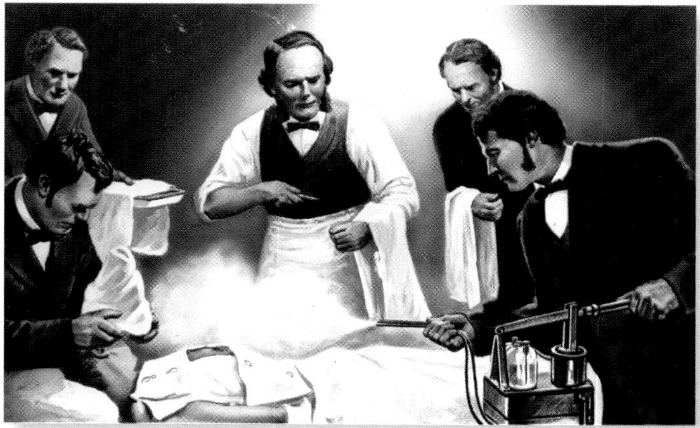

Figure 1-1. Joseph Lister pioneered the study and practice of eliminating as many microorganisms as possible during medical procedures.

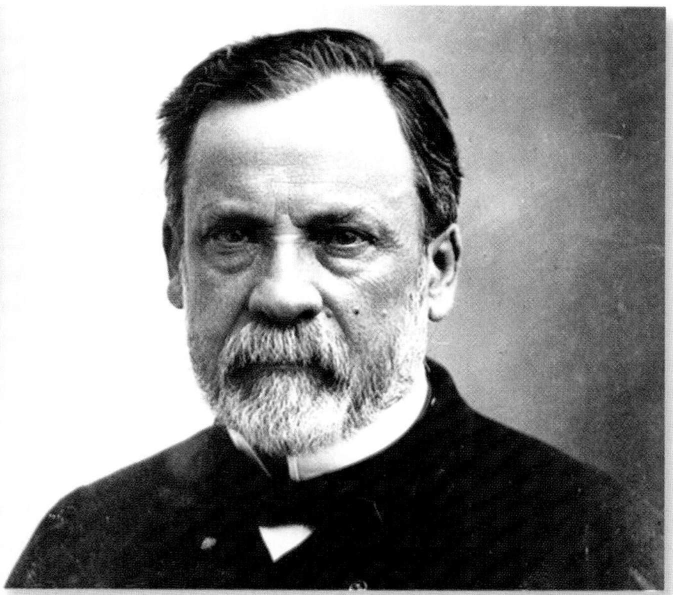

Figure 1-2. Louis Pasteur developed the germ theory and suggested that germs (microorganisms) might cause disease in humans.

organisms are so small that they can be seen only through a microscope.

Lister practiced in the Glasgow Royal Infirmary in Scotland, where 45% to 50% of people who had amputations died as a result of infection. The device used for amputations was simply wiped with a towel or on someone's sleeve and put back in its case. At the time, even simple operations had similar rates of infection and death, and surgery was often fatal. Because people did not yet understand that microorganisms cause infection, almost no one made an effort to destroy the organisms, much less keep a sterile environment and/or sterile surgical instruments.

Lister worked to lower the rate of infection and death. He had heard of the work of Louis Pasteur (1822–1895), the French chemist and microbiologist who had developed the germ theory. Pasteur, shown in Figure 1-2, had discovered that microorganisms, which he called germs, cause particular types of fermentation in certain liquids, such as milk and wine. He suggested that specific germs might also grow in humans and cause specific diseases. He believed that all microorganisms multiply from previously existing ones (biogenesis) rather than spontaneously growing or coming to life from nowhere (abiogenesis). Pasteur worked to increase the practices of hygiene, sanitation, and direct means of destroying microorganisms as ways to fight the spread of disease.

Joseph Lister used Pasteur's germ theory to conclude that microorganisms caused the infection of surgical wounds. He thought that the key was to keep germs from getting into a wound.

In 1865 Lister tried treating wounds with a type of carbolic acid that had been shown to cure infections in cattle. Unsatisfied with the results, he tried a purer form of carbolic acid. Like Pasteur, Lister believed that germs travel mainly through the air, so he tried spraying the acid into the air above the wounds. Later he realized that the germs that come into direct contact with a wound through hands and instruments did more damage than germs in the air. He then applied the acid directly on wounds, cleansing and dressing them with it. As a result, the death rate among the amputees dropped to 15%. Eventually, the death rate from operations went down to 2% to 3%, and surgeons were able to perform a wider variety of operations more safely.

Lister also used antiseptics to disinfect surgical equipment and supplies. His work led to the practice of sterile technique: making an operating room germ-free. This technique included such measures as having workers wear protective, sterile clothing and draping patients to expose only the area being operated on.

Oliver Wendell Holmes and Ignaz Semmelweis

The American physician and essayist Oliver Wendell Holmes (1809–1894) was another key figure in solving the puzzle of infection. In 1843 he published *The Contagiousness of Puerperal Fever.* This paper demonstrated that puerperal fever, a disease that was responsible for the deaths of many women in childbirth, was carried from patient to patient by doctors. This concept was harshly criticized, but Holmes did not back down. He reprinted the paper, with additions, in 1855, after serving as the dean of Harvard Medical School.

About the same time, in Vienna a Hungarian physician, Ignaz Semmelweis (1818–1865), also concluded that puerperal fever was a communicable disease. He ordered students in his hospital ward to scrub their hands with a chlorinated lime solution before moving from one patient to another. Although the hospital's mortality rate from puerperal fever fell dramatically, Semmelweis's views were not widely accepted during his lifetime.

These and other contributions to knowledge about infection have evolved into the current techniques for keeping infectious microorganisms out of the medical office and operating room. These techniques are now widely accepted and are legally required in the practice of medicine. You will apply these techniques in your daily work as a medical assistant.

Microorganisms and Disease

Microorganisms live all around us. They are found in and on our bodies, in the air we breathe, in the water we drink, and on almost every surface we touch. Types of microorganisms include:

- Viruses, the smallest infectious agents, many of which cause disease
- Bacteria, single-celled organisms that reproduce quickly and are a major cause of disease
- Protozoans, single-celled organisms found in soil and water, most of which do not cause disease
- Fungi, organisms with a complex cell structure, most of which do not cause disease
- Very small multicellular organisms, a few of which are parasitic (living on or in another organism) and cause disease

Although everyone is surrounded by microorganisms, people are able to escape infection most of the time for the following three reasons:

1. The majority of microorganisms are either beneficial or harmless. **Pathogens,** microorganisms capable of causing disease, comprise only a small portion of the total number of microorganisms that exist in a given environment.
2. The human body has a wide variety of defenses that allow people to resist infection.
3. Conditions must be favorable for a pathogen to grow and to be transmitted to a person who is susceptible (sensitive) to infection.

The Disease Process

Many types of diseases affect humans. An infectious disease is one that is caused by the action of a microorganism. An infection begins when the microorganism finds a human host, that is, a body in which it can survive, multiply, and thrive. To grow, a microorganism requires specific conditions, which include the proper temperature, pH (a measure of the body's acid-base balance), and moisture level. The temperature within the human body (98.6°F, or 37°C), the body's neutral pH, and the body's dark, moist environment are prime conditions for the growth of microorganisms.

Some pathogens nearly always cause disease, whereas others cause disease less often or only under certain circumstances. A microorganism's disease-producing power is called **virulence.** When microorganisms damage the body, they do so in many ways:

- By depleting nutrients or other materials needed by the cells and tissues they invade
- By reproducing themselves within body cells
- By making body cells the targets of the body's own defenses
- By producing toxins, or poisons, that damage cells and tissues

The Body's Defenses

Daily life constantly exposes people to multitudes of pathogens, but the bodies of healthy individuals have built-in defenses against them. The condition of being resistant to pathogens and the diseases they cause is called **immunity.** When these defenses are not functioning properly (as when individuals have poor health, inadequate nutrition, or poor hygiene habits), people become particularly susceptible to invasion, setting the stage for infection to occur.

There are other reasons that a person's defenses may be weak. A break in the skin caused by injury can leave a person especially vulnerable to microorganisms. This type of opening in the body provides the organisms with an unprotected point of entry. Drugs can also weaken the body's ability to fight infection. For example, anticancer drugs may kill healthy cells along with the cancer cells. Disorders of the immune system, such as AIDS, interfere with the body's natural ability to fight infection.

Because people are constantly, and quite literally, surrounded by pathogens, the body's natural defenses against pathogens are crucial to survival. If people do not have these defenses, they are potentially vulnerable to infection by every microorganism they encounter, including those naturally found in the body. Infections by microorganisms that can cause disease only when a host's resistance is low are called **opportunistic infections.** Examples of opportunistic infections are pneumonia caused by *Pneumocystis carinii* (a protozoan) and oral candidiasis, caused by *Candida* (a yeastlike fungus found commonly in the mouth as well as the intestinal tract and vagina). Both of these infections are common in AIDS patients.

The human body has many types of defense mechanisms that work to fight off pathogens. **Normal flora** are beneficial bacteria found in the body that create a barrier against pathogens. These bacteria produce substances that can harm invaders and starve them by using up the resources pathogens need to live. Normal flora colonize the skin, nose, mouth, vagina, rectum, and intestines. For example, some staphylococci bacteria are normally present on the skin and in the upper respiratory tract. The normal flora in any given area are specific (endogenous) to those areas, different from flora in or on other parts of the body.

Intact skin is the best first-line defense people have against disease. Skin secretions also serve as a barrier to

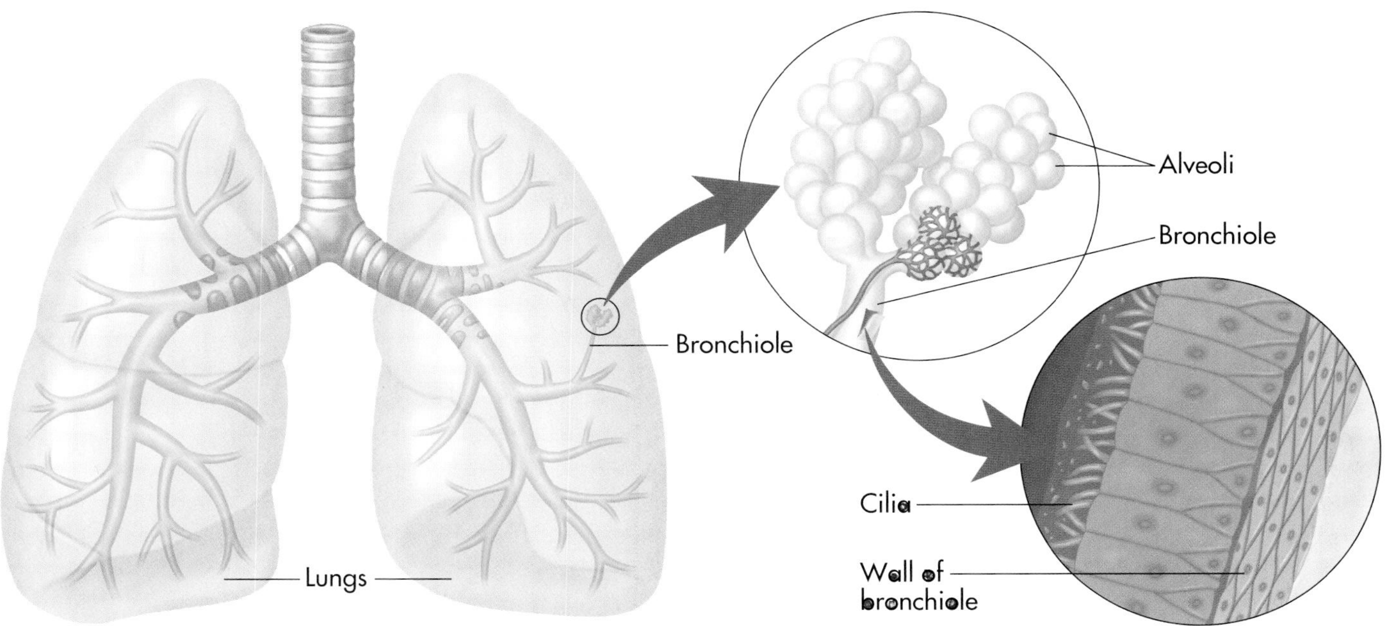

Figure 1-3. The sweeping motion of cilia that line the respiratory tract helps rid the body of foreign particles and some microorganisms.

invaders. Other body fluids and functions protect people from disease as well. Tears, saliva, and internal secretions such as prostatic fluid and cervical mucus have a mild germ-killing acidity. The respiratory tract is lined with cilia, tiny projections that continuously beat upward to expel foreign substances trapped in mucus (Figure 1-3). Coughing and sneezing rid the respiratory tract of excess mucus. Normally high acidic levels of the stomach and urine help to prevent or inhibit bacterial growth. Contractions of smooth muscle along the intestinal tract help rid the body of infectious microorganisms as well.

When microorganisms successfully invade body tissues, the immune system immediately begins to neutralize and destroy them. The immune system includes nonspecific defenses, which are often used in conjunction with the two main types of specific defenses: humoral defenses (fluid mechanisms) and cell-mediated defenses. The immune system also involves the spleen, lymph nodes, tonsils, thymus, lungs, liver, and kidneys, all of which contain lymphatic tissue. Lymphatic tissue is a filtering network of connective tissue containing large numbers of lymphocytes. Lymphocytes are specialized white blood cells that combat infectious agents.

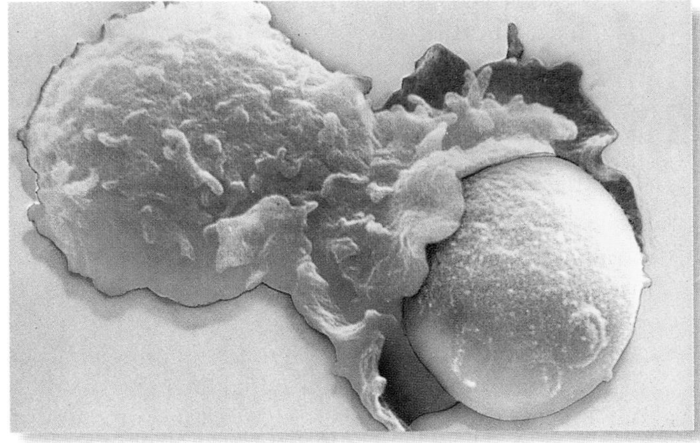

Figure 1-4. Phagocytes protect the body from infection by finding, surrounding, and digesting intruding microorganisms.

Nonspecific Defense

One type of nonspecific defense is the process known as phagocytosis, which occurs when special white blood cells called **phagocytes** engulf and digest pathogens. (Figure 1-4 shows how a phagocyte "swallows" a pathogen.) A pouch forms around the pathogen as it is engulfed. The phagocyte secretes enzymes and metabolites into the pouch, destroying the trapped material. Phagocytes are the cells that form pus as they go to the site of infection to help destroy microorganisms.

There are several varieties of phagocytes, two of which are of particular importance. Neutrophils are phagocytes that move on their own and can act quickly to destroy an invading microorganism. **Macrophages,** which are known as monocytes while in the bloodstream, are phagocytes found in the lymph nodes, liver, spleen, lungs, bone marrow, and connective tissue. They are larger and generally slower-moving than neutrophils, but they live longer. Macrophages also play several roles in humoral and cell-mediated immunity, including presenting the antigens to the lymphocytes involved in these defenses.

Humoral Immunity

One type of humoral protection is provided by **antibodies,** highly specific proteins that attach themselves to foreign substances. This defense involves two types of lymphocytes: B cells (also called B lymphocytes) and T cells (also known as T lymphocytes). When the body is invaded by **antigens** (foreign substances), helper T cells activate B cells to produce antibodies, which combine with the antigens to neutralize them. Although the initial response to a major invasion by an antigen may not be a highly effective defense, memory B cells are produced for the appropriate antibody. A later invasion by the same antigen will be quickly and effectively countered. Specific antibodies are produced in response to specific antigens. These antibodies act as a homing device to attract phagocytes, which then engulf and destroy the antigen.

The formation of antibodies gives the body immunity from a particular disease. Immunity can be natural or artificial, active or passive (Figure 1-5).

- Active immunity is a long-term immunity in which the body produces its own antibodies. Active immunity can be natural or artificial.
- Passive immunity results when antibodies produced outside the body enter the body. Passive immunity can be natural or artificial.
- Natural active immunity results from exposure to organisms that cause a disease, such as mumps. Although the person becomes sick with the disease, the body produces antibodies that prevent the individual from having the disease again if reexposed. A fetus acquires natural passive immunity when the mother's antibodies move across the placenta. Natural passive immunity lasts only a short time, usually a few weeks after birth.
- Artificial active immunity results from administration of an immunization or vaccine with killed or weakened organisms. These organisms induce the formation of antibodies without causing the disease. Artificial passive immunity occurs as a result of some types of immunizations (injections of antibodies) that provide temporary protection for people who have been exposed to serious diseases, such as hepatitis and tetanus. Artificial passive immunity lasts only a short time, usually a few weeks.

The other type of humoral defense is called complement. Complement is a group of proteins that circulates in the blood and body fluids and is always present in low amounts. When it is activated by antibodies, however, complement can multiply rapidly and destroy pathogens. It helps the white blood cells ingest microorganisms, sometimes making a hole in the microorganisms' cells that causes the cells to rupture and consequently be destroyed. The main reason that most bacteria do not cause disease is that these proteins can destroy many species of bacteria.

Cell-Mediated Immunity

In addition to their role in humoral immunity, T cells are instrumental in cell-mediated immunity. Cell-mediated immunity differs from humoral immunity in that T cells do not form antibodies to combat antigens. Instead, they directly attack the invader. Several different types of T cells are involved in the attack process. Helper T cells activate the killer T cells, which bind with the antigen and kill it. Suppressor T cells slow down or stop the attack after the antigen is destroyed. Memory T cells are formed and will respond quickly to another attack by the same antigen.

Cell-mediated defenses against infection often result in inflammation of the affected area. Inflammation occurs when phagocytes enter the area, stick to the lining of the blood vessels, and come out of the vessels to attack the infecting agent. Small blood vessels then dilate and leak fluid, resulting in swelling, redness, and warmth. This process often causes fever, which is a common response to many infections and may play a part in fighting infection.

Immunity

Active Immunity	**Passive Immunity**
Body produces its own antibodies; provides long-term immunity	Antibodies produced outside of the body are introduced into the body; provides only temporary immunity
Natural Active Immunity	**Natural Passive Immunity**
Results from exposure to disease-causing organism	Results when antibodies from the mother cross the placenta to the fetus
Artificial Active Immunity	**Artificial Passive Immunity**
Results from administration of a vaccine with killed or weakened organisms	Results from immunization with antibodies to a disease-causing organism

Figure 1-5. Immunity to a disease can be acquired in a variety of ways: naturally, artificially, actively, and passively.

PROCEDURE 1.1

Aseptic Hand Washing

Objective: To remove dirt and microorganisms from under the fingernails and from the surface of the skin, hair follicles, and oil glands of the hands

OSHA Guidelines: This procedure does not involve exposure to blood, body fluids, or tissues.

Materials: Liquid soap, nailbrush or orange stick, paper towels

Method

1. Remove all jewelry (plain wedding bands may be left on and scrubbed).
2. Turn on the faucets using a paper towel, and adjust the water temperature to moderately warm. (Sinks with knee-operated faucet controls prevent contact of the surface with the hands.)
3. Wet your hands and apply liquid soap. (Liquid soap, especially when dispensed with a foot pump, is preferable to bar soap. There is less available area for dirt to accumulate on a liquid soap dispenser than on bar soap, and there is a smaller chance of dropping the soap dispenser into the sink or onto the floor.)
4. Work the soap into a lather, making sure that all of both hands are lathered. Rub vigorously in a circular motion for 2 minutes. Keep your hands lower than your forearms so that dirty water flows into the sink instead of back onto your arms. The fingertips should be pointing down. Interlace your fingers to clean between them, and use the palm of one hand to clean the back of the other (Figure 1-10).
5. Use a nailbrush or orange stick to dislodge dirt around your nails and cuticles (Figure 1-11).
6. Rinse your hands well, keeping the hands lower than your forearms and not touching the sink or faucets.
7. With the water still running, dry your hands thoroughly with clean, dry paper towels, and then turn off the faucets using a clean, dry paper towel. Discard the towels.

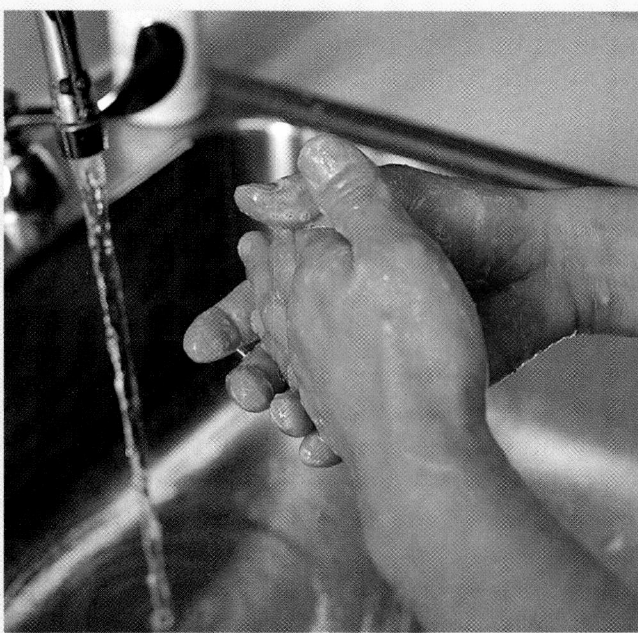

Figure 1-10. When you wash your hands, be sure to clean all surfaces, including the palms, between the fingers, and under the fingernails.

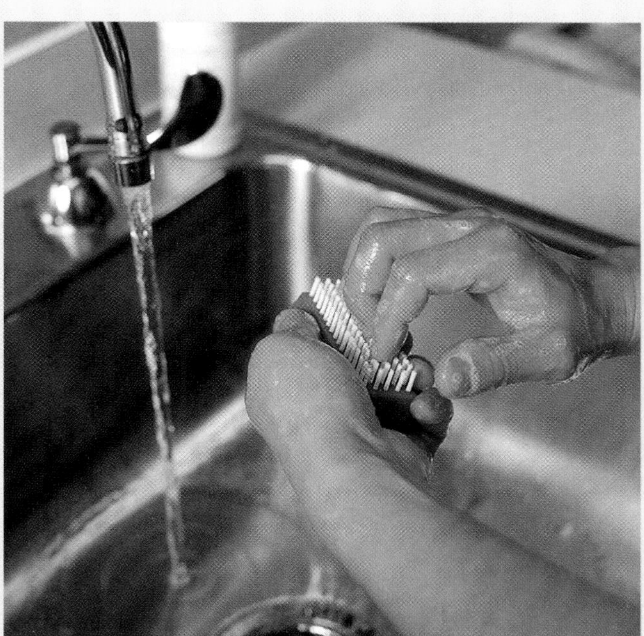

Figure 1-11. The nails and cuticles require additional attention to ensure that all dirt is removed.

either sterile or not sterile, and if there is any question, you must consider the object or area contaminated. To prevent interruptions in the technique, you must also ensure that when objects touch one another, clean goes against clean, unclean goes against unclean, and sterile goes against sterile.

The surgical scrub is of primary importance in surgical asepsis. Surgical scrub procedures are similar to those for aseptic hand washing, but there are several distinctions. Differences include the following:

- A sterile scrub brush is used instead of a nailbrush.
- Both hands and forearms are washed.
- The hands are kept above the elbows to prevent water from running from the arms onto washed areas.
- Sterile towels are used instead of paper towels.
- Sterile gloves are put on immediately after the hands are dried.

Surgical Asepsis During a Surgical Procedure. Chapter 23 describes assisting with minor surgery. Several points concerning surgical asepsis, however, are introduced here. Before performing a surgical procedure, the doctor may ask you to help prepare the skin. Your goal is to remove as many microorganisms as possible from around the area that is to undergo surgery so that you reduce the chances of these organisms entering the surgical opening. The skin and body openings, particularly the nose, mouth, and perineum, cannot be considered sterile. Nevertheless, the principles of aseptic technique require that you try to keep the area as contamination-free as possible.

Asepsis also involves keeping instruments and supplies sterile for use during the surgical procedure. After the sterile field has been created, handle items as little as possible to minimize the chance of contamination. Cover items that are not being used immediately with a sterile towel. If you are not wearing sterile gloves during a procedure (as when you are the only medical assistant and you must hand the doctor items from outside the sterile field), you must use transfer forceps to handle a sterile instrument. Transfer forceps look like big scissors or tweezers. Although the handles are not sterile, the tips that touch the instruments are.

If you are wearing sterile gloves, you handle sterile items directly and carefully avoid touching anything that is not sterile. Throughout the procedure, you are responsible for maintaining the sterile field (in this case, the area of surgery).

After the procedure, you continue using aseptic technique in caring for the patient's surgical wound. Typically, you need to apply dressings and keep the wound clean in an aseptic manner to prevent infection. You will also instruct the patient in how to care for the wound.

After you instruct the patient and guide the person out of the room, immediately place any supplies and disposable instruments that were used during the surgery into the appropriate **biohazardous waste containers.** These are leakproof containers that are color-coded red or labeled with a special biohazard symbol to show that they contain **biohazardous materials** (biological agents that can spread disease to living things). These containers are used to store and dispose of contaminated supplies and equipment in a way that preserves aseptic techniques and complies with the law.

Sanitizing, Disinfecting, and Sterilizing Instruments

After disposing of biohazardous waste, you must sanitize, disinfect, and sterilize reusable surgical instruments. **Sanitization** involves reducing the number of microorganisms on an object or a surface to a fairly safe level. To sanitize instruments after surgery, rinse them under warm, running water. If you cannot rinse them with water immediately, soak them in a disinfectant solution that has anticoagulant properties.

After rinsing the instruments, scrub them using hot, soapy water. Use a neutral-pH detergent that does not cause stains, corrosion, scratching, or a high level of suds and that is an effective blood solvent. Always wear utility gloves, use plastic brushes (never steel wool or wire), and keep different types of instruments (sharp, hinged, or of different metals) apart from each other when sanitizing them. After removing all visible stains and residue, rinse the instruments under running water, and roll them in a clean towel to dry them. Examine all instruments closely to make sure that they are in working order.

Disinfection is the destruction of infectious agents on an object or surface by direct application of chemical or physical means. Common disinfectants include chemical germicides, boiling water, and steam. You use disinfectants only on objects and surfaces because they are too strong to use on human tissue. Although disinfection kills a great many pathogens, **bacterial spores** (primitive, thick-walled reproductive bodies capable of developing into new individuals) and some viruses are not eliminated through disinfection.

To kill spores and viruses resistant to disinfection on instruments, you must sterilize them. **Sterilization** is the destruction of all microorganisms, including bacterial spores, by specific means. (For detailed information and procedures on instrument sanitization, disinfection, and sterilization, see Chapter 2.)

Disinfecting Work Surfaces

Another postsurgical aseptic procedure you will perform is disinfecting all work surfaces that were exposed to contamination (Figure 1-12). For this process, you must use bleach or a germ-killing solution approved by the U.S. government's Environmental Protection Agency (EPA). If protective coverings on surfaces or equipment were exposed to contamination during a procedure, they must be replaced.

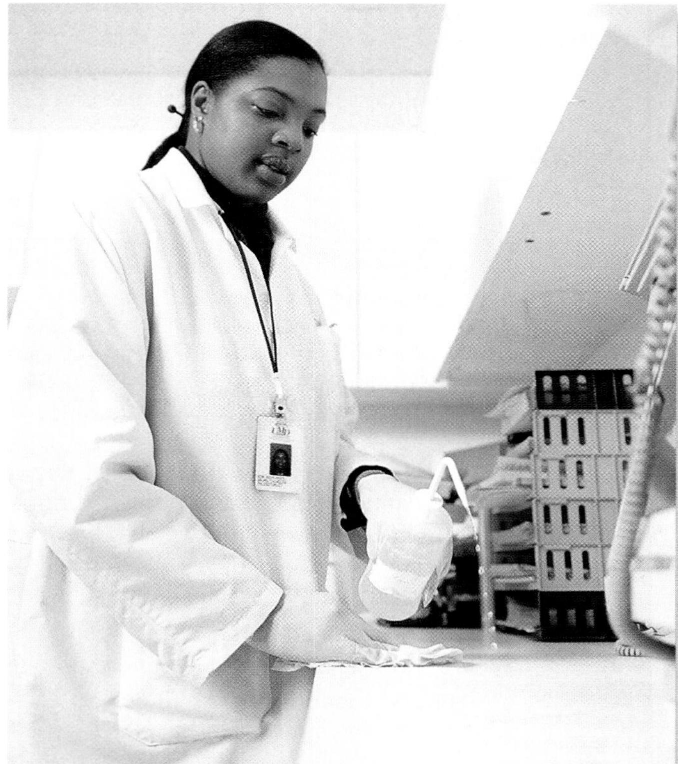

Figure 1-12. Work surfaces must be thoroughly cleaned with an EPA-approved chemical disinfectant.

Medical asepsis and surgical asepsis are required by law. Each individual who works in a medical setting must recognize the importance of asepsis and strictly adhere to aseptic procedures in daily routines.

OSHA Blood-borne Pathogens Standard and Universal Precautions

You must know the laws that require basic practices of infection control in a medical office. You must also know how to apply these laws in your office. Federal regulations related to infection control and asepsis were developed by the Department of Labor's Occupational Safety and Health Administration (OSHA) and described in the OSHA Blood-borne Pathogens Standard of 1991. These laws protect health-care workers from health hazards on the job, particularly from accidentally acquiring infections. They also help protect from health hazards patients and any other people who may come into the medical office.

OSHA Blood-borne Pathogens Standard

To ensure that biohazardous materials do not endanger people or the environment, laws set forth in the OSHA Blood-borne Pathogens Standard of 1991 dictate how you must handle infectious or potentially infectious waste generated during medical or surgical procedures. According to these rules, any potentially infectious waste materials must be discarded or held for processing in biohazardous waste containers. These wastes include the following:

- Blood products
- Body fluids
- Human tissues
- Vaccines
- Table paper, linen, towels, and gauze with body fluids on them
- Used scalpels, needles, sutures with needles attached, and other sharp instruments (known as sharps)
- Used gloves, disposable instruments, cotton swabs, and disposable applicators

Many medical offices today use only disposable paper gowns, drapes, coverings, and towels. Some offices, however, use cloth linens, which must be laundered. Certain rules apply to the laundering of cloth linens that are soiled with potentially infectious materials.

Medical offices use outside, licensed waste management services approved by the EPA to dispose of medical waste. A waste management service can provide instructions for preparing items before they are taken away.

The disposition and handling of contaminated sharps are of special concern because these instruments can easily puncture the skin and expose you to extremely dangerous viruses. Used sharps must never be bent, broken, recapped, or otherwise tampered with. After use, place them in a rigid, leakproof, puncture-resistant biohazardous waste container for sharps. Disposable and reusable sharps are kept in separate containers. Metal basins containing disinfectant are often used to store reusable sharps until they can be processed. The outside waste management company may supply containers for the disposable items, sterilize them on its premises, and discard them in the city trash dump or incinerate them. You may sanitize, disinfect, and sterilize reusable sharps in your office, particularly if the practice is in a rural area without an outside waste management company nearby. See the Caution: Handle With Care section for a discussion of the guidelines you must follow when disposing of biohazardous waste and potentially infectious laundry waste.

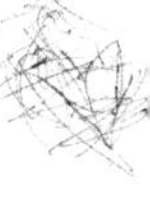

OSHA's laws for hazardous waste disposal, as well as other OSHA regulations about measures to prevent the spread of infection, provide a margin of safety, ensuring that medical facilities meet at least the minimal criteria for asepsis. These laws include requirements for training personnel, keeping records, housekeeping, wearing protective gear, and other measures.

Although federal laws exist, individual states have some discretion in applying them. You should become familiar with the laws in your state to ensure that you are helping your medical office comply. Penalties for failing to comply with regulations can be severe (see Table 1-1).

CAUTION *Handle With Care*

Proper Use of Biohazardous Waste Containers and Handling of Infectious Laundry Waste

Biohazardous waste containers are available in a variety of designs. Frequently, more than one design is used in the clinical setting. These containers are often provided by outside sterilization and waste management companies. Examples of biohazardous waste containers include:

- Bags or containers that are red or have a biohazardous waste label (for any material contaminated with blood or body fluids, such as used dressings or gloves)
- Boxes with biohazardous waste labels (sometimes lined with red bags and used for disposable gowns, examination table covers, and similar items that may be contaminated with blood or body fluids)
- Rigid, leakproof sharps containers that are red or have a biohazardous waste label (for lancets, needles, and other sharp objects)

Every biohazardous waste container has a lid that you must replace immediately after use. In addition, you may not overfill the container, and you must replace it when it is two-thirds full. All biohazardous waste containers must have a fluorescent orange or orange-red label with the biohazard symbol and the word *BIOHAZARD* in a contrasting color (Figure 1-13). Red bags or red containers may be substituted for containers with biohazardous waste labels.

You must follow these guidelines when handling hazardous waste.

- Always wear gloves
- Place hazardous waste in the appropriate biohazardous waste container immediately or as soon as possible
- Keep biohazardous waste containers close to the place where the waste material is generated
- Keep the containers closed when not in use, close them before removing them from the area of use, and keep them upright to avoid any spills

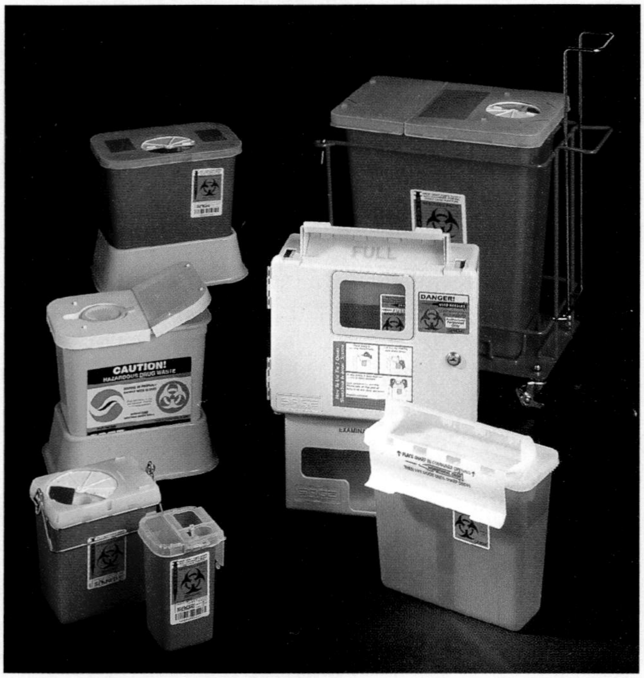

Figure 1-13. All biohazardous sharps containers must be rigid, leakproof, and labeled with the biohazard symbol.

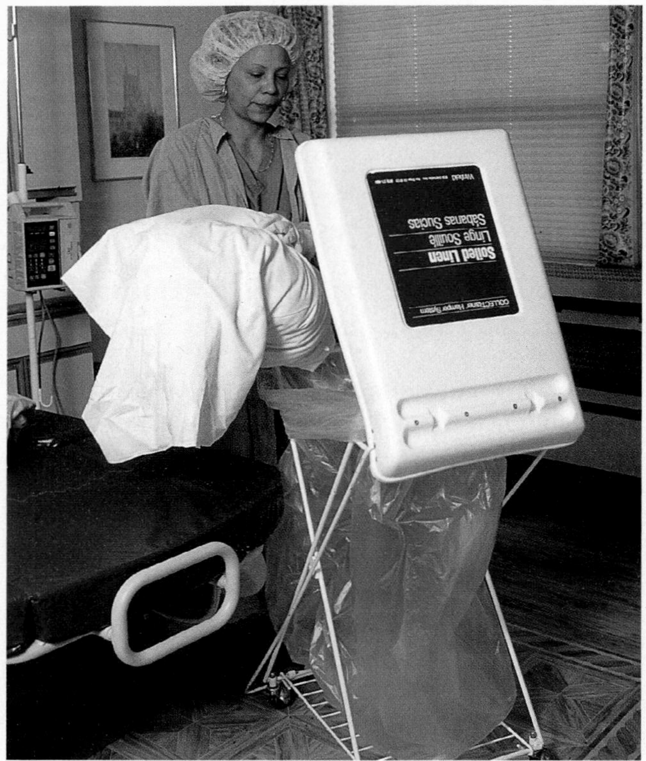

Figure 1-14. Place soiled linens and other laundry in an appropriate bag as soon as possible.

continued ⟶

CAUTION *Handle With Care*

Proper Use of Biohazardous Waste Containers and Handling of Infectious Laundry Waste *(continued)*

- If outside contamination of the primary container occurs, place that container in a secondary container to prevent leakage during handling, processing, storage, and transport
- Drop—do not push—intact contaminated needles into the biohazardous waste container for sharps
- To avoid accidental puncture wounds, never break off, recap, reuse, or handle needles after use
- If there is a danger of hazardous waste puncturing the primary container, place that container in a secondary container
- Do not open, empty, or clean reusable sharps containers by hand
- When they are two-thirds full, discard disposable sharps containers in large biohazardous waste containers

When cleaning up spills, place the resulting contaminated material in a biohazardous waste bag. The bag must be leakproof on the sides and bottom and be closed tightly. Then place the plastic bag in a cardboard box also marked with the biohazard symbol. The outside waste management agency will pick up the box for incineration before disposing of it in a public landfill.

Potentially infectious laundry waste must also be handled in a specific manner. OSHA has issued regulations for handling this type of waste. You must be sure to:

- Place contaminated laundry in a laundry bag that is red, marked with the biohazard symbol, or recognizable to facility employees as contaminated material to be handled using Universal Precautions (Figure 1-14)
- Pack any laundry to be transported so that it does not leak in transit
- Have the laundry washed in a designated area on-site or at a professional laundry facility

Any laundry service the medical office uses should abide by all OSHA regulations. For example, anyone handling laundry must wear gloves and handle contaminated materials as little as possible.

TABLE 1-1 Infectious Waste Disposal: Penalties for Not Following Regulations, as Set Forth by OSHA

Type of Violation	Characteristics of Violation	Penalties for Violation
Other than serious violation	Direct relationship to job safety and health but would probably not result in death or serious physical harm	Fine of up to $7,000 (discretionary)
Serious violation	Substantial probability that death or serious physical harm could result; employer knew, or should have known, of the hazard	Fine of up to $7,000 (mandatory)
Willful violation	Violation committed intentionally and knowingly	Fine of up to $70,000, with a $5,000 minimum; if violation resulted in death of employee, additional fine and/or up to 6 months' imprisonment
Repeated violation	Substantially similar (but not the same) violation found upon reinspection; not applicable if initial citation is under contest	Fine of up to $70,000
Failure to correct prior violation	Initial violation was not corrected	Fine of up to $7,000 for each day the violation continues past the date it was supposed to stop

Universal Precautions

OSHA requires medical professionals to follow specific "universal blood and body fluid precautions" as set forth by the Department of Health and Human Services' Centers for Disease Control and Prevention (CDC). These **Universal Precautions** prevent health-care workers from exposing themselves and others to infections. Following Universal Precautions means assuming that all blood and body fluids are infected with blood-borne pathogens. Universal Precautions apply to:

- Blood and blood products
- Human tissue
- Semen and vaginal secretions
- Saliva from dental procedures
- Cerebrospinal, synovial, pleural, peritoneal, pericardial, and amniotic fluids, which bathe various internal structures in the body
- Other body fluids, if visibly contaminated with blood or of questionable origin in the body

Breast milk, while not on the list of fluids covered by Universal Precautions, is generally treated as such because it has been shown that mothers can pass along the human immunodeficiency virus (HIV) to their infants through breast milk.

Hospitals now use **Standard Precautions,** which are a combination of Universal Precautions and rules to reduce the risk of disease transmission by means of moist body substances (known as Body Substance Isolation guidelines). Standard Precautions apply to:

- Blood
- All body fluids, secretions, and excretions except sweat
- Nonintact skin
- Mucous membranes

Standard Precautions are used in hospitals for the care of all patients. They are an important measure for preventing the transmission of disease in the hospital setting. In medical offices, Universal Precautions are used when dealing with patients. The application of Universal Precautions is expanding, in practice, to include all body fluids, secretions, and excretions and moist body surfaces.

As mentioned earlier, some types of pathogens can be transmitted when the host's infected blood comes in contact with another person's skin. Skin that has been broken from a needle puncture or other wound and mucous membranes, such as those lining the nose and throat, are the areas that need the most protection. If a patient's (or coworker's) blood or body fluids come in contact with such areas, pathogens can be transferred from the patient's body to that of the medical worker.

OSHA outlines the routine safeguards to take when performing each medical procedure or task, depending on that task's level of risk. The degree of risk is determined by how much exposure to potentially infectious substances you are likely to encounter. When a procedure is explained, particular icons will be used to represent each of the OSHA guidelines. These icons are shown in Figure 1-15.

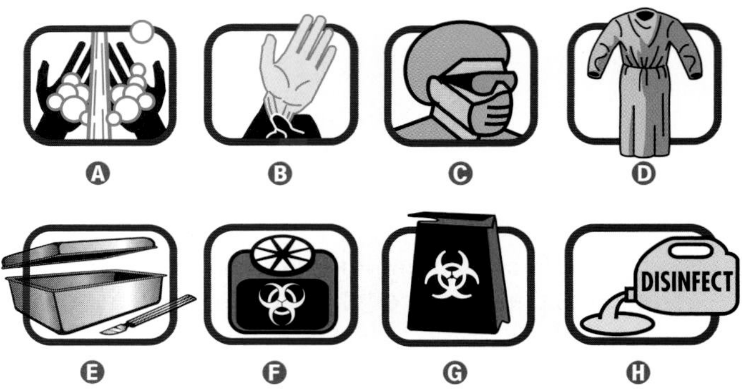

Figure 1-15. These icons will appear at the beginning of each Procedure to let you know which OSHA guidelines you should follow. They represent (a) hand washing, (b) gloves, (c) mask and protective eyewear or face shield, (d) laboratory coat or gown, (e) reusable sharps container, (f) sharps disposal, (g) biohazardous waste container, and (h) disinfection.

OSHA divides tasks into the following three categories.

1. Category I tasks are those that expose a worker to blood, body fluids, or tissues or those that have a chance of spills or splashes. These tasks always require specific protective measures.
2. Category II tasks do not usually involve risk of exposure. Because they may involve exposure in certain situations, however, OSHA requires that precautions be taken.
3. Category III tasks do not require any special protection. These tasks, such as taking a patient's blood pressure, involve no exposure to blood, body fluids, or tissues. (Observe patients for open wounds before you touch them to perform such tasks.)

Category I Tasks

A Category I task you might perform would be assisting with a minor surgical procedure in the office, such as the removal of a cyst. This procedure requires that you wash your hands before and after the procedure and that you wear protective gloves, a mask and protective eyewear or a face shield, and protective clothing. After the procedure, you must follow the guidelines for dealing with disposable and nondisposable sharp equipment and decontaminating work surfaces.

Category II Tasks

A Category II task you might perform would be giving mouth-to-mouth resuscitation to a patient. Because blood is usually not visible in such situations, the task is not

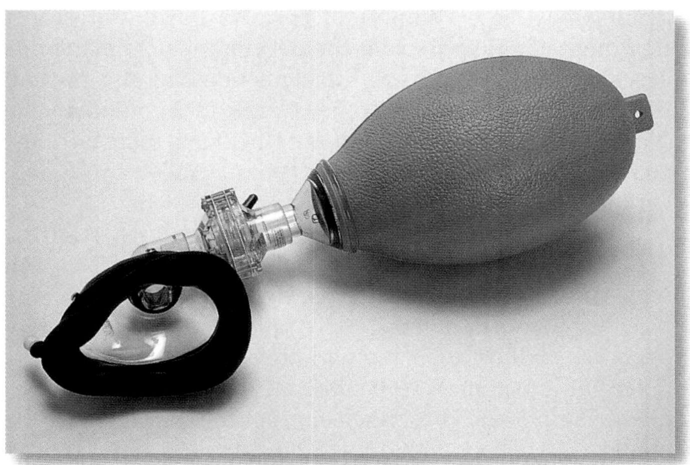

Figure 1-16. Resuscitation bags are sometimes used when a person requires mouth-to-mouth resuscitation. You must use one of these bags if blood is visible in the person's mouth or airway.

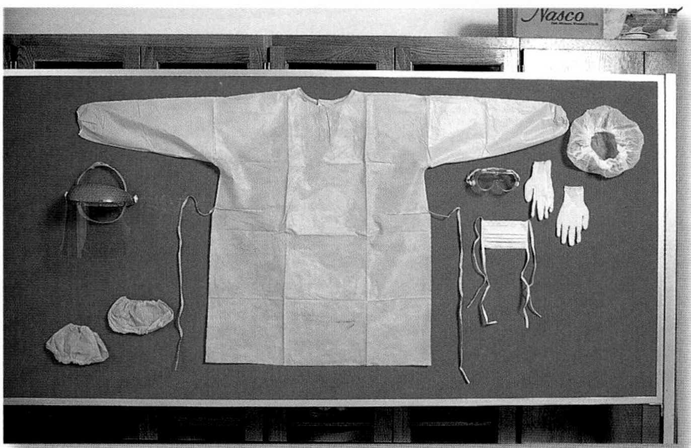

Figure 1-17. Health-care workers may need to use various types of personal protective equipment including gloves, masks and protective eyewear or face shields, gowns, and other protective clothing.

classified as Category I. Gloves are still recommended, however, although you may not have time to get them in an emergency. Because you will be exposed to saliva in such a procedure, OSHA recommends using disposable airway equipment and resuscitation bags (shown in Figure 1-16), which medical offices are required to supply.

OSHA recommends taking these precautions to decrease the risk of transmitting infectious diseases through mouth-to-mouth resuscitation. Of particular concern to health-care workers is HIV, which causes AIDS, and the hepatitis B virus (HBV).

AIDS damages the body's ability to fight disease, and it is ultimately fatal in most instances. Hepatitis B is a highly contagious and potentially fatal disease that causes inflammation of the liver and sometimes liver failure. Health-care workers become infected with these viruses at work every year. Hepatitis B infection occurs far more frequently on the job than does HIV infection. (See Chapter 3 for detailed information on these and other blood-borne pathogens.)

Category III Tasks

A Category III procedure you may perform is giving a patient medicated nose drops. This task involves tilting the patient's head and holding the dropper above the patient's nostril. Although you must perform aseptic hand washing before and after the procedure, there are no other protective requirements. Some Category III tasks require no precautions. Examples of these tasks are instructing a patient in how to use a heating pad or how to take care of a cast for a broken leg.

Personal Protective Equipment

Employers are required by law to supply personal protective equipment (PPE) at no charge to their employees. Health-care workers require many kinds of personal protective equipment to do their jobs, including gloves, masks and protective eyewear or face shields, and protective clothing (Figure 1-17). During each procedure, keep in mind that the greater your chances of exposure to blood, the more protective equipment you need to wear.

Gloves. You must wear gloves for all procedures that involve exposure to blood, other body fluids, or broken skin. There are several kinds of gloves for different situations.

- Disposable gloves are worn once and then discarded. They cannot be used if they are torn, punctured, or otherwise damaged. Both examination and sterile gloves are disposable.
- Examination gloves are worn during procedures that do not require a sterile environment.
- Sterile gloves are used for sterile procedures such as minor surgery or urinary catheterization.
- Utility gloves (used when cleaning up) are stronger than disposable gloves and may be decontaminated and reused if they show no signs of deterioration (including discoloration) after use.

Masks and Protective Eyewear or Face Shields. You must wear appropriate masks and protective eyewear or face shields for procedures in which your eyes, nose, and mouth may be exposed. These procedures are ones that have a potential for spraying or splashing blood, such as surgery or the collection or examination of blood.

Protective Clothing. If you are likely to have blood or body fluids sprayed or splashed on your clothing during a procedure, you must wear a protective laboratory coat, gown, or apron. You may also wear a hair covering and/or shoe coverings for such procedures. You should always have a change of work clothing available in the event that blood or body fluids penetrate your regular clothes around or through the protective clothing.

OSHA Procedures for Postprocedure Cleanup

After a procedure, personnel in every medical office must follow specific steps to clean and decontaminate the environment. The cleanup steps that OSHA requires are as follows:

1. Decontaminate all exposed work surfaces with bleach or a germ-killing solution approved by the EPA.
2. Replace protective coverings on surfaces or equipment if they have been exposed.
3. Decontaminate receptacles, such as bins, pails, and cans, on a regular basis as part of routine housekeeping procedures.
4. Pick up any broken glass with tongs—never by hand—even when wearing gloves, because the sharp edges may cut the gloves and expose the skin to infecting organisms. Never use a vacuum to pick up broken glass.
5. Discard all potentially infectious waste materials in appropriate biohazardous waste containers.

Applying the Law to Daily Work

In the course of daily work, you and other medical personnel may come in contact with patients who carry dangerous or fatal infectious disease. You are at risk for accidental exposure to these types of disease with every patient. Pathogens may be present in a patient's blood or other body fluids.

A patient or anyone who comes in contact with infectious waste generated by another patient or a health-care worker is at risk for infection. To minimize the risk of cross contamination, you need to become familiar with the OSHA regulations that describe the precautions medical office personnel must take in matters such as clothing, housekeeping, record keeping, and training.

Exposure Incidents

The OSHA Blood-borne Pathogens Standard also specifies what to do in case of an exposure incident. An exposure incident is one in which a worker, despite all precautions, has reason to believe that he has come in contact with a substance that may transmit infection. Contact may occur when a medical worker accidentally sticks himself with a used needle. This "puncture exposure incident" is the most common kind of exposure.

The basic rules covering exposure incidents apply to all serious infections, such as HBV and HIV. The rules covering HBV also include vaccination.

When an exposure incident occurs, the physician or employer must be notified immediately. This prompt action is extremely important because quick and proper treatment can help prevent the development of many diseases, such as hepatitis B. Timely action can also prevent the worker from exposing other people to a potentially acquired infection. Reporting the incident increases the chance of preventing the same type of accident from happening again.

After such an exposure, the employer must offer the exposed employee a free medical evaluation. The employer must refer the employee to a licensed health-care provider who can counsel the employee about what happened as well as about how to prevent the spread of any potential infection. The health-care provider also takes a blood sample and prescribes appropriate treatment. If the employee does not want to participate in the medical evaluation and treatment, he has the right to refuse it. (The employee's refusal should be documented.)

If an employee who has not received the HBV vaccination and is not known to be immune is exposed to any infected person—especially someone who is HBV-positive or at high risk—it is recommended that the employee be tested for HBV and receive the vaccination if necessary. This vaccination may prevent infection. When the source person's HBV status is unknown and the person does not wish to be tested, the employee should be tested. If the source person agrees to be tested, the law requires that the employee be informed of the test results. The employee may agree to give blood but not to be tested. In such a case, the blood sample must be kept for 90 days in case the employee later develops symptoms of HBV or HIV infection and decides to be tested then.

The health-care provider who performs the postexposure evaluation must give the employer a written report stating whether HBV vaccination was recommended and received and that the employee was informed of the results of any blood tests. Any additional information must be kept confidential.

Other OSHA Requirements

OSHA also requires that all health-care workers who have occupational exposure to blood or other potentially infectious materials have the opportunity to receive the HBV vaccine, free of charge, as needed throughout employment. Within 10 days of a medical worker's starting a job, the doctor or employer is required to offer the worker the opportunity to receive this vaccination. The vaccine is recommended for all health-care workers unless:

- They have received it in the past
- A blood test shows them to be immune to the virus
- There are medical reasons for which the vaccine is contraindicated

In most cases, the employee is permitted to decline the vaccination if he signs a form accepting all the conditions. (A few employers require HBV vaccination as a condition for employment.) Even if the health-care worker declines the vaccination when beginning employment, he still has the opportunity to receive the free vaccine and any necessary booster shots throughout his employment.

Transmission From Health-Care Workers to Patients

There may be times when a health-care worker has a serious infection that could be transmitted to a patient. For this reason, OSHA has special recommendations for workers who perform procedures that could result in a patient's exposure to disease. Although the risk of a health-care worker's transmitting an infection to a patient is small if OSHA standards are followed, these additional precautions are advised for high-risk procedures. High-risk procedures include the following:

- Those that are thought to have caused the transmission of infection from a medical worker to a patient in the past
- Those that may carry that risk, such as oral or obstetric or gynecologic procedures
- Those that involve needles, especially if a needle is in a body cavity or a body space that is difficult to see and the health-care worker's fingers are nearby (if the worker's skin was cut, the patient could be exposed to the worker's blood)

Workers who perform high-risk procedures should know their HIV and HBV status. HBV vaccination is strongly recommended. Also, workers who have skin conditions characterized by sores that secrete fluid should forgo direct patient care and the handling of equipment used for exposure-prone procedures until their condition has healed.

A member of the medical staff who is infected with HIV or HBV should not perform procedures that might result in exposure for the patient without the advice of an expert review panel. This panel could include the health-care worker's own physician, someone with expert knowledge about the transmission of infectious disease, a medical professional with expert knowledge about the procedures in question, public health officials, and a member of the infection-control committee of the institution, if applicable.

The panel advises the worker on whether procedures may be performed. The advice includes requiring the worker to inform potential patients of the infection before the procedure. The panel must otherwise protect the health-care worker's confidentiality.

Although great controversy has surrounded the subject of required testing of all health-care workers for HIV or HBV, no recommendations are in place for such testing. The risk of infection transmission from worker to patient is not considered great enough to justify the extensive resources that mandatory testing would require.

Educating Patients About Preventing Disease Transmission

As a medical assistant, you can be influential in educating patients about ways to protect themselves from disease. Whenever you have the opportunity for patient education, you should stress the basic principles of hygiene and disease prevention.

- Wash your hands frequently, especially before eating and after using the toilet, touching dirty objects, coming into contact with bodily fluids (including one's own), and touching doorknobs, railings, and handles
- Take a daily shower or bath, maintain daily dental care, and use clean clothes and bedding
- Thoroughly wash dirty drinking glasses, dishes, and utensils, especially when someone in the household is ill
- Use tissues when coughing or sneezing, and discard them properly after one use
- Maintain adequate light and ventilation in the home
- Routinely use a commercial disinfectant to clean rooms in the home, especially the bathroom and kitchen
- Use condoms if you have sexual intercourse with more than one partner or with people whose HIV or HBV status is unknown
- Adhere to immunization schedules
- Eat nutritious foods and keep physically fit
- Avoid stress
- Protect against exposure to potentially harmful insects or animals

Educating patients about health promotion and disease prevention is an important part of your job. Patients with adequate knowledge can work to keep their defenses functioning properly. They can also avoid exposing themselves to infections and transmitting infections when they are ill. In addition, they are more likely to have a successful recovery from illness. To provide patients with the knowledge they need, you should educate them in the following subjects:

- Nutrition and diet
- Exercise and weight control
- Prevention of sexually transmitted diseases
- Smoking cessation
- Alcohol and drug abuse prevention and treatment
- Proper use of medications and prescribed treatments for an infection already acquired
- Stress-reduction techniques

The goal of patient education is to help patients take care of themselves. In fact, many patients expect this kind of education along with their treatment. Thus, you should

Educating the Patient

Following the Doctor's Instructions

Patients' visits do not always end with the doctor's diagnosis. Occasionally, you will need to clarify the doctor's instructions or explain procedures that patients will need to perform at home. As you take part in patient education, follow these steps when you begin and end procedures.

1. Begin by identifying yourself as a medical assistant, and identify patients by name.
2. Ask patients to repeat the highlights of their sessions to determine their level of understanding.
3. As patients are leaving, encourage them to call the office with any problems or questions. Briefly document educational sessions and their topics in patients' records, dating and initialing each entry.

Patient compliance with treatment is often a problem, particularly for treatment of infection. After the physician informs a patient that medication is being prescribed, you should emphasize the importance of completing the course of treatment in the exact way it was prescribed. Explain that even if symptoms of the illness disappear before the treatment is finished, the patient must complete the full course of medication. Also instruct patients to do the following.

- Call the office immediately if you experience any unexpected reaction
- Eat a balanced diet and drink plenty of fluids
- Avoid sharing medication
- Keep medication out of the reach of children
- Refrain from activities that will interfere with healing
- Stay away from substances that would interact poorly with the prescribed medication

Teach patients any relevant procedures, such as how to take a temperature. After teaching sessions, have patients demonstrate the procedures to ensure that they are performing them correctly. For patients who have had minor surgery, teach simple concepts of asepsis to use in caring for the surgical wound at home.

encourage patients to play an active part in their own health care. A variety of patient education tools are available to help with this task. Charts, diagrams, brochures, videotapes, audiotapes, and anatomical models can be excellent teaching resources. You may find it helpful to develop or design some resources that deal with issues of particular importance to the patients with whom you work routinely. Figure 1-18 shows examples of brochures you could use to educate patients about infection control.

In addition to educating patients about disease prevention, you will also need to educate them about disease treatment. Some patients do not follow their doctor's instructions, and they may prolong their illness or experience a relapse as a result. You will need to stress to patients the important role they play in their own treatment. See the Educating the Patient section for more information about patient compliance.

Your extensive interaction with patients and your key role in managing the office provide you with many opportunities for patient education. You will share the responsibility for educating patients with the doctor and other health-care personnel. On average, doctors spend 25% of their total office time providing information to, instructing, and counseling patients. Your role is to reinforce and explain the doctor's instructions. If you encounter patient concerns, questions, or problems that you are not equipped to deal with, refer them to the doctor.

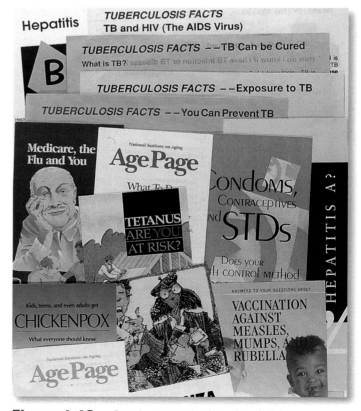

Figure 1-18. Brochures and other visual aids are effective means of educating patients about infection control.

Summary

As doctors and scientists have learned more about the causes of infection, they have developed principles and practices of asepsis. You will be responsible for using these techniques to keep patients, yourself, and your workplace free from contamination. The two levels of asepsis used today are medical asepsis and surgical asepsis. You must also follow federal regulations related to infection control and asepsis, including the OSHA Blood-borne Pathogens Standard, Universal Precautions, and Standard Precautions (if you work in a hospital).

To protect patients and yourself, you need to know how pathogens cause disease, how disease is transmitted, and how to prevent the spread of infection. You will also use this knowledge to help your employer educate patients about ways they can remain healthy and reduce their risk of contracting diseases.

REVIEW

CHAPTER 1

CASE STUDY QUESTIONS

Now that you have completed this chapter, review the case study at the beginning of the chapter and answer the following questions:

1. What part of the cycle of infection caused the problem for the medical assistant?
2. How did the patient become infected?
3. How does the Blood-borne Pathogens Standard apply to the medical assistant?
4. Because the medical assistant did not observe the regulation, what penalties, if any, could be imposed by OSHA?

Discussion Questions

1. A patient expresses concern about the possibility of acquiring HIV from other patients who may be HIV-positive. What could you say about your office to reassure this patient?
2. Differentiate between active, passive, and natural active immunity.
3. Discuss the differences between medical asepsis and surgical asepsis.

Critical Thinking Questions

1. Why are people, as a rule, able to escape infections?
2. What special areas or situations at home or in public need extra aseptic precautions?
3. In your opinion, which is better: Universal Precautions or Standard Precautions? Explain your reasoning.

Application Activities

1. Rub your fingers across a culture plate. Then perform aseptic hand washing. Rub your fingers across another culture plate. Place the two plates in a warm area. After 24 hours, compare the microorganisms that have grown on each plate. Record your results.
2. Make a chart showing specific types of procedures that you might perform and what safeguards you should take to protect yourself from exposure to potentially infectious substances during those procedures. Below the chart, list general precautions you should take during or after procedures.
3. With another student, role-play a scenario involving a medical assistant and a patient. The medical assistant should use various media to explain and teach the patient about a specific infectious disease.

CHAPTER 2

Infection-Control Techniques

AREAS OF COMPETENCE

2003 Role Delineation Study

CLINICAL

Fundamental Principles

- Apply principles of aseptic technique and infection control

GENERAL

Legal Concepts

- Document accurately
- Implement and maintain federal and state health-care legislation and regulations
- Comply with established risk management and safety procedures

Instruction

- Teach methods of health promotion and disease prevention

KEY TERMS

antiseptic
autoclave
contraindication
disinfectant
immunization
induration
nosocomial infection
sterilization indicator
ultrasonic cleaning

CHAPTER OUTLINE

- The Medical Assistant's Role in Infection Control
- The Three Levels of Infection Control
- Sanitization: The First Level of Infection Control
- Disinfection: The Second Level of Infection Control
- Sterilization: The Third Level of Infection Control
- Some Infectious Diseases
- Drug-Resistant Microorganisms
- Reporting Guidelines
- Guideline for Isolation Precautions in Hospitals
- Immunizations: Another Way to Control Infection

OBJECTIVES

After completing Chapter 2, you will be able to:

2.1 Describe the three levels of infection control.
2.2 Compare and contrast the procedures for sanitization, disinfection, and sterilization.
2.3 Describe measures used in sanitization.
2.4 List various methods used in disinfection and the advantages and disadvantages of each.
2.5 Explain what an autoclave is and how it operates.
2.6 List the steps in the general autoclave procedures.
2.7 Explain how to wrap and label items for sterilization in an autoclave.

OBJECTIVES *(Continued)*

2.8 Describe how to complete the sterilization procedure using an autoclave.

2.9 Describe four other methods for sterilizing instruments.

2.10 List some infectious diseases, and identify their signs and symptoms.

2.11 Describe Centers for Disease Control and Prevention (CDC) requirements for reporting cases of infectious disease.

2.12 Describe CDC guidelines for patient isolation.

2.13 Explain the purpose of immunization.

2.14 Describe your role in educating patients about immunizations.

Introduction

Although our bodies ordinarily are quite capable in their defense against pathogens, patients coming into an office for treatment may be more susceptible to infections. In this chapter you will learn the three levels of infection control and their respective processes. You will also be introduced to the identification of infectious diseases, the reporting guidelines established by the CDC (Centers for Disease Control and Prevention), and the procedures for isolating patients. The importance of immunizations and patient education regarding immunizations will be stressed as a method of infection control.

CASE STUDY

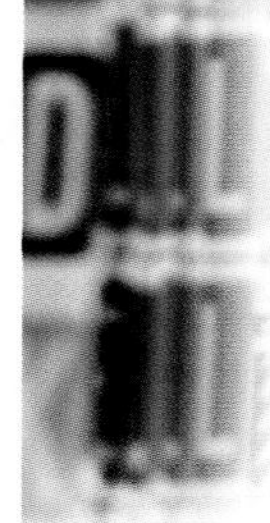

An 18-year-old female patient comes into an obstetrical office for a routine visit to obtain birth control pills. There are other women in the waiting room, many of them in various trimesters of pregnancy. While performing the patient screening, you find that she has a low-grade fever, an itchy rash, and is not up-to-date on her childhood immunizations. You discover later that she was diagnosed with rubella.

While reading this chapter, consider the following questions:

1. What is the common, or lay, term for rubella?
2. How is it transmitted?
3. Since pregnant women were probably exposed, is there a concern for their fetuses?
4. Does the disease have any reporting guidelines?

The Medical Assistant's Role in Infection Control

As you learned in Chapter 1, the cycle of infection is one in which pathogens grow and are transmitted from one host to another. To control infectious diseases, this cycle must be broken. You can help break the cycle by applying information you have learned to specific tasks in the office setting. These tasks include:

- Following correct sanitization, disinfection, and sterilization procedures
- Helping patients understand basic disease prevention techniques and recognize infectious diseases
- Administering immunizations and educating patients about the importance of immunizations and schedules for obtaining them

The Three Levels of Infection Control

Three levels of infection control are used in a medical office setting. The following are the three levels and guidelines for determining which level to use:

1. Sanitization is the process of cleaning and scrubbing instruments and equipment, generally by washing with detergents and scrubbing as needed. Sanitization removes contaminated materials and some microorganisms from surfaces. It is often utilized as the first step for preparation of instruments for disinfection and sterilization.
2. Disinfection is the second level of infection control. It is used on instruments and equipment that come in contact with intact mucous membranes or other surfaces

not considered sterile. Disinfection kills many, but not all, microorganisms on surfaces. (It does not destroy spore-forming organisms.) To disinfect instruments such as nasal specula and endotracheal tubes, you would use a chemical approved by the Environmental Protection Agency (EPA).

3. Sterilization is the complete destruction of all microorganisms—pathogenic, beneficial, and harmless—from the surface of instruments and equipment. It is required for all instruments that penetrate the skin (needles) or that come in contact with normally sterile areas of the body, such as muscle tissue and internal organs. Specialized equipment, such as an autoclave, is used to sterilize equipment.

Sanitization: The First Level of Infection Control

Sanitization is the scrubbing of instruments and equipment with special brushes and detergent to remove blood, mucus, and other contaminants or media where pathogens can grow. Sanitization is used to clean items that touch only healthy, intact skin. For other equipment, sanitization is the first step before disinfection and sterilization. Instruments and equipment that you can sanitize and reuse without further disinfection or sterilization include the following:

- Blood pressure cuff
- Ophthalmoscope (an instrument containing a mirror and lenses used to examine the interior of the eye)
- Otoscope (an instrument used for inspecting the ear)
- Penlight
- Reflex hammer
- Stethoscope
- Tape measure
- Tuning fork

Collecting Instruments for Sanitization

Sanitize instruments as soon as possible after use. If you cannot sanitize them immediately, place them in a sink or container filled with water and a neutral-pH detergent solution that has anticoagulant properties. In a surgical setting, use a special receptacle of disinfectant solution for collecting contaminated instruments. In an examination setting, place instruments in a sink or a container that can be transported to a sink. Take care when placing instruments in sinks or basins. You can damage pieces of equipment if you drop them carelessly into a receptacle. Nicks or scratches can affect their function and can provide opportunities for bacterial contamination.

When you are ready to begin the sanitization procedure, put on properly fitting, intact utility gloves. They are the barrier between your skin and any infectious material on the instruments and equipment to be cleaned. When you work with instruments that may be contaminated with blood, body fluids, or tissue, you may want the additional protection of a mask, eye protection, or protective clothing.

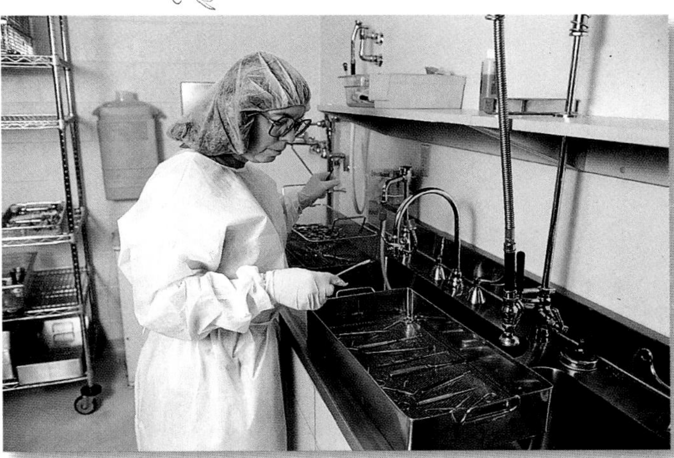

Figure 2-1. When working with instruments and equipment, separate pointed or sharp-edged instruments from all others.

Separate the sharp instruments from all other equipment (Figure 2-1). Separating them reduces the risk of blunting sharp edges or points, damaging other equipment, and injuring yourself.

Scrubbing Instruments and Equipment

Begin by draining the disinfectant or detergent solution in which the equipment was soaking. Rinse each piece of equipment in hot running water, and handle only one item at a time (by its handles where applicable). Scrub each item using hot, soapy water and a small plastic scrub brush. Never use metal brushes or steel wool, which can scratch and damage instruments. Pay careful attention to hinges, ratchets, and other nooks and crannies where it is possible for contaminated material to collect (Figure 2-2). Use brushes of different sizes to clean all areas of each item.

Use a detergent specially formulated for medical instruments and equipment. This type of detergent is low-sudsing, has a neutral pH, and is formulated to dissolve blood and blood products. Equipment and instrument manufacturers provide guidelines for sanitizing various types of products. For example, stainless steel items must be sanitized differently from chrome-plated instruments. Follow manufacturers' guidelines when you are working with their products.

After scrubbing all surfaces and removing all visible stains and residue, rinse instruments individually, and place each one on a clean towel. Roll the instrument in the towel to remove most of the moisture. Then dry the instrument thoroughly, and examine it closely to be sure that it is operating correctly. Be sure that all moving parts operate smoothly and that surfaces are free from nicks, scratches, and other imperfections. Instruments that need only to be sanitized can be returned to trays or bins for

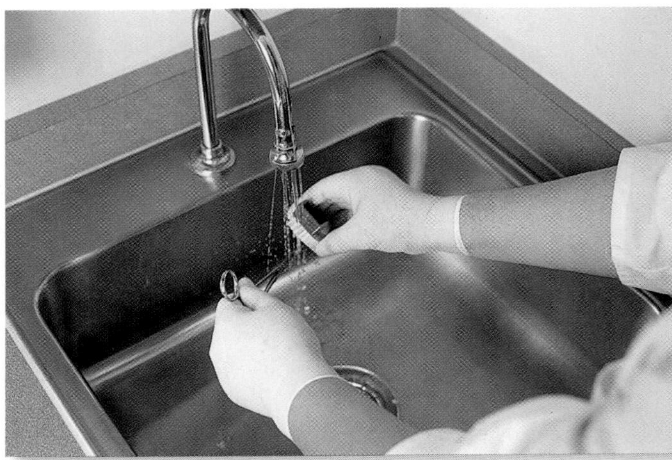

Figure 2-2. Clean all areas of an instrument, using a brush for hard-to-reach surfaces.

storage. Wrap items that require disinfection and sterilization in a clean covering, and set them aside for those processes.

Rubber and Plastic Products

To sanitize rubber and plastic products, you may need to soak them only for a short period or not at all. Some rubber and plastic products fade or discolor if left in a detergent solution. When you sanitize these products, be sure to follow manufacturers' guidelines.

Syringes and Needles

Disposable syringes and needles have replaced reusable ones in medical offices. Using disposable instruments helps reduce the risk of infection to both patients and health-care personnel.

Ultrasonic Cleaning

Delicate instruments or those with moving parts should be sanitized by using ultrasonic cleaners. **Ultrasonic cleaning** involves placing instruments in a special bath. The cleaner generates sound waves through a cleaning solution, loosening contaminants. Ultrasonic cleaning is safe for even very fragile instruments. If your medical office sanitizes instruments with an ultrasonic cleaner, follow the manufacturer's guidelines for operating the device.

Instruments with points or sharp edges and instruments made of different types of metal should be separated from other equipment. The ultrasonic cleaning process can cause one metal to disintegrate and fuse with another metal, rendering all instruments useless. Place all instruments with hinges or ratchets in the ultrasonic cleaner in the open position. If such an instrument is placed in the cleaner in the closed position, contaminated material can become trapped between the two surfaces.

After the instruments have been in the ultrasonic cleaner for the recommended cleaning time, remove them and rinse them under cool running water. Be sure to remove all the ultrasonic cleaning fluid. Then dry the instruments, and wrap them for storage or for disinfection and sterilization.

You can reuse ultrasonic cleaning solution for several cleaning baths. Replace it according to the care and maintenance procedures outlined by the manufacturer of the cleaning device.

Disinfection: The Second Level of Infection Control

Sanitization is often only the beginning of the process of eliminating microorganisms. After sanitization, some instruments and equipment require only disinfection before being used again. Disinfection of other items, however, is merely the second step in infection control, performed before the process of sterilization. You must wear gloves when handling instruments during disinfection procedures because instruments requiring disinfection are considered to be contaminated.

To destroy microorganisms, a disinfectant solution must reach every surface of an instrument; however, disinfection cannot kill all microorganisms. Bacterial spores and certain viruses have been known to survive disinfection with strong chemicals and boiling water. It is essential to understand this limitation of disinfection when you work with instruments and equipment.

Disinfection is usually sufficient for instruments that do not penetrate a patient's skin or that come in contact only with a patient's mucous membranes or other surfaces not considered sterile. Instruments and equipment that you can disinfect and reuse without sterilization include the following:

- Enamelware
- Endotracheal tubes (tubes used to establish an artificial airway through the nose, mouth, or direct tracheal route)
- Glassware
- Laryngoscopes (tubes equipped with lighting and used to examine the interior of the larynx through the mouth)
- Nasal specula (instruments used to enlarge the opening of the nose to permit viewing)

Note that you must sterilize any instrument or piece of equipment—including those just listed—if there is visible contamination with blood or blood products before another use, even if disinfection is commonly considered sufficient. Sterilization is the only reliable measure you can take to eliminate blood-borne pathogens.

Using Disinfectants

Disinfectants are cleaning products applied particularly to instruments and equipment to reduce or eliminate infectious organisms. They are used primarily on inanimate materials. In contrast, cleaning products that are used on human tissues as anti-infection agents are called **antiseptics.**

There are no clear indications that an item has been properly and completely disinfected. To ensure optimum effectiveness of disinfectants, follow the manufacturers' guidelines carefully when using them.

Other factors may also have an impact on the effectiveness of a disinfectant. For example, if the disinfectant solution has been used many times, it may not be as powerful as a fresh solution. When wet items are put in the disinfectant bath, the surface moisture may dilute the solution. Traces of the soap used in the sanitization process can alter the chemical makeup of the disinfectant, making it nonlethal to pathogens. Evaporation can also alter the chemical makeup of the solution.

Choosing the Correct Disinfectant

Manufacturers' guidelines are the most accurate and up-to-date sources of information about the type of disinfectant to use on a given product. Generally, disinfect instruments and equipment by using one or more of the following agents:

- Boiling water
- Germicidal soap products
- Alcohol
- Acid products
- Formaldehyde
- Glutaraldehyde
- Household bleach
- Iodine and iodine compounds

Each of these disinfectants has advantages and disadvantages. Before using any disinfectant product or procedure, it is important to understand some general guidelines about disinfectant use as well as specific concerns with each approach.

Boiling Water. It was long considered sufficient to boil instruments and equipment to achieve sterilization. Research has proved that boiling water is not sufficient to sterilize a surface. Boiling water is, however, an effective means of disinfection. A special unit is used for boiling instruments and equipment for disinfection purposes.

When boiling items, place them in the unit in the open position. Do not preheat the instruments. Place them in the unit at room temperature. Use distilled water in the unit to reduce the formation of mineral deposits on the instruments as well as on the unit itself. Empty the unit, and clean it according to the manufacturer's instructions.

After boiling, allow the instruments to cool. Then remove them, using sterile transfer forceps. Store the instruments carefully according to recommended procedures to prevent contamination.

Germicidal Soap Products. Research has shown that the use of soap in the process of disinfection is less important than the scrubbing and rinsing steps. Germ-killing additives may increase the effectiveness of soap products, however, and a soap-and-water disinfection may be sufficient for items that do not come in contact with a patient's skin or mucous membranes.

Alcohol. Alcohol (70% isopropyl) is commonly used to clean instruments and equipment that would be damaged by immersion in soap and water or other disinfectant solutions. It is a corrosive product, however, and can cause damage to the skin if it is used excessively.

Acid Products. The killing power of concentrated acid products such as phenol (carbolic acid) is quite high. In a concentrated form, acid products are also extremely corrosive and toxic to tissue and should be used with care.

Formaldehyde. Formaldehyde is a corrosive and an irritant to body tissue. It is commonly used as a preservative in a 10% solution, whereas in a 5% solution it can be used as a germicidal agent and a sporicidal agent. Formaldehyde must be used at room temperature because its effectiveness is reduced in cooler environments. After disinfecting items with formaldehyde, rinse them thoroughly with distilled or sterile water before using them on patients.

Glutaraldehyde. Glutaraldehyde (known more commonly by the trade names Cidex, Cidexplus, and Glutarex) is used in chemical sterilization processes, but you can also use it as a disinfectant. Immersing instruments or equipment in a bath of glutaraldehyde for 10 to 30 minutes is sufficient for disinfection. Any chemical used in this "cold disinfection" method must be rated as a sterilant and registered with the EPA.

Household Bleach. Bleach (sodium hypochlorite) is commonly used in laboratory settings to provide a measure of protection against transmission of the human immunodeficiency virus (HIV). It is an effective disinfectant when used in a 10% solution. Bleach is used to disinfect surfaces and to soak rubber equipment before sanitization. Ventilation may be necessary when you use bleach because the fumes should not be inhaled for a prolonged period.

Iodine and Iodine Compounds. Iodine products are used as both disinfectants (solutions stronger than 2%) and antiseptics (solutions weaker than 2%). They are somewhat corrosive, however, and their effectiveness is limited by the presence of blood products, mucus, or soap.

Handling Disinfected Supplies

After disinfecting equipment, handle it with care to prevent contamination of any surface that may later come in contact with a patient. Use sterile transfer forceps, or sterilizing forceps, to remove items from whatever disinfection unit is used. Always wear gloves to handle disinfected items, and make sure you store disinfected equipment in a clean, moisture-free environment.

Sterilization: The Third Level of Infection Control

Sterilization is required for all instruments or supplies that will penetrate a patient's skin or come in contact with any other normally sterile areas of the body. Sterilization is also required for all instruments that will be used in a sterile field, even if they will not actually be used on a patient. An item is considered either sterile or unsterile. If you doubt the status of an item, consider it unsterile.

Before sterilizing an item, you must first sanitize it and, sometimes, disinfect it. Instruments and equipment that need to be sterilized include the following:

- Curettes (spoon-shaped instruments for removing material from the wall of a cavity or other surface)
- Needles
- Syringes
- Vaginal specula (instruments used to enlarge the opening of the vagina and allow examination of the vagina and cervix)

Sterilize instruments and equipment by one of the following methods:

- Autoclaving
- Chemical (cold) processes
- Dry heat processes
- Gas processes
- Microwave processes

The Autoclave

The primary method for sterilizing instruments and equipment is the use of pressurized steam in an **autoclave** (Figure 2-3). This device forces the temperature of steam above the boiling point of water (212°F, or 100°C). There are two reasons why sterilization by autoclave is such a widely accepted method of sterilization. First, steam autoclaves can operate at a lower temperature than is required for dry heat sterilization. The moist heat from steam more quickly permeates the clean, porous wrappings in which all instruments are placed prior to loading them into the unit. Second, the moisture causes coagulation of proteins within microorganisms at a much lower temperature than is possible with dry heat. When cells containing coagulated protein cool, their cell walls burst, resulting in the death of the microorganisms.

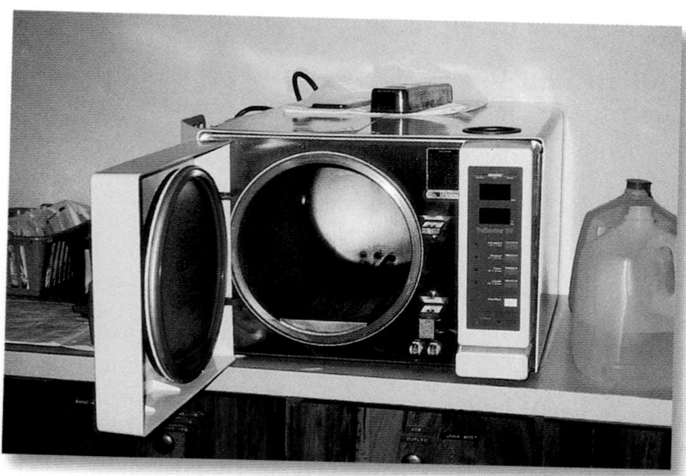

Figure 2-3. Steam autoclaving is the most common method of sterilizing instruments and equipment.

General Autoclave Procedures. In general, the autoclave process involves your taking the following steps.

1. Prepare sanitized and disinfected instruments and equipment for loading into the autoclave by wrapping them in muslin or special porous paper or plastic bags or envelopes and labeling each pack. (Include sterilization indicators.)
2. Preheat the autoclave according to the manufacturer's guidelines. (Some models require putting instruments in before preheating.)
3. Perform any required quality control procedures (besides including sterilization indicators in instrument packs).
4. Load the instruments and equipment into the autoclave. Allow adequate space around the items to ensure that steam reaches all areas.
5. Set the autoclave for the correct time after the correct temperature and pressure have been reached.
6. Run the autoclave through the sterilization cycle, including drying time.
7. Remove the instruments and equipment from the autoclave.
8. Store the instruments and equipment properly for the next use. Rotate stored items so that packages with the oldest date are used first.
9. Clean the autoclave and the surrounding work area.

During each step of the process, assume that the instruments and equipment are contaminated, and follow Universal Precautions.

- Wear gloves to avoid contamination by blood, body fluids, or tissues
- Take measures to protect against needlesticks or cuts—for example, by using forceps to handle sharps
- Wash your hands thoroughly after all cleaning procedures

Wrapping and Labeling All Items. Wrap items in porous fabric, paper, or plastic when placing them in the autoclave. This material helps surround the items with the correct levels of moisture and heat. Instruments and equipment that are to be used immediately after autoclaving can be placed on trays with material above and below the items. Items that are to be stored or that must be sterile when used must be wrapped and sealed before autoclaving. Refer to Procedure 2-1 for wrapping and labeling instructions.

PROCEDURE 2.1

Wrapping and Labeling Instruments for Sterilization in the Autoclave

Objective: To enclose instruments and equipment to be sterilized in appropriate wrapping materials to ensure sterilization and to protect supplies from contamination after sterilization

OSHA Guidelines

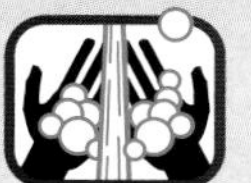
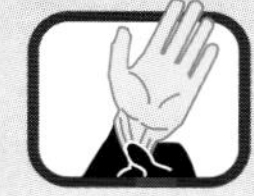
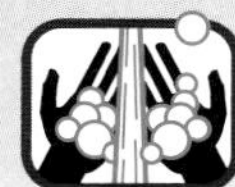

Materials: Dry, sanitized, and disinfected instruments and equipment; wrapping material (paper, muslin, gauze, bags, envelopes); sterilization indicators; autoclave tape; labels (if wrapping does not include space for labeling); pen

Method

For wrapping instruments or equipment in pieces of paper or fabric:

1. Wash your hands and put on gloves before beginning to wrap the items to be sterilized.
2. Place a square of paper or muslin on the table with one point toward you. With muslin, use a double thickness. The paper or fabric must be large enough to allow all four points to cover the instruments or equipment you will be wrapping and to provide an overlap, which will be used as a handling flap.
3. Place each item to be included in the pack in the center area of the paper or fabric "diamond" (Figure 2-4a). Items that will be used together should be wrapped together. Take care, however, that surfaces of the items do not touch each other inside the pack. Inspect each item to make sure it is operating correctly. Place hinged instruments in the pack in the open position. Wrap a small piece of paper, muslin, or gauze around delicate edges or points to protect against damage to other instruments or to the pack wrapping.
4. Place a sterilization indicator inside the pack with the instruments. Position the indicator correctly, following the manufacturer's guidelines.
5. Fold the bottom point of the diamond up and over the instruments in to the center (Figure 2-4b). Fold back a small portion of the point (Figure 2-4c). This "handle" will be used later, when the sterile pack is opened.

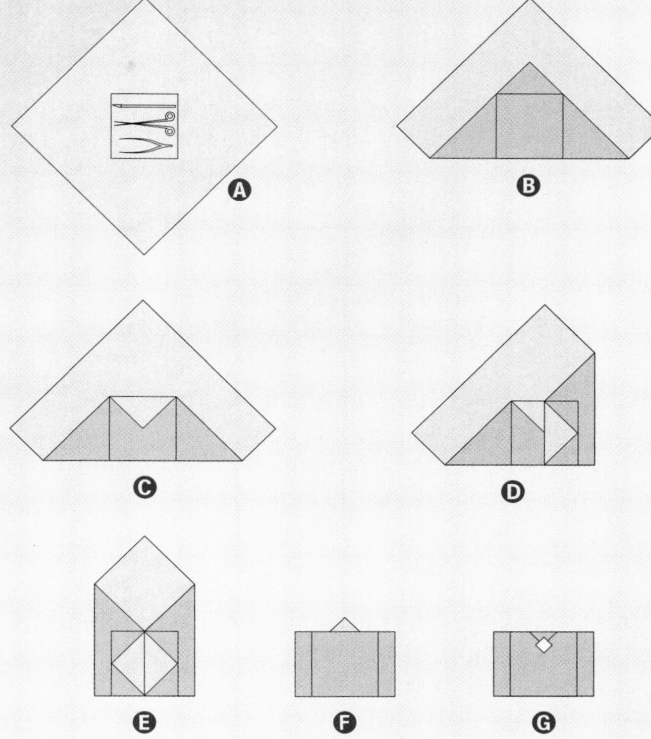

Figure 2-4. Follow this sequence when you wrap instruments in a paper or fabric pack for sterilization in an autoclave.

6. Fold the right point of the diamond in to the center. Again, fold back a small portion of the point to be used as a handle (Figure 2-4d).
7. Fold the left point of the diamond in to the center, folding back a small portion to form a handle. The pack should now resemble an open envelope (Figure 2-4e).
8. Grasp the covered instruments (the bottom of the envelope) and fold this portion up, toward the top point (Figure 2-4f). Fold the top point down over the pack, making sure the pack is snug but not too tight.
9. Secure the pack with autoclave tape (Figure 2-4g). A "quick-opening tab" can be created by folding a small portion of the tape back onto itself. The pack must be snug enough to prevent instruments from slipping out of the wrapping or damaging each other

continued ⟶

PROCEDURE 2.1

Wrapping and Labeling Instruments for Sterilization in the Autoclave *(continued)*

inside the pack but loose enough to allow adequate circulation of steam through the pack.

10. Label the pack with your initials and the date. List the contents of the pack as well. If the pack contains syringes, be sure to identify the syringe size(s).
11. Place the pack aside for loading into the autoclave.
12. Remove gloves, dispose of them in the appropriate waste container, and wash your hands.

For wrapping instruments and equipment in bags or envelopes:

1. Wash your hands and put on gloves before beginning to wrap the items to be sterilized.
2. Insert the items into the bag or envelope as indicated by the manufacturer's directions. Hinged instruments should be opened before insertion into the package.
3. Close and seal the pack. Make sure the sterilization indicator is not damaged or already exposed.
4. Label the pack with your initials and the date. List the contents of the pack as well. The pens or pencils used to label the pack must be waterproof; otherwise, the contents of the pack and date of sterilization will be obliterated.
5. Place the pack aside for loading into the autoclave.
6. Remove gloves, dispose of them in the appropriate waste container, and wash your hands.

A number of products are available for wrapping items for sterilization. Muslin (140 count) is the most commonly used wrapping fabric. Other products include permeable paper or plastic bags or envelopes, disposable nonwoven fabric, and clear plastic envelopes with one side made of permeable material. Figure 2-5 shows several common wrapping products.

Instruments that will be used together must be wrapped together to form a sterile pack. Take care to wrap the pack loosely so that the steam can reach the instruments inside. Position the instruments so they do not touch each other inside the pack. After using a pack later, consider all items (even those not used) unsterile, and return them for sanitization, disinfection, and sterilization.

Clearly label each pack to identify the item or items inside the wrapping and the person who completed the procedure. The label must also include the date so that packs are not used after their expiration dates. A 30-day period is generally considered the maximum shelf life for a sterile pack wrapped in cloth (6 months for airtight pouches).

Preheating the Autoclave. Be careful to check for solution that may have boiled over and for the formation of deposits on any of the inner surfaces. Make sure the water reservoir is filled to the proper level with distilled water. Also check the discharge lines and valves to make sure there are no obstructions. If lines or valves are blocked, air may remain trapped inside the chamber, rendering the load unsterile.

Following this inspection, preheat the unit according to the manufacturer's guidelines. Loading cold instruments into an overheated chamber can cause excess condensation, so be sure to understand and follow the preheating instructions.

Understanding Autoclave Settings. Modern autoclaves are designed to operate as automatically as possible. Because you are responsible for the sterility of the items

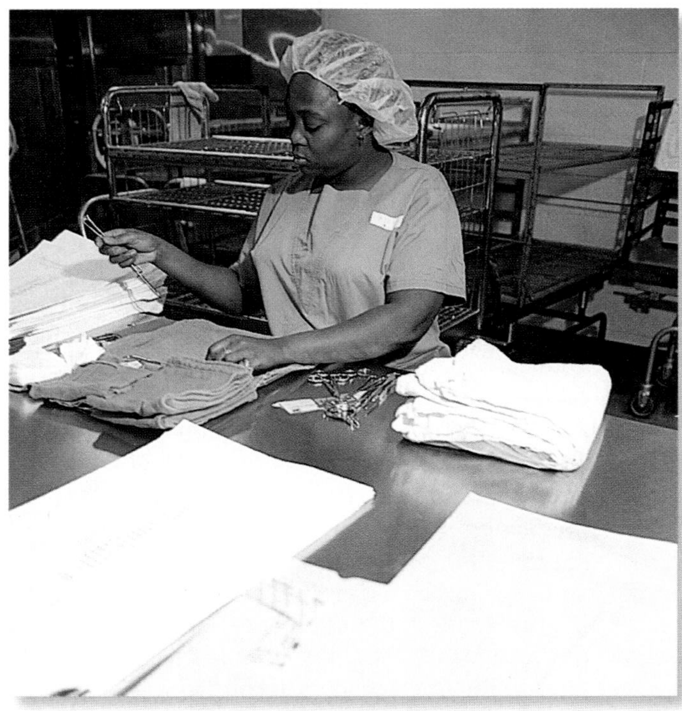

Figure 2-5. Many wrapping products are available for use when instruments or equipment are autoclaved.

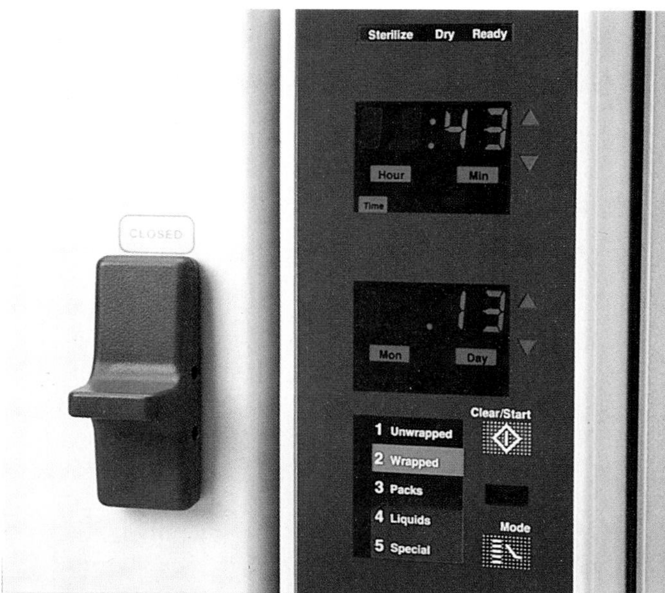

Figure 2-6. Understanding the gauges and timer is essential to proper operation of an autoclave.

processed by the autoclave, however, you must be able to identify the various gauges and interpret their readings correctly.

Most autoclaves have three gauges and a timer (Figure 2-6). The jacket pressure gauge shows the outer chamber's steam pressure. The chamber pressure gauge shows the inner chamber's steam pressure. The temperature gauge shows the temperature inside the inner, or sterilization, chamber. The timer allows you to control the number of minutes that the load is exposed to the high-temperature, pressurized steam.

Exact temperature and pressure requirements vary with the model and type of autoclave as well as with the instruments and packaging in the load. In general, the temperature must reach 250° to 270°F (121° to 132°C), and the chamber pressure gauge must show 15 to 30 pounds of pressure. Follow the manufacturer's instructions precisely for each autoclave load. Procedure 2-2 describes the general steps to follow for running a load through the preheated autoclave.

Storing Sterilized Supplies. After packs and instruments are sterilized in the autoclave, you must store them in a clean, dry location. The method you use to wrap an item for sterilization determines the item's sterile shelf life. As a general rule, double-layer, fabric- or paper-wrapped packages are considered sterile for 30 days. The manufacturers of other wrapping products provide their own guidelines for sterile shelf life.

Return items for sanitization, disinfection, and sterilization after the sterile shelf life period has elapsed. Do not reuse any wrapping or labeling products. Instead, process each item as if it had never been cleaned.

Cleaning the Autoclave and Work Area. Clean the autoclave after each use to prevent accumulation of deposits that might affect the unit's operation. You may use an all-purpose cleaner, although specific cleaning products are available for use with autoclaves.

You are responsible for ensuring that routine cleaning is done correctly and thoroughly. When you clean the unit, also check for signs of cracking or wear in gaskets, drain valves, and tubing. Check the level of distilled water in the reservoir. Service representatives who specialize in the maintenance of your unit should periodically clean and check all seals and gauges.

The work area around the autoclave unit should be divided into two areas: one for unsterile, not-yet-autoclaved items and one for sterile equipment as it is removed from the unit. Each area should be clearly marked. Do not use supplies from one area in the other. Be sure to move any sterile packs or equipment to the correct storage areas when cleaning the counters and other work surfaces. If anything is spilled on a sterile pack or instrument, return the item for sanitization, disinfection, and sterilization.

Performing Quality Control. From time to time, personnel at an independent testing facility should check the operation of the autoclave. Commonly, this check is done by running a regular load through the complete cycle and sending one or more samples from the load to a testing laboratory. The laboratory examines the articles and tests them for sterility. You may be required to process the test load and prepare it for submission to the test facility.

Preventing Incomplete Sterilization. Although the autoclave is generally considered the simplest and most effective method for sterilizing instruments and equipment, certain pitfalls can cause incomplete sterilization. The four leading factors that cause incomplete sterilization are incorrect timing, insufficient temperature, overcrowding of packs and inadequate steam levels. Once again, the manufacturer's guidelines provided with the autoclave unit are the best source for accurate information about how to operate it correctly.

Timing Guidelines. After loading the autoclave, make sure the heating cycle lasts long enough to allow the steam to permeate all wrappings to reach the instruments and equipment inside. Timing for items to be sterilized should not be started until the unit has reached the proper temperature. Although following timing guidelines helps ensure sterilization, you should also use sterilization indicators. **Sterilization indicators** are tags, inserts, tapes, tubes, or strips that confirm that the items in the autoclave have been exposed to the correct volume of steam at the correct temperature for the correct length of time. Several types of indicators are available (Figure 2-8).

You place tags or inserts within the load, whereas you affix tapes to the outside of wrapped instrument packs. These types of indicators have designated areas or words that change color when the correct temperature has been reached. Some also show when the proper temperature, pressure, and duration have occurred. Although it is generally acceptable to rely on these indicators as a guarantee

PROCEDURE 2.2

Running a Load Through the Autoclave

Objective: To run a load of instruments and equipment through an autoclave, ensuring sterilization of items by properly loading, drying, and unloading them

OSHA Guidelines

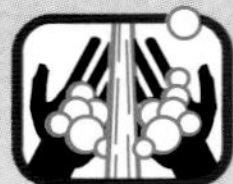 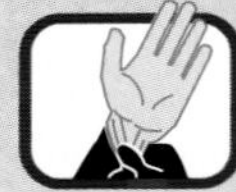 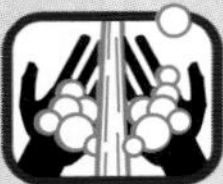

Materials: Dry, sanitized, and disinfected instruments and equipment, both individual pieces and packs; oven mitts; sterile transfer forceps; storage containers for individual items

Method

1. Wash your hands and put on gloves before beginning to load items into the autoclave.
2. Rest packs on their edges, and place jars and containers on their sides.
3. Place lids for jars and containers with their sterile sides down.
4. If the load includes plastic items, make sure no other item leans against them. (Pressure that results from the high temperatures can cause plastic items to bend or warp.)
5. If your load is mixed—containing both wrapped packs and individual instruments—place the tray containing the instruments below the tray containing the wrapped packs (Figure 2-7). (This arrangement prevents any condensation that forms on the instruments from dripping onto the wrapped packs, saturating the wrapping.)
6. Close the door and start the unit.
7. Start the timer when the indicators show the recommended temperature and pressure.
8. Right after the end of the steam cycle and just before the start of the drying cycle, open the door to the autoclave slightly (between ¼ and ½ inch). (Opening the door more than ½ inch causes cold air to enter the autoclave, possibly resulting in excessive condensation in the chamber. This condensation would cause incomplete drying.)
9. Dry according to the manufacturer's recommendations. (Packs and large items may require up to 45 minutes to dry completely.)

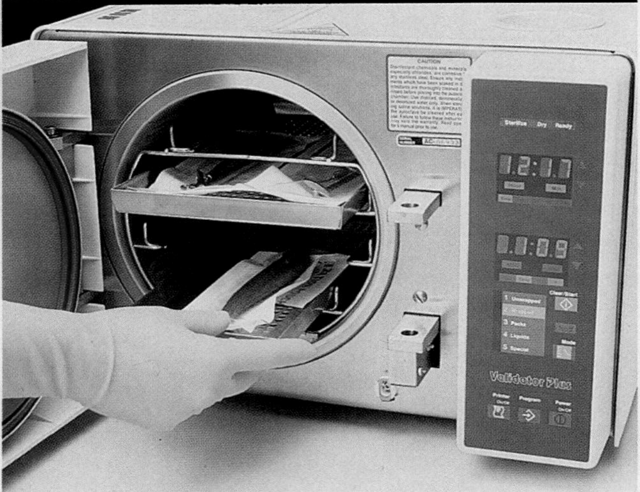

Figure 2-7. Properly loaded trays allow steam to reach all instruments and equipment.

10. Unload the autoclave after the drying cycle is finished. (Do not unload any packs or instruments with wet wrappings, or the object inside will be considered unsterile and must be processed again.)
11. Unload each package carefully. Wear oven mitts to protect yourself from burns when removing wrapped packs. Use sterile transfer forceps to unload unwrapped individual objects.
12. Inspect each package or item, looking for moisture on the wrapping, underexposed sterilization indicators, and tears or breaks in the wrapping. (Consider the pack unsterile if any of these conditions is present.)
13. Place sterile packs aside for transfer to storage.
14. Place individual items that are not required to be sterile in clean containers.
15. Place items that must remain sterile in sterile containers, being sure to close the container covers tightly.
16. As you unload items, avoid placing them in an overly cool location because the cool temperature could cause condensation on the instruments or packs.
17. Remove gloves, dispose of them in the appropriate waste container, and wash your hands.

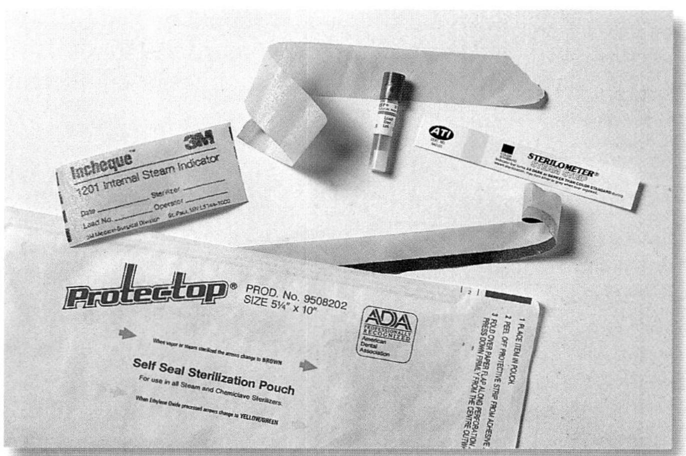

Figure 2-8. Sterilization indicators are manufactured in many sizes and shapes.

of sterility, they are, in reality, only indicators that the load has been exposed to conditions that usually result in sterile surfaces. They do not guarantee that the contents of the autoclave are actually sterile.

Other sterilization indicators are bioindicator tubes and strips. These tubes and strips contain live microorganisms or bacterial spores. After being run through a sterilization cycle, the microorganisms in the indicator should be dead. If they are still alive, you know that the sterilization cycle is not working. Some of these indicators must be sent to a laboratory for testing, whereas others can be cultured in the office. It is important to remember that although these indicators show more conclusively than others that bacteria have been killed, items in a given load may still be unsterile.

In general, place indicators in a sufficient number of places in the load so that you can be reasonably confident of the sterility of all items in the chamber. The following locations are suitable for indicator positioning:

- Within instrument packs
- On the outside of wrapped instrument packs
- Inside containers, especially those that cannot be positioned so that steam surrounds the item
- Near the air exhaust valve
- In any other areas into which steam might not be able to flow freely

If you have any doubt about the sterility of an instrument or piece of equipment, do not use it. Instead, put it aside for another cycle of sanitization, disinfection, and sterilization. The risks to patients and to you are too great to take chances.

Temperature Guidelines. The length of the sterilization cycle is only one factor that has an impact on the final quality of autoclave operations. You must also be sure that the unit is operating at the correct temperature. Unit thermometers and sterilization indicators help confirm that correct temperatures have been reached.

Temperatures that are too high can cause problems as easily as those that are too low. If the temperature is too high inside the autoclave compartment, the steam does not have the correct level of moisture. The heat and moisture will not penetrate wrapped packs of instruments, and the result will be an unsterilized load.

If the temperature is too low, the steam contains too much moisture. Packs will be oversaturated, and the drying cycle will be insufficient. Wet packs can easily pick up contaminants from surfaces they touch after you unload them from the autoclave. Common causes of low temperature are failing to preheat the autoclave chamber, loading cold instruments into an overheated chamber, opening the unit door too wide during drying, and overfilling the water reservoir.

Overcrowding. Packs or instruments placed in too close proximity in the autoclave chamber may not be sterilized because of the inability of the steam to penetrate or reach all surfaces.

Steam Level Guidelines. If the correct level of steam is not present during the autoclave cycle, items will not be sterile at the end of the cycle. It is vital that the unit force all air out of the chamber at the beginning of the sterilization cycle. It is also essential that you place items in the chamber in positions that will not cause formation of air pockets.

To help ensure proper operation of the unit, check all release valves and discharge lines to make sure they are free from obstruction. Clogged valves and lines may prevent elimination of all air from the chamber.

To prevent the formation of air pockets, load items in the autoclave so that the steam can circulate freely around all sides of the items. Place containers on their sides to avoid trapping air. Besides allowing the free flow of steam, careful positioning helps ensure that all items dry thoroughly before you remove them from the autoclave.

Other Methods of Sterilization

Although steam autoclaving is the most common method of instrument and equipment sterilization, other methods may be used. In fact, the autoclave is not recommended for some instruments because of the extreme temperatures used.

Chemical Processes. Sterilization using chemical solutions is sometimes called cold sterilization because this method does not use heat to kill microorganisms. The chemical sterilization process is generally used on instruments that can be damaged by prolonged exposure to the high temperatures of a steam autoclave. The time required for cold sterilization can extend from 20 minutes to 10 hours, however, and you must be sure to follow the manufacturer's guidelines exactly to ensure sterilization.

One chemical process uses an unsaturated chemical vapor sterilizer, or as it is known by its trade name, the Chemiclave (Figure 2-9). This unit combines chemical sterilization with steam autoclaving techniques. A measured amount of bactericidal solution is released into a cleaning

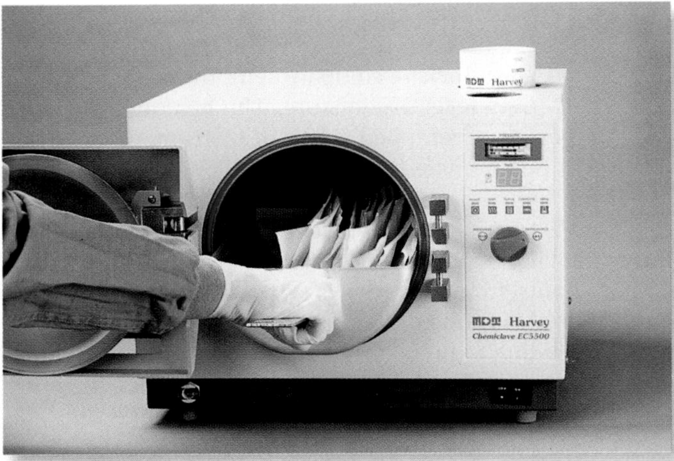

Figure 2-9. The Chemiclave is an unsaturated chemical vapor sterilizer.

chamber. The temperature inside the unit is raised to 270°F (132°C), and the pressure is raised to 20 to 40 pounds. This unit has the advantage of fast operation (about 20 minutes) because there is no need to preheat the inner chamber.

Dry Heat Processes. Dry heat processes are used when the items to be sterilized would be damaged by immersion in chemical solutions or by exposure to steam. Operating essentially the same way as a household oven, the dry heat unit raises the temperature in the sterilizing chamber to 250° to 320°F (121° to 160°C). Sterilization is accomplished in about an hour at the upper end of the temperature range; however, time requirements increase dramatically for lower temperatures (about 9 hours at 250°F).

Gas Processes. Gas sterilization uses ethylene oxide, a gas that is hazardous to humans and to the environment. Because of this potential danger, gas sterilization is commonly used only in hospital and manufacturing environments. Instruments that can be damaged by exposure to heat and moisture can be effectively sterilized by this method. Gas sterilization usually takes longer than steam autoclaving (about 2 to 3 hours) because the gas process includes a mandatory aeration step to remove residual gas from the items being cleaned.

Microwave Processes. The newest method of instrument sterilization is microwaving. This method uses low-pressure steam with radiation to produce localized heat that kills microorganisms. The cycle, which may be as short as 30 seconds, is faster than other methods of sterilization. Current models, however, have a small chamber size: 1 to 3 cubic feet. You can sterilize metal instruments in a microwave unit by placing them under a partial vacuum in a glass container.

Waste Disposal

The sanitization, disinfection, and sterilization processes generate some waste products. If you are resterilizing equipment whose shelf life has expired, the old wrappings should be considered unsterile and should be handled appropriately. Follow correct disposal procedures for biohazardous waste when discarding any supplies or equipment during the sterilization process.

Some Infectious Diseases

Sanitization, disinfection, and sterilization are crucial to infection control. Infection control is not limited to these procedures, however. Identifying signs and symptoms of some infectious diseases can also help protect health-care workers and patients from exposure to pathogens. Signs are objective findings as measured or perceived by an examiner. They may include a fever or a rash. Symptoms are subjective indications of a disease or a change in condition as perceived by the patient. Nausea and dizziness are examples of symptoms. Table 2-1 summarizes characteristics of some infectious diseases.

You can help break the cycle of infection by recommending guidelines for patients to follow to limit the spread of infectious disease in general. In Chapter 1, you learned about ways to educate patients in the prevention of disease transmission. It is also helpful to teach patients to recognize the symptoms of infectious diseases they may encounter. Early recognition may prompt early treatment and measures to protect others who are vulnerable to transmission of the disease from the infected patient. In a hospital setting, follow additional guidelines to prevent hospital-related, or **nosocomial, infection.** Several guidelines to follow in hospitals are discussed in the Diseases and Disorders section.

Chickenpox (Varicella)

Chickenpox, or varicella, is a contagious viral infection with an incubation period of 7 to 21 days. Patients with chickenpox experience an itchy rash that begins as tiny, red bumps and eventually becomes fluid-filled blisters. The blisters break and dry into scabs, usually within a few days. The rash may cover most of the body. Patients may also run a slight fever, have a headache, and experience general malaise. The infection is spread through direct or indirect transmission as well as by droplets, or airborne secretions. Patients should be isolated for about a week following the initial eruption of the rash, until all the blisters have scabbed over. In 1996 the Food and Drug Administration (FDA) approved a live vaccine for chickenpox, and it was recently added to the immunization schedule for children. Many states require reporting chickenpox cases to the state or county department of health, although there are no national requirements for reporting them.

Common Cold

Common colds are viral infections of the upper respiratory tract. They are transmitted from person to person through direct or indirect contact. The patient does not have to be isolated. It is important, however, that commonsense precautions be taken to avoid spreading the infection to

TABLE 2-1 Characteristics of Some Infectious Diseases

Disease	Infecting Agent	Transmission Method	Incubation Period	Isolation Period	Reporting Required
Chickenpox	Virus	D/I/DR	7–21 days	Until all blisters have scabbed over	By some states
Common cold	Various viruses	D/I	2–3 days	None	No
Croup	Various bacteria, viruses	D/I	2–3 days	None	No
Diphtheria	Bacteria	D/I/DR	2–5 days	Two negative tissue samples	Yes
Hib infections	Bacteria	D/I/DR	3 days	Varies	No
Influenza	Various viruses	D/I	1–3 days	As patient can be isolated	No
Measles	Virus	D/DR	8–14 days, until rash appears	7 days after rash onset	Yes
Meningitis	Various bacteria, viruses	D/DR	1–3 days	None	Yes
Mumps	Virus	D/DR	2–3 weeks	Until swelling stops	Yes
Pertussis	Bacteria	D/I/DR	1 week	3 weeks after cough onset	Yes
Poliomyelitis	Virus	D	Usually 7–14 days	1 week after onset	Yes
Roseola	Possibly virus	Unknown	5–15 days	Unknown	No
Rubella	Virus	D/DR	Usually 16–18 days	None except to protect pregnant women	Yes
Scarlet fever	Bacteria	D/DR	1–3 days	7 days	No
Tetanus	Bacteria	D (through contamination of puncture wound)	3–21 days	None	Yes
Tuberculosis	Bacteria	DR	4–12 weeks	Variable	Yes

Note: D = direct; I = indirect; DR = droplet

others. For example, advise the patient to use tissues when coughing or sneezing, and have the patient and family wash their hands frequently and, if possible, use disposable dishware while the patient is ill. Incubation normally lasts for 2 to 3 days.

Croup

Croup is a condition that occurs when an allergy, a foreign body, an infection, or a new growth obstructs the upper airway. It is characterized by a harsh, barking cough, difficulty breathing, hoarseness, and low-grade fever. Croup is most common in infants and young children. Symptoms of croup may be lessened by humidifying the air in the child's room, encouraging rest, and giving clear, warm fluids. If croup accompanies a bacterial respiratory infection, the doctor may prescribe antibiotics. As with the common cold, have the patient and family take commonsense precautions to prevent spreading the respiratory infection to others.

Diphtheria

Diphtheria is a bacterial infection, primarily of the nose, throat, and larynx. The patient may experience pain, fever, and respiratory obstruction. Untreated, diphtheria is generally fatal. The incubation period is between 2 and 5 days.

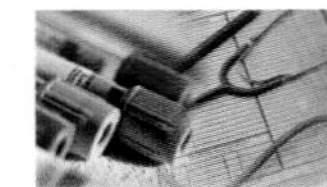

Diseases and Disorders

Preventing Nosocomial Infections

Patients in hospital settings are at risk not only from the disease or injury that caused the hospitalization but also from nosocomial, or hospital-related, infection. The Centers for Disease Control and Prevention (CDC) publishes a seven-part series discussing techniques for control of nosocomial infections. The guidelines cover the following topics:

- Catheter-associated urinary tract infections
- Hand washing and environmental control
- Infection control in hospital personnel
- Intravascular device-related infections
- Isolation precautions in hospitals (discussed later in this chapter)
- Nosocomial pneumonia
- Surgical wound infections

Researchers at the CDC have found that if hospital personnel pay careful attention to the care of instruments and devices used to deliver care to patients, significant improvements can be made regarding patients' chances for avoiding infection. In addition, new, less-invasive techniques for delivering medications are promising an even greater reduction in patient risk.

To obtain a copy of these guidelines, contact:

National Technical Information Service (NTIS)
5285 Port Royal Road
Springfield, VA 22161
703-487-4650

The CDC can also be found on the World Wide Web at http://www.cdc.gov.

The patient must be isolated from others and undergo antibiotic therapy until tissue cells taken from the nose and the throat show negative results. Once a leading cause of death among young children, diphtheria is now rare in the United States because of widespread immunization. Cases of diphtheria must be reported to the state or county health department.

Haemophilus Influenzae Type B

Haemophilus influenzae type B (Hib) is a frequent cause of bacterial infections—including blood infections, epiglottitis, and pneumonia—in infants and young children in the United States. It is spread through direct, indirect, and droplet transmission. The incubation period is approximately 3 days. The patient may experience upper respiratory symptoms, fever, drowsiness, body aches, and diminished appetite. The infection can also cause bacterial meningitis (a swelling or inflammation of the tissue covering the spinal cord and brain) and should be carefully monitored.

Influenza (Flu)

Nearly everyone has experienced symptoms of influenza, or the flu: fever, chills, headaches, body aches, and upper respiratory congestion. Isolation and other commonsense precautions can greatly reduce transmission of this viral infection.

Measles (Rubeola)

Measles, also called rubeola, is an infectious viral disease spread through droplets or direct transmission. Normally, the disease requires 8 to 13 days for the initial symptom of fever to appear. The characteristic itchy rash appears 14 days after exposure. Patients should follow isolation procedures for 7 days after the rash first appears. Children under the age of 3 are especially at risk for contagion and should be kept apart from family members who have contracted the disease. The CDC requires reporting measles to the state or county health department.

Meningitis

Meningitis is an inflammation and infection of the protective coverings of the brain and spinal cord, and the fluid that surrounds these tissues. Meningitis is usually caused by an infection with a virus or bacteria. Viral meningitis is usually relatively mild. It clears up in a week or two without specific treatment. Viral meningitis is also called aseptic meningitis.

Bacterial meningitis is a serious, life-threatening condition that requires immediate medical treatment. Severe bacterial meningitis can result in brain damage and even death. It affects more men than women. At highest risk are the elderly, children under age 5, and people with chronic illnesses. Risk groups include children in daycare, schools, and college students living in dorms or other close environments.

Between 5% and 20% of the population normally carry the bacteria that cause meningitis. These bacteria are commonly found in the nose and throat. Occasionally, a person who carries these bacteria develops meningitis. A person with an ear or sinus infection is at greater risk for meningitis. In addition, persons who have certain types of skull fractures also have a higher risk for developing meningitis.

For patients over the age of 2, symptoms may include a red, blotchy rash; confusion and delirium (delusions or hallucinations); coma (in severe cases); discomfort looking into bright lights; headache; high fever and chills; nausea and vomiting; pain in the arms, legs, and abdomen; sleepiness; and a stiff neck and back. The classic symptoms of fever, headache, and neck stiffness may be absent or difficult to detect in newborns and small infants. The infant may only appear slow or inactive, be irritable, have vomiting, or be feeding poorly.

Some forms of bacterial meningitis are contagious. The bacteria are spread through the exchange of respiratory and throat secretions (for example, coughing, kissing, laughing, or sneezing). It can also be spread to individuals who have had close or prolonged contact with an infectious patient who has meningitis caused by *Neisseria meningitidis* (also called meningococcal meningitis) or Hib. Any health-care worker who has had direct contact with an infectious patient's oral secretions would be considered at increased risk of acquiring the infection. The CDC requires reporting meningitis to the state or county health department.

Mumps

Mumps is a viral infection that primarily affects the salivary glands. The incubation period lasts from 2 to 3 weeks. The patient may experience pain, especially related to parotitis (inflammation of the parotid gland near the ear), and fever. Isolation procedures should be followed until glandular swelling stops. You must report all cases of mumps to the state or county health department.

Pertussis (Whooping Cough)

Pertussis, or whooping cough, is an acute, highly contagious bacterial infection of the respiratory tract. Symptoms include slight fever, sneezing, runny nose, and quick, short coughs. The characteristic "whoop" occurs during the inhaled breath that follows a severe coughing fit. The patient should be isolated for 3 weeks after the onset of the spasmodic coughs. Whooping cough cases must be reported to the state or county health department.

Poliomyelitis (Polio)

Poliomyelitis, also called polio, is an acute viral disease involving the gray matter of the spinal cord. It is caused by any of three related viruses, and it occurs in three different forms:

1. Inapparent, in which a patient may experience fever, sore throat, headache, and vomiting
2. Nonparalytic, in which a patient experiences the same symptoms as with the inapparent type, but in a more severe form, and in which pain and stiffness occur in the neck, back, and legs
3. Paralytic, in which a patient has the same symptoms as with the nonparalytic form, followed by recovery and then signs of central nervous system paralysis

Although polio outbreaks occur worldwide, polio's current incidence in the United States is limited to fewer than ten cases each year. Since the 1950s, the incidence of polio has decreased as a result of the routine immunization of most children. Vaccinations may be administered orally or by injection to protect against all three types of polio viruses. There is no drug treatment once the disease begins. Report all cases of polio to the state or county health department.

Roseola

Roseola is a rose-colored rash thought to be caused by a human herpes virus. The disease affects infants and young children; its incubation period lasts between 5 and 15 days. Symptoms include sudden, high fever; sore throat; swollen lymph nodes; and after several days, a rash. Although seizures may sometimes accompany cases involving a very high fever, the disease is usually not serious.

Rubella (German Measles)

Rubella, or German measles, is a highly contagious viral disease. It is transmitted through direct or droplet transmission, and incubation normally occurs in 16 to 18 days, although periods as long as 23 days have been recorded. Symptoms are mild and include fever and an itchy rash. Because of effective vaccination programs, the occurrence of rubella is diminishing. Fetuses of pregnant women who are not immune to rubella are at the greatest risk because the disease can cause birth defects in a fetus during the first trimester of pregnancy. Report rubella to the state or county department of health.

Scarlet Fever (Scarlatina)

Scarlet fever, also known as scarlatina, commonly accompanies strep throat (a bacterial infection). In addition to the symptoms of strep throat (fever, sore throat, and swollen glands), the patient experiences the characteristic "strawberry rash" (tiny, bright-red spots) that progresses from the trunk and neck to the face and extremities, along with nausea and vomiting. Incubation occurs in 1 to 3 days, and the patient may be kept isolated for 7 days, although a shorter period may be allowed if symptoms indicate the infection is not severe.

Tetanus

Tetanus is an acute, often fatal infectious bacterial disease. The infection follows the introduction of pathogenic spores, which enter the body through a contaminated puncture wound. If the disease process is not halted, the patient can experience lockjaw (a motor disturbance resulting in difficulty opening the mouth) and, eventually, paralysis. Incubation of the disease is normally 3 to 21 days. Patients with tetanus do not need to be isolated, but you must report cases to the state or county health department.

Tuberculosis

Tuberculosis, also called TB, is an infectious bacterial disease that mainly affects the lungs but can also involve other organs. TB is the leading infectious killer of adults worldwide. A patient infected with tuberculosis may not have any symptoms. The body's immune system often destroys the bacteria, leaving only a scar or spot on the lungs. Sometimes, however, the infection spreads, and the patient exhibits these symptoms:

- Night sweats
- Productive and prolonged cough
- Fever
- Chills
- Fatigue
- Unexplained weight loss
- Diminished appetite
- Bloody sputum

Incidence of Tuberculosis. After a rise in the nationwide number of tuberculosis cases between 1985 and 1992, the incidence in the United States began to decline. Incidence remains high or on the increase in many states, however, particularly in some urban centers. You may encounter patients with tuberculosis, and you can never relax your vigilance when working in environments where there is any risk of infection.

Many factors contribute to the continued high incidence of tuberculosis. You may work with patients who are affected by some or all of these factors:

- Infection with HIV increases the risk for developing tuberculosis after exposure to the pathogen
- The population of the United States is shifting to include a larger percentage of people from countries where there is a higher incidence of tuberculosis
- The number of people living in environments known to pose increased risk, such as long-term institutional settings, homeless centers, and medically underserved neighborhoods, has increased
- The public health-care system is unable to meet the needs of its constituents, resulting in patients who remain untreated
- New drug-resistant strains of the tuberculosis pathogen are appearing, requiring longer and more potent therapy regimens, which are harder to enforce and with which many patients do not comply

Understanding how tuberculosis is transmitted and managed will help you apply the principles of infection control.

Transmission of Tuberculosis. *Mycobacterium tuberculosis,* the microorganism responsible for tuberculosis infection, is spread through droplet transmission. The bacteria can spread through the air near an infected person when the person breathes, coughs, sneezes, or talks. When another person inhales the bacteria, they travel through that person's respiratory system to lodge in the alveoli. From there, the bacteria can eventually spread throughout the body.

The most effective way to break the growth cycle of the tuberculosis pathogen is to contain the bacteria at the source. Containing the pathogen at this point prevents its entrance into another host. Containment measures include the following:

- Instruct patients in the correct procedure for covering the mouth when sneezing, coughing, laughing, or yawning. Explain that patients should properly dispose of tissues or other materials that have been used to block a sneeze or a cough and should thoroughly wash their hands afterward.
- When you must perform a procedure that induces coughing, conduct the procedure in an area with negative air pressure, such as inside a protective booth. Negative air pressure acts to draw contaminated air out of the immediate area and into a filtration system.
- When you work with a patient who is infectious, wear a personal respirator to prevent inhalation of the bacteria. Be sure also to apply standard sanitization, disinfection, and sterilization techniques to instruments and equipment.

Increasing Resistance to Tuberculosis. Another way to break the pathogenic growth cycle is to decrease the susceptibility of the host. Early diagnosis, prompt treatment, and compliance with the treatment regimen have a positive impact on the outcome of tuberculosis. Risk factors for infection include the following:

- HIV infection or any disease state that weakens the immune system
- Intravenous drug use
- Previous tuberculosis infection
- Diabetes mellitus, a disorder characterized by a deficiency of the hormone insulin
- End-stage renal disease, a type of kidney disease
- Low body weight

Treating Tuberculosis. Tuberculosis infection must be confirmed by a Mantoux tuberculin skin test, in which you administer tuberculin intradermally with a needle and syringe. If the test results are positive, the skin area turns red and becomes raised and hard, which is termed **induration.** A positive test result reveals that a patient has had previous exposure to tuberculosis, either from immunization (common outside the United States) or from coming in contact with the tuberculosis bacteria. If a patient tests positive for tuberculin sensitivity, further tests, including chest x-rays and sputum examination, are performed.

The specific treatment of a patient with active tuberculosis depends on the part of the body affected and the type of tuberculosis involved. In all cases, however, drug therapy must be initiated immediately. Emphasize to patients the importance of completing the entire course of treatment (12 to 18 months on medication). Help patients comply with the treatment by providing education about the disease, the expected course of treatment, the anticipated outcome, and measures patients can take to prevent the spread of the disease.

Patients with active pulmonary tuberculosis should be hospitalized in a facility approved for treating the disease. They should also be placed in an isolation room with negative air pressure. Visitors should be kept to a minimum. Patients may be discharged to their homes after starting TB therapy, even though they may still be infectious. Transmission is less likely to occur after treatment has begun.

Drug-Resistant Microorganisms

Resistance to antimicrobial agents is a severe problem. Drug-resistant pathogens are the cause of many infections. It is the responsibility of physicians, medical staff, and patients to use antibiotics wisely. Becteria and other microorganisms that have developed resistance to antimicrobial drugs include the following:

- **MRSA**—methicillin/oxacillin-resistant *Staphylococcus aureus*
- **VRE**—vancomycin-resistant enterococci
- **VISA**—vancomycin-intermediate *Staphylococcus aureus*
- **VRSA**—vancomycin-resistant *Staphylococcus aureus*
- **ESBLs**—extended-spectrum beta-lactamases, which are resistant to cephalosporins and monobactams
- **PRSP**—penicillin-resistant *Streptococcus pneumoniae*

MRSA and VRE are the most common multidrug-resistant organisms in patients who reside in non-hospital health-care facilities, such as nursing homes and other long-term care facilities. PRSP are more common in patients seeking care in physicians' offices and clinics, especially in pediatric settings.

Risk Factors

There are a number of risk factors for both the development and infection of drug-resistant organisms. These risk factors include the following:

- Advanced age
- Invasive procedures, which include dialysis, the presence of invasive devices, and urinary catheterization
- Previous exposure to antimicrobial agents
- Repeated contact with the health-care system
- Severity of the illness
- Underlying diseases or conditions, especially chronic renal disease, insulin-dependent diabetes mellitus, peripheral vascular disease, and dermatitis or skin lesions.

Reporting Guidelines

The CDC requires reporting of certain diseases to the state or county department of health. This information, which is forwarded to the CDC, helps research epidemiologists control the spread of infection. Figure 2-10 lists diseases that must be reported.

The Notifiable Disease Surveillance System

Acquired immunodeficiency syndrome (AIDS)
Amebiasis
Anthrax
Aseptic meningitis
Botulism, food-borne
Botulism, infant
Botulism, wound
Botulism, unspecified
Brucellosis
Chancroid
Cholera
Congenital rubella syndrome
Diphtheria
Encephalitis, post-chickenpox
Encephalitis, postmumps
Encephalitis, postother
Encephalitis, primary
Gonorrhea
Granuloma inguinale
Hansen disease
Hepatitis A
Hepatitis B
Hepatitis C
Hepatitis, unspecified
Legionellosis
Leptospirosis
Lyme disease
Lymphogranuloma venereum
Malaria
Measles
Meningococcal infections
Mumps
Pertussis
Plague
Poliomyelitis, paralytic
Psittacosis
Rabies, animal
Rabies, human
Rheumatic fever
Rocky Mountain spotted fever
Rubella
Salmonellosis
Shigellosis
Syphilis, all stages
Syphilis, primary and secondary
Syphilis, congenital
Tetanus
Toxic shock syndrome
Trichinosis
Tuberculosis
Tularemia
Typhoid fever
Yellow fever

Note: The National Notifiable Disease Surveillance System does not require the reporting of varicella (chickenpox) cases. Many state agencies do, however, and the Council of State and Territorial Epidemiologists recommends the reporting of varicella cases to the CDC.

Figure 2-10. These diseases must be reported to the National Notifiable Disease Surveillance System of the CDC, through your state or county health department.

Guideline for Isolation Precautions in Hospitals

In early 1996 the CDC issued the current Guideline for Isolation Precautions in Hospitals. If you work in a hospital, it is essential to understand and apply these precautions. You must always ensure that you create an environment that protects people from disease-causing microorganisms. The guideline is made up of three major parts.

1. The first part combines the important features of Universal Precautions and Body Substance Isolation guidelines into one comprehensive set of precautions. This combined guideline is called Standard Precautions, and it is required in hospital settings.
2. The second part lists precautions designed to prevent the spread of infection through droplet, airborne, or contact transmission. These guidelines, called Transmission-Based Precautions, must be applied when you know the infectious status of patients. These Transmission-Based Precautions are applied in addition to Standard Precautions.
3. The third part describes specific syndromes you may encounter that are highly indicative of infection. When you do not know a patient's status but observe characteristics of infectious disease, follow the precautions described in this section of the guideline to prevent droplet, airborne, or contact transmission of pathogens until a diagnosis can be made.

Immunizations: Another Way to Control Infection

One of the necessary elements in the cycle of infection is the transmission of the pathogen to a susceptible host. You have already learned how to reduce the risk of infection by altering environmental conditions so that microorganisms find it difficult or impossible to survive. In addition, the risk of infection can be decreased by reducing the susceptibility of the host to infection. This reduction can be accomplished through **immunization** (administration of a vaccine or toxoid to protect susceptible individuals from infectious diseases).

When a healthy patient is vaccinated with a weakened strain of a virus, the lymphocytes manufacture antibodies against that virus. These antibodies remain in the body, making it immune to that virus in the future. Live-virus vaccines are used to immunize against measles and poliomyelitis. Immunization with a related virus can also be effective against some diseases. For example, immunization with cowpox virus has completely eradicated the incidence of smallpox, a contagious disease that leaves permanent scars on the skin.

Killed-virus vaccines, which are used to immunize against influenza and typhoid fever, do not provide protection for as long a period as that provided by live-virus vaccines. Weakened toxins, called toxoids, are used to produce active immunity against diseases such as tetanus and diphtheria.

Immunization Recommendations

The Advisory Committee on Immunization Practices, the American Academy of Pediatrics, and the American Academy of Family Physicians jointly publish immunization schedules for children. The National Coalition for Adult Immunization (NCAI) publishes similar schedules for adults. You should be familiar with the current guidelines regarding these vaccination schedules. The pediatric schedule is shown in Figure 2-11. The adult schedule is shown in Figure 2-12.

Many patients think of immunization requirements as existing only for children; however, there are also immunizations every adult should have. According to the NCAI, more than half of Americans over the age of 50 are not properly immunized against two potent diseases: tetanus and diphtheria.

Administering Immunizations

In many states, medical assistants may administer immunizations. Most immunizations are given as injections. (Chapter 33 describes administration of various types of injections.) Some vaccines, such as live polio, are given orally.

Whether or not you administer vaccines, you must explain the need for immunization to patients as well as describe what side effects, if any, they may experience. Common side effects of immunizations include soreness near the injection site, low-grade fever, and general malaise.

Special Immunization Concerns

Patients who are young, pregnant, or elderly, as well as those who have a weakened immune system, may require special handling related to immunizations. Health-care workers have special immunization needs too.

Pediatric Patients. Encourage parents to bring their children to the office at the recommended times for all immunizations. If a child has a fever, however, postpone the immunization until the fever has subsided. Do not postpone the visit if the child has an upper respiratory infection *without* a fever. Remember that the child does not need to restart a series of immunizations. He can simply receive the next scheduled immunization as soon as possible.

Informed Consent. As with any drug, the physician may ask you to explain the benefits and risks of immunization. For a pediatric patient, provide this information to the parents. Explain that the side effects of immunizations are usually mild, such as a slight fever or soreness, and of short duration. Advise parents that the benefits of immunity greatly outweigh the risks. Then obtain informed

Recommended Childhood and Adolescent Immunization Schedule — United States, January – June 2004

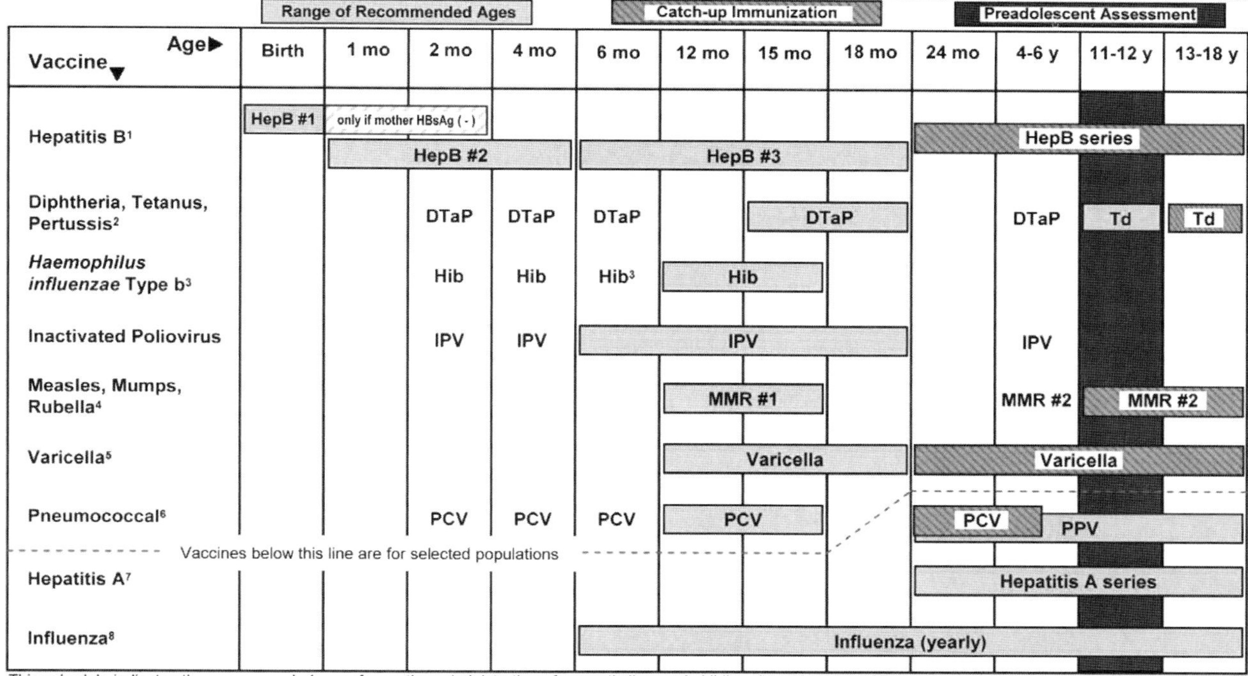

Range of Recommended Ages | Catch-up Immunization | Preadolescent Assessment

Vaccine ▼ / Age ►	Birth	1 mo	2 mo	4 mo	6 mo	12 mo	15 mo	18 mo	24 mo	4-6 y	11-12 y	13-18 y
Hepatitis B[1]	HepB #1	only if mother HBsAg (-)										
		HepB #2	HepB #2	HepB #2	HepB #3	HepB #3	HepB #3	HepB #3	HepB series	HepB series	HepB series	HepB series
Diphtheria, Tetanus, Pertussis[2]			DTaP	DTaP	DTaP		DTaP	DTaP		DTaP	Td	Td
Haemophilus influenzae Type b[3]			Hib	Hib	Hib[3]	Hib	Hib					
Inactivated Poliovirus			IPV	IPV	IPV	IPV	IPV	IPV		IPV		
Measles, Mumps, Rubella[4]						MMR #1	MMR #1			MMR #2	MMR #2	MMR #2
Varicella[5]						Varicella	Varicella	Varicella	Varicella	Varicella	Varicella	Varicella
Pneumococcal[6]			PCV	PCV	PCV	PCV	PCV		PCV	PCV		
									PPV	PPV	PPV	PPV
Vaccines below this line are for selected populations												
Hepatitis A[7]									Hepatitis A series	Hepatitis A series	Hepatitis A series	Hepatitis A series
Influenza[8]					Influenza (yearly)	Influenza (yearly)	Influenza (yearly)	Influenza (yearly)	Influenza (yearly)	Influenza (yearly)	Influenza (yearly)	Influenza (yearly)

This schedule indicates the recommended ages for routine administration of currently licensed childhood vaccines, as of December 1, 2003, for children through age 18 years. Any dose not given at the recommended age should be given at any subsequent visit when indicated and feasible. ▨ Indicates age groups that warrant special effort to administer those vaccines not previously given. Additional vaccines may be licensed and recommended during the year. Licensed combination vaccines may be used whenever any components of the combination are indicated and the vaccine's other components are not contraindicated. Providers should consult the manufacturers' package inserts for detailed recommendations. Clinically significant adverse events that follow immunization should be reported to the Vaccine Adverse Event Reporting System (VAERS). Guidance about how to obtain and complete a VAERS form can be found on the Internet: http://www.vaers.org/ or by calling 1-800-822-7967.

1. Hepatitis B (HepB) vaccine. All infants should receive the first dose of hepatitis B vaccine soon after birth and before hospital discharge; the first dose may also be given by age 2 months if the infant's mother is hepatitis B surface antigen (HBsAg) negative. Only monovalent HepB can be used for the birth dose. Monovalent or combination vaccine containing HepB may be used to complete the series. Four doses of vaccine may be administered when a birth dose is given. The second dose should be given at least 4 weeks after the first dose, except for combination vaccines which cannot be administered before age 6 weeks. The third dose should be given at least 16 weeks after the first dose and at least 8 weeks after the second dose. The last dose in the vaccination series (third or fourth dose) should not be administered before age 24 weeks.

Infants born to HBsAg-positive mothers should receive HepB and 0.5 mL of Hepatitis B Immune Globulin (HBIG) within 12 hours of birth at separate sites. The second dose is recommended at age 1 to 2 months. The last dose in the immunization series should not be administered before age 24 weeks. These infants should be tested for HBsAg and antibody to HBsAg (anti-HBs) at age 9 to 15 months.

Infants born to mothers whose HBsAg status is unknown should receive the first dose of the HepB series within 12 hours of birth. Maternal blood should be drawn as soon as possible to determine the mother's HBsAg status; if the HBsAg test is positive, the infant should receive HBIG as soon as possible (no later than age 1 week). The second dose is recommended at age 1 to 2 months. The last dose in the immunization series should not be administered before age 24 weeks.

2. Diphtheria and tetanus toxoids and acellular pertussis (DTaP) vaccine. The fourth dose of DTaP may be administered as early as age 12 months, provided 6 months have elapsed since the third dose and the child is unlikely to return at age 15 to 18 months. The final dose in the series should be given at age ≥4 years. **Tetanus and diphtheria toxoids (Td)** is recommended at age 11 to 12 years if at least 5 years have elapsed since the last dose of tetanus and diphtheria toxoid-containing vaccine. Subsequent routine Td boosters are recommended every 10 years.

3. *Haemophilus influenzae* type b (Hib) conjugate vaccine. Three Hib conjugate vaccines are licensed for infant use. If PRP-OMP (PedvaxHIB or ComVax [Merck]) is administered at ages 2 and 4 months, a dose at age 6 months is not required. DTaP/Hib combination products should not be used for primary immunization in infants at ages 2, 4 or 6 months but can be used as boosters following any Hib vaccine. The final dose in the series should be given at age ≥12 months.

4. Measles, mumps, and rubella vaccine (MMR). The second dose of MMR is recommended routinely at age 4 to 6 years but may be administered during any visit, provided at least 4 weeks have elapsed since the first dose and both doses are administered beginning at or after age 12 months. Those who have not previously received the second dose should complete the schedule by the 11- to 12-year-old visit.

5. Varicella vaccine. Varicella vaccine is recommended at any visit at or after age 12 months for susceptible children (i.e., those who lack a reliable history of chickenpox). Susceptible persons age ≥13 years should receive 2 doses, given at least 4 weeks apart.

6. Pneumococcal vaccine. The heptavalent **pneumococcal conjugate vaccine (PCV)** is recommended for all children age 2 to 23 months. It is also recommended for certain children age 24 to 59 months. The final dose in the series should be given at age ≥12 months. **Pneumococcal polysaccharide vaccine (PPV)** is recommended in addition to PCV for certain high-risk groups. See *MMWR* 2000;49(RR-9):1-38.

7. Hepatitis A vaccine. Hepatitis A vaccine is recommended for children and adolescents in selected states and regions and for certain high-risk groups; consult your local public health authority. Children and adolescents in these states, regions, and high-risk groups who have not been immunized against hepatitis A can begin the hepatitis A immunization series during any visit. The 2 doses in the series should be administered at least 6 months apart. See *MMWR* 1999;48(RR-12):1-37.

8. Influenza vaccine. Influenza vaccine is recommended annually for children age ≥6 months with certain risk factors (including but not limited to children with asthma, cardiac disease, sickle cell disease, human immunodeficiency virus infection, and diabetes; and household members of persons in high-risk groups [see *MMWR* 2003;52(RR-8):1-36]) and can be administered to all others wishing to obtain immunity. In addition, healthy children age 6 to 23 months are encouraged to receive influenza vaccine if feasible, because children in this age group are at substantially increased risk of influenza-related hospitalizations. For healthy persons age 5 to 49 years, the intranasally administered live-attenuated influenza vaccine (LAIV) is an acceptable alternative to the intramuscular trivalent inactivated influenza vaccine (TIV). See *MMWR* 2003;52(RR-13):1-8. Children receiving TIV should be administered a dosage appropriate for their age (0.25 mL if age 6 to 35 months or 0.5 mL if age ≥3 years). Children age ≤8 years who are receiving influenza vaccine for the first time should receive 2 doses (separated by at least 4 weeks for TIV and at least 6 weeks for LAIV).

For additional information about vaccines, including precautions and contraindications for immunization and vaccine shortages, please visit the National Immunization Program Web site at www.cdc.gov/nip/ or call the National Immunization Information Hotline at 800-232-2522 (English) or 800-232-0233 (Spanish).

Approved by the Advisory Committee on Immunization Practices (www.cdc.gov/nip/acip), the American Academy of Pediatrics (www.aap.org), and the American Academy of Family Physicians (www.aafp.org).

Figure 2-11. This schedule shows recommended ages for various childhood immunizations.

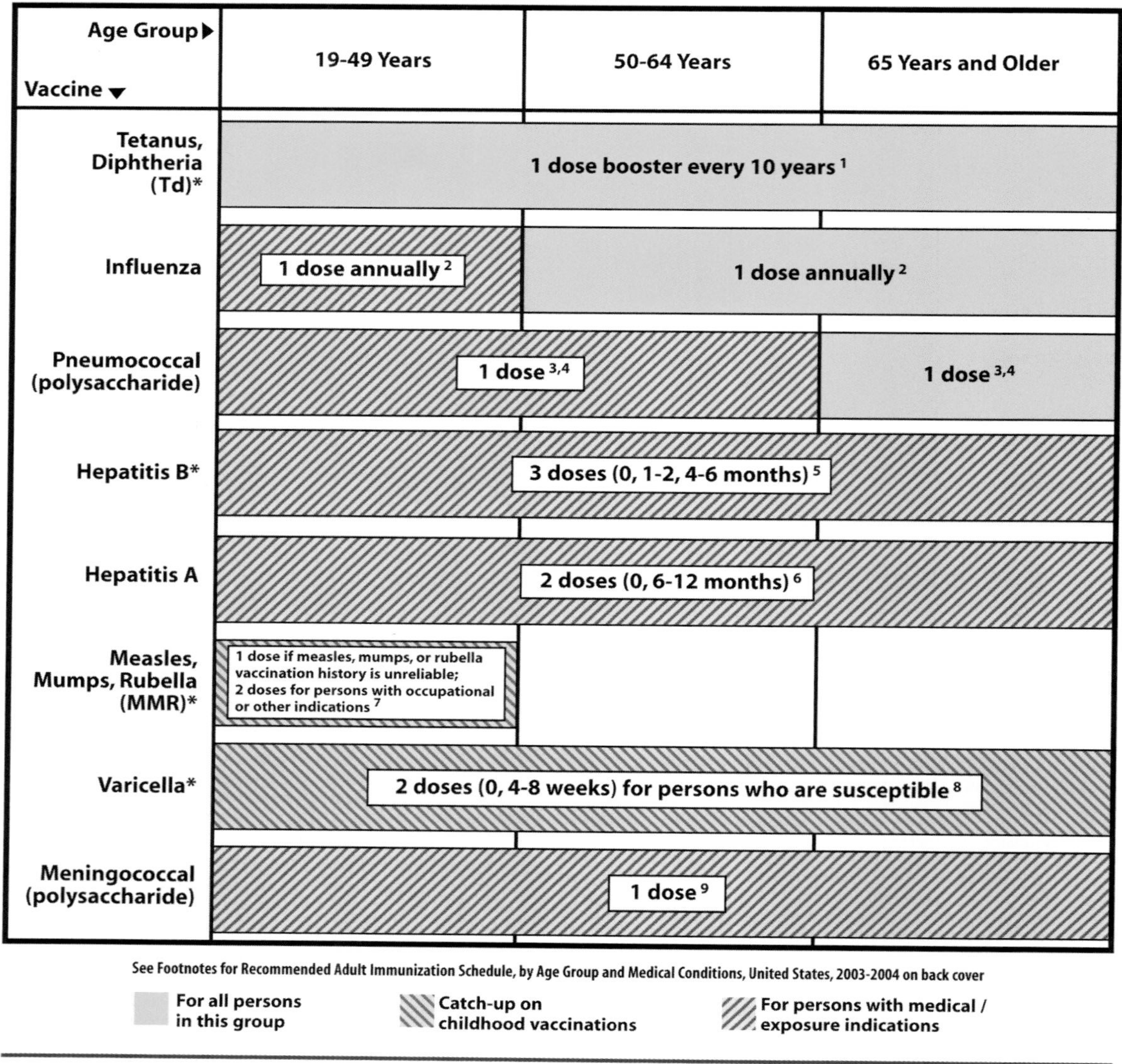

Recommended Adult Immunization Schedule, United States, 2003-2004
by Age Group

Age Group ▶ / Vaccine ▼	19-49 Years	50-64 Years	65 Years and Older
Tetanus, Diphtheria (Td)*	1 dose booster every 10 years[1]		
Influenza	1 dose annually[2]	1 dose annually[2]	
Pneumococcal (polysaccharide)	1 dose[3,4]		1 dose[3,4]
Hepatitis B*	3 doses (0, 1-2, 4-6 months)[5]		
Hepatitis A	2 doses (0, 6-12 months)[6]		
Measles, Mumps, Rubella (MMR)*	1 dose if measles, mumps, or rubella vaccination history is unreliable; 2 doses for persons with occupational or other indications[7]		
Varicella*	2 doses (0, 4-8 weeks) for persons who are susceptible[8]		
Meningococcal (polysaccharide)	1 dose[9]		

See Footnotes for Recommended Adult Immunization Schedule, by Age Group and Medical Conditions, United States, 2003-2004 on back cover

For all persons in this group

Catch-up on childhood vaccinations

For persons with medical / exposure indications

*Covered by the Vaccine Injury Compensation Program. For information on how to file a claim call 800-338-2382. Please also visit www.hrsa.gov/osp/vicp To file a claim for vaccine injury contact: U.S. Court of Federal Claims, 717 Madison Place, N.W., Washington D.C. 20005, 202-219-9657.

This schedule indicates the recommended age groups for routine administration of currently licensed vaccines for persons 19 years of age and older. Licensed combination vaccines may be used whenever any components of the combination are indicated and the vaccine's other components are not contraindicated. Providers should consult the manufacturers' package inserts for detailed recommendations.

Report all clinically significant post-vaccination reactions to the Vaccine Adverse Event Reporting System (VAERS). Reporting forms and instructions on filing a VAERS report are available by calling 800-822-7967 or from the VAERS website at www.vaers.org.

For additional information about the vaccines listed above and contraindications for immunization, visit the National Immunization Program Website at www.cdc.gov/nip/ or call the National Immunization Hotline at 800-232-2522 (English) or 800-232-0233 (Spanish).

Approved by the Advisory Committee on Immunization Practices (ACIP), and accepted by the American College of Obstetricians and Gynecologists (ACOG) and the American Academy of Family Physicians (AAFP)

Figure 2-12. Adult immunizations are recommended for adults who did not receive vaccines as children and for older adults with chronic illnesses. (National Coalition for Adult Immunization. Reprinted with permission.)

consent for the child's immunization. Remember that religious beliefs may prohibit parents from consenting to immunizations for their child. Record this information in the patient's chart.

Contraindications. Before administering a childhood immunization, check for any contraindications to its use. A **contraindication** is a symptom that renders use of a remedy or procedure inadvisable, usually because of risk. For example, pertussis vaccine must not be given to a child with a progressive neurological disorder. It also must not be administered to a child who developed seizures, persistent crying, or a fever of 104°F or higher after receiving a previous pertussis vaccine. In such a situation, the doctor would direct you to administer diphtheria and tetanus toxoids instead of diphtheria and tetanus toxoid and pertussis vaccine (DTP).

Immunization Records. Under the National Childhood Vaccine Injury Act of 1988, you must record certain information about immunizations in a child's permanent medical record. Required information includes:

- The vaccine's type, manufacturer, and lot number
- The date of administration
- The name, address, and title of the health-care professional who administered the vaccine

You must also document:

- The administration site and route
- The vaccine's expiration date

Parents should maintain an accurate, up-to-date immunization record for each child. Each state issues an immunization record form, which may be available in languages other than English, depending on the state. You can obtain copies from your state's department of health. Complete a form after each child's first immunization. Instruct the parents to keep the form and bring it with the child for each subsequent immunization so that you can update the record.

Advise parents that this record is important to keep because it acts as proof of immunization, required by day-care centers, schools, the military, and other organizations. This record may also be helpful when parents consult another doctor, in case of emergency, or when moving to a new location.

Pregnant Patients. Because pregnancy may increase a woman's susceptibility to diseases and because some maternal diseases can endanger the fetus, certain immunizations may be recommended during pregnancy. Other immunizations, such as that for rubella, however, should not be administered to pregnant women because they can cause fetal defects. In general, vaccines that are based on a live virus should not be given to pregnant patients.

Before administering any immunization or other drug to a pregnant patient, determine the fetal risks associated with it. One method is to find out the drug's pregnancy risk category. The FDA has established five categories to indicate the results of clinical tests performed on animals and humans:

- Category A indicates that there is no known risk to the fetus
- Categories B, C, and D indicate some potential risk, which may be outweighed by the benefits of the drug
- Category X indicates an unacceptable degree of risk to the fetus

For a more detailed discussion of pregnancy risk categories, see Table 33-7 in Chapter 33. Each drug's package insert should indicate its pregnancy risk category and specific contraindications or precautions for taking the drug during pregnancy.

Elderly Patients. Influenza and influenza-related pneumonia represent a serious health risk for patients over the age of 65. Although elderly patients can be immunized against influenza each year and influenza-related pneumonia one time, they may have common misconceptions about vaccinations. They may worry about the expense, about getting the disease from the vaccine, or about the need for vaccination when they do not feel ill.

Explain to patients who are concerned about the cost of vaccinations that if they are not enrolled in one of the many insurance plans that covers immunization, Medicare Part B covers the cost. For those worried about the potential side effects of immunization, describe the mild symptoms they may encounter, and emphasize that the symptoms are short-lived. You might also mention that compared to the potential dangers of contracting a serious infection, the symptoms are quite mild.

Because older patients are much more likely than younger patients to develop side effects as a result of immunizations, instruct older patients so that they recognize and immediately report any adverse effects. That way, the physician can treat elderly patients before their illness becomes severe.

Immunocompromised Patients. Patients who have an impaired or weakened immune system (are immunocompromised) include those with acquired immunodeficiency syndrome (AIDS) or other immune disorders and those undergoing chemotherapy. Infants may also be considered immunocompromised if they have mothers who are infected with HIV or have AIDS or an unknown immune status.

All immunizations affect the immune system. A patient with a compromised immune system can experience minimal to dangerous effects, depending on the vaccine. Before administration of any immunization, the physician should check the patient's medical history. If the patient is immunocompromised, the dosage may need to be adjusted or administration postponed.

Immunization for immunocompromised patients depends on exactly what disease is present. For example, inactive poliomyelitis vaccinations should be given to patients with altered immune systems, whereas the oral form that is based on the live virus can be given to patients with healthy immune systems. Also consider the immunization status of the patients' families and caregivers. All family members and caregivers of patients with AIDS should receive only inactive poliomyelitis vaccinations and should receive annual flu vaccinations.

Health-Care Workers. Health-care workers are at risk of contracting infectious diseases and should pay careful attention to their own immunization status. Regulations of the Occupational Safety and Health Administration (OSHA) require employers to offer medical workers vaccination against hepatitis B at no cost to employees. Healthcare workers may choose to decline this service under certain circumstances, but if they do, a waiver must be signed and maintained in the personnel file. If the employee chooses to take the vaccine at a later date, it must be offered at no charge.

Summary

You have many opportunities to break the cycle of infectious disease transmission while carrying out your duties as a medical assistant. Your own safety and the safety of both patients and colleagues depend on your knowledge and skills as you handle instruments and equipment, recognize symptoms of infectious diseases, and teach patients about the importance of immunization.

Sanitization, disinfection, and sterilization break the pathogen growth cycle by eliminating microorganisms on the surface of instruments and equipment. The steam autoclave is the most effective method for controlling infections transmitted by unsterile instruments. Familiarity with all aspects of the autoclave operation is essential, including preparing instruments for sterilization, running the load through the autoclave, removing and inspecting sterilized items, and storing supplies to ensure sterility.

In addition to recognizing the symptoms of infectious diseases, you can teach patients about symptoms of infectious diseases that are likely to affect them. Informed patients are more likely than the uninformed to seek medical aid quickly and less likely to spread illness to others. You can play a vital role in reducing patient vulnerability by encouraging patients to maintain a correct immunization status and by remaining aware of special immunization concerns for certain patients.

REVIEW

CHAPTER 2

CASE STUDY QUESTIONS

Now that you have completed this chapter, review the case study at the beginning of the chapter and answer the following questions:

1. What is the common, or lay, term for rubella?
2. How is it transmitted?
3. Since pregnant women were probably exposed, is there a concern for their fetuses?
4. Does the disease have any reporting guidelines?

Discussion Questions

1. A coworker responsible for autoclaving instruments is in a hurry to leave for the day; at the end of the autoclave sterilization cycle, the coworker does not allow time for the drying process. What significance, if any, does omitting the drying step have?
2. You are preparing to disinfect a tray of assorted equipment. At the bottom of the tray, you discover several pieces of gauze stained with what appears to be dried blood. What should you do with the instruments? What should you do with the gauze?
3. Identify several common childhood illnesses that must be reported to the state or county department of health. What might occur if you were to neglect reporting such illnesses?

Critical Thinking Questions

1. You are taking the general history of a 13-year-old female patient. You discover that she never had a second measles-mumps-rubella (MMR) vaccination. What special considerations, if any, should be taken into account before administering the vaccination?
2. The autoclave was not allowed to come up to its proper temperature before the timing of the cycle was started. What impact does this have on the sterilization?
3. Discuss the instructions that should be explained to a patient diagnosed with tuberculosis in order to minimize the risk of transmission.

Application Activities

1. Prepare a receptacle of sanitized and disinfected instruments and equipment for steam autoclaving. Demonstrate the correct method for handling instruments with hinges or ratchets.
2. Load an autoclave with wrapped instrument packs and other equipment. Demonstrate the correct placement of open glass containers, plastic items, instrument packs, and a tray of loose instruments.
3. Work with another student to role-play a situation in which you explain the recommended immunizations for the following people: a 4-month-old baby, a 5-year-old boy who has never received any immunizations, a 15-year-old boy who has never had chickenpox, and an adult female who was born in 1958 and was never immunized for measles, mumps, and rubella.

CHAPTER 3

HIV, Hepatitis, and Other Blood-Borne Pathogens

KEY TERMS

anergic reaction
blood-borne pathogen
chancre
clinical drug trial
enzyme-linked immunosorbent assay (ELISA) test
hairy leukoplakia
helper T cell
immunocompromised
immunofluorescent antibody (IFA) test
jaundice
Kaposi's sarcoma
mucocutaneous exposure
percutaneous exposure
terminal
Western blot test

AREAS OF COMPETENCE

2003 Role Delineation Study

CLINICAL

Fundamental Principles

- Apply principles of aseptic technique and infection control
- Screen and follow up patient test results

GENERAL

Professionalism

- Treat all patients with compassion and empathy

Legal Concepts

- Perform within legal and ethical boundaries
- Implement and maintain federal and state health-care legislation and regulations

Instruction

- Instruct individuals according to their needs
- Teach methods of health promotion and disease prevention
- Locate community resources and disseminate information

CHAPTER OUTLINE

- Transmission of Blood-Borne Pathogens
- Universal Precautions
- Disease Profiles
- AIDS Patients
- Other Blood-Borne Infections
- Reporting Guidelines
- Patient Education
- Special Issues With Terminal Illness

OBJECTIVES

After completing Chapter 3, you will be able to:

3.1 Describe ways in which blood-borne pathogens can be transmitted.
3.2 Explain why strict adherence to Universal Precautions is essential in preventing the spread of infection.
3.3 Describe the symptoms of hepatitis and AIDS.
3.4 List and describe the blood tests used to diagnose HIV infection.

OBJECTIVES *(Continued)*

3.5 Identify chronic disorders often found in patients who have AIDS.

3.6 Compare and contrast drugs used to treat AIDS/HIV infection.

3.7 Describe the symptoms of infection by other common blood-borne pathogens.

3.8 Explain how to educate patients about minimizing the risks of transmitting blood-borne infections to others.

3.9 Describe special issues you may encounter when dealing with patients who have terminal illnesses.

Introduction

This chapter expands on the OSHA Blood-borne Pathogen Standard and explains how you should reduce your risk of exposure to blood-borne pathogens. You will learn about HIV, hepatitis, and other blood-borne infections, about reporting guidelines, and about educating patients on minimizing the risk of transmission. You will also be introduced to issues associated with terminal illnesses such as AIDS.

CASE STUDY

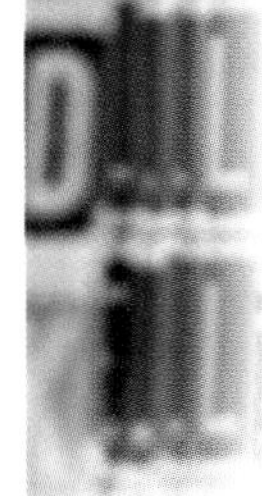

An anxious 34-year-old nurse currently employed at the local hospital comes into the office with complaints of fatigue, stomach pain, and vomiting. While talking with the patient, you notice a yellowish color to her skin and eyes. The patient confides in you that the required vaccination for her job description was never administered. The physician diagnoses the patient with hepatitis.

As you read this chapter, consider the following questions:

1. Which type of hepatitis does this patient probably have?
2. What are two medical terms for the yellowish discoloration you observed?
3. How long might the patient expect to suffer from the symptoms of the acute phase of the illness?
4. Could this disease have been prevented? If so, how?

Transmission of Blood-Borne Pathogens

As discussed in Chapter 1, infectious diseases are spread through a cycle that involves transmission of pathogens from host to host. When you use medical and surgical asepsis and various techniques and procedures to sanitize, disinfect, and sterilize instruments, equipment, and surfaces, you help prevent the transmission of all types of pathogens. You also need to know about specific types of pathogens—how they are transmitted and what measures you can take to prevent their transmission. **Blood-borne pathogens** are disease-causing microorganisms carried in the host's blood. They are transmitted from one host to another through contact with infected blood, tissue, body fluids, or mucous membranes.

The Centers for Disease Control and Prevention (CDC) has identified specific substances that can serve as transmission agents for blood-borne diseases. (Although breast milk is not included, it has been implicated in the transmission of the human immunodeficiency virus [HIV]. Breast-feeding is contraindicated for women who have HIV infection.) The following substances can serve as transmission agents:

- Blood
- Blood products (such as plasma)
- Human tissue
- Semen
- Vaginal secretions
- Saliva from dental procedures
- Cerebrospinal fluid (from around the brain and spinal cord)
- Synovial fluid (from joints and around tendons)
- Pleural fluid (from around the lungs)
- Peritoneal fluid (from the abdominal cavity)
- Pericardial fluid (from around the heart)
- Amniotic fluid (from the sac containing a fetus)

Some substances are not considered a viable means for transmitting blood-borne disease, even though they may transmit other types of disease. If any of these substances contain visible traces of blood, however, their status shifts because they may then serve as transmission agents for blood-borne diseases. The substances are as follows:

- Feces
- Nasal secretions
- Perspiration
- Sputum
- Tears
- Urine
- Vomitus
- Saliva

The growth cycle of pathogenic microorganisms requires a means of exit from the host. In the case of a blood-borne disease, the means of exit can be any of the substances identified as transmission agents or potential transmission agents. The cycle also requires a means of entrance into a new host. Blood-borne pathogens can be introduced into a new host through several routes, including:

- Needlesticks from needles used on an infected patient
- Cuts or abrasions on the skin of the uninfected person
- Any body opening of an uninfected person
- A transfusion with infected blood

People at Increased Risk

People who are at increased risk for developing an infectious disease caused by blood-borne pathogens are those who come in contact with substances that may harbor the

TABLE 3-1 Cases of Health-care Workers With AIDS/HIV Infection

Cases of U.S. health-care workers with documented and possible occupationally acquired AIDS or HIV infection, reported through December 2001.[1]

Occupation	Documented Occupational Transmission[2] Number	Possible Occupational Transmission[3] Number
Dental worker, including dentist	–	6
Embalmer/morgue technician	1	2
Emergency medical technician/paramedic	–	12
Health aide/attendant	1	15
Housekeeper/maintenance worker	2	13
Laboratory technician, clinical	16	17
Laboratory technician, nonclinical	3	–
Nurse	24	35
Physician, nonsurgical	6	12
Physician, surgical	–	6
Respiratory therapist	1	2
Technician, dialysis	1	3
Technician, surgical	2	2
Technician/therapist, other than those listed above	–	9
Other health-care occupations	–	5
Total	**57**	**139**

Source: Centers for Disease Control and Prevention.

[1]Health-care workers are defined as those persons, including students and trainees, who have worked in a health-care, clinical, or HIV laboratory setting at any time since 1978. See *MMWR* (1992) 41:823–25.

[2]Health-care workers who had documented HIV seroconversion after occupational exposure or had other laboratory evidence of occupational infection: 48 had percutaneous exposure, 5 had mucocutaneous exposure, 2 had both percutaneous and mucocutaneous exposures, and 2 had an unknown route of exposure. Forty-nine exposures were to blood from an HIV-infected person, 1 to visibly bloody fluid, 4 to an unspecified fluid, and 3 to concentrated virus in a laboratory. Twenty-four of these health-care workers developed AIDS.

[3]These health-care workers have been investigated and are without identifiable behavioral or transfusion risks; each reported percutaneous or mucocutaneous occupational exposures to blood or body fluids, or laboratory solutions containing HIV, but HIV seroconversion specifically resulting from an occupational exposure was not documented.

pathogens. Besides health-care professionals, people in certain other careers are at increased risk for exposure to blood-borne pathogens, including members of these groups:

- Law enforcement officers
- Mortuary or morgue attendants
- Firefighters
- Medical equipment service technicians
- Barbers
- Cosmetologists

Of all the blood-borne microorganisms, the pathogens posing the greatest risk are two variants of the hepatitis virus (hepatitis B virus [HBV] and hepatitis C virus [HCV]) and HIV, which can lead to acquired immunodeficiency syndrome (AIDS). The CDC records information about the occurrence of many blood-borne diseases, including AIDS/HIV infection and hepatitis. Table 3-1 shows reported cases of AIDS/HIV infection in health-care workers to whom the virus was or may have been transmitted during the performance of their jobs.

Researching the Spread of Infectious Diseases

Health-care workers across the country file reports on the incidence of infectious diseases, such as AIDS and hepatitis, to state health departments. These state health departments pass the information on to the CDC. Epidemiologists at the CDC use this information to research trends in the spread of infectious diseases. Their research into the trends and patterns of disease outbreaks helps identify effective disease control tactics and allocate resources to especially hard-hit areas.

Career Opportunities

HIV/AIDS Instructor

To gain medical assistant credentials, you must fulfill the requirements of either the American Association of Medical Assistants (for a Certified Medical Assistant) or the American Medical Technologists (for a Registered Medical Assistant). After obtaining your medical assistant certification or registration, you may wish to acquire additional skills in specialty areas through course work or on-the-job training. Although this course work or training may not lead to an additional certification or degree, it will enable you to expand your role in the medical office and advance your career as the demand for skilled health professionals increases.

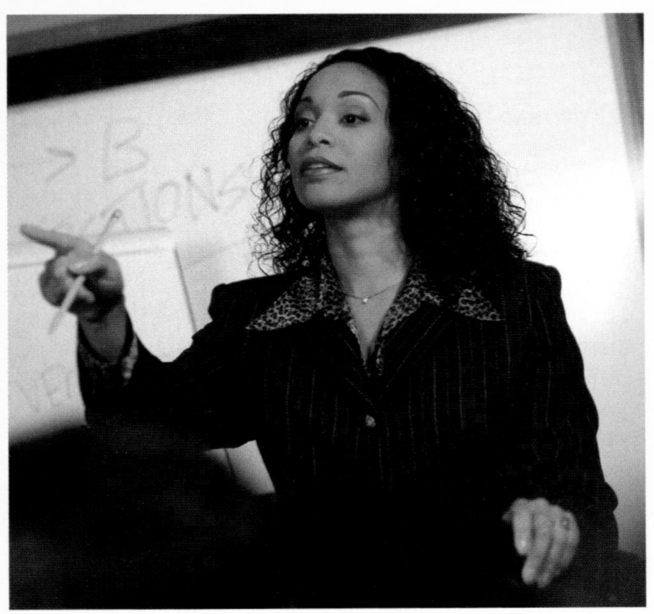

Skills and Duties

An HIV/AIDS instructor educates people about HIV infection and AIDS. Trained and certified by the American Red Cross, the HIV/AIDS instructor presents factual information in an age-appropriate, nonjudgmental, and culturally sensitive manner. She educates the community about HIV transmission and prevention and personalizes the facts about HIV and AIDS. She also emphasizes the importance of showing compassion toward people who are living with HIV or whose family members, friends, or partners may be HIV-positive.

The HIV/AIDS instructor may be certified in a number of Red Cross programs, including:

- The Basic HIV/AIDS Program, which presents a variety of interactive educational activities to educate the community.
- The African American HIV/AIDS Program, which was developed by African American staff of the Red Cross in partnership with the National Urban League to present culturally affirming information.
- The Hispanic HIV/AIDS Program, which was developed by the Red Cross with national Hispanic organizations and is available in both Spanish and English.

continued ⟶

Career Opportunities

HIV/AIDS Instructor *(continued)*

- The Workplace HIV/AIDS Program, which is tailored for each specific work site and covers topics such as rights and responsibilities, disability laws, local resources, and other issues of interest to employers and employees.
- Act SMART, developed by the Red Cross and the Boys & Girls Clubs of America to provide prevention knowledge and skills through age-appropriate activities for people ages 6 through 17.

Workplace Settings

HIV/AIDS instructors work in a variety of settings. They may run programs in schools, universities, offices, places of worship, community meeting rooms, clinics, hospitals, and people's homes.

Education

To become an HIV/AIDS instructor, you must be trained and certified by your local American Red Cross chapter. There are no specific educational requirements to be eligible for the training. This is often an unpaid volunteer position.

More than 26,000 instructors were teaching one or more of the Red Cross HIV/AIDS programs in 1995. To date, instructors trained by the Red Cross have reached more than 12 million people through HIV/AIDS education sessions. With the increasing awareness of AIDS and other sexually transmitted diseases, this field is expected to grow.

Where to Go for More Information

The American Red Cross
HIV/AIDS Education, Health and Safety Services
8111 Gatehouse Road, 6th Floor
Falls Church, VA 22042
703-206-7180

Universal Precautions

The most effective means of preventing the spread of HIV, hepatitis, and other blood-borne pathogens is to avoid contamination. As a medical assistant, you have a responsibility to help prevent infection in your patients, yourself, and your coworkers.

Following Universal Precautions, as required by the Department of Labor's Occupational Safety and Health Administration (OSHA), is critical to fulfillment of that responsibility. In recent years the application of Universal Precautions has been broadened in medical offices to include all body fluids, secretions, excretions, and moist body surfaces. This broadening is more like the application of Standard Precautions, which must be used in hospitals. (See Chapter 1 for more information on Universal Precautions and Standard Precautions.) Your best course of action is to assume that every patient is contaminated with blood-borne pathogens. Procedure 3-1 explains how to apply Universal Precautions to prevent transmission of blood-borne pathogens during any procedure or treatment in your medical facility.

Disease Profiles

You must understand infectious diseases, especially hepatitis and AIDS, to help prevent their spread. Because researchers continue to identify new diseases, you need to keep up-to-date on developments in the area of infectious diseases to perform your job effectively. This knowledge about diseases is useful to you for several reasons.

- You can identify symptoms that may indicate patients are infected with a blood-borne disease
- You can provide patients with education they can use to limit their risk of contracting such a disease
- You can identify habits your patients have that may increase their risk of spreading disease and educate them in different techniques to limit their risk

Hepatitis

Hepatitis is a viral infection of the liver that can lead to cirrhosis and death. There are several hepatitis virus variants that differ in their means of transmission as well as in the presenting symptoms of infection. These variations include the following:

- Hepatitis A, caused by hepatitis A virus (HAV). Hepatitis A is spread mainly through the fecal-oral route. People can be infected with HAV by drinking contaminated water, eating contaminated food, or having intimate contact with an infected person. HAV can spread in day-care settings when an attendant changes the diaper of an infected child, then helps another child with feeding before performing adequate hand washing. The disease is rarely fatal (the recovery rate is 99%), and there is a vaccine that prevents infection.

PROCEDURE 3.1

Applying Universal Precautions

Objective: To take specific protective measures when performing tasks in which a worker may be exposed to blood, body fluids, or tissues

OSHA Guidelines

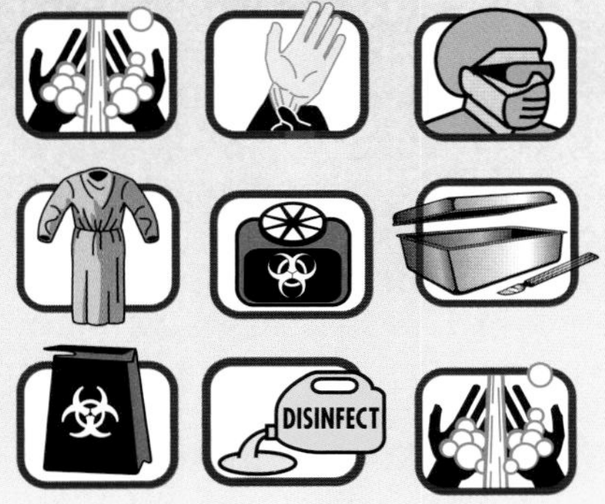

Materials: Items needed for the specific treatment or procedure being performed

Method

1. Perform aseptic hand washing. (See Procedure 1-1 in Chapter 1.)
2. Put on gloves and a gown or a laboratory coat and, if required, eye protection and a mask or a face shield.
3. Assist with the treatment or procedure as your office policy dictates.
4. Follow OSHA procedures (outlined in Chapter 1) to clean and decontaminate the treatment area (Figure 3-1).
5. Place reusable instruments in appropriate containers for sanitizing, disinfecting, and sterilizing, as appropriate (see Chapter 2).
6. Remove your gloves and all personal protective equipment. Place them in waste containers or laundry receptacles, according to OSHA guidelines (see Chapter 1).
7. Wash your hands.

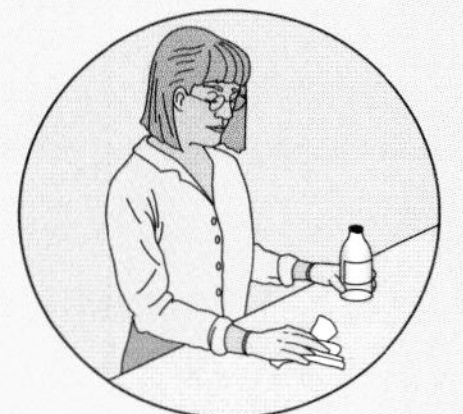

❶ Decontaminate exposed work areas.

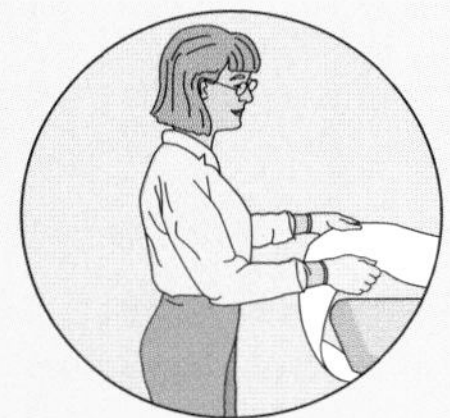

❷ Replace exposed protective coverings.

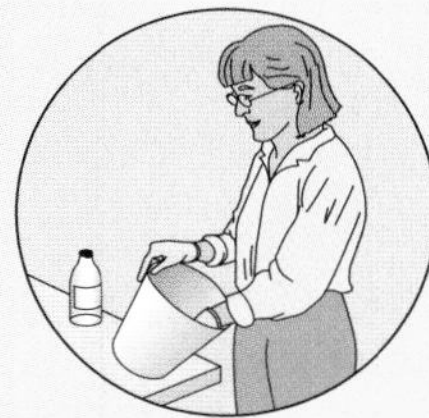

❸ Decontaminate receptacles.

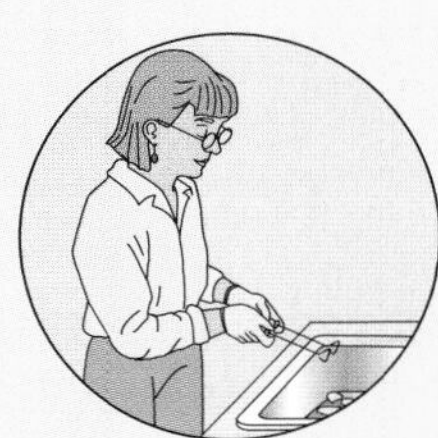

❹ Pick up broken glass.

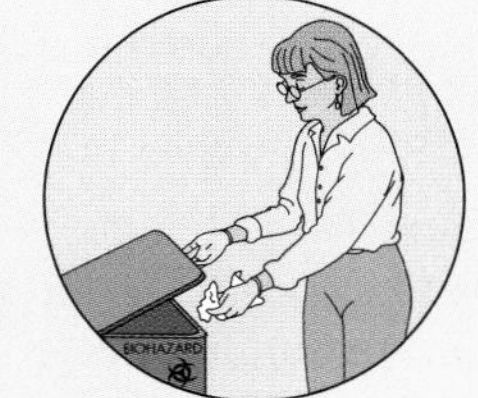

❺ Discard infectious waste.

Figure 3-1. Follow these OSHA guidelines to clean and decontaminate the medical environment after each procedure or treatment.

- Hepatitis B, which is the most common blood-borne hazard health-care workers face. It is spread through contact with contaminated blood or body fluids and through sexual contact. Most patients recover fully from HBV infection, but some patients develop chronic infection or remain carriers of the pathogen for the rest of their lives. Adults and children with hepatitis B who develop lifelong infections may experience serious health problems, including cirrhosis (scarring of the liver), liver cancer, liver failure, and death. Preventing the spread of the infection is the most effective means of combating the disease. Following Universal Precautions and receiving HBV vaccination are the most effective ways to control the spread of the infection.
- Hepatitis C (also referred to as non-A/non-B), which is also spread through contact with contaminated blood or body fluids and through sexual contact. There is no cure for this variant, which has resulted in more deaths than hepatitis A and hepatitis B combined. Many people become carriers of hepatitis C without knowing it, because they do not experience any symptoms of the virus. If the infection causes immediate symptoms, they often resemble the flu. Although treatment exists to suppress the virus, nothing can prevent or stop the virus from replicating. Over time, it is likely to damage the liver, causing cirrhosis, liver failure, and cancer. As with hepatitis B, preventing the spread of the infection is the best way to combat the disease.

CAUTION *Handle With Care*

Preventing Transmission of Viruses in the Health-Care Setting

Certain procedures are thought to cause the transmission of infection from a medical worker to a patient, and other procedures may also carry that risk. For example, skin-puncture injuries in medical workers are not uncommon. Therefore, many procedures involving needles are considered exposure-prone. If the worker's skin is cut or punctured, the patient could be exposed to the worker's blood.

The risk that a health-care worker will transmit an infection to a patient is small, if proper precautions are taken. Workers participating in high-risk procedures, however, should take extra precautions. Workers with skin conditions characterized by sores that secrete fluid should forgo direct patient care and the handling of equipment used for exposure-prone procedures until the condition has healed. Workers performing high-risk procedures should know their HIV and HBV status. (HIV refers to the virus that causes AIDS; HBV refers to the hepatitis B virus.) HBV vaccination is strongly recommended.

A health-care worker who is infected with HIV or HBV should not perform procedures that might result in exposure without the advice of an expert review panel. This panel might include the health-care worker's own physician, someone with expert knowledge about the transmission of infectious disease, a medical professional with expert knowledge about the procedures in question, public health officials, and a member of the infection control committee of the institution.

The panel will advise the worker about when she will be allowed to perform certain procedures. The panel will require her to inform potential patients of the infection before the procedure. The panel must, however, otherwise protect the health-care worker's confidentiality.

Although there has been great controversy on the subject, there are no recommendations in place for required testing of all health-care workers for HIV or HBV because the risk of transmission from worker to patient is not considered great enough to justify the expense. Educational and training activities can help reinforce the extra precautions exposure-prone workers should take.

- Hepatitis D (delta agent hepatitis), which occurs only in people infected with HBV. Delta agent infection may make the symptoms of hepatitis B more severe, and it is associated with liver cancer. The HBV vaccine also prevents delta agent infection.
- Hepatitis E, caused by hepatitis E virus (HEV). Hepatitis E is transmitted by the fecal-oral route, usually through contaminated water. Chronic infection does not occur, but acute hepatitis E may be fatal in pregnant women.

Risk Factors. Risk factors for HBV and HCV infection are the same. Although both infections can be spread through sexual contact—and high-risk sexual activity is a risk factor for hepatitis—the main risk factor is working in an occupation that requires exposure to human blood and body fluids. Other risk factors include:

- Using intravenous drugs
- Having hemophilia, a disorder characterized by a permanent tendency to bleed and requiring blood transfusions
- Traveling internationally to areas with a high prevalence of hepatitis B
- Having received blood transfusions before screening for HBV/HCV was in place
- Receiving hemodialysis, a procedure in which toxic wastes are removed from a patient's blood
- Living with a partner who has hepatitis B or hepatitis C
- Having multiple sexual partners

Risk in the Medical Community. As described, the primary risk factor for HBV and HCV infection is occupational exposure to the virus. In fact, although exposure to HIV has received more publicity and causes the greatest fear, your risk of contracting hepatitis, particularly hepatitis B, is actually considerably greater. Studies show that the risk of contracting HIV from a single needlestick exposure is approximately 0.5%, whereas the risk of contracting hepatitis B from a single needlestick exposure varies from 6% to as much as 33%. Several variables are responsible for the broad range of measured risk in HBV infection, including the immune status of the recipient and the efficiency of the virus transmission.

Progress of the Infection. Infection with hepatitis is a multistage process. The stages are as follows:

1. The prodromal stage, in which patients may experience general malaise, specific symptoms such as nausea and vomiting, or no symptoms at all
2. The icteric, or **jaundice,** stage, characterized by yellowness of the skin, eyes, mucous membranes, and

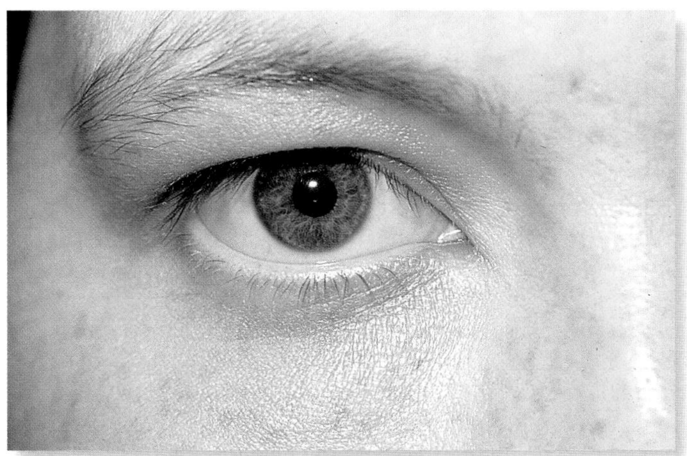

Figure 3-2. Jaundice is caused by excess bilirubin, which is produced in the liver and deposited throughout the body and which results in the yellow appearance of the patient's eyes and skin.

excretions (Figure 3-2), which usually appears 5 to 10 days after initial infection

3. The convalescent stage, which occurs after the two acute infection stages and can last from 2 to 3 weeks as symptoms gradually abate

The acute illness lasts approximately 16 weeks for hepatitis B and hepatitis C. Although patients recover, they may remain infected with the virus for life.

Symptoms. People infected with hepatitis may show no symptoms, may experience such mild or subtle symptoms that they do not realize they are seriously ill, or may experience severe symptoms. When you treat patients with hepatitis infection, any of these signs and symptoms may be present:

- Jaundice
- Diminished appetite
- Fatigue
- Nausea
- Vomiting
- Joint pain or tenderness
- Stomach pain
- General malaise

Diagnosis. Diagnosis of hepatitis is made through an investigation of risk factors and exposure incidents as well as through several blood tests. Most of the blood tests indicate the presence of antigen-antibody systems that relate to infection by hepatitis. They can also be used to determine the stage of the disease.

Preventive Measures. The best prevention against hepatitis is avoiding contact with contaminated substances. Follow Universal Precautions when working with all patients, and be especially careful with patients who have unknown or hepatitis-positive status.

A vaccine is available to prevent HBV infection. In fact, OSHA has established guidelines that require your employer to offer you this vaccine at no charge. If you decline the offer, you must sign a waiver. Current standard medical practice recommends against declining the vaccine. (For more information on this vaccination, see Chapter 1.)

Vaccination against HBV does not protect you from other strains of hepatitis. There are currently no vaccines for HCV, for example.

In the past, HBV vaccination was recommended only for high-risk individuals, such as medical personnel, dialysis patients, homosexual men, and intravenous drug users. This program of vaccinating only selected individuals did not greatly reduce the incidence of infection. Today the CDC recommends routine vaccination for everyone.

If you are exposed to hepatitis B and have not been vaccinated, you can receive a postexposure inoculation of hepatitis B immune globulin (HBIG). HBIG is given in large doses during the 7-day period after exposure. Shortly after beginning the treatment, you would also receive HBV vaccination. The HBIG inoculation is also used for infants born to HBV-infected mothers.

AIDS/HIV Infection

HIV is a virus that infects and gradually destroys components of the immune system. AIDS is the condition that results from the advanced stages of this viral infection.

Over a period of time and in most cases, HIV infection develops into AIDS, which results in death. The pathogen gradually destroys helper T cells. **Helper T cells** are white blood cells that are a key component of the body's immune system and that work in coordination with other white blood cells (B cells, macrophages, and so on) to combat infection.

The virus also attacks neurons, causing demyelination (destruction of the myelin sheath of a nerve), which results in neurological problems, including dementia. Most patients with AIDS acquire various opportunistic infections. Opportunistic microorganisms do not ordinarily cause disease in a person with a properly functioning immune system. Examples of opportunistic infections are *Pneumocystis carinii* pneumonia and oral candidiasis.

Virtually everyone is at risk for contracting AIDS. Although the initial outbreak of the disease in the United States appeared in the male homosexual population and currently homosexual and bisexual men comprise a large percentage of AIDS cases, the disease knows no limits. The incidence of HIV infection in homosexual men, however, has leveled off and even declined slightly in some areas of the United States. At the same time, the incidence of infection in heterosexual men and women and teenagers is increasing rapidly. The incubation period in adults is between 8 and 15 years, and the majority of adults with the disease are between the ages of 25 and 45.

Risk Factors. The greatest risk factor for contracting HIV infection is unprotected sexual activity. The virus can be found in blood, semen, and vaginal secretions and can be transmitted to an uninfected person through mucous membranes in the vagina, rectum, or mouth, especially if there are cuts or open sores in those areas. Some strains of the virus are more likely to infect the cells in the female reproductive tract (Langerhans cells). The HIV strain most common in the United States, however, targets the monocyte or lymphocyte white blood cells and is more prone to being passed along through anal sex and blood-to-blood contact.

The virus can also be spread by the sharing of needles used by intravenous drug users. The minute amount of blood left on a needle after injection provides an ample supply of the virus to transmit the infection to another host. Needles used in tattooing and ear piercing can also pose a risk. In all cases needles should be new and sterile.

The virus can pass from mother to fetus during pregnancy, as well as to an infant during delivery or through breast-feeding. Not every infant born to an infected mother contracts the disease, and some infected infants have cleared the virus from their systems within a year after birth. Scientists are studying these children in an effort to determine how their immune systems allow them to escape infection altogether or to eradicate the virus after infection. Scientists suspect that either the immune systems of the infants in the study fought off an HIV invasion or the infants developed a permanent tolerance for it.

At one time the virus was also being spread through the nation's blood supply. Transmission was occurring through transfusion of HIV-contaminated blood products. This form of transmission has virtually stopped as a result of an aggressive screening program that began in 1985. All blood donations are tested for the virus, and contaminated donations are destroyed. People who received blood prior to 1986 (especially between 1978 and 1985) were at risk for coming down with AIDS. Because of the long incubation period of the virus (8 to 15 years), infected people may not have exhibited any symptoms of infection.

Risk in the Medical Community. Health-care workers have contracted HIV infection as a direct result of occupational activities (see Table 3-1). Investigations showed that infection in most of the cases occurred as a result of **percutaneous exposure,** that is, exposure through a puncture wound or needlestick. **Mucocutaneous exposure,** or exposure through a mucous membrane, resulted in infection in a few cases.

Further analysis identified that in most cases the infecting substance was HIV-infected blood. Concentrated virus cultures in the laboratory and visibly bloody body fluid caused a few of the cases.

Progress of the Infection. Current research has shown that development of AIDS occurs in three main stages:

1. Initial infection
2. Incubation period
3. Full-blown AIDS

Initial infection by the virus can occur years before any symptoms appear to arouse suspicions about HIV infection. In some cases the initial infection is marked by severe flulike symptoms. Identification of the initial infection, however, is almost always through hindsight. The virus attacks helper T cells during this initial phase.

During the initial phase of infection by HIV, the virus enters the cell, and the host cell produces multiple copies of the virus. As a result helper T cells die or are disabled. The body's immune system responds to the attack at this point, cleansing the blood supply of the virus, and the virus enters an inactive phase.

The incubation period begins when the virus incorporates its genetic material into the genetic material of the helper T cells. The virus is trapped within the lymph system, and the host experiences few, if any, symptoms of the disease. Many doctors discover the infection in patients during this period when treating them for other illnesses. This incubation period, in which people are HIV-positive but do not have AIDS, generally lasts 8 to 15 years.

Sometime during the incubation period, HIV becomes active again and continues to attack and destroy helper T cells. As the number of helper T cells dwindles, the patient becomes more prone to opportunistic infections.

The threshold at which a patient is officially diagnosed with AIDS is the point at which there are 200 or fewer helper T cells per milliliter of blood. Once a person has full-blown AIDS—the third phase of infection—opportunistic infections take hold as the overall immune system undergoes deterioration. Neurons are destroyed, resulting in neurological problems, including dementia.

Diagnosis. To know for certain whether a person is infected with HIV, that person must have blood tested specifically for HIV infection. (All HIV testing is anonymous.) The **enzyme-linked immunosorbent assay (ELISA) test** confirms the presence of antibodies developed by the body's immune system in response to an initial HIV infection. ELISA is only about 85% accurate because of cross-reactivity from other viruses. Therefore, positive specimens are confirmed by a different method—the **Western blot test** or the **immunofluorescent antibody (IFA) test.** These tests are more accurate because they are specific to individual viruses.

These HIV tests were first developed for use on blood samples, but the ELISA and Western blot tests can also be run on oral fluid samples obtained in the medical office. Positive results from two of the three HIV tests (ELISA plus one other) yield an accurate diagnosis in almost 100% of patients tested.

Home tests are available that involve an ELISA test followed by either a Western blot test or an IFA test if the ELISA results are positive. These tests are performed on a drop of the patient's blood, which is collected on a specially treated card. Patients are identified only by a number, which they use to obtain their test results. (Keep in mind that people who perform home tests may not report positive results to the proper authorities.)

In all cases involving testing for HIV, you must follow measures to ensure protection of the patient's confidentiality. Knowledge about a patient's test results should be limited to those who will be treating the patient and appropriate authorities as required by law. The patient's decision on whether or not to reveal test results to family and friends should be respected at all times.

Symptoms. HIV infection can cause a variety of problems as it progresses to AIDS. Patients with AIDS may complain of any of the following symptoms:

- Systemic complaints, such as weight loss, fatigue, fever, chills, and night sweats
- Respiratory complaints, such as sinus fullness, dry cough, shortness of breath, difficulty swallowing, and sinus drainage
- Oral complaints, such as gingivitis, oral lesions, and **hairy leukoplakia,** which is a white lesion on the tongue
- Gastrointestinal complaints, such as diarrhea and bloody stool
- Central nervous system complaints, such as depression, personality changes, concentration difficulties, and confusion or dementia
- Peripheral nervous system complaints, such as tingling, numbness, pain, and weakness in the extremities
- Skin-related complaints, such as rashes, dry skin, and changes in the nail bed
- **Kaposi's sarcoma,** an unusual malignancy occurring in the skin and sometimes in the lymph nodes and organs manifested by reddish purple to dark blue patches or spots on the skin

Because many other diseases can cause these symptoms, the occurrence of any one symptom is not necessarily indicative of AIDS. Be aware, however, that patients exhibiting a combination of symptoms should be tested. The two symptoms most indicative of AIDS are hairy leukoplakia and Kaposi's sarcoma.

Preventive Measures. The only way to prevent the spread of HIV infection is to avoid specific activities or to take safety precautions when engaging in these activities. Activities requiring preventive measures can be divided into three groups, based on the means of transmission of the disease:

1. Sexual contact
2. Sharing of intravenous needles
3. Medical procedures

Prevention and Sexual Contact. The most effective method for preventing the spread of AIDS/HIV infection through sexual contact is to avoid high-risk sexual activity. Such high-risk activities or situations include:

- Having unprotected vaginal, oral, or anal sex, either homosexual or heterosexual, *unless* the individuals are involved in a long-term, monogamous relationship, they both have been tested and received negative results, and they have not engaged in any unsafe sexual activity 6 months before the test or anytime after the test
- Having multiple sexual partners, even when using protection against infection
- Experiencing a concurrent infection with another sexually transmitted disease

In addition, precautions must be taken when using a condom as a means of protection against infection. Proper use of a condom requires adherence to the following guidelines.

- A condom must be used every time the individual has sex and must never be reused.
- Only latex condoms provide protection against spread of the HIV pathogen. Lambskin condoms provide birth control only, not protection against disease.
- If lubrication is required, the lubricant must be water-based, not petroleum-based (such as petroleum jelly). Lubricants other than those specifically formulated for use with latex condoms can damage the condom, rendering it permeable and eliminating its usefulness as a barrier against disease.
- Condoms should be placed on the penis before any risk of leakage of seminal fluid occurs. Space should be left at the tip to act as a reservoir for ejaculated semen.
- Intercourse should not be attempted unless the penis is fully erect, and the penis should be withdrawn while it is still erect.
- The condom must remain in place from the beginning to the end of intercourse and should be held in place during withdrawal to prevent slippage. After withdrawal the condom should be disposed of properly.

Prevention and Intravenous Drug Use. Intravenous drug users are at risk for infection when they share needles. The most effective means of preventing the spread of the pathogen among drug users is to avoid sharing or reusing needles.

Prevention and Medical Procedures. Preventing the spread of AIDS/HIV infection in the medical environment involves taking many precautions. You must take precautions to prevent the spread of infection between patients, between yourself and the patient, and when you are working with equipment, supplies, or instruments that may be contaminated.

Strict adherence to Universal Precautions (Standard Precautions in a hospital) when working with patients is the best method for preventing the spread of disease among patients and between the patient and you. You must use gloves whenever there is a risk of contact with blood, tissue, or body fluids, and you must dispose of gloves properly after use. (See Chapter 1 for specific disposal guidelines.)

You must wash your hands carefully and thoroughly between patients. Wear additional personal protective equipment in situations where there is a risk of being splashed or sprayed by blood or body fluids.

Although gloves and other personal protective equipment provide adequate protection in many situations, they provide only limited protection against injury. Be especially careful when handling pointed or sharp-edged instruments or equipment. Needles must be disposed of in a puncture-proof biohazardous waste container. Pick up broken glass with tongs, and dispose of it in a puncture-proof biohazardous waste container.

Education as Prevention. As a medical assistant, you will encounter many opportunities to inform and educate patients about the dangers of HIV infection and AIDS, the ways in which the disease is spread, the ways in which it is not spread, and methods for preventing its spread. Use these opportunities to educate patients, because one of the best preventive measures is providing accurate and thorough information to people.

AIDS Patients

Treating patients infected with HIV and those who have developed AIDS is one of today's most challenging areas of medicine. New research findings occur frequently and may change treatment and diagnostic procedures. Because HIV infection is nearly always fatal, patients—and their families and caregivers—usually experience extreme psychological stress.

The AIDS Patient Profile

Although there are certain high-risk populations, such as intravenous drug users and homosexual men, virtually no one is immune to AIDS. Research evidence shows that HIV has been in the United States since approximately 1970. This conclusion is based on knowledge about the incubation period of the disease and the initial reports of *Pneumocystis carinii* pneumonia and Kaposi's sarcoma in homosexual men beginning in 1978. These diseases, which had been quite rare, are now considered hallmarks of HIV infection.

Because the infection seemed to occur exclusively in homosexual men, it was originally called gay-related infectious disease, or GRID. Rapidly, however, it became apparent that the disease could be passed not only through male-to-male sexual contact but also through blood transfusion, through the sharing of intravenous drug paraphernalia, through occupational exposure, through male-to-female sexual contact, through female-to-female sexual contact, and from mother to fetus as well as from mother to infant during breast-feeding.

As of December 1996, 22.6 million men, women, and children were HIV-infected worldwide. That number increased to approximately 200 million by the year 2000.

Homosexual men still constitute a large percentage of people with HIV infection and AIDS in the United States. Growth in infection of people in this group has slowed, however, as a result of educational campaigns and the population's adherence to "safer sex" practices. Data show that the disease occurs primarily among young people, especially those in large metropolitan areas. AIDS incidence rates for large metropolitan areas are approximately three times as high as rates for small metropolitan areas and nearly five times as high as rates in rural areas. Rural areas are, however, starting to show an increase in incidence.

Two groups of people who are contracting HIV infection in increasing numbers are intravenous drug users (especially African Americans and Hispanics in large metropolitan areas) and women. Because of the increase in infection among women, there has also been an increase in the number of infected children.

The CDC publishes a quarterly report, *The HIV/AIDS Surveillance Report,* which contains data about the incidence of HIV infection and AIDS nationwide. Information about age, gender, sexual orientation, race, occupation, residence, and source of infection are some of the facts collected in an effort to help epidemiologists generate an accurate picture of the patterns of the disease. Data also help identify the prevention programs most likely to succeed with a given population and help community leaders make decisions about the care of people with HIV infection and AIDS.

Chronic Disorders of the AIDS Patient

The impaired immune system of the AIDS patient permits opportunistic infections, which further reduce the body's ability to fight off infection. These infections attack many different parts of the body (Figure 3-3).

One of the cornerstones of the care of patients who have AIDS is to prevent opportunistic infections and identify such infections as quickly as possible when they occur. Identifying malignancies, if they occur, is also of utmost importance. If you are familiar with the common disorders an AIDS patient faces, you will be better able to identify early signs of infection or malignancy and point them out to the doctor, in turn initiating early treatment, which is usually most effective. You can help patients who have been diagnosed with HIV to understand the risks they face as well as the measures best suited to preventing particular infections.

***Pneumocystis Carinii* Pneumonia.** The most common opportunistic infection in AIDS patients is *Pneumocystis carinii* pneumonia, or PCP. Nearly 75% of AIDS patients experience this protozoal infection, with symptoms of fever, cough, and breathing difficulties. These symptoms are often very general, may not be very severe, and can be overlooked or attributed to other problems. Diagnosis is made through chest radiographs (x-ray film records of the chest), the Wright-Giesma sputum stain (substances that impart color so sputum can be studied), and bronchoalveolar lavage (a technique by which cells and fluid from alveoli, tiny sacs in the lungs, are removed for diagnosis).

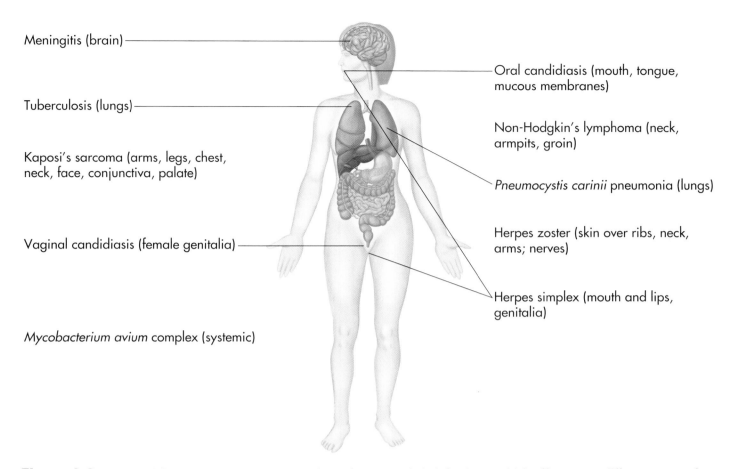

Meningitis (brain)

Oral candidiasis (mouth, tongue, mucous membranes)

Tuberculosis (lungs)

Non-Hodgkin's lymphoma (neck, armpits, groin)

Kaposi's sarcoma (arms, legs, chest, neck, face, conjunctiva, palate)

Pneumocystis carinii pneumonia (lungs)

Herpes zoster (skin over ribs, neck, arms; nerves)

Vaginal candidiasis (female genitalia)

Herpes simplex (mouth and lips, genitalia)

Mycobacterium avium complex (systemic)

Figure 3-3. The AIDS patient may contract a variety of opportunistic infections, which affect many different parts of the body.

AIDS patients should avoid contact with people who have colds or the flu. If contact is unavoidable, ill people should wear surgical masks to reduce the risk of spreading infection to AIDS patients. Everyone who comes in regular contact with AIDS patients should have a current flu immunization. Flu immunizations must be renewed every year.

Treatments for *Pneumocystis carinii* pneumonia can cause side effects. Some of the side effects are measurable only through laboratory tests, whereas some may be reported by the patient. Side effects include the following:

- Nausea
- Rash
- Hypotension (abnormally low blood pressure)
- Anemia
- Neutropenia (diminished number of neutrophils in the blood)
- Hepatitis
- Colitis (inflammation of the colon)
- Leukopenia (reduction in the number of leukocytes in the blood)

Kaposi's Sarcoma. Kaposi's sarcoma is a particularly aggressive form of tumor. Although it is uncommon in the general population (it is found in males averaging age 89 in the Mediterranean Sea region), it is the most common HIV-related malignancy. Kaposi's sarcoma appears as reddish purple to dark blue skin lesions that are found anywhere on the body (Figure 3-4). They are usually first found on the arms and legs, then on the chest, neck, and face. The lesions may appear in areas such as

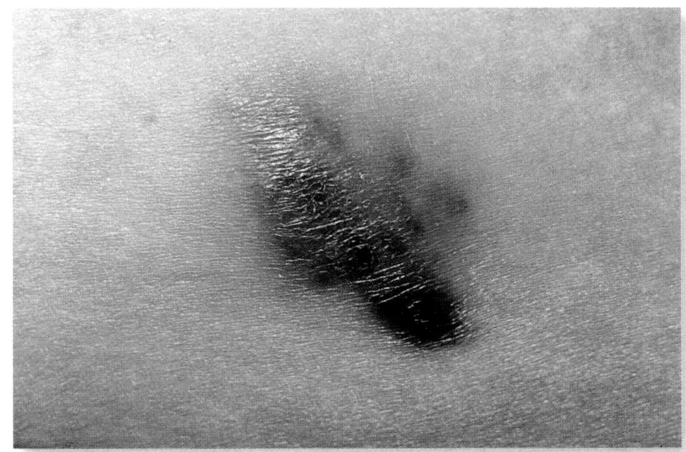

Figure 3-4. Kaposi's sarcoma is a rare form of skin cancer associated with AIDS.

the conjunctiva or the eyelids, between the toes, behind the ears, and on the palate.

Treatment for Kaposi's sarcoma includes chemotherapy. Chemotherapy may cause flulike symptoms accompanied by fever.

Non-Hodgkin's Lymphoma. The second most common malignancy associated with HIV infection is non-Hodgkin's lymphoma (NHL). Because NHL can appear in multiple sites, it is difficult to predict the problems HIV-infected patients will encounter with it. The symptoms vary, depending on which, if any, opportunistic infections are present. Other considerations are the rate of tumor growth and the location of the malignancy.

Tuberculosis. Tuberculosis is often a curable disease when treatment regimens are followed exactly and completely. (See Chapter 2 for more information on tuberculosis.) There has, however, been a rise in the number of cases in recent years as a result of HIV infection and antibiotic resistance. HIV infection is by far the single largest risk factor for the development of tuberculosis infection into the active form of the disease. HIV infection reduces the effectiveness of the immune system and makes it possible for tuberculosis bacilli to multiply and spread infection more easily. AIDS patients who have symptoms of tuberculosis should receive the Mantoux skin test (TB scratch test), a chest x-ray, and possibly a sputum culture. These tests are the only means of definitive diagnosis. AIDS patients should be tested yearly for tuberculosis infection. If they suspect they have been exposed to the pathogen through contact with a known or suspected source, they should undergo testing at the earliest opportunity.

The Mantoux skin test yields false negative results in some people with AIDS. In fact, as the number of helper T cells decreases, the more likely it is for patients to exhibit negative results. When two or more other antigens are combined with the tuberculin units used in the Mantoux test, a more accurate picture of infection emerges.

If patients do not respond to any of the substances injected for the test, they are considered to have an **anergic reaction.** An anergic reaction occurs when the body is unable to mount a normal response to invasion by a pathogen. Patients who respond to the other substances but not to the tuberculin units are considered free of tuberculosis infection. People with AIDS who exhibit an anergic reaction to the test should be considered for preventive therapy designed to halt development of the tuberculosis infection into disease.

***Mycobacterium Avium* Complex (MAC) Infection.** *Mycobacterium avium* complex (MAC) is responsible for 97% of the nontuberculous bacterial infections in AIDS patients, although it is difficult to detect in these patients. Postmortem studies of AIDS patients indicate that the disease is undetected in more than 50% of cases. The pathogen can be acquired orally or through inhalation. Symptoms include the following:

- Systemic illness
- Fever
- Night sweats
- Fatigue
- Weight loss
- Diarrhea
- Stomach pain

Meningitis. The pathogens that cause many of the common opportunistic infections in patients with AIDS can result in several forms of meningitis. Diagnosis is often difficult because the presenting symptoms and laboratory results are not always consistent with those found in patients without compromised immune systems. Infection of the central nervous system in an AIDS patient can lead to AIDS dementia complex, in which the patient's mental and motor functions gradually and irreversibly decline.

Oral Candidiasis. More than half the patients diagnosed with AIDS develop oral candidiasis *(Candida albicans)*, or thrush. The infection in an AIDS patient takes one of three primary forms:

1. Reddened, atrophic patches on the hard mucous membranes
2. Coating of the tongue
3. Patches on the tongue, soft palate, tonsils, and mucous membranes toward the cheek

Vaginal Candidiasis. Women who have AIDS are predisposed to vaginal candidiasis. Those who develop the infection often experience a severe case that is difficult to cure. Symptoms include these:

- Pruritus (extreme itching)
- Dysuria (painful or difficult urination)
- Labial excoriations (abrasions of the genital labia)
- Thick, adherent discharge

Herpes Simplex. One of the most common infections experienced by humans, herpes simplex virus (HSV), can manifest in a range of forms, from mild to life-threatening. People with compromised immune systems are especially at risk for infection by HSV. There are two forms of the virus: HSV-1 and HSV-2. HSV-2 is transmitted primarily through sexual exposure, whereas HSV-1 is transmitted primarily through exposure to oral secretions. It is possible, however, for HSV-2 to be transmitted through oral contact and for HSV-1 to be transmitted sexually.

Herpes Zoster. The herpes virus that causes chickenpox may become dormant in the body and may return as shingles, or herpes zoster. Generally the patient experiences pain followed by the appearance of reddened, raised lesions on one side of the body. In a patient who has a healthy immune system, the lesions last from 3 to 5 days and clear up within 15 days, although it can take an additional month for the patient's skin to return to its preinfection condition. In a patient who is **immunocompromised** (having an impaired or weakened immune system), however, the formation of lesions can last as long as 2 weeks, and clearing may not occur for 21 to 28 days. Herpes zoster rarely proves fatal, even in immunocompromised patients.

Treating Opportunistic Infections

The wide variety of opportunistic infections that may afflict AIDS patients makes treatment management a challenge. In some instances drug side effects that patients with intact immune systems would easily tolerate pose major problems for the immunocompromised patient. Repeated episodes of infection can leave a patient allergic to treatment medication or with a tolerance to the medication, requiring higher and higher doses for effectiveness. The pathogen itself may mutate into a strain that is resistant to treatment. Treatment for one set of symptoms may conflict with treatment for another set or may exacerbate other symptoms.

Testing Regulations

Currently the CDC does not recommend mandatory HIV testing for health-care workers. Health-care professionals emphasize that a health-care worker's chances of being infected by a patient are much higher than a patient's chances of being infected by a health-care worker. Although there have been well-publicized incidents of infection from health-care worker to patient, no required testing programs exist today. (Refer to Chapter 1 for additional precautions for avoiding transmission of disease from health-care workers to patients.)

Drug Treatments

A growing number of drugs are available for the treatment of HIV and AIDS. Billions of dollars are spent each year for research into HIV/AIDS treatments and vaccines. There is no cure for either of these diseases; however, pharmaceutical companies are making great strides in creating new drugs that slow the reproduction of the virus. A patient with HIV or AIDS is no longer limited to one or two therapies. Because more than 20 drugs are available for treatment, an individual with HIV or AIDS who has had no success with one regimen or treatment might find success with another. This is important for increasing life expectancy. Table 3-2 identifies different classifications of drugs currently approved by the FDA for the treatment of diseases associated with HIV infection and AIDS.

Treatment Goals. The goals of drug treatment for HIV and AIDS include the following:

- Increasing the time between infection and symptomatic disease (AIDS)
- Improving the quality of life of those diagnosed with AIDS
- Reducing transmission of HIV to uninfected persons
- Reducing maternal-infant transmission
- Reducing the number of HIV-related deaths

Treatment Guidelines. Some basic guidelines for implementing HIV/AIDS treatment were developed by the Panel on Clinical Practices for Treatment of HIV Infection (the Panel). These guidelines include initial and follow-up testing of viral load and $CD4^+$ T cell count and drug resistance testing. Drug resistance testing is especially useful for patients who have failed initial therapy. Viral load and $CD4^+$ T cell counts are good indicators of the overall effectiveness of the treatment.

FDA-approved pharmaceutical agents used in the treatment of HIV/AIDS are divided into four classes: (1) fusion inhibitors, (2) nonnucleoside reverse transcriptase inhibitors (NNRTIs), (3) nucleoside reverse transcriptase inhibitors (NRTIs), and (4) protease inhibitors (PIs). Each of these classes of drugs has a different manner of working against the HIV virus. Fusion inhibitors block the entrance of the virus into the human cell. NNRTIs, NRTIs, and PIs all act to limit the HIV virus from making copies of itself, each acting in a slightly different way. All of these classes, used in combination, are important weapons in the arsenal of treatments used to combat HIV/AIDS.

The Panel recommends a combination of drug treatment called highly active anti-retroviral therapy (HAART). This therapy combines three or more HIV drugs. Taking three or more drugs has proven to be more effective than taking two or fewer, because viral load decrease is only temporary in those taking one or two HIV drugs. Treatment during pregnancy is the only exception to this. Because many HIV/AIDS drugs are contraindicated during pregnancy (with some exceptions), pregnant patients will be offered a single drug in order to limit passing HIV to their infants.

Initiating Therapy. When therapy should begin is an important decision that must be made by both the patient and the physician. To assist in making this decision, the Panel has made several recommendations. These recommendations are based on a combination of $CD4^+$T cell count, viral load, and the presence or absence of symptoms. Starting therapy immediately is recommended if patients have severe symptoms (AIDS diagnosis) or if their $CD4^+$T cell count is less than 200 cells/mm^3. The physician should consider treatment if the $CD4^+$T cell count is between 200 and 350 cells/mm^3. In patients with a $CD4^+$T cell count greater than 350 cells/mm^3, no symptoms, and a viral load greater than 55,000 copies/mL, observation of the patient is recommended with a delay of treatment. The patient and physician should decide whether to take an aggressive approach or a conservative one. If a conservative approach is taken, the patient should have routine $CD4^+$T cell and viral load counts.

TABLE 3-2 FDA-Approved Drugs for HIV/AIDS Infection (Antiretroviral Drugs)

Classification & Function	Generic Name (Trade Name)	Major Side Effects
Fusion Inhibitor Blocks viral entrance into the human cell	Enfuvirtide; 2003 (Fuzeon)	Bacterial pneumonia, allergic reaction, injection site infections
Nonnucleoside Reverse Transcriptase Inhibitors (NNRTIs) Block the ability of HIV to make copies of itself	Delavirdine; 1997 (Rescriptor)	Skin rash, eye inflammation, fever, joint or muscle pain, oral lesions, swelling
	Efavirenz; 1998 (Sustiva)	Skin rash, depression
	Nevirapine; 1996 (Viramune)	Skin rash, liver disease, chills and fever, sore throat, oral lesions
Nucleoside Reverse Transcriptase Inhibitors (NRTIs) Block the ability of HIV to make copies of itself	Abacavir sulfate; 1998 (Ziagen)	Fatal hypersensitivity reaction, liver disease
	Abacavir + lamivudine + Zidovudine; 2000 (Trizivir)	Fatal hypersensitivity reaction, liver disease
	Didanosine; 1991 (Videx)	Severe gastralgia, nausea, vomiting; burning, numbness, or tingling of the hands, arms, feet or legs; visual disturbances
	Emtricitabine; 2003 (Emtirva)	Nausea, vomiting, abdominal pain, anorexia, weight loss, dyspnea, fatigue
	Lamivudine; 1995 (Epivir)	Burning, numbness, pain, or tingling in the hands, arms, feet, or legs; fever muscle aches, nausea, vomiting, skin rash
	Lamivudine + zidovudine; 1997 (Combivir)	Burning, numbness, pain, or tingling in the hands, arms, feet, or legs; fever, muscle aches, nausea, vomiting, skin rash, unusual tiredness or weakness
	Stavudine; 1994 (Zerit)	Burning, numbness, pain, or tingling in the hands, arms, feet, or legs; fever, muscle aches, nausea, vomiting, skin rash
	Tenofovir disoproxil fumarate; 2001 (Viread)	Liver or kidney failure, lactic acidosis, pancreatitis
	Zalcitabine; 1992 (HIVID)	Gastralgia, nausea, vomiting; burning, numbness, pain, or tingling in the hands, arms, feet, or legs; skin rash, ulcerative stomatitis
	Zidovudine; 1987 (Retrovir, AZT, ZDV)	Fatigue, weakness, fever, chills, sore throat

continued ⟶

TABLE 3-2 FDA-Approved Drugs for HIV/AIDS Infection (Antiretroviral Drugs) *(continued)*		
Classification & Function	**Generic Name (Trade Name)**	**Major Side Effects**
Protease Inhibitors (PIs) Block the ability of HIV to make copies of itself	Amprenavir; 1999 (Agenerase)	Severe rash, changes in body fat, increased cholesterol, hyperglycemia
	Atazanavir; 2003 (Reyataz)	Jaundice, heart block, hyperglycemia, diarrhea, nausea; infection, hematuria
	Fosamprenavir; 2003 (Lexiva)	Severe rash, changes in body fat, increased cholesterol, hyperglycemia
	Indinavir; 1996 (Crixivan)	Nephrolithiasis, changes in body fat, hyperglycemia
	Lopinavir + ritonavir; 2000 (Kaletra)	Pancreatitis, hyperglycemia, nephrolithiasis
	Nelfinavir; 1997 (Viracept)	Changes in body fat, hypercholesterolemia, hyperglycemia
	Ritonavir; 1996 (Norvir)	Pancreatitis, hyperglycemia, hyperlipidemia
	Saquinavir; 1997 (Fortovase)	Changes in body fat, hyperglycemia

Note: The number following the generic drug name represents the date or dates the drugs were approved for the specified purpose.
Source: US Department of Health and Human Services; Food and Drug Administration and AIDSInfo

Delayed Treatment. There are advantages and disadvantages to delaying therapy. The benefits of delaying treatment include postponing drug-related adverse affects, delaying the development of drug resistance, and preserving treatment options for the future. The risks of delaying treatment include irreversible immune system damage and an increased risk of the patient transmitting HIV to others.

Early Treatment. There are also advantages and disadvantages to beginning treatment early. The benefits of early treatment include the suppression of viral replication (that is, the spread of the virus within the patient's system), thus preserving immune function; a reduction in the risk of the patient's transmitting HIV to others; and helping the patient live symptom-free longer. The disadvantages of early treatment are:

- Development of drug toxicity
- Drug resistance and the subsequent transmission of drug-resistant HIV strains to others
- Adverse effects on the quality of life
- Loss of treatment options in the future

Each of these advantages and disadvantages must be carefully weighed by the patient and physician based on the patient's symptoms, lifestyle, and ability to comply with the treatment.

Treating Complications. In addition to treating the patient for the HIV virus, it is often necessary to treat the opportunistic infections and associated complications acquired by the patient. Individuals with a compromised immune system are more prone to bacterial, protozoal, viral, and fungal infections as well as to certain types of malignancies. See Table 3-2 for a list of drugs used in the treatment of these HIV- and AIDS-related complications.

Continuing Research. Researchers continue with their efforts to develop an effective vaccine. Until a vaccine is found, it is important to prevent new HIV infections and to effectively treat persons who are already infected. The U.S. Department of Health and Human Services has allocated billions of dollars for vaccine and treatment research, monitoring those with HIV/AIDS, caring for those who are infected, and fighting the disease on a global level. As a medical assistant, it is your responsibility to remain informed regarding new treatments and prevention methods and to assist in educating patients regarding these advances.

Other Blood-Borne Infections

Hepatitis and HIV infections are the best known of the blood-borne pathogens you may encounter working in the medical field. There are also several other blood-borne diseases of which you should be aware. Some of these diseases pose particular risk to patients already infected with HIV. For this reason, you should advise HIV-positive patients about symptoms and preventive measures related to the diseases.

Cytomegalovirus

People with compromised, or impaired, immune systems and infants (whose immune systems undergo additional development after birth) are especially at risk for cytomegalovirus (CMV). CMV is an extremely common infection. Blood tests show that nearly 80% of adults tested have antibodies for the virus. The presence of these antibodies indicates an infection at some point in the person's life. The infection rarely causes noticeable symptoms in adults with normal immune systems.

The disease sometimes takes a form similar to infectious mononucleosis in otherwise healthy adults, however. It may develop into severe lung disease in immunocompromised adults. Symptoms of the infection may include swollen glands, fever, and fatigue.

Pregnant women can pass the disease on to their newborns. Infants with CMV present signs of jaundice, a rash, and low birth weight. In severe cases CMV can cause brain damage, mental retardation, deafness, blindness, and death.

Erythema Infectiosum (Parvovirus B19)

Erythema infectiosum, or fifth disease, is a moderately contagious disease seen mainly in children and caused by human parvovirus B19. The term *fifth disease* was assigned to this "fifth" eruptive disease found in children in the late 1800s. (Sources vary on which diseases were considered first through fourth, but all include measles and rubella. Popular knowledge adds mumps and chickenpox to the list, while some more formal sources include scarlet fever and Dukes' disease.) The disease is characterized by the abrupt onset of a rash. The virus may be transmitted from mother to fetus, and although it does not cause birth defects, there is some risk of fetal death from infection. More severe signs of infection may be seen in immunocompromised patients.

Human T-Cell Lymphotrophic Virus

Infection with the human T-cell lymphotrophic virus (HTLV-1) often appears in intravenous drug users, in people who have received multiple blood transfusions, and in the sexual partners, children, and household contacts of infected people. The virus attacks T cells, an important component of the body's immune system, by penetrating the cells and incorporating its genetic material into the cells' genetic material.

Some people who are infected with HTLV-1 show no symptoms, while others exhibit severe symptoms. Infection with HTLV-1 most commonly leads to adult T-cell leukemia/lymphoma (ATLL), although patients can also contract disturbances of the spinal cord or partial paralysis.

Physical findings in cases of ATLL include skin lesions, disease of the lymph nodes, fever, abdominal distress, arthritis, and sometimes hypercalcemia (an excess of calcium in the blood). Diagnosis is confirmed when the virus is found in blood or other body tissues.

Listeriosis

Listeriosis is an infectious disease caused by the bacterium *Listeria monocytogenes.* Once infected, an individual can pass the infection to others through contact with blood or blood products, and a pregnant woman can pass the infection to her fetus.

If the infection is passed to a fetus during the later stages of pregnancy, the infant may be stillborn. Infected infants who survive may develop meningitis, pneumonia, or septicemia (blood poisoning).

Symptoms in infected adults may include fever, shock, rash, and generalized aches, but most people do not notice any symptoms. The disease can rapidly cause death in elderly or immunocompromised patients through circulatory collapse.

Listeriosis is diagnosed by blood tests. If symptoms are present and the patient is at high risk, however, antibiotic therapy is sometimes initiated before positive identification of the pathogen.

Malaria

Malarial infection is spread from person to person primarily through the bite of infected mosquitoes. There have also been cases of transmission from mother to fetus as well as from an infected to an uninfected person through an accidental needlestick. Malaria is mainly a tropical infection present in parts of Africa, Asia, and Central and South America.

The parasite usually enters the bloodstream through the mosquito's bite. It invades the liver, moving from there into red blood cells. Within a red blood cell, the parasite multiplies and eventually causes rupture of the cell. When the cell ruptures, new parasites are released to continue the cycle of infection, growth, rupture, and release. An infected person does not exhibit symptoms until several of these cycles have occurred. Symptoms are caused by the pigments released from the red blood cells and metabolic toxins from the parasites.

A 4- to 8-hour, three-part cycle marks infection with malaria. In the first stage of the cycle, the patient experiences shaking chills. In the second stage, the patient experiences high fever that spikes as high as 104° or 105°F. The third stage is marked by excessive perspiration. The patient may also report nausea, vomiting, headache, and gastrointestinal symptoms and may exhibit an enlarged spleen and liver tenderness. Laboratory results will show normal or decreased white blood cell counts and decreased platelet count.

Avoidance of infection is the best means of preventing the spread of malaria. Once infected, most people recover from the disease if treated quickly. When malaria is suspected, blood tests are performed every few hours until the diagnosis is confirmed or another reason is discovered for the patient's symptoms.

Syphilis

Syphilis is a sexually transmitted disease caused by the spirochete *Treponema pallidum.* A pregnant woman can pass this disease to her fetus. An affected infant experiences the most severe form of syphilis. An infant born with congenital syphilis may exhibit nail exfoliation (the nails falling off), hair loss, rhinitis (inflammation of the nose), lesions, anemia, failure to thrive, and paralysis of one or more limbs.

Syphilis in adults and adolescents occurs in the following three stages.

1. In the first stage, infection is indicated by the initial appearance of a painless ulcer, called a **chancre.** This ulcer may appear on the tongue, lips, genitalia, rectum, or elsewhere. In females, the chancre may not be visible, and the first stage could be missed.
2. Patients in the second stage may experience nontender swelling of the lymph nodes. This stage may also include a generalized skin rash, fever, and the presence of mucous-membrane lesions. Condylomas (wartlike lesions of the skin) may appear in areas of moist skin.
3. The third stage may occur between several years and 2 or 3 decades after initial infection. During this stage, the patient may exhibit tumors of the skin, bones, and liver as well as central nervous system manifestations such as dementia, abnormal reflexes, and psychosis.

Between the first two stages and the final stage is a period of latency during which the patient exhibits no symptoms and appears to be disease-free. Blood tests will still show indications of infection, and treatment is usually administered in an effort to prevent the disease from reaching the late stage.

Identifying and treating syphilis in an HIV-positive individual are difficult tasks. Because the presence of the HIV pathogen alters the function of the immune system, test results that normally indicate the presence of syphilis may yield false-negative findings. Additional tests are required to confirm diagnosis. With the presence of HIV, the course of the syphilis infection may be accelerated, and the benefits of drug therapy to combat the infection may be reduced.

Toxoplasmosis

The primary source of the pathogen *Toxoplasma gondii* is cat feces. Although undercooked meat products are another source, most cases appear in people who have handled cat litter boxes. For that reason pregnant women and those with compromised immune systems, such as patients with AIDS, should not handle cat litter boxes.

Most people infected with toxoplasmosis experience no symptoms. Symptoms may, however, include fever, malaise, sore throat, rash, stiff neck, disease of the lymph nodes, and fatigue. A pregnant woman may pass the infection to her fetus, and the infection may result in spontaneous abortion, malformation, or retardation (depending on the trimester in which the organism enters). Infants who survive may also suffer from deafness, blindness, brain damage, and seizures. Diagnosis is confirmed through blood tests.

Reporting Guidelines

Each state formulates requirements for reporting HIV infection and AIDS. That information is then sent to the Centers for Disease Control and Prevention. Table 3-3 lists states that require reporting of HIV infection by name of patient, states that accept anonymous reporting, and states that do not require reporting. Follow your employer's guidelines or procedures when you must report cases of HIV infection.

When you report a communicable disease, you must fill out a report form. Your state health department may have a different form for each reportable disease. You must obtain the correct form and a disease identification number from the health department every time you report a communicable disease. To fill out such a form, you need access to the following information:

- Disease identification (usually a code number as well as the name of the disease)
- Patient identification (including name, address, date of birth, sex, ethnic origin, and occupational or educational status) if required (as already noted, some states require only anonymous reporting of some diseases)
- Infection history (date of onset, vaccination history, laboratory results)
- Reporting-institution information (name of person completing report, title, contact information)

Each state and each medical facility has specific guidelines to which you must adhere when filling out such a form. Procedure 3-2 describes, in general, how to notify state and county agencies about reportable diseases.

Reporting guidelines must also be followed if a worker comes in contact with a substance that may transmit infection. These guidelines, which are explained in OSHA's

TABLE 3-3 States' Reporting Guidelines for HIV Infection

States Requiring Name-Based Reports	States Requiring Code-Based Reports[1]	States Required Name-to-Code-Based Reports[2]
Alabama	California	Delaware
Alaska	District of Columbia	Maine
Arizona	Hawaii	Montana
Arkansas	Illinois	Oregon
Colorado	Kentucky	Washington
Connecticut	Maryland	
Florida	Massachusetts	
Idaho	Rhode Island	
Indiana	Vermont	
Iowa		
Kansas		
Louisiana		
Michigan		
Minnesota		
Mississippi		
Missouri		
Nebraska		
Nevada		
New Jersey		
New Mexico		
New York		
North Carolina		
North Dakota		
Ohio		
Oklahoma		
Pennsylvania		
South Carolina		
South Dakota		
Tennessee		
Texas		
Utah		
Virginia		
West Virginia		
Wisconsin		
Wyoming		

[1]Code-Based Reporting: Coded identifiers are used in place of names.

[2]Name-to-Code-Based Reporting: Initially reported by name and then converted to a coded identifier

Notes: New Hampshire allows reporting to be either Name-Based or Code-Based. Georgia does not conduct follow-up reporting. HIV reporting is anonymous in Georgia.

Source: The Henry J. Kaiser Family Foundation. 2400 Sand Hill Road, Menlo Park, CA 94025; http://www.statehealthfacts.kff.org/

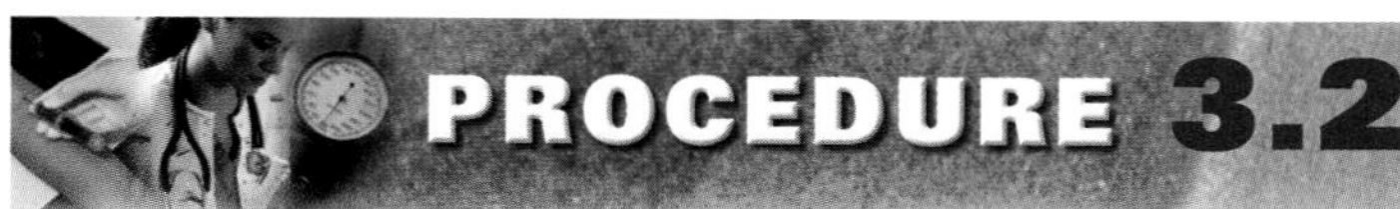

PROCEDURE 3.2

Notifying State and County Agencies About Reportable Diseases

MICHIGAN DEPARTMENT OF PUBLIC HEALTH
Division of Disease Surveillance

ENTERIC ILLNESS CASE INVESTIGATION
(Please check appropriate illness)

_______Shigellosis
_______Non-typhoid Salmonellosis
_______Campylobacter enteritis
_______Giardiasis
_______Amebiasis

CASE INFORMATION

Name: ______________ Age or Birthdate: ______________ Sex: ________ Race: ________

Address: ______________ (Street) (City) (County) (Zip) Phone: ______________

Occupation: ______________ (What) (Where) *High Risk: Y N

(If infant or student list school, nursery or day care center)

Attending Physician: ______________ Address or Phone: ______________ Was the patient hospitalized: Y N

Hospital: ______________ Dates: ______________ (Admission) (Discharge)

Onset: ______________ Date recovered: ______________ Symptom Summary: ______________

Suspected Causative Agent: ______________
(include species or serotype if known)

HOUSEHOLD CONTACTS INFORMATION

Name	Age	Family Relationship	Occupation	*High Risk Y N	Provide date of onset for all household members with concurrent similar illness
1)					
2)					
3)					
4)					
5)					
6)					
7)					
8)					
9)					
10)					

*"High Risk" = occupation as food handler, direct patient care worker, day care center worker or person attending day care or who is institutionalized. Stool specimens should be obtained on "high risk" cases and "high risk" household contacts as appropriate for the illness. Results may be recorded in Laboratory Information Section of this form (see over).

Name of the person who completed this form: ______________ County: ________

Information obtained from: ______________ Date: ______________

Telephone Interview: ________ Home Visit: ________ Outbreak Investigation: ________

C-30 Rev. 10/83 AUTH: Act 368, P.A. 1978

Figure 3-5. Some states have specific forms for use with particular communicable diseases or diseases of a certain type.

continued ⟶

PROCEDURE 3.2

Notifying State and County Agencies About Reportable Diseases *(continued)*

Objective: To report cases of infection with reportable disease to the proper state or county health department

OSHA Guidelines: This procedure does not involve exposure to blood, body fluids, or tissues.

Materials: Communicable disease report form, pen, envelope, stamp

Method

1. Check to be sure you have the correct form. Some states have specific forms for each reportable infectious disease or type of disease (Figure 3-5), as well as a general form (Figure 3-6). CDC forms may also be used for reporting specific diseases.
2. Fill in all blank areas unless they are shaded (generally for local health department use).
3. Follow office procedures for submitting the report to a supervisor or physician before sending it out.
4. Sign and date the form. Address the envelope, put a stamp on it, and place it in the mail.

NON-HOUSEHOLD CONTACTS WITH A CONCURRENT SIMILAR ILLNESS

Name	Approximate date of onset of symptoms	Address and/or Phone	Relationship to case (Nature of contact)
1)			
2)			
3)			
4)			
5)			

ADDITIONAL EXPOSURES OR COMMENTS

Home Sewage System: Municipal Septic Tank Other

Home drinking Water Type: Municipal Private Well Other

As appropriate for the illness, ask about meals eaten away from home, stores where groceries bought, brand of poultry, meat, dairy products consumed, overnight travel, recent foreign travel, group functions, exposure to raw milk, untreated water, animals, etc. within one incubation period before onset.

(shigellosis to 7 days, salmonellosis - up to 3 days, Campylobacter enteritis - up to 10 days)

Be specific, provide place name(s) and date(s).

FOLLOW-UP FECAL CULTURE RESULTS FOR "HIGH RISK" CASE AND/OR CONTACTS.

Name or Initials	Date(s) Obtained and Findings
1)	
2)	
3)	
4)	
5)	

Figure 3-5. Continuation of form.

continued ⟶

PROCEDURE 3.2

ARIZONA DEPARTMENT OF HEALTH SERVICES
COMMUNICABLE DISEASE REPORT
Important Instructions on Reverse Side
PLEASE PRINT OR TYPE

County/IHS ID Number/Chapter

State ID Number

PATIENT'S NAME (Last) (First)

DATE OF BIRTH

SEX
☐ Male
☐ Female

ETHNICITY
☐ Hispanic
☐ Non-Hispanic

STREET ADDRESS

CENSUS TRACT

CITY

RACE
☐ White
☐ Am. Indian
☐ Asian
☐ Black
☐ Other
☐ Unknown

COUNTY

STATE

ZIP CODE

PHONE NO.

DIAGNOSIS OR SUSPECT REPORTABLE CONDITION

COUNTY USE ONLY:

LAB CONFIRMATION DATE:________

☐ Negative
☐ Positive
☐ Not Done
☐ Unknown

DATE ONSET

DATE OF DIAGNOSIS

LAB RESULTS

PATIENT OCCUPATION OR SCHOOL

PHYSICIAN OR OTHER REPORTING SOURCE

PHONE NUMBER

COUNTY USE ONLY:
☐ Confirmed case
☐ Probable case
☐ Outbreak Associated
☐ Ruled Out

STREET ADDRESS

CITY

STATE

ZIP CODE

Original and 1st copy to County Health Department ☐ CHECK IF ADDITIONAL FORMS ARE NEEDED (Quantity)________

REPORTABLE DISEASES

Arizona Revised Statutes and Arizona Administrative Code require the following diseases to be reported to the County Health Department or Indian Health Services within 5 business days of diagnosis or treatment.

AIDS[3]
Amebiasis[1]
Anthrax
Aseptic meningitis
Botulism*
Brucellosis
Campylobacteriosis[1]
Chancroid[3]
Chlamydial infections (genital)[3]
Cholera*
Coccidioidomycosis
Colorado tick fever
Conjunctivitis, acute[2]
Cryptosporidiosis
Dengue
Diphtheria*
Ehrlichiosis
Encephalitis, viral
Foodborne illness/ Waterborne illness*
Giardiasis[1]
Gonorrhea[3]
Haemophilus influenzae*
Hemolytic Uremic Syndrome[1]
Hepatitis A[1]
Hepatitis B, Delta Hepatitis
Hepatitis Non-A, Non-B
Herpes Genitalis[3]
HIV[3]
Lead Poisoning[3]
Legionellosis
Leprosy
Listeriosis
Lyme Disease
Malaria
Measles*
Meningococcal disease*
Mumps
Pediculosis[2]
Pertussis*
Pesticide poisoning[3]
Plague*
Poliomyelitis*
Psittacosis
Q Fever
Rabies in humans*
Relapsing fever
Reye's Syndrome
Rocky Mt. spotted fever
Rubella*
Congenital rubella syn.
Salmonellosis[1]
Scabies[2]
Shigellosis[1]
Staphylococcal disease[1,2]
Streptococcal diseases[1,2]
Syphilis[3]
Tetanus
Toxic Shock Syndrome
Trichinosis
Tuberculosis[3]
Tuberculosis infection in children <6 yrs of age
Tularemia
Typhoid Fever[1]
Typhus fever
Varicella
Yellow Fever*

*Telephone report required to the County Health Department or Indian Health Services within 24 hours.

[1] Report within 24 hours of diagnosis if in food handler.

[2] Outbreak reports only

[3] These conditions are reported on other forms, call 1-800-334-1540 for a supply

ADHS/DPS/OIDS/IDES-1 (Rev. 11-94)

Figure 3-6. Each state has its own communicable disease report.

Blood-borne Pathogens Standard, include reporting exposure incidents to employers immediately. (See Chapter 1 for specific guidelines on handling exposure incidents.)

Patient Education

Patient education is one of the most effective means of preventing disease transmission. As a medical assistant, you are in a pivotal position in relation to your patients. You can assess patients' understanding of their risk for infection, measures they must take to eradicate an infection (if possible), potential dangers posed by treatments, and methods for controlling an infection's spread. Staying up-to-date on new information will help you provide patients with effective, relevant education.

Drug Trials

New drug treatments for HIV infection and AIDS are being tested every day. Some patients may be interested in information about clinical drug trials. **Clinical drug trials** are internationally recognized research protocols designed to evaluate the efficacy or safety of drugs and to produce scientifically valid results. According to your institution's protocol, you may be required to introduce certain patients to such programs or to monitor patients involved in drug trial programs. You can obtain information about drug trials from the AIDS Clinical Trials Information Service at 800-874-2572.

Patients With Special Concerns

You will be responsible for educating patients with a variety of needs and concerns. Some patients, particularly teenagers and patients about to be discharged from the hospital, may have specific concerns involving HIV and HBV infection.

Teenagers. You may work with teenagers who have come in to obtain a means of birth control or receive treatment for sexually transmitted diseases (STDs). During the patient interview, you are in a position to educate the teenagers about the dangers of HIV and HBV infection. Most teenagers think that they are invincible and that disease happens only to "other people." You can effectively educate teenagers about HIV and HBV infection by helping them realize that disease can happen to anyone. Begin by establishing a trusting relationship with them and by providing them with facts rather than lectures or moral appeals. Figure 3-7 shows the various risk factors, or exposure categories, that are commonly implicated in the transmission of AIDS to male adolescents aged 13 to 19. Figure 3-8 provides similar information for females aged

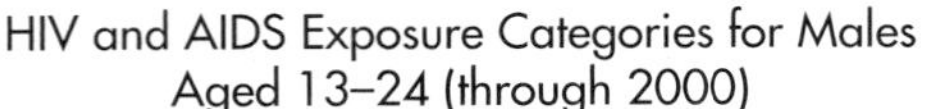

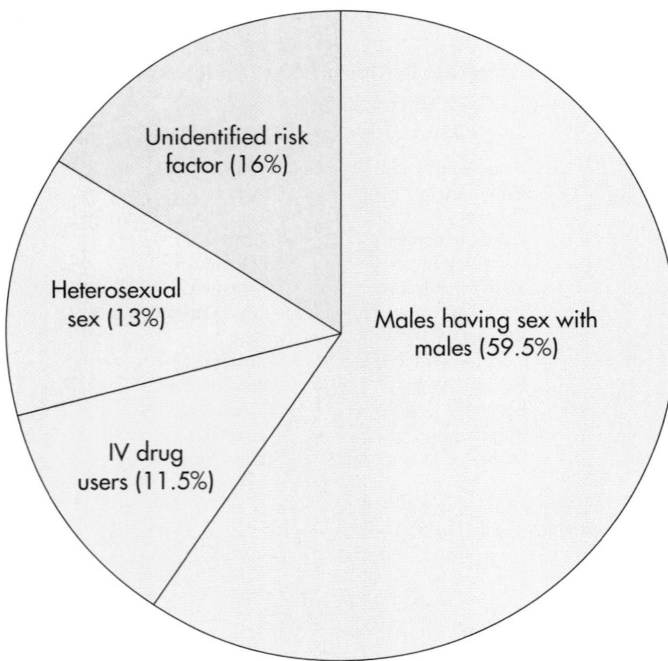

Figure 3-7. These percentages provide insight into the types of exposure male teenagers should guard against.

Source: HIV/AIDS Surveillance Report, Vol. 14. Atlanta, GA: Centers for Disease Control and Prevention, November 2003 http://www.cdc.gov/hiv/stats/hasr1402/2002SurveillanceReport.pdf

HIV and AIDS Exposure Categories for Females
Aged 13–24 (through 2000)

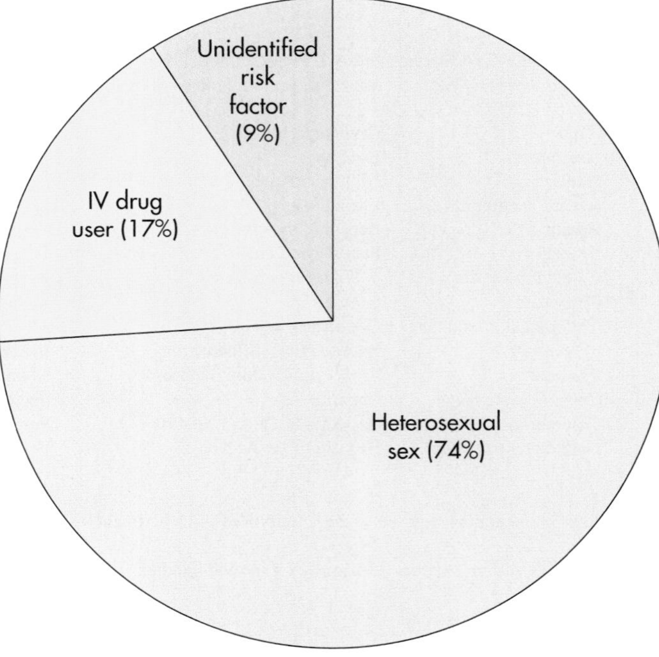

Figure 3-8. Female teenagers face a greater risk of HIV infection from heterosexual contact than male teenagers do.

Source: HIV/AIDS Surveillance Report, Vol. 14. Atlanta, GA: Centers for Disease Control and Prevention, November 2003 http://www.cdc.gov/hiv/stats/hasr1402/2002SurveillanceReport.pdf

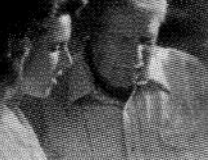

Educating the Patient

Obtaining Information About AIDS and Hepatitis

Some patients who have AIDS or hepatitis may want additional information about care options, drug treatments and clinical trials, prevention guidelines, risk factors, and therapy management. Many high-quality resources are available for these patients.

One of the best places to direct patients is to the Centers for Disease Control and Prevention, located in Atlanta, Georgia. The CDC offers a variety of services, such as the following:

- CDC National AIDS Clearinghouse (800-458-5231)
- CDC National AIDS Hotline (800-342-2437)
- AIDS Clinical Trials Information Service (800-874-2572)
- HIV/AIDS Treatment Information Service (800-448-0440)

The Consumer Information Center (CIC), in Pueblo, Colorado, offers a variety of free and low-cost booklets about many health matters, including topics such as HIV/AIDS, hepatitis, and other sexually transmitted diseases. The CIC can be reached at:

Consumer Information Center
Pueblo, CO 81009
303-544-5277, Ext. 370

Patients who are comfortable using computers and who have access to the World Wide Web can find a variety of resources there. The Web sites for both the CDC (www.cdc.gov) and the CIC (www.pueblo.gsa.gov) are very comprehensive.

Many local support and resource organizations may also be available to the patient. In your position you can serve both the patient, by helping him contact these organizations, and the organizations, by publicizing their efforts.

13 to 19. In addition, the number of new HIV infections for male and female adolescents aged 13 to 19 can be found in Figure 3-9. Armed with data such as these, you can stress to teenage patients the importance of preventive behaviors in avoiding HIV infection.

The Patient About to Be Discharged. When a patient has been hospitalized with HBV or HIV infection, the disruption in his life often lingers long past the discharge date. He must make changes and continue some treatment when he goes home. Your job as a medical assistant is to make sure that the patient comes to the medical office for follow-up care, reports any adverse reactions to therapy or treatment, and knows which signs and symptoms to report to the doctor. You must also ensure that the patient knows what precautions to take to avoid transmitting the infection to others.

As part of the education process, the patient may request additional information from you, or you may need to provide information to the patient's family members or other caregivers. See the Educating the Patient section for suggestions on where to obtain information for patients and their families.

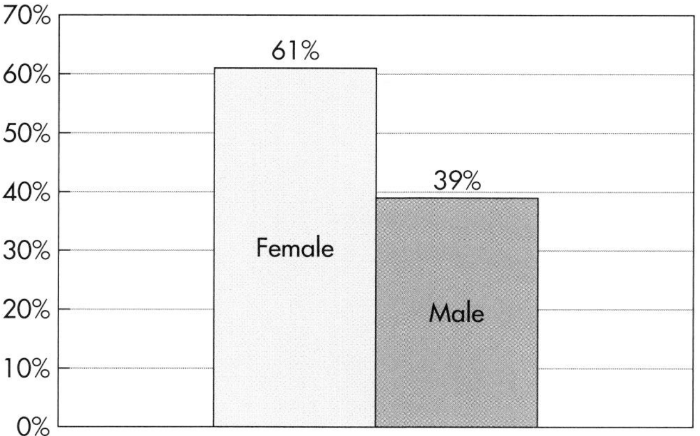

Figure 3-9. Female adolescents are at a much higher risk of developing HIV than their male counterparts are. *Source:* HIV/AIDS Surveillance Report, Vol. 14. Atlanta, GA: Centers for Disease Control and Prevention, November 2003 http://www.cdc.gov/hiv/stats/hasr1402/2002SurveillanceReport.pdf

Multicultural Concerns

Although you must be sensitive to and respectful toward patients from all backgrounds, you may need to target your education efforts toward certain groups. For example, according to the CDC's quarterly report, the incidence of HIV infection is increasing more in some groups than in others. Data in the report on the pattern of the disease can help you ascertain which groups need improved education. If you work with patients who are in these high-risk groups or who know people in them, you are in a unique position to provide them with information on preventive measures they can follow to avoid exposure to blood-borne pathogens. Because some patients may be reluctant to discuss sensitive subjects, be sure to have brochures available (in several languages) for them to take home and read.

Special Issues With Terminal Illness

In this chapter you have learned about a variety of blood-borne diseases. One of these diseases is almost always fatal, and others may be fatal in certain situations. Just as you need to educate patients about preventing such diseases and about methods of treatment, you need to provide support and counsel to patients, their families, and their loved ones when they are informed that their illnesses are **terminal,** or fatal. You must understand something of people's reactions to a terminal diagnosis to help them cope with the situation.

Patients react to the idea of dying in different ways. Some are angry that death is coming to them. Others are grateful that relief from pain and suffering is near. Many terminal patients respond by denying that they are dying. After patients fully realize that they are going to die, depression is a common reaction. The only thing you can be certain of is that no two patients respond to a terminal diagnosis in exactly the same way.

You can help patients come to terms with the fact that they are going to die by:

- Supporting and accepting them no matter how they react
- Encouraging them to express their feelings and thoughts freely
- Communicating respect through your use of nonverbal communication, including your posture and touch
- Meeting reasonable needs and demands as quickly as possible
- Providing referrals to hospices, which offer a variety of services, including personal care for patients who are dying and emotional support for them and their families

Summary

Infectious diseases are transmitted in many different ways. Medical and surgical asepsis and various techniques and procedures for sanitizing, disinfecting, and sterilizing instruments, equipment, and surfaces all help prevent disease transmission. Specific transmission methods dictate which approaches work best for which diseases. The focus of this chapter has been blood-borne transmission.

The transmission of blood-borne pathogens is a particular concern for medical assistants as well as for people in many other professions. The pathogens that pose the greatest risk are HIV, HBV, and HCV. Infection with these pathogens can result in death or chronic disease.

Your role as a medical assistant is to help prevent the spread of such infectious diseases. The preventive measures you will take at work include following Universal Precautions, watching patients for signs of infectious diseases, and educating patients about the risk factors associated with blood-borne diseases.

Information about infectious diseases changes constantly. You can best serve your patients and your employer if you keep up-to-date on research, advances in treatment, and general information. Your efforts with patient education may include information about preventive measures, drug trials, follow-up care, and hospices for terminally ill patients.

REVIEW

CHAPTER 3

CASE STUDY QUESTIONS

Now that you have completed this chapter, review the case study at the beginning of the chapter and answer the following questions:

1. Which type of hepatitis does this patient probably have?
2. What are two medical terms for the yellowish discoloration you observed?
3. How long might the patient expect to suffer from the symptoms of the acute phase of the illness?
4. Could this disease have been prevented? If so, how?

Discussion Questions

1. Describe the differences between the various forms of hepatitis and ways to prevent the transmission of each.
2. As a medical worker, what preventive measures can you take to avoid acquiring HBV infection? HCV infection?
3. Why do opportunistic infections pose such a risk to the HIV-infected patient?

Critical Thinking Questions

1. Hemophilia is a disease that requires blood transfusions. What reassurance can you give to patients regarding AIDS and hepatitis transmission associated with transfusions?
2. Accidental needlesticks are a risk to the medical community. Which disease, HIV or hepatitis, is more likely to be contracted from an accidental needlestick from an infected patient? What can you do to protect yourself?
3. While talking with one of your patients, an HIV-positive individual, you learn that friends have recently purchased a kitten for her. What will you do or say?

Application Activities

1. Working in a small group, have all members role-play a situation in which a patient and his family have just learned that he has HIV infection. Have one member of the group assume the role of the medical assistant and offer support and understanding to them. Then have other students in the class critique your approach.
2. Contact your local legislature to determine what, if any, pertinent legislation is being considered that would have an impact on HIV-positive patients. Present your findings to the class in an oral report.
3. Identify resources in your area that a person might use if she is exposed to HIV. Explore what is available to patients at various points in the disease process. Prepare a brochure in which you identify the resources and what they provide

CHAPTER 4

Preparing the Examination and Treatment Areas

KEY TERMS

accessibility
consumable
fixative
general physical examination
occult blood
transcutaneous absorption

AREAS OF COMPETENCE

2003 Role Delineation Study

CLINICAL

Fundamental Principles

- Apply principles of aseptic technique and infection control

PATIENT CARE

- Prepare and maintain examination and treatment areas
- Assist with examinations, procedures, and treatments

GENERAL

Legal Concepts

- Comply with established risk management and safety procedures

CHAPTER OUTLINE

- The Medical Assistant's Role in Preparing the Examination Room
- The Examination Room
- Cleanliness in the Examination Room
- Room Temperature, Lighting, and Ventilation
- Medical Instruments and Supplies
- Physical Safety in the Examination Room

OBJECTIVES

After completing Chapter 4, you will be able to:

4.1 Explain the medical assistant's role in preparing the examination room.
4.2 Describe the layout and features of a typical examination room.
4.3 Describe steps to prevent the spread of infection in the examination room.
4.4 Explain how and when to disinfect examination room surfaces.
4.5 Describe the importance of such factors as temperature, lighting, and ventilation in the examination room.
4.6 Identify instruments and supplies used in a general physical examination, and tell how to arrange and prepare them.
4.7 Explain how to eliminate hazards to physical safety in the examination room.

Introduction

One of the most important tasks you encounter as a practicing medical assistant is the preparation of the examination room and treatment area. In this chapter you will learn about the common layouts of examination rooms; keeping the rooms clean and stocked with instruments, disposable, and consumable supplies; maintaining the comfort of the room; and making the room safe for patients and coworkers. You will also be introduced to the requirements for accessibility established by the Americans With Disabilities Act.

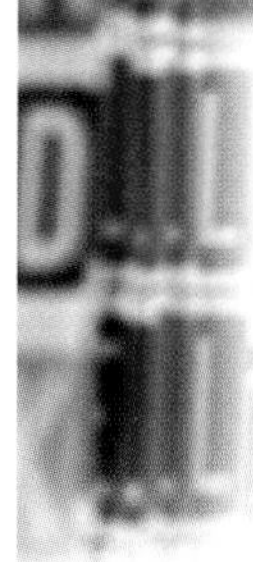

CASE STUDY

As a medical assistant, you are reviewing the charts as you prepare for the next day's appointments, and you notice that a female patient who is scheduled for her routine gynecological checkup has a flag on her chart because she has bilateral cataracts.

As you read this chapter, consider the following questions:

1. What are bilateral cataracts, and why would this condition be a consideration when you come in contact with this patient?
2. What instruments should be assembled for the physician to use during the examination?
3. What disposable and consumable supplies may reasonably be anticipated for use?
4. What measures can you take to ensure the patient's comfort and safety?

The Medical Assistant's Role in Preparing the Examination Room

When a patient enters an examination room, the patient expects to find it clean and neat. The doctor assumes that all medical instruments and supplies necessary for an examination or treatment are ready to use. Preparing the examination room for patients and doctors is your responsibility. You must keep this room not only spotlessly clean and in good order but also free from obstacles that might cause an accidental injury. Safety, efficiency, and comfort are the main concerns in the examination room.

The Examination Room

The examination room is the area where the physician observes the patient, listens to the patient's description of symptoms, performs a general physical examination, and dispenses treatment. A physician performs a **general physical examination** to confirm a patient's health or diagnose a medical problem. Figure 4-1 shows a typical examination room.

Number and Size of Rooms

The number of examination rooms in a medical office depends on the number of doctors who work there and on each doctor's patient load. Ideally, each doctor in a medical office has at least two examination rooms for her or his exclusive use. A minimum of two rooms per doctor enables the medical assistant to prepare one room while the doctor examines a patient in the other room.

The customary size for an examination room is 8 by 12 feet. The room should be large enough to accommodate the doctor, the patient, and one assistant comfortably. At the same time, it should be small enough that instruments and supplies will be within easy reach. Doors and interior walls should be soundproofed to ensure privacy for patients.

Some examination rooms have dressing cubicles in one corner. Other rooms have screens in one corner, behind which the patient may disrobe. Regardless of a room's layout, you should provide privacy for patients whenever they need to disrobe and put on gowns.

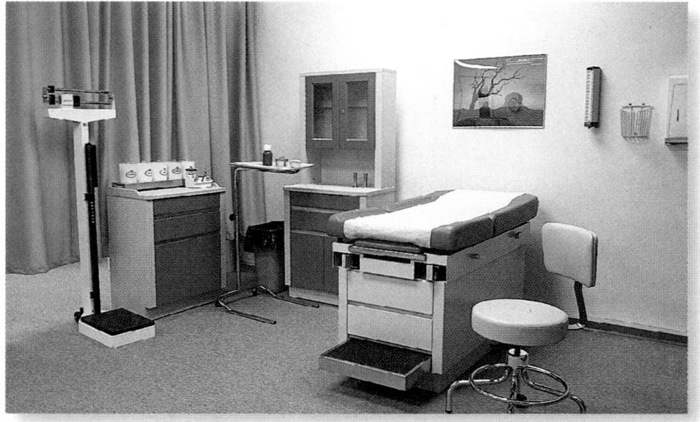

Figure 4-1. You are responsible for making sure the examination room is clean and orderly.

A rack for the patient's medical records usually hangs on the wall directly outside the examination room or on the outside of the door. A light or other device on the wall or door may be used to signal that the room is occupied.

Furnishings

Furnishings should be arranged for efficiency, the convenience of the physician, and the comfort of the patient. The examining table is the key piece of equipment in the examination room. It should be positioned in the center of the room or coming out from the wall. This arrangement allows the physician and an assistant to attend to the patient on at least three sides. The examining table usually contains a pullout step for the patient to use when getting onto the table. It may also contain drawers for storing instruments and table coverings.

Examining tables are usually adjustable to enable the patient to assume the various positions that the physical examination may require. The physician will probably tell you beforehand if you need to adjust the table in a particular way.

Most examination rooms also have a sink, a countertop, and a writing surface large enough to spread out the patient's records. Shelves, cupboards, and drawers store routine supplies such as dressings, adhesive tape, and bandages.

The examination room may also include the following items:

- One or more chairs
- A rolling stool
- A weight scale with height bar
- A metal wastebasket with a lid
- Biohazardous waste containers for disposal of biohazardous materials (biological agents that can spread disease to living things)
- Puncture-proof containers for disposal of biohazardous sharps
- A high-intensity lamp
- Wall brackets for hanging instruments

Special Features

The Americans With Disabilities Act of 1990 (ADA) requires that businesses, services, and public transportation provide "reasonable accommodations" for the disabled. To comply with this act, the examination room in a medical office must have features that make the area accessible to patients who use wheelchairs or who have visual or other types of physical impairments. **Accessibility** refers to the ease with which people can move in and out of a space. The ADA accessibility guidelines require the following:

- A doorway at least 36 inches (915 mm) wide to allow a person in a wheelchair to pass through
- A clearance space in rooms and hallways that is 60 inches (1525 mm) in diameter to allow a person in a wheelchair to make a 180° turn
- Stable, firm, slip-resistant flooring
- Door-opening hardware that can be grasped with one hand and does not require the twisting of the wrist to use
- Door closers adjusted to allow time for a person in a wheelchair to enter or exit through the door
- Grab bars in the lavatory

Cleanliness in the Examination Room

As you learned in Chapter 1, you can follow specific measures to achieve medical asepsis and prevent the spread of pathogenic microorganisms in the medical office. These measures involve strict housekeeping standards and adherence to government guidelines.

A clean examination room is extremely important in preventing the spread of infectious diseases to patients and health-care workers. Part of your job is to carefully follow infection-control procedures in the medical office and to keep the examination room clean and neat.

Infection Control

People with a variety of contagious diseases visit medical offices every day. The potential for the spread of infection is thus higher in medical offices than in most other places. For that reason, you must be especially careful to follow infection-control procedures at work. You can safeguard the health of staff members and patients by:

- Making hand washing a priority
- Keeping the examining table clean
- Disinfecting all work surfaces

Hand Washing. Clean hands are the first step in preventing infection transmission in the examination room. Wash your hands with disinfectant soap and warm water at the following times:

- At the beginning of the day
- Before and after having contact with each patient
- Before and after using gloves or performing any procedure
- Before handling clean or sterile supplies
- Before and after eating or taking a break
- Before and after using the bathroom
- After blowing your nose, coughing, or sneezing
- Before and after handling specimens or waste
- Before leaving for the day

After washing your hands, use a clean paper towel to handle faucets or doorknobs. The paper towel helps you

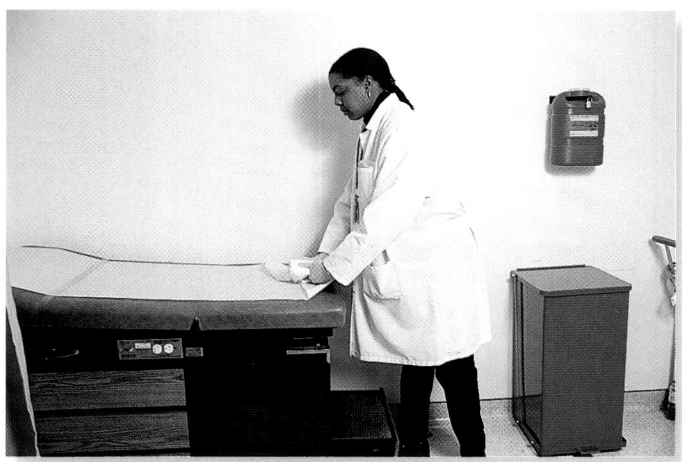

Figure 4-2. When you remove the cover from the examining table, roll it up tightly and quickly. Then carefully prepare it for disposal.

avoid contaminating your clean hands with microorganisms. (See Procedure 1-1 in Chapter 1 for the steps in performing aseptic hand washing.)

Examining Table. The disposable paper that covers the examining table provides a barrier to infection during an examination. Always change the covering after each use (Figure 4-2). Your office might use precut lengths, or you might need to tear off a piece from a roll of paper. Cover pillows with fresh paper. Also, provide paper towels for patients who need to wipe away excess lubricants after certain procedures.

When you remove the used covering from the examining table, roll it up quickly and carefully. You should have a small, tight bundle of paper when you finish. Crumpling the paper haphazardly or shaking it in the air stirs up dust and microorganisms and can spread infection.

Dispose of used paper coverings soiled by body fluids, especially blood, in a biohazardous waste container. (Refer to Chapter 1 for specific guidelines for disposing of hazardous items.) Used coverings with no visible fluids may be disposed of according to the procedures established by your office. Place soiled linen cloths and pillowcases in biohazard-labeled bags for sending to a laundry for cleaning.

Surfaces. You are responsible for disinfecting work surfaces in the examination room, including the examining table, sink, and countertop. As you learned in Chapter 2, disinfection involves exposing all parts of a surface to a disinfectant such as a 10% solution of household bleach in water or a product approved by the Environmental Protection Agency (EPA). Surfaces must be disinfected at the following times:

- After an examination or treatment during which surfaces have become visibly contaminated with tissue, blood, or other body fluids
- Immediately following accidental blood or body fluid spills or splatter
- At the end of your work shift

Clean and disinfect the toilet and sink in the patient lavatory, and inspect and disinfect reusable receptacles such as wastebaskets on a regular basis. In most offices these tasks are performed once a day. You must, however, follow the schedule established by your office. Procedure 4-1 describes how to disinfect work surfaces, floors, and equipment in the examination room. Replace protective coverings on equipment or surfaces that were exposed to blood, other body fluids, or tissue during the examination.

Storage. During the examination, you may need to collect biohazardous specimens, such as blood or urine, from the patient for testing. You are responsible for storing these specimens properly. See the Caution: Handle With Care section for guidelines to follow when storing biohazardous materials.

Storage of testing kits and specimens often involves refrigeration as a means of preservation. Adequate preservation requires maintaining careful control of the temperature in a refrigerator. Read the Caution: Handle With Care section for more information on preventing spoilage by controlling refrigerator temperature.

Putting the Room in Order

After ensuring that the examining table is clean, all surfaces are properly disinfected, and all necessary items are stored, take time to straighten the examination room and put things in order. A neatly arranged room boosts patient confidence and supports the impression of a well-run office. It also contributes to the physical safety of patients and staff. Tasks include the following:

- Putting the rolling stool in its place
- Pushing in the examining-table step
- Returning supplies to containers
- Putting away prescription pads and sample medications that may have been left out

Housekeeping

Medical offices usually contract with a janitorial service for after-hours cleaning. Janitorial services perform general cleaning tasks such as emptying wastebaskets, vacuuming carpets, scrubbing floors, dusting furniture, washing windows, and cleaning blinds. To be sure that the service cleans and sanitizes all areas adequately, you need to work with your employer to develop and implement a cleaning schedule. Take into account the types of surfaces to be cleaned, the type of contamination present, and the tasks or procedures to be performed.

You may be responsible for assigning housekeeping chores to janitorial workers. If so, you will need to monitor their work and let the service know if there are any lapses in cleanliness. You may also do some housekeeping chores yourself, such as damp dusting an open shelf. Because dust harbors bacteria and allergens, it is important to keep the examination rooms as dust-free as possible.

PROCEDURE 4.1

Guidelines for Disinfecting Examination Room Surfaces

Objective: To reduce the risk of exposure to potentially infectious microorganisms in the examination room

OSHA Guidelines

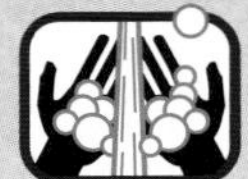
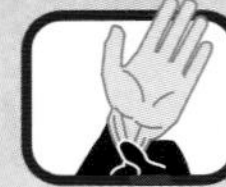
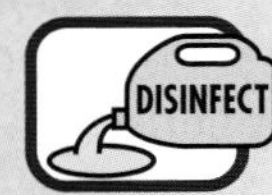

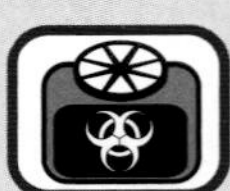

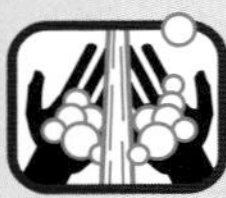

Materials: Utility gloves, disinfectant (10% bleach solution or EPA-approved disinfecting product), paper towels, dustpan and brush, tongs, forceps, clean sponge or heavy rag

Method

1. Wash your hands and put on utility gloves.
2. Remove any visible soil from examination room surfaces with disposable paper towels or a rag.
3. Thoroughly wipe all surfaces with the disinfectant.
4. In the event of an accident involving a broken glass container, use tongs, a dustpan and brush, or forceps to pick up shattered glass, which may be contaminated (Figure 4-3).
5. Remove and replace protective coverings, such as plastic wrap or aluminum foil, on equipment if the equipment or the coverings have become contaminated. After removing the coverings, disinfect the equipment and allow it to air-dry. (Follow office procedures for the routine changing of protective coverings.)
6. When you finish cleaning, dispose of the paper towels or rags in a biohazardous waste receptacle. (This step is especially important if you are cleaning surfaces contaminated with blood, body fluids, or tissue.)
7. Remove the gloves and wash your hands.
8. If you keep a container of 10% bleach solution on hand for disinfection purposes, replace the solution daily to ensure its disinfecting potency (Figure 4-4).

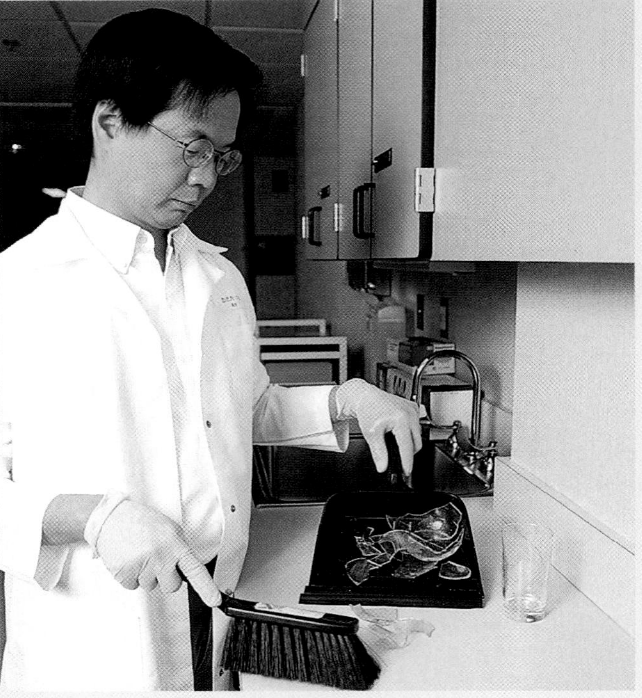

Figure 4-3. Because broken glass may be contaminated, never pick it up directly with your hands. Use a brush and dustpan, tongs, or forceps to clean it up.

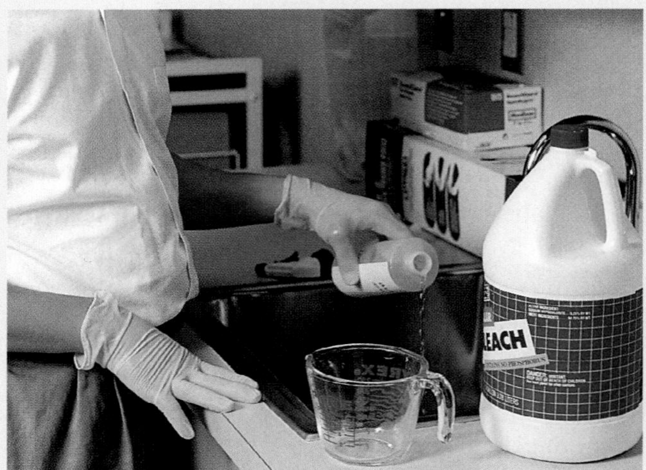

Figure 4-4. Replace the bleach solution each day to ensure its disinfecting potency.

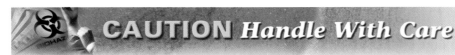

CAUTION *Handle With Care*

Storing Biohazardous Materials

During a general physical examination, the physician may ask you to collect various types of specimens from the patient for testing in the laboratory. These specimens must be handled and stored properly because they have the potential to be biohazards. Exposure that can spread disease may occur through the following routes:

- Inhalation (breathing)
- Ingestion (swallowing)
- **Transcutaneous absorption** (absorption through a cut or crack in the skin)

Occupational Safety and Health Administration (OSHA) regulations require storing biohazardous materials separately from food and beverages. You must not place food and beverages in refrigerators, freezers, or cabinets where blood or other potentially infectious materials are present or put specimens in a refrigerator that is otherwise used to store food and beverages.

There are several reasons why it is dangerous to put food or beverages in the laboratory refrigerator. If a biohazardous substance is not clearly labeled and you are in a hurry, you might accidentally ingest it. There is always the possibility that containers of biohazardous substances might leak or spill or that residue from the hazardous material might not have been thoroughly cleaned from the outside of containers. This residue could lead to contamination of food or beverages.

OSHA regulations require that a warning label containing the biohazard symbol be clearly and securely posted on the outside of refrigerators, freezers, and cabinets where biohazardous materials are stored. The government also recommends keeping the laboratory refrigerator and the refrigerator for the employees' personal use in separate rooms. These measures help prevent employees from accidentally putting food and beverages in the wrong place.

OSHA regulations also prohibit medical personnel from doing any of the following activities in a room where potentially infectious materials are present:

- Eating
- Drinking
- Smoking
- Chewing gum
- Applying cosmetics
- Handling contact lenses
- Chewing pencils or pens
- Rubbing eyes

These work practice controls, like all OSHA regulations, represent safeguards to protect workers against the health hazards of blood-borne pathogens.

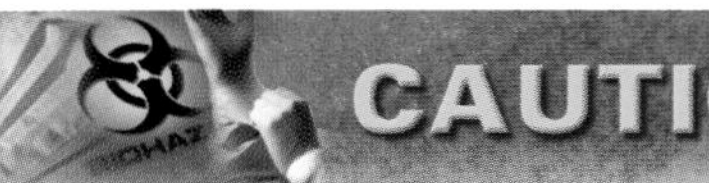

CAUTION *Handle With Care*

Refrigerator Temperature Control

Health inspectors visit medical facilities periodically to check that health and safety standards are being upheld. One of the first things they check is the temperature of refrigerators. To prevent spoilage or deterioration of testing kits, blood specimens, and other stored materials, the temperature of the laboratory refrigerator should be maintained between 36° and 46°F (2° and 8°C). Keep a thermometer in the laboratory refrigerator to monitor the temperature.

Similar guidelines apply to the refrigerator in the employee area. Food spoils quickly in a refrigerator if the temperature is not low enough. The temperature of the food refrigerator should be maintained between 32° and 40°F (0° and 4.4°C). In addition to monitoring the temperature, make sure that food is not stored in the refrigerator too long. All food containers—including brown bags containing lunches—should be dated and thrown out when their freshness has expired. You can prevent the growth of bacteria by wiping up food spills immediately and cleaning the interior and exterior of the refrigerator routinely.

Follow office procedures for the routine cleaning of both laboratory and food refrigerators and for the proper maintenance of the temperature of the refrigerators' contents while the refrigerators' interiors are cleaned. Specimens, for example, must be kept at a specific temperature at all times. For documentation purposes, keep a log of dates when the laboratory refrigerator is cleaned.

Room Temperature, Lighting, and Ventilation

No patient wants to sit in an examination room that looks unkempt. Nor do patients feel comfortable in a room that is cold, dimly lit, or stuffy. Adjusting the temperature, lighting, and ventilation is part of keeping the examination room in good order and fit for use.

Room Temperature

Because patients may be wearing only a thin paper gown or drape while in the examination room, you must be sure the examination room is warm enough. Set the thermostat to maintain the temperature at approximately 72°F, and make sure there are no drafts from windows or doors. Patients often feel anxious while waiting for the doctor, and a warm room can help them relax.

Lighting

Good lighting is required to make accurate diagnoses, to correctly carry out medical procedures, and to read orders and instructions. A well-lit room also helps prevent accidents.

Adjust room lights and blinds or drapes as necessary in preparation for an examination. If there is an examination lamp with a movable arm, be sure the arm is positioned appropriately. Replace all burned-out lightbulbs as soon as possible.

Ventilation

The air in the examination area should smell fresh and clean. From time to time, you may have to deal with offensive odors from urine, vomitus, body odors, or laboratory chemicals. First you must eliminate the source of the odor, especially if the source is potentially infectious or toxic. Then you can take steps to remove the odor.

Some examination rooms have a ventilation system with a filter that absorbs odors. If the rooms in your office do not, you may be able to turn on a high-speed blower to vent room air to the outside. In some cases an open window and a fan may be sufficient to freshen the air. Remember to check the room temperature after using fresh-air approaches to odor control.

If necessary, you can temporarily mask unpleasant odors with a room deodorizer or spray. Some sprays also help kill germs.

Medical Instruments and Supplies

Doctors require various instruments and supplies to perform an examination or procedure. Instruments are tools or implements doctors use for particular purposes. Disposable instruments are often referred to as supplies.

You must maintain all instruments and supplies needed in the examination room. This responsibility involves the following three tasks:

1. Ordering and stocking all supplies needed for examinations and treatment procedures
2. Keeping the instruments sanitized, disinfected, or sterilized (as appropriate) and in working order
3. Ensuring that all instruments and supplies are placed where the doctor can easily reach them

Instruments Used in a General Physical Examination

Many of the instruments physicians use are made of fine-grade stainless steel and are reusable. Some of these instruments may have disposable parts.

Physicians also use a number of disposable instruments, such as curettes and needles, because these instruments are both convenient and sanitary. As discussed in Chapter 1, you must discard used disposable instruments and supplies according to OSHA guidelines. Place any such items contaminated with blood or other body fluids in biohazardous waste containers.

Commonly used instruments are shown in Figure 4-5.

- An anoscope is used to open the anus for examination.
- An examination light provides an additional source of light during the examination. It is usually on a flexible arm to permit light to be directed to the area being examined.
- A laryngeal mirror reflects the inside of the mouth and throat for examination purposes.
- A nasal speculum is used to enlarge the opening of the nose to permit viewing. This type of speculum may consist of a reusable handle with a disposable speculum tip, or it may be a disposable one-piece unit.
- An ophthalmoscope is a lighted instrument that is used to examine the inner structures of the eye.
- An otoscope is used to examine the ear canal and the tympanic membrane. The otoscope consists of a light source, a magnifying lens, and an ear speculum. An otoscope may also be used to examine the nostrils and the anterior sinuses.
- A penlight is a small flashlight used when additional light is necessary in a small area. It may also be used to check pupil response in the eye.
- A reflex hammer has a hard-rubber triangular head. It is used to check a patient's reflexes.
- A sphygmomanometer is a piece of equipment used to measure blood pressure and is commonly referred to as a blood pressure cuff.
- A stethoscope is used to listen to body sounds. It is described in more detail in Chapter 19.
- A tape measure is a long, narrow strip of fabric, marked off in inches and sometimes in centimeters,

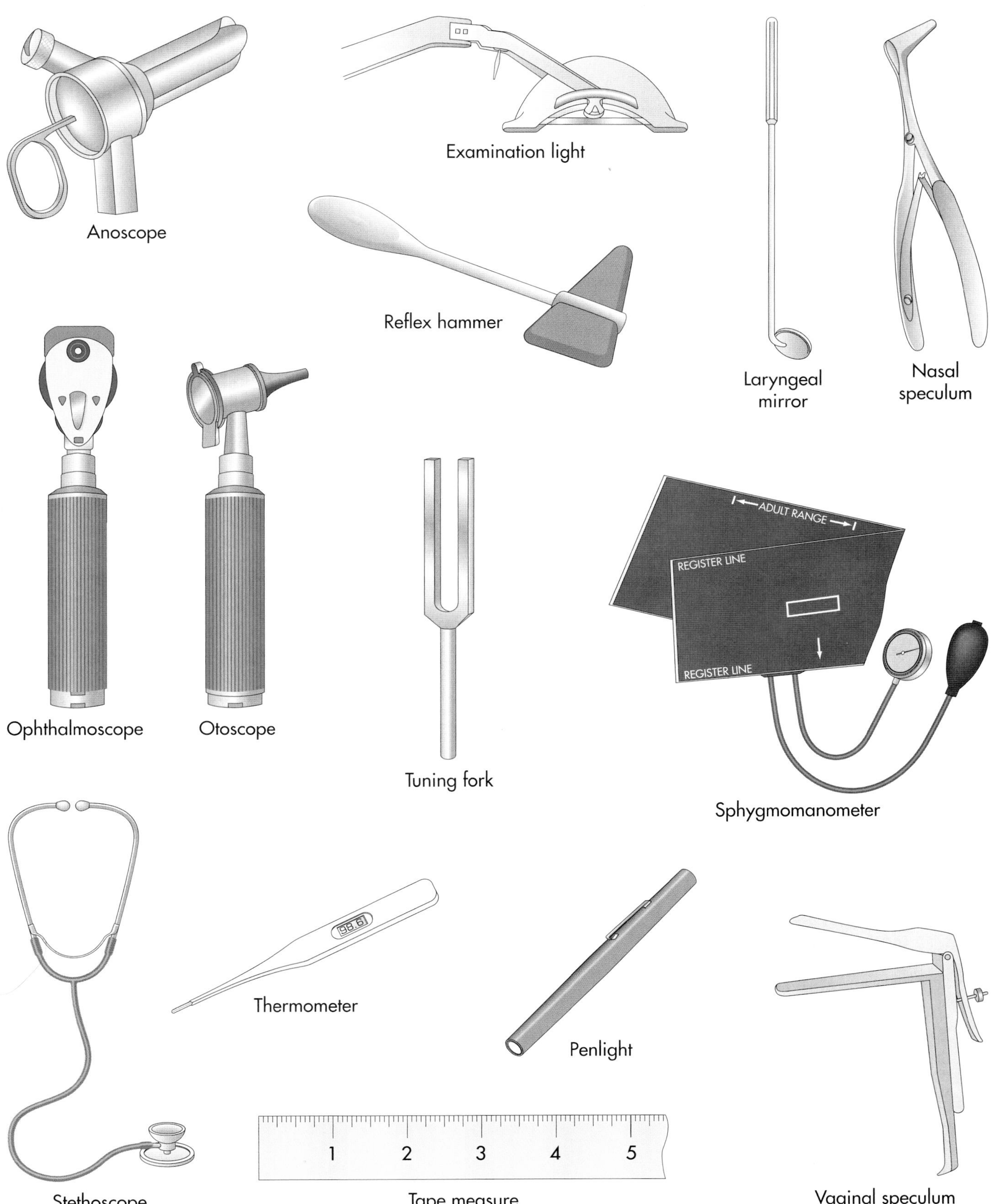

Figure 4-5. These instruments may be used in a general physical examination.

used to measure size or development of an area or part of the body.

- A thermometer is used to measure body temperature.
- A tuning fork tests patients' hearing.
- A vaginal speculum is used to enlarge the vagina to make the vagina and the cervix accessible for visual examination and specimen collection.

Inspecting and Maintaining Instruments. Prior to the examination, make sure that all instruments are sanitized, disinfected, or sterilized (as appropriate) and that they are in good working order. (See Chapter 2 for a description of the types of instruments requiring sanitization, disinfection, or sterilization and of the methods used for each.) For example, test the lights on the otoscope and ophthalmoscope to make sure that the lights work. Place all rechargeable batteries in a battery charger when the instruments are not in use.

Medical instruments are expensive and are designed to work in precise ways. Read the manufacturers' directions so that you are familiar with the care and maintenance of various instruments. Routinely check instruments for chipping and rusting, and report to the doctor any instruments that need repair or replacement.

Arranging Instruments. The doctor must be able to find and reach instruments easily during an examination. You can assist by placing instruments in the same place for every examination or by arranging them in the order the doctor will use them.

Doctors usually begin a general physical examination by examining the patient's head and face and working down the body. They may want instruments placed in that order. Other doctors may have individual preferences about how they want instruments arranged. In any case, make certain you know each doctor's preferences.

With the exception of the stethoscope, which most doctors carry with them, instruments are kept in one of three places during an examination:

1. Mounted on the wall (sphygmomanometer, some otoscopes and ophthalmoscopes)
2. Set out on the countertop (penlight, reflex hammer, tape measure, tuning fork, thermometer, some otoscopes and ophthalmoscopes)
3. Set on a clean (or sterile, if appropriate) towel or tray (anoscope, laryngeal mirror, nasal speculum, vaginal speculum)

Preparing Instruments. You must prepare some instruments before they can be used. For example, you may need to warm a vaginal speculum by holding it under warm water just prior to the examination. You might warm the mirrored end of the laryngeal mirror with water or over an alcohol lamp. You can also spray it with a special spray that prevents fogging. Any time you will be handling instruments, you must first wash your hands. If the instruments are sterile, you must also wear sterile gloves.

Cleaning Instruments. After the examination, put used instruments in a container, and take them to the cleaning area. Always handle instruments carefully, because mishandling can alter their precision. Dispose of supplies in the appropriate containers, and use approved procedures for sanitizing, disinfecting, and sterilizing reusable instruments and equipment. Refer to Table 4-1 for

TABLE 4-1 General Guidelines for Cleaning Instruments

Process	Guidelines*	Instruments
Sanitization	• Use detergent, or as indicated by the manufacturer • Applies to instruments that do not touch the patient or that touch only intact skin • Disinfect these instruments if contaminated with blood or body fluids	Ophthalmoscope Otoscope Penlight Reflex hammer Sphygmomanometer Stethoscope Tape measure Tuning fork
Disinfection	• Use an EPA-approved chemical or a 10% bleach solution to kill infectious agents outside the body • Applies to instruments that touch intact mucous membranes but do not penetrate the patient's body surfaces	Laryngeal mirror Nasal speculum
Sterilization	• Use an autoclave or other approved method to kill all microorganisms • Applies to instruments that penetrate the skin or contact normally sterile areas of the body	Anoscope Curette Needle Syringe Vaginal speculum

*Keep in mind that these guidelines are general. Each office may have its own methods and schedule for cleaning instruments, depending on the office's specialty.

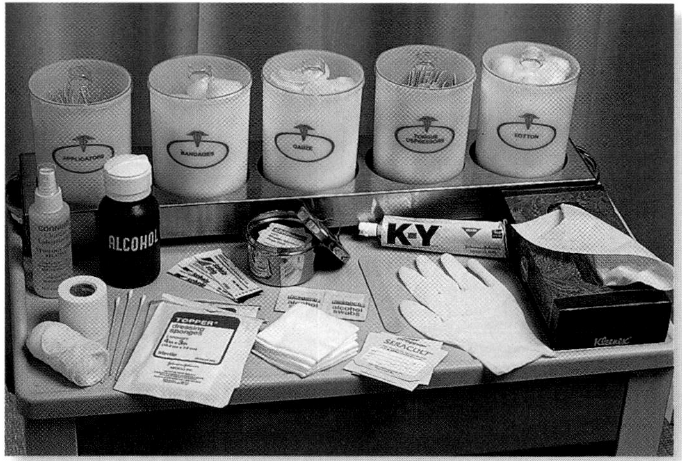

Figure 4-6. These supplies may be used in a general physical examination.

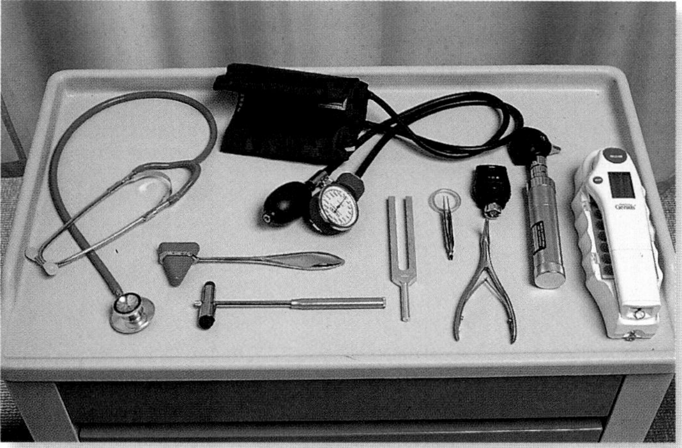

Figure 4-7. Arrange the instruments for a general physical examination so that they are convenient for the doctor.

general guidelines on cleaning instruments. (See Chapter 2 for detailed information on this topic.)

Supplies for a General Physical Examination

Supplies for a general physical examination may be either disposable or consumable. Figure 4-6 shows various types of supplies.

Disposable supplies are items that are used once and discarded. They include the following:

- Cervical scraper (a wooden scraper used to obtain samples of cervical secretions)
- Cotton balls
- Cotton-tipped applicators
- Curettes
- Disposable needles
- Disposable syringes
- Gauze, dressings, and bandages
- Glass slides
- Gloves, both sterile and examination (nonsterile) types
- Paper tissues
- Prepared paper slides used to test the stool for the presence of **occult blood** (blood not visible to the naked eye)
- Specimen containers
- Tongue depressors

Consumable supplies are items that can be emptied or used up in an examination. These items include the following:

- **Fixative** (a chemical spray used for preserving a specimen obtained from the body for pathologic examination)
- Isopropyl alcohol (for cleansing skin)
- Lubricant (a water-soluble gel used during examination of the rectum or vaginal cavity)

As they do with instruments, doctors may have a preferred arrangement of supplies for the general physical examination. Figure 4-7 shows a typical arrangement of instruments.

Keep supplies such as prescription blanks, drugs (especially narcotics), and needles in a locked cabinet away from the patient examination areas. Make sure that patients do not have access to these items.

Storing Supplies. You can use the cabinets and drawers in the examination room to store nonperishable supplies. You should store every item in its own place so that you can find it quickly. You might even color-code or label drawers so that you can easily locate items. You should store supplies that come in various sizes, such as bandages, according to size. You need to routinely straighten and clean the insides of all cabinets and drawers in the examination room.

Restocking Supplies. To be sure you have a sufficient quantity of items on hand, order new supplies well in advance of needing them. A good guideline to follow is to order a new supply when the first half of a box, tube, or bottle has been used up. A record-keeping system will help you determine which supplies you need to restock most frequently and how long it takes for new supplies to arrive. The information you should keep track of to develop such a system includes the following:

- The types of supplies your office uses
- The quantities of each type of supply you use in a given amount of time, such as a month
- The frequency with which you must reorder particular supplies
- The names of various suppliers, along with the amount of time it takes to receive your orders

Physical Safety in the Examination Room

Accidents can happen in the examination room. For example, patients and staff members can fall or cut themselves. You have an important responsibility to remove or correct hazards that might cause injury to patients, physicians, or staff members. This responsibility constitutes an integral part of a risk management plan.

Maintaining a Safe Environment

It is easier to maintain a safe environment if you pay special attention to the following areas in the examination room:

- Floor
- Cabinets and drawers
- Furniture
- Cords and cables

Floor. You can take several measures to prevent falls. Wipe or mop up spills immediately. Clear the floor of dropped objects. If the floor is carpeted, make sure there are no snags or tears that could cause someone to trip and fall. Spilled medications, chemicals, and other substances pose a threat to young children, who may ingest anything they find on the floor. Destroy and dispose of medications that are accidentally dropped on the floor.

Cabinets and Drawers. Close overhead cabinet doors promptly after removing supplies. Leaving cabinet doors open can result in injury. In addition, an open cabinet door leaves supplies exposed to patients. Make sure drawers are kept closed so that no one bumps into them.

Furniture. Routinely inspect the furniture in the examination room and reception area. Make sure there are no rough edges or sharp corners on the examining table, countertop, chairs, or other furniture. If you are not authorized to repair or replace unsafe pieces of furniture, bring them to the attention of your supervisor.

Cords and Cables. Electrical cords and medical and office equipment cables should run along the walls and should be taped or fastened down securely. Replace tape on cords and cables when it becomes worn.

Special Safety Precautions

Some patients, such as children and people with disabilities, may be particularly susceptible to accidents in your office. You need to take special precautions to ensure their safety.

Children. Keep sharp instruments out of the reach of children, and store toxic items in high cabinets. Also, keep all medications and objects out of the reach of young children, because children are likely to pick up items and put them in their mouths and could choke or be poisoned.

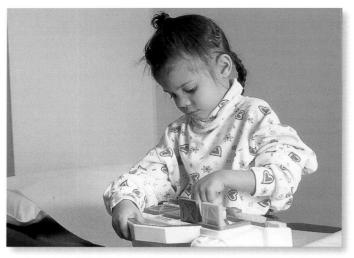

Figure 4-8. Toys provided must be safe for children of all ages.

If children's toys and books are kept in the reception area or examination room, make sure they are picked up when not in use and stored safely. Toys should be washable and made of safe materials. (Sanitize daily those toys that children put in their mouths; sanitize other toys weekly. If well children and sick children use the same reception area or examination room, sanitize and disinfect toys after sick children play with them.) Periodically check toys for sharp edges that might cause cuts. Make sure toys do not have small parts or pieces that could cause choking if swallowed. Figure 4-8 shows an appropriate toy for the medical office reception area or examination room.

Patients With Physical Disabilities. Patients with disabilities are more likely than other patients to fall. Some patients may use walkers or canes for support, whereas others may simply be unsteady on their feet. Patients with vision impairments may have difficulty seeing obstacles, stairs, and other potential hazards. Safe flooring and handrails in the reception area, bathroom, hallways, and examination room help ensure the safety of patients with impaired mobility or vision. Procedure 4-2 explains how to make the examination room safe for visually impaired patients.

Fire Safety

Fire is a safety hazard anywhere, but it is especially likely where there is sophisticated, high-voltage medical equipment—such as an x-ray machine. Any electrical instrument in the examination room, however, is a potential fire hazard. Other potentially hazardous items are gas tanks and flammable chemicals.

Fire Prevention. Be aware of anything that might cause a fire in the examination room. If you cannot correct the situation yourself, report the hazard to your supervisor.

Be alert to the following potential hazards:

- Frayed electrical wires, overloaded outlets, and improperly grounded plugs. These present a danger of

PROCEDURE 4.2

Making the Examination Room Safe for Patients With Visual Impairments

Objective: To ensure that patients with visual impairments are safe in the examination room

OSHA Guidelines: This procedure does not involve exposure to blood, body fluids, or tissue.

Materials: Reflective tape, if needed

Method

1. Make sure the hallway leading to the examination room is clear of obstacles.
2. Increase the amount of lighting in the room. Adjust the shades on windows in the room—if there are any windows—to allow for maximum natural light. Turn on all lights, especially those under cabinets, to dispel shadows.
3. Clear a path along which the patient can walk through the room. Make sure the chairs are out of the way. If there is a scale in the room, position it out of the path. If there is a step stool for the examining table, place it right up against the table.
4. Make sure the floor is not slippery.
5. Remove furniture that might be easily tipped over, such as a visitors' chair that is lightweight. If the physician will use an examination chair, push it out of the way.
6. Provide a sturdy chair with arms and a straight back to make it easier for the patient to sit down and stand up.
7. A wide strip of reflective tape will make the examining-table step visible for all patients. Apply it to the step's edge if tape is not there already. If your office uses a step stool instead of a step, make sure the tape on the stool is facing out.
8. Alert the patient to protruding equipment or furnishings.
9. Arrange the supplies for the patient, such as gowns or drapes, with the following guideline in mind: It is easier to see light objects against dark objects or dark objects against light objects than light objects against light objects or dark objects against dark objects. If, for example, there is a dressing cubicle, lay the light-colored gown or drape against a dark bench instead of hanging the gown or drape against a light wall.

electric shock and fire. Contact a licensed electrician to remedy these problems.

- Materials that are extremely flammable, including alcohol and some disinfectants. Supplies such as paper table coverings can also ignite and spread flames quickly in the event of a fire. Check to make sure that all such items are stored and disposed of properly to minimize the fire danger. Flammable liquids should never be kept near a heat source. If you are not sure whether a chemical is flammable, read the manufacturer's label or Material Safety Data Sheet. (Material Safety Data Sheets are discussed in Chapter 27.)
- Smoking. Smoking should not be permitted anywhere in a medical facility. In addition to causing health problems, smoking is a fire hazard. "No Smoking" signs should be posted prominently throughout the office.
- Inoperative smoke detectors. Make sure that smoke detectors throughout the office are working properly. Replace batteries promptly. If smoke detectors are wired into the building's electrical system, report any malfunction to the building manager.

In Case of Fire. Despite the precautions that you and your coworkers take, a fire may break out. Be prepared to use fire safety equipment and to evacuate the building safely.

Using Safety Equipment. The number of fire extinguishers in the office depends on the size and number of rooms in the office. Regardless of the total number of extinguishers, you should locate an all-purpose fire extinguisher in or close to each examination room. Figure 4-9 shows how to operate a typical fire extinguisher. Have the fire extinguisher professionally serviced once a year to ensure its effectiveness.

If there is a fire blanket in the examination room, be sure that you know how to use it and that it is stored so as to be easily accessible in an emergency. To use a fire blanket to smother burning clothing, wrap the victim in the blanket and roll him on the floor.

Planning an Evacuation Route. An evacuation route provides a safe way out of a building during an emergency. Learn the location of fire alarms, fire doors, and fire escapes in relation to the examination room. Use exit signs

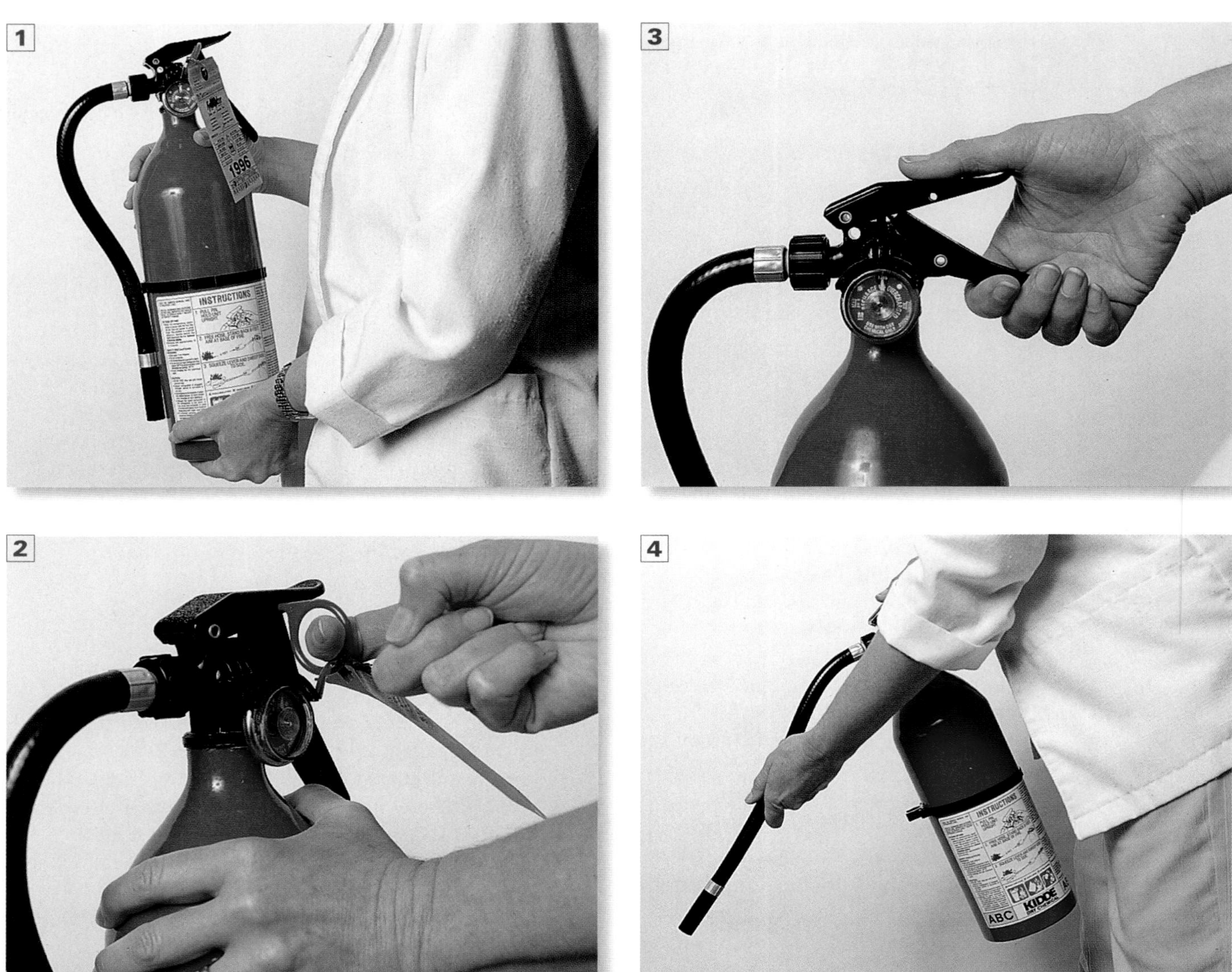

Figure 4-9. To use a fire extinguisher, (1) hold it upright, (2) remove the safety pin, (3) push the top handle down, and (4) direct the hose at the base of the fire.

as a guide in unfamiliar areas of the building. Stage fire drills with your coworkers so that you can evacuate the facility and lead patients to safety. Plan what you will do if your route becomes blocked.

Summary

Preparing the examination and treatment area for doctors and patients is part of your responsibility as a medical assistant. Room readiness involves making sure the room is clean, neat, and orderly and has adequate lighting, heat, and ventilation. You must select the instruments each doctor requires and make sure they are sanitized, disinfected, or sterilized (as appropriate) and ready for use. Room preparation also includes removing obstacles to physical safety, taking safety precautions, and following fire safety guidelines.

Your role in preparing the area is an important one for several reasons. First, you reduce the chance that infections will spread. Second, you help make the examination proceed efficiently. Third, you contribute to the comfort and safety of patients, doctors, and coworkers. Perform these tasks well, and you will inspire patients' confidence in the quality of the medical care provided at the facility.

REVIEW

CHAPTER 4

CASE STUDY QUESTIONS

Now that you have completed this chapter, review the case study at the beginning of the chapter and answer the following questions:

1. What are bilateral cataracts, and why would this condition be a consideration when you come in contact with this patient?
2. What instruments should be assembled for the physician to use during the examination?
3. What disposable and consumable supplies may reasonably be anticipated for use?
4. What measures can you take to ensure the patient's comfort and safety?

Discussion Questions

1. Inadequate hand washing has been identified as a primary cause for transmitting infections. List the circumstances in a medical office when you should wash your hands.
2. Identify instruments that are commonly used for patient examinations.
3. List four areas that require special attention in order to maintain a safe environment for patients and employees.

Critical Thinking Questions

1. The Americans With Disabilities Act of 1990 enacted a provision for "reasonable accommodations" for accessibility for the disabled. Identify the accessibility guidelines, and explain why each is important.
2. Risk management is essential in the medical office. What types of problems can occur in the examination room, and what can you do to help prevent them?
3. The Occupational Safety and Health Administration mandates that biohazardous materials must be stored in a separate refrigerator. What is the rationale for this requirement?

Application Activities

1. Make a checklist of steps for preparing the examination room. List tasks in the following categories: before/after an examination, daily, weekly, and monthly.
2. Working in small groups, prepare a tip sheet explaining how a patient could apply methods of infection control in the home. Have everyone in the group contribute at least one idea.
3. Go through the classroom, noting any safety hazards and listing solutions to the problems. Discuss hazards with classmates to make a master list of solutions.

SECTION 2

ANATOMY AND PHYSIOLOGY

CHAPTER 5

Organization of the Body

CHAPTER OUTLINE

- The Study of the Body
- Organization of the Body
- Body Organs and Systems
- Anatomical Terminology
- Body Cavities and Abdominal Regions
- Chemistry of Life
- Cell Characteristics
- Movement Through Cell Membranes
- Cell Division
- Genetic Techniques
- Heredity
- Major Tissue Types

OBJECTIVES

After completing Chapter 5, you will be able to:

5.1 Describe how the body is organized from simple to more complex levels.
5.2 List all body organ systems, their general functions, and the major organs contained in each.
5.3 Define the anatomical position and explain its importance.
5.4 Use anatomical terminology correctly.
5.5 Name the body cavities and the organs contained in each.
5.6 Explain the abdominal regions.
5.7 Explain why a basic understanding of chemistry is important in studying the body.
5.8 Describe important molecules and compounds of the human body.
5.9 Label the parts of a cell and list their functions.
5.10 List and describe the ways substances move across a cell membrane.
5.11 Describe the stages of cell division.
5.12 Describe the uses of the genetic techniques, DNA fingerprinting, and the polymerase chain reaction.
5.13 Explain how mutations occur and what effects they may produce.
5.14 Describe the different patterns of inheritance.
5.15 Describe the signs and symptoms of various genetic conditions.
5.16 Describe the locations and characteristics of the four main tissue types.

KEY TERMS

acids
active transport
allele
anatomical position
anatomy
anterior
atoms
autosome
bases
biochemistry
caudal
cell membrane
cells
chemistry
chromosome
complex inheritance
compound
connective tissue
cranial
cytokinesis
cytoplasm
deep
diaphragm
diffusion
distal
DNA
dorsal
electrolytes
endocrine gland
epithelial tissue
exocrine gland
femoral
filtration
frontal
gene

KEY TERMS *(Continued)*

homologous chromosome	metabolism	organelle	sagittal
inferior	midsagittal	organ	sex chromosome
inorganic	mitosis	organ systems	sex-linked trait
interphase	molecule	organic	superficial
ions	muscle tissue	organism	superior
lateral	mutation	osmosis	tissue
matrix	nervous tissue	physiology	transverse
matter	neuroglial cells	posterior	ventral
medial	neurons	proximal	
meiosis	nucleus	RNA	

Introduction

The human body is complex in its structure and function. This chapter provides an overview of the human body. It introduces you to the way the body is organized from the chemical level all the way up to the organ system level. You will also learn important terminology used in the clinical setting to describe body positions and parts. This chapter also focuses on how diseases develop at the genetic level.

CASE STUDY

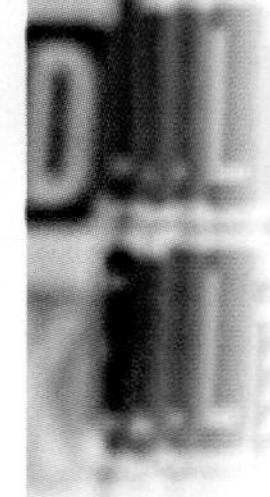

Last week a 12-year-old boy came to the doctor's office complaining of severe abdominal pains and nausea. He was diagnosed with appendicitis, requiring the removal of his appendix. The boy's medical chart indicates that he was diagnosed with *situs inversus,* a condition in which the organs of the thoracic and abdominal cavities are reversed from left to right. He has returned to the office for suture removal and bandage change.

As you read this chapter, consider the following questions:

1. On what side of the body is the appendix normally located?
2. If the medical assistant observes the boy's right lower abdominal quadrant for the bandage, is this correct? Why or why not?
3. Where should the bandage be found?
4. What precautions should this patient take given his diagnosis of *situs inversus?*

The Study of the Body

Anatomy is the scientific term for the study of body structure. For example, in discussing the structure or anatomy of the heart, it may be described as a hollow, cone-shaped organ with an average size of 14 centimeters in length and 9 centimeters in width. It is also very important to know the position of normal body structures and how to describe these positions precisely and correctly. **Physiology** is the term used for the study of function. For example, the physiology of the heart can be described by saying that the heart pumps blood into blood vessels for the transportation of nutrients throughout the body. Anatomy and physiology are commonly studied together because they are always related. For example, the anatomy of the heart (a hollow, muscular organ) allows it to do its function (pump blood into tubular blood vessels). If the heart was not hollow, it could not allow blood to flow into it. If the heart was not muscular, it not could pump blood.

Knowledge of anatomy and physiology will help you grasp the meaning of diagnostic and procedural codes and can help you understand the clinical procedures you will perform as a medical assistant. It will also make it easier to see how and why certain diseases develop. Disease states develop in the body when homeostasis is not maintained. **Homeostasis** is defined as the maintenance of stable internal conditions. Conditions in the body that must remain stable include body temperature, blood pressure, and the concentration of various chemicals within the blood. Individual cells must also maintain homeostasis. For example, if chemicals within a cell change the DNA or genetic makeup of the cell, that cell can become cancerous.

Organization of the Body

The structure of the body can be divided into different levels of organization. The chemical level is the simplest level and refers to the billions of atoms and molecules in the body. **Atoms** are the simplest units of all matter, and many are essential to life. **Matter** is anything that takes up space and has weight. The four most common atoms in the human body are carbon, hydrogen, oxygen, and nitrogen. **Molecules** are made up of atoms that bond together. For example, water is formed when two hydrogen atoms bond to an oxygen atom, which is an example of a small but very important molecule. Proteins and carbohydrates are examples of much larger molecules that consist of hundreds of atoms.

Molecules join together to form **organelles,** which can be thought of as cell parts. Organelles combine to form cells such as leukocytes (white blood cells), erythrocytes (red blood cells), neurons (nerve cells), and adipocytes (fat cells). **Cells** are considered the smallest living units of structure and function in the body. When cells of the same type organize together, they form **tissues.** The four major types of body tissue are epithelia, connective, nervous, and muscle. Two or more tissue types combine to form **organs,** and organs arrange to form **organ systems.** Finally, organ systems combine to form the **organism** called the human body (Figure 5-1).

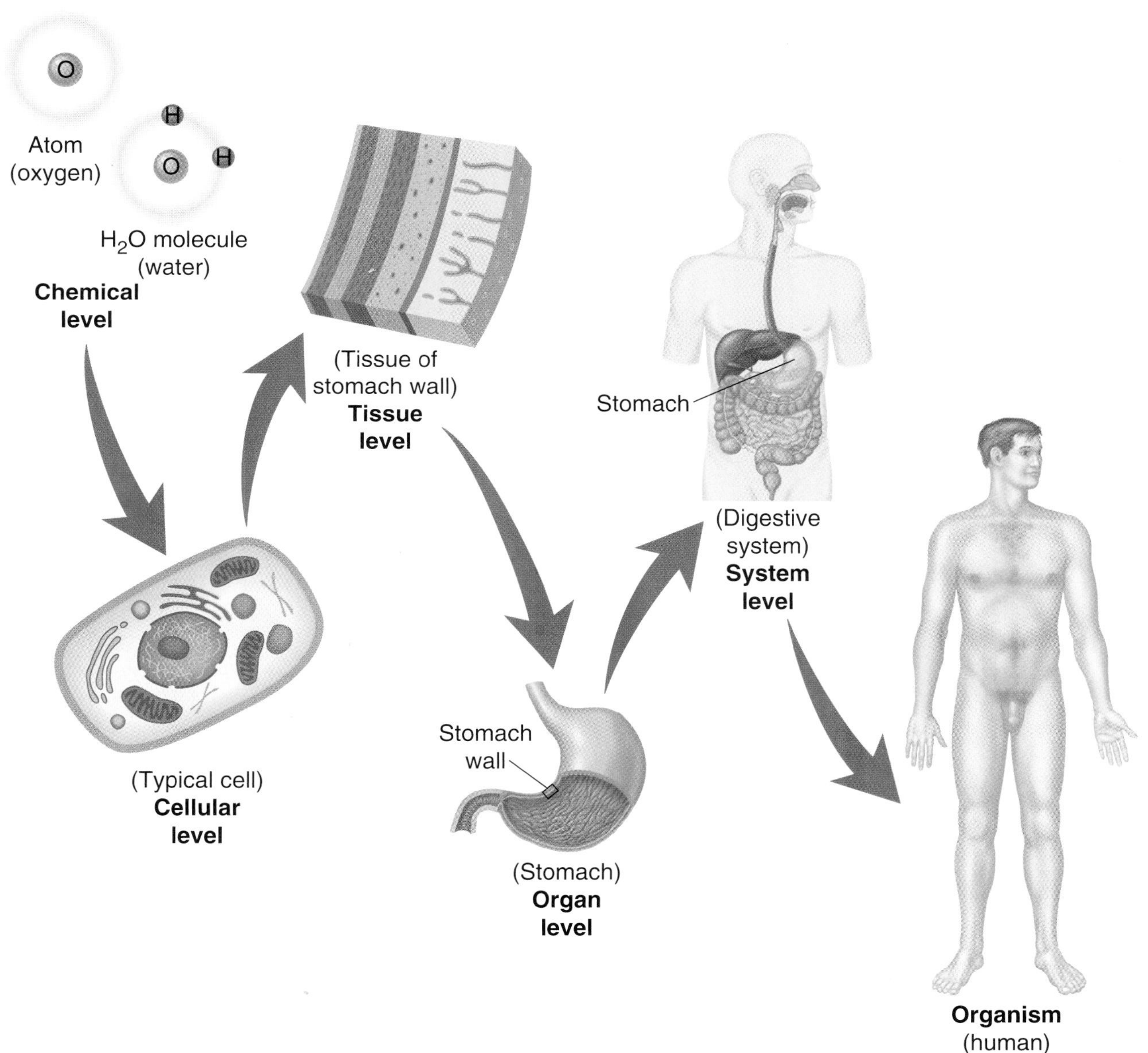

Figure 5-1. The human body is organized in levels, beginning with the chemical level and progressing to the cellular, tissue, organ, system, and organism (whole body) levels.

Body Organs and Systems

Organs can be defined as structures formed by the organization of two or more different tissue types that work together to carry out specific functions. For example, the heart is composed of a wall of cardiac muscle tissue and connective tissue and is lined with an epithelial tissue. These tissues work together to carry out the function of the heart, which is to effectively pump blood into blood vessels. Organ systems are formed when organs join together to carry out vital functions. For example, the heart and blood vessels unite to form the cardiovascular system. The organs of the cardiovascular system function to circulate blood throughout the body to ensure that all body cells receive an adequate supply of nutrients. See Figure 5-2 for a summary of the organ systems of the

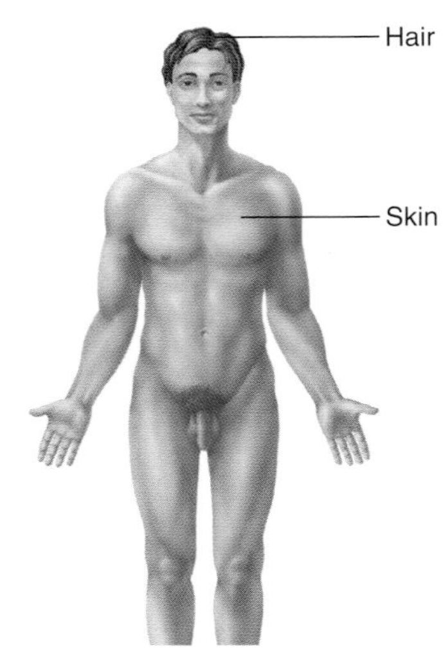

Integumentary System

Provides protection, regulates temperature, prevents water loss, and produces vitamin D precursors. Consists of skin, hair, nails, and sweat glands.

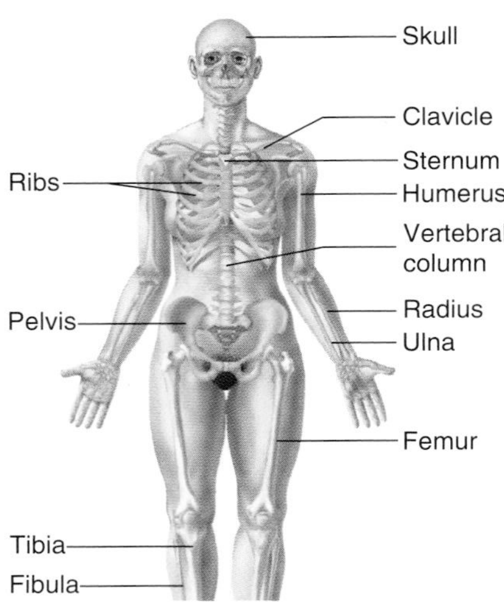

Skeletal System

Provides protection and support, allows body movements, produces blood cells, and stores minerals and fat. Consists of bones, associated cartilages, ligaments, and joints.

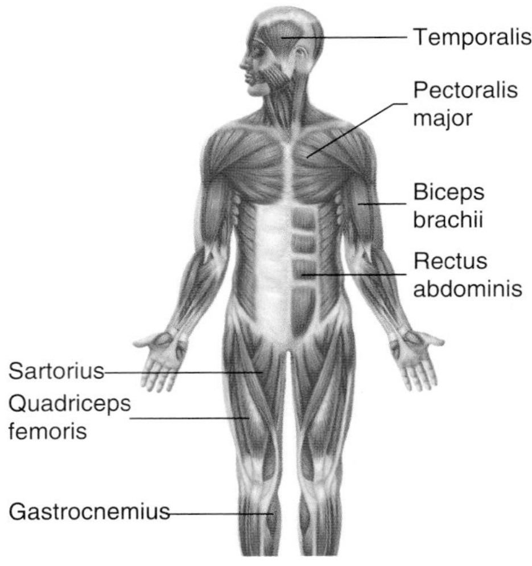

Muscular System

Produces body movements, maintains posture, and produces body heat. Consists of muscles attached to the skeleton by tendons.

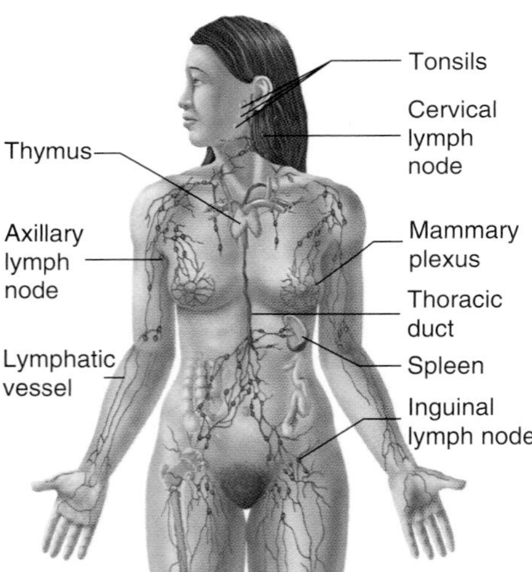

Lymphatic System

Removes foreign substances from the blood and lymph, combats disease, maintains tissue fluid balance, and absorbs fats from the digestive tract. Consists of the lymphatic vessels, lymph nodes, and other lymphatic organs.

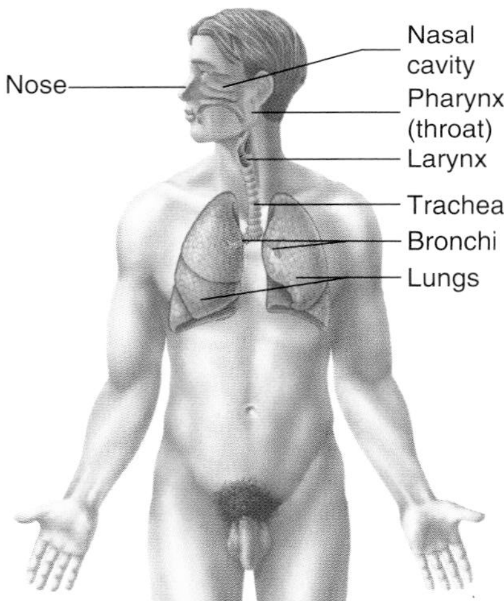

Respiratory System

Exchanges oxygen and carbon dioxide between the blood and air and regulates blood pH. Consists of the lungs and respiratory passages.

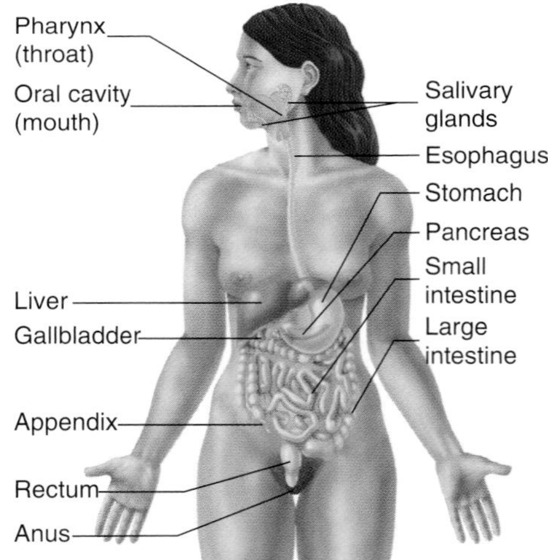

Digestive System

Performs the mechanical and chemical processes of digestion, absorption of nutrients, and elimination of wastes. Consists of the mouth, esophagus, stomach, intestines, and accessory organs.

Figure 5-2. Organ systems of the body.

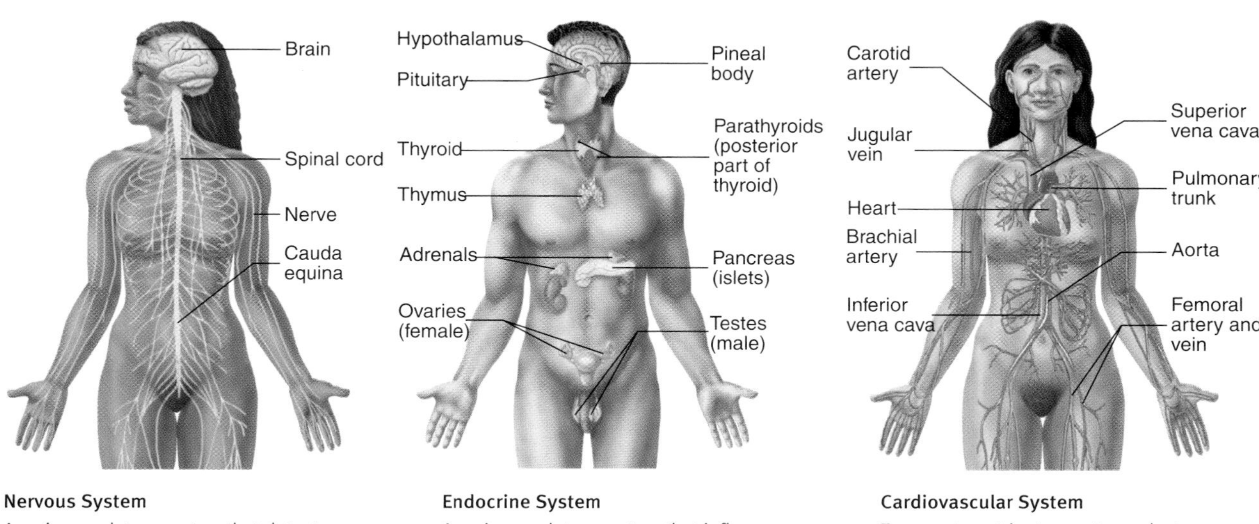

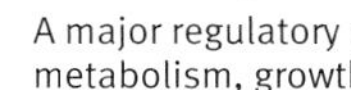

Nervous System

A major regulatory system that detects sensations and controls movements, physiologic processes, and intellectual functions. Consists of the brain, spinal cord, nerves, and sensory receptors.

Endocrine System

A major regulatory system that influences metabolism, growth, reproduction, and many other functions. Consists of glands, such as the pituitary, that secrete hormones.

Cardiovascular System

Transports nutrients, waste products, gases, and hormones throughout the body; plays a role in the immune response and the regulation of body temperature. Consists of the heart, blood vessels, and blood.

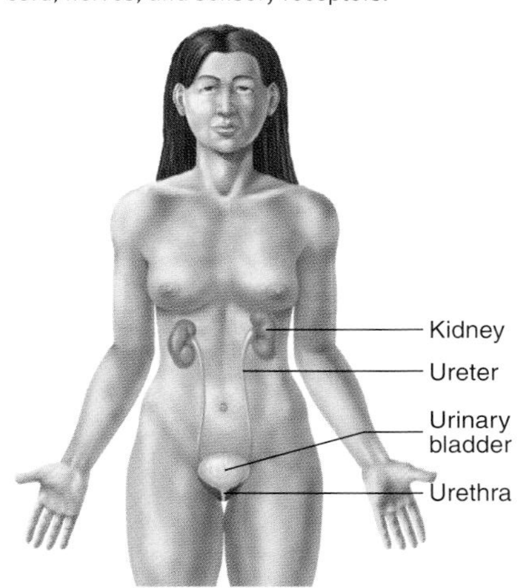

Urinary System

Removes waste products from the blood and regulates blood pH, ion balance, and water balance. Consists of the kidneys, urinary bladder, and ducts that carry urine.

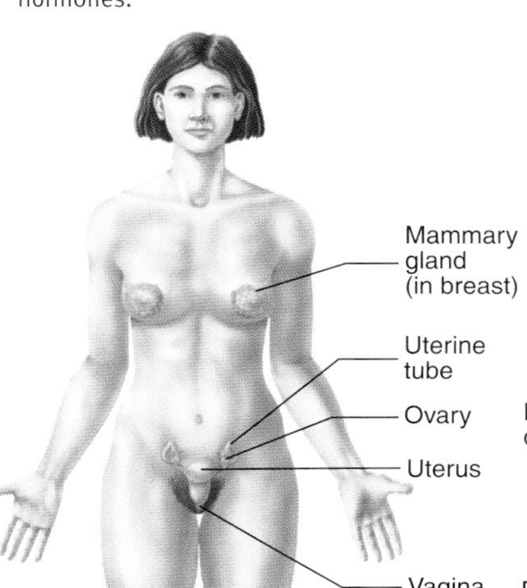

Female Reproductive System

Produces oocytes and is the site of fertilization and fetal development; produces milk for the newborn; produces hormones that influence sexual function and behaviors. Consists of the ovaries, vagina, uterus, mammary glands, and associated structures.

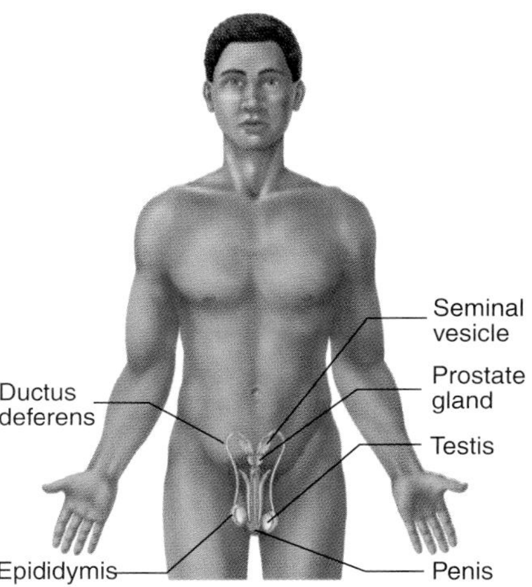

Male Reproductive System

Produces and transfers sperm cells to the female and produces hormones that influence sexual functions and behaviors. Consists of the testes, accessory structures, ducts, and penis.

Figure 5-2. (continued)

body, their general functions, and the organs contained in each.

Anatomical Terminology

Anatomical terms are a group of universal terms used to describe the location of body parts and various body regions. In order to correctly use these terms, it is assumed that the body is in the anatomical position. In the **anatomical position,** a body is standing upright and facing forward with the arms at the sides and the palms of the hands facing forward. Even if patients are lying down, for consistency and correct communication when you use anatomical terms, always refer to patients as if they are in the anatomical position.

Directional Anatomical Terms

The directional anatomical terms are **cranial, caudal, ventral, dorsal, medial, lateral, proximal, distal, superficial,** and **deep.** They are used to identify the position of body structures compared to other body structures. For example, the eyes are medial to the ears but lateral to the nose. See Table 5-1 and Figure 5-3 for an explanation and illustration of these important directional terms.

TABLE 5-1 Directional Anatomical Terms

Term	Definition	Example
Superior (cranial)	Above or close to the head	The thoracic cavity is superior to the abdominal cavity.
Inferior (caudal)	Below or close to the feet	The neck is inferior to the head.
Anterior (ventral)	Toward the front of the body	The nose is anterior to the ears.
Posterior (dorsal)	Toward the back of the body	The brain is posterior to the eyes.
Medial	Close to the midline of the body	The nose is medial to the ear.
Lateral	Farther away from the midline of the body	The ears are lateral to the nose.
Proximal	Close to a point of attachment or to the trunk of the body	The knee is proximal to the toes.
Distal	Farther away from a point of attachment or from the trunk of the body	The fingers are distal to the elbow.
Superficial	Close to the surface of the body	Skin is superficial to muscles.
Deep	More internal	Bones are deep to skin.

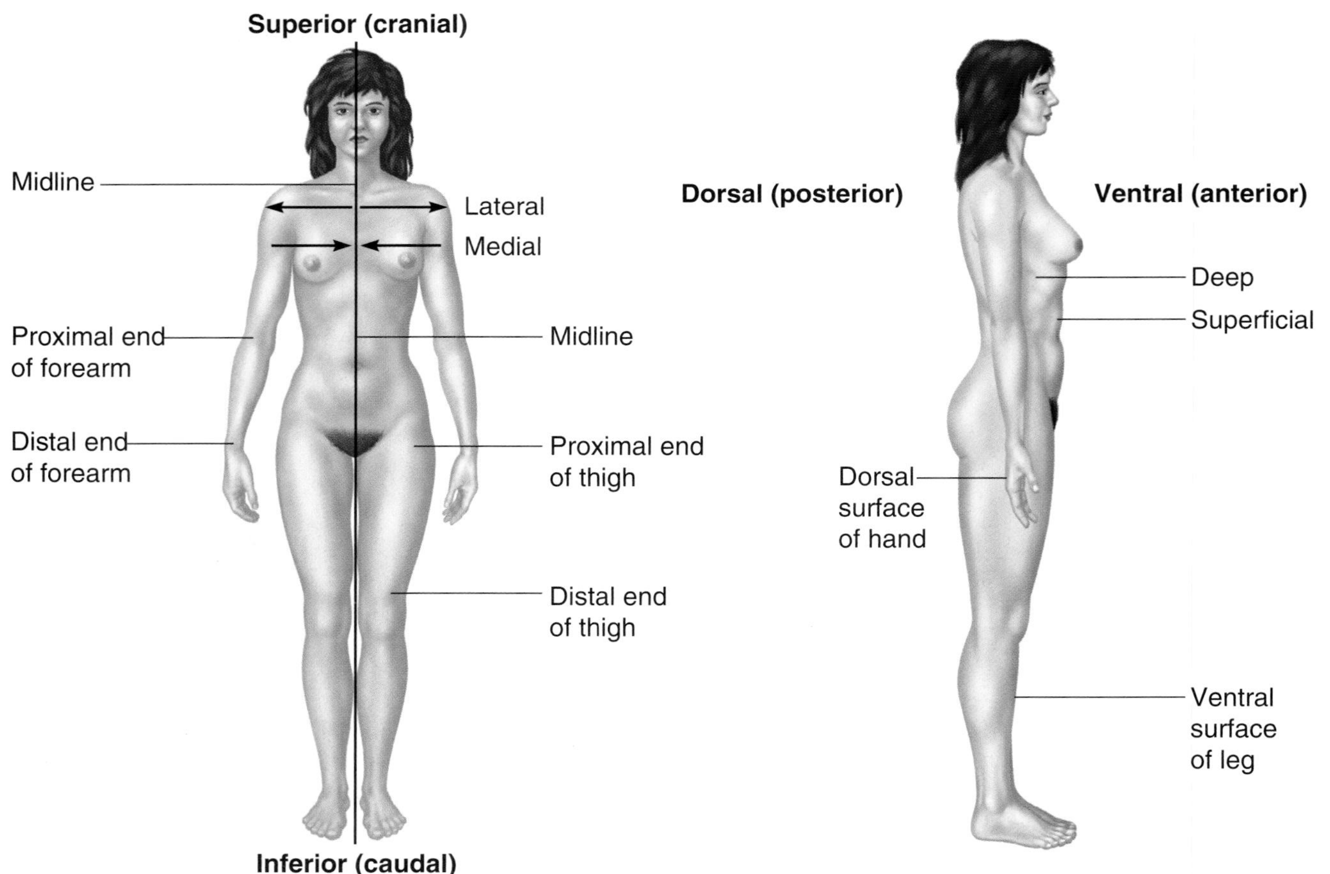

Figure 5-3. Directional terms provide mapping instructions for locating organs and body parts.

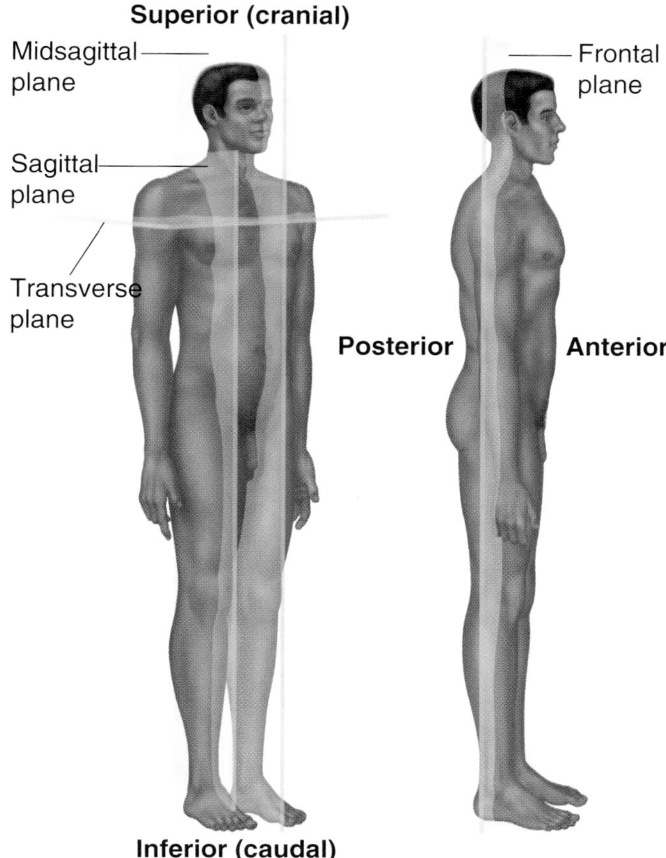

Figure 5-4. Spatial terms are based on imaginary cuts or planes through the body.

Anatomical Terms Used to Describe Body Sections

Sometimes in order to study internal body parts, the body has to be imagined as being divided into sections. It is useful to use the following terms to describe how the body is divided into sections: sagittal, transverse, and frontal (coronal).

A **sagittal** plane divides the body into left and right portions. A **midsagittal** plane runs lengthwise down the midline of the body and divides it into equal left and right halves. A **transverse** plane divides the body into **superior** (upper) and **inferior** (lower) portions. A **frontal,** or coronal, plane divides the body into **anterior** (frontal) and **posterior** (rear) portions. Figure 5-4 illustrates these planes.

Anatomical Terms Used to Describe Body Parts

Many other anatomical terms are used to describe different regions or parts of the body. For example, the term *brachium* refers to the arm and the term **femoral** refers to the thigh. Figure 5-5 illustrates many of the common anatomical terms used to describe body parts.

Body Cavities and Abdominal Regions

The largest body cavities are the dorsal cavity and the ventral cavity. The dorsal cavity is divided into the cranial cavity and the spinal cavity. The cranial cavity houses the brain, and the spinal cavity contains the spinal cord. The ventral cavity is divided into the thoracic cavity and the abdominopelvic cavity. The muscle called the **diaphragm** separates the thoracic and abdominopelvic cavities from each other. The lungs, heart, esophagus, and trachea are contained in the thoracic cavity. The abdominopelvic cavity is divided into a superior abdominal cavity and an inferior pelvic cavity. Most of the organs of digestion are found in the abdominal cavity, and the bladder and internal reproductive organs are located in the pelvic cavity. Figure 5-6 depicts these cavities. The abdominal area is further divided into nine regions or four quadrants, which are illustrated in Figure 5-7.

Chemistry of Life

The lowest level of organization is the chemical level, which includes all the chemical elements that make up matter. Liquids, solids, and gases are all matter. **Chemistry** is the study of what matter is composed of and how matter changes. It is important to have a basic understanding of chemistry when studying anatomy and physiology because body structures and functions result from chemical changes that occur within body cells or fluids.

When two or more atoms are chemically combined, a molecule is formed. Molecules are the basic units of compounds. A **compound** is formed when two or more atoms of more than one element are combined. An example of a molecule is water, which is composed of two hydrogen atoms and one oxygen atom. Water is also an example of a compound because its molecules are made up of atoms of two different elements—hydrogen and oxygen. Water is critical to both chemical and physical processes in human physiology, and it accounts for approximately two-thirds of a person's body weight.

Metabolism is the overall chemical functioning of the body. Metabolism includes all the processes that build small molecules into large ones (anabolism) and break down large molecules into small ones (catabolism).

Electrolytes

When put into water, some substances release **ions,** which are either positively or negatively charged particles; these substances are called **electrolytes.** For example, NaCl (sodium chloride) is an electrolyte. When you put NaCl in water, it releases the sodium ion (Na^+) and the chloride ion (Cl^-). Electrolytes are critical because the movements of ions into and out of body structures regulate or trigger many physiologic states and activities in the body. For

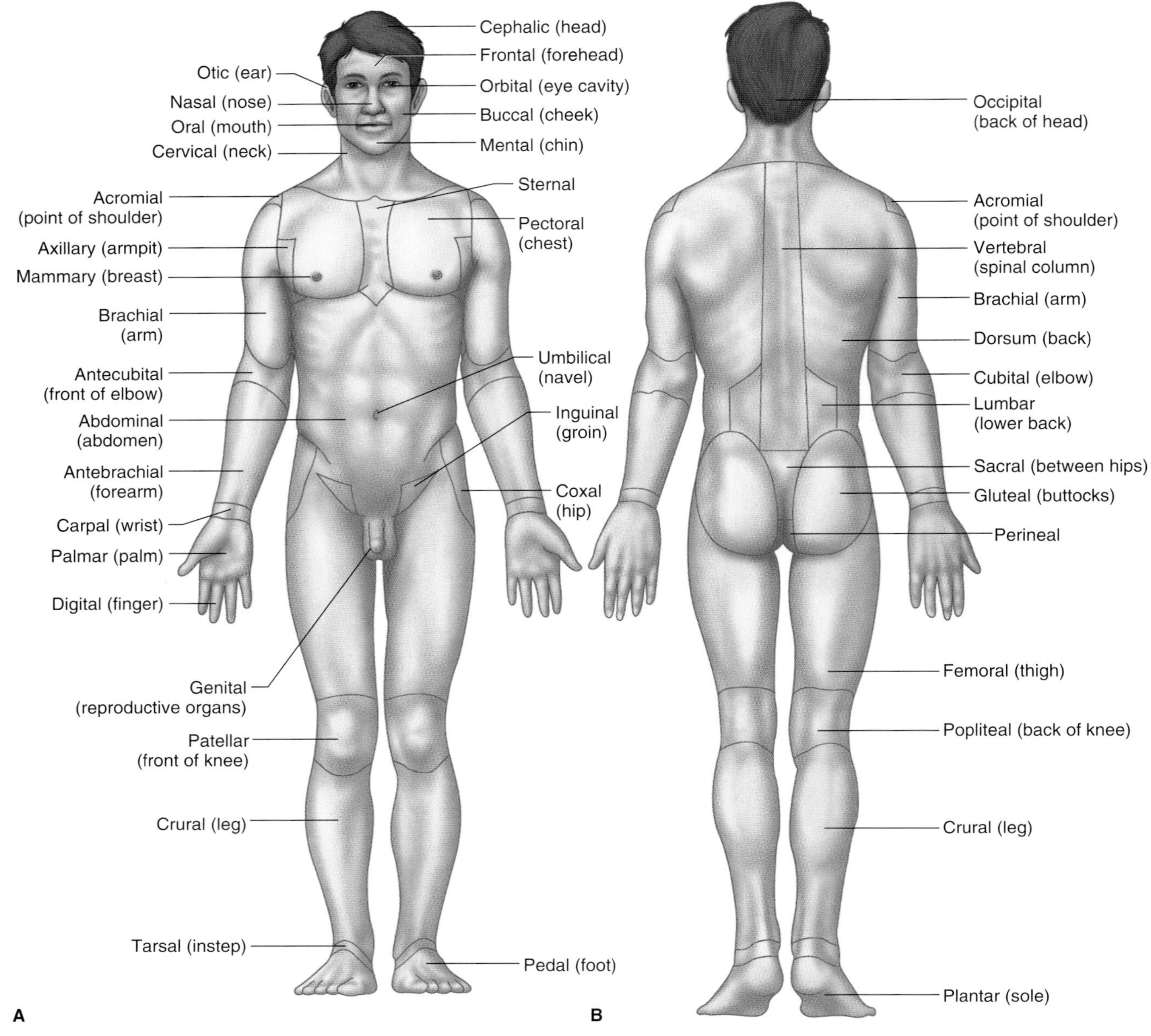

Figure 5-5. Numerous anatomical terms are used to describe regions of the body: (a) anterior view and (b) posterior view.

example, electrolytes are essential to fluid balance, muscle contraction, and nerve impulse conduction.

Acids. **Acids** are a type of electrolytes. They are defined as electrolytes that release hydrogen ions (H^+) in water. For example, hydrochloric acid (HCl) will release hydrogen ions when you put it in water. Therefore, it is acidic. It is also an electrolyte because it releases ions. Many acids, such as lemon juice and vinegar, have a sour taste.

Bases. **Bases** are also a type of electrolytes. They release hydroxyl ions (OH^-) in water. Sodium hydroxide (NaOH) is an example of a base because in water, it releases hydroxyl ions. A basic substance may also be referred to as an alkali. Many basic substances are slippery and bitter to the taste. Detergents are examples of basic substances.

Testing Acids and Bases. In the clinical setting, litmus paper or a pH meter is often used to determine if a substance is acidic or basic. An acidic substance will turn blue litmus paper red, and a basic substance will turn red litmus paper blue. The pH scale runs from 0 to 14. If a solution has a pH of 7, the solution is neutral, which means that it is neither acidic nor basic. If a solution has a pH less than 7, the solution is acidic. If a solution has a pH greater than 7, it is basic, or alkaline. The more acidic a solution is, the higher the concentration of hydrogen ions it contains. The pH values of some common substances are shown in Figure 5-8.

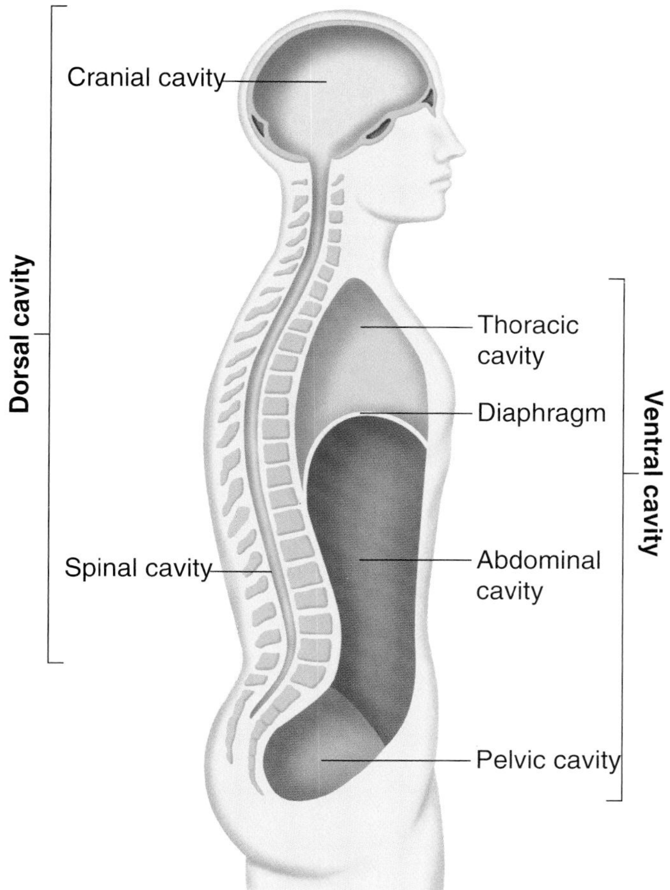

Figure 5-6. The two main body cavities are dorsal and ventral.

Biochemistry

The study of matter and chemical reactions in the body is called **biochemistry.** Matter can be divided into two large categories—organic and inorganic matter. **Organic** matter contains carbon and hydrogen. **Inorganic** matter generally does not contain carbon and hydrogen. Organic molecules tend to be large, whereas inorganic molecules tend to be small. Examples of inorganic substances are water, oxygen, carbon dioxide, and salts such as sodium chloride. Water is the most abundant inorganic compound in the body. The four major classes of organic matter in the body are carbohydrates, lipids, proteins, and nucleic acids.

Carbohydrates. Body cells depend on carbohydrate molecules primarily to make energy. The most common carbohydrate used by body cells is glucose. Glucose can also be stored in the body as a more complex carbohydrate called glycogen. Starches are a type of carbohydrate commonly found in potatoes, pastas, and breads.

Lipids. Three types of lipids found in the body are triglycerides, phospholipids, and steroids. Triglycerides are used to store energy for cells, and phospholipids are primarily used to make cell membranes. Butter and oils are composed of triglycerides, and the body stores these molecules in adipose tissue (fat). Steroids are very large lipid molecules used to make cell membranes and some hormones. Cholesterol is an example of an essential steroid for body cells.

Proteins. Proteins have many functions in the body. Many proteins act as structural materials for the building

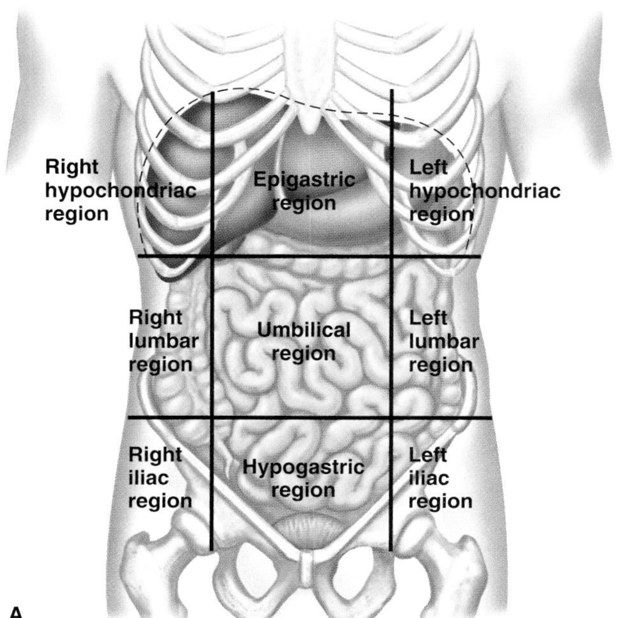

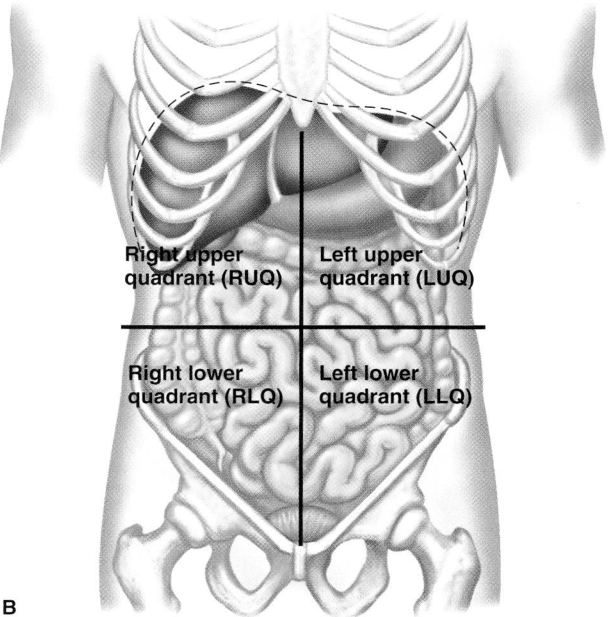

Figure 5-7. (a) The abdominal area divided into nine regions and (b) the abdominal area divided into four quadrants.

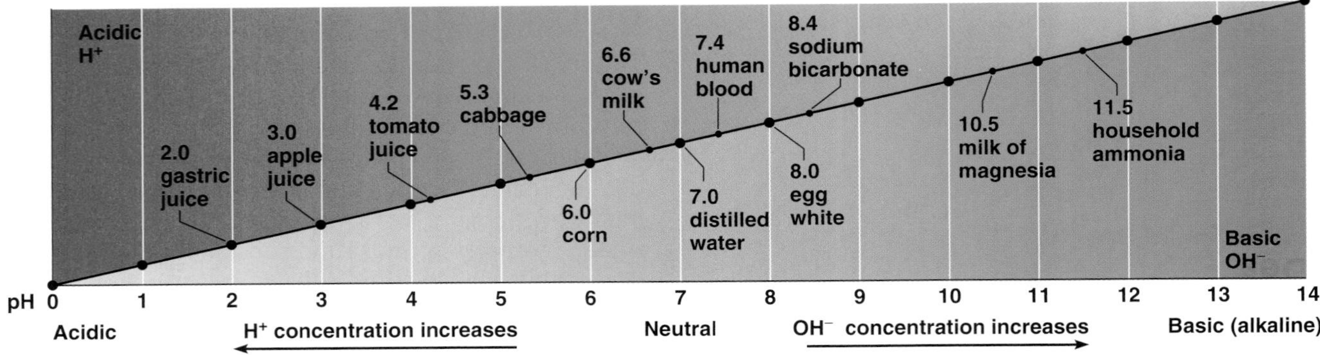

Figure 5-8. pH scale. As the concentration of hydrogen ions (H^+) increases, a solution becomes more acidic and the pH decreases. As the concentration of hydroxyl ions (OH^-) increases, a solution becomes more basic and the pH increases.

of solid body parts. Other proteins act as hormones, enzymes, receptors, and antibodies.

Nucleic Acids. **DNA** (deoxyribonucleic acid) and **RNA** (ribonucleic acid) are two examples of nucleic acids. DNA contains the genetic information of cells, and RNA is used to make proteins.

Cell Characteristics

Chemicals react to form the complex substances that make up cells, the basic unit of life. The human body is composed of millions of cells. There are many kinds of cells, and each type has a specific function. Most cells have three main parts: cell membrane, cytoplasm, and nucleus. Figure 5-9 shows the structure of a composite cell.

Cell Membrane

The **cell membrane** is the outer limit of a cell. It is very thin and is described as being selectively permeable, which means that it allows some substances to pass through it while preventing other substances from passing through. The cell membrane is composed of two layers of phospholipids, different types of proteins, cholesterol, and a few carbohydrates.

Cytoplasm

The **cytoplasm** of a cell can be imagined as the "inside" of the cell. It is mostly made up of water, proteins, ions, and nutrients.

Nucleus

The **nucleus** of a cell is typically round in structure and is placed near the center of a cell. It is enclosed by a nuclear membrane that contains nuclear pores so that larger substances can move into and out of the nucleus. It contains **chromosomes,** which are threadlike structures made up of DNA.

Movement Through Cell Membranes

The cell membrane controls what moves into and out of cells. Some substances move across the cell membrane without the use of energy. These movements are called passive mechanisms. Sometimes the cell has to use energy to move a substance across its membrane. In this case, the substances move through active mechanisms.

Diffusion

Diffusion is the movement of a substance from an area of high concentration to an area of low concentration—it can be described as the spreading out of a substance. Substances that easily diffuse across the cell membrane include gases such as oxygen and carbon dioxide.

Osmosis

Osmosis refers to the diffusion or movement of water across a semipermeable membrane, such as a cell membrane. You should remember that water will always try to diffuse or move toward the higher concentration of solutes (solids in solution).

Filtration

In **filtration,** some type of pressure, such as gravity or blood pressure, forces substances across a membrane that acts like a filter. Filtration separates substances in solutions. For example, you could separate sand from water by pouring the sand/water mixture through a filter. In the body, capillaries in the kidneys act as filters to separate components in blood.

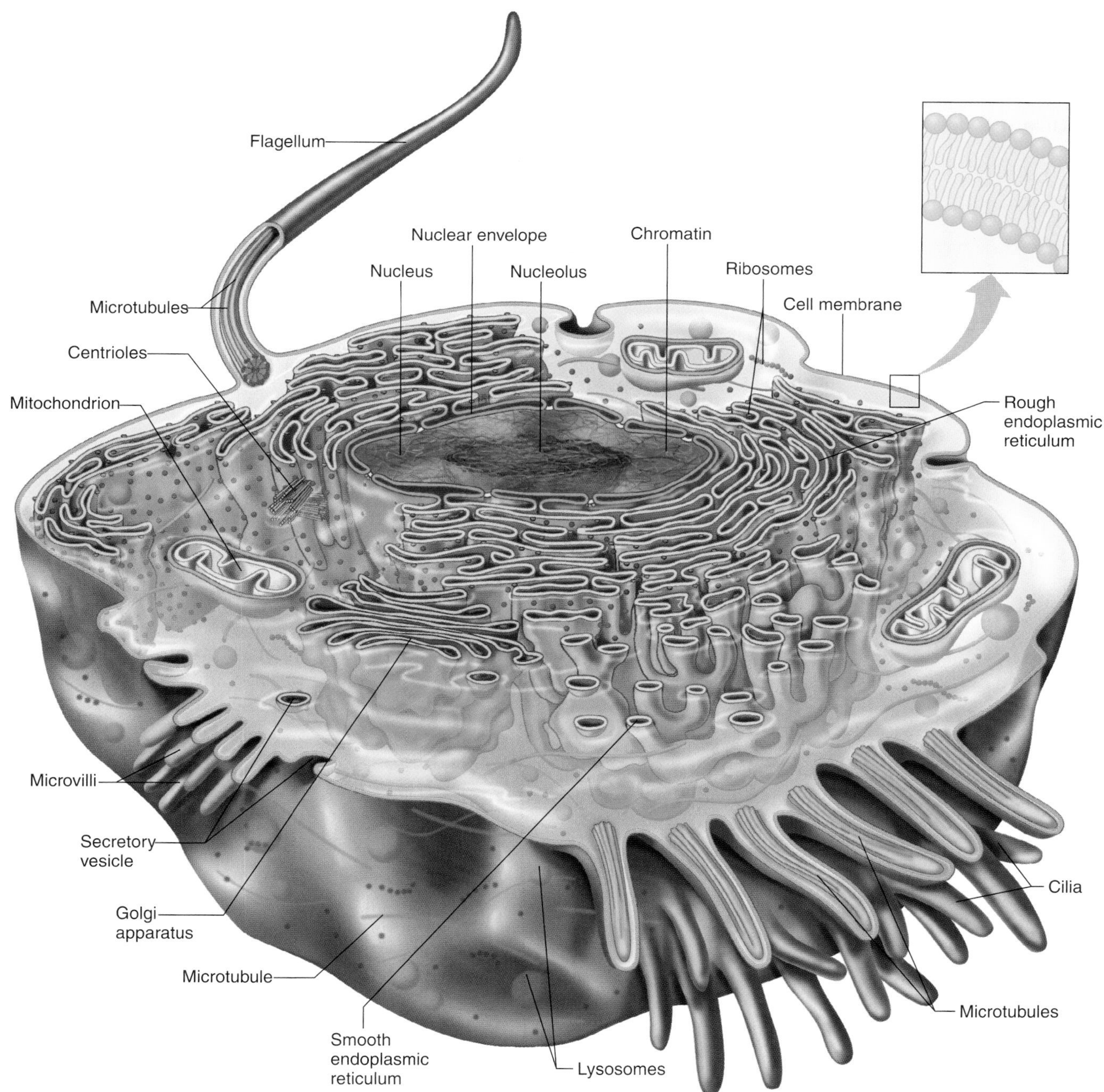

Figure 5-9. Composite cell.

Active Transport

In **active transport,** substances move across the cell membrane with the help of carrier molecules from an area of low concentration to an area of high concentration. In other words, substances are gathered together, which is the opposite of diffusion. Some substances that are moved across the cell membrane through active transport include sugars, amino acids, potassium, calcium, and hydrogen ions.

Cell Division

Cells can become damaged, diseased, or worn out, and replacements must be made. Also, new cells are needed for normal growth. Cells reproduce by cell division, a process that involves splitting the nucleus, through **mitosis** or **meiosis,** and splitting the cytoplasm, called **cytokinesis.**

A cell that carries out its normal daily functions and is not dividing is said to be in **interphase.** For example, if a liver cell is in interphase, it is making liver enzymes, detoxifying blood, and processing nutrients. During interphase, a cell prepares for cell division by duplicating its DNA and cytoplasmic organelles. For most body cells, each daughter cell will have the exact same copy of DNA and organelles as the original mother cell. Sometimes when the DNA is duplicated, errors called **mutations** occur. These mutations will be passed on to the descendants (daughter cells) of that cell and may or may not affect the cells in harmful ways.

Mitosis

Following interphase, a cell may enter mitosis, a part of cell division in which the nucleus divides. When mitosis is almost complete, cytoplasmic division (cytokinesis) occurs. During this process, the cell membrane constricts to divide the cytoplasm of the cell. The result is that the organelles of the original cell get distributed almost evenly into the two new cells.

During mitosis, the nucleus makes a complete copy of all 23 of its chromosome pairs (46 chromosomes altogether). As the cell divides, each new cell receives a complete set of chromosome pairs. The resulting cells are identical to each other.

Meiosis

Reproductive cell division, or meiosis, takes place only in the reproductive organs when the male and female sex cells are formed. During meiosis, the nucleus copies all 23 chromosome pairs, but two divisions take place. The four cells that are formed each contain only one of each chromosome pair, for a total of 23 chromosomes. This type of cell division must occur so that when the sex cells combine during fertilization, the resulting cell contains the usual number of chromosomes (46).

Genetic Techniques

DNA is the primary component of genes and is found in the nucleus of most cells within the body. A segment of DNA that determines a body trait is called a **gene.** Genetic techniques involve using or manipulating genes.

DNA molecules are made up of a linear sequence of compounds called nucleotides, and each nucleotide contains one of four different nitrogen bases. The chemical structure of every person's DNA is the same. The only difference among people is the order of the nitrogen bases. The unique sequence of the nucleotides determines the characteristics of an individual. One DNA molecule will contain hundreds or thousands of genes. Each gene occupies a particular location on the DNA molecule, making it possible to compare the same gene in a number of different samples. Two widely used genetic techniques in the clinical setting are the polymerase chain reaction and DNA fingerprinting.

Polymerase Chain Reaction

The polymerase chain reaction, PCR, is a quick, easy method for making millions of copies of any fragment of DNA. This technique has been revolutionary in the study of genetics and has very quickly become a necessary tool for improving human health.

Because PCR can produce millions of gene copies from tiny amounts of DNA, even from just one cell, the method is especially useful for detecting disease-causing organisms that are impossible to culture, such as many kinds of bacteria, fungi, and viruses. It can, for example, detect the AIDS virus sooner—during the first few weeks after infection—than other tests. PCR is also more accurate than standard tests. The technique can detect bacterial DNA in children's middle ear fluid, which indicates an infection, even when culture methods fail to detect bacteria. Other diseases diagnosed through PCR include Lyme disease, stomach ulcers, viral meningitis, hepatitis, tuberculosis, and many sexually transmitted diseases, including herpes and chlamydia.

PCR is also leading to new kinds of genetic testing because it can easily distinguish among the tiny variations in DNA that all people possess. This testing can diagnose people who have inherited disorders or who carry mutations that could be passed to their children. PCR is also used in tests that determine who may develop common disorders such as heart disease and various types of cancer. This knowledge helps individuals take steps to prevent those diseases.

DNA Fingerprinting

A DNA "fingerprint" refers to the unique sequences of nucleotides in a person's DNA and is the same for every cell, tissue, and organ of that person. It cannot be altered by any known method. Consequently, DNA fingerprinting is a reliable method for identifying and distinguishing among human beings, such as in a criminal case.

DNA fingerprinting is also used to diagnosis genetic disorders; it can be used to detect inherited disorders in unborn babies. These disorders include cystic fibrosis, hemophilia, Huntington's disease, familial Alzheimer's, sickle cell anemia, thalassemia, and many others. Detecting genetic diseases early allows patients and medical staff to prepare for proper treatment. Also, studying the DNA fingerprints of groups of individuals with the same disease allow researchers to identify DNA patterns associated with genetic diseases.

Another important use of DNA fingerprints is to establish paternity for custody and child support issues. The biological father has a DNA fingerprint that is very similar to the DNA fingerprint of his child. If the DNA fingerprints are not similar, the paternity test is negative.

Heredity

Heredity is the transfer of genetic traits from parent to child. When a sperm cell and an egg unite, a cell called a zygote forms. The zygote has 46 chromosomes, or 23 chromosomal pairs. One half of each pair came from the sperm, and the other half from the egg. Two chromosomes in each pair are called **homologous chromosomes.** The chromosomes of the first 22 pairs are called **autosomes,** and those of the 23rd pair are called **sex chromosomes.** If the sex chromosomes are an X chromosome and a Y chromosome, the child is a male. If the sex chromosomes are both X chromosomes, the child is a female. Although the sex chromosomes determine the gender of the child, they also determine other body traits. However, the autosomes determine most body traits.

Each chromosome possesses many genes. Homologous chromosomes carry the same genes that code for a particular trait, but the genes may be of different forms, which are called **alleles.** Many times only one allele is actually expressed as a trait even if another allele is present. The allele that is always expressed over the other is called a dominant allele. The one that is not expressed is called recessive. The only way a recessive allele can be expressed is if there is no dominant allele present.

Detached earlobes are an example of a trait that is determine by a dominant allele. If a child inherits a dominant allele for this trait from one parent but inherits the recessive allele from the other parent, the child will have detached earlobes. If the child inherits recessive alleles from both parents, then he will have attached earlobes.

Most traits in the body are determined by multiple alleles. For example, hair color, height, skin tone, eye color, and body build are each determined by many different genes. **Complex inheritance** is the term used to describe inherited traits that are determined by multiple genes. It explains why different children within the same family can each have different characteristics.

Sex-linked traits are carried on the sex chromosomes, X and Y. The Y chromosome is much smaller than the X chromosome and does not carry many genes. Therefore, if the X chromosome carries a recessive allele, it is likely to be expressed because there is usually no corresponding allele on the Y chromosome. For example, red-green color blindness is determined by the presence of a recessive allele that is always found on the X chromosome. This disorder (like most sex-linked disorders) primarily affects males because the corresponding Y chromosome does not have any allele to prevent the expression of the recessive allele.

Genetic influences are known to contribute to many thousands of different health conditions. See the Pathophysiology section for a description of some of the more common genetic disorders.

Pathophysiology

Common Genetic Disorders

Albinism is a condition in which a person is born with little or no pigmentation in the skin, eyes, or hair. Albinism affects all races, and in most cases there is no family history.

- **Causes.** At least six different genes are involved with pigment production. This condition develops when a person inherits one or more faulty genes that do not produce the usual amounts of a pigment.
- **Signs and symptoms.** People with the condition experience visual problems and sun-sensitive skin.
- **Treatment.** Although there is no cure, treatments are available to help the symptoms. Prenatal testing for the condition is available.

Attention deficit hyperactivity disorder (ADHD) is the most common behavioral disorder. It usually begins in childhood.

- **Causes.** Although ADHD is not normally considered a genetic disorder, there is evidence that genetic factors play a role in increasing the susceptibility to this condition. Twin and genetic studies show that several genes are likely to be involved.
- **Signs and symptoms.** People with this disorder have difficulty paying attention without being distracted and find it difficult to control impulsive physical actions. Children with ADHD have normal intelligence but are more likely to be depressed and anxious as well as to have problems with speech and language. Hyperactivity usually improves when the child reaches puberty.
- **Treatment.** There is no cure for ADHD, but treatments such as the drug Ritalin or behavior modification are available.

Cleft lip and *cleft palate* are gaps or depressions in the upper lip or palate (roof of the mouth). These conditions commonly occur together.

- **Causes.** These conditions develop when separate areas of a developing fetus's face and head do not join together during early fetal development. Although genes may play a role in the development of these conditions, other causes include maternal rubella (German measles) or the use of certain medications during pregnancy.
- **Signs and symptoms.** Cleft lip or palate may lead to problems with feeding, recurrent ear infections, aspiration pneumonia, and speech problems later in life.
- **Treatment.** Surgery is usually very successful in repairing these conditions.

continued →

Common Genetic Disorders *(continued)*

Cystic fibrosis is a life-threatening disease that mainly affects the lungs and pancreas. This disease is one of the most common inherited life-threatening disorders among white people in the United States.

- **Causes.** Inheritance is autosomal recessive, so if both parents are carriers, there is a 25% chance that each child born to them will develop cystic fibrosis.
- **Signs and symptoms.** Patients with this disorder have increasing problems with breathing. Thick secretions eventually block passageways in the air, and these secretions may become infected.
- **Treatment.** There is no cure, but treatments are available to help patients live with the complications associated with this disorder. Newborn babies are commonly screened for the disease because the sooner treatment begins, the healthier the child can be. Parents are also commonly screened for the gene to determine the likelihood of having a child with cystic fibrosis.

Down syndrome is a disorder that causes mental retardation and physical abnormalities.

- **Causes.** This disorder occurs when a person has three copies of chromosome 21 instead of two. This condition can be diagnosed through prenatal tests such as amniocentesis. The risk of having a child with Down syndrome increases with the age of the mother.
- **Signs and symptoms.** The signs of Down syndrome include a flat facial profile, protruding tongue, oblique slanting eyes, abundant neck skin, short broad hands, and poor muscle tone. Heart, digestive, hearing, and visual problems are also common in people with this condition. Learning difficulties are common in Down syndrome and can range from moderate to severe.
- **Treatment.** There is no cure, but support programs and the treatment of health problems allow many patients with Down syndrome to live a relatively normal life.

Fragile X syndrome is the most common inherited cause of learning disability. All races and ethnic groups seem to be affected equally by this syndrome.

- **Causes.** In this disorder, one of the genes on the X chromosome is defective and makes the chromosome susceptible to breakage. This sex-linked disorder affects boys more severely than girls. It is estimated that approximately 1 in 300 females are carriers for this disorder.
- **Signs and symptoms.** Mental impairment, learning disabilities, attention deficit disorder, a long face, large ears, and flat feet are some of the signs and symptoms. Fragile X syndrome can be easily diagnosed using prenatal tests such as amniocentesis.
- **Treatment.** There is no cure, but some treatments and support groups are available to patients with this disorder.

Hemophilia is a group of inheritable blood disorders. Each condition may be severe to mild.

- **Causes.** In each type, an essential clotting factor is low or missing. Most types of hemophilia are X-linked recessive disorders; therefore, this disorder primarily affects males. Carriers of the gene can be identified with a blood test, and prenatal tests can diagnose the condition in the fetus.
- **Signs and symptoms.** Symptoms include easy bruising, spontaneous bleeding, and prolonged bleeding. Repeated bleeding in the joints leads to arthritis and permanent joint damage.
- **Treatment.** Treatments include injections of the missing clotting factors.

Klinefelter's syndrome is a chromosomal abnormality that affects males.

- **Causes.** People with this disorder have an extra X chromosome.
- **Signs and symptoms.** Tall stature, pear-shaped fat distribution, small testes, sparse body hair, and infertility are the most common signs and symptoms. Thyroid problems, diabetes, and osteoporosis are also common in patients with this syndrome.
- **Treatment.** There is no cure, but treatments such as testosterone replacement therapy can decrease the risk of osteoporosis and produce more male characteristics.

Muscular dystrophy is a group of genetic disorders that primarily affect the muscular and nervous systems. It most often affects males.

- **Causes.** Most types involve mutations in the genes responsible for producing muscle proteins. Some types of muscular dystrophy are inherited as an X-linked disorder, but some are caused by gene mutations.
- **Signs and symptoms.** In this disorder, muscle cells gradually break down, causing progressive muscle weakness.
- **Treatment.** There is no cure, and few treatments are available to slow down the loss of muscle cells. Prenatal genetic tests are available for some types of muscular dystrophies.

Phenylketonuria (PKU) develops if a person cannot synthesize the enzyme that converts phenylalanine to tyrosine. Phenylalanine is an essential amino acid, but too much of it can be harmful, so the body regularly converts it to tyrosine.

- **Causes.** This condition is inherited as an autosomal recessive disorder.
- **Signs and symptoms.** If phenylalanine builds up in the blood, it can lead to the irreversible damage of organs, including the brain.

continued ⟶

Common Genetic Disorders *(continued)*

- **Treatment.** Phenylalanine is found in many proteins, so meats and other protein-rich foods must be avoided. The early detection of PKU is important in order to prevent developmental delays. There is no cure for PKU, but special diets allow a person to lead a normal life. Most newborns are tested for PKU, and prenatal diagnosis is also available.

Sickle cell anemia is an inheritable genetic condition in which abnormal hemoglobin is produced in red blood cells. Normal hemoglobin carries most of the oxygen in the blood. Patients with sickle cell anemia produce an abnormal type of hemoglobin that cannot carry oxygen and that also causes red blood cells to become rigid and have a sickle shape. These rigid red blood cells are less able to squeeze through small blood vessels, so these blood vessels become blocked. It primarily affects people of African or Caribbean descent.

- **Causes.** This disease is inherited as an autosomal recessive disorder.
- **Signs and symptoms.** Blood vessels can become blocked in organs such as the liver, kidney, lungs, heart, and spleen and can cause severe pain. The red blood cells also break down easily, which leads to anemia.
- **Treatment.** There is no cure for sickle cell anemia, but treatments have been successful in preventing the complications associated with this disease. This condition can be diagnosed with prenatal tests.

Spina bifida occurs when one or more vertebrae do not form properly, leaving a gap in the spinal column and leading to damage of the spinal cord.

- **Causes.** This condition is thought to be caused by a combination of genetic and environmental factors.
- **Signs and symptoms.** Signs and symptoms will vary greatly, depending on the level of the gap in the spinal column. In the most severe forms, paralysis of many body muscles can result. Hydrocephalus (increased pressure in the fluid of the brain) often accompanies spina bifida, which can lead to brain damage. Prenatal tests can sometimes diagnose the condition. Folic acid supplements are believed to reduce the risk of the development of this disorder.
- **Treatment.** The treatment primarily consists of physical therapy, which helps to keep muscles strong.

Turner's syndrome is a disorder that almost exclusively affects females.

- **Causes.** This disease results when an X chromosome is completely or partially missing.
- **Signs and symptoms.** The signs and symptoms may include web neck, broad chest, widely spaced nipples, low hairline, short stature, and infertility. Prenatal tests can diagnose the condition, but most girls are diagnosed in late childhood when they fail to start menstruating.
- **Treatment.** There is no cure for Turner's syndrome, but treatments with growth hormone replacements can increase the height of the patient.

Major Tissue Types

As you learned earlier in the chapter, tissues are groups of cells that have similar structures and functions. The four major tissue types in the body are **epithelial, connective, muscle,** and **nervous.**

Epithelial Tissue

When you think of epithelial tissue, you should think of a covering, lining, or gland. Epithelial tissue covers the body and most organs. Epithelial tissue lines tubes of the body such as blood vessels and the esophagus as well as hollow organs of the body such as the stomach and heart. This type of tissue also lines body cavities (such as the thoracic cavity and the abdominopelvic cavity). Glandular tissue is also classified as a type of epithelial tissue.

Glandular epithelium is composed of cells that make and secrete (give off) substances. If a gland secretes its product into a duct, it is called an **exocrine gland.** If a gland secretes its product directly into tissue fluids or blood, it is called an **endocrine gland.** Endocrine glands do not have ducts, so they have to secrete their products into surrounding tissue fluids or blood.

Epithelial tissues are avascular, which means that they lack blood vessels. However, these tissues have a nerve supply and are very mitotic—they divide constantly. In addition, the cells within epithelial tissues are packed together tightly. Epithelial tissues possess many functions, depending on their location in the body. For example, those covering the body provide protection against invading pathogens and toxins. Those that line the digestive tract secrete a variety of enzymes needed for digestion and often possess microvilli, which allow the body to absorb nutrients. Epithelial tissues lining the respiratory tract have cilia and goblet cells. The goblet cells produce mucus that traps small particles that enter the respiratory tract. The cilia constantly push the mucus and trapped particles away from the lungs (Figure 5-10). Epithelial cells within the kidneys act as filters that help to remove waste products from blood.

Connective Tissue

Connective tissues are the most abundant tissues in the body. The cells of connective tissues do not pack together tightly. Instead, a **matrix** separates the cells. Think of the matrix simply as the matter that is between the cells of

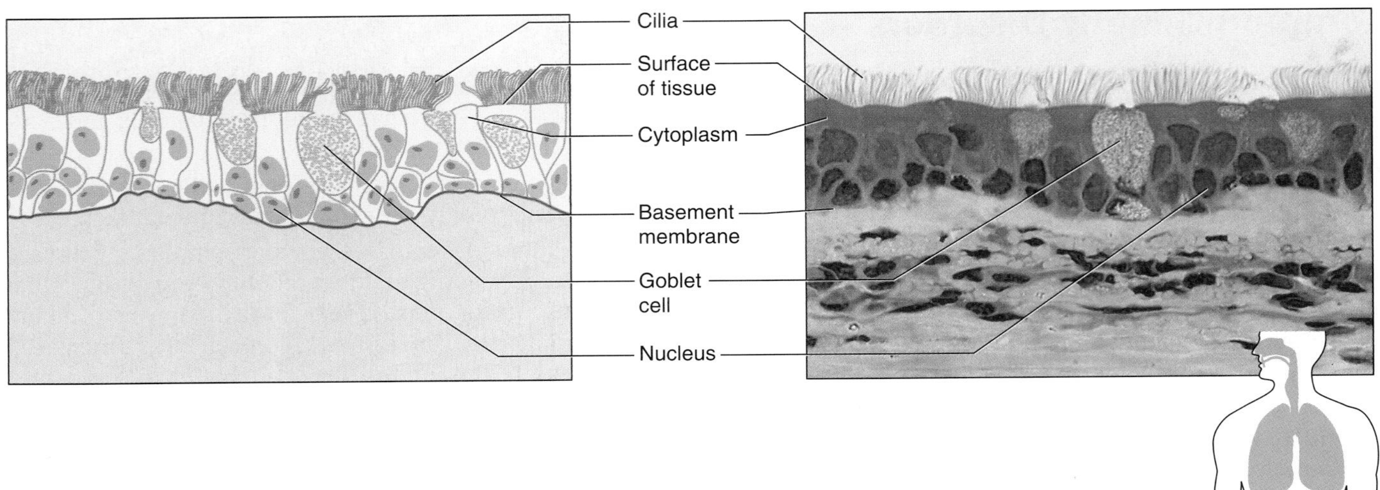

Figure 5-10. Epithelial tissue lining the respiratory tract.

connective tissue. It contains fibers, water, proteins, inorganic salts, and other substances. The components of the matrix vary, depending on the type of connective tissue. Connective tissues generally have a rich blood supply, except for cartilage and some dense connective tissues that contain a very poor blood supply.

There are many different cell types located in connective tissues. The most common cell types are fibroblasts, mast cells, and macrophages. Fibroblasts make fibers, and mast cells secrete substances such as heparin and histamine that promote inflammation during times of tissue damage. Macrophages are cells that destroy unwanted material such as bacteria or toxins.

Blood. This tissue is composed of red blood cells, white blood cells, and plasma. Plasma is the matrix of blood. Unlike other connective tissues, this matrix does not contain fibers. Blood functions to transport substances throughout the body.

Osseous (Bone) Tissue. The matrix of osseous tissue contains mineral salts that make it a very hard tissue. Contrary to popular belief, bone tissue is metabolically active.

Cartilage. The matrix of cartilage is rigid, although it is not as hard as osseous tissue. Cartilage gives shape to structures such as the ears and nose. It also protects the ends of long bones and forms the discs between the vertebrae of the neck and spine.

Dense Connective Tissue. The matrix of dense connective tissue is packed with tough fibers that make it a soft but very strong tissue. Ligaments, tendons, and joint capsules have large amounts of this tissue type. Ligaments

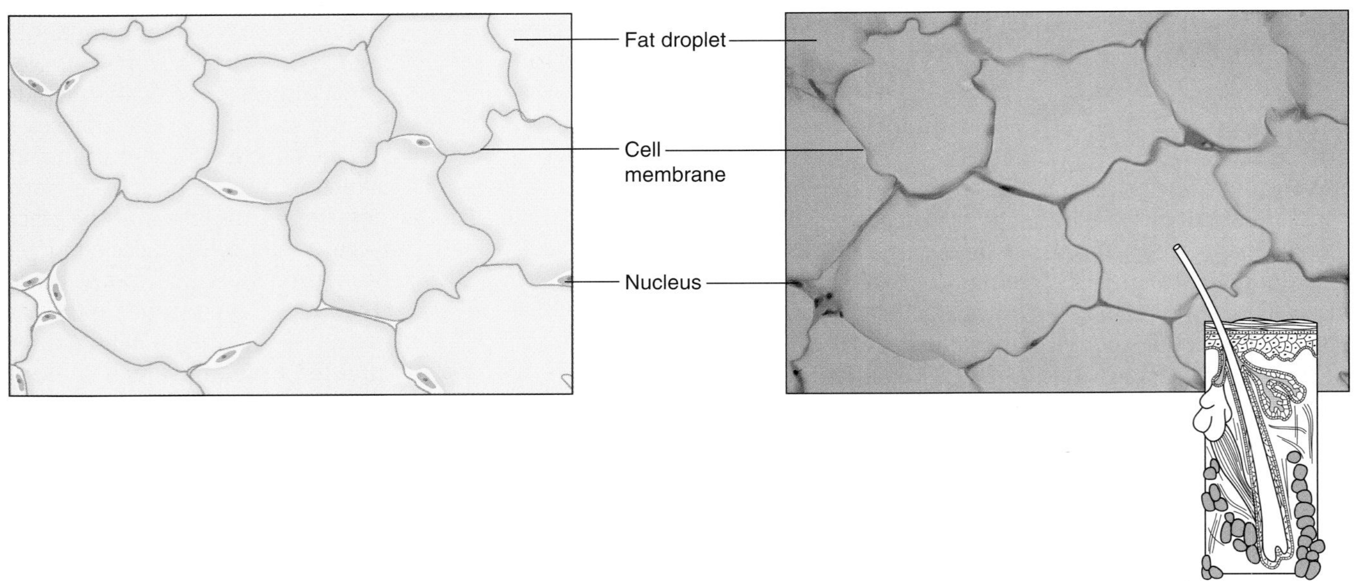

Figure 5-11. Adipose tissue.

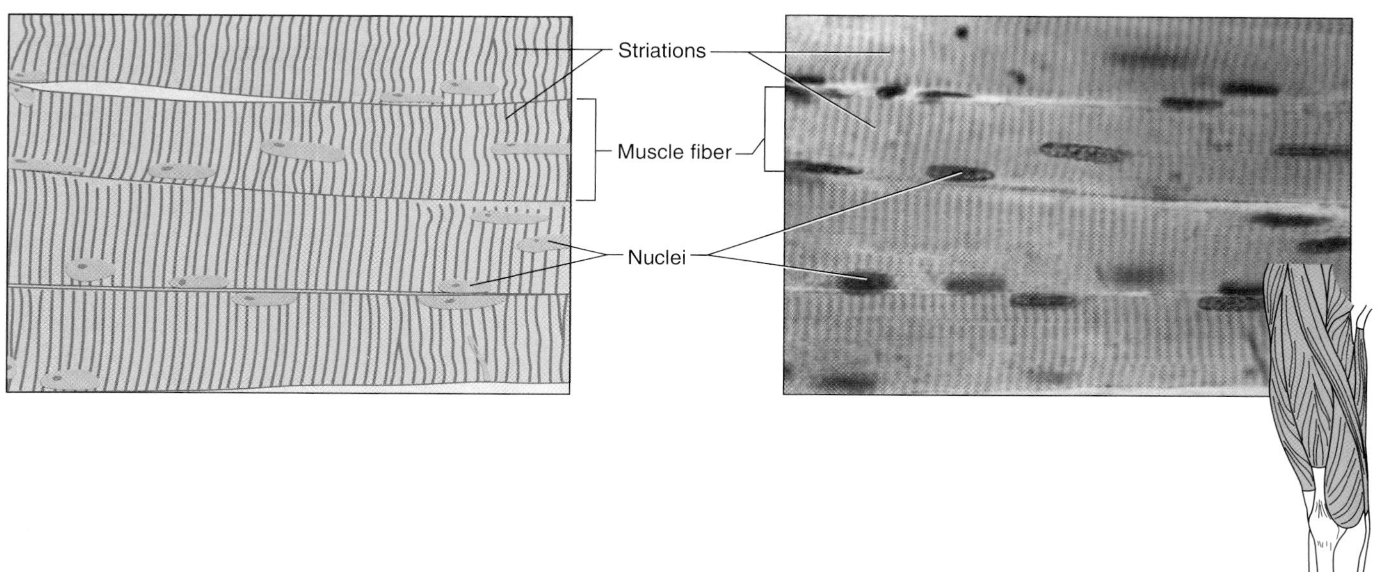

Figure 5-12. Skeletal muscle tissue.

connect bones to bones, tendons connect bones to muscles, and joint capsules surround moveable joints in the body. Dense connective tissues also make up a large part of the dermis of skin. When skin is damaged, this tissue "fills" in the space of damage and forms a scar.

Adipose (Fat) Tissue. Within adipose tissue, unique cells—adipocytes—store fats. The functions of this tissue type include storing energy for cells of the body, cushioning body parts and organs, and insulating the body against excessive heat or cold (Figure 5-11).

Muscle Tissue

Muscle tissue is a specialized type of tissue that shortens and elongates; in other words, it contracts and relaxes. The three types of muscle tissue are skeletal, smooth, and cardiac. Skeletal muscle tissue, as its name suggests, is attached to the skeleton. This type of muscle tissue is described as voluntary because we can consciously control its movement. For example, we can consciously decide to contract the skeletal muscles attached to our arm bones and make them move. It is also referred to as being striated because the cells of this muscle tissue type have striations or stripes in their cytoplasm (Figure 5-12).

Smooth muscle tissue is located in the walls of hollow organs (except the heart), the walls of blood vessels, and the dermis of skin. It is not voluntary because we cannot consciously control its movement. For example, you do not consciously decide when the smooth muscle of your stomach contacts. This tissue is called smooth because its cells do not possess striations in their cytoplasm.

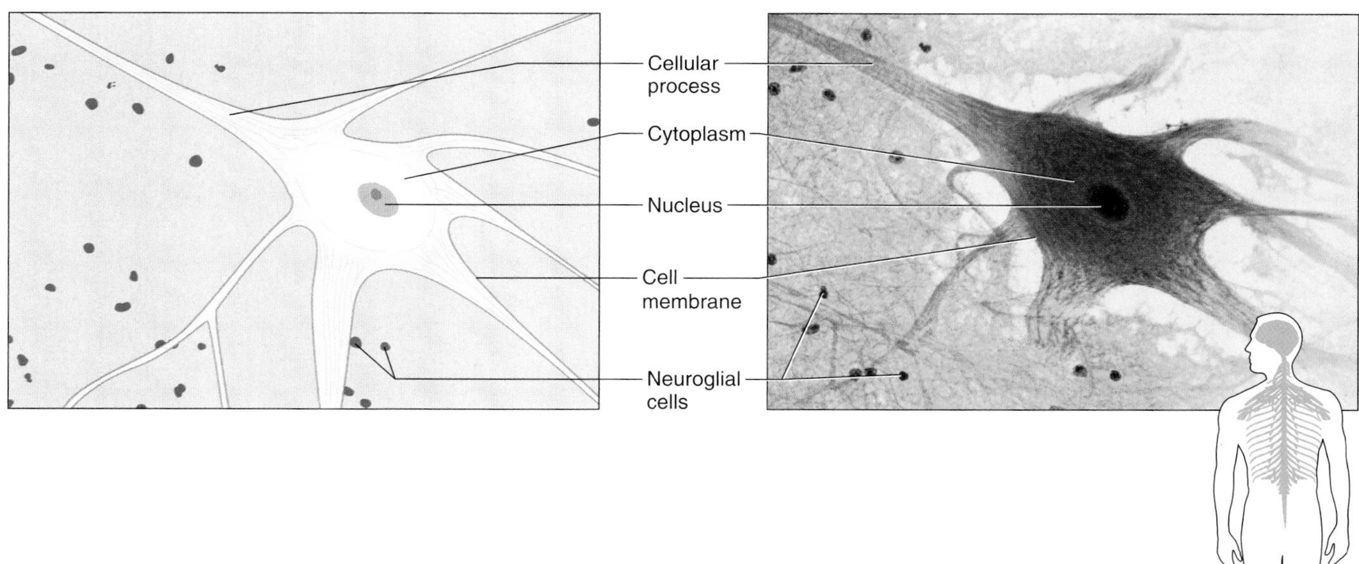

Figure 5-13. Nervous tissue.

Cardiac muscle tissue is located in the wall of the heart. Like skeletal muscle tissue, it is striated and like smooth muscle tissue, it is not under voluntary control.

Nervous Tissue

Nervous tissue is located in the brain, spinal cord, and peripheral nerves. This tissue specializes in sending impulses or electrical messages to the neurons, muscles, and glands in the body. Nervous tissue contains two types of cells: **neurons** and **neuroglial cells.** Neurons are the largest cells and possess characteristic cellular processes. Although neuroglial cells are smaller, they are more abundant and support neurons (Figure 5-13).

Summary

The human body is divided into several levels of organization, from the simplest to the most complex. These levels are chemical, cellular, tissue, organ, organ system, and organism. Anatomy is the study of the structure of the human body. Physiology is the study of its functions. Directional terms are used to describe the location of body parts and regions. These terms always relate to the anatomic position. It is important to understand the basics of the organization of the human body before studying the individual systems.

REVIEW

CHAPTER 5

CASE STUDY QUESTIONS

Now that you have completed this chapter, review the case study at the beginning of the chapter and answer the following questions:

1. On what side of the body is the appendix normally located?
2. If the medical assistant observes the boy's right lower abdominal quadrant for the bandage, is this correct? Why or why not?
3. Where should the bandage be found?
4. What precautions should this patient take given his diagnosis of *situs inversus*?

Discussion Questions

1. Explain the function of the four types of tissues in one of the body systems.
2. Describe the four abdominal quadrants and the nine abdominal regions. What is the importance of knowing these areas in the clinical setting?
3. What are acids and bases? Describe the pH scale.

Critical Thinking Questions

1. Diseases develop when homeostasis is not maintained. What treatments can bring the following conditions back to normal: high body temperature, dehydration, and high blood pressure?
2. What clinical laboratory tests have you encountered that require a knowledge of chemistry to interpret?
3. Moveable joints like elbows and knees always contain cartilage and dense connective tissues. Why are they so slow to heal once they have been injured?

Application Activities

1. Referring to figures in the chapter, name an organ or part of the body that is located:
   a. Distal to the elbow
   b. Proximal to the ankle
   c. In the thoracic cavity
   d. In the pelvic cavity
   e. Medial to the acromial region
2. What organs would you expect to see if you were looking at a transverse plane cut at the level of the umbilicus?

Internet Activity

1. Go to the Web site for the Centers for Disease Control and Prevention (**http:www.cdc.gov**) and answer the following questions:
   a. What are the Centers for Disease Control and Prevention?
   b. Click on Health Topics A–Z, and then click on Spina Bifida. How are spina bifida and folic acid related?
   c. Each year in the United States, about how many infants are born with spina bifida or anencephaly?
   d. What are the annual medical care and surgical costs for persons with spina bifida in the United States?
2. Find an interactive periodic table of elements, and answer the following questions:
   a. Carbon, hydrogen, oxygen, and nitrogen are the four most abundant elements of the human body. What are the atomic symbols for each of these elements?
   b. Who discovered hydrogen?
   c. What is the name origin of oxygen?
   d. When was nitrogen discovered?
   e. How many protons does one carbon atom contain?

CHAPTER 6

The Integumentary System

KEY TERMS

alopecia
apocrine gland
arrector pili
cellulitis
cyanosis
dermatitis
dermis
eccrine gland
eczema
epidermis
follicle
folliculitis
hemoglobin
herpes simplex
herpes zoster
hypodermis
impetigo
keratin
keratinocyte
lunula
melanin
melanocyte
nail bed
psoriasis
rosacea
scabies
sebaceous
sebum
stratum basale
stratum corneum
subcutaneous
warts

CHAPTER OUTLINE

- Functions of the Integumentary System
- Skin Structure
- Skin Color
- Accessory Organs
- Skin Healing

OBJECTIVES

After completing Chapter 6, you will be able to:

6.1 List the functions of skin.
6.2 Explain the role of skin in regulating body temperature.
6.3 Describe the layers of skin and the characteristics of each layer.
6.4 Explain the factors that affect skin color.
6.5 List the accessory organs of skin and describe their structures and functions.
6.6 Describe the appearance, causes, and treatments of various types of skin cancer.
6.7 Describe the appearance, causes, and treatment of common skin disorders.
6.8 Explain the ABCD rule and its use in evaluating melanoma.
6.9 List the different types of burns and describe their appearances and treatments.
6.10 Describe the signs, symptoms, causes, and treatments of other skin disorders and diseases.

Introduction

The integumentary system consists of skin and its accessory organs. The accessory organs of skin are hair follicles, nails, and skin glands. Skin is the body's outer covering and its largest organ.

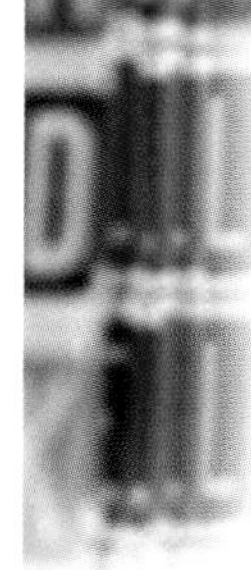

CASE STUDY

Last New Year's Eve, a 23-year-old man came to the urgent care facility where you work as a medical assistant. He had been in an accident involving fireworks and was diagnosed with second-degree burns to his anterior torso.

As you read this chapter, consider the following questions:

1. Using the rule of nines, estimate the percentage of the patient's body surface that was affected by this burn.
2. What layers of skin has the burn affected?
3. What functions of the skin are lost by this injury?
4. What types of treatments does this burn require?

Functions of the Integumentary System

People are often interested in the appearance of their skin but rarely consider its functions. The integumentary system serves many purposes, including these important functions:

- Protection. As long as skin is intact and not inflamed, it provides very good protection against the entry of bacteria and viruses. It also protects underlying structures from ultraviolet radiation and dehydration.
- Body temperature regulation. Skin plays a major role in regulating body temperature. When a person is hot, dermal blood vessels dilate, which is why a person's skin becomes pinkish. Because the dermal blood vessels are dilated, more blood than normal passes through the skin. This is beneficial because blood carries a lot of the heat in the body. When the blood gets close to the surface of the body (to skin), the heat can escape. Conversely, if a person is cold, the dermal blood vessels constrict, preventing the heat in blood from escaping.
- Vitamin D production. When exposed to sunlight, the skin produces a molecule that is turned into vitamin D. The body needs vitamin D for calcium absorption.
- Sensation. The skin is packed with sensory receptors that can detect touch, heat, cold, and pain.
- Excretion. Small amounts of waste products are lost through skin when a person perspires.

Skin Structure

The skin is a complex organ consisting of two layers, the **epidermis** and the **dermis.** Skin sits on a third layer called the **hypodermis,** also called the **subcutaneous** layer (Figure 6-1).

Epidermis

The epidermis is the most superficial layer of skin. It is made up of many layers of tightly packed cells. The epidermis can be divided into two layers, the stratum corneum and the stratum basale.

The **stratum corneum** is the most superficial layer of the epidermis. Most of the cells in this layer are dead and very flat. Because they have accumulated keratin, the cells in this layer stick together and form an impermeable layer for skin. Most bacteria, viruses, and water cannot penetrate the stratum corneum.

The **stratum basale** is the deepest layer of the epidermis. The cells in this layer are constantly dividing, and older cells are constantly pushed up toward the stratum corneum.

The most common cell type in the epidermis is the **keratinocyte.** This cell makes and accumulates the protein keratin. **Keratin** is a durable protein that makes the epidermis waterproof and resistant to bacteria and viruses. Another cell type of the epidermis is the **melanocyte,** which makes the pigment **melanin.** Melanin is deposited throughout the layers of the epidermis. This pigment traps ultraviolet (UV) radiation from sunlight and prevents the radiation from harming structures in the underlying layers of the skin.

Dermis

The dermis is the deep layer of skin and is the most complex layer. The dermis contains all the major tissue types, including epithelial tissue, connective tissues, muscle tissue, and nervous tissue. The dermis contains sweat glands, sebaceous (oil) glands, hair follicles, the arrector pili muscles, collagen fibers, elastic fibers, nerve fibers, and many blood vessels. The dermis binds the epidermis to the hypodermis.

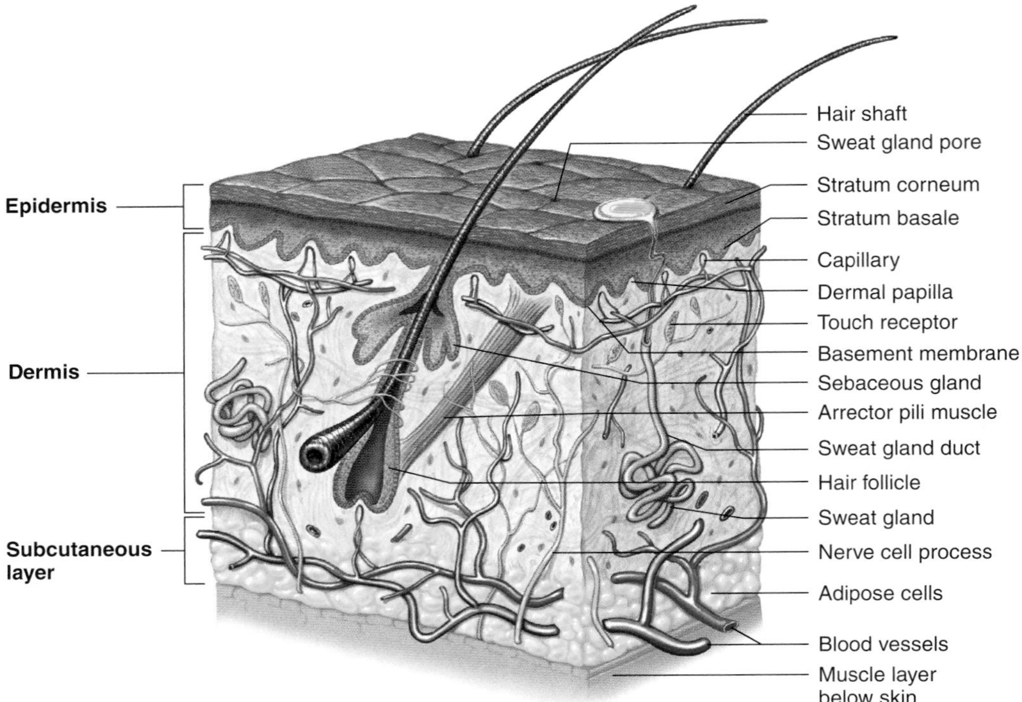

Figure 6-1. Section of skin.

Hypodermis

The subcutaneous layer of skin, the hypodermis, is largely made of adipose tissue. In fact, most adipose tissue in the body is found in your hypodermis. This layer also contains blood vessels and nerves.

Skin Color

Skin color is largely determined by the amount of melanin in the epidermis of skin. Melanin can range in color from yellowish to brownish. The more melanin a person has in the skin, the darker the skin color. All people have about the same number of melanocytes regardless of skin color. What varies from person to person is how active the melanocytes are in producing melanin. A person with dark skin has very active melanocytes.

Another factor that determines skin color is the amount of oxygenated blood in the dermis of skin. **Hemoglobin** is a pigment in blood that is bright red when it is oxygenated. Hemoglobin that is not oxygenated is a dark red color. A person with a rich supply of oxygenated blood will have skin that is a pinkish hue. When the supply of oxygen in the blood is low, the skin looks rather pale or bluish. A bluish color of skin is called **cyanosis.**

Pathophysiology

Skin Cancer and Common Skin Disorders

Skin is vulnerable to many disorders because it is the most exposed of all body organs.

SKIN CANCER

Skin cancer develops from cells in the epidermis of skin. It is more common in people who have light-colored skin and who have had excessive exposure to sunlight. It can occur anywhere on the body but is most likely to appear on skin that is readily exposed to sunlight. The two most common types of skin cancer are basal cell carcinoma and squamous cell carcinoma, but the most deadly type is melanoma (Figure 6-2).

Basal cell carcinoma accounts for approximately 90% of all skin cancers in the United States. Fortunately, it progresses slowly and rarely spreads to other body parts. It is derived from cells of the stratum basale of the epidermis.

continued ⟶

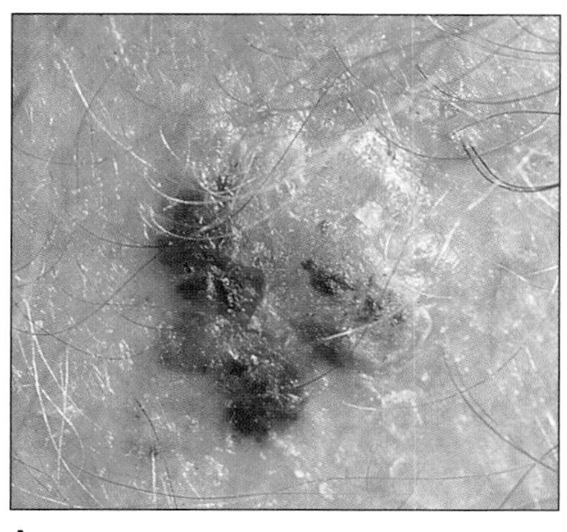
A

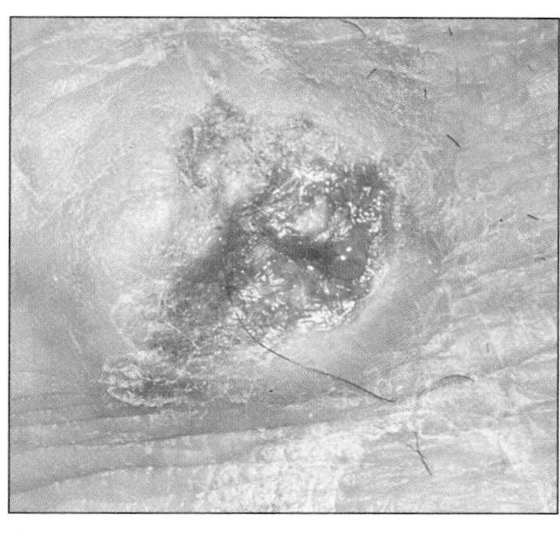
B

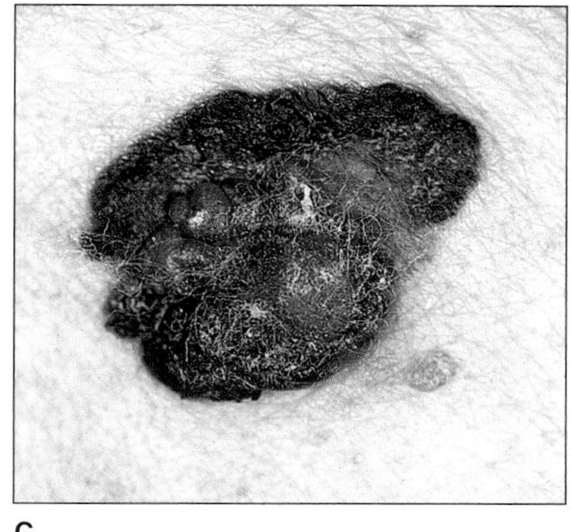
C

Figure 6-2. Types of skin cancer: (a) squamous cell carcinoma, (b) basal cell carcinoma, and (c) malignant melanoma.

- **Signs and symptoms.** Signs and symptoms include changes on the skin and a new growth or sore on the skin that does not heal. Its appearance may be waxy, smooth, red, pale, flat, or lumpy, and it may or may not bleed.
- **Treatment.** Several forms of treatment are available:
  - Curettage and electrodessication. In curettage, a sharp instrument is used to scoop out the cancerous spot. Electrodessication uses electrical currents to minimize bleeding as well as to kill any remaining cancer cells.
  - Mohs' surgery. The cancerous spot is shaved off one layer at a time.
  - Cryosurgery. Freezing is used to kill cancer cells.
  - Laser Therapy. A beam of light destroys cancer cells.

Squamous cell carcinoma is much less common than basal cell carcinoma but is more likely to spread to surrounding tissues. It arises from flat cells of the epidermis. The signs and symptoms and the treatments for this type of cancer are the same as for basal cell carcinoma.

Melanoma is much more aggressive than both basal cell and squamous cell carcinomas. Melanoma can occur anywhere on the body but most often appears on the trunk, head, and neck in men and on the arms and legs in women. Melanoma is cancer that arises from melanocytes.

- **Signs and symptoms.** A mole that itches or bleeds is a common symptom. New moles may develop near it. It may change to have any sign of the ABCD rule:
  - Asymmetry. The mole should not become asymmetrical.
  - Border. The border of the mole should not become irregular.
  - Color. The mole should not change color or become a mixture of colors.
  - Diameter. The mole should not grow larger than the diameter of a pencil eraser.
- **Treatment.** The treatment will depend on the staging of this cancer. Available treatments include the following:
  - Surgery to remove the melanoma
  - Lymph node biopsy to determine if the cancer has spread
  - Removal of cancerous lymph nodes
  - Chemotherapy for advanced stages of cancer
  - Radiation therapy for advanced stages of cancer
  - Immunotherapy to boost the patient's immune system
- **Stages of melanoma.** Melanoma has five different stages, which are described from the least to the most serious:
  - Stage 0. Melanoma is found only in the epidermis
  - Stage I. Melanoma has spread to the epidermis and dermis and has a thickness of 1 to 2 millimeters.
  - Stage II. Melanoma has a thickness of 2 to 4 millimeters and may have ulceration.
  - Stage III. Melanoma has spread to one or more nearby lymph nodes.
  - Stage IV. Melanoma has spread to other body organs or other lymph nodes far away from the original melanoma site.

COMMON SKIN AND HAIR DISORDERS

Alopecia is a disorder that specifically targets hair. This disorder results in hair loss.

- **Causes.** Most of the time, alopecia is inherited. Other common causes include hormonal changes, chemotherapy, stress, burns, and fungal infections of the skin.
- **Signs and symptoms.** Alopecia is more commonly called baldness, but it may occur on areas of skin other than the scalp.

continued ⟶

Skin Cancer and Common Skin Disorders *(continued)*

- **Treatment.** If due to heredity, this disorder is not curable. Hair transplants and some drugs may slow down hair loss. Hair loss caused by other factors is usually temporary.

Cellulitis is an inflammation of connective tissues in skin and primarily occurs on the face and legs.

- **Causes.** This skin disease is caused by staphylococcal and streptococcal bacteria.
- **Signs and symptoms.** Skin appears red and tight and is often painful. The inflammation may trigger a fever.
- **Treatment.** Treatment is with antibiotics.

Dermatitis is a general term defined as inflammation of skin or a rash. It has many causes and is a sign of many types of skin disorders.

Eczema is one type of chronic dermatitis. This condition most commonly occurs in infants but it may also occur in adults.

- **Causes.** Causes of eczema are mostly unknown, but it is thought to be a type of allergy. Environmental irritants, stress, and dry skin can bring about episodes of this disease.
- **Signs and symptoms.** The rashes of eczema are scaly and itchy.
- **Treatment.** Treatments include steroids and other types of anti-inflammatory drugs. Of course, avoiding factors that trigger eczema are also helpful.

Folliculitis, which is a disorder specific to hair, is an inflammation of hair follicles.

- **Causes.** This disorder usually results from shaving or excess rubbing of skin areas. It may also be caused by bacteria and fungi.
- **Signs and symptoms.** Follicles become red and itchy and often look like pimples.
- **Treatment.** Treatments include regular cleansing of skin, topical antibiotics, and use of electric razors instead of razor blades.

Herpes simplex types 1 and 2 are the most common types of herpes simplex.

- **Causes.** Herpes simplex types 1 and 2 are both caused by a virus. Herpes simplex type 1 is very contagious and is spread through saliva. Herpes simplex type 2 is sexually transmitted.
- **Signs and symptoms.** Herpes simplex type 1 causes painful sores on the lips, mouth, and face. Herpes simplex type 2 normally causes painful sores on genital areas.
- **Treatment.** There is no cure for herpes simplex, and its skin lesions usually recur throughout life. However, antiviral drugs prevent frequent outbreaks.

Herpes zoster is a disorder commonly known as shingles.

- **Causes.** Herpes zoster is caused by the same virus that causes chickenpox. After a person has chickenpox, the virus becomes inactive but can become active again later in life to cause shingles.
- **Signs and symptoms.** Herpes zoster causes inflammation that affects the nerves on one side of the body and results in very painful skin blisters.
- **Treatment.** Some antiviral medications shorten the duration of the disease, but normally it is treated only with pain medications. Recovery is usually complete, and reoccurrences of the disease are rare. It is uncertain whether the chickenpox vaccine prevents herpes zoster.

Impetigo causes the formation of oozing skin lesions that eventually crust over.

- **Causes.** This disease is caused by staphylococcal and streptococcal bacteria.
- **Signs and symptoms.** The skin develops oozing lesions that eventually crust over.
- **Treatment.** This condition is treated with antibiotics.

Psoriasis is a common skin problem.

- **Causes.** This skin disorder is most likely an inherited autoimmune disorder.
- **Signs and symptoms.** Patients with psoriasis have frequent episodes of itching and redness and have outbreaks of scaly skin lesions. Some people also have joint pain.
- **Treatment.** Mild cases are treated with anti-inflammatory drugs and special ointments. Severe cases require hospitalization.

Rosacea is a skin disorder that commonly appears as facial redness.

- **Causes.** Rosacea's causes are unknown, but it occurs most frequently in fair-skinned people.
- **Signs and symptoms.** Redness and acne-like symptoms on the face are the most common symptoms.
- **Treatment.** Although it is not curable, rosacea is usually managed well with various medications.

Scabies is a very contagious skin condition.

- **Causes.** Scabies is caused by mites that burrow beneath skin. Sometimes the burrows of the mites, which look like red pencil marks, can be seen.
- **Signs and symptoms.** Redness and severe itching are usually the only symptoms of scabies.
- **Treatment.** Most cases are easily treated with prescription medications. Because scabies is contagious, it is wise to treat an entire family if one member is infected.

continued ⟶

Warts (verrucae) are harmless skin growths that can appear almost anywhere on the body surface but most commonly occur on the hands, feet, and face.

- **Causes.** These growths are caused by a virus.
- **Signs and symptoms.** Warts vary greatly in appearance; they can be smooth, flat, rough, raised, dark, small, or large.
- **Treatment.** Warts are often removed with over-the-counter medications but can also be treated through surgery, lasers, freezing, or burning.

Accessory Organs

The accessory organs of the skin include hair follicles, oil glands, nails, and sweat glands.

Hair Follicles

Hair **follicles** are tube-like depressions in the dermis of skin. Hair follicles are made of epithelial tissue and function to generate hairs (Figure 6-3). Cells called keratinocytes make up most of the hair follicle. As new keratinocytes are produced in the base of the hair follicles, old ones are pushed toward the surface of skin. The old keratinocytes stick together to produce a hair. The portion of the hair embedded in skin is called the root, and the portion of the hair extending from the surface of skin is called the shaft.

Melanocytes are also found in hair follicles. They produce and distribute pigments to create hair color. A person develops gray hair when these melanocytes produce less pigment than normal.

When a hair follicle goes into a resting cycle, the hair falls out. Most of the time, the hair follicle will begin a growing cycle again and produce a new hair. However, sometimes hair follicles completely die, and baldness (alopecia) develops.

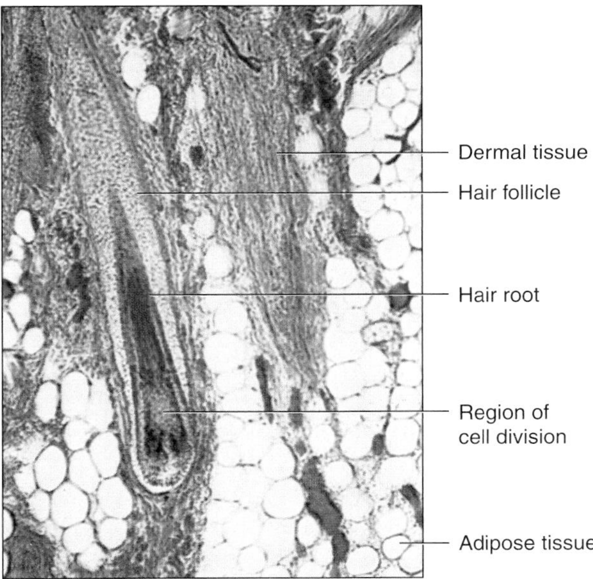

Figure 6-3. Hair follicle.

Arrector pili muscles are attached to most hair follicles. When a person is cold or nervous, these muscles pull on hair follicles and cause hairs to stand erect. These muscles also pull on fibers in the dermis of skin, causing goose bumps to form (see Figure 6-1).

Sebaceous Glands

Sebaceous glands are more commonly called oil glands. They produce an oily substance called **sebum.** Sebum is secreted onto hairs to keep them soft and pliable. Sebum eventually is deposited onto skin to keep it soft as well. Sebum also prevents bacteria from growing on skin (see Figures 6-1 and 6-3).

Nails

Nails function to protect the ends of the fingers and toes. The portion of a nail that you can see is the nail body, and the portion embedded in skin is called the nail root. The nail root contains active keratinocytes that constantly divide to produce nail growth. The white half-moon–shaped area at the base of a nail is called a **lunula.** The lunula also contains very active keratinocytes. Beneath each nail is a layer called the **nail bed.** The nail bed holds the nail down to underlying skin and provides nutrients to the nail (Figure 6-4).

Sweat Glands

Most sweat glands are located in the dermis of skin. However, their ducts open onto the epidermis of skin. There are two types of sweat glands—eccrine and apocrine.

Eccrine sweat glands are the most numerous type. They produce a watery type of sweat and are activated primarily by heat. Once sweat is deposited onto skin, it evaporates and carries heat away from the body. Eccrine sweat glands are most concentrated on the forehead, neck, and back.

Apocrine sweat glands produce a thicker type of sweat that contains more proteins than the type of sweat produced by eccrine sweat glands. Apocrine glands are most concentrated in areas of skin with course hair, such

Educating the Patient

Preventing Acne

Acne is a clinical term used to describe pimples and blackheads. This skin condition occurs when excess oil and dead skin cells clog pores. Bacteria easily accumulate in the clogged pores, which results in pimples or whiteheads. Acne is not the result of poor hygiene or diet. If patients have acne, you can instruct them to follow these steps to help minimize it:

- Use skin-care products that are *noncomedogenic*, meaning that they will not clog pores
- Wash the face twice a day
- Keep hands away from the face
- Remove all makeup daily
- Use makeup or lotion that contains sunscreen
- Wash hair frequently because oils from hair can end up on the face

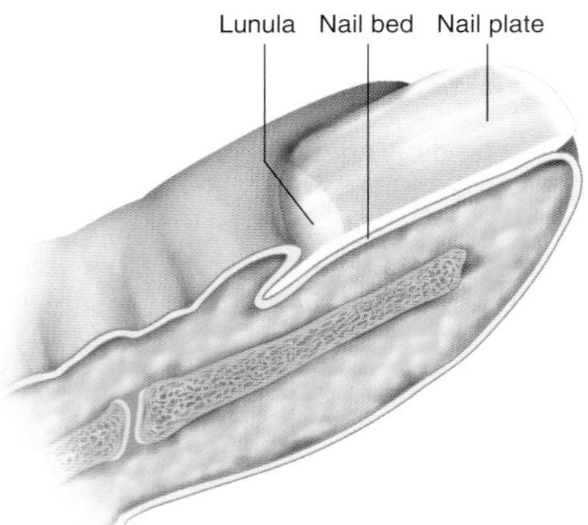

Figure 6-4. Section of a nail.

as the armpit and groin areas. They are primarily activated by nervousness or stress but can also be activated by heat. These are the glands responsible for producing a cold sweat. Bacteria often break down the proteins in the sweat produced by apocrine glands. As the proteins are digested, the bacteria release a foul-smelling waste product that is responsible for the smell of body odor.

Skin Healing

When skin is injured, it becomes inflamed. An inflamed area looks red because nearby blood vessels dilate. The inflamed area also swells because the dilated blood vessels "leak" and fluids seep into spaces between cells. Inflamed areas are often painful because the excess fluid activates pain receptors. However, inflammation promotes healing because more blood is delivered to the area. The extra blood carries more nutrients needed for skin repair as well as defensive cells to clear up the cause of inflammation.

When structures and blood vessels of the dermis are injured, a blood clot initially forms. The blood clot is eventually replaced by a scab, which is basically clotted blood and other dried tissue fluids. The scab is normally replaced by collagen fibers that act to bind the edges of the wound together. Collagen fibers are whitish and the major component of scars. Sometimes skin scars are replaced with new skin, but if the wound is extensive, a scar will persist. Scars cannot carry out most functions of skin so their formation leads to the loss of certain functions.

Pathophysiology

Burns

The second leading cause of accidental death in the United States, after motor vehicle accidents, is burn injuries. There are more than 200 special burn care centers in the United States. More than 2 million burn injuries are reported each year, and more than 11,000 patients die annually from burn injuries. This year, about 1 million people will suffer a burn injury that causes a significant or permanent disability.

The extent of the body surface area affected and the severity (degree) of a burn are the most important factors in predicting the risk of death associated with burn injuries. The rule of nines is a quick way to estimate the

continued ⟶

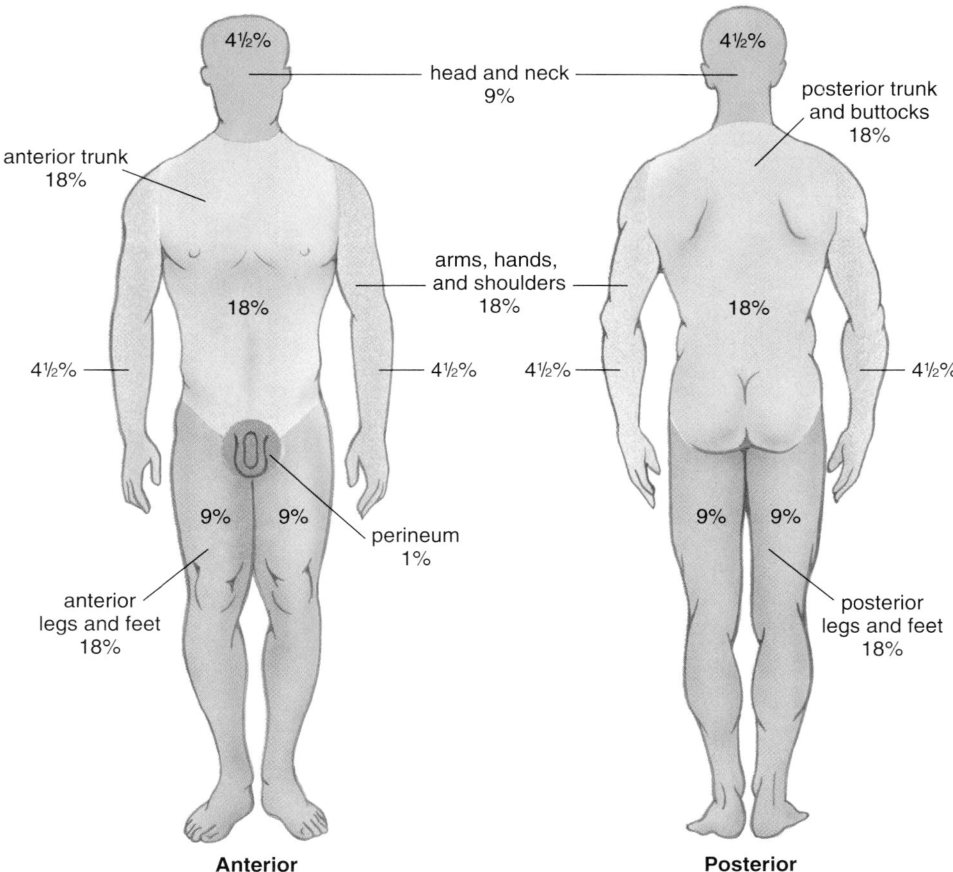

Figure 6-5. Using the rule of nines aids in estimating the extent of burns.

extent of body surface area affected by burns. This method divides the body into 11 areas, each accounting for 9% of the total body surface. The genital area accounts for 1% (Figure 6-5).

- Rule of nines. The 11 body areas of the rule of nines are identified as follows:
  - Head
  - Right arm
  - Left arm
  - Front of right leg
  - Front of left leg
  - Back of right leg
  - Back of left leg
  - Front of body trunk is two areas
  - Back of body trunk is two areas
- Burn severity. The severity of burns indicates the thickness of the injury (Figure 6-6). The following terms are used to report burn severity:
  - *First-degree.* These burns are also called superficial burns. They involve only the epidermis and are characterized by pain, redness, and swelling. Unless they are extensive, they do not require medical attention and usually heal well.
  - *Second-degree.* These burns are also called partial-thickness burns and involve the epidermis and dermis. Pain, redness, swelling, and blisters characterize them. Medical staff should treat any second-degree burn that affects 1% or more of the body surface. A body surface area of 1% is about the size of a person's hand. Shock is likely to develop in second-degree burn injuries that affect 9% or more of the body surface. Second-degree burns can be life-threatening, depending on their extent.
  - *Third-degree.* These burns are also called full-thickness burns. They involve all layers of skin and often underlying structures such as muscles and bones. The skin often looks black or charred in these burns. They always require medical attention regardless of the extent. A full-thickness burn of any size should always be medically treated.
- General Guidelines for Treating Burns
  - Anything sticking to the burn should not be removed.
  - Butter, lotions, or ointments should not be applied to the burn. Only ointments prescribed by a doctor or recommended by a pharmacist should be used.

continued ⟶

Burns *(continued)*

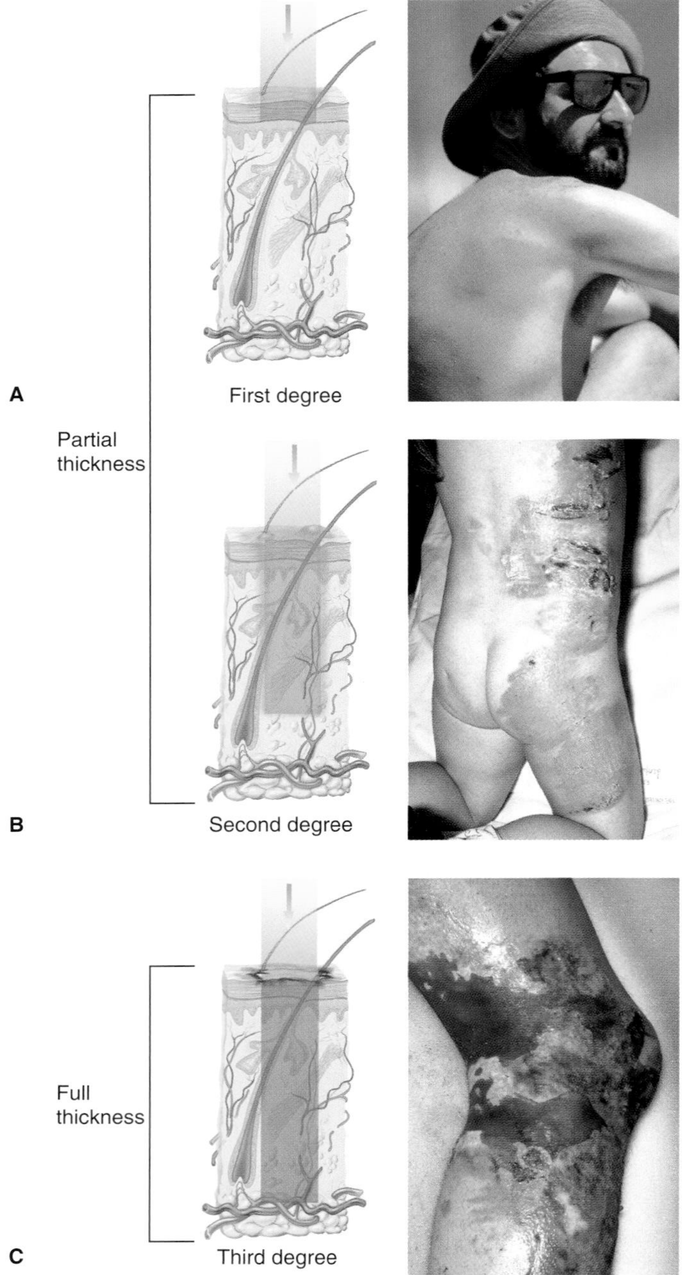

Figure 6-6. The degrees of burn severity include (a) first-degree (superficial burns), (b) second-degree (partial-thickness burns), and (c) third-degree (full-thickness burns).

- The burn should be cooled with large amounts of cold water.
- The burn should be covered with a sterile sheet or plastic bag. Burns to the face, however, should not be covered.
- Emergency medical personnel should be contacted for serious burns.
- In burns to the mouth and throat, the airways should be checked to see if there is any swelling. Burns to the head are always more serious than burns to other body parts. They almost always require emergency medical treatment.

Summary

The integumentary system is the first line of defense for the body. The skin covers the surface of the body, protecting it from invading organisms, chemicals, UV light, and water loss. Hair and nails also serve as protective barriers. In addition, the skin helps regulate body temperature. This system plays an important role in diagnostic testing, including allergy testing and tuberculosis screening. Understanding this system can help you be more effective in your role as a medical assistant.

REVIEW

CHAPTER 6

CASE STUDY QUESTIONS

Now that you have completed this chapter, review the case study at the beginning of the chapter and answer the following questions:

1. Using the rule of nines, estimate the percentage of the patient's body surface that was affected by this burn.
2. What layers of skin has the burn affected?
3. What functions of the skin are lost by this injury?
4. What types of treatments does this burn require?

Discussion Questions

1. Describe the factors that determine skin color.
2. Name the two layers of the epidermis and tell how they differ.
3. Name two types of sweat glands. Where is each located, and how do their secretions differ?

Critical Thinking Questions

1. Why do anti-inflammatory drugs reduce pain? Are these drugs likely to prevent healing or promote healing?
2. Which is more serious, a cat born without arrector pili muscles or a human? Why?
3. Albinos lack melanin. What body structures are affected by this? What precautions must an albino take that non-albinos do not have to worry about?

Application Activities

1. Describe the functions of the following cell types of the epidermis:
   a. Keratinocyte
   b. Melanocyte
2. Describe the role of skin in the following functions:
   a. Protection
   b. Sensation
   c. Body temperature regulation
   d. Excretion
   e. Vitamin D production
3. Describe the following parts of a nail:
   a. Nail root
   b. Lunula
   c. Nail bed
   d. Nail body

CHAPTER 7

The Skeletal System

KEY TERMS

appendicular
articular cartilage
atlas
axial
axis
bursitis
calcaneus
canaliculi
carpal
carpal tunnel syndrome
clavicle
coccyx
condyle
costal
coxal
diaphysis
ear ossicle
endochondral
endosteum
epiphyseal disk
epiphysis
ethmoid
femur
fibula
fontanel
foramen magnum
gout
humerus
hyoid
ilium
intramembranous
ischium
lacunae
lamella
ligament
mandible
marrow
mastoid process

CHAPTER OUTLINE

- Bone Structure
- Functions of Bones
- Bone Growth
- The Skull
- The Spinal Column
- The Rib Cage
- Bones of the Shoulders, Arms, and Hands
- Bones of the Hips, Legs, and Feet
- Bone Fractures
- Joints

OBJECTIVES

After completing Chapter 7, you will be able to:

7.1 Describe the parts of a long bone.
7.2 List the substances that make up bone tissue.
7.3 List the functions of bones.
7.4 Describe how long bones grow.
7.5 List the bones of the skull, spinal column, rib cage, shoulders, arms, hands, hips, legs, and feet. Describe the location of each bone.
7.6 Define fontanels and explain their importance.
7.7 List different types of bone fractures and describe their characteristics.
7.8 Explain how fractures heal.
7.9 Describe the three major types of joints and give examples of each.
7.10 Describe the structure of a synovial joint.
7.11 Describe the characteristics, causes, and treatments of various diseases and disorders of the skeleton.

KEY TERMS *(Continued)*

maxillae
medullary cavity
metacarpal
metatarsal
nasal
occipital
ossification
osteoblast
osteoclast
osteocyte
osteon
osteoporosis
osteosarcoma
palatine
parietal
patella
pectoral girdle
pelvic girdle
periosteum
phalanges
pubis
radius
sacrum
scapula
scoliosis
sella turcica
sphenoid
sternum
suture
synovial
tarsal
temporal
tibia
ulna
vomer
zygomatic

Introduction

Bones provide the body with structure and support. In this chapter you will learn about the bones of the body, their structure, and how the joints of the body work. The skeletal system is composed of 206 bones as well as joints and related connective tissues. The skeleton has two major divisions—the **axial** skeleton and the **appendicular** skeleton. The axial skeleton contains 80 bones. It includes the bones of the skull, vertebral column, and rib cage. It functions to support the head, neck, and trunk and protects the brain, spinal cord, and the organs in the thorax. The **hyoid** bone, which anchors the tongue, is also included in the axial skeleton. The appendicular skeleton includes the bones of the arms, the legs, the **pectoral girdle** and the **pelvic girdle.** The pectoral girdle attaches the arms to the axial skeleton, and the pelvic girdle attaches the legs to the axial skeleton (Figure 7-1).

CASE STUDY

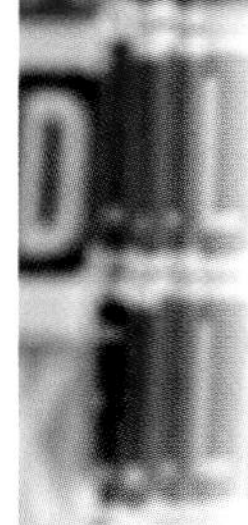

Yesterday afternoon, an 11-year-old boy came to the orthopedic clinic with a closed fracture at the distal end of his left radius (Colles fracture). His chart also notes that the distal epiphyseal plate was damaged as a result of the break.

As you read this chapter, consider the following questions:

1. Where is the distal end of the left radius?
2. Will this patient need surgery?
3. Have other tissues been damaged besides bone?
4. Why is the damage to the epiphyseal plate of special concern?

Bone Structure

Bones contain various kinds of tissues, including osseous tissue, blood vessels, and nerves. Osseous tissue can appear compact or spongy (Figure 7-2). At the microscopic level, spongy bone has more spaces within it than compact bone does. These spaces are filled with red marrow. Compact bone looks solid; however, the following structures can be observed with a microscope (Figure 7-3):

- **Osteons.** Osteons are elongated cylinders that run up and down the long axis of the bone. Each osteon has a central canal that contains blood vessels and nerves.
- Bone matrix. The matrix is the substance between bone cells. Bone cells are called **osteocytes.** The components of the matrix are inorganic salts, collagen fibers, and proteins. The primary salt of the matrix is calcium phosphate. This salt makes the matrix of bone very hard.
- **Lamella.** Lamella are layers of bone surrounding the canals of osteons.
- **Lacunae.** Lacunae are holes in the matrix of bone that hold osteocytes.
- **Canaliculi.** These tiny canals connect lacunae to each other. They allow osteocytes to spread nutrients to each other.

All bones are made up of both compact and spongy bone. They are classified according to their shape:

- Long bones. Long bones are located primarily in the arms and legs. Examples include the **femur** (thigh bone) and the **humerus** (upper arm bone). Long bones have the following parts (Figure 7-4):
  - **Diaphysis**—the shaft of a long bone. It is tubular and consists of a thick collar of compact bone that surrounds a central medullary cavity.
  - **Epiphysis**—the expanded end of a long bone. It consists of a thin layer of compact bone surrounding spongy bone. Long bones have an epiphysis at both ends.
  - **Articular cartilage**—the cartilage that covers the epiphyses of long bones. It functions to cushion bones and to absorb stress during bone movements.
  - **Medullary cavity**—a canal that runs through the center of the diaphysis. In adults it contains yellow bone **marrow,** which is mostly fat.
  - **Periosteum**—a membrane that surrounds the diaphysis. It contains bone-forming cells, dense fibrous connective tissue, nerves, and blood vessels.
  - **Endosteum**—a membrane that lines the medullary cavity and the holes of spongy bone. It contains bone-forming cells.

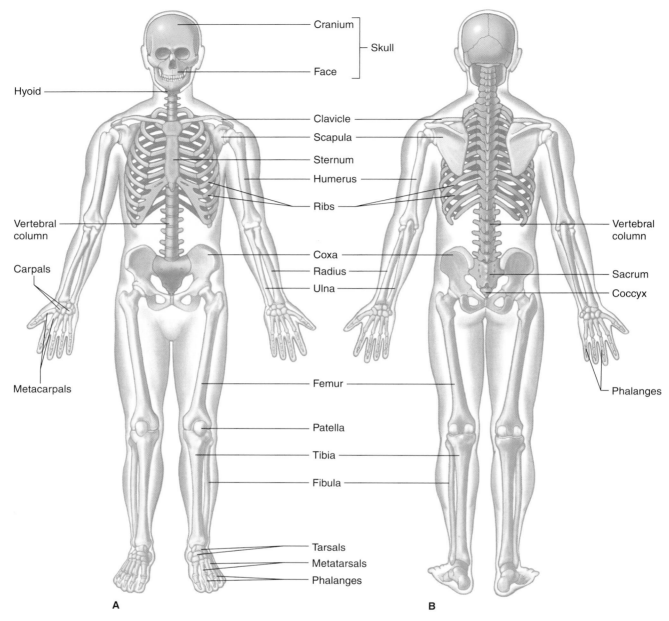

Figure 7-1. Major bones of the skeleton: (a) anterior view and (b) posterior view. The axial skeleton is shown in orange and the appendicular skeleton is shown in yellow.

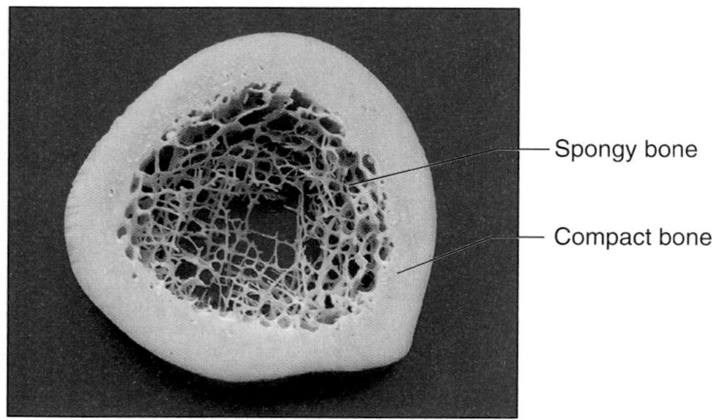

Figure 7-2. Cross section of bone showing compact and spongy bone tissue.

- Short bones. The small bones are located in the wrists and ankles. Examples include the **carpals** (wrist bones) and some of the **tarsals** (ankle bones).
- Flat bones. Flat bones are primarily located in the skull and rib cage. Examples include the ribs and frontal bone.
- Irregular bones. Irregular bones include the vertebrae and the bones of the pelvic girdle.

Functions of Bones

Bones have many functions. They give shape to body parts such as the head, legs, arms, and trunk. Bones also support and protect soft structures in the body. For

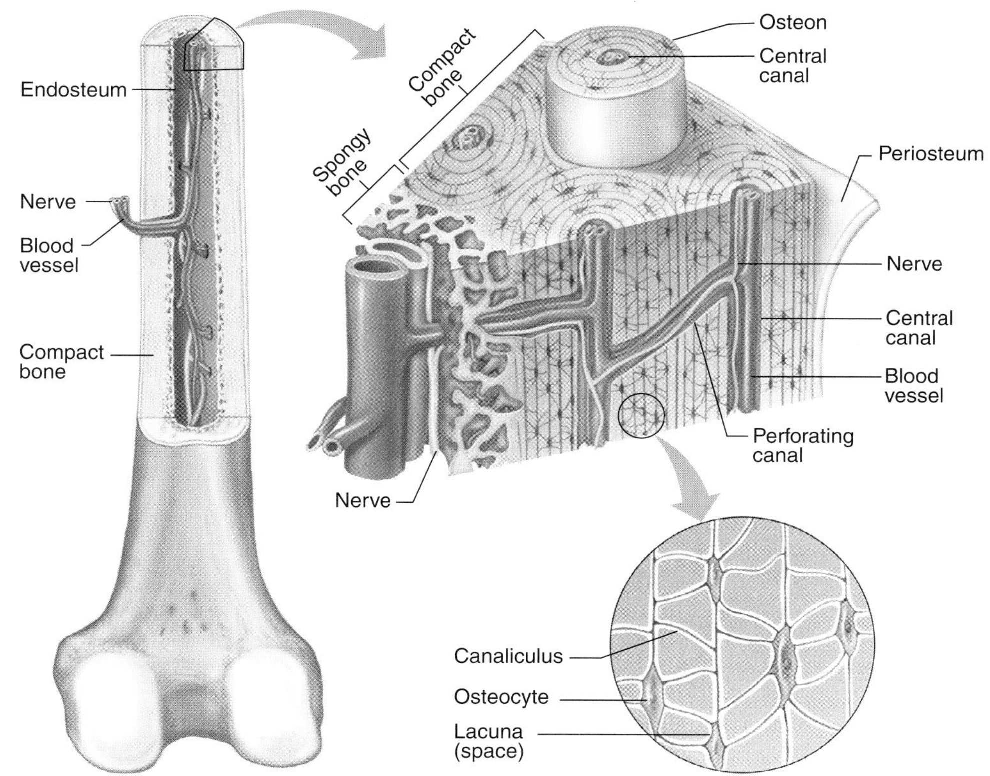

Figure 7-3. Compact bone at the microscopic level.

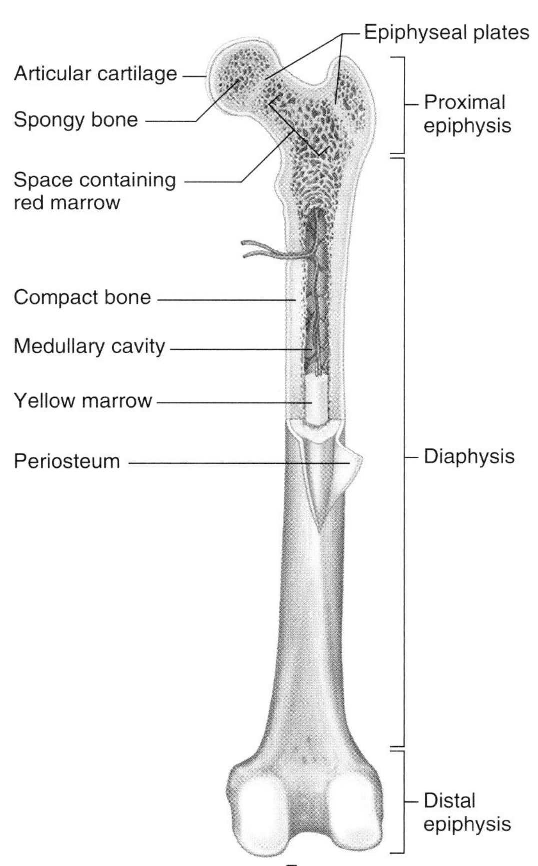

Figure 7-4. Parts of a long bone.

example, the skull protects the brain. Bones also function in body movement because skeletal muscles attach to them.

The red marrow of bone produces new blood cells. Red bone marrow is normally found in spaces of spongy bone. Bones also store calcium for the body. Every cell in the body needs calcium, so the body must have a large supply readily available.

Bone Growth

Bones grow through a process called **ossification.** Two types of ossification are intramembranous and endochondral.

In **intramembranous** ossification, bones begin as tough, fibrous membranes. Eventually, bone-forming cells called **osteoblasts** turn the membrane to bone. Intramembranous bones are found in the skull, except for the lower jawbone.

In **endochondral** ossification, bones start out as cartilage models. Eventually, the osteoblasts form a bone collar around the diaphysis of the cartilage model. Then bone is formed in the diaphysis of the bone. This area is called the primary ossification center. Later, the epiphyses turn to bone (secondary ossification centers), and the medullary cavity and spaces in spongy bone are formed. The cells that form holes in bone are called **osteoclasts.** As long as a bone contains some cartilage between an

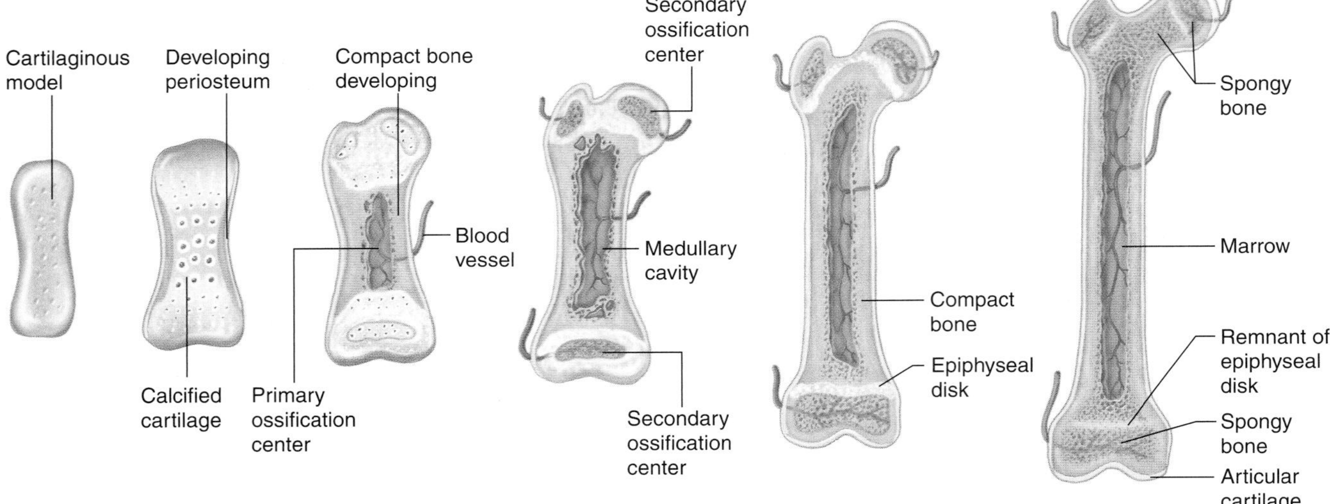

Figure 7-5. Steps in endochondral ossification.

epiphysis and the diaphysis, it can continue to grow in length. This plate of cartilage is called an **epiphyseal disk.** Once the cartilage is gone, bone growth stops. For most people, bone growth stops between the ages of 18 and 25 (Figure 7-5).

Even after bone growth stops, osteoclasts and osteoblasts continually remodel bone tissue. Throughout life, osteoclasts break down bone when the body needs more calcium in the blood, and osteoblasts replace the bone when there is excess calcium in the blood.

Pathophysiology

Common Diseases and Disorders of Bone

Bursitis is inflammation of a bursa, which is a fluid-filled sac that cushions tendons. It occurs most commonly in the elbow, knee, shoulder, and hip.

- **Causes.** Overuse of and trauma to joints are the most common causes of this condition. Bacterial infections can also cause bursitis.
- **Signs and symptoms.** Signs and symptoms include joint pain and swelling as well as tenderness in the structures surrounding the joint.
- **Treatment.** The most common treatments are bed rest, pain medications, steroid injections, aspiration of excess fluid from the bursa, and antibiotics.

Carpal tunnel syndrome occurs when the median nerve in the wrist is excessively compressed. Typists, assembly-line workers, painters, and people who play sports such as racquetball are most likely to develop carpal tunnel syndrome.

- **Causes.** Overuse of the wrist is a common cause of this syndrome.
- **Signs and symptoms.** Weakness and numbness in the hand, and pain in the wrist, hand, or elbow are common symptoms.
- **Treatment.** This condition can be treated with wrist splints, pain medications, and steroid injections and by having the patient change work habits to better position and support the wrists. If these treatments do not improve the patient's condition, surgery to reduce pressure on the nerves may be needed.

Ewing's family of tumors (EFT) is a group of tumors that affect different tissue types. However, the tumors primarily affect bone.

- **Causes.** Causes of EFT are not clear, but it most often affects Caucasians, the long bones of the body, and people between the ages of 10 and 20.
- **Signs and symptoms.** Fever, pain in the tumor location, fractures, and bruises in the tumor location are the primary symptoms.

continued ⟶

Common Diseases and Disorders of Bone *(continued)*

- **Treatment.** Treatment options include surgery, chemotherapy, radiation therapy, a bone marrow transplant, or a stem cell transplant.

Gout is a type of arthritis that usually occurs more frequently with age.

- **Causes.** Gout is caused by deposits of uric acid crystals in the joints. People with gout cannot break down uric acid properly and remove it from their bloodstream.
- **Signs and symptoms.** Symptoms include sudden or chronic joint pain, joint swelling and stiffness, and fever.
- **Treatment.** The most common treatments are pain medications and changes to the patient's diet. Patients should eliminate from their diet certain foods that cause the formation of uric acid (meats, fish, beer, or wine).

Osteogenesis imperfecta is more commonly called brittle-bone disease. People with this disease have decreased amounts of collagen in their bones, which leads to very fragile bones. There are four types of this disease: type 1 is the most common, and type 2 is the most severe.

- **Causes.** The disorder is hereditary and very often runs in a family.
- **Signs and symptoms.** Signs and symptoms include fractures (all types), blue sclera (type 1), dental problems (types 1 and 4), hearing loss (type 1), a triangular face (type 1), abnormal spinal curves (types 1 and 4), very small stature (types 2 and 3), a small chest (type 2), a barrel-shaped chest (type 3), fractures at birth (type 3), loose joints (types 3 and 4), and small muscles (type 3).
- **Treatment.** Because there are many symptoms of this disease, the list of treatments is extensive and includes the following: fractures, surgery to strengthen bones by inserting metal rods into them, dental procedures, physical therapy, braces to prevent bone deformities, wheelchairs and other supportive aids, medications, and counseling. Other surgeries may be required to treat lung and heart problems that sometimes occur with this disease.

Osteoporosis is a condition in which bones become thinned over time. It is a very common disorder in the United States and affects women more than men and Caucasians more than any other race. This condition occurs when bone is broken down to release calcium into the blood but it is not sufficiently replaced.

- **Causes.** The causes include hormone deficiencies (estrogen in women and testosterone in men), a sedentary lifestyle, a lack of calcium and vitamin D in the diet, bone cancers, corticosteroid excess (usually as a result of endocrine diseases), smoking, excess alcohol consumption, and the use of steroids.
- **Signs and symptoms.** There are usually no symptoms in the early stages of this disease. Patients may later experience fractures (usually in spine, wrists, or hips), back and neck pain, a loss of height over time, and an abnormal curving of the spine.
- **Treatment.** The most common treatments include medications to prevent bone loss and relieve bone pain, estrogen replacement therapy, lifestyle changes to prevent bone loss (including regular exercise and diets or supplements that include calcium, phosphorous, and vitamin D), moderation in use of alcohol, and stopping smoking.

Osteosarcoma is a type of bone cancer that originates from osteoblasts, the cells that make bony tissue. It occurs most often in children, teens, and young adults and more often in males than females. Usually this type of cancer affects bones of the legs.

- **Causes.** The causes of this type of cancer are unclear.
- **Signs and symptoms.** Primary symptoms include pain in affected bones (usually the legs), swelling around affected bones, and an increase in pain with movement of the affected bones.
- **Treatment.** Treatments include surgery, chemotherapy, and radiation therapy. Amputation of the affected limb, followed by a prosthesis fitting, may be needed in some cases.

Paget's disease causes bones to enlarge and become deformed and weak. It usually affects people over the age of 40.

- **Causes.** This disease may be caused by a virus or various hereditary factors.
- **Signs and symptoms.** Bone pain, deformed bones, and fractures are common symptoms. Patients may experience headaches and hearing loss if the disease affects skull bones.
- **Treatment.** Treatments include surgery to remodel bones, hip replacements, medications to prevent bone weakening, and physical therapy.

Scoliosis is an abnormal curvature of the spine.

- **Causes.** This disorder can develop prenatally when vertebrae do not fuse together. It can also result from diseases that cause weakness of the muscles that hold vertebrae together. Other causes of scoliosis are unknown but they may be genetic.
- **Signs and symptoms.** A patient with scoliosis usually has a spine that looks bent to one side, with one shoulder or hip appearing to be higher than the other. Patients often experience back pain.
- **Treatment.** Treatment includes different types of back braces, surgery to correct spinal curves, and physical therapy.

Educating the Patient

Building Better Bones

Bone health is influenced by many factors, including diet, exercise, and a person's overall lifestyle. You can help patients improve or maintain their bone health by teaching them about behaviors that will support bone health.

Bone-Healthy Diet

Good nutrition is essential for proper bone growth during childhood and the teen years. It is equally important in adulthood in order to maintain healthy bones. Bone-building nutrients are found in dairy products, broccoli, kale, spinach, salmon, sardines, egg yolks, whole grains, and fruits—especially bananas and oranges. Calcium and vitamin D are particularly important for healthy bones. Without vitamin D, calcium cannot be absorbed from the digestive tract into the bloodstream. Without calcium, bone tissue will slowly wear away. Supplements can always be taken if a person's diet does not include adequate amounts of calcium and vitamin D.

Bone-Healthy Exercises

Weight-bearing and strength-training exercises are best for bone health. When your muscles contract, they pull on your bones. This tension stimulates bones to thicken and strengthen. Lifting weights is an effective way to increase the tension on bones. Other activities such as jogging, walking briskly, or playing a sport regularly will also stimulate bones to increase in density.

Bone-Healthy Lifestyle

A person with a bone-healthy lifestyle avoids smoking and alcohol. Smoking rids the body of calcium, which is necessary for bone growth. Alcohol prevents calcium absorption in the digestive tract. People who smoke are almost twice as likely to develop osteoporosis as nonsmokers.

Bone Tests

Bone-density tests and bone scans are currently the most useful tools in determining bone health. Bone-density tests are painless procedures used to determine the density of a person's bones. Because osteoporosis shows no symptoms in early stages, these tests are important to have done when your doctor recommends them. Bone scans help diagnose the causes of bone pain, arthritis, bone infections, and bone cancers. These scans use radioactive dyes that are injected into the patient and that concentrate in bone tissue.

The Skull

Skull bones are divided into two types: cranial and facial bones. Cranial bones form the top, sides, and back of the skull. Facial bones form the face (Figure 7-6). The skull bones of an infant are not completely formed. The "soft spots" felt on an infant's skull are actually **fontanels,** which are tough membranes that connect the incompletely developed bones.

The major cranial bones are the following:

- The frontal bone forms the anterior portion of the cranium. It is also called the forehead bone.
- **Parietal** bones form most of the top and sides of the skull.
- The **occipital** bone forms the back of the skull. A large hole in the occipital bone is called the **foramen magnum.** It allows the brain to connect to the spinal cord. Two bumps called occipital **condyles** are on either side of the foramen magnum. They sit on top of the first vertebra. When you nod your head, your occipital condyles are rocking back and forth on the first vertebra of the spinal column.
- Two **temporal** bones form the lower sides of the skull. A canal called the external auditory meatus runs through each temporal bone. This canal is commonly called the ear canal. A large bump called the **mastoid process** is located on each temporal bone just behind each ear. Mastoid processes are where major neck muscles attach to your skull.
- A **sphenoid** bone forms part of the floor of the cranium. It is shaped like a butterfly. In the center of this bone is a deep depression called the **sella turcica.** The pituitary gland sits in this deep depression.
- **Ethmoid** bones are between the sphenoid bone and the nasal bones. They also form part of the floor of the cranium.
- **Ear ossicles** are the smallest bones of the body. They are the malleus, incus, and stapes and are in the middle ear cavities of the temporal bones.

The following are major facial bones:

- The **mandible** is the lower jawbone and is the only moveable bone in the skull. It anchors the lower teeth and forms the chin.
- The **maxillae** form the upper jawbone. They anchor the upper teeth to form the central portion of the facial skeleton.
- The **zygomatic** bones form the prominence of the cheeks.

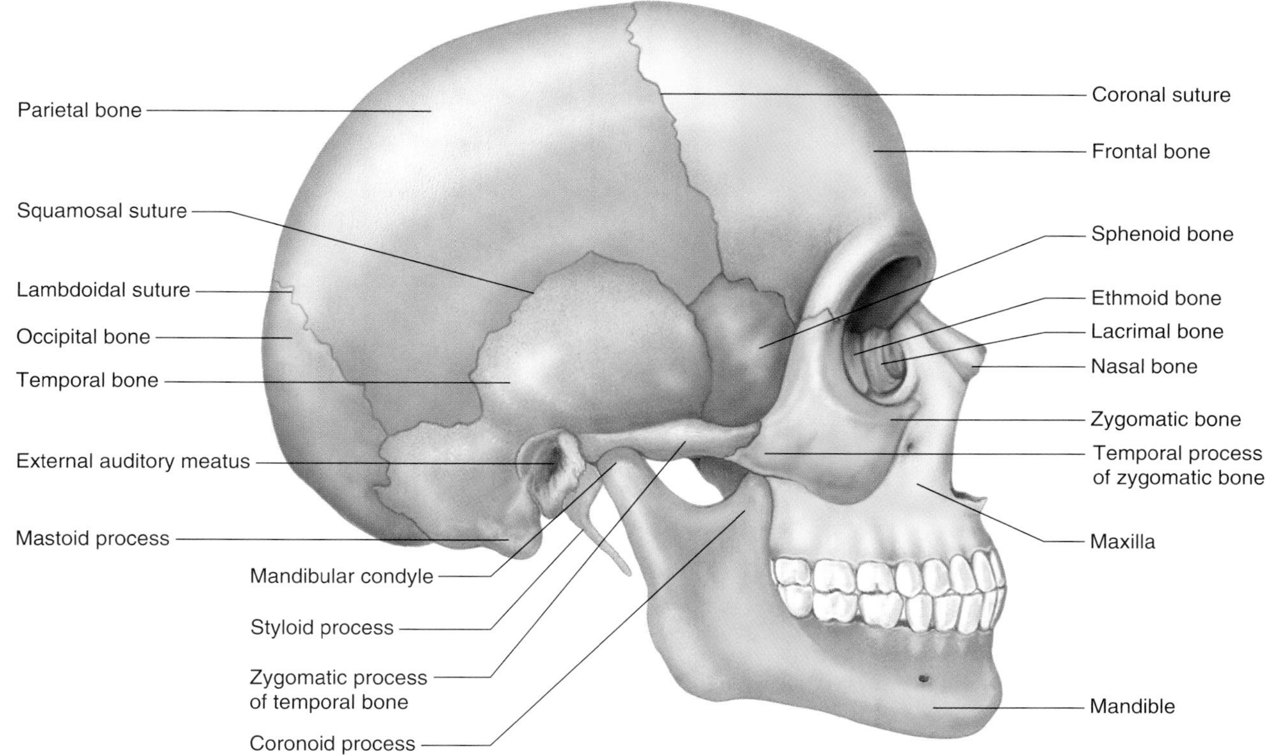

Figure 7-6. Lateral view of the skull.

- Several thin **nasal** bones fuse together to form the bridge of the nose.
- **Palatine** bones form the anterior portion of the palate, which is the roof of the mouth.
- The **vomer** is a thin bone that divides the nasal cavity.

The Spinal Column

The spinal column consists of 7 cervical vertebrae, 12 thoracic vertebrae, 5 lumbar vertebrae, a sacrum, and a coccyx (Figure 7-7):

- Cervical vertebrae are the smallest and lightest of the vertebrae and are located in the neck region. The first cervical vertebra is called the **atlas** and the second is called the **axis.** When you turn your head from side to side, your atlas is pivoting around your axis.
- Thoracic vertebrae join the 12 pairs of ribs. They have long, sharp, spinous processes that you can feel when you run your finger down someone's spine.
- Lumbar vertebrae have very sturdy structures. They form the small of the back and bear the most weight of all the vertebrae.
- The **sacrum** is a triangular-shaped bone that consists of five fused vertebrae. The **coccyx** is a small, triangular-shaped bone made up of three to five fused vertebrae and is considered unnecessary. It is more commonly called the tailbone.

The Rib Cage

The rib cage is made of 12 pairs of ribs and the **sternum** (Figure 7-8). The sternum forms the front, middle portion of the rib cage. It is often called the breastplate. The sternum joins with the clavicles and most ribs. All 12 pairs of ribs are attached posteriorly to thoracic vertebrae. Most ribs are also attached to structures anteriorly. Based on what ribs attach to anteriorly, they can be classified as follows:

- True. The first seven pairs of ribs are true ribs. They attach directly to the sternum through pieces of cartilage called **costal** cartilages.
- False. Rib pairs 8, 9 and 10 are called false ribs. They attach to the costal cartilage of rib pair number 7.
- Floating. Rib pairs 11 and 12 are called floating ribs because they do not attach anteriorly to any structure.

Bones of the Shoulders, Arms, and Hands

The bones of the shoulders are called pectoral girdles and include **clavicles** and **scapulae.** They function to attach the arm to the trunk of the body. The clavicles are commonly known as the collarbones. They are slender in shape and each joins with the sternum and a scapula. Clavicles are very commonly broken bones in body.

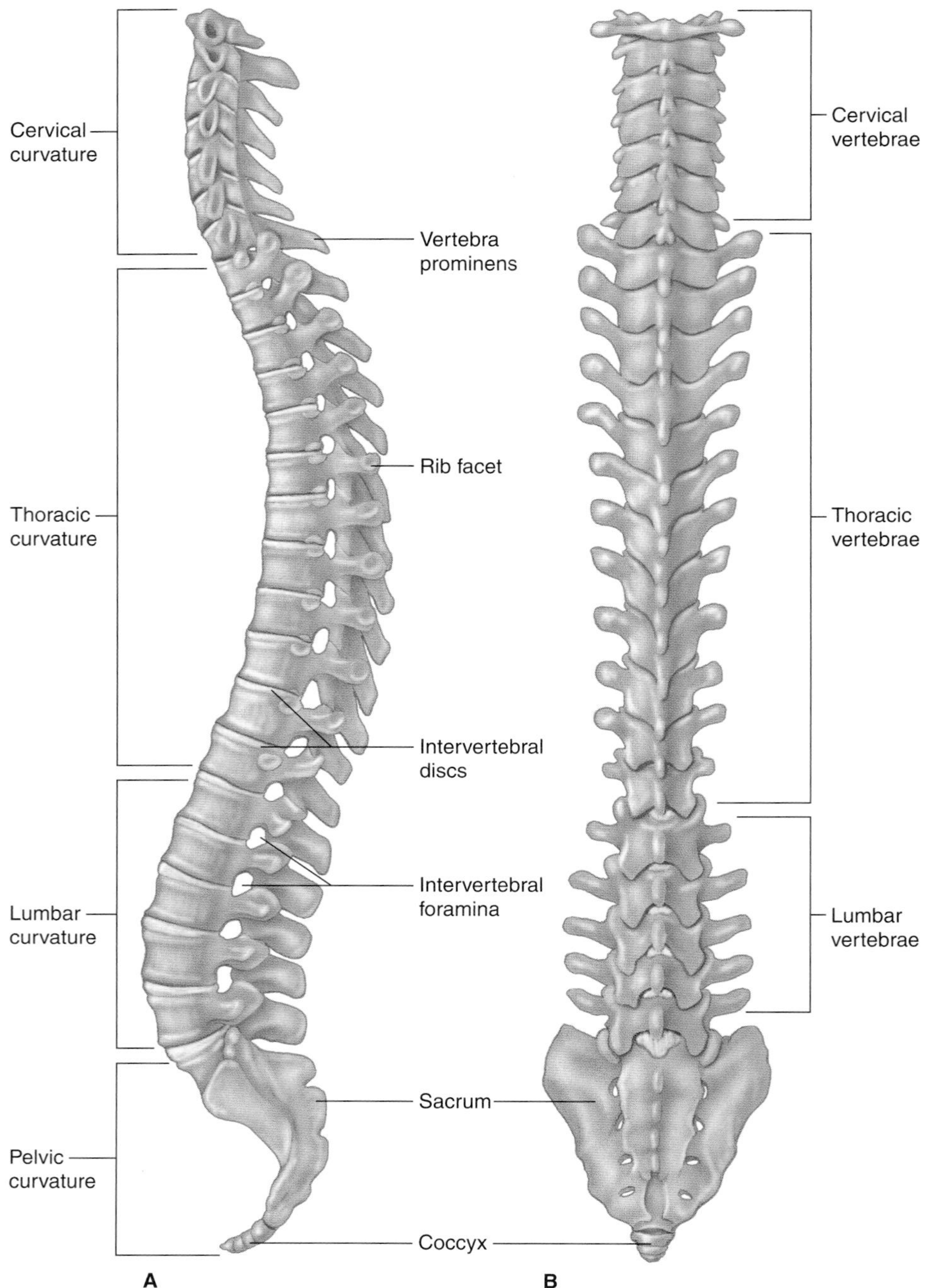

Figure 7-7. Vertebral column: (a) lateral view and (b) posterior view.

Scapulae are thin, triangular-shaped flat bones. They are also called shoulder blades and are located on the dorsal surface of the rib cage. Each scapula joins with the head of a humerus and a clavicle.

The upper limb, or arm, bones include the humerus, radius, and ulna. The humerus is located in the upper part of the arm. It joins with the scapula, the radius, and the ulna. The **radius** is the lateral bone of the forearm. It is on the same side of the arm as your thumb. It joins with the humerus, the ulna, and the wrist bones. The **ulna** is the medial bone of the lower arm. It joins with the humerus to form the elbow joint. It also joins with the radius and some of the bones of the wrist.

The bones of the hand include carpals, metacarpals, and phalanges. Carpals are wrist bones. Each wrist contains eight marble-sized carpal bones. **Metacarpals** form the palms of the hands. Each hand has five metacarpals. **Phalanges** are the bones of the fingers. There are 14 phalanges in each hand—three for each finger and two per thumb.

Refer to Figure 7-1 for the bones of the shoulders, arms, and hands.

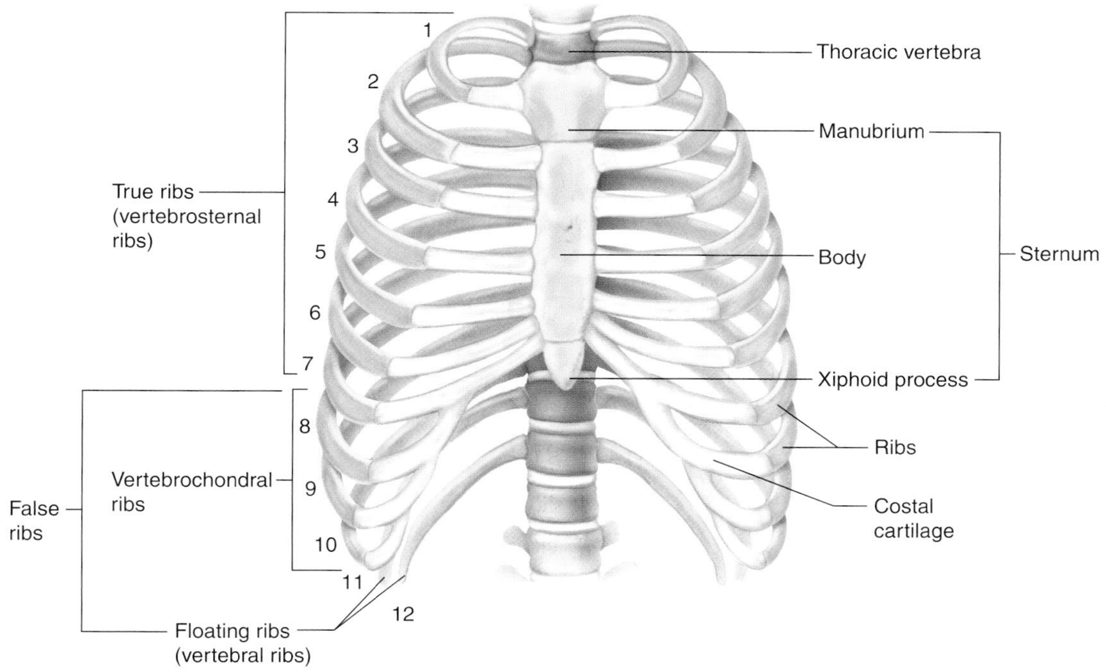

Figure 7-8. Rib cage.

Bones of the Hips, Legs, and Feet

The hipbones are also called **coxal** bones. They attach the leg to the axial skeleton. They also protect pelvic organs. Each coxal bone has three parts: the ilium, the ischium, and the pubis. The **ilium** is the most superior part of a coxal bone. When you put your hands on your hips, you are touching the ilium. The **ischium** forms the lower part of a coxal bone and the pubis forms the front. The **pubis** bones of each coxal bone join together to form the pubic symphysis, which is also referred to as the pelvic girdle (Figure 7-9).

The bones of the lower limb, or leg, include the femur, the patella, the tibia, and the fibula. The femur is the thighbone and the largest bone in the body. It joins with the hipbone, the tibia, and the **patella** (kneecap). The **tibia** is the

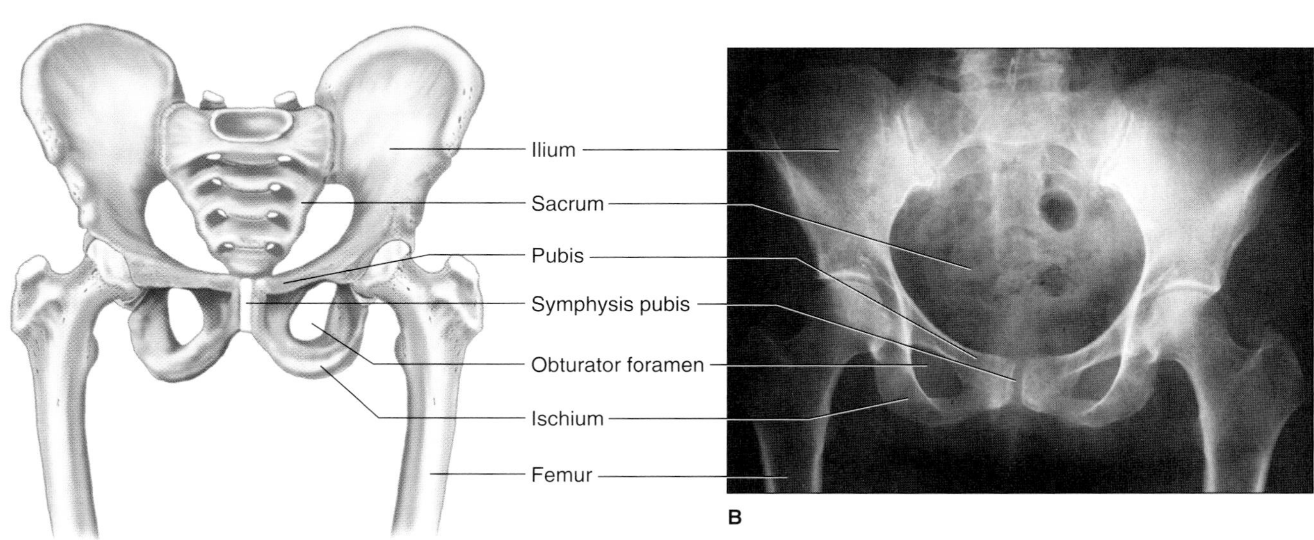

Figure 7-9. (a) Pelvic girdle. (b) Radiograph of the pelvic girdle.

medial bone of the lower leg. It is commonly called the shinbone. It joins with the femur, the fibula, and the anklebones. The **fibula** is the lateral bone of the lower leg. It is much thinner than the tibia. It joins with the anklebones.

The bones of the foot include the tarsals, the metatarsals, and the phalanges. The tarsal bones form the back of the foot. The **calcaneus,** or heel bone, is the largest tarsal bone. There are seven tarsal bones per foot. **Metatarsals** are bones that form the front of the foot. There are five metatarsals per foot. The bones of the toes are called phalanges. Each foot contains 14—two for each big toe and three in all the other toes.

Refer to Figure 7-1 for the bones of the hips, legs, and feet.

Bone Fractures

Bone fractures can be classified in many ways. For example, if a bone breaks because of trauma such as a car accident or sports injury, it is called a stress fracture. If a bone breaks because of some disease process, it is called a pathologic fracture. Table 7-1 defines some other commonly used terms to describe various types of fractures (also see Figure 7-10).

A broken bone may take three months or longer to heal, depending on the type of fracture and the general health of the patient. Fractures must be reduced, or set back into their normal position. If surgery is required to reduce the fracture, this procedure is called an open reduction. Pins, screws, or plates are often used to hold the bone fragments together. If surgery is not required to set the bones, the procedure is called a closed reduction. Once fractures are reduced, it is important to immobilize the bone with braces or casts while the bone heals.

When a bone breaks, the following steps occur in the body's repair of the bone (Figure 7-11):

1. A hematoma (blood clot) forms around the fracture.
2. Granulation tissue slowly replaces the hematoma. Granulation tissue is a very delicate tissue made up of capillaries and various cells. The cells include macrophages, which help to prevent microbes from invading the broken bone. Other cells include fibroblasts that produce collagen fibers to help hold the bone ends together and osteoblasts that will start to make new bone tissue.
3. A soft callus is formed that replaces the granulation tissue. The soft callus contains cartilage that holds the broken ends of the bones securely together.
4. A hard callus replaces the soft callus. Bone tissue makes up the hard callus, and this is the structure that cements the broken ends back together most securely.
5. The hard callus is remodeled so that it takes on the shape of the original bone.

TABLE 7-1 Types of Fractures

Type	Description
Closed (simple)	Ends of fractured bone do not break through skin
Open (compound)	Ends of fractured bone break through skin
Complete	Bone is completely broken into two or more pieces
Incomplete	Bone is partially broken
Greenstick	Bone is bent on one side and has an incomplete fracture on the opposite side
Hairline	Bone has fine cracks but bone sections remain in place
Comminuted	Bone is broken into three or more pieces
Displaced	Ends of fractured bone move out of the normal position
Nondisplaced	Ends of fractured bone stay in the normal position
Impacted	Piece of broken bone is forced into a space of another bone fragment
Depressed	Fractured bone forms a concavity; mostly seen in skull fractures
Linear	Fracture is parallel to the long axis of the bone
Transverse	Fracture is perpendicular to the long axis of the bone
Oblique	Fracture runs diagonally across the bone
Spiral	Fracture spirals around long axis of bone, usually the result of twisting a bone
Colles	Fracture is at the distal end of the radius and ulna
Potts	Fracture is at the distal end of the tibia or fibula

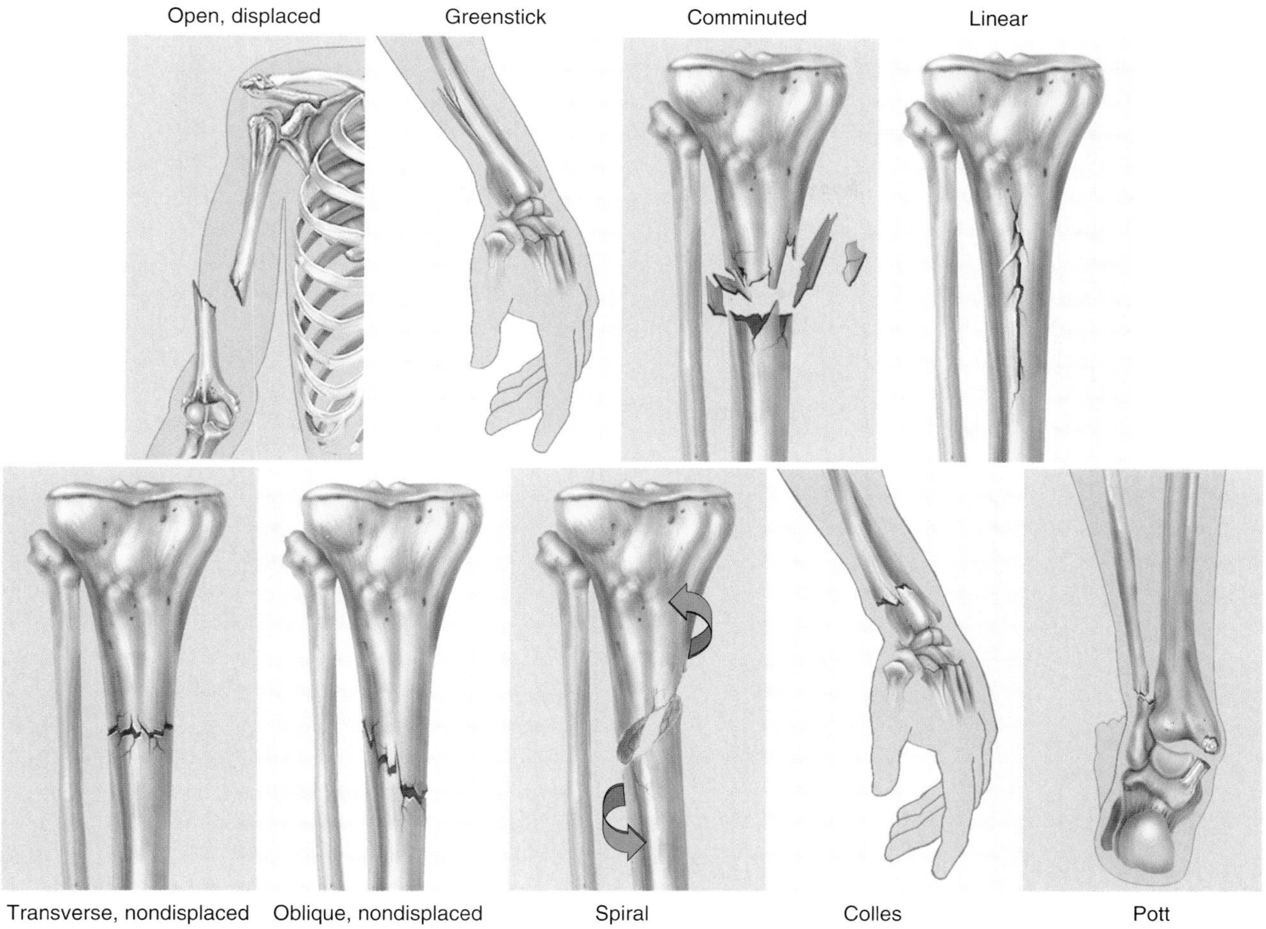

Open, displaced
Greenstick
Comminuted
Linear
Transverse, nondisplaced
Oblique, nondisplaced
Spiral
Colles
Pott

Figure 7-10. Types of bone fractures.

Medullary cavity
Hematoma
Compact bone
Fibrocartilage
Soft callus
New blood vessels
Hard callus
Spongy bone
A
B
C
D

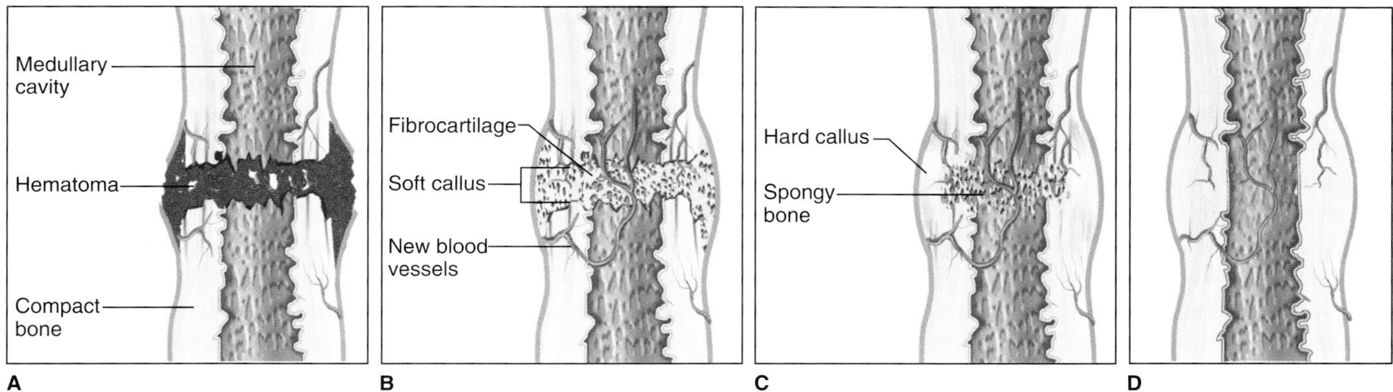

Figure 7-11. The healing of a bone fracture includes (a) hematoma formation, (b) soft callus formation, (c) hard callus formation, and (d) the remodeling of bone.

Joints

Joints are the junctions between bones. Based on their structure, joints can be classified as fibrous, cartilaginous, or synovial.

The bones of fibrous joints are connected together with short fibers. Therefore, the bones of this type of joint do not normally move against each other. Most fibrous joints are found between cranial bones and facial bones. Fibrous joints in the skull are called **sutures.**

Educating the Patient

Falls and Fractures

Falls account for about 50% of all fractures, so it is important to teach patients about preventing falls. Although most fractures are not life-threatening, some are. For example, hip fractures in the elderly can result in complications such as pneumonia. Approximately half of all patients who suffer hip fractures will use some type of walking aid for the rest of their lives.

Persons most at risk for falling are those with the following conditions:

- Muscle weakness
- Difficulty walking
- Poor vision
- Dependence on bifocals
- Hearing loss
- Dependence on medications that cause dizziness or drowsiness
- Alzheimer's disease
- Parkinson's disease

Falls can be prevented through the following steps:

- Awareness. Educate patients to try not to climb or stretch for items that they use regularly. Instead, they should move these items to easy-to-reach places.
- Balance. Patients should stand up gradually, especially from a lying-down position. They should stand for a few seconds before walking. This allows time for blood flow to reach the brain, preventing dizziness.
- Lifestyle. Patients should drink alcohol in moderation in order to prevent falls that result from intoxication. They should also avoid foods high in sugar to prevent dizziness caused by sudden surges of blood sugar. You can also recommend that patients clean up any clutter in their living space so that they are less likely to trip on items.

When a fall can't be prevented, the following steps may be helpful:

- Falling backward, instead of forward or sideways, is less risky.
- Breaking the fall with one's hands is better than not breaking the fall at all. Wrist fractures are painful but are not life-threatening like hip or skull fractures.
- Grabbing onto anything to help break the fall.
- Wearing soft shoes or padded clothing if prone to falls. Hip padding is available from doctors.

The bones of cartilaginous joints are connected together with a disc of cartilage. This type of joint is slightly moveable. The joints between vertebrae are cartilaginous joints.

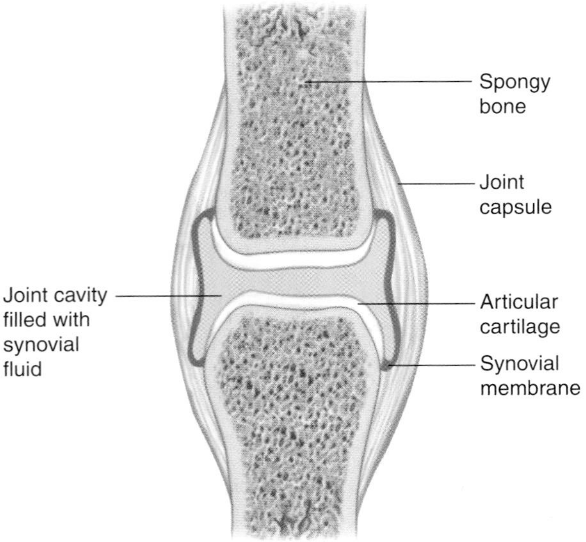

Figure 7-12. Structure of a synovial joint.

The bones of **synovial** joints are covered with hyaline cartilage and are held together by a fibrous joint capsule (Figure 7-12). The joint capsule is lined with a synovial membrane. The membrane secretes a slippery fluid called synovial fluid, which allows the bones to move easily against each other. Bones are also held together through tough, cord-like structures called **ligaments.** Synovial joints are freely moveable. Examples of synovial joints are the elbows, knees, shoulders, and knuckles.

Summary

The bones of the skeletal system are divided into two major divisions: the axial and the appendicular skeletons. In addition to bones, the skeletal system consists of cartilage, tendons, and ligaments. The skeletal system provides support for the body, protects internal organs, serves as attachments for muscles to produce movement, stores minerals such as calcium, and produces new blood cells. Bones are used as landmarks for procedures such as injections, electrocardiograms, and x-rays. It is important for medical assistants to have knowledge of this system in order to effectively perform their duties.

REVIEW

CHAPTER 7

CASE STUDY QUESTIONS

Now that you have completed this chapter, review the case study at the beginning of the chapter and answer the following questions:

1. Where is the distal end of the left radius?
2. Will this patient need surgery?
3. Have other tissues been damaged besides bone?
4. Why is the damage to the epiphyseal plate of special concern?

Discussion Questions

1. List and describe the functions of bone.
2. Describe how joints are classified. Give examples of each classification.
3. What are the bones and functions of the pectoral and pelvic girdles?

Critical Thinking Questions

1. If a 32-year-old woman developed arthritis, what type is she likely to have? Why?
2. If a physician needed a red bone marrow sample from a patient, from where is he likely to get the sample?
3. Tarsal bones are often called anklebones. Why is this term not entirely correct?

Application Activities

1. State whether each of the following is a bone of the axial skeleton or the appendicular skeleton.
   a. Humerus
   b. Femur
   c. Clavicle
   d. Parietal bone
   e. Nasal bone
   f. Ear ossicles
2. Name the bone that forms the following:
   a. Forehead
   b. Chin
   c. Palms of the hands
   d. Fingers
   e. Hip
   f. Cheekbone
3. Name the bone that contains the following:
   a. External auditory meatus
   b. Foramen magnum
   c. Sella turcica
   d. Mastoid process

Internet Activity

1. Go to the University of Maryland Web site **http://www.umm.edu/bone/** and choose Diagnostic Procedures. Answer the following questions:
   a. What is the role of MRI in diagnosing bone diseases?
   b. What are the two types of biopsy used?
   c. What is bone densitometry and what is it used for?

CHAPTER 8

The Muscular System

KEY TERMS

abduction
acetylcholine
acetylcholinesterase
adduction
aerobic respiration
antagonist
aponeurosis
botulism
circumduction
creatine phosphate
depression
dorsiflexion
elevation
endomysium
epimysium
eversion
extension
fascia
fascicle
fibromyalgia
flexion
hyperextension
insertion
intercalated disc
inversion
Krebs cycle
lactic acid
multiunit smooth muscle
muscle fatigue
muscle fiber
muscular dystrophy
myasthenia gravis
myofibrils
myoglobin

CHAPTER OUTLINE

- Functions of Muscle
- Types of Muscle Tissue
- Production of Energy for Muscle
- Structure of Skeletal Muscles
- Attachments and Actions of Skeletal Muscles
- Major Skeletal Muscles

OBJECTIVES

After completing Chapter 8, you will be able to:

8.1 List the functions of muscle.
8.2 Explain how muscle tissue generates energy.
8.3 List the three types of muscle tissue and describe the locations and characteristics of each.
8.4 Describe how smooth muscle produces peristalsis.
8.5 Describe the structure of a skeletal muscle.
8.6 List and define the various types of body movements produced by skeletal muscles.
8.7 Define the terms *origin* and *insertion.*
8.8 List the major skeletal muscles of the body and give the action of each.
8.9 Describe various disorders and diseases of the muscular system.

KEY TERMS *(Continued)*

norepinephrine
origin
oxygen debt
perimysium
peristalsis
plantar flexion
prime mover
pronation
protraction
retraction
rhabdomyolysis
rotation
sarcolemma
sarcoplasm
sarcoplasmic reticulum
sphincter
striations
supination
synergist
tendon
tetanus
trichinosis
visceral smooth muscle

Introduction

Bones and joints do not themselves produce movement. By alternating between contraction and relaxation, muscles cause bones and supported structures to move. The human body has more than 600 individual muscles. Although each muscle is a distinct structure, muscles act in groups to perform particular movements. This chapter focuses on the differences among three muscle tissue types, the structure of skeletal muscles, muscle actions, and the names of skeletal muscles.

CASE STUDY

Five days ago, a 40-year-old woman came to the doctor's office where you work as a medical assistant. She complained about pain in her back and right leg. Because this patient had a history of disc damage in her spine, she was sent home with pain medication and an order for bed rest for a 24-hour period. Two days later, she returned to the office with nausea, a severe headache, muscle twitching in her legs and arms, severe back pain, and tightness in her chest. The doctor once more asked the patient to elaborate on her activities the day before she fell ill. He was told that she had sprayed her furniture and carpets with an organophosphate insecticide to get rid of fleas in her house. She had also dipped her cats and dogs with the same insecticide. The doctor explained that organophosphates block acetylcholinesterase and immediately transferred her to the hospital for respiratory therapy and medicine to combat the insecticide poisoning.

As you read this chapter, consider the following questions:

1. What is the function of acetylcholinesterase?
2. Why does this patient exhibit muscle twitching and back pain?
3. What type of respiratory therapy will this patient require?
4. What precautions should a person take when using insecticides that contain organophosphates?
5. Why is it important for patients to give their doctor a complete account of their activities prior to an illness?

Functions of Muscle

Muscle tissue is unique because it has the ability to contract. It is this contraction that allows muscles to perform various functions. In addition to allowing the human body to move, muscles provide stability, the control of body openings and passages, and warming of the body.

Movement

Because skeletal muscles are attached to bones, when they contract, the bones attached to them move. This allows for various body motions, such as walking or waving your hand. Facial muscles are attached to the skin of the face, so when they contract, different facial expressions are produced, such as smiling or frowning. Smooth muscle is found in the walls of various organs, such as the stomach, intestines, and uterus. The contraction of smooth muscle in these organs produces movements of their contents, such as the movement of food material through the intestine. Cardiac muscle in the heart produces the pumping of blood into blood vessels.

Stability

You rarely think about it but muscles are holding your bones tightly together so that your joints remain stable. There are also very small muscles holding your vertebrae together to make your spinal column stable.

Control of Body Openings and Passages

Muscles form valve-like structures called **sphincters** around various body openings and passages. These sphincters control the movement of substances into and out of these passages. For example, a urethral sphincter prevents urination, or it can be relaxed to permit urination.

Heat Production

When muscles contract, heat is released, which helps the body maintain a normal temperature. This is why moving your body can make you warmer if you are cold.

Types of Muscle Tissue

There are three types of muscle tissue: skeletal, smooth, and cardiac. Study Table 8-1 to review their locations and features.

Muscle cells are called **muscle fibers** because of their long lengths. The cell membrane of a muscle fiber is called a **sarcolemma.** The cytoplasm of this cell type is called **sarcoplasm,** and the endoplasmic reticulum is called **sarcoplasmic reticulum.** Most of the sarcoplasm is filled with long structures called **myofibrils.** The arrangement of filaments in myofibrils produce the **striations** observed in skeletal and cardiac muscle cells. Muscle fibers are controlled by motor neurons that release neurotransmitters onto the fibers. See Figure 8-1 for an illustration of the structure of a skeletal muscle.

Skeletal Muscle

Skeletal muscle fibers respond only to the neurotransmitter **acetylcholine.** Acetylcholine causes skeletal muscle to contract. Once contraction has occurred, skeletal muscles release an enzyme called **acetylcholinesterase,** which breaks down acetylcholine. This allows the muscle to relax.

Smooth Muscle

There are two types of smooth muscle—multiunit and visceral. **Multiunit smooth muscle** is found in the iris of the eye and the walls of blood vessels. This muscle type contracts in response to neurotransmitters and hormones. **Visceral smooth muscle** contains sheets of muscle cells that closely contact each other. It is found in the walls of hollow organs such as the stomach, intestines, bladder, and uterus. Muscle fibers in visceral smooth muscle respond to neurotransmitters, but they also stimulate each other to contract; therefore, the muscle fibers tend to contract and relax together. This type of muscle produces an action called peristalsis. **Peristalsis** is a rhythmic contraction that pushes substances through tubes of the body.

Two neurotransmitters are involved in smooth muscle contraction—acetylcholine and **norepinephrine.** Depending on the smooth muscle type, these neurotransmitters cause or inhibit contraction.

Cardiac Muscle

Groups of cardiac muscle are connected to each other through **intercalated discs.** These discs allow the fibers in that group to contact and relax together. This design allows the heart to work as a pump. Cardiac muscle is also self-exciting, which means that it does not need nerve stimulation to contract. Nerves only speed up or slow down the contraction of the heart. Like smooth muscle, cardiac muscle responds to two neurotransmitters—acetylcholine and norepinephrine. Acetylcholine slows the heart rate, and norepinephrine speeds it up.

Production of Energy for Muscle

Because a lot of ATP (adenosine triphosphate), which is a type of chemical energy, is needed for sustained or repeated muscle contractions, a muscle cell must have multiple ways to store or make this substance. There are three ways through which muscle cells make this energy:

1. **Creatine phosphate** production. Creatine phosphate is a protein that stores extra phosphate groups. When ATP is used to produce work, it loses a phosphate and energy. Creatine phosphate can then donate a phosphate group to the resulting molecule to restore its energy potential. This is a very rapid way for muscles to produce energy.
2. **Aerobic respiration** of glucose. When a cell wants to make a lot of ATP, it turns to its glucose stores. A cell will break down glucose into pyruvic acid. As long as oxygen is available, the pyruvic acid is converted to a substance called acetyl coenzyme A. Acetyl coenzyme A starts a series of reactions called the **Krebs cycle,** which is also known as the citric acid cycle. This cycle

TABLE 8-1 Types of Muscle Tissue

Muscle Group	Major Location	Major Function	Mode of Control	Rate of Contraction	Intercalated Discs
Skeletal Muscle	Attached to bones and skin of the face	Produces body movements and facial expressions	Voluntary	Fast to contract and relax	No
Smooth Muscle	Walls of hollow organs, blood vessels, and iris	Moves contents through organs; vasoconstriction	Involuntary	Slow to contract and relax	No
Cardiac Muscle	Wall of the heart	Pumps blood through heart	Involuntary	Groups of muscle fibers contract as a unit	Yes

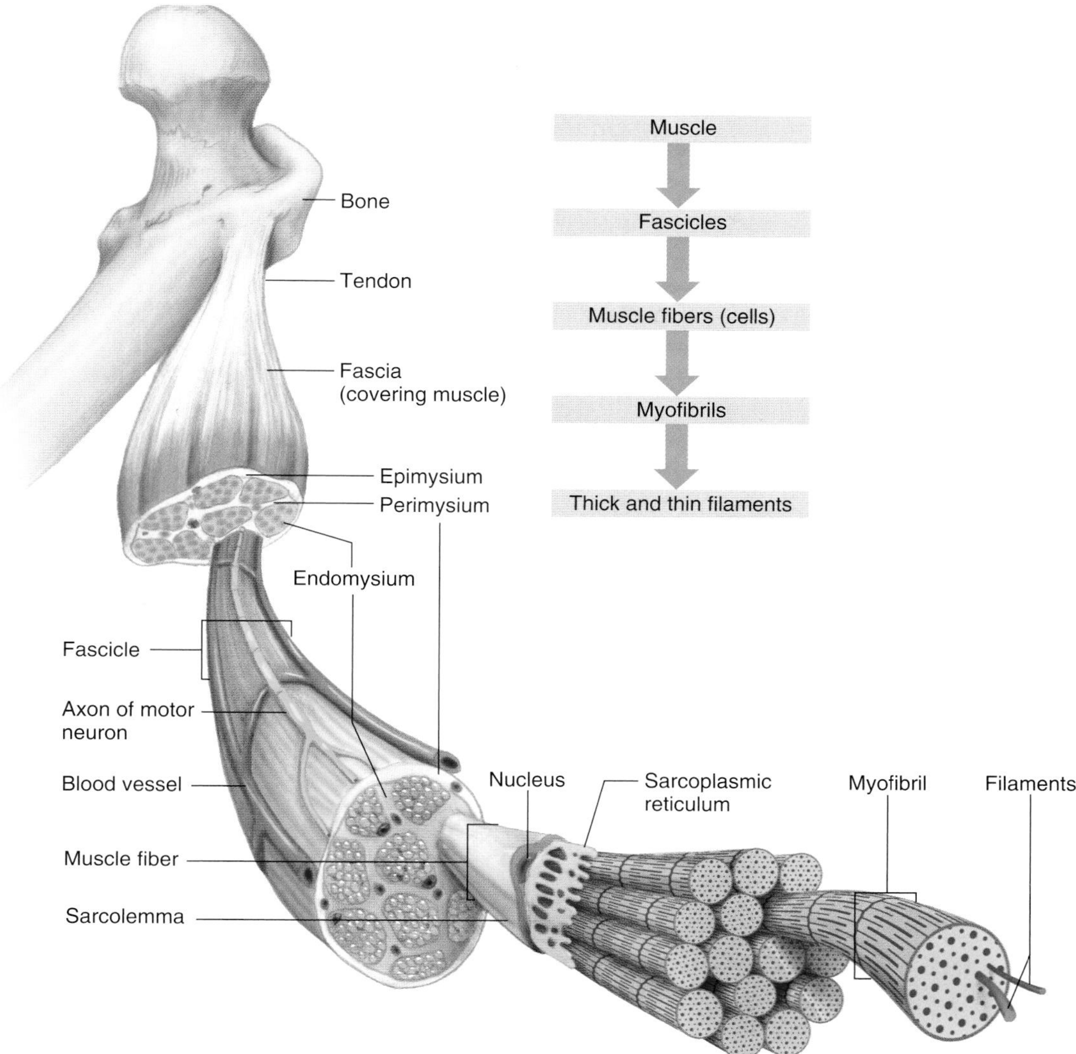

Figure 8-1. Structure of a skeletal muscle.

generates a lot of ATP for the muscle cell. The use of glucose to make ATP is called aerobic respiration because oxygen is required for this production. Because this process requires large amounts of oxygen, muscle cells contain a pigment called **myoglobin,** which stores extra oxygen. This pigment is pinkish in color and is responsible for giving muscles their color.

3. **Lactic acid** production. When a cell is low on oxygen, it must convert pyruvic acid to lactic acid. This reaction generates a small amount of ATP for the cell, but the lactic acid is a waste product that must be released from the cell.

Oxygen Debt

When skeletal muscles are used strenuously for a minute or two, **oxygen debt** develops. This condition occurs when oxygen supplies in the muscle are low and the aerobic respiration of glucose can no longer be used to produce ATP. When oxygen is low, muscle fibers must convert pyruvic acid to lactic acid to produce energy. The buildup of lactic acid causes muscle fatigue. Lactic acid is then carried by the bloodstream to the liver where it can be converted back into glucose. However, this process requires energy. The oxygen debt is the amount of oxygen the liver cells need to make enough ATP to convert lactic acid into glucose. This process explains why your body still burns energy even after you are done exercising.

Muscle Fatigue

Muscle fatigue is a condition in which a muscle has lost its ability to contract. It usually develops because of an accumulation of lactic acid. It can occur also if the blood supply to a muscle is interrupted or if a motor neuron loses its ability to release acetylcholine onto muscle fibers. Cramps—which are painful, involuntary contractions of muscles—can accompany muscle fatigue.

Structure of Skeletal Muscles

Skeletal muscles are the major organs that make up the muscular system. A skeletal muscle consists of connective tissues, skeletal muscle tissue, blood vessels, and nerves. When you see marbling in a steak, you are actually viewing connective tissues in the steak. The red portion of the steak is the muscle tissue.

The following connective tissue coverings are associated with skeletal muscles (see Figure 8-1):

- **Fascia.** This structure covers entire skeletal muscles and separates them from each other.
- **Tendon.** This tough, cord-like structure is made of fibrous connective tissue that connects muscles to bones.
- **Aponeurosis.** This tough, sheet-like structure is made of fibrous connective tissue. It typically attaches muscles to other muscles.
- **Epimysium.** This tissue is a thin covering that is just deep to the fascia of a muscle. It surrounds the entire muscle.
- **Perimysium.** This connective tissue divides a muscle into sections called **fascicles.**
- **Endomysium.** This covering of connective tissue surrounds individual muscle cells.

Pathophysiology

Common Diseases and Disorders of the Muscular System

Botulism is usually thought of as a disease that affect the gastrointestinal tract, but it can also affect various muscle groups. This disease most commonly affects infants. Although a person can survive this disease, its affects may be long-lasting.

- **Causes.** This disease is a rare but very serious disorder caused by the bacterium *Clostridium botulinum,* which normally lives in soil and water. If this bacterium gets on food, it can produce a toxin that can lead to a type of food poisoning. The foods most likely to contain *Clostridium botulinum* are canned vegetables, cured pork, raw fish, honey, and corn syrup. A person can also acquire this bacterium through open wounds that are not cleaned properly.
- **Signs and symptoms.** This disease causes many symptoms, including difficulty swallowing, paralysis, weak muscles, nausea and vomiting, abdominal cramps, double vision, difficulty breathing, poor feeding and suckling in infants, the inability to urinate, the absence of reflexes, and constipation. The signs and symptoms usually appear 8 to 40 hours after the toxin is ingested. The diagnosis is usually made by either a blood test to identify the toxin or an analysis of the suspected food.
- **Treatment.** Treatment includes emergency hospitalization, intubation to open airways, mechanical ventilation if respiratory muscles are impaired, intravenous fluids or nasogastric feeding if swallowing is impaired, and the administration of an antitoxin.
- **Prevention tips.** You can instruct patients to prevent botulism by observing the following guidelines:
  - Never give honey or corn syrup to infants
  - Sterilize home-canned foods properly (250°F for 35 minutes)
  - Do not use foods from bent or bulging cans
  - Never eat foods that smell as if they may have spoiled
  - Cook and store foods properly

Fibromyalgia is a fairly common condition that results in chronic pain primarily in joints, muscles, and tendons. It most commonly affects women between the ages of 20 and 50.

- **Causes.** The causes of this disorder are poorly understood. Fibromyalgia may be caused by sleep disturbance, emotional distress, a decreased blood flow to muscles, a virus, or any combination of these factors.
- **Signs and symptoms.** Symptoms include fatigue, tenderness in different areas of the body, sleep disturbances, and chronic facial pain. The diagnosis is usually made by ruling out other possible diseases. It is not normally diagnosed unless a person has muscle and joint pain for at least three months in certain body areas.
- **Treatment.** Treatment is varied and includes antidepressants, anti-inflammatory medications, physical therapy, lifestyle changes to reduce stress, counseling to improve coping skills, reduction or elimination of caffeine to improve sleeping, and diet supplements to improve nutrition.

Muscular dystrophy is a group of inherited disorders characterized by muscle weakness and a loss of muscle tissue. There are at least seven types of muscular dystrophy, and they are distinguished from each other by types of symptoms, the age at when symptoms appeared, and the cause.

- **Causes.** The causes of this disorder are primarily hereditary. Genetic fetal testing is available.

continued ⟶

- **Signs and symptoms.** The signs and symptoms vary widely and depend on the type of muscular dystrophy. The symptoms of Duchenne muscular dystrophy progress steadily and are eventually fatal. Other types cause mild symptoms, and patients usually have normal life expectancies. Specific signs and symptoms include muscle weakness in various muscle groups, depending on the type; difficulty walking; drooling; a delayed development of motor skills; frequent falls; mental retardation in some types; a curved spine; the formation of a claw hand or clubfoot; a loss of muscle mass; the accumulation of fat or fibrous connective tissue in muscles; and arrhythmias in some types. The diagnosis is primarily made through a muscle biopsy. Other tests include DNA testing; an EMG (electromyography) test, which tests muscle weakness; or an ECG (electrocardiogram), which tests cardiac function.
- **Treatment.** Treatment includes physical therapy to maintain muscle function, the use of braces and wheelchairs, various medications based on the type, and spinal surgery.

Myasthenia gravis is a condition in which affected persons experience muscle weakness. In this condition, a person produces antibodies that prevent muscles from receiving neurotransmitters from neurons. It most commonly affects young women and older men, especially if they have other autoimmune disorders.

- **Causes.** This disease is usually considered an autoimmune disorder.
- **Signs and symptoms.** The signs and symptoms usually get better with rest and worsen with activity. They include double vision; muscle weakness; difficulty swallowing, talking, chewing, lifting, or walking; fatigue; drooling; and difficulty breathing. The diagnosis may be difficult, but a single-fiber EMG test is often useful. This test measures the response of a muscle fiber to nervous stimulation. Other tests include acetylcholine receptors antibody tests and the Tensilon test. In a positive Tensilon test, muscle activity increases after medication is given that blocks the breakdown of acetylcholine.
- **Treatment.** Treatments include lifestyle changes to avoid excessive stress and heat, the use of an eye patch to treat double vision, medications to improve communication between nerves and muscles, medications to suppress the immune system, plasmapheresis to remove harmful antibodies from blood, and removal of the thymus.

Rhabdomyolysis is a condition in which the kidneys have been damaged and is related to serious muscle injuries.

- **Causes.** Kidneys become damaged because of toxins released from muscle cells. When muscles are damaged, excessive amounts of the pigment myoglobin are released, which is then broken down into harmful chemicals. Muscles are most often damaged through trauma; excessive use (for example, marathon running); overdoses of cocaine, heroine, and other drugs; alcoholism; and a blockage of the blood supply to the muscles.
- **Signs and symptoms.** Symptoms include dark urine, muscle tenderness, muscle weakness, muscle stiffness, seizures, joint pain, and fatigue. The diagnosis includes urinalysis for the presence of myoglobin, creatine phosphokinase (CPK), and creatinine; blood is also tested for the presence of myoglobin, CPK, or high levels of potassium. CPK is an enzyme released into the blood when muscles are damaged. Creatinine is a protein released by the breakdown of muscle tissue.
- **Treatment.** Treatment includes hydration to rapidly eliminate toxins from the kidneys, diuretics to help flush toxins from the body, medications to flush excess potassium from the body, and therapy for kidney failure.

Tetanus is commonly called lockjaw. This disease has a high mortality rate, especially in infants. Immediate treatment is necessary to prevent death or long-lasting effects. However, this disease is completely preventable through regular vaccinations.

- **Causes.** A toxin produced by the bacterium *Clostridium tetani,* which lives naturally in soil and water, causes this disease. People most commonly acquire this bacterium through open wounds caused by objects contaminated with soil.
- **Signs and symptoms.** Symptoms usually appear between 5 and 10 days after infection. Muscle spasms in the jaw, neck, and facial muscles are usually the first signs. Other signs and symptoms include severe spasms of muscles that spread to other body locations; muscles spasms that may cause bone fractures; breathing difficulties; irritability; fever; profuse sweating; and drooling. The diagnosis is usually based on the type of wound and the characteristic signs and symptoms of the disease. Tetanus antibody tests can also be used in diagnosis, but cultures of the wound site often produce false-negative findings.
- **Treatment.** Administering antitoxin and antibiotics is a key treatment. Others include wound cleaning, muscle relaxants, sedation, and bed rest. The insertion of an endotracheal tube and mechanical ventilation may be needed for patients with severe breathing difficulties.

Trichinosis is an infection caused by parasites (worms).

- **Causes.** This disease is caused by worms that are usually ingested by eating undercooked meat. Once ingested, the worms can leave the digestive tract and infect skeletal muscles, the heart, the lungs, and the brain. This disease is preventable by not eating meat

continued ⟶

from wild animals. Proper cooking will also prevent trichinosis. There is no cure for this disease once the worms leave the digestive tract and infect other tissues.

- **Signs and symptoms.** Common symptoms include abdominal pain, diarrhea, muscle pain, fever, and pneumonia. In more serious cases, arrhythmias (irregular heart rhythms), heart failure, and encephalitis (swelling of the brain) can result. The diagnosis is usually based on the symptoms, a blood test to determine if there is an increase in eosinophils in blood, or by a muscle biopsy that reveals the presence of the worm.
- **Treatment.** Patients with this disease are treated with medications to kill worms in the digestive tract and with anti-inflammatory drugs to reduce muscle pain and swelling.

Attachments and Actions of Skeletal Muscles

The actions of skeletal muscles depend largely on what the skeletal muscles are attached to. Insertions and origins are sites of attachments for skeletal muscles. An **insertion** is an attachment site that moves when a muscle contracts. An **origin** is an attachment site that does not move when a muscle contracts. For example, the biceps brachii (the muscle on the front of the upper arm) attaches to two places on the scapula and to one site on the radius. When the biceps brachii contracts, the radius moves and the arm bends at the elbow. Therefore, the insertion site of the biceps brachii is its attachment site on the radius. The origin of the biceps brachii is where it attaches to the scapula (Figure 8-2).

Most of the time a body movement is produced not just by one muscle but by a group of muscles. However, one muscle is responsible for most of the movement; this muscle is called the **prime mover.** Other muscles help the prime mover by stabilizing joints; these muscles are called **synergists.** An **antagonist** is a muscle that produces a movement opposite to the prime mover. When the prime mover contracts, the antagonist must relax in order to produce a smooth body movement. For example, when you bend your arm at the elbow, the prime mover is the biceps brachii. The synergist muscles are the brachialis and brachioradialis. The antagonist is the triceps brachii because its action is to extend the arm at the elbow.

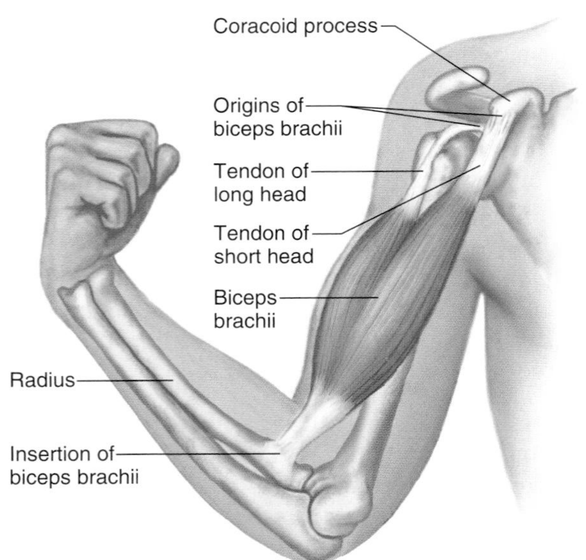

Figure 8-2. Origins and insertion of biceps brachii.

The body movements produced by skeletal muscles include the following:

- **Flexion**—bending a body part
- **Extension**—straightening a body part
- **Hyperextension**—extending a body part past the normal anatomical position
- **Dorsiflexion**—pointing the toes up
- **Plantar flexion**—pointing the toes down
- **Abduction**—moving a body part away from its position in the anatomical position
- **Adduction**—moving a body part toward its position in the anatomical position
- **Rotation**—twisting a body part; for example, turning your head from side to side
- **Circumduction**—moving a body part in a circle; for example, moving your arm in a circular motion
- **Pronation**—turning the palm of the hand down
- **Supination**—turning the palm of the hand up
- **Inversion**—turning the sole of the foot medially
- **Eversion**—turning the sole of the foot laterally
- **Retraction**—moving a body part posteriorly
- **Protraction**—moving a body part anteriorly
- **Elevation**—lifting a body part; for example, elevating your shoulders as in a shrugging expression
- **Depression**—lowering a body part; for example, lowering your shoulders

See Figures 8-3, 8-4, and 8-5 for illustrations of these types of movements.

Major Skeletal Muscles

The name of a skeletal muscle often describes it in some way. Usually the name indicates the location, size, action, shape, or number of attachments of the muscle. For

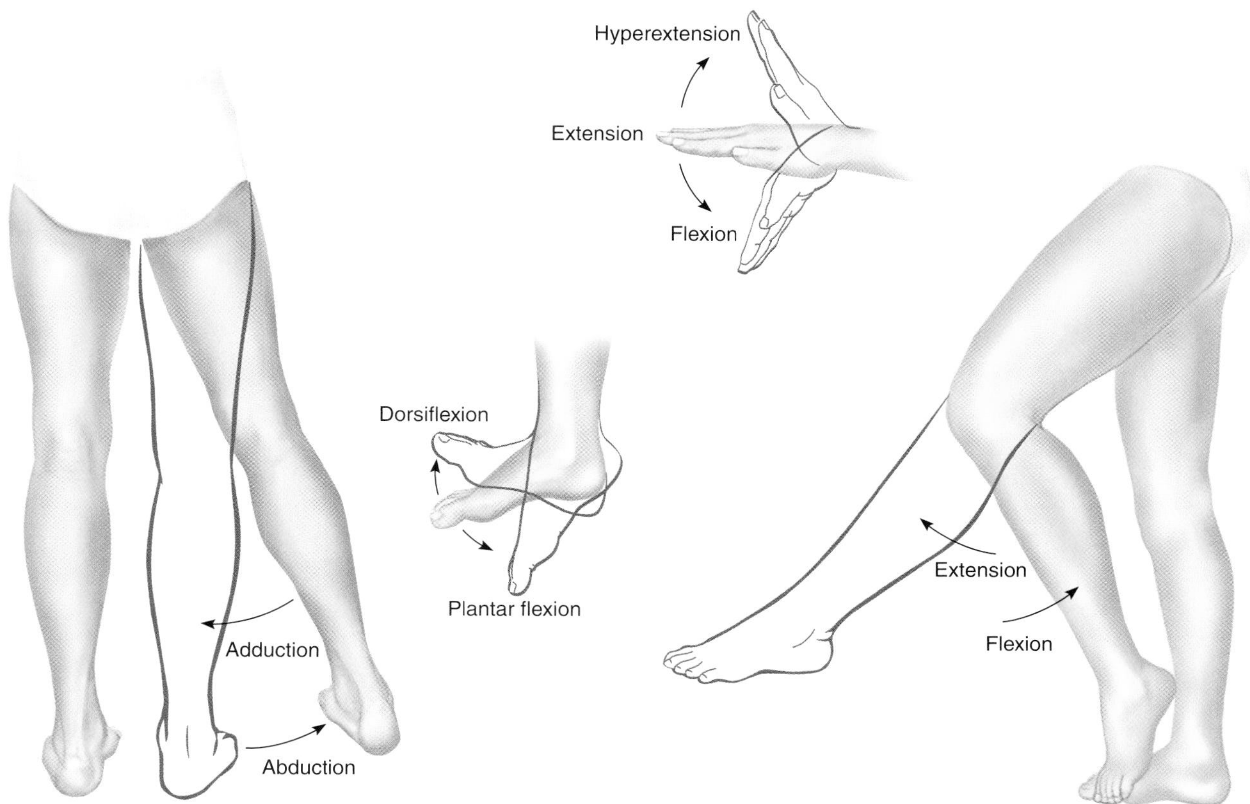

Figure 8-3. Adduction, abduction, dorsiflexion, plantar flexion, hyperextension, extension, and flexion.

example, the pectoralis major is named for its large size (major) and its location (pectoral, or chest, region). The sternocleidomastoid is named for its attachment sites—*sterno* (sternum), *cleido* (clavicle), and *mastoid* (the mastoid process of the temporal bone). As you study muscles, you will find it easier to remember them if you think about what the name describes.

Muscles of the Head

The muscles of the head include those that move the head, provide facial expression, and move the jaw. See Figures 8-6 and 8-7 for illustrations of these various muscles.

Muscles that move the head include the following:

- Sternocleidomastoid. This muscle pulls the head to one side and also pulls the head to the chest.
- Splenius capitis. This muscle rotates the head and allows it to bend to the side.

Muscles of facial expression include the following:

- Frontalis. This muscle raises the eyebrows.
- Orbicularis oris. This muscle allows the lips to pucker.
- Orbicularis oculi. This muscle allows the eyes to close.
- Zygomaticus. This muscle pulls the corners of the mouth up.
- Platysma. This muscle pulls the corners of the mouth down.

The muscles of the jaw allow for mastication (chewing) and include the following:

- Masseter and temporalis. These muscles close the jaw.

Arm Muscles

Muscles that move the arm include muscles of the arm and forearm (see Figures 8-6, 8-7, and 8-8). The muscles of the arm include the following:

- Pectoralis major. This muscle pulls the arm across the chest; it also rotates and adducts the arms.
- Latissimus dorsi. This muscle acts to extend, adduct, and rotate the arm inwardly.
- Deltoid. This muscle acts to abduct and extend the arm at the shoulder.
- Subscapularis. This muscle rotates the arm medially.
- Infraspinatus. This muscle rotates the arm laterally.

Muscles that move the forearm include the following:

- Biceps brachii. This muscle flexes the arm at the elbow and rotates the hand laterally.
- Brachialis. This muscle flexes the arm at the elbow.
- Brachioradialis. This muscle flexes the forearm at the elbow.
- Triceps brachii. This muscle extends the arm at the elbow.

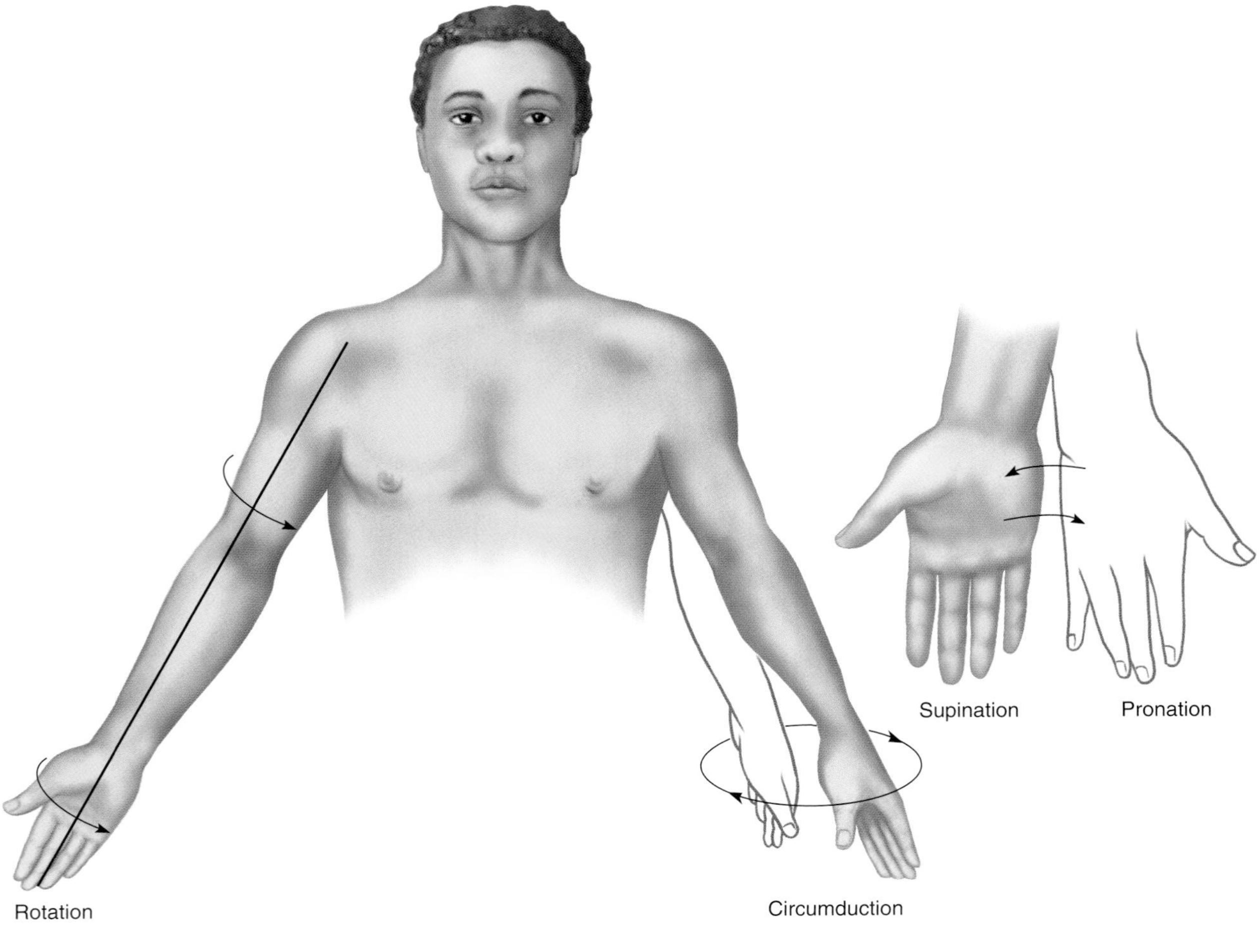

Supination
Pronation
Rotation
Circumduction

Figure 8-4. Rotation, circumduction, supination, and pronation.

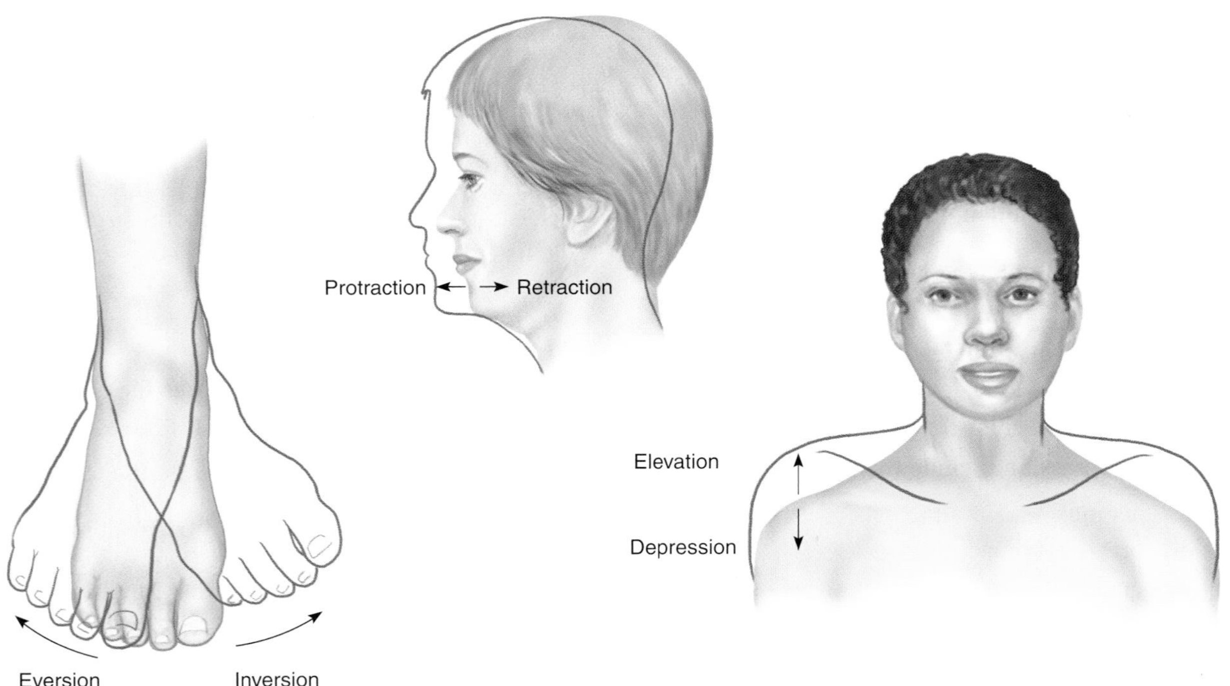

Figure 8-5. Eversion, inversion, protraction, retraction, elevation, and depression.

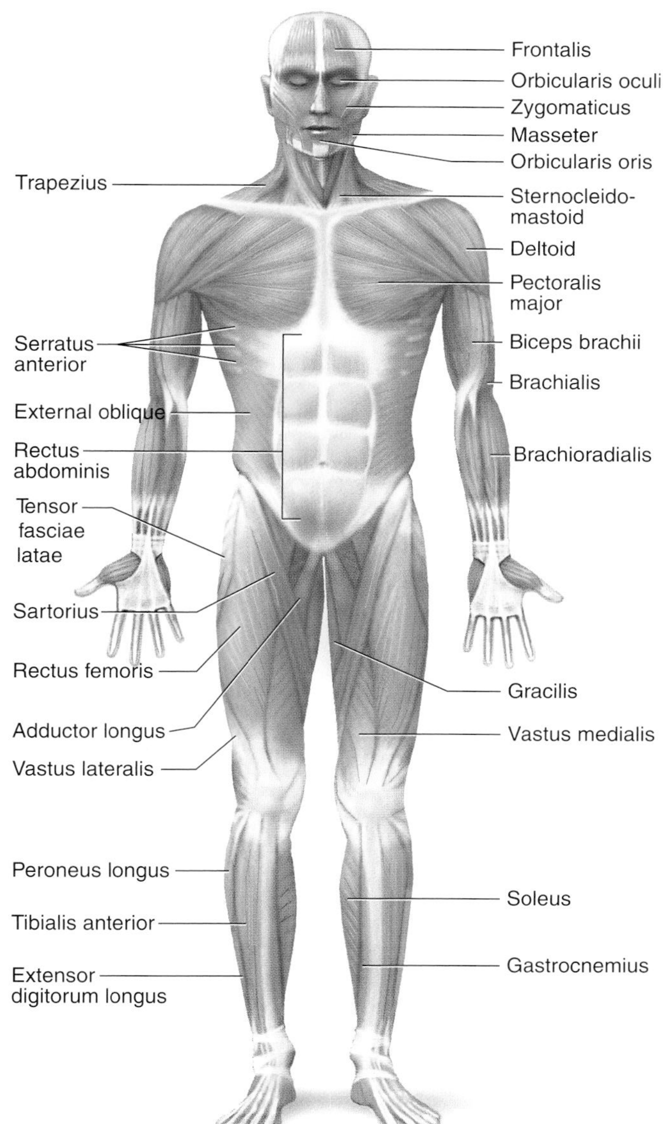

Figure 8-6. Anterior view of superficial skeletal muscles.

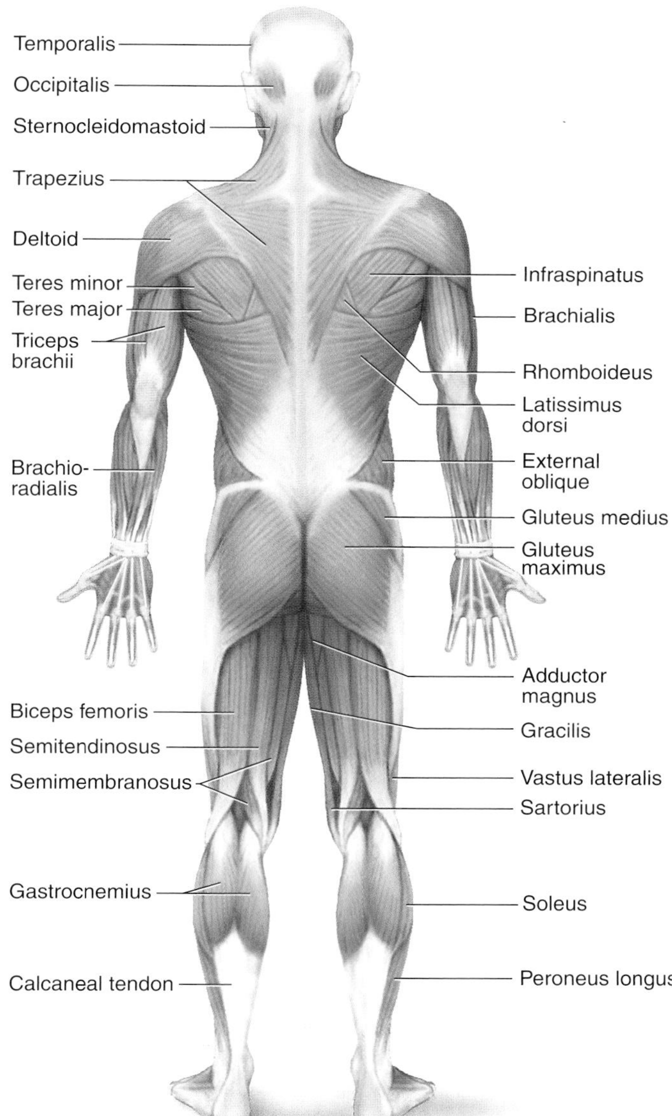

Figure 8-7. Posterior view of superficial skeletal muscles.

- Supinator. This muscle rotates the forearm laterally (supination).
- Pronator teres. This muscle rotates the forearm medially (pronation).

Muscles of the Wrist, Hand, and Fingers

Muscles that move the wrist, hand, and fingers can be seen in Figures 8-6, 8-7 and 8-8. These muscles include the following:

- Flexor carpi radialis and flexor carpi ulnaris. These muscles flex and abduct the wrist.
- Palmaris longus. This muscle flexes the wrist.
- Flexor digitorum profundus. This muscle flexes the distal joints of the fingers but not the thumb.
- Extensor carpi radialis longus and brevis. These muscles extend the wrist and abduct the hand.
- Extensor carpi ulnaris. This muscle extends the wrist.
- Extensor digitorum. This muscle extends the fingers but not the thumb.

Respiratory Muscles

The muscles of respiration include the following:

- Diaphragm. This muscle separates the thoracic cavity from the abdominal cavity; its contraction causes inspiration.
- External and internal intercostals. The contraction of these muscles expands and lowers the ribs during breathing. See Figure 8-9 for an illustration of the internal intercostal muscle.

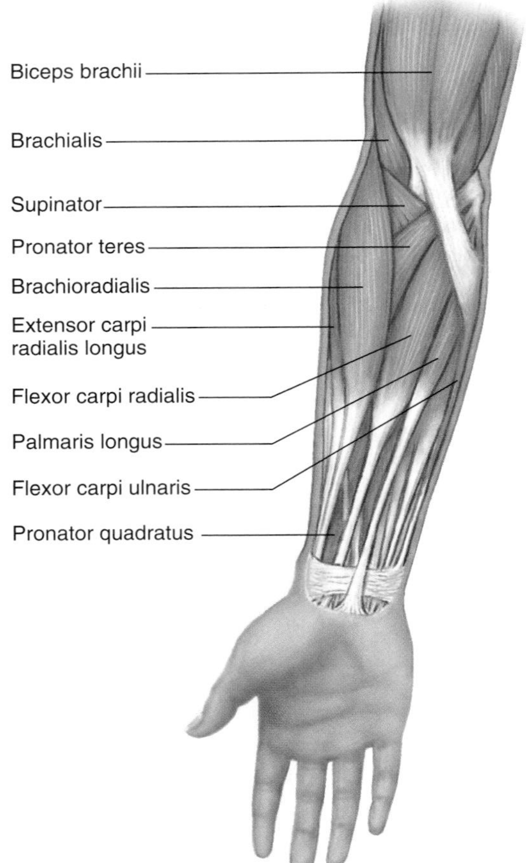

Figure 8-8. Muscles of the anterior forearm.

Abdominal Muscles

The muscles of the abdominal wall include the following:

- External and internal obliques. These muscles compress the abdominal wall.
- Transverse abdominis. This muscle also compresses the abdominal wall.
- Rectus abdominis. This muscle acts to flex the vertebral column and compress the abdominal wall.

See Figures 8-6, 8-7, and 8-9 for illustrations of these muscles.

Muscles of the Pectoral Girdle

The muscles that move the pectoral girdle (shoulder) include these muscles:

- Trapezius. This muscle raises the arms and pulls the shoulders downward.
- Pectoralis minor. This muscle pulls the scapula downward and raises the ribs.

See Figures 8-6, 8-7, and 8-9 for illustrations of these muscles.

Leg Muscles

The leg muscles include muscles of the thigh and lower leg (see Figures 8-6 and 8-7). Muscles that move the thigh include the following:

- Psoas major. This muscle flexes the thigh.
- Iliacus. This muscle also flexes the thigh.
- Gluteus maximus. This muscle extends the thigh.

Educating the Patient

Muscle Strains and Sprains

Muscle strains are injuries that excessively stretch muscles or tendons. Muscle sprains are more serious injuries that result in tears to muscles, tendons, ligaments, or cartilage. You can teach patients to prevent these types of injuries by doing the following:

- Warm up. Warming up muscles for just a few minutes before an intense activity raises muscle temperature. This increase in temperature prevents injuries by making muscle tissue more pliable.
- Stretch. Stretching improves muscle performance and should always be done after the warm-up or after exercising. A person should never stretch further than he can hold for 10 seconds.
- Cool down. Slowing down the exercise before completely stopping prevents dizziness and fainting. If a person suddenly stops exercising, blood can pool in the legs and is prevented from reaching the brain. Cooling down also helps to remove lactic acid from muscles.

If sprains or strains do occur, immediate RICE treatment is recommended:

- R is for rest. Resting minimizes bleeding, further injury, and swelling.
- I is for ice. Ice minimizes swelling and pain. A bag that is filled with crushed ice conforms better to a body part than one filled with ice cubes. A bag full of frozen peas or other small

continued ⟶

Educating the Patient

Muscle Strains and Sprains *(continued)*

vegetables can also be used. The ice should be applied for 10 minutes and then removed for 10 minutes. This should be kept up for about an hour and repeated several times during a 24-hour period. Ice can be applied for a shorter period of time if blood vessels dilate during its application.

- C is for compression, which minimizes swelling. A bandage should be loosely wrapped around the injured area and the bag of ice. Compression should be applied and removed along with the ice.
- E is for elevation. The injured muscle should be elevated, which minimizes swelling, and elevation should be continued as long as swelling is present.

- Gluteus medius and minimus. These muscles abduct the thighs and rotate them medially.
- Adductor longus and magnus. These muscles adduct the thighs and rotate them laterally.
- Biceps femoris, semitendinosus, and semimembranosus. These three muscles are known as the hamstring group. They act to flex the leg at the knee and extend the leg at the thigh.
- Rectus femoris, vastus lateralis, vastus medialis, and vastus intermedius. These four muscles are known as the quadriceps group; they act to extend the leg at the knee.
- Sartorius. This muscle flexes the leg at the knee and thigh. It also abducts the thigh, rotating the thigh laterally but rotating the lower leg medially; it carries out the act of sitting cross-legged.

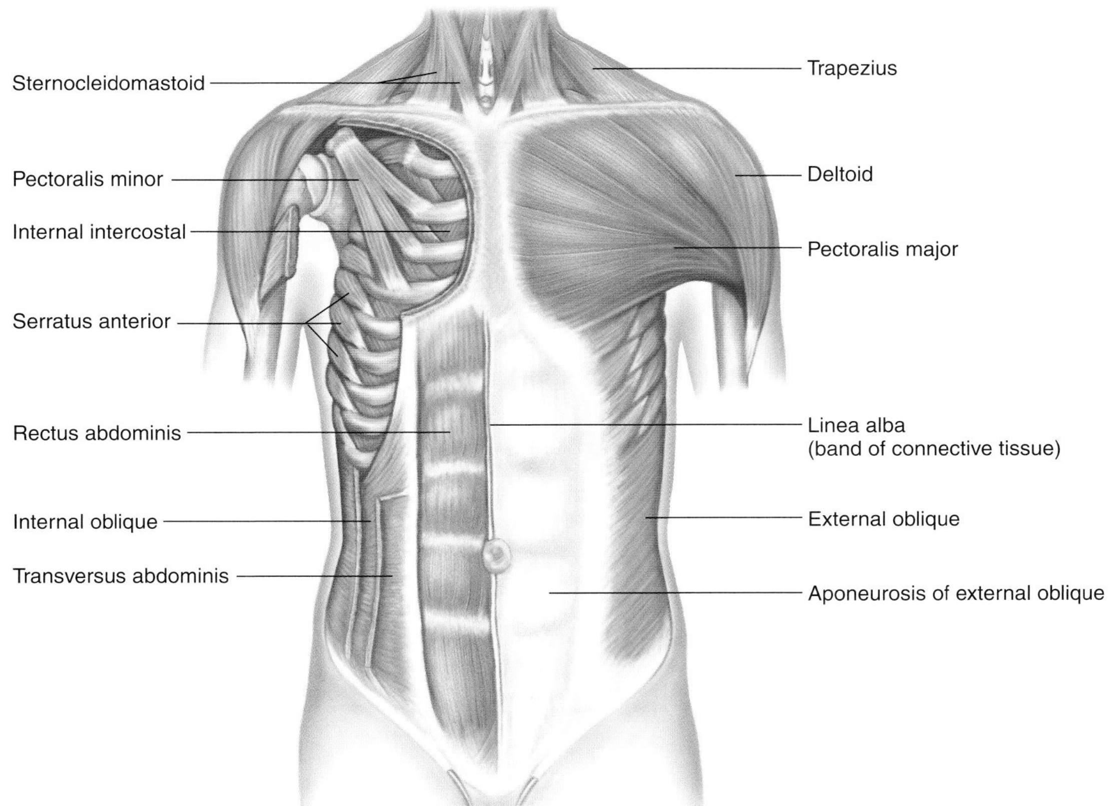

Figure 8-9. Muscles of the anterior chest and abdominal wall.

Muscles of the Ankle, Foot, and Toes

Muscles that move the ankle, foot, and toes include the following:

- Tibialis anterior. This muscle inverts the foot and points the foot up (dorsiflexion).
- Extensor digitorum longus. This muscle extends the toes and points the foot up.
- Gastrocnemius. This muscle flexes the foot and flexes the leg at the knee.
- Soleus. This muscle also flexes the foot.
- Flexor digitorum longus. This muscle flexes the foot and toes.

See Figures 8-6 and 8-7 for illustrations of these muscles.

Summary

Skeletal muscle works in conjunction with the skeletal system to produce movement. This movement is accomplished voluntarily. In addition, skeletal muscles help stabilize joints and are important in heat production. Muscles under involuntary control include smooth and cardiac muscle. Smooth muscles control body openings and passages. Cardiac muscle is responsible for the pumping action of the heart. Medical assistants should understand the muscular system in order to give muscular injections, prepare patients for massage therapy, demonstrate ambulatory techniques, and assist in the care of sprains and strains.

REVIEW

CHAPTER 8

CASE STUDY QUESTIONS

Now that you have completed this chapter, review the case study at the beginning of the chapter and answer the following questions:

1. What is the function of acetylcholinesterase?
2. Why does this patient exhibit muscle twitching and back pain?
3. What type of respiratory therapy will this patient require?
4. What precautions should a person take when using insecticides that contain organophosphates?
5. Why is it important for patients to give their doctor a complete account of their activities prior to an illness?

Discussion Questions

1. Name the muscles used for facial expression. Tell what facial expression each produces.
2. How are muscles named? Give examples for each method of naming a muscle.
3. What are the functions of muscles?
4. What is oxygen debt, and how does it develop?

Critical Thinking Questions

1. Why is it important to do warm-up activities before participating in sporting events?
2. What steps can be taken to minimize muscle wasting or decline in the legs of patients who are dependent on wheelchairs?
3. How does the application of heat ease the pain associated with muscle soreness?
4. If a workout buddy at the gym told you his muscles were getting bigger because he was growing more muscle cells, would he be correct? What actually makes a muscle larger?

Application Activities

1. Define the following terms related to muscle structure:
   a. Fascia
   b. Epimysium
   c. Fascicle
   d. Perimysium
   e. Aponeurosis
   f. Tendon
2. Describe the following actions:
   a. Flexion
   b. Extension
   c. Pronation
   d. Supination
   e. Abduction
   f. Adduction
   g. Rotation
   h. Circumduction
3. Describe the actions of the following muscles:
   a. Biceps brachii
   b. Triceps brachii
   c. Orbicularis oris
   d. Hamstring group
   e. Quadricep group
   f. Deltoid
   g. Gastrocnemius
4. Give the locations of each of the following muscle types:
   a. Cardiac muscle
   b. Visceral smooth muscle
   c. Multiunit smooth muscle
   d. Skeletal muscle

CHAPTER 9

The Nervous System

KEY TERMS

action potential
areflexia
ascending tracts
autonomic
axon
blood-brain barrier
brain stem
cell body
central nervous system (CNS)
cerebellum
cerebrospinal fluid (CSF)
cerebrum
cervical enlargement
convolutions
corpus callosum
cortex
cranial nerves
dendrite
depolarized
descending tracts
diencephalon
dorsal root
effectors
epilepsy
ganglia
gray matter
gyri
hyperreflexia
hyporeflexia
hypothalamus
interneuron
lobe
lumbar enlargement
membrane potential
meninges
meningitis

CHAPTER OUTLINE

- General Functions of the Nervous System
- Neuron Structure
- Nerve Impulse and Synapse
- Central Nervous System
- Peripheral Nervous System
- Neurologic Testing

OBJECTIVES

After completing Chapter 9, you will be able to:

9.1 Explain the difference between the central nervous system and the peripheral nervous system.
9.2 Describe the functions of the nervous system.
9.3 Describe the structure of a neuron.
9.4 Describe the function of a nerve impulse and how a nerve impulse is created.
9.5 Describe the structure and function of a synapse.
9.6 Describe the function of the blood-brain barrier.
9.7 Describe the structure and functions of meninges.
9.8 Describe the structure and functions of the spinal cord.
9.9 Define reflex and list the parts of a reflex arc.
9.10 List the major divisions of the brain and give the general functions of each.
9.11 Describe the differences between the somatic nervous system and autonomic nervous system.
9.12 Explain the two divisions of the autonomic nervous system.
9.13 Explain the functions of the cranial and spinal nerves.
9.14 Describe the location and function of cerebrospinal fluid.
9.15 Describe various disorders of the nervous system and how they are diagnosed and treated.

KEY TERMS *(Continued)*

motor
myelin
nerve fiber
nerve impulse
neuralgia
neurotransmitter
parasympathetic
paresthesias
peripheral nervous system
plexus
polarized
reflex
repolarization
Schwann cell
sciatica
seizure
sensory
somatic
spinal nerves
subarachnoid space
sulci
sympathetic
synaptic knob
thalamus
ventral root
ventricle
vesicles
white matter

Introduction

The nervous system is a highly complex system. It controls all other organ systems and is important for maintaining balance within those systems. Disorders of the nervous system are numerous and often very difficult to diagnose and treat because of the complexity of this system.

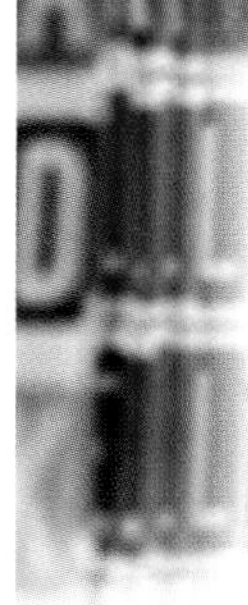

CASE STUDY

A 22-year-old woman comes to the family practice office where you work. She complains of tingling sensations in her fingers and toes. She also states that even though she wears thick mittens during cold weather, her fingers and toes turn blue and she experiences a lot of pain. A doctor diagnoses her with Raynaud's disease and tells her that it is an overreaction of the sympathetic nerves in her fingers and toes. She is scheduled for a regional sympathectomy, which will cut the sympathetic fibers to her fingers and toes.

As you read this chapter, consider the following questions:

1. What effect do sympathetic nerves have on blood vessels?
2. Why does Raynaud's disease produce pain and blue coloration in the fingers and toes?
3. How is a sympathectomy going to help this patient's condition?

General Functions of the Nervous System

The nervous system is divided into two major parts—the **central nervous system (CNS)** and the **peripheral nervous system.** The CNS consists of the brain and the spinal cord, and the peripheral nervous system consists of peripheral nerves.

The three functions of the nervous system are to (1) detect and interpret **sensory** information, (2) make decisions about the sensory information that is received, and (3) carry out **motor** functions based on the decisions made.

Sensory receptors at the ends of peripheral nerves pick up information about the body's internal and external environment. For example, when you feel pain, a sensory receptor identifies that information. When you see images, special types of sensory receptors called visual receptors detect those images. All sensory information is picked up in the peripheral nervous system and sent to the CNS for interpretation. When sensory information reaches a part of the brain called the cerebral cortex, a person actually perceives the sensory information.

The decision-making function (also called the integrative function) takes place in the brain or spinal cord. These organs receive sensory information and make decisions regarding the information. For example, if you feel pain your brain might decide you need to move away from the painful stimulus. If you see a red light, your brain might decide you need to stop your car.

Once decisions are made, the nervous system carries out motor functions. A motor function is the stimulation of a muscle (skeletal, smooth, or cardiac) or a gland. For example, if your brain interpreted that you are touching something hot and decided you should move away from the painful stimulus, the motor function would be stimulation of the skeletal muscles in your arm that allow you to pull your finger away from the painful stimulus. If you see a red light and your brain decided that you need to stop the car, the motor function would be activating the muscles in the leg that allow you to push a brake pedal. Muscles and glands are called **effectors** of the nervous system.

Neuron Structure

Neurons are the functional cells of the nervous system. They transmit electrochemical messages called **nerve impulses** to other neurons and effectors (muscles or glands). An important characteristic about neurons is that they lose their ability to divide. Therefore, when neurons are destroyed by disease, they cannot be replaced. However, the neuroglial cells that surround and support neurons never lose their ability to divide. All neurons have a **cell body** and processes called **nerve fibers** that extend from the cell body (Figure 9-1).

The cell body is the portion of the neuron that contains the nucleus and typical organelles such as rough endoplasmic reticulum, mitochondria, lysosomes, and a Golgi apparatus. It is responsible for generating the large amount of proteins and energy that the neuron needs to carry out its important functions.

Extending from the cell body are nerve fibers. The two types of nerve fibers are axons and dendrites. A neuron may have one or more dendrites but typically has only one axon. **Dendrites** are usually short and branch profusely near the cell body. Their function is to receive information for the neuron. **Axons** are typically long and branch profusely after they have extended far away from the cell body.

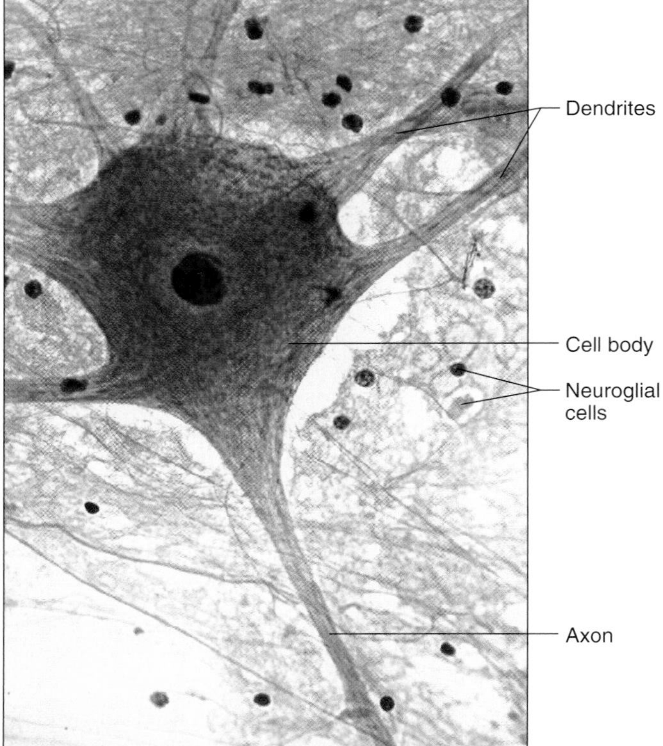

Figure 9-1. A typical neuron surrounded by neuroglial cells.

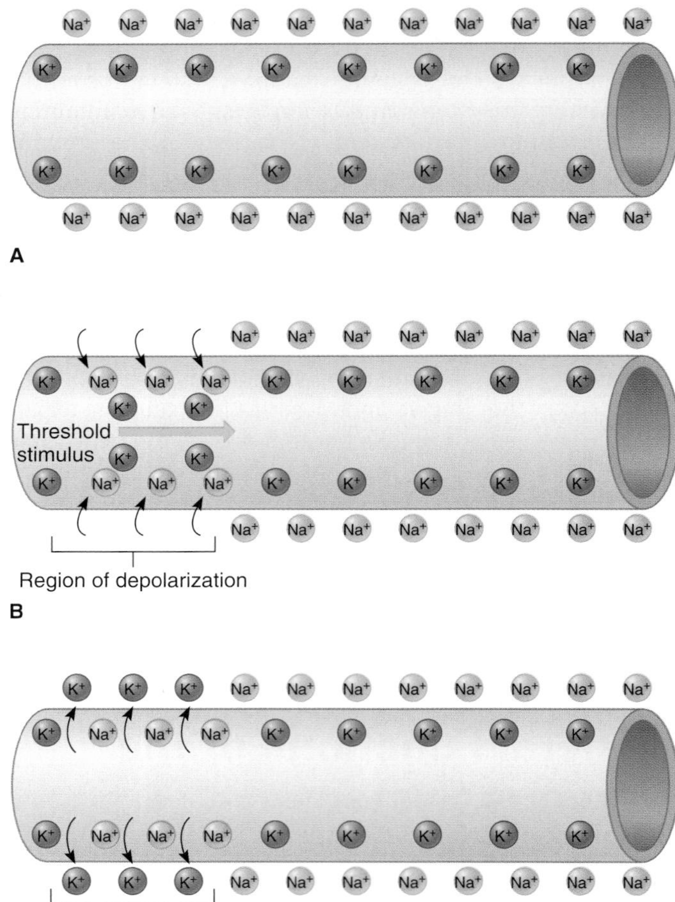

Figure 9-2. Nerve impulse. (a) At rest, or in its polar state, more Na^+ is on the outside of the membrane, which makes the outside positive and the inside negative (less positive). (b) When Na^+ moves into the cell, the membrane depolarizes, meaning that the inside becomes more positive. (c) The membrane repolarizes when K^+ and later Na^+ move to the outside of the cell membrane.

Their function is to send information (nerve impulses) away from the cell body.

In the peripheral nervous system, neuroglial cells, called **Schwann cells,** wrap themselves around axons; the axons are coated by the cell membranes of the Schwann cells. The cell membranes contain large amounts of **myelin,** which is a fatty substance. Myelin insulates the axons and allows them to send nerve impulses quickly.

Neurons can be classified as sensory neurons, **interneurons,** or motor neurons based on their functions. Sensory (afferent) neurons carry sensory information from the periphery to the CNS. These neurons pick up sensory information from their receptors, which are usually at the tips of their dendrites. Interneurons are found only in the CNS, and they function to link neurons together. Interneurons also transmit impulses from one part of the spinal cord or brain to another. They are involved in the decision-making function of the nervous system, and they direct information to motor neurons. Motor (efferent) neurons carry information from the CNS to effectors (muscles or glands) in the peripheral nervous system. They are responsible for stimulating muscles to contract or glands to secrete their products.

Nerve Impulse and Synapse

Neuron cell membranes have a cell **membrane potential.** This means the membrane is polarized. Just like a battery is polar—one end is negative and the other end is positive—neuron cell membranes are polar because the inside is negatively charged and the outside is positively charged. In most of the cells in the body, the outside of cell membranes is positively charged because more positive ions are on the outside. The inside of cell membranes is negatively charged because more negative ions are on the inside. This membrane potential is very important for the function of neurons (Figure 9-2).

Potassium and sodium ions are both positively charged and play important roles in generating nerve impulses. When a neuron is at rest or without stimulation, the outside of its membrane is positively charged and the inside is negatively charged because the total of sodium and potassium ions is greater outside the membrane. As long as the neuron is at rest, it remains in this **polarized** state.

However, a neuron will respond to stimuli such as heat, pressure, and chemicals by changing the amount of polarization across its membrane. For example, it can respond to a stimulus by making the outside of its membrane less positive. When this happens, the neuron has **depolarized.** In other words, it has become less polar. To make the outside of the membrane less positive, some of the sodium ions flow to the inside of the cell membrane. If the membrane of an axon becomes depolarized enough, a nerve impulse (**action potential**) is created. A nerve impulse is the flow of electric current along the axon membrane. Eventually, the axon membrane becomes polar again by the return of positively charged ions to the outside of the cell membrane. The return to the original polar (resting) state is called **repolarization.**

An unmyelinated axon does not conduct a nerve impulse as quickly as a myelinated axon does. Also, the speed of the nerve impulse is related to the diameter of the axon. The larger the diameter, the faster the nerve impulse travels to the end of the axon.

When a nerve impulse travels down an axon, the impulse eventually reaches the ends of axon branches, called **synaptic knobs.** These synaptic knobs contact dendrites, cell bodies, and the axons of other neurons. Whatever the synaptic knob is contacting is called a postsynaptic structure. Within synaptic knobs are **vesicles,** or small sacs that contain chemicals called **neurotransmitters.** When the nerve impulse reaches the synaptic knobs, the neurotransmitters are released onto postsynaptic structures (Figure 9-3).

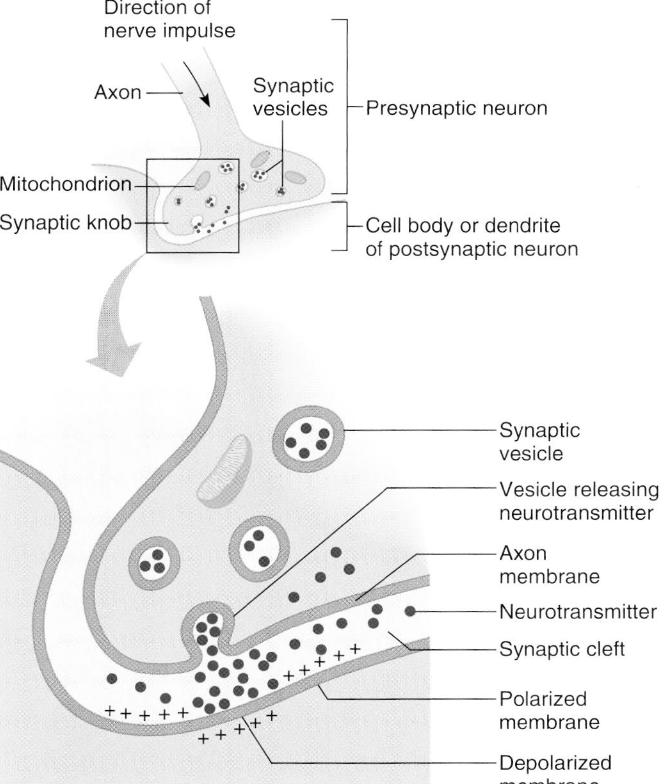

Figure 9-3. Synapse. When a nerve impulse reaches a synaptic knob, it releases a neurotransmitter onto the postsynaptic structure.

There are about 50 different neurotransmitters. Most neurons release only one type of neurotransmitter but some will release more than one type. Neurotransmitters are released through exocytosis. Their functions include causing muscles to contract or relax, causing glands to secrete products, activating neurons to send nerve impulses, or inhibiting neurons from sending nerve impulses.

Central Nervous System

The central nervous system includes the spinal cord and brain (Figure 9-4). The tissues of the CNS are so delicate that a **blood-brain barrier** and layers of membranes protect them. Tight capillaries form the blood-brain barrier. This barrier prevents certain substances from entering the tissues of the CNS. For example, various waste products and drugs do not cross the blood-brain barrier very well. Inflammation, however, can make this barrier more permeable.

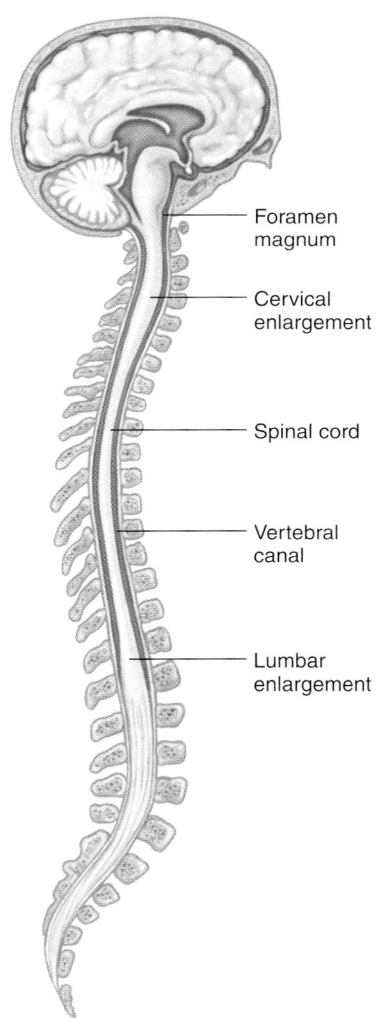

Figure 9-4. The central nervous system(CNS) consists of the brain and spinal cord. The spinal cord ends at the level of third lumbar vertebra.

Meninges are membranes that protect the brain and spinal cord. The three layers of meninges are dura mater, arachnoid mater, and pia mater. Dura mater is the toughest and outermost layer of the meninges. Arachnoid mater is the middle layer and is wispy in appearance (much like a spider's web—hence the name arachnoid, which means spider). Pia mater is the innermost and most delicate layer. It sits directly on top of the brain and spinal cord and holds blood vessels onto the surface of these structures. Between the arachnoid mater and pia mater is an area called the **subarachnoid space.** It contains **cerebrospinal fluid (CSF),** which cushions the CNS.

Spinal Cord

The spinal cord is a slender structure that is continuous with the brain. The spinal cord descends into the vertebral canal and ends around the level of the first or second lumbar vertebra. The spinal cord is divided into 31 spinal segments: 8 cervical segments, 12 thoracic segments, 5 lumbar segments, 5 sacral segments, and 1 coccygeal segment. The thickening of the spinal cord in the neck region is called the **cervical enlargement** and contains the motor neurons that control the muscles of the arms. Another thickening of the spinal cord occurs in the lumbar region. This thickening is called the **lumbar enlargement** and contains the motor neurons that control the muscles of the legs (Figure 9-4).

Gray and White Matter. When you view a cross section of the spinal cord, you observe two differently colored areas. The inner tissue is termed **gray matter** because its color is darker than the outer tissue, which is termed **white matter.** The gray matter contains neuron cell bodies and their dendrites, whereas the white matter contains myelinated axons. The divisions of the gray matter are called horns, and the divisions of the white matter are called columns (funiculi). The columns contain groups of axons called nerve tracts. A canal runs down the entire length of the spinal cord through the center of the gray matter. This canal is called the central canal and contains CSF (Figure 9-5).

Ascending and Descending Tracts. One function of the spinal cord is to carry sensory information up to the brain. The tracts that carry sensory information up to the brain are called **ascending tracts.** Another function of the spinal cord is to carry motor information down from the brain to muscles and glands. These tracts are called **descending tracts.**

Reflexes. Another important function of the spinal cord is to participate in reflexes. A **reflex** is a predictable, automatic response to stimuli. For example, if you touch something very hot, the predictable response is that you will pull your finger away from the hot surface; this type of reflex is called a withdrawal reflex. The information that flows through a typical reflex moves in the following order: from receptors to sensory neurons to interneurons

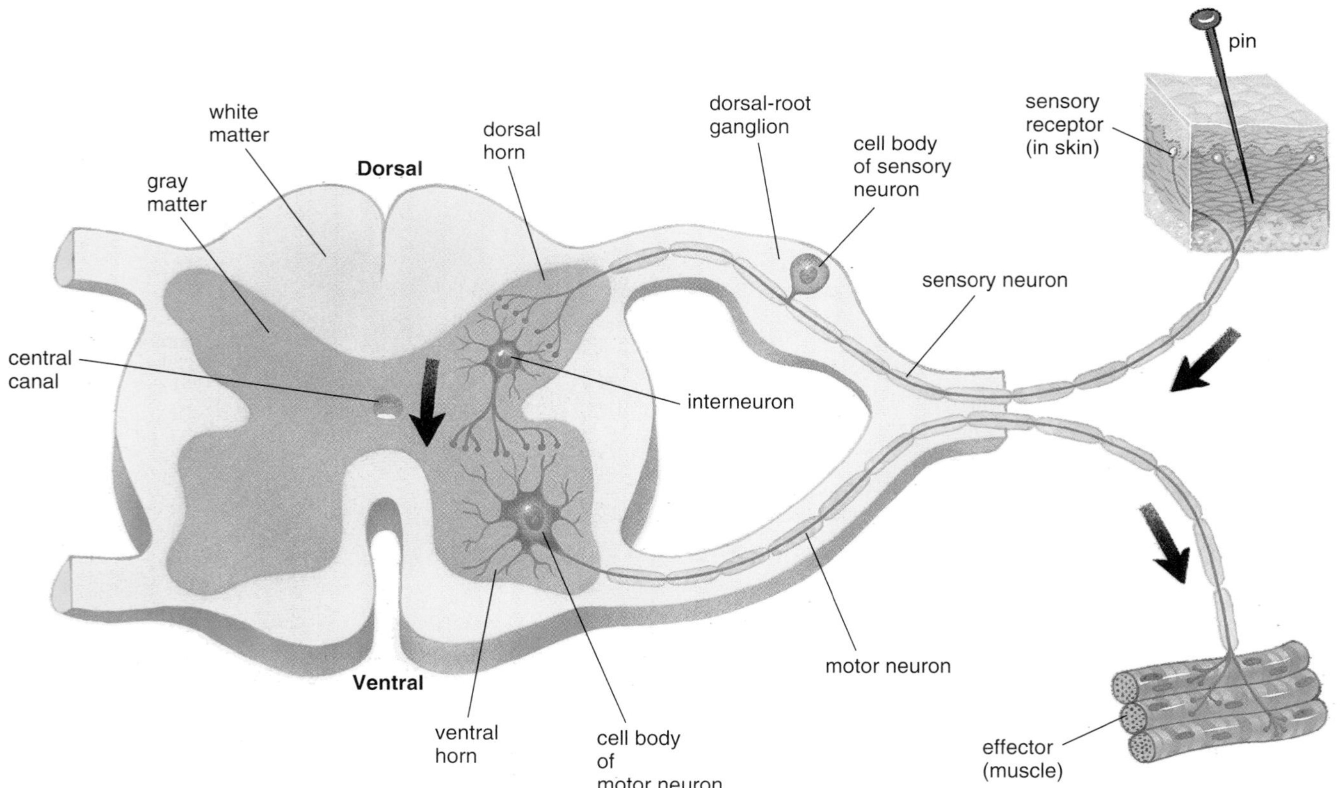

Figure 9-5. This cross section of the spinal cord and a spinal nerve illustrates a reflex arc.

to motor neurons to effectors. In this example of the withdrawal reflex, the receptors are in the skin at the tips of the fingers. These receptors send their information to sensory neurons that relay the information to interneurons in the spinal cord. The interneurons immediately relay the information to motor neurons that activate the muscles (effectors) in the arm. The muscles in the arm coordinate the movement of pulling your finger away from the painful stimulus. A person can consciously inhibit a reflex because the information also goes to the cerebral cortex where a person makes conscious decisions.

Brain

The brain can be divided into four major areas: the cerebrum, the diencephalons, the brain stem, and the cerebellum (Figure 9-6).

Cerebrum. The **cerebrum** is the largest part of the brain. It is divided into two halves called cerebral hemispheres. A thick bundle of nerve fibers called the **corpus callosum** connects the two hemispheres. The grooves on the surface of the cerebrum are called **sulci.** The "bumps" of brain matter between the sulci are called **gyri,** or **convolutions.** A deep groove called the longitudinal fissure runs between the two longitudinal hemispheres.

Lobes. Each cerebral hemisphere is divided into **lobes**—frontal, parietal, temporal, and occipital. The frontal lobes contain motor areas that allow a person to consciously decide to produce a body movement such as walking or tapping a pencil. Somatosensory areas are located in parietal lobes. These areas interpret sensations felt on or within the body. For example, if you feel a light touch on your right hand, the somatosensory area interprets the sensation and

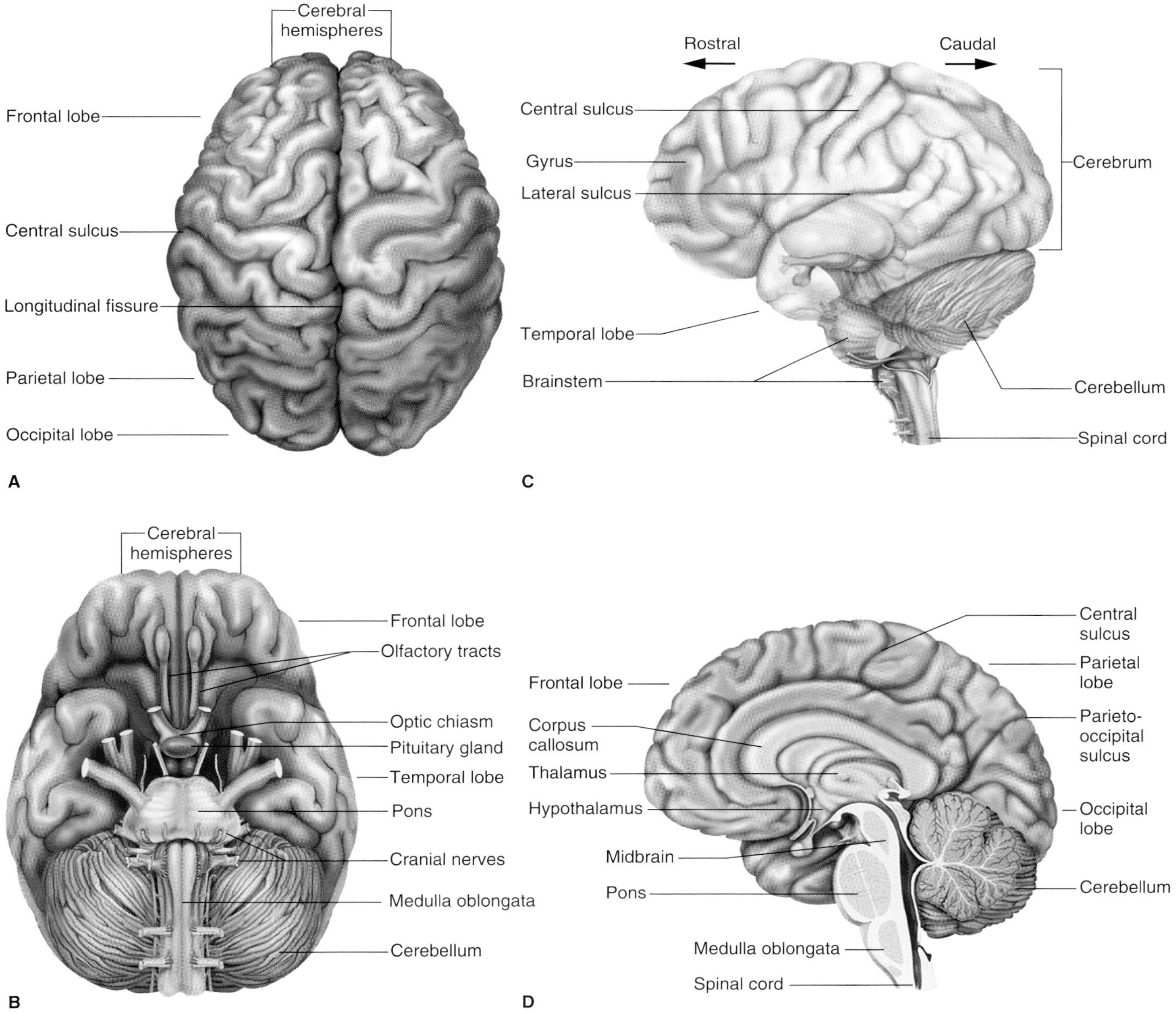

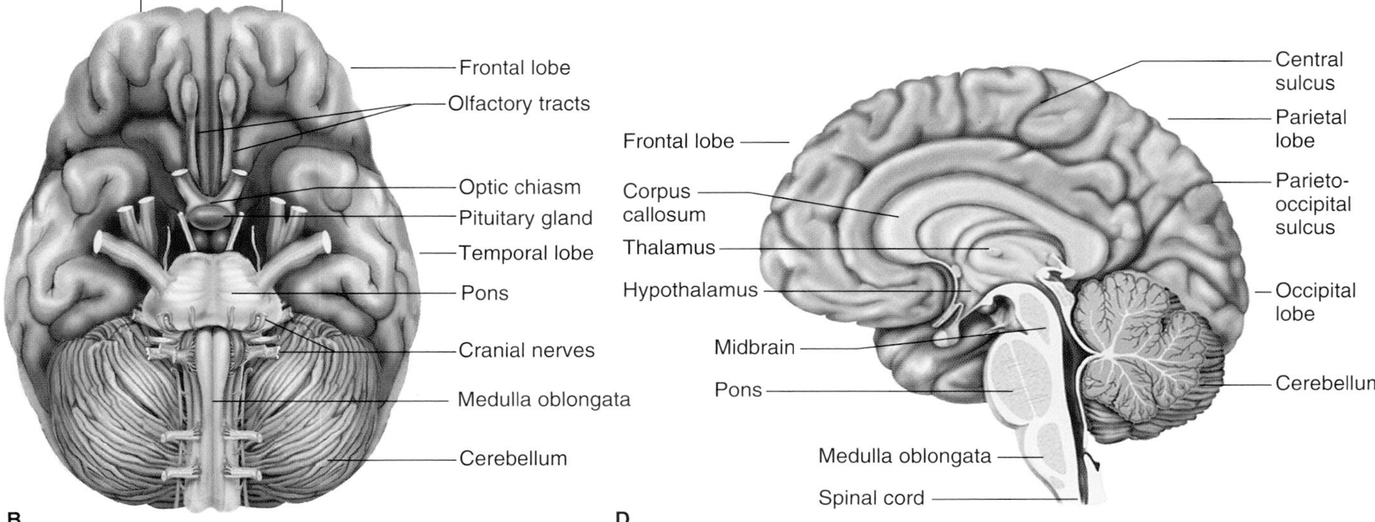

Figure 9-6. Four views of the brain: (a) superior, (b) inferior, (c) left lateral, and (d) sagittal section.

where it is occurring. The temporal lobes contain auditory areas that interpret sounds. Visual areas are located in the occipital lobes, and they interpret what a person sees.

Cortex. The outermost layer of the cerebrum is called the cerebral **cortex.** It is composed of gray matter and therefore contains neuron cell bodies and dendrites. This layer contains nearly 75% of all neurons in the entire nervous system. Beneath the cerebral cortex is white matter. Besides interpreting sensory information and initiating body movements, the cortex also stores memories and creates emotions.

Ventricles. **Ventricles** are interconnected cavities within the brain. They are filled with CSF. Recall that this fluid is also found in the subarachnoid space of the meninges and the central canal of the spinal cord. Therefore, CSF is located within the brain and spinal cord and also around the brain and spinal cord. This fluid protects and cushions the central nervous system.

Diencephalon. The **diencephalon** is located between the cerebral hemispheres and is superior to the brain stem. The diencephalon includes the thalamus and hypothalamus. The **thalamus** serves as a relay station for sensory information that heads to the cerebral cortex for interpretation. If sensory information does not pass through the thalamus before it reaches the cerebral cortex, it cannot be interpreted correctly. For example, say you are feeling pain in your left forearm. This information goes up the spinal cord and through the thalamus and then to the cerebral cortex for interpretation. If the information did not go through the thalamus, the cerebral cortex may interpret that you are feeling cold instead of pain in your left forearm. The **hypothalamus** maintains balance by regulating many vital activities such as heart rate, blood pressure, and breathing rate.

Brain Stem. The **brain stem** is a structure that connects the cerebrum to the spinal cord. The three parts of the brain stem are the midbrain, the pons, and the medulla oblongata. The midbrain lies just beneath the diencephalon. It controls both visual and auditory reflexes. An example of a visual reflex is when you see something in your peripheral vision and you automatically turn your head to view it more clearly.

The pons is a rounded bulge on the underside of the brain stem situated between the midbrain and the medulla oblongata. It contains nerve tracts to connect the cerebrum to the cerebellum. The pons also regulates breathing.

The medulla oblongata is the most inferior portion of the brain stem and is directly connected to the spinal cord. It controls many vital activities such as heart rate, blood pressure, and breathing. It also controls reflexes associated with coughing, sneezing, and vomiting.

Educating the Patient

Preventing Brain and Spinal Cord Injuries

In the United States alone, almost half a million people a year suffer brain and spinal cord injuries. The most common causes of these injuries are motor vehicle accidents, sports and recreational accidents—especially diving—and violence. People at the highest risk for spinal cord injuries are children and teens. However, most brain and spinal cord injuries can be prevented. You can use the following tips to educate patients on preventing these types of injuries.

Prevention Tips

- Know the depth of water into which you are diving. More than 90% of diving injuries occur in 5 feet of water or less.
- Explore diving areas before diving. For example, know where rocks are located before you dive.
- Do not drive or do any recreational activity while intoxicated. Alcohol affects good judgment and control. Alcohol-related traffic crashes are the leading cause of disabling brain and spinal cord injuries.
- Always wear a helmet when riding a bike or motorcycle. Your risk of brain injury is 85% greater during a biking accident if you are not wearing a helmet. Make sure your helmet fits properly.
- Always wear appropriate protective gear while playing any sport.
- Avoid surfing headfirst.
- Always wear your safety belt.
- Make sure children use car seats that appropriate for their age and weight.
- Be familiar with ways to get help quickly in emergencies.
- Follow traffic rules and signs while walking, biking, or driving.
- Follow safety rules on playgrounds.
- Store firearms and ammunition in separate and locked places.
- Teach children the safety rules to follow if they find a gun.

Cerebellum. The **cerebellum** is inferior to the occipital lobes of the cerebrum and posterior to the pons and medulla oblongata. It coordinates complex skeletal muscle contractions that are needed for body movements. For example, when you walk, many muscles have to contract and relax at appropriate times. Your cerebellum coordinates these activities. The cerebellum also coordinates fine movements such as threading a needle, playing an instrument, and writing.

Peripheral Nervous System

The peripheral nervous system consists of nerves that branch off the CNS. These nerves are called peripheral nerves and are classified in two types—**cranial nerves** and **spinal nerves.**

Cranial Nerves

Cranial nerves are peripheral nerves that originate from the brain. Roman numerals and names designate the twelve different cranial nerves.

I. *Olfactory nerves* carry smell information to the brain for interpretation.
II. *Optic nerves* carry visual information to the brain for interpretation.
III. *Oculomotor nerves* are found within the muscles that move the eyeball, eyelid, and iris.
IV. *Trochlear nerves* act in the muscles that move the eyeball.
V. *Trigeminal nerves* carry sensory information from the surface of the eye, the scalp, facial skin, the lining of the gums, and the palate to the brain for interpretation. They also are found within the muscles needed for chewing.
VI. *Abducens nerves* act in the muscles that move the eyeball.
VII. *Facial nerves* are found in the muscles of facial expression as well as in the salivary and tear glands. These nerves also carry sensory information from the tongue.
VIII. *Vestibulocochlear nerves* carry hearing and equilibrium information from the inner ear to the brain for interpretation.
IX. *Glossopharyngeal nerves* carry sensory information from the throat and tongue to the brain for interpretation. They also act in the muscles of the throat.
X. *Vagus nerves* carry sensory information from the thoracic and abdominal organs to the brain for interpretation. These nerves are also found within the muscles in the throat, stomach, intestines, and heart.
XI. *Accessory nerves* are found within the muscles of the throat, neck, back, and voice box.
XII. *Hypoglossal nerves* are found within the muscles of the tongue.

Spinal Nerves

Spinal nerves are peripheral nerves that originate from the spinal cord (Figure 9-7). There are 31 pairs of spinal nerves: 8 pairs of cervical nerves (numbered C1 through C8), 12 pairs of thoracic nerves (numbered T1 through T12), 5 pairs of lumbar nerves (numbered L1 through L5), 5 pairs of sacral nerves (numbered S1 through S5), and one pair of coccygeal nerves (Co).

Two roots, a ventral root and a dorsal root, form each spinal nerve (see Figure 9-5). The **ventral root** contains axons of motor neurons only, and the dorsal root contains axons of sensory neurons only. The **dorsal root** also contains a dorsal root ganglion, which contains the cell bodies of sensory neurons.

Except in the thoracic region, the main portions of spinal nerves fuse together to form nerve **plexuses.** The major nerve plexuses are the cervical, brachial, and lumbosacral. Nerves coming off the cervical plexus supply the skin and the muscles of the neck. The phrenic nerve also originates from the plexus. This nerve controls the diaphragm, which is a muscle that is needed for breathing.

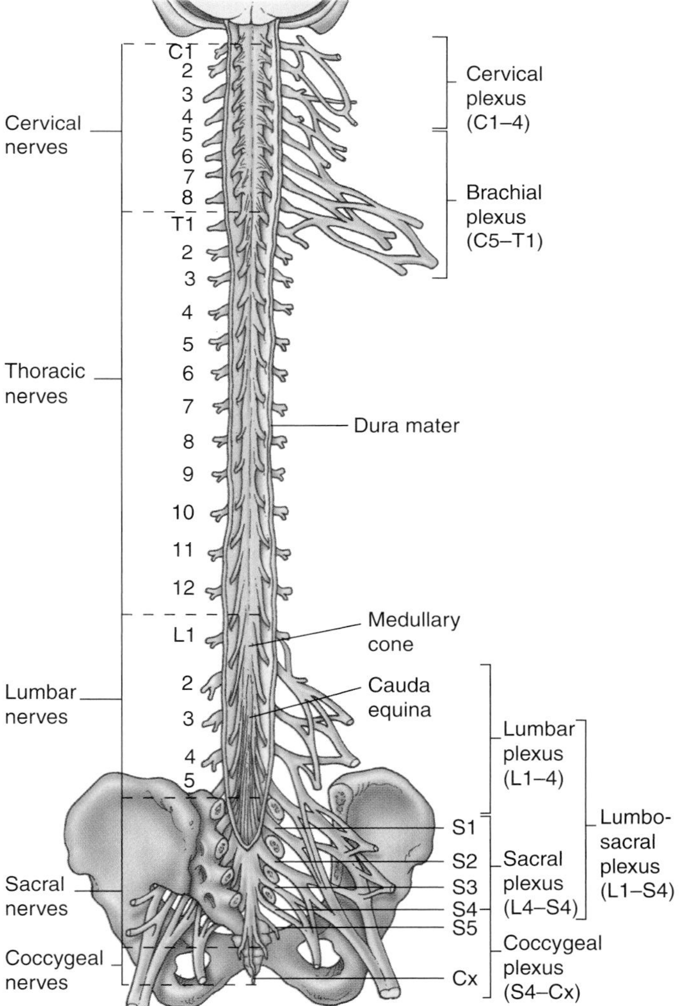

Figure 9-7. Spinal cord, spinal nerves, and plexuses.

The brachial plexus forms nerves that control muscles in the arms. The lumbosacral plexus supplies the lower abdominal wall, external genitalia, buttocks, thighs, legs, and feet. The largest nerve of the body, the sciatic nerve, originates from this plexus. This nerve controls the muscles of the legs.

Somatic and Autonomic Nervous Systems

The peripheral nervous system is divided into a somatic nervous system and an autonomic nervous system. The **somatic** nervous system consists of nerves that connect the CNS to skin and skeletal muscle. The somatic nervous system is often called the "voluntary" nervous system because it controls skeletal muscles, which are under voluntary control. The **autonomic** nervous system consists of nerves that connect the CNS to organs and other structures such as the heart, stomach, intestines, glands, blood vessels, and bladder (among others). The autonomic nervous system controls organs not under voluntary control, so it is often referred to as the "involuntary" nervous system.

In the autonomic nervous system, motor neurons from the brain and spinal cord communicate to other motor neurons that are located in ganglia. **Ganglia** are collections of neuron cell bodies outside the CNS. The motor neurons of ganglia then communicate to various organs and blood vessels.

The two divisions of the autonomic nervous system are the sympathetic and the parasympathetic (Figure 9-8). The **sympathetic** division prepares organs for "fight-or-flight" situations. In other words, it prepares them for stressful or emergency situations. For example, the sympathetic division prepares the heart for a stressful or frightening situation by increasing the heart rate. The **parasympathetic** division prepares the body for resting and digesting. For example, the parasympathetic division prepares the heart for resting by keeping the heart rate relatively low. Notice that sympathetic and parasympathetic actions are antagonistic, meaning that they function in opposite ways. Most of the body's organs are under parasympathetic control.

Many neurons of the sympathetic division are located in the thoracic and lumbar regions of the spinal cord. For this reason, this division is also called the thoracolumbar division. The sympathetic neurons usually release the neurotransmitter norepinephrine into organs and glands. Norepinephrine increases the heart and breathing rates, slows down the activity of the digestive glands, slows down the muscles of the stomach and the intestines, and dilates the pupils. Sympathetic nerves also control the constriction of blood vessels. When blood vessels constrict, blood pressure increases, which is a needed response during an emergency situation.

Many neurons of the parasympathetic division are located in the brain stem and the sacral regions of the spinal

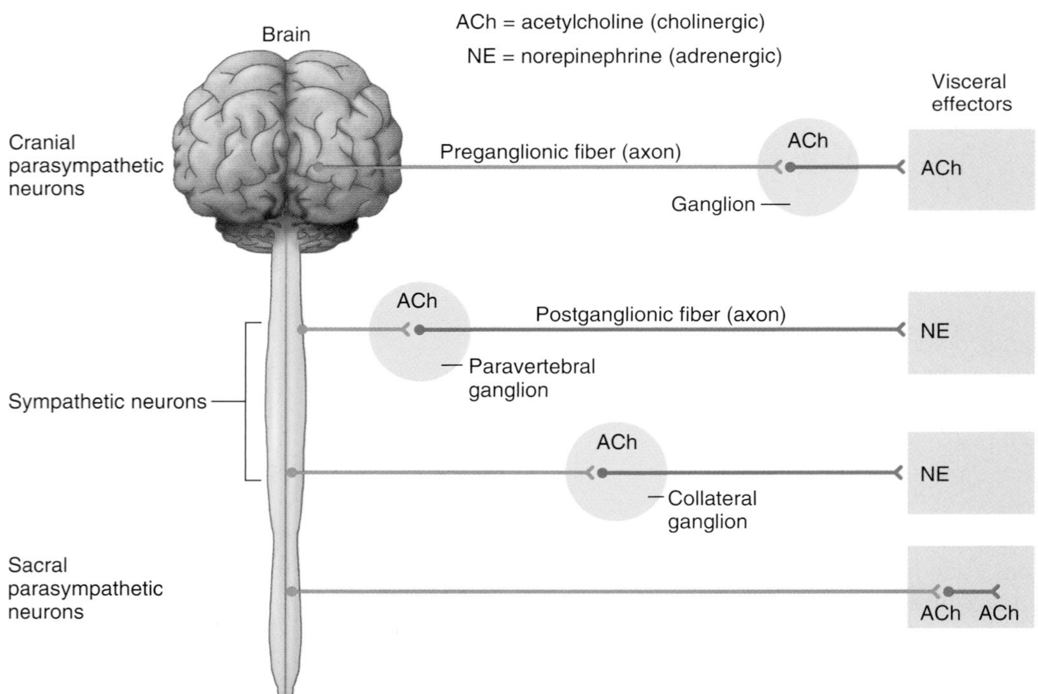

Figure 9-8. Divisions of the autonomic nervous system. Most parasympathetic fibers release acetylcholine onto visceral effectors. Most sympathetic fibers release norepinephrine onto visceral effectors.

cord. For this reason, this division is also referred to as the craniosacral division. All parasympathetic neurons release acetylcholine onto organs and glands. Acetylcholine is a neurotransmitter that slows the heart and breathing rates, constricts the pupils, activates digestive glands, and activates the muscles of the stomach and intestines. Most blood vessels in the body do not receive communication from parasympathetic nerves.

Neurologic Testing

Patients with nervous system disorders may have a wide variety of signs and symptoms, but the most common are headache, muscle weakness, and **paresthesias** (loss of feeling). A typical neurologic examination can determine the following:

- State of consciousness. This state can vary from normal to a state of coma. A patient in a coma cannot respond to stimuli and cannot be awakened. Other terms used to describe states of consciousness include *stupor* (difficulty being awakened), *delirium* (being confused or having hallucinations), *vegetative* (having no cortical function), and *asleep* (can be aroused with normal stimulation).
- Reflex activity. Reflex tests primarily determine the health of the peripheral nervous system.
- Speech patterns. Abnormal speech patterns include a loss of the ability to form words correctly or to form sentences that make sense.
- Motor patterns. Abnormal motor patterns include the loss of balance, abnormal posture, or inappropriate movements of the body. For example, chorea is an exaggerated and sudden jerking of a body part.

Diagnostic Procedures

Common diagnostic procedures to determine neurologic disorders include the following specialized tests:

- Lumbar puncture. Whenever a physician needs to examine CSF, a lumbar puncture is performed. A needle is used to remove CSF from the subarachnoid space usually below the third lumbar vertebra of the spinal column. Analysis of this fluid provides a great deal about the health of a patient. For example, cancer cells in CSF often indicate a brain or spinal cord tumor. White blood cells in this fluid indicate infections such as meningitis. Red blood cells indicate abnormal bleeding.
- Magnetic resonance imaging (MRI). This procedure allows for the brain and spinal cord to be visualized from many angles. It uses powerful magnets to generate images and is useful at detecting tumors, bleeding, or other abnormalities.
- Positron emission tomography (PET) scan. This procedure uses radioactive chemicals that collect in specific areas of the brain. These chemicals allow images of those specific areas to be generated. This test is useful in detecting blood flow to areas of the brain, brain tumors, and the diagnosis of such diseases as Parkinson's and Alzheimer's.
- Cerebral angiography. This procedure uses dyes that can be visualized in the blood vessels of the brain. It is useful in detecting aneurysms (abnormally dilated blood vessels).
- Computerized tomography (CT) scan. This very common procedure produces images that provide more information than a standard x-ray. It is useful in detecting tumors and other abnormal structures.
- Electroencephalogram (EEG). This test detects electrical activity in the brain. It is useful in diagnosing various states of consciousness.
- X-ray. This procedure is useful in detecting skull or vertebral fractures.

Cranial Nerve Tests

Disorders of the cranial nerves can be determined using the following tests:

- The olfactory nerves (I) are tested by asking a patient to smell various substances.
- Cranial nerves III, IV, and VI are tested by asking a patient to track the movement of the physician's finger. If a patient cannot move her eyeballs properly, there may be damage to one of these nerves. Recall that these nerves control the muscles that move the eyeballs.
- Cranial nerve V controls the muscles needed for chewing. To assess this nerve, a patient is asked to clench his teeth. The physician then feels the jaw muscles. If they feel limp or weak, this nerve may be damaged.
- If a person can no longer make facial expressions, then cranial nerve VII may be damaged. This nerve controls the muscles needed to make facial expressions.
- If a patient cannot extend his tongue and move it from side to side, cranial nerve XII may be damaged. This nerve controls tongue movement.

Reflex Testing

Testing a patient's reflexes allows a physician to evaluate the components of a reflex as well as the overall health of the individual's nervous system. The absence of a reflex is called **areflexia. Hyporeflexia** is a decreased reflex, and **hyperreflexia** is a stronger than normal reflex. The following are common reflex tests:

- Biceps reflex. The absence of this reflex may indicate spinal cord damage in the cervical region.
- Knee reflex. The absence of this reflex may indicate damage to lumbar or femoral nerves.
- Abdominal reflexes. These reflexes are used to evaluate damage to thoracic spinal nerves.

Pathophysiology

Common Diseases and Disorders of the Nervous System

Alzheimer's disease is a progressive, degenerative disease that occurs in the brain.

- **Causes.** Fiber tangles within neurons, degenerating nerve fibers, and a decreased production of neurotransmitters cause the symptoms of this disorder. This disease is associated with advanced age, family history, certain genes, and possibly some environmental factors. Many causes have not yet been determined.
- **Signs and symptoms.** Common symptoms include a loss of memory, confusion, personality changes, language deterioration, impaired judgment, and restlessness.
- **Treatment.** There is no cure, but proper nutrition, physical exercise, social activity, and calm environments help to manage the disease.

Amyotrophic lateral sclerosis (ALS) is a fatal disorder characterized by the degeneration of neurons in the spinal cord and brain.

- **Causes.** Most causes are unknown but they are likely to involve hereditary and environmental factors.
- **Signs and symptoms.** Early symptoms include cramping of hand and feet muscles, persistent tripping and falling, chronic fatigue, and slurred speech. Signs and symptoms that appear in later stages include breathing difficulty and muscle paralysis.
- **Treatment.** There is no cure for this disorder; however, physical, speech, and respiratory therapies help to manage the symptoms. Some medications relieve muscle cramping, and one drug that prolongs the life of ALS patients has been approved by the FDA.

Bell's palsy is a disorder in which facial muscles are very weak or totally paralyzed.

- **Causes.** This condition can result from damage to cranial nerve VII (the facial nerve), but many times the cause is unknown. It is more common in people with diabetes, the flu, or a cold.
- **Signs and symptoms.** The most common signs and symptoms are a loss of feeling in the face, the inability to produce facial expressions, headache, and excessive tearing or drooling.
- **Treatment.** Treatments include the use of eyedrops, anti-inflammatory medications, and pain relievers. Symptoms usually diminish or go away within 5 to 10 days.

Brain tumors and cancers are abnormal growths in the brain. A brain tumor with cancer cells is termed malignant. Malignant tumors that start in any tissue of the brain are called primary brain cancers. Those that start in body parts and spread to the brain are classified as secondary brain cancers. The most common primary brain tumors are gliomas that arise from neuroglial cells.

- **Causes.** Like most cancers, the causes are gene mutations. Factors associated with gene mutations include exposure to toxins, an impaired immune system, and hereditary factors.
- **Signs and symptoms.** The signs and symptoms depend on size and location of the tumor. Common symptoms include headache, seizures, nausea, weakness in the arms or legs, fatigue, changes in speech patterns, and a loss of memory.
- **Treatment.** Treatment often includes surgery, radiation therapy, chemotherapy, and gene therapy. The success of the treatment depends on the type of tumor, the extent of the diseases, the location of the tumor, the tumor's response to treatment, and the overall health of the patient.

Epilepsy and **seizures** occur when parts of the brain receive a burst of electrical signals that disrupt normal brain functioning. Seizures may be either partial or generalized. Partial seizures occur on one side of the brain, and generalized seizures occur on both sides. Epilepsy is the condition of having repeated, long-term seizures.

- **Causes.** Causes vary but may include birth trauma, high fevers, alcohol and drug withdrawal, head trauma, infections, brain tumors, and certain medications. Many causes are unknown.
- **Signs and symptoms.** The signs and symptoms may include visual disturbances, nausea, generalized abnormal feelings, a loss of consciousness, and uncontrolled muscle contractions and tremors.
- **Treatment.** The primary treatment is medication to prevent seizures. Surgery is sometimes an option in patients with partial seizures.

Guillain-Barré syndrome is a disorder in which the body's immune system attacks part of the peripheral nervous system. It usually has a sudden and unexpected onset.

- **Causes.** The destruction of myelin by the body's immune system produces the signs and symptoms. Viral infections, immunizations, and pregnancy sometimes trigger the disease.
- **Signs and symptoms.** Symptoms may include weakness or tingling sensations in the legs or arms that can progress to paralysis. Difficulty breathing and an abnormal heart rate are dangerous signs and symptoms. The disease normally runs its course, and with proper medical treatment, it is not fatal.

continued ⟶

- **Treatment.** Various supportive therapies, such as the use of respirators and heart machines, are necessary until the disease subsides. Physical therapy is used to keep muscles strong.

Headaches affect almost everyone at some point in life. They can affect the very young to the very old. A wide variety of factors produce headaches. Most headaches do not require medical attention, but a physician should evaluate repetitive and severe headaches. Headaches commonly include tension headaches, migraines, and cluster headaches.

Tension headaches are classified as either episodic (occurring randomly) or chronic (occurring frequently):

Episodic tension headaches are the most common type of tension headache.

- **Causes.** This type of headache occurs randomly and is often the result of temporary stress or anger.
- **Signs and symptoms.** Symptoms include pain or soreness in the temples and the contraction of head and neck muscles.
- **Treatment.** Most of these headaches can be managed by taking an over-the-counter (OTC) medicine, and relief usually occurs in 1 or 2 hours. A person who takes medication daily or almost daily for headaches, should see a physician.

Chronic tension headaches occur almost every day and persist for weeks or months.

- **Causes.** This type of headache may be the result of stress or fatigue, but it may also be associated with physical problems, psychological issues, or depression.
- **Signs and symptoms.** As with episodic tension headaches, the symptoms include pain or soreness in the temples and the contraction of head and neck muscles.
- **Treatment.** People who suffer from chronic headaches should seek medical treatment.

Migraines are the most severe type of headache. They are responsible for more "sick days" than any other headache type. Almost 30 million people in the United States suffer from migraines.

- **Causes.** Hormones may influence migraines, which may explain why women experience migraines at least three times more often than men do. Migraine headaches are considered vascular headaches because they are associated with the distension of the arteries of the brain.
- **Signs and symptoms.** Migraines often begin as dull pains that develop into throbbing pains accompanied by nausea and a sensitivity to light and noise. There are many types of migraines but the two most common are *migraine with aura* and *migraine without aura.* Some patients have migraines that begin with an aura. Auras may include the appearance of jagged lines or flashing lights, tunnel vision, hallucinations, or the detection of strange odors. The auras may last up to an hour and usually go away as the headache begins. Most migraine headaches last about 4 hours but some can last up to a week.
- **Treatment.** When treating migraines, a physician will prescribe a drug to relieve the pain but will also try to identify the factors that trigger it. There are many medicines available to treat migraines.

Cluster headaches are so named because the attacks come in groups. They are the most severe type of migraines. More men than women experience these types of headaches.

- **Causes.** Some research indicates that alcohol consumption can bring on attacks of cluster headaches.
- **Signs and symptoms.** Common symptoms include a runny nose, watery eyes, and swelling below the eyes. Cluster headaches normally last about 45 minutes to an hour, although they can last longer. It is common for a patient with this disorder to experience 1 to 4 headaches a day during a cluster time span. Cluster time spans can last weeks or months.
- **Treatment.** Various drugs are available for the treatment of these headaches.

Meningitis is an inflammation of the meninges.

- **Causes.** Causes may include bacterial, viral, and fungal infections. Some types of meningitis can be prevented with vaccines.
- **Signs and symptoms.** Fever, headache, vomiting, stiffness in the neck, sensitivity to light, drowsiness, and joint pain usually accompany this disorder.
- **Treatment.** The treatment varies depending on the type of meningitis. Intravenous antibiotics are used for bacterial meningitis, supportive therapy for viral meningitis, and antifungal drugs for fungal meningitis.

Multiple sclerosis (MS) is a chronic disease of the central nervous system in which myelin is destroyed.

- **Causes.** The causes are mostly unknown, but some known causes are viruses, genetic factors, and immune system abnormalities.
- **Signs and symptoms.** Depending on the type of MS, symptoms can range from mild to severe. In severe cases, a person will lose the ability to walk or speak.
- **Treatment.** There is no cure for MS, but supportive treatments can lessen the symptoms. Some medications are also available to treat symptoms.

Neuralgias are a group of disorders commonly referred to as nerve pain. They most frequently occur in the nerves, of the face.

- **Causes.** There are many causes of neuralgia, including trauma, chemical irritation of the nerves, bacterial

continued ⟶

infections, and diabetes. Many times the causes are unknown.

- **Signs and symptoms.** Sudden and severe skin pain are the most common symptoms. The pain repeatedly occurs in the same body area. Numbness of skin areas is also common.
- **Treatment.** Many times the disorder goes away by itself, and treatment, other than pain medication, is not needed. Other treatments include injections of anesthetics or surgery to remove the affected nerves.

Parkinson's disease is a motor system disorder. It is slowly progressive and degenerative.

- **Causes.** Most causes are undetermined, although it is known that patients with this disease lack certain chemicals in the brain. Brain tumors, certain drugs, carbon monoxide, or repeated head trauma may produce Parkinson's disease.
- **Signs and symptoms.** The most common signs and symptoms include trembling and stiffness of the arms and legs as well as a lack of coordination and balance.
- **Treatment.** There is no cure, but medications alleviate some symptoms and slow down the progression of this disease. Surgery is useful in some cases of Parkinson's.

Sciatica occurs when the sciatic nerve is damaged.

- **Causes.** The sciatic nerve is commonly damaged by excessive pressure on the nerve from prolonged sitting or lying down. It is also easily damaged from trauma to the pelvis, buttocks, or thighs.
- **Signs and symptoms.** The most usual symptoms include numbness, pain, or tingling sensations on the back of a leg or foot. Weakness of leg and foot muscles can also develop.
- **Treatment.** This disorder is usually treated with pain medication and steroids. Physical therapy is also needed following trauma to the nerve.

Stroke occurs when brain cells die because of an inadequate blood flow. Stroke is sometimes referred to as a "brain attack."

- **Causes.** Most strokes are caused by the blockage of an artery in the neck or brain. They may also be caused by aneurisms that burst.
- **Signs and symptoms.** Signs and symptoms may include paralysis, speech problems, memory and reasoning deficits, coma, and possibly death. Symptoms will vary depending on the location of the stroke within the brain.
- **Treatment.** Because neurons in the brain cannot be replaced, the effects of a stroke can be permanent. However, physical and speech therapy are often very useful in lessening the effects of a stroke.

Summary

The functions of the nervous system include detecting and interpreting sensory information, making decisions about that information, and responding to and carrying out motor functions based on those decisions. The cells responsible for these functions are neurons.

There are two divisions of the nervous system. The CNS consists of the brain and spinal cord. The peripheral nervous system is made up of cranial nerves and spinal nerves. All organs are under the control of the nervous system. Knowledge of this system is essential when assisting the physician during a neurologic exam.

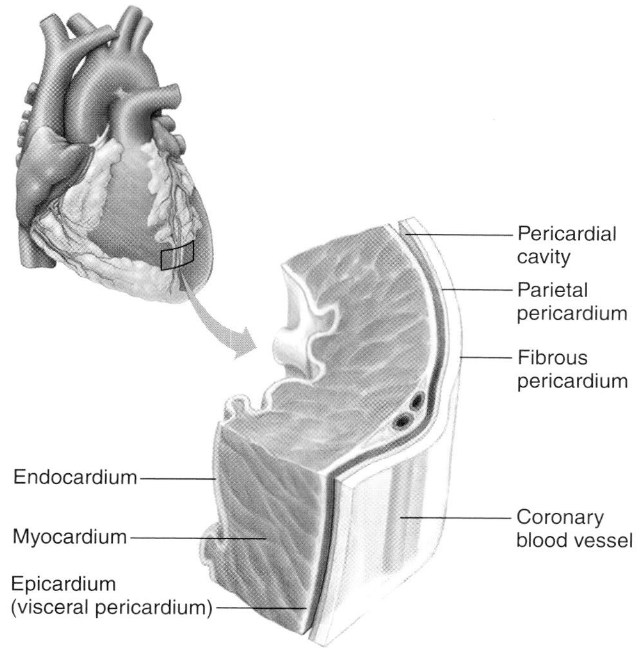

Figure 10-2. Layers of the wall of the heart.

Bicuspid Valve. The **bicuspid valve** has two cusps and is located between the left atrium and the left ventricle. It prevents blood from flowing back into the left atrium when the left ventricle contracts. This valve is known as the **mitral valve** and the left AV valve. Like the tricuspid valve, the bicuspid valve also has chordae tendineae attached to papillary muscles.

Pulmonary Valve. The **pulmonary valve** is situated between the right ventricle and the pulmonary trunk. It prevents blood from flowing back into the right ventricle. Because its cusps are shaped like a half moon, this valve is called a semilunar valve.

Aortic Valve. The **aortic valve** is situated between the left ventricle and the aorta. It prevents blood from flowing back into the left ventricle and is also known as a semilunar valve.

Blood Flow Through the Heart

Blood that is low in oxygen and rich in carbon dioxide enters the right atrium of the heart through large veins called the inferior and superior vena cavae. From the right atrium, the blood flows over the tricuspid valve into the right ventricle. When the right ventricle contracts, blood is pushed over the pulmonary valve into a larger artery called the **pulmonary trunk.** The pulmonary trunk branches into pulmonary arteries, which carry blood to the lungs. In the lungs, blood picks up oxygen and gets rid of carbon dioxide. Blood rich in oxygen and low in carbon dioxide then returns to the heart through four veins called the pulmonary veins. The pulmonary veins empty the blood into

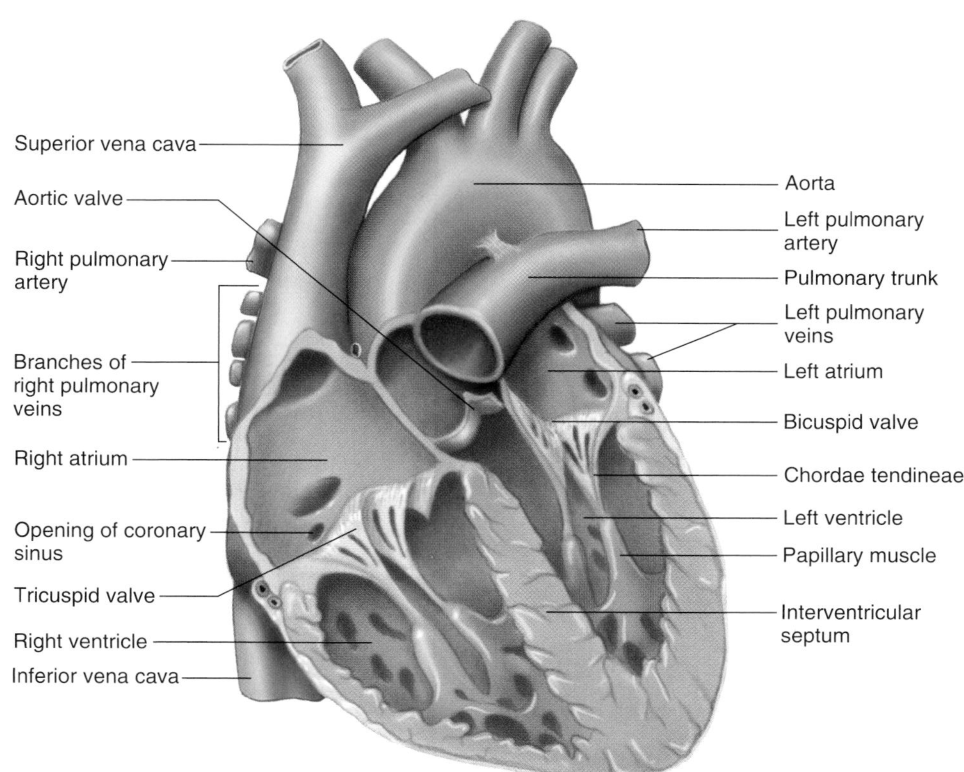

Figure 10-3. Coronal section of the heart.

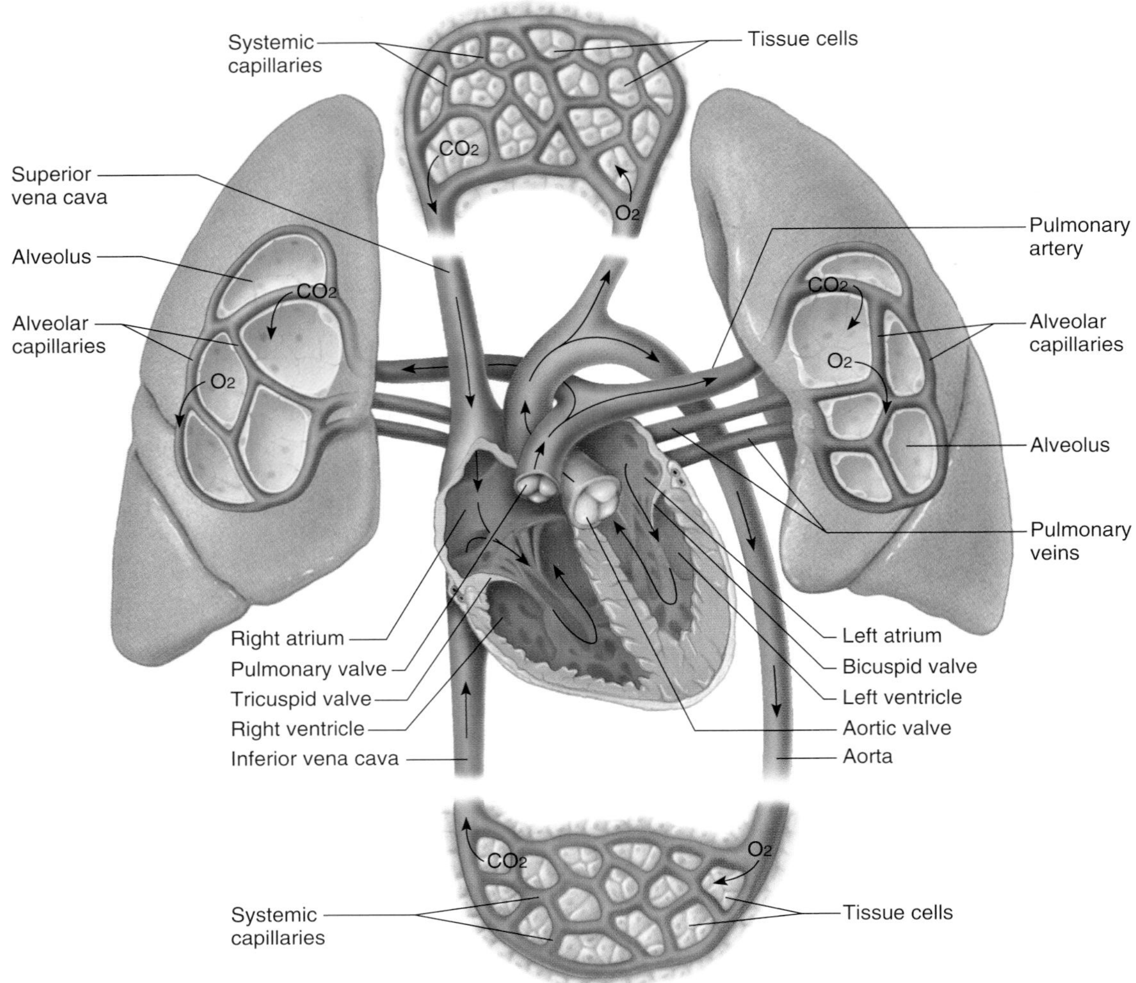

Figure 10-4. Pathway of blood through the heart and lungs and on to other body parts. The right side of the heart delivers blood to the lungs and the left side delivers blood to all other body parts.

the left atrium. From the left atrium, blood flows over the bicuspid valve into the left ventricle. When the left ventricle contracts, blood is pushed over the aortic valve into the aorta. The aorta distributes blood into its branches and throughout the body.

In the body, the blood gives oxygen to cells and picks up carbon dioxide. Veins of the body pick up the oxygen-poor blood and empty it into the vena cavae, and the whole circuit starts all over again. Note that arteries carry blood away from the heart and veins carry blood to the heart (Figure 10-4).

Cardiac Cycle

One heartbeat makes up one cardiac cycle. In one cardiac cycle, the top chambers (atria) of the heart contract and relax together and then the bottom chambers (ventricles) of the heart contract and relax together. When the right atrium contracts, the tricuspid valve opens and blood flows into the right ventricle. Likewise, when the left atrium contracts, the bicuspid valve opens and blood flows into the left ventricle. When the right ventricle contracts, the tricuspid valve must close, the pulmonary valve opens, and blood is pushed into the pulmonary trunk. When the left ventricle contracts, the bicuspid valve must close, the aortic valve opens, and blood is pushed into the aorta.

The following factors influence the cardiac cycle:

- Exercise. Strenuous exercise increases the heart rate because skeletal muscles need more oxygen.
- Parasympathetic nerves. The parasympathetic nerve to the heart is the vagus nerve, and it generally keeps the heart rate relatively low.
- Sympathetic nerves. The sympathetic nerves increase the heart rate during times of stress.
- Cardiac control center. This center is located in the medulla oblongata. When blood pressure rises, this control center sends impulses to decrease the heart rate. When blood pressure falls, it sends impulses to increase the heart rate.

- Body temperature. An increase in body temperature usually increases the heart rate. This explains the high heart rate when a person runs a fever.
- Potassium ions. Low concentrations of potassium ions in the blood decrease the heart rate, but a high concentration causes an arrhythmia (abnormal heart rate).
- Calcium ions. Low concentrations of calcium ions in the blood depress heart actions, but high concentrations cause heart contractions called titanic contractions, which are longer than normal heart contractions.

Heart Sounds

During one cardiac cycle you can hear two heart sounds. The sounds are called *lubb* and *dupp*. These sounds are generated when valves in the heart snap shut. Lubb is the first heart sound and occurs when the ventricles contract and the tricuspid and bicuspid valves snap shut. Dupp is the second heart sound and occurs when the atria contract and the pulmonary and aortic valves snap shut.

Physicians will listen to heart sounds in order to diagnose certain conditions. For example, if AV valves are damaged, they will not close completely. This allows blood to leak back into atria when the ventricles contract and produces an abnormal heart sound called a **murmur.** Murmurs may indicate serious heart conditions, although many times heart murmurs are harmless.

Cardiac Conduction System

The cardiac conduction system consists of a group of structures that send electrical impulses through the heart. When cardiac muscle receives an electrical impulse, it contracts (Figure 10-5). The components of the cardiac conduction system are as follows:

- **Sinoatrial node** (SA node). This node is located in the wall of the right atrium and generates an impulse that flows to the atrioventricular node. The SA node is also called the pacemaker of the heart because it generates the heart's rhythmic contractions.
- **Atrioventricular node** (AV node). This node is located between the atria. After the impulse reaches the AV node, the atria contract and the impulse is sent to the atrioventricular bundle.
- **Atrioventricular bundle** (AV bundle). This structure is located between the ventricles and sends an electrical impulse to the Purkinje fibers.
- **Purkinje fibers.** These fibers are located in the lateral walls of the ventricles. After the impulse flows through the Purkinje fibers, the ventricles contract and the SA node will start the flow of a new impulse.

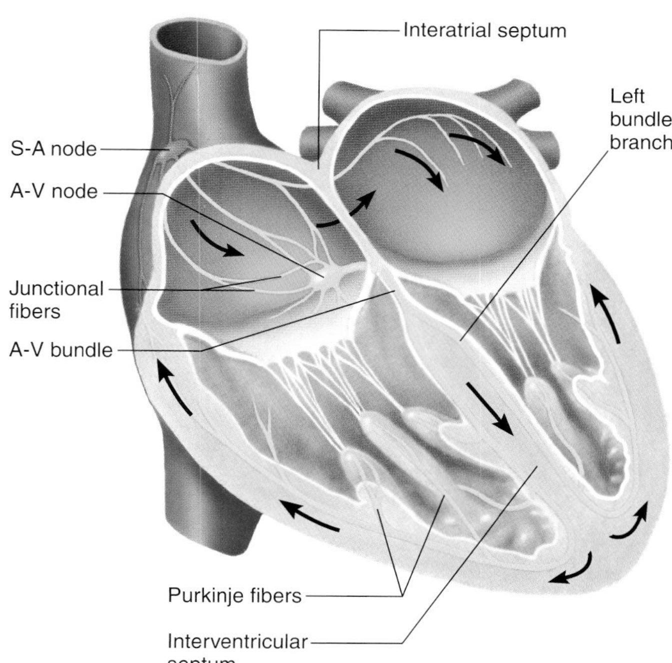

Figure 10-5. Cardiac conduction system.

Physicians use a test called an electrocardiogram (ECG or EKG) to tell if the cardiac conduction system is working properly. In a normal ECG, three waves are produced (Figure 10-6). The first wave (P wave) indicates that an electrical impulse was sent through the atria, which causes them to contract. The second wave (the QRS wave) is the largest of the three and indicates that an electrical impulse

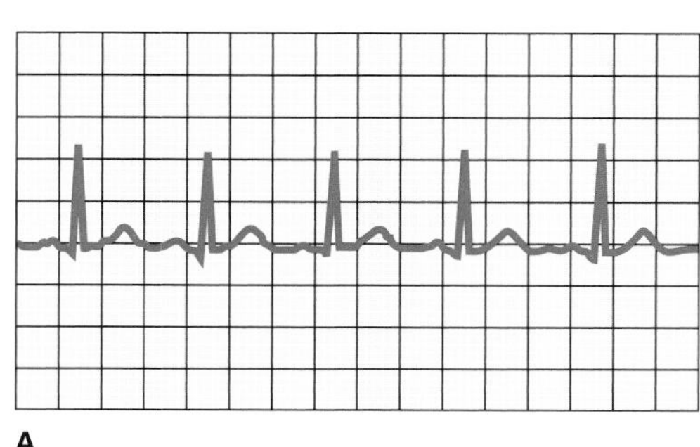

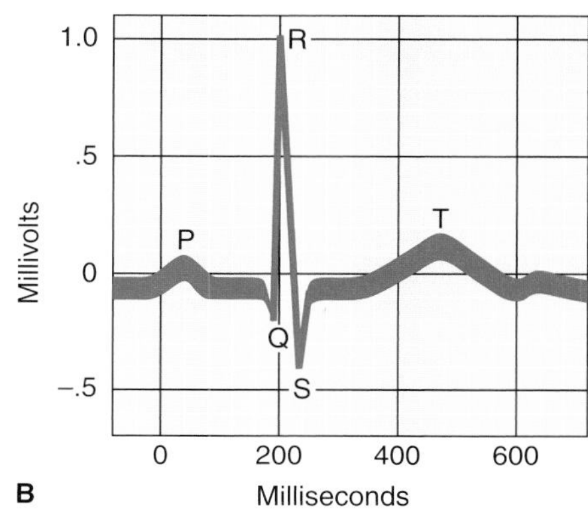

Figure 10-6. Electrocardiogram. (a) A normal ECG and (b) waves of a normal ECG pattern.

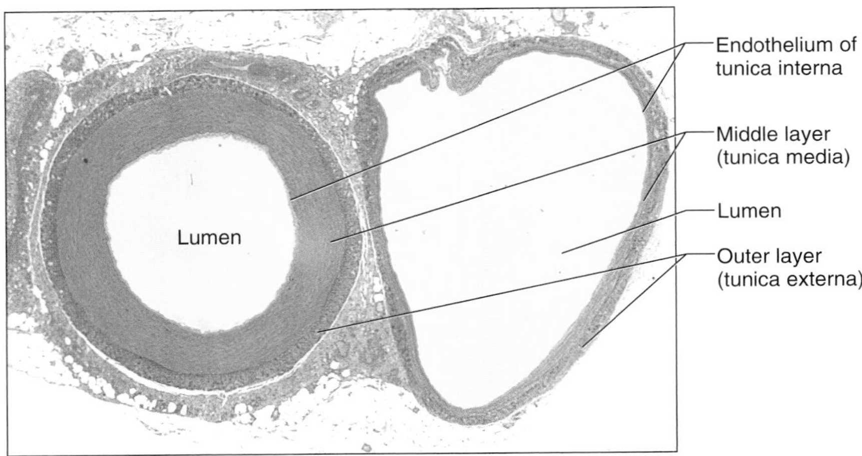

Figure 10-7. Cross sections of an artery (left) and a vein (right).

was sent through the ventricles, which causes them to contract. The third wave (T wave) indicates electrical changes that are occurring in the ventricles as they relax.

Blood Vessels

Blood vessels form a closed pathway that carries blood from the heart to cells and back again. These vessels include arteries, arterioles, veins, venules, and capillaries.

Arteries and Arterioles

Arteries are the strongest of the blood vessels. The muscular layer of arteries contains smooth muscle and is thicker than the muscular layer of other types of blood vessels (Figure 10-7). Arteries carry blood away from the heart and are under high pressure, which is the main reason they need to have thick walls. The muscular wall of an artery can constrict **(vasoconstriction)** to increase blood pressure or it can dilate **(vasodilation)** to decrease blood pressure. Small branches of arteries are called arterioles.

The tissues of the heart receive their blood supply through coronary arteries. Branches of the coronary arteries eventually give rise to very small blood vessels called capillaries. The capillaries of the heart are in the myocardium and allow oxygen to diffuse into the cardiac muscle cells. Blood leaving capillaries in the heart go to cardiac veins. Cardiac veins eventually deliver the oxygen-poor blood to a large vein called the **coronary sinus.** The coronary sinus empties the blood into the right atrium. A heart attack or myocardial infarction often involves the blocking of one of the coronary arteries.

Veins and Venules

Blood is under no pressure in veins and does not move very easily. Therefore, the movement of blood through veins requires skeletal muscle contractions and valves. When skeletal muscles contract, they squeeze the veins and blood is pushed through them, much like the way toothpaste is pushed out of a tube. The valves in veins prevent blood from flowing backward (Figure 10-8). **Varicose veins** occur when valves are destroyed and blood pools in veins, causing them to become dilated or expanded.

The sympathetic nervous system also influences the flow of blood through veins. The sympathetic nervous system causes vein walls to constrict, which forces blood through the veins. This only happens if blood pressure gets abnormally low in arteries.

Venules are very small blood vessels that are formed when capillaries merge together (Figure 10-9). Venules merge together to make veins, and veins carry blood toward the heart. The muscular layer in the walls of veins is thinner than the layer found in arteries.

Capillaries

Capillaries are branches of arterioles and are the smallest type of blood vessel. They connect arterioles to venules and have very thin walls that are only about one cell layer

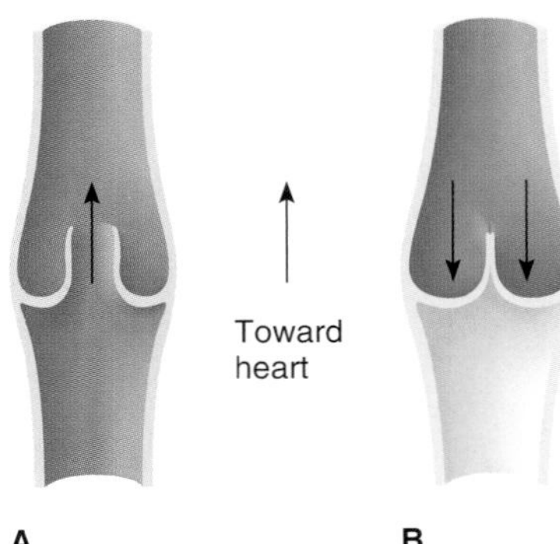

Figure 10-8. Venous valve. (a) Valve opens when blood is flowing toward the heart. (b) Valve closes to prevent blood from flowing away from the heart.

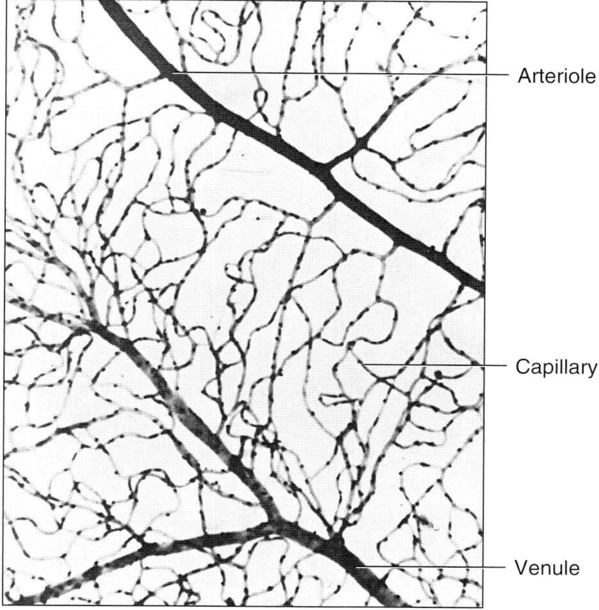

Figure 10-9. Light micrograph of a capillary network.

thick. These thin walls allow substances to pass into and out of capillaries (Figures 10-9 and 10-10). For example, oxygen and nutrients can pass out of a capillary into a body cell, and carbon dioxide and other waste products can pass out of a body cell into a capillary. In fact, capillaries are the only type of blood vessel that allows substances to move in and out of the blood.

Tissues that require a lot of oxygen, such as muscle and nervous tissues, will have a lot of capillaries. Capillary openings have precapillary sphincters that control the amount of blood that flows into them. When the sphincter relaxes, more blood flows into the capillary.

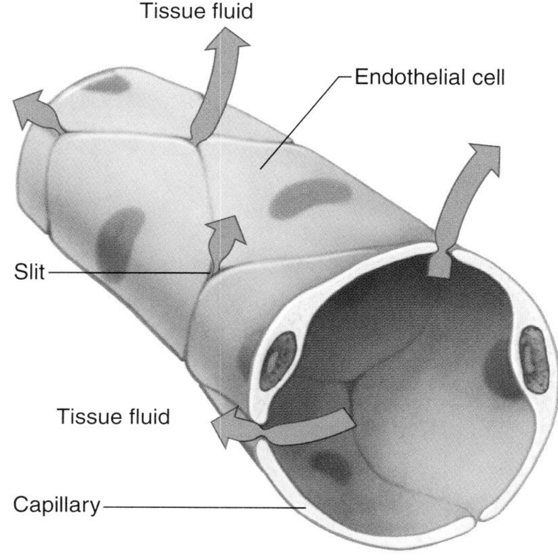

Figure 10-10. Structure of a capillary wall.

The substances that move through the capillary wall (oxygen, carbon dioxide, nutrients, water, and metabolic wastes) do so through diffusion, filtration, and osmosis. When blood first enters a capillary, it has high concentrations of oxygen and nutrients. The body cells surrounding the capillary usually have low concentrations of oxygen and nutrients but high concentrations of carbon dioxide and other waste products. Substances naturally diffuse from an area of high concentration to an area of low concentration. Therefore, oxygen and nutrients diffuse out of the capillary and into body cells. At the same time, carbon dioxide and waste products diffuse out of the body cells and into the capillary.

Because blood is under pressure as it enters the capillary, water is forced through the capillary wall via filtration. This allows water to enter a body cell. By the time blood leaves a capillary, it has a high solid concentration and a low water concentration; water therefore moves back into the capillary through osmosis. Water always moves toward the greater concentration of solids, if possible.

Blood Pressure

Blood pressure is defined as the force that blood exerts on the inner walls of blood vessels. Blood pressure is highest in arteries and lowest in veins. In the clinical setting, blood pressure refers to the pressure in arteries.

Arterial blood pressure rises and falls as the ventricles of the heart contract and relax. When the ventricles contract, blood pressure is greatest in the arteries. This pressure is called the **systolic pressure.** When the ventricles relax, blood pressure in arteries is at its lowest. This pressure is called the **diastolic pressure.** Blood pressure is usually reported as the systolic number over the diastolic number.

You can feel the surge of blood through arteries when you take a pulse. The pulse is created as the artery expands when pressure increases and then subsequently relaxes as blood pressure decreases. Common places to feel a pulse are the carotid and radial arteries.

Many factors affect blood pressure, the most common being cardiac output, blood volume, vasoconstriction, and blood viscosity. Cardiac output is the total amount of blood pumped out of the heart in one minute. As cardiac output increases and decreases, blood pressure increases and decreases. When a person loses a large amount of blood, his blood pressure significantly decreases. If blood pressure falls too low, vasoconstriction, which is the tightening of blood vessel walls, helps to raise blood pressure. In contrast, if blood pressure is too high, vasodilation, which is the widening of blood vessels, decreases the blood pressure. Under certain circumstances, such as dehydration, blood becomes more viscous, or thicker, than normal. This also decreases blood pressure.

Blood pressure is controlled to a large extent by the amount of blood pumped out of the heart. The amount of blood entering the heart should be equal to the amount of blood pumped out of the heart. The heart has a way to ensure that this happens. When blood enters the left ventricle, the wall of the ventricle is stretched. The more the wall is stretched, the harder it will contract and the more blood it will pump out. This is referred to as *Starling's law of the heart*. If only a small amount of blood enters the left ventricle, it will not be stretched very much and therefore will not contract very forcefully. In this case, not much blood is pumped out of the heart.

Baroreceptors also help regulate blood pressure. Baroreceptors measure blood pressure and are located in the aorta and carotid arteries. If pressure increases in these blood vessels, this information is sent to the cardiac center in the medulla oblongata. The cardiac center then knows to decrease the heart rate, which lowers blood pressure. If pressure gets too low in the aorta, baroreceptors pick up this information and relay it to the cardiac center. The cardiac center then increases the heart rate to raise blood pressure.

Circulation

Pulmonary Circuit

The **pulmonary circuit** is the route that blood takes from the heart to the lungs and back to the heart again. The function of this circuit is to oxygenate blood. It also allows carbon dioxide to leave blood and enter the lungs (see Figure 10-4). The pulmonary circuit can be summarized as follows:

right atrium → right ventricle → pulmonary trunk → pulmonary arteries → lungs → pulmonary veins → heart (left atrium)

Systemic Circuit

The **systemic circuit** is the route blood takes from the heart through the body and back to the heart. The function of this circuit is to deliver oxygen and nutrients to body cells. It also picks up carbon dioxide and waste products from body cells (see Figure 10-4). The systemic circuit can be summarized as follows:

left atrium → left ventricle → aorta → arteries → arterioles → capillaries → venules → veins → vena cavae → heart (right atrium)

Arterial System

Arteries carry blood away from the heart. Most of them carry oxygen-rich blood, although pulmonary arteries carry oxygen-poor blood. Many arteries in the body are also paired, meaning that there is a left and a right artery of the same name. The aorta comes directly off the left ventricle and is the largest artery in the body. It has many branches that supply blood to various parts of the body. Other arteries are summarized in Table 10-1. Also see Figure 10-11.

TABLE 10-1 Major Arteries of the Body

Artery	Anatomic Location or Organ Supplied
Lingual	Tongue
Facial	Face
Occipital	Back of scalp and neck
Maxillary	Teeth, jaw, and eyelids
Ophthalmic	Eye
Axillary	Armpit area
Brachial	Upper arm
Ulnar	Forearm and hand
Radial	Forearm and hand
Intercostals	Rib area
Lumbar	Posterior abdominal wall
External iliac	Anterior abdominal wall
Common iliac	Legs, gluteal area, and pelvic organs
Femoral	Thigh
Popliteal	Posterior knee
Tibial	Lower leg and foot

Venous System

Veins are blood vessels that carry blood toward the heart. Most veins in the body carry oxygen-poor blood, but the pulmonary veins are exceptions. Large veins often have the same names as the arteries they run next to. However, there are exceptions to this rule as well. For example, the veins next to carotid arteries are called jugular veins.

Large veins empty blood into vena cavae, which are the largest veins of the body. The superior vena cava generally collects blood from veins above the heart and the inferior vena cava collects blood from veins below the heart. The major veins of the body are summarized in Table 10-2. Also see Figure 10-12.

Veins of digestive organs carry blood from the digestive tract to the liver. The liver then processes nutrients in the blood and returns it to general circulation through hepatic veins. The collection of veins carrying blood to the liver is called the **hepatic portal system.**

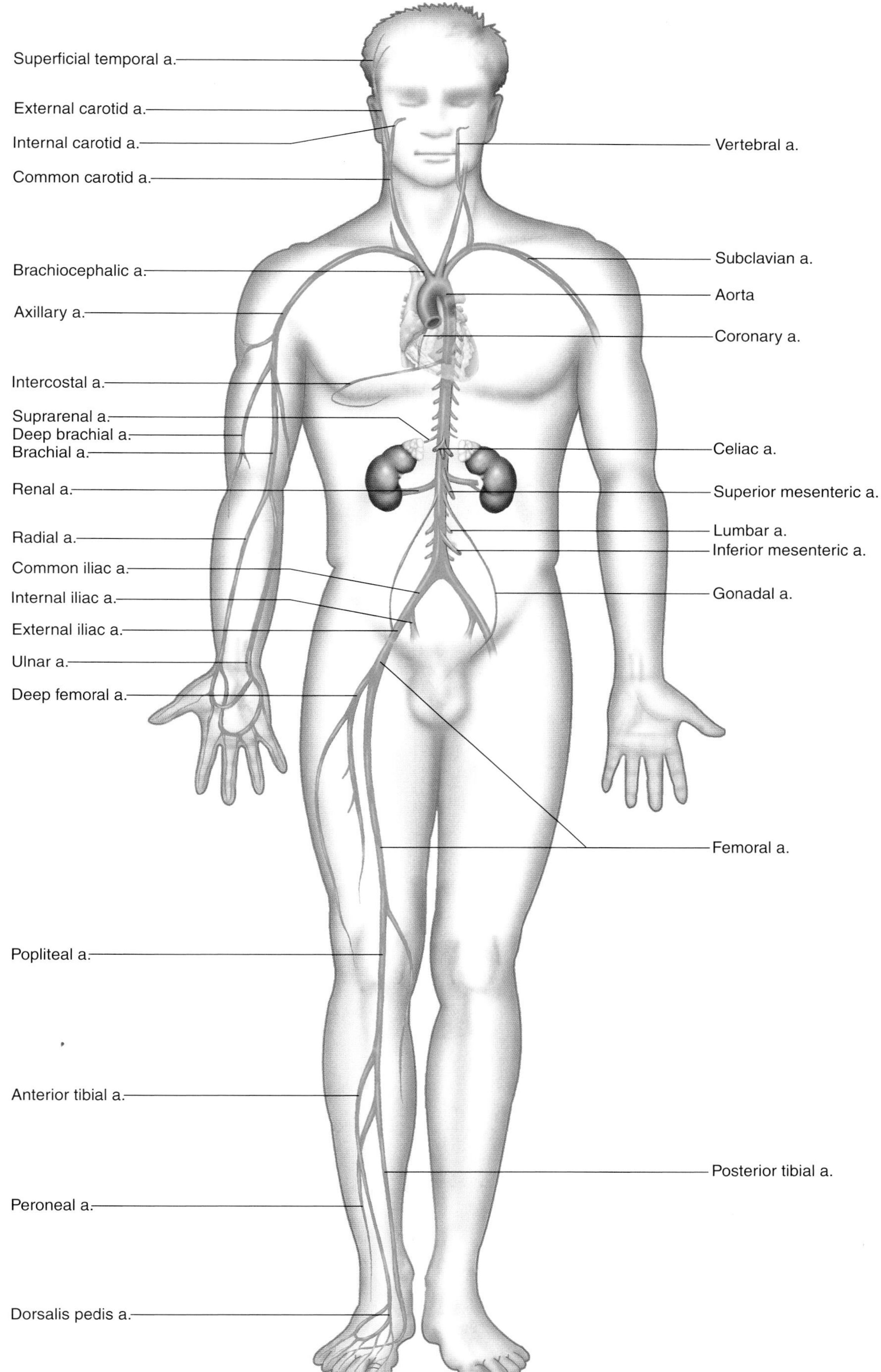

Figure 10-11. Major arteries of the body. (*a.* stands for *artery.*)

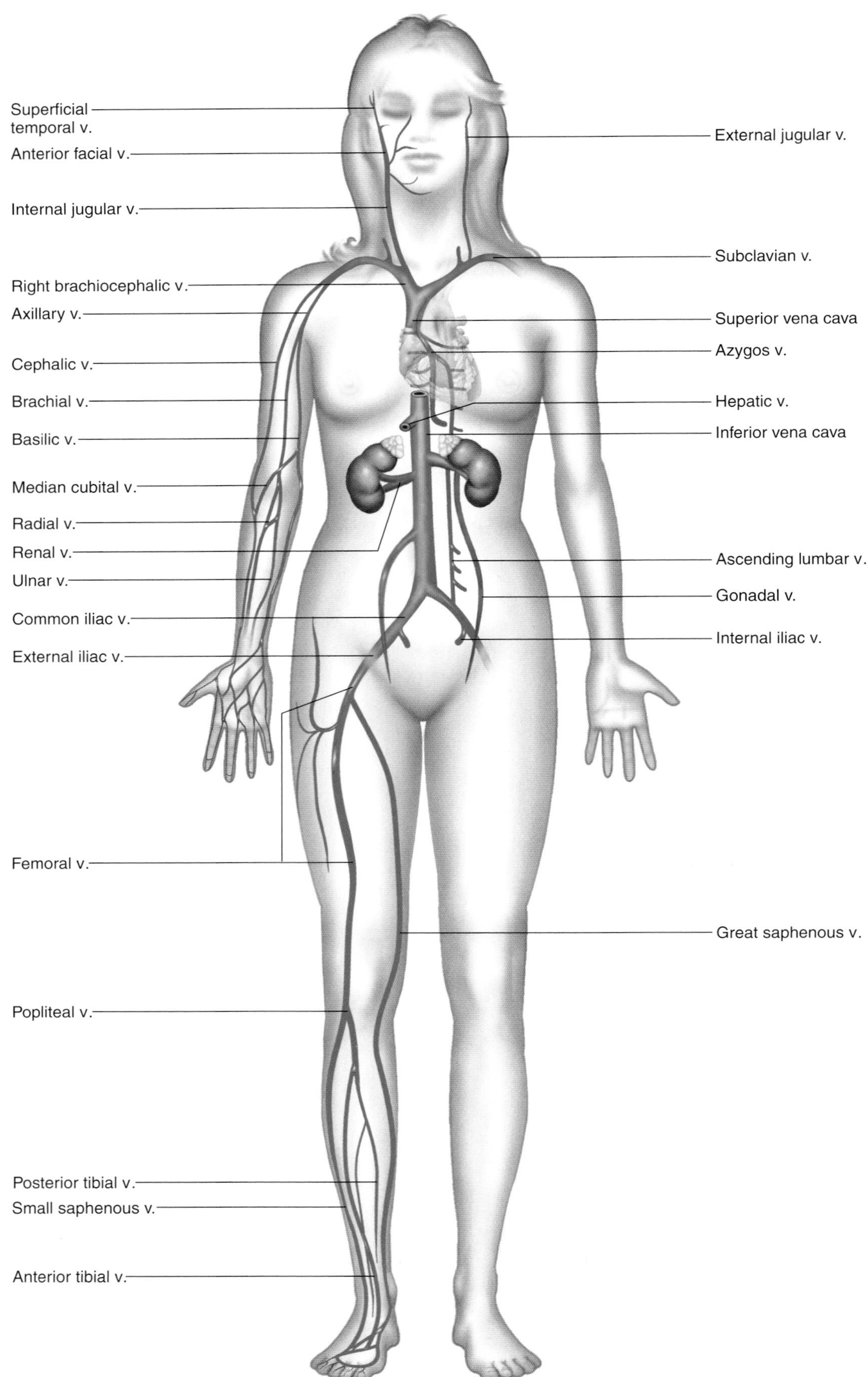

Figure 10-12. Major veins of the body. (*v.* stands for *vein.*)

TABLE 10-2 Major Veins of the Body

Vein	Anatomic Location or Organ Drained
Jugular	Head and neck
Brachiocephalic	Head and neck
Axillary	Armpit area
Brachial	Upper arm
Ulnar	Lower arm and hand
Radial	Lower arm and hand
Intercostal	Thorax
Azygos	Thorax and abdomen
Gastric—part of the hepatic portal system	Stomach to the liver
Splenic—part of the hepatic portal system	Spleen, pancreas, and stomach to the liver
Mesenteric—part of the hepatic portal system	Intestines to the liver
Hepatic portal—part of the hepatic portal system	Gastric, splenic, and mesenteric veins to the liver
Hepatic	Liver to the inferior vena cava
Iliac	Pelvic organs, legs, and gluteal areas
Femoral	Thighs
Popliteal	Knees
Saphenous	Legs

Blood

Blood is a type of connective tissue that is made up of various parts, including red and white blood cells, cell fragments called platelets, and plasma (the fluid part of the blood). An average-sized adult contains approximately 5 liters of blood. However, blood volume varies from person to person depending on the person's size, the amount of adipose tissue, and the concentrations of certain ions in the blood.

Components of Blood

The percentage of red blood cells in a sample of blood is referred to as **hematocrit.** A healthy person normally has a hematocrit level of about 45%. Most of the cells are red blood cells, and only about 1% are white blood cells and platelets. The rest of blood (approximately 55%) is plasma (Figure 10-13).

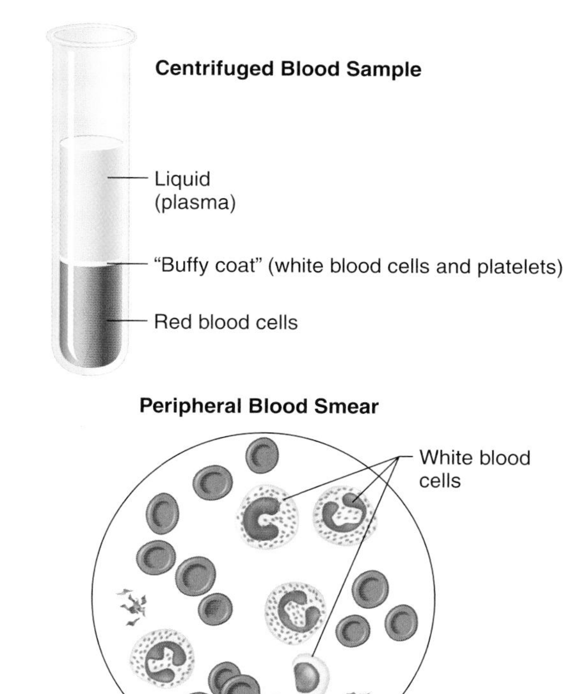

Figure 10-13. Centrifuged blood sample and peripheral blood smear showing blood components.

Red Blood Cells. Red blood cells, called **erythrocytes,** are biconcave-shaped cells that are small enough to pass through capillaries (Figure 10-14). Mature red blood cells do not contain nuclei because they must lose their nuclei in order to make room for a pigment called hemoglobin. Hemoglobin's function is to carry oxygen. Hemoglobin that carries oxygen is called **oxyhemoglobin** and is bright red in color; hemoglobin that does not carry oxygen is called **deoxyhemoglobin** and has a darker red color.

A red blood cell count is the number of red blood cells in one cubic millimeter of blood (a cubic millimeter of blood is roughly 20 drops of blood). This count is normally between 4 million and 6.5 million red blood cells. Because the function of a red blood cell is to transport oxygen throughout the body, a low count reflects a decreased ability to carry oxygen. This condition is known as **anemia.**

When red blood cells age, macrophages in the liver and spleen destroy them. When a red blood cell is destroyed, a pigment called **biliverdin** is released from the cell. The liver usually converts biliverdin into an orange-colored pigment called **bilirubin.** Bilirubin is used to make bile, which is needed for the digestion of fats. However, sometimes bilirubin is not used to make bile; instead, it persists in the bloodstream. This causes a person's skin to appear yellowish, which is a condition known as **jaundice.**

During development, red blood cells are made in the fetal yolk sac, the liver, and the spleen. However, once a baby is born, most red blood cells are produced in red

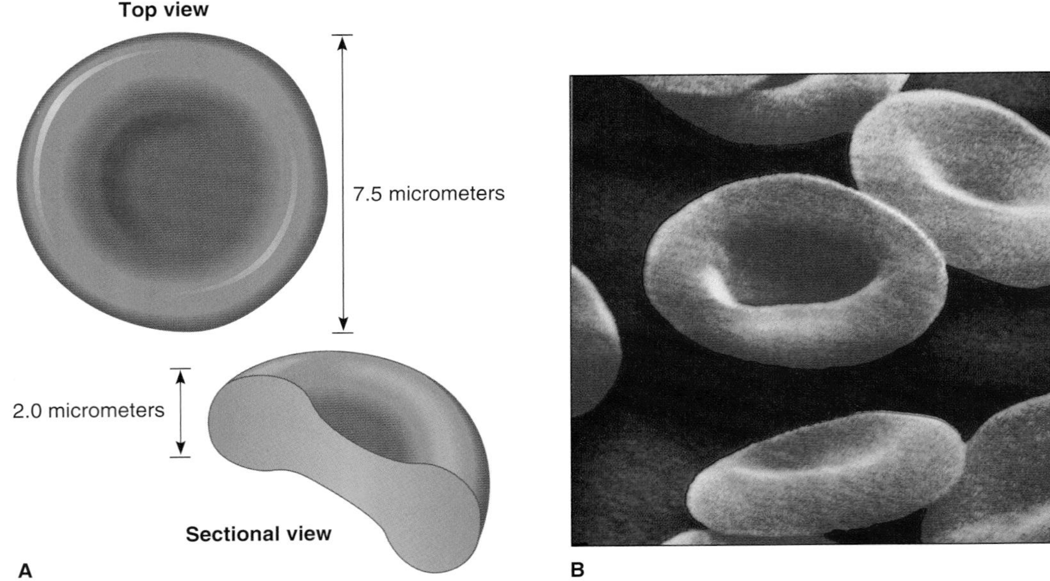

Figure 10-14. Red blood cells. (a) Biconcave shape of red blood cells and (b) scanning electron micrograph of red blood cells.

Educating the Patient

Chest Pain

Chest pain is a common reason people go to the emergency room every year. Although all chest pains should be taken seriously, they do not always indicate life-threatening heart conditions. There are two primary causes of chest pain—cardiac and noncardiac. Use the information in this box to teach patients about the conditions that cause chest pain.

The cardiac causes of chest pain include the following:

- Heart attack. Heart attacks are caused by the complete blockage of coronary arteries and are life-threatening conditions. The pain associated with a heart attack feels like pressure or fullness in the chest. Sometimes pain also occurs in the back, neck, face (especially jaw), shoulder, or arms (the left arm more than the right). Other signs and symptoms include shortness of breath, sweating, nausea, and dizziness.
- Angina. Angina is caused by a narrowing of coronary arteries and is not immediately life-threatening. The pain of angina is usually described as a tight feeling in the chest and is often brought about by stress or physical activity. This type of chest pain usually goes away after the stress or physical activity stops. A doctor should monitor patients with angina regularly.
- Pericarditis. This condition is characterized by inflammation of the sac surrounding the heart. It usually produces a sharp and localized pain in the chest. It is not immediately life-threatening but should be treated. This condition often produces a fever.
- Coronary spasms. In this condition, coronary arteries temporarily spasm and limit blood flow to cardiac muscle tissue. The pain accompanied by coronary spasms is similar to that of angina. It should be treated as soon as possible.

The noncardiac causes of chest pain include the following:

- Heartburn. Heartburn occurs when acids from the stomach are pushed into the esophagus. Heartburn pain is described as a burning sensation. This pain usually follows a meal and gets worse if a patient bends forward.
- Panic attacks. During times of intense stress or fear, chest pains can occur and are often accompanied by increased heart and breathing rates as well as excessive sweating.

continued ⟶

Educating the Patient

Chest Pain *(continued)*

- Pleurisy. This condition occurs when the membranes surrounding the lungs become inflamed. Pleurisy produces a sharp chest pain that usually feels worse when a patient coughs or inhales.
- Costochondritis. This condition occurs when the cartilage attached to ribs becomes inflamed. The chest pain associated with this condition feels much like the pain of a heart attack but generally occurs only when someone pushes on the patient's chest.
- Pulmonary embolism. This condition occurs when a blood clot blocks an artery in the lungs. The pain associated with it is severe, sharp, and increases when a patient inhales deeply or coughs. A pulmonary embolism can also produce shortness of breath, an increased heart rate, and dizziness. This condition is life-threatening.
- Sore muscles. Chest pain from sore muscles usually occurs only during body movements such as raising the arms.
- Broken ribs. Fractures of the ribs tend to produce sharp and localized chest pains.
- Shingles. This disease is caused by the chickenpox virus. It appears in adulthood during periods of sickness or stress. Shingles produces blisters on the skin, but a burning type of chest pain can occur days before the blisters appear.
- Inflammation of the gallbladder or pancreas. Pain associated with these conditions usually begins in the abdomen and spreads to the chest.

Tests used to determine the cause of chest pain include the following:

- Electrocardiogram (ECG). This test is useful in determining if a heart attack is occurring or has already occurred.
- Stress tests. Stress tests are ECGs performed while a patient is exercising or has been given drugs to increase her heart rate. Stress tests are useful for determining the health of coronary blood vessels.
- Blood tests. These tests are useful in determining if a heart attack has occurred. When heart tissue is damaged, certain enzymes are found in the blood.
- Chest x-ray. X-rays show the size and shape of the lungs and heart and can therefore indicate any serious conditions.
- Nuclear scan. These scans follow radioactive substances through the blood vessels of the heart and lungs. They can reveal narrow or obstructed arteries.
- Electron beam computerized tomography (EBCT). This procedure is much like a CT scan of the arteries. It is useful for finding narrowed arteries.
- Coronary catheterization. This procedure uses a dye that is followed through coronary arteries. It can also show narrowing of the arteries.
- Echocardiogram. This procedure uses sound waves to visualize the shape of the heart.
- Endoscopy. This procedure involves inserting a tube with a tiny camera down the throat and into the stomach. It helps to diagnose disorders of the stomach or esophagus that might produce chest pains.

bone marrow by cells called **hemocytoblasts.** The average life span of a red blood cell is only about 120 days, so red bone marrow is constantly making new cells. The hormone **erythropoietin** is responsible for regulating the production of red blood cells. This hormone is produced by the kidneys and stimulates the red bone marrow to produce new red blood cells. The kidneys release this hormone when oxygen concentrations in the blood get low.

Vitamin B_{12} and folic acid are two dietary factors that affect red blood cell production. These vitamins are necessary for DNA synthesis, so any actively dividing tissue such as red bone marrow is affected when DNA cannot be produced. Iron is also necessary to make hemoglobin. Too few red blood cells or too little hemoglobin can result in anemia.

White Blood Cells. White blood cells, which are called **leukocytes,** are divided into two categories: granulocytes and agranulocytes. **Granulocytes** have granules in their cytoplasm and include neutrophils, eosinophils, and basophils. **Agranulocytes** do not have granules in their cytoplasm and include monocytes and lymphocytes.

Neutrophils account for about 55% of all white blood cells (Figure 10-15). They are important for destroying bacteria, viruses, and toxins in the blood. **Eosinophils**

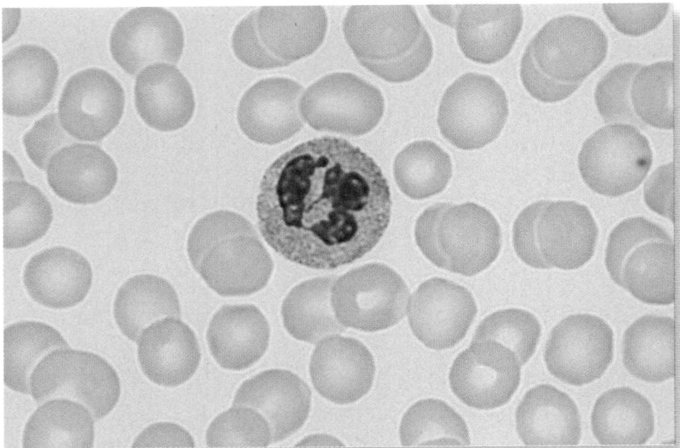

Figure 10-15. Neutrophils have distinct nuclei with many lobes.

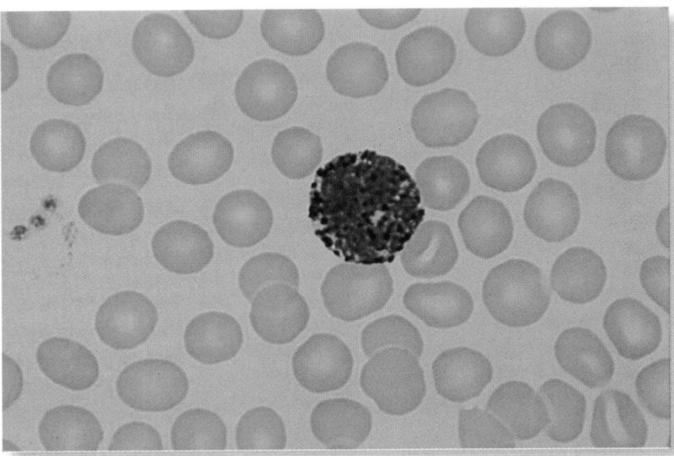

Figure 10-17. Basophils have cytoplasmic granules that stain deep blue.

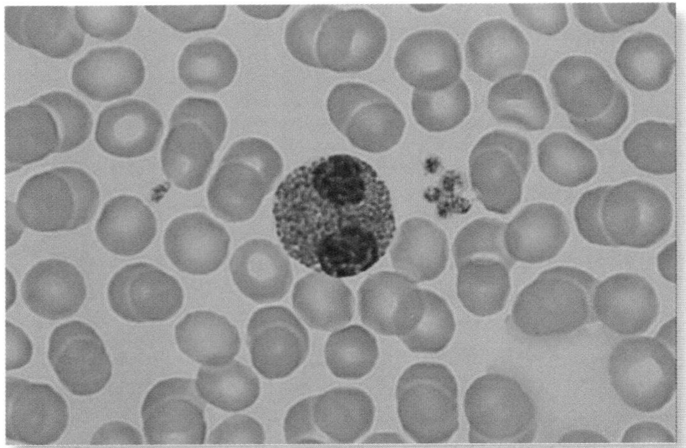

Figure 10-16. Eosinophils have cytoplasmic granules that stain red.

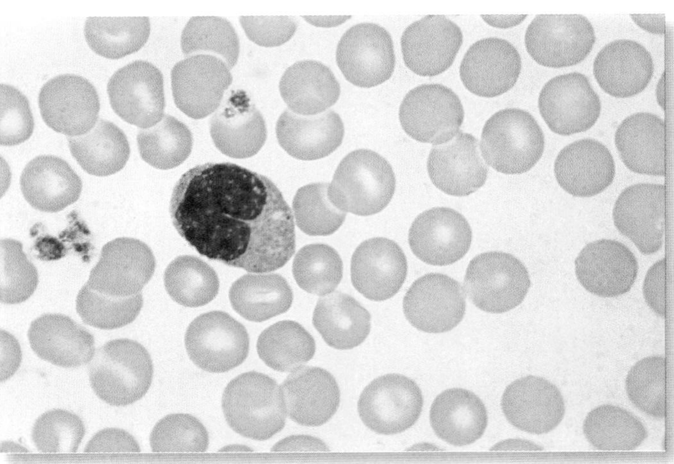

Figure 10-18. Monocytes have large kidney-shaped nuclei. They do not have cytoplasmic granules.

account for about 3% of all white blood cells and are effective in getting rid of parasitic infections such as worms (Figure 10-16). Eosinophils also help control inflammation and allergic reactions. **Basophils** account for less than 1% of all white blood cells. They release substances such as histamine and heparin, which promote inflammation (Figure 10-17).

Monocytes account for about 8% of all white blood cells. They are important for destroying bacteria, viruses, and toxins in the blood (Figure 10-18). **Lymphocytes** account for about 33% of all white blood cells and provide immunity for the body (Figure 10-19).

A white blood cell count is the number of white blood cells in 1 cubic millimeter of blood. This count is normally between 5000 and 10,000 cells. A white blood cell count above normal is termed **leukocytosis.** This condition often results from bacterial infections. A white blood cell count below normal is called **leukopenia,** which is caused by some viral infections and various other conditions.

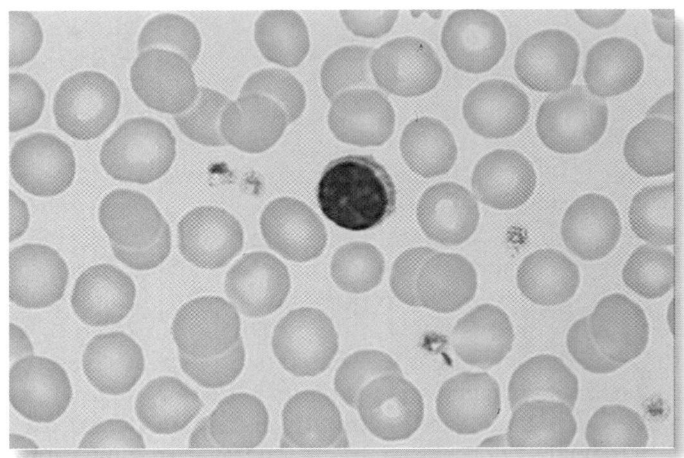

Figure 10-19. Lymphocytes have large round nuclei.

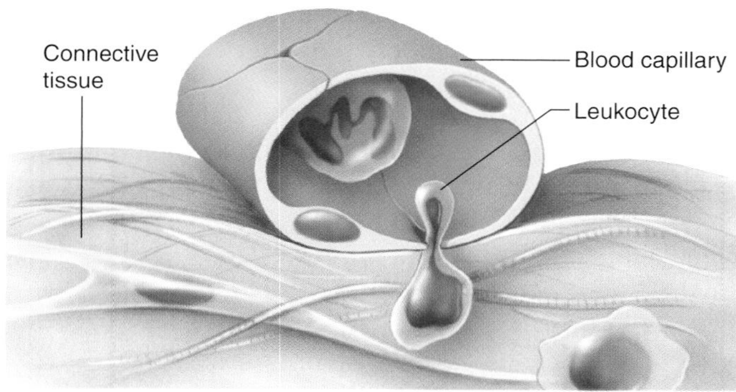

Figure 10-20. Diapedesis of a white blood cell into surrounding tissue.

A differential white blood cell count lists the percentages of the different types of leukocytes in a sample of blood. This is a useful test because the numbers of different white blood cells change in certain diseases. For example, neutrophil numbers increase at the beginning of a bacterial infection but monocyte numbers will not increase until about two weeks after a bacterial infection. Eosinophil numbers increase during worm infections. In AIDS, lymphocyte numbers fall.

Some white blood cells stay in the bloodstream to fight infections while others leave the bloodstream by squeezing through blood vessel walls to reach other tissues. The squeezing of a cell through a blood vessel wall is called **diapedesis** (Figure 10-20).

Blood Platelets. **Platelets** are fragments of cells that are found in the bloodstream (Figure 10-13). Platelets are also called **thrombocytes** and are important in the clotting of blood. Platelets come from cells called **megakaryocytes** that are in red bone marrow. A normal platelet count is between 130,000 and 360,000 platelets per cubic millimeter of blood.

Blood Plasma. Plasma is the liquid portion of blood. It is mostly water but also contains a mixture of proteins, nutrients, gases, electrolytes, and waste products. The three major types of proteins found in plasma are albumins, globulins, and fibrinogen. **Albumins** are the smallest of the plasma proteins and are important for pulling water into the bloodstream to help maintain blood pressure. **Globulins** transport lipids and some vitamins in plasma. Some globulins become antibodies. **Fibrinogen** is important for blood clotting.

Nutrients in plasma include amino acids, glucose, nucleotides, and lipids that have all been absorbed from the digestive tract. Because lipids are not water soluble and because plasma is mostly water, lipids must combine with molecules called **lipoproteins** to be transported. The different types of lipoproteins are **chylomicrons,** very low-density lipoproteins (VLDL), low-density lipoproteins (LDL), and high-density lipoproteins (HDL).

The gases dissolved in plasma include oxygen, carbon dioxide, and nitrogen. Many electrolytes are dissolved in plasma. They include sodium, potassium, calcium, magnesium, chloride, bicarbonate, phosphate, and sulfate. Molecules that contain nitrogen but are not proteins make up a group called nonprotein nitrogenous substances. They include amino acids, urea, and uric acid. Urea and uric acid are waste products produced by cells.

Bleeding Control

Hemostasis refers to the stoppage of bleeding. This is important when blood vessels are damaged and bleeding begins. Three processes occur in hemostasis: (1) blood vessel spasm, (2) platelet plug formation, and (3) blood coagulation.

When a blood vessel breaks, the smooth muscle at the site of the damage in its wall contracts and causes the blood vessel to spasm. This spasm reduces the amount of blood lost through the vessel. Platelets also begin to stick to the broken area and to each other to form a platelet plug. The platelet plug stops the bleeding temporarily (Figure 10-21).

A blood clot eventually replaces the platelet plug. The formation of a blood clot is called blood **coagulation.** In this process, the plasma protein fibrinogen is converted to fibrin. Once fibrin forms, it sticks to the damaged area of

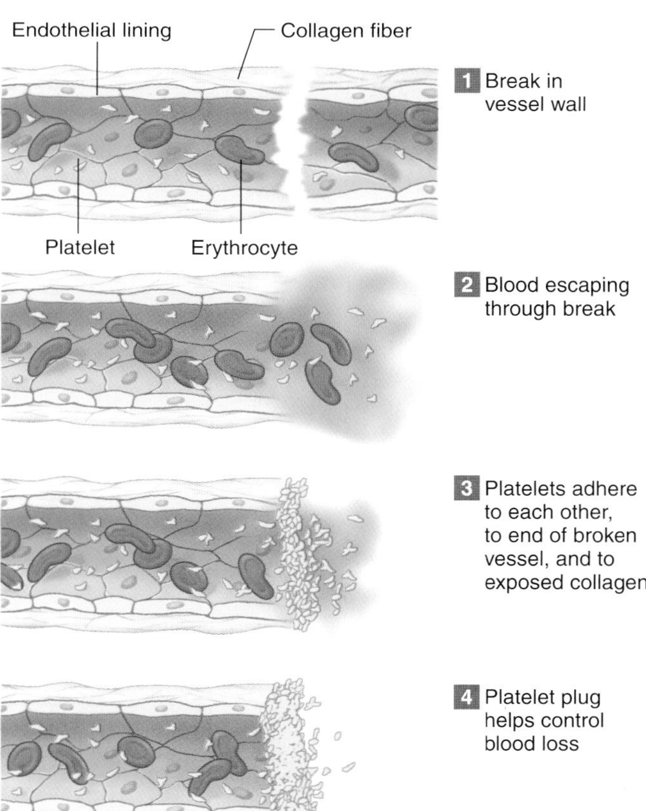

Figure 10-21. Steps in platelet plug formation.

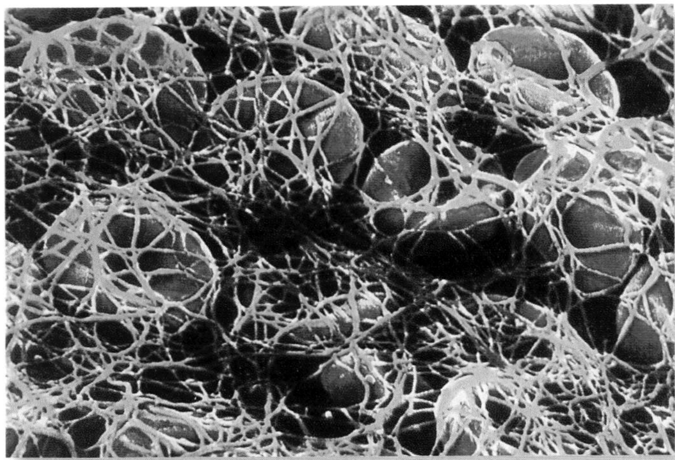

Figure 10-22. Scanning electron micrograph of a blood clot. Yellow fibrin threads are covering red blood cells.

the blood vessel, creating a meshwork that entraps blood cells and platelets. The resulting mass, the blood clot, stops bleeding until the vessel has repaired itself (Figure 10-22).

When a blood vessel is injured, it is normal for a blood clot to form. However, sometimes blood clots form on the side of a blood vessel with no known injury; this abnormal blood clot is called a **thrombus.** The danger of a thrombus is that a portion of it can break off and start moving through the bloodstream. The moving portion of the thrombus is called an **embolus.** An embolus is dangerous because it will eventually block a small artery. An embolus that originates in the vein of a leg travels to the right atrium of the heart through the inferior vena cava and is pumped by the right ventricle to the lungs. Here the embolus gets stuck in a small artery and causes pulmonary embolism, a fatal condition if not treated.

Blood Types

The ABO blood group consists of four different blood types: A, B, AB, and O. They are distinguished from each other in part by their antigens and antibodies.

Agglutination is the clumping of red blood cells following a blood transfusion. This clumping is not desirable because it leads to severe anemia. Agglutination occurs because proteins called *antigens* on the surface of red blood cells bind to antibodies in plasma (Figure 10-23). To prevent agglutination, antigens should not be mixed with antibodies that will bind to them. Fortunately, most antibodies do not bind to antigens on blood cells; only very specific ones bind to them.

Type A. People with type A blood have antigen A on the surface of their red blood cells. They also have antibody B in their plasma. Antibody B will only bind to antigen B.

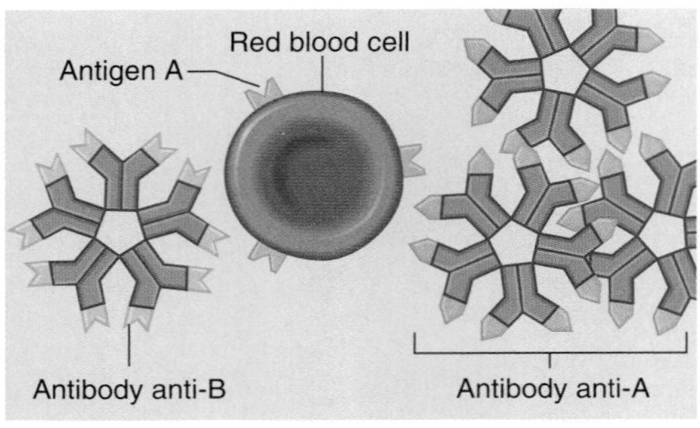

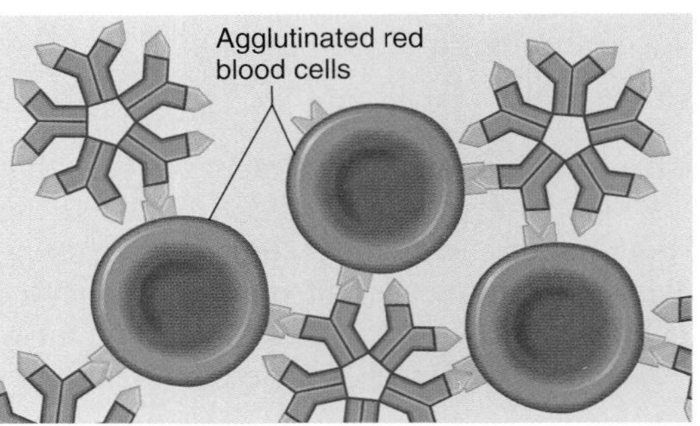

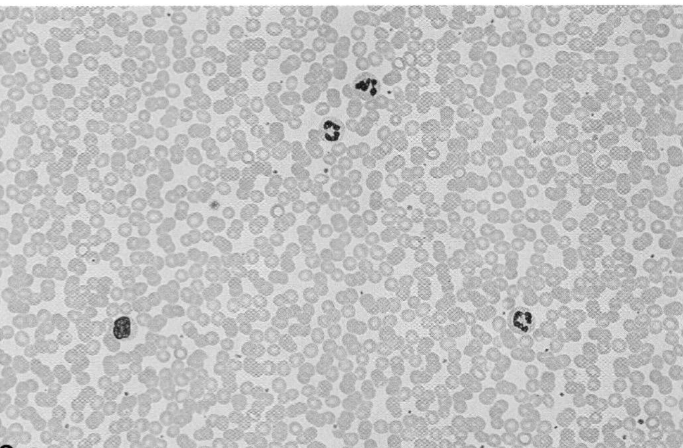

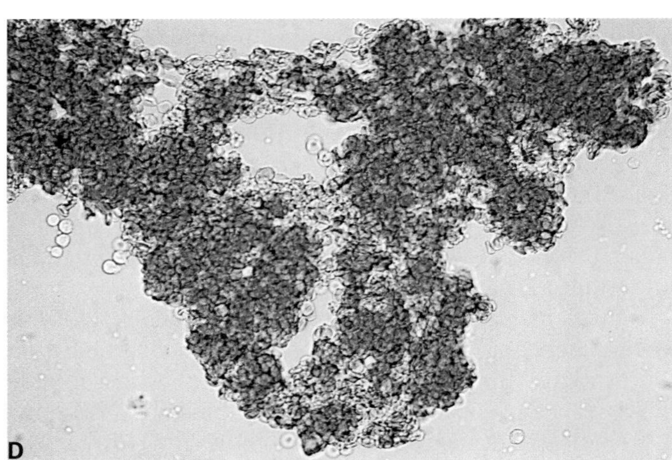

Figure 10-23. Agglutination. (a) Red blood cells with antigen A are added to blood that contains antibody anti-A. (b) Antibody anti-A reacts with antigen A, causing the agglutination of blood. (c) Normal blood. (d) Agglutinated blood.

TABLE 10-3 ABO Blood Group

Blood Type	Antigen Present	Antibody Present	Blood That Can Be Received
A	A	B	A and O
B	B	A	B and O
AB	AB	None	A, B, AB, and O
O	None	A and B	O

Type B. People with type B blood have antigen B on the surface of their red blood cells. They also have antibody A in their plasma.

If a person with type A blood is given type B blood, then the antibody B in the recipient's blood will bind with the red blood cells of the donor blood because those cells have antigen B on their surfaces. Therefore, agglutination occurs, and the donated red blood cells are destroyed. This is why a person with type A blood should not be given type B blood (and vice versa).

Type AB. People with type AB blood have both antigen A and antigen B on the surface of their red blood cells. They have neither antibody A nor antibody B in their plasma. People with type AB blood are called universal recipients, because most of them can receive all ABO blood types. They can receive these blood types because they lack antibody A and antibody B in their plasma, so there is no reaction with antigens A and B of the donor blood.

Type O. People with type O blood have neither antigen A nor antigen B on the surface of their red blood cells. However, they do have both antibody A and antibody B in their plasma. People with type O blood are called universal donors because their blood can be given to most people regardless of recipients' blood type. Type O blood will not agglutinate when given to other people because it does not have the antigens to bind to antibody A or antibody B. Table 10-3 summarizes the ABO blood group. Also see Figure 10-24.

The Rh Factor. The **Rh antigen** is a protein first discovered on red blood cells of the Rhesus monkey, hence the name Rh. People who are Rh-positive have red blood cells that contain the Rh antigen. People who are Rh-negative have red blood cells that do not contain the Rh antigen. If a person who is Rh-negative is given Rh-positive blood, then the Rh-negative person's blood will make antibodies that bind to the Rh antigens. If the Rh-negative person is given Rh-positive blood a second time, the antibodies will bind to the donor cells and agglutination will occur.

Clinically, it is very important for a female to know her Rh type. If an Rh-negative female mates with an Rh-positive male, there is a fifty-fifty chance that her fetus will be Rh-positive. When the blood of a fetus who is Rh-positive mixes with the blood of a mother who is Rh-negative, the

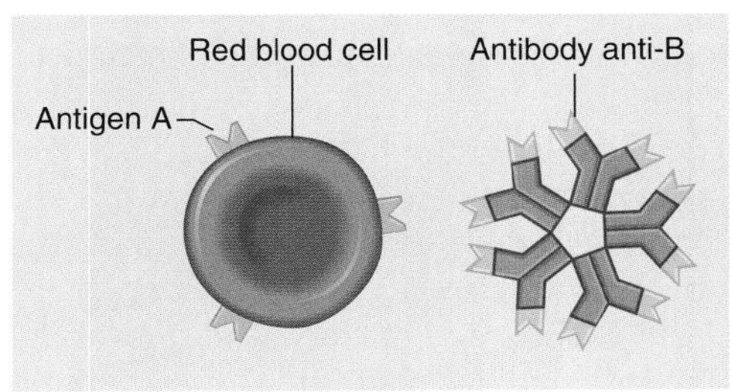

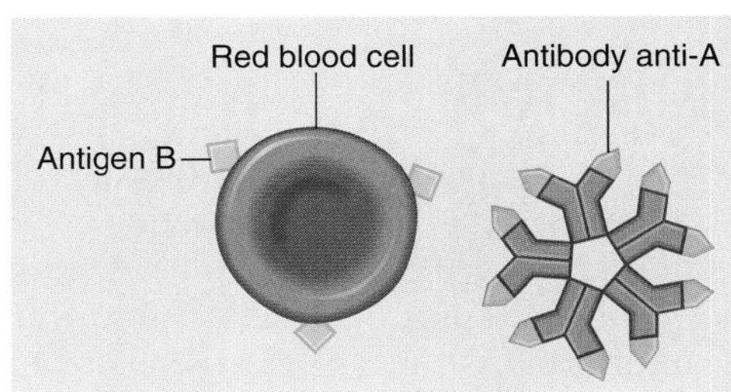

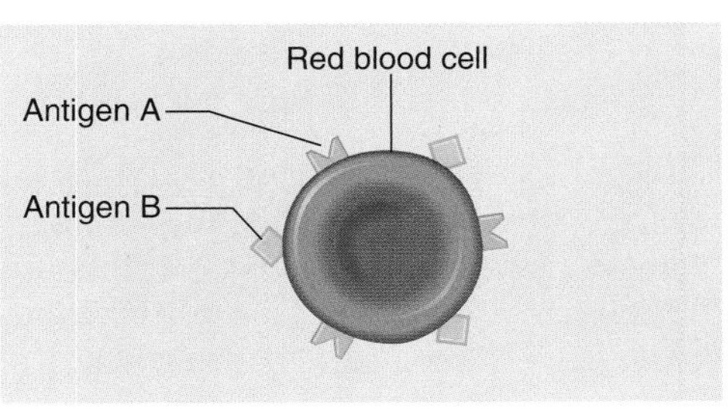

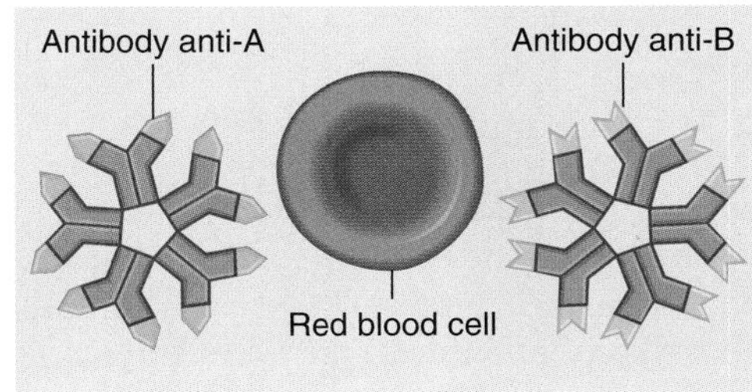

Figure 10-24. A, B, AB, and O blood types.

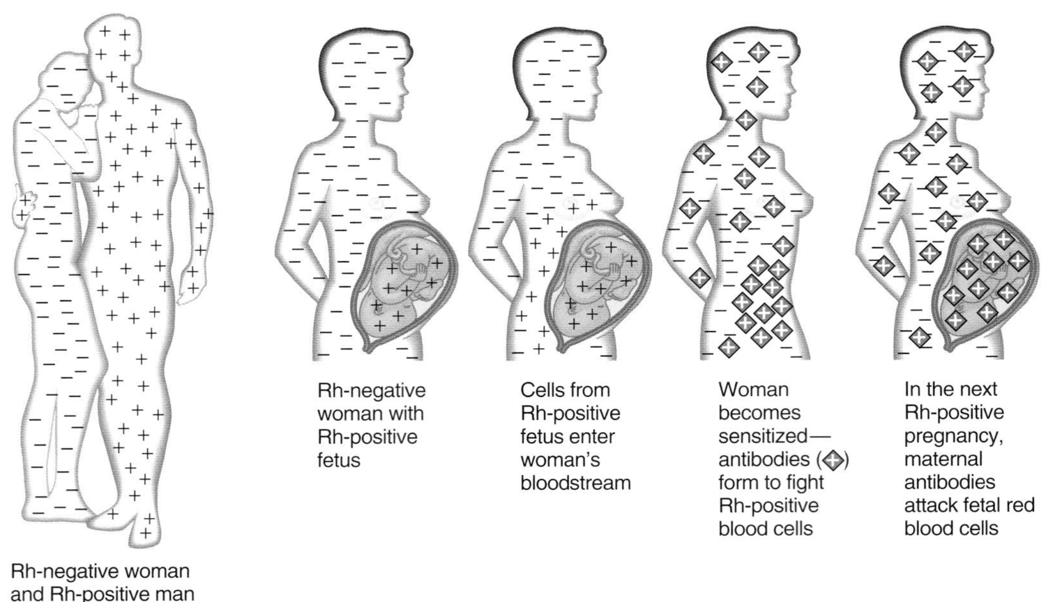
Rh-negative woman and Rh-positive man conceive a child
Rh-negative woman with Rh-positive fetus
Cells from Rh-positive fetus enter woman's bloodstream
Woman becomes sensitized— antibodies (⊕) form to fight Rh-positive blood cells
In the next Rh-positive pregnancy, maternal antibodies attack fetal red blood cells

Figure 10-25. Development of antibodies in an Rh-negative woman in relation to the blood of her Rh-positive fetus.

mother develops antibodies against the fetus's red blood cells. The first Rh-positive fetus usually does not suffer from these antibodies because it takes so long for the mother's body to generate them. However, if the mother conceives a second Rh-positive fetus, the fetus's blood will be attacked by the antibodies right away. The second fetus then develops a condition called **erythroblastosis fetalis,** and the baby is born severely anemic (Figure 10-25). Erythroblastosis fetalis is prevented by giving an Rh-negative woman the drug **RhoGAM.** RhoGAM prevents an Rh-negative mother from making antibodies against the Rh antigen.

The Lymphatic System

The lymphatic system is a network of connecting vessels that collects fluids between cells. These lymphatic vessels then return this fluid, called **lymph,** to the bloodstream. The lymphatic system also picks up lipids from the digestive organs and transports them to the bloodstream. Finally, the lymphatic system functions to defend the body against disease-causing agents called **pathogens.** (See Chapter 11 for more information about this function.)

Lymphatic Pathways

Lymphatic pathways start with tiny vessels called lymphatic capillaries. The lymphatic capillaries merge together to make lymphatic vessels. Lymphatic vessels eventually merge together to make lymphatic trunks, and the trunks merge into lymphatic collecting ducts.

Lymphatic capillaries extend into the spaces between cells called interstitial spaces. Lymphatic capillaries have very permeable, thin walls that are designed to pick up fluids in interstitial spaces. Once fluid enters the lymphatic capillaries, it is called lymph. Lymphatic capillaries deliver lymph to lymphatic vessels, and lymphatic vessels deliver the fluid to lymph nodes. The cells inside lymph nodes can remove pathogens from lymph or start an immune response against the pathogen.

Lymph leaves lymph nodes through efferent lymphatic vessels. Efferent lymphatic vessels eventually deliver lymph to lymphatic trunks, and the trunks deliver the lymph to lymphatic collecting ducts. There are two major lymphatic collecting ducts in the body—the thoracic duct and the right lymphatic duct. Both of these ducts empty lymph into the bloodstream, usually near the right and left subclavian veins in the thoracic cavity. See Figures 10-26, 10-27, and 10-28.

The right lymphatic duct is much smaller than the thoracic duct. The right lymphatic duct collects all the lymph from the right side of the head and neck, the right arm, and the right side of the chest. The thoracic duct collects lymph from the left side of the head and neck, the left arm, the left side of the thorax, the entire abdominopelvic area, and both legs (Figure 10-28).

Tissue Fluid and Lymph

Fluid constantly leaks out of blood capillaries into the spaces between cells. This fluid is high in nutrients, oxygen, and small proteins. Most of this fluid is picked up by body cells. However, some of the fluid persists between cells. This fluid is called tissue fluid and is destined to become lymph.

Once lymph enters lymphatic vessels, it is pushed through the vessels by the squeezing action of neighboring

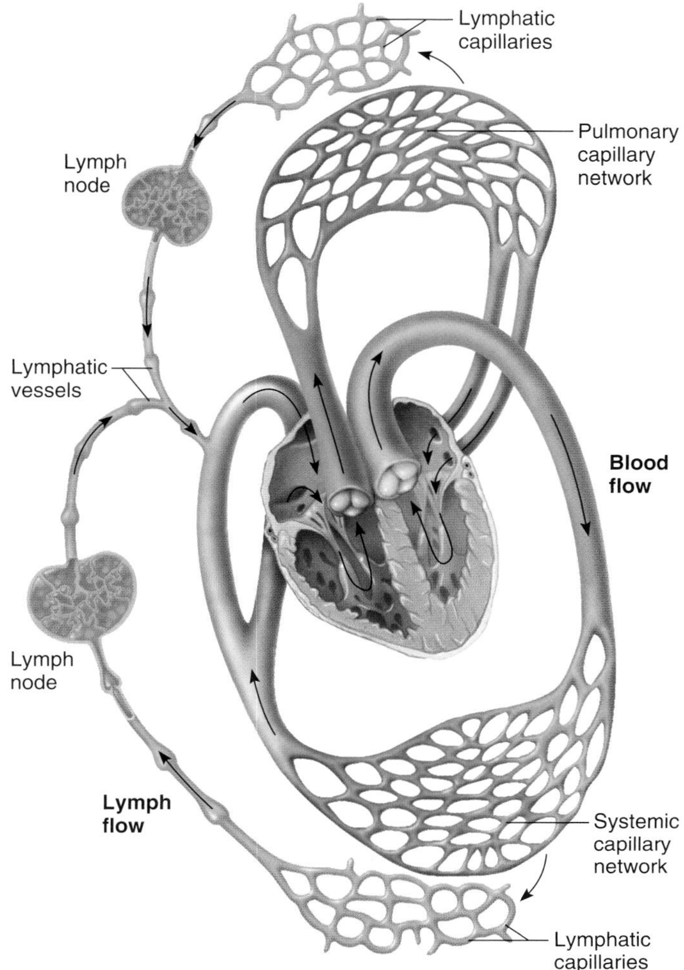

Figure 10-26. Schematic flow of lymph from the lymphatic capillaries to the bloodstream.

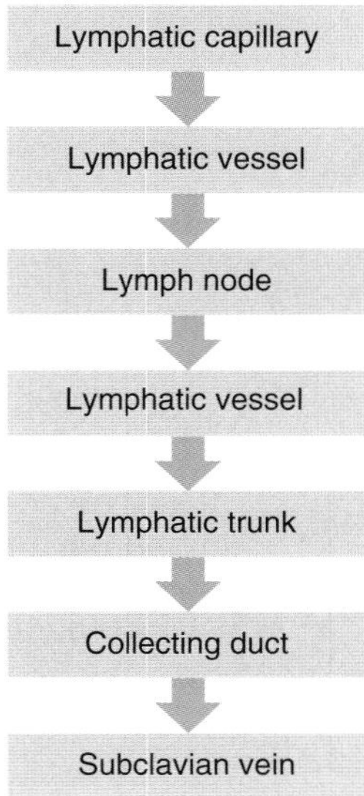

Figure 10-27. Lymphatic pathway.

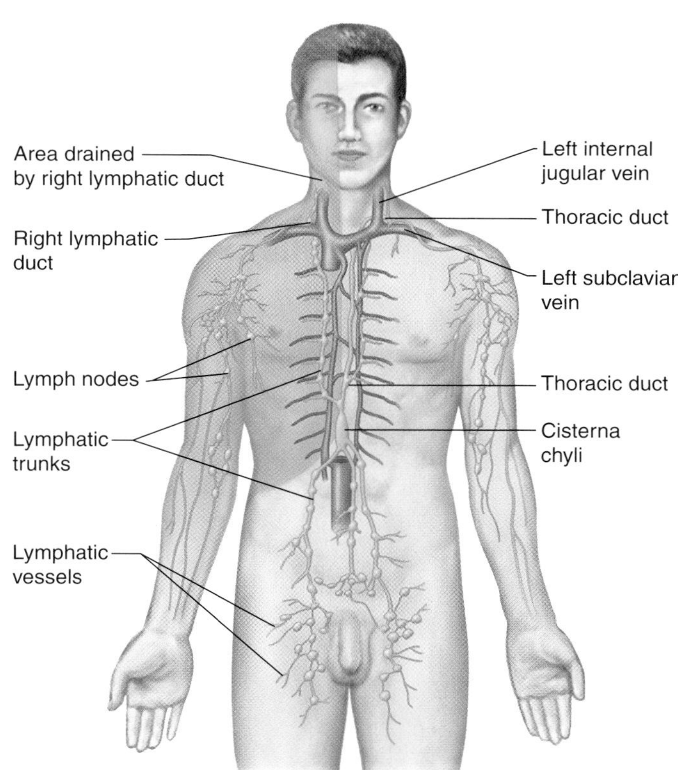

Figure 10-28. Areas drained by the right lymphatic duct (shaded) and thoracic duct (not shaded).

skeletal muscles. Lymphatic vessels contain valves that prevent the backflow of lymph. Breathing movements also squeeze lymphatic vessels and therefore promote lymph movement. If lymph is not pushed through a lymphatic vessel, it will leak back out of the lymphatic capillaries. When this happens, swelling of the surrounding tissue occurs. This condition is called **edema.**

Lymph Nodes

Lymph nodes are very small, glandular structures that usually cannot be felt very easily. They are located along the paths of larger lymphatic vessels and are spread throughout the body, but they do not occur in the nervous system. One side of a lymph node, called the **hilum,** is indented. Nerves and blood vessels enter the node through the hilum.

Some lymphatic vessels carry lymph to a lymph node on the side away from the hilum. These vessels are called afferent lymphatic vessels (afferent, meaning "to"). About four or five afferent vessels are associated with each node. Lymphatic vessels that carry lymph out of a node are called efferent vessels (efferent, meaning "away from"). A lymph node usually has only one or two efferent vessels. Because more lymph enters the node than can exit at one time, lymph tends to pool, or stay, in the node for some period of time.

Two important cell types are found inside the node—macrophages and lymphocytes. Macrophages digest unwanted pathogens in the lymph as it sits in the node, and the lymphocytes start an immune response against the pathogen. Lymph nodes are also responsible for the generation of some lymphocytes. See Figure 10-29.

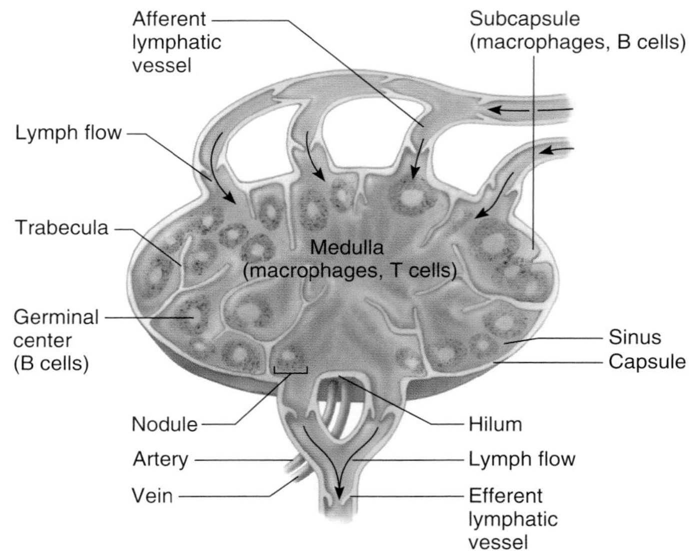

Figure 10-29. Section of a lymph node.

The Thymus and Spleen

The thymus is a soft, bilobed organ located just above the heart. As a person ages, the thymus shrinks. The thymus carries out the same functions as a lymph node but is also responsible for the production of lymphocytes and the hormone called thymosin. Thymosin stimulates the production of mature lymphocytes.

The spleen is the largest lymphatic organ. It is located in upper left portion of the abdominal cavity. The spleen is filled with blood, macrophages, and lymphocytes. It filters blood in much the same way that lymph nodes filter lymph. The spleen also removes worn-out red blood cells from the bloodstream.

Pathophysiology

Common Diseases and Disorders of the Circulatory System

Anemia is a condition in which a person does not have enough red blood cells or hemoglobin in the blood to carry an adequate amount of oxygen to the body's cells. It is the most common blood disorder in the United States and can be a sign of a more serious disorder. It generally affects more women than men.

- **Causes.** The causes of this condition are many and include the following:
  - Iron deficiency. Iron deficiency is the most common cause of anemia. Iron is needed to make hemoglobin, which is the pigment that carries most oxygen in the blood. Pregnant women and women with heavy menstrual cycles are most susceptible to this type of anemia.
  - Chronic blood loss. Slow blood loss can occur in conditions such as ulcers, colon polyps, or colon cancer.
  - Vitamin deficiency. Vitamin B_{12} and folic acid are needed to make enough red blood cells.
  - Inability to absorb vitamin B_{12}. This condition is called *pernicious anemia*. Some intestinal disorders prevent the absorption of vitamin B_{12}.
  - Side effect of medication. Some oral contraceptives, seizure medications, and drugs used to treat cancer can cause anemia.
  - Chronic illness. Chronic diseases such as AIDS, cancer, rheumatoid arthritis, leukemia, and kidney failure can cause anemia.
  - Bone marrow disorder. When the bone marrow fails to produce enough blood cells, aplastic anemia results. This is a life-threatening type of anemia. Toxins, chemotherapy, and radiation therapy can destroy bone marrow.
  - Destruction of red blood cells. Some blood diseases, such as sickle cell disease, cause red blood cells to be destroyed faster than they can be made.

Anemia can be prevented through a healthy diet high in iron, vitamin B_{12}, and folic acid.

- **Signs and symptoms.** Signs and symptoms include tiredness, weakness, pale skin, rapid heartbeat, numb or cold hands and feet, dizziness, headache, and jaundice.
- **Treatment.** Injections of vitamin B_{12} may be necessary. Treatment often begins with addressing the underlying causes, such as an ulcer or colon polyps. Other treatment options include administering various medications, discontinuing the use of medications that can cause anemia, and blood transfusions if defective bone marrow is the cause.

An **aneurysm** is defined as a ballooning of an artery wall that results when the wall of the blood vessel becomes weak. The most common locations of aneurysms are the aorta and arteries in the brain, legs, intestines, and spleen. An aortic aneurysm is a bulge in the wall of the aorta. Most aortic aneurysms occur in the abdominal aorta but some occur in the thoracic aorta. Most aortic aneurysms do not rupture; however, when they do, serious life-threatening emergencies result.

continued ⟶

Common Diseases and Disorders of the Circulatory System *(continued)*

- **Causes.** Most causes are unknown. One identified risk to developing an aneurysm is **artherosclerosis,** which is a hardening of the arteries usually associated with a diet high in cholesterol. Smoking and obesity also increase the risk of atherosclerosis. Congenital conditions may cause an aneurysm—some individuals are born with weak aortic walls. A traumatic injury to the chest may also be a risk factor. The risk of developing an aneurysm can be reduced by not smoking, by losing excess weight, and by having a diet low in cholesterol. Periodic screening is an option for patients with a family history of aortic aneurysms.
- **Signs and symptoms.** There are usually no signs and symptoms of an aneurysm, although hypertension can be a sign. When symptoms do exist, a pulsation in the abdomen and back pain are the most commonly seen. A sudden pain in the abdomen or back, dizziness, a fast pulse, or a loss of consciousness are signs that an aneurysm has burst.
- **Treatment.** The primary treatment is surgery to repair the aneurysm.

Arrhythmias are abnormal heart rhythms in which the heart beats too quickly (tachycardia) or too slowly (bradycardia). The most common type of heart arrhythmia is atrial fibrillation, which is a sporadic and quick beating of the atria. The most serious type of heart arrhythmia is ventricular fibrillation, which produces ineffective contractions of the ventricles. Most sudden cardiac deaths are caused by ventricular fibrillation.

- **Causes.** These abnormal rhythms usually result when electrical impulses of the cardiac conduction system do not flow correctly through the heart. The list of risk factors and causes is long and includes electrical shock, certain drugs (for example, over-the-counter cough medicines that contain pseudoephedrine), herbal supplements containing ephedra, high blood pressure, a previous heart attack, decreased blood flow to the heart, coronary artery disease, heart valve disorders, weakening of the heart muscle (cardiomyopathy), some genetic diseases such as Wolff-Parkison-White syndrome, thyroid problems, diabetes, sleep apnea, electrolyte imbalances (including potassium, sodium, and calcium), excess alcohol consumption, smoking, caffeine consumption, and drugs such as amphetamines or cocaine.
- **Signs and symptoms.** Symptoms include shortness of breath, dizziness or fainting, an uncharacteristically rapid or slow heart rate, a fluttering feeling in the chest, and chest pain.
- **Treatment.** The first management of arrhythmias should be to treat the underlying cause. Other treatment options include the following:
  - Pacemakers.
  - Various medications.
  - Cardiopulmonary resuscitation if there is no evidence of blood flow.
  - Vagal maneuvers to slow the heart rate. These include holding the breath, straining (bearing down as when a person is having a bowel movement), or putting one's face in cold water.
  - Electrical shock to reset heart rhythms.
  - Radiofrequency catheter ablation, a procedure that destroys a small amount of heart tissue in order to change the flow of the electrical current through the heart.
  - Implantation of an ICD (implantable cardioverter defibrillator), a device that regulates heart rhythms.
  - Maze procedure, which is an operation to form scars in the atria. These scars correct the electrical flow through the heart.
  - Surgery to correct heart defects such as narrow coronary arteries.

Carditis is an inflammation of the heart. It is more specifically referred to as *endocarditis, myocarditis,* or *pericarditis,* depending on the layer of the heart that is affected.

Endocarditis is an inflammation of the lining of the heart, including the heart valves.

- **Causes.** Bacterial infections are the most common cause of endocarditis. Patients are more susceptible to this condition if they have abnormal heart valves.
- **Signs and symptoms.** Common signs and symptoms include weakness, fever, excessive sweating, general body aches, difficulty breathing, and blood in the urine.
- **Treatment.** The treatment for this condition is intravenous antibiotics followed by oral antibiotics for up to 6 weeks.

Myocarditis is an inflammation of the muscular layer of the heart. It is relatively uncommon but very serious because it leads to weakening of the heart wall.

- **Causes.** The most common cause of myocarditis is a viral infection, but it may also be caused by exposure to certain chemicals, allergens, and bacteria.
- **Signs and symptoms.** Signs and symptoms include fever as well as chest pains that feel like a heart attack. Difficulty breathing, decreased urine output, fatigue, and fainting may also accompany myocarditis.
- **Treatment.** Treatment normally includes steroids to reduce inflammation, bed rest, and a low-salt diet.

Pericarditis is inflammation of the pericardium, which is a group of membranes that surround the heart.

- **Causes.** This condition is most commonly caused by complications of viral or bacterial infections. However, heart attacks and chest injuries can also lead to pericarditis.
- **Signs and symptoms.** Symptoms include sharp, stabbing chest pains, especially during deep breaths.

continued ⟶

Fever, fatigue, and difficulty breathing while lying down are also common symptoms.

- **Treatment.** The treatment usually includes painkillers. Diuretics are used to remove excess fluids around the heart. If pericarditis is caused by bacteria, antibiotics are used. In chronic cases, surgery may be required to remove part of the membranes surrounding the heart.

Congestive heart failure is a slowly developing condition in which the heart weakens over time. Eventually, the heart is no longer able to pump enough blood to meet the body's needs.

- **Causes.** There are many risk factors for this condition, including smoking, being overweight, a diet high in cholesterol, a lack of exercise, atherosclerosis, a heart attack, high blood pressure, a damaged heart valve, excessive alcohol consumption, and diabetes. Congenital heart defects, present at birth, and drugs that weaken the heart (especially cocaine, heroin, and some cancer drugs) may also contribute to the development of this disorder. This condition may be prevented by controlling high blood pressure and high cholesterol, not smoking, having a healthy diet, engaging in regular exercise, and treating any existing atherosclerosis or diabetes.
- **Signs and symptoms.** Signs and symptoms include shortness of breath, constant wheezing, prominent veins in the neck, swelling in the legs or feet, swelling of the abdomen, fluid retention, nausea, dizziness, and an irregular or rapid heartbeat.
- **Treatment.** Common treatment options include medications to slow a rapid heartbeat, diuretics to decrease fluid accumulation in the lungs, and medications to reduce blood pressure. In more serious cases, surgery to repair defective heart valves or other heart defects, a heart transplant, or the implantation of a cardiac pacemaker may be needed.

Coronary artery disease is also known as atherosclerosis. It affects more Americans than any other type of heart disease. Males and African Americans are more likely to develop coronary artery disease than are women or Caucasians.

- **Causes.** This condition is characterized by the narrowing of coronary arteries. Usually the narrowing is produced by the buildup of fat, cholesterol, and calcium in the arteries. The risk factors for developing this condition include high levels of LDL cholesterol in the blood, a diet high in fat and cholesterol, smoking, high blood pressure, obesity, a lack of exercise, and diabetes. As with congestive heart failure, this condition may be prevented by controlling high blood pressure and high cholesterol, not smoking, having a healthy diet, engaging in regular exercise, and treating any existing diabetes.
- **Signs and Symptoms.** There are often no signs or symptoms until a heart attack occurs. The most common symptoms include angina (a type of chest pain caused by a decreased flow of blood to the heart), shortness of breath, tightness in the chest, fatigue, and swelling in the legs or feet.
- **Treatment.** Treatment includes aspirin therapy and medications to slow a rapid heartbeat. Surgery to repair or widen narrowed coronary arteries may be needed in more serious cases.

Hypertension, commonly known as high blood pressure, is defined as a consistent resting blood pressure measured at 140/90 mm Hg or higher. This condition increases a person's risk of heart attack, stroke, heart failure, and kidney failure. African Americans are twice as likely to have high blood pressure as Caucasians are.

- **Causes.** Many of the causes are unknown. Known causes and risk factors include narrowing of the arteries, various medications such as oral contraceptives and cold medicines, kidney disease, endocrine disorders, pregnancy, drug use (especially cocaine and amphetamines), sleep apnea, obesity, smoking, a high-sodium diet, excessive alcohol consumption, stress, and diabetes.
- **Signs and symptoms.** There are usually no symptoms to hypertension. When symptoms do present, they include excessive sweating, muscle cramps, fatigue, frequent urination, and an irregular heart rate.
- **Treatment.** The first management of hypertension should be to treat the underlying causes. Other common treatments include a diet low in sodium and cholesterol, regular exercise, various medications to slow the heart rate and dilate blood vessels, diuretics to reduce blood volume, and lifestyle changes such as managing stress and stopping smoking.

Leukemia is a condition in which the bone marrow produces a large number of white blood cells that are not normal. These abnormal cells prevent normal white blood cells from carrying out their defensive functions. This disorder is sometimes referred to as cancer of the white blood cells. There are several different kinds of leukemia.

- **Causes.** Causes include mutations (changes) in white blood cells, chemotherapy for the treatment of other cancers, genetic factors (for example, the inheritance of abnormal genes), and exposure to agents that cause changes in the white blood cells.
- **Signs and symptoms.** The signs and symptoms are many and include fatigue, difficulty breathing during physical activity, an enlarged liver or spleen, swollen lymph nodes, abnormal bruising, cuts that heal slowly, frequent infections, nosebleeds, bleeding gums, chronic fever, unexplained weight loss, and excessive sweating.

continued ⟶

- **Treatment.** Treatment options include chemotherapy, bone marrow transplant, medications to strengthen the immune system, a stem cell transplant, radiation therapy, and antibodies to destroy mutated white blood cells.

Murmurs are simply defined as abnormal heart sounds. Normally, heart sounds are clear and strong, as valves close completely, and smooth, as blood flows over the lining of the heart with no resistance. Not all murmurs indicate a heart disorder. Murmurs are graded from 1 to 6, 1 being barely audible (and the least serious).

- **Causes.** Not all the causes of heart murmurs are known. In children, the failure of the foramen ovale or ductus arteriosis to close completely after birth can cause murmurs. Other causes include stress and defective heart valves that cannot close completely.
- **Signs and symptoms.** The signs and symptoms vary considerably depending on the cause and severity of the heart murmur. Severe symptoms include weakness, pale skin, edema (fluid retention), and other common signs associated with heart failure.
- **Treatment.** Many times, no treatment is required. Surgery to correct valve defects or other heart defects may be needed in more serious cases.

A **myocardial infarction,** which is the term used for a heart attack, is characterized by damage to cardiac muscle due to a lack of blood supply. Heart attacks are often fatal or can leave permanent damage because cardiac muscle does not grow back once it is lost.

- **Causes.** The causes and contributing factors include blockage of the coronary artery due to atherosclerosis or a blood clot, or drugs such as cocaine that cause coronary arteries to spasm. Preventing a heart attack includes treating or reducing the risk of atherosclerosis. This condition may be further prevented by controlling high blood pressure and high cholesterol, not smoking, having a healthy diet, and engaging in regular exercise.
- **Signs and symptoms.** Common symptoms include recurring chest pain; a squeezing pain in the chest; pain in the shoulder, arm, back, teeth, or jaw; chronic pain in the upper abdomen; shortness of breath; sweating; dizziness or fainting; and nausea or vomiting.
- **Treatment.** The first treatment, if possible, is chewing an aspirin at the onset of the heart attack. In an unconscious patient, CPR (cardiopulmonary resuscitation) should be administered. Other treatment options include the use of a defibrillator (if available), thrombolytic drugs to destroy the blood clots that block a coronary artery, medications to thin the blood and slow the heart rate, and surgery to replace or repair blocked coronary arteries.

Sickle cell anemia is a condition in which abnormal hemoglobin causes red blood cells to change to a sickle (crescent) shape. These sickle-shaped red blood cells get stuck in capillaries. Sickle cell anemia affects about 1 in every 500 African Americans and 1 in every 1400 Hispanics born in the United States.

- **Causes.** The primary cause is hereditary. A person with this disease must inherit a sickle cell gene from both parents. If only one sickle cell gene is inherited, the person is said to have sickle cell trait and may have mild symptoms of the disease. This condition may be prevented through genetic screening.
- **Signs and symptoms.** The signs and symptoms are many and include anemia, periodic episodes of pain called *crises*, chest pain, numbness in the hands or legs, fainting, fatigue, swollen hands and feet, jaundice, frequent infections, sores on the skin, delayed growth, stroke, seizures, and breathing difficulties. Retina damage, which causes visual problems, and spleen, liver, or kidney damage may also be seen.
- **Treatment.** Treatment includes antibiotics to treat infections, blood transfusions, pain medications, bone marrow transplants, supplemental oxygen, and medications to promote the development of normal hemoglobin.

Thrombophlebitis is a condition in which a blood clot and inflammation develop in a vein. It most commonly occurs in the veins of the legs. The danger of this disorder is that the blood clot may break loose. Once it reaches the heart, it is pumped to the lungs and is likely to block a blood vessel, causing a pulmonary embolism (an obstruction in the lungs). If the blood clot reaches the aorta and is pumped into arterial circulation, it can block either a coronary artery, causing a heart attack, or an artery in the brain, causing a stroke.

- **Causes.** The causes and risk factors include prolonged inactivity, oral contraceptives, hormone replacement therapy for estrogen, certain types of cancer, paralysis in the arms or legs, the presence of a catheter in a vein, a family history of this condition, varicose veins, and trauma to veins.
- **Signs and symptoms.** The most common symptoms are tenderness and pain in the affected area, redness, swelling, and fever.
- **Treatment.** This disorder is most often treated by the application of heat to the affected area, elevation of the legs, anti-inflammatory drugs, blood-thinning medications, the wearing of support stockings, and the removal of varicose veins. Surgery to remove the clot may be needed in some cases.

Varicose veins are dilated veins that are usually seen in the legs. They affect women more often than men.

- **Causes.** Varicose veins may be caused by prolonged sitting or standing, damage to valves in the veins, a loss of elasticity in the veins, obesity, pregnancy, oral

continued ⟶

Common Diseases and Disorders of the Circulatory System *(continued)*

contraceptives, or hormone replacement therapy. Varicose veins may be prevented through exercise and elevation of the legs.

- **Signs and symptoms.** Signs and symptoms include discomfort in the legs, discolorations around the ankles, clusters of veins, and enlarged, dark veins that are seen through skin.
- **Treatment.** The treatment of varicose veins includes the following:
  - Sclerotherapy, which is a procedure that prevents blood from flowing through varicose veins.
  - Laser surgery to prevent blood from flowing through affected veins.
  - Vein stripping, which involves removing affected veins.
  - Insertion of a catheter in the affected veins in order to destroy them.
  - Endoscopic vein surgery to close off affected veins.

Summary

The circulatory system acts as the transport system for the body. It brings oxygen to tissues and carries carbon dioxide away. Nutrients are picked up from the digestive system and delivered throughout the body, while waste products are carried away so that certain organs may remove them. The circulatory system consists of the heart and blood vessels and includes arteries, veins, and capillaries.

Blood is the transport medium that is pumped throughout the body. It is a liquid tissue that consists of plasma and formed elements (red blood cells, white blood cells, and platelets). It is important for the medical assistant to have an understanding of this system in order to effectively perform electrocardiograms, phlebotomy, and blood tests.

REVIEW

CHAPTER 10

CASE STUDY QUESTIONS

Now that you have completed this chapter, review the case study at the beginning of the chapter and answer the following questions:

1. What symptoms suggest that this patient is suffering from coronary artery disease and not some other disorder?
2. Why is it important to test the heart under stress rather than obtaining a resting echocardiogram?
3. What lifestyle changes should this patient make to prevent future heart attacks?
4. Why is a cardiac catheterization needed in addition to the stress echocardiogram?
5. What are the treatment options for this patient?

Discussion Questions

1. Trace the flow of blood from the right atrium and back.
2. List the components of plasma and give the importance of each.
3. Define hemostasis and describe the three events involved in this process.

Critical Thinking Questions

1. Why is it important for a woman to know her Rh blood type either before she gets pregnant or early into her pregnancy?
2. If an embolism begins in a saphenous vein, where is it most likely to block a blood vessel?
3. What is the difference between a white blood cell count and a differential white blood cell count? If monocyte numbers came back high on a differential count, what would be the significance?

Application Activities

1. For each blood type, give the antigen present on the red blood cells and the antibody present in plasma:
   - **a.** Type A
   - **b.** Type B
   - **c.** Type AB
   - **d.** Type O
2. Give the area of the body supplied by each of the following arteries:
   - **a.** Brachial
   - **b.** Femoral
   - **c.** Renal
   - **d.** Coronary
   - **e.** Iliac
   - **f.** Carotid
3. Give the area of the body drained by each of the following veins:
   - **a.** Jugular
   - **b.** Gastric
   - **c.** Popliteal
   - **d.** Mesenteric
4. Tell how the following affect systemic blood pressure:
   - **a.** An increase in stroke volume
   - **b.** A decrease in peripheral resistance
   - **c.** A decrease in blood volume
   - **d.** Vasoconstriction of systemic arteries

Internet Activity

Go to the Web site **http:www.americanheart.org/**, the American Heart Association, and choose Health Tools on the left menu bar. Then click Risk Assessment. Fill in the form to determine your risk of developing a heart disorder.

CHAPTER 11

The Immune System

KEY TERMS

acquired immunodeficiency syndrome (AIDS)
allergens
anaphylaxis
antihistamines
biopsy
carcinogen
complement
cytokines
epinephrine
hapten
human immunodeficiency virus (HIV)
humors
immunoglobulins
infection
inflammation
interferon
lupus erythematosus
lymphedema
lysozyme
major histocompatibility complex (MHC)
malignant
natural killer (NK) cells
phagocytosis

CHAPTER OUTLINE

- Defenses Against Disease
- Antibodies
- Immune Responses and Acquired Immunities
- Major Immune System Disorders

OBJECTIVES

After completing Chapter 11, you will be able to:

11.1 Define the terms *infection, pathogen,* and *antigen.*
11.2 List and describe the nonspecific body defense mechanisms.
11.3 Explain the signs and causes of inflammation.
11.4 Explain what is meant by specific body defenses.
11.5 Define B cells and T cells and describe their locations and functions.
11.6 Explain the importance of MHC proteins.
11.7 List the different types of T cells and describe their functions.
11.8 List the different types of antibodies and tell how they differ.
11.9 Explain how antibodies fight infection.
11.10 Define complement proteins and give their function.
11.11 Explain the difference between the primary immune response and secondary immune response.
11.12 Describe the function of a vaccine.
11.13 Explain the four different types of acquired immunities.
11.14 Describe how allergies develop.
11.15 Explain how the AIDS virus affects the immune system.
11.16 Identify the ways a person acquires the AIDS virus.
11.17 Define the terms *cancer* and *carcinogen.*
11.18 Explain how cancers are classified.
11.19 Describe how cancers are diagnosed and treated.
11.20 Describe the signs and symptoms of other common immune disorders.

Introduction

The immune system is responsible for protecting the body against bacteria, viruses, fungi, toxins, parasites, and cancer. It works with the organs of the lymphatic system to clear the body of these disease-causing agents.

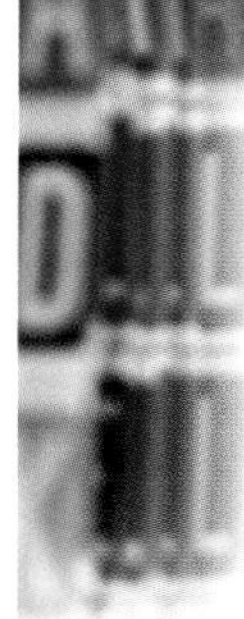

CASE STUDY

A few days ago a 17-year-old female came to the doctor's office convinced that she had AIDS. She had been running a slight fever for the past week, had been very tired, had tender lymph nodes in her neck, and had been losing weight without dieting. Her chart indicated that she had never been sexually active, had never used intravenous drugs, and had never received a blood transfusion.

As you read this chapter, consider the following questions:

1. Why is the 17-year-old female not likely to have AIDS?
2. What test can be done to assure the patient that she does not have AIDS?
3. What other diseases can cause the signs and symptoms of AIDS?
4. Based on her symptoms, what disease—beside AIDS—is this patient least likely to have?

Defenses Against Disease

An **infection** is the presence of a pathogen in or on the body. A **pathogen** is a disease-causing agent such as a bacterium, virus, toxin, fungus, or protozoan. The body has mechanisms to protect itself against pathogens in general; these mechanisms are called nonspecific defenses. The body also has mechanisms to protect itself against very specific pathogens; these mechanisms are called immunities and are considered specific defenses.

Nonspecific Defenses

The nonspecific mechanisms that protect bodies against pathogens include species resistance, mechanical and chemical barriers, and **phagocytosis.** Fever and **inflammation** are also effective in protecting the body from invading organisms.

Species Resistance. Species resistance simply means that a species typically gets only diseases that are unique to that species. For example, humans do not get diseases that affect plants. Humans also do not get most diseases that affect animals.

Mechanical Barriers. The covering of the body (skin) and the linings of the tubes of the body (mucous membranes) provide mechanical barriers against pathogens. Intact skin is impermeable to most pathogens. Intact mucous membranes, although generally impermeable, do permit the entry of a few pathogens.

Chemical Barriers. Chemicals and enzymes in body fluids provide chemical barriers that destroy pathogens. For example, acids in the stomach destroy pathogens that are swallowed. **Lysozymes** in tears destroy pathogens on the surface of the eye. Salt in sweat also kills bacteria, and **interferon** in blood blocks viruses from infecting cells.

Phagocytosis. Neutrophils and monocytes are the most active phagocytes in blood. They can also leave the bloodstream to attack pathogens in other tissues. When a monocyte leaves the bloodstream, it becomes a macrophage, which is simply a larger phagocytic cell.

Fever. An elevated body temperature is a fever. Fever causes the liver and spleen to take iron out of the bloodstream. Many pathogens need iron to survive in a body, so when their iron sources are gone, they die. Fever also activates phagocytic cells in the body to attack pathogens.

Inflammation. When an area of the body becomes injured or infected with a pathogen, inflammation can result. In inflammation, blood vessels in the injured area dilate and become leaky. Because blood vessels dilate, more blood enters the area, bringing phagocytic white blood cells to the area to attack the pathogen. The blood also brings proteins to replace injured tissues and clotting factors to stop any bleeding. The clotting factors also "wall off" the area so that pathogens cannot spread. Because blood vessels become leaky, more fluid accumulates in the injured area, which leads to edema. The excess fluid often irritates pain receptors. The four cardinal signs of inflammation are redness, heat, swelling, and pain.

Specific Defenses

Specific defenses are called immunities. They protect the body against very specific pathogens. For example, a person who has chickenpox develops a specific defense that prevents that person from getting chickenpox again. However, this specific defense does not protect the person from any other disease.

Antigens are very simply defined as foreign substances in the body. Pathogens have many antigens on their surfaces. The immune system is programmed to recognize antigens in the body. Foreign substances in the body too small to start an immune response by themselves are called **haptens.** Many times, haptens join to proteins in the blood where they are then able to trigger an immune response. Penicillin is an example of a hapten.

Antibodies and **complements** are the major proteins involved in specific defenses. **Lymphocytes** and **macrophages** are the major white blood cells involved in specific defenses.

B Cells and T Cells. Two major types of lymphocytes are B cells and T cells. Although both B cells and T cells circulate in the blood, most of the lymphocytes in blood are T cells. B cells and T cells are also found in lymph nodes, the spleen, the thymus, the lining of digestive organs, and bone marrow.

Both T cells and B cells recognize antigens in the body; however, they respond to antigens in different ways. T cells bind to antigens on cells and attack them directly. This type of response is called a cell-mediated response. T cells also respond to antigens by secreting different type of chemicals called **cytokines.** Cytokines increase T cell production, increase B cell production, directly kill cells that have antigens, and stimulate red bone marrow to produce more white blood cells.

B cells do not attack antigens directly. B cells respond to antigens by becoming plasma cells. The plasma cells then make antibodies against the specific antigen. The antibodies end up attaching to antigens in the **humors** (fluids) of the body; this response is called a humoral response.

B cells become activated when a specific antigen binds to receptors on their surfaces. Each group of B cells only recognizes one type of antigen. Once activated, B cells divide to make plasma cells and memory B cells. Plasma cells make antibodies. Antibodies go out into the fluids of the body and bind to the antigens that activated the B cells. Memory B cells trigger a stronger immune response the next time the person is exposed to the same antigen (Figures 11-1 and 11-2).

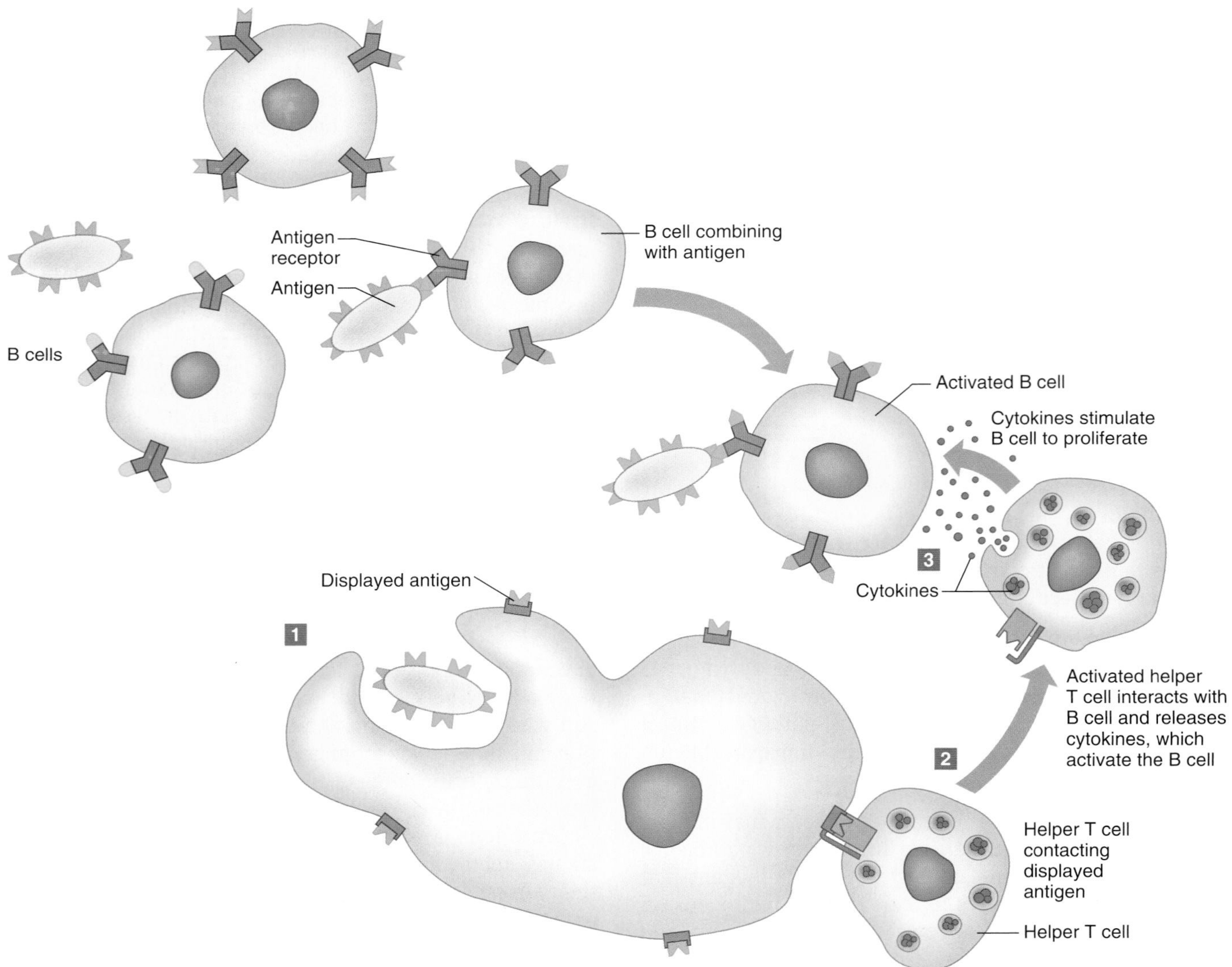

Figure 11-1. T cell and B cell activation. (1) A macrophage displays an antigen on its cell membrane. (2) A helper T cell binds to the antigen on the macrophage and becomes activated. (3) An activated helper T cell releases cytokines to help an activated B cell proliferate. Notice that the B cell must also bind to an antigen to become activated.

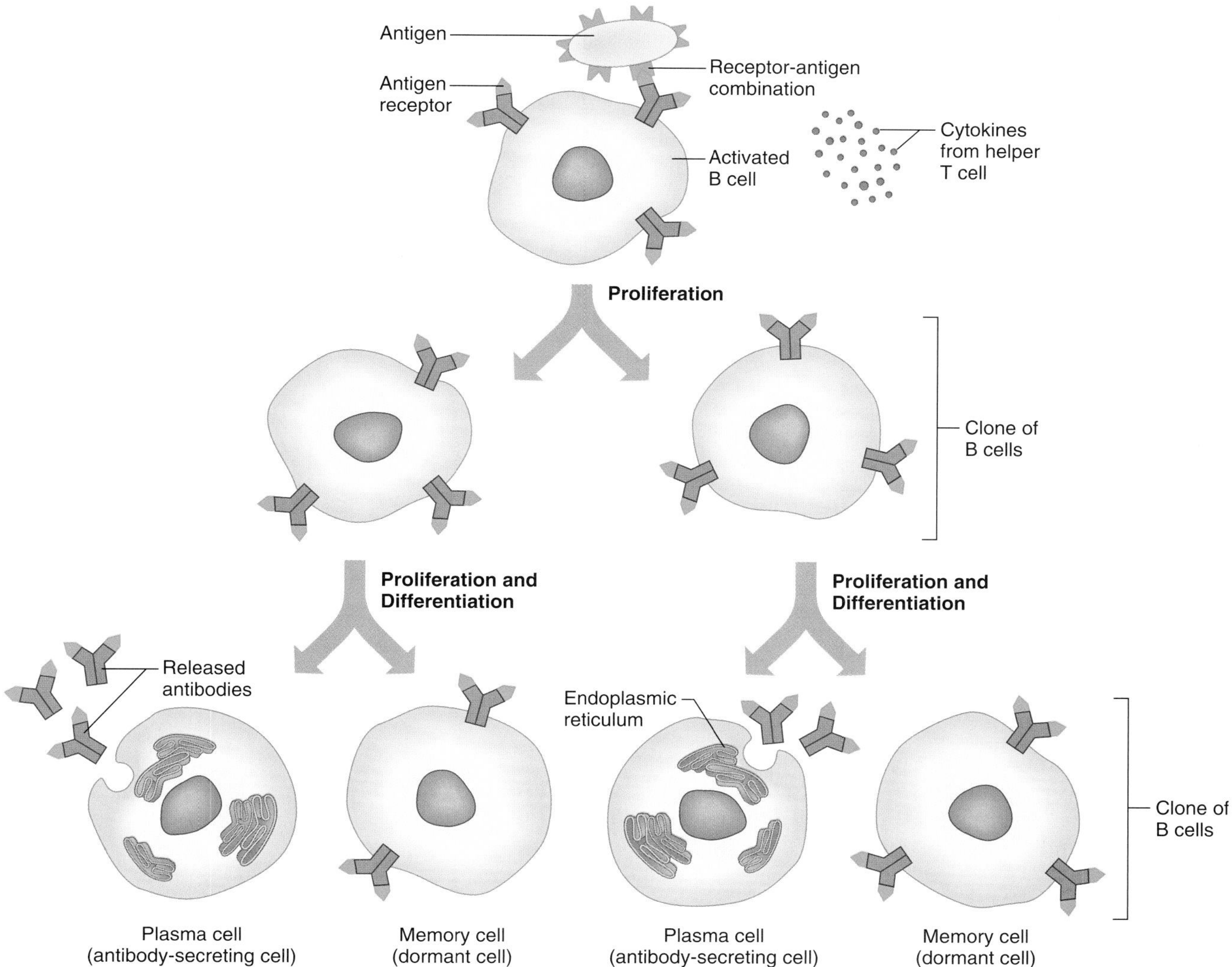

Figure 11-2. An activated B cell multiplies to become memory cells and plasma cells. Plasma cells secrete antibodies.

Before a T cell can respond to an antigen, it must be activated. T cell activation begins when a macrophage ingests and digests a pathogen that has antigens on it. The macrophage then takes some of the antigens from the pathogen and puts them on its cell membrane next to a large protein complex called a **major histocompatibility complex (MHC).** A T cell that has a receptor for the antigen recognizes and binds to the antigen and the MHC on the surface of the macrophage. The T cell is now activated and begins to divide to form other types of T cells and T memory cells. It is important to note that T cells cannot be activated without macrophages and MHC proteins.

Some activated T cells form cytotoxic T cells. This type of T cell is important in protecting the body against viruses and cancer cells. Other activated T cells become helper T cells, which carry out many important roles in immunity. Helper T cells increase antibody formation, memory cell formation, B cell formation, and phagocytosis. Some activated T cells become memory T cells. The memory cells "remember" the pathogen that activated the original T cell. When a person is later exposed to the same pathogen, memory cells trigger an immune response that is more effective than the first immune response. The production of memory cells prevents a person from suffering from the same disease twice.

Natural Killer (NK) Cells. **Natural killer (NK) cells** are another type of lymphocyte. They primarily target cancer cells but also protect the body against many types of pathogens. Like cytotoxic T cells, NK cells kill harmful cells on contact. They secrete chemicals that produce holes in the membranes of harmful cells, which cause the cells to burst. Unlike B cells and T cells, NK cells do not have to recognize a specific antigen to start destroying pathogens.

Antibodies

Antibodies are also called **immunoglobulins.** The following is a list of different types of immunoglobulins (Ig):

- IgG. This antibody primarily recognizes bacteria, viruses, and toxins. It can also activate complements, which are proteins in serum that attack pathogens.
- IgA. This antibody is found in secretions of the body such as breast milk, sweat, tears, saliva, and mucus. It prevents pathogens from entering the body.
- IgM. This antibody is very large and primarily binds to antigens on food, bacteria, or incompatible blood cells. It also activates complements.
- IgE. This antibody is found wherever IgA is located. It is involved in triggering allergic reactions.

When antibodies bind to antigens, they take one of the following actions:

- They allow phagocytes to recognize and destroy antigens.
- They make antigens clump together, causing them to be destroyed by macrophages. This is how incompatible blood cells are destroyed.
- They cover the toxic portions of antigens to make them harmless.
- They activate complements. Complements are proteins in serum that attack pathogens by forming holes in them. Complement proteins also attract macrophages to pathogens and can stimulate inflammation.

Immune Responses and Acquired Immunities

A primary immune response occurs the first time a person is exposed to an antigen. This response is slow and takes several weeks to occur. In this response, memory cells are made. A secondary immune response occurs the next time a person is exposed to the same antigen. This response is very quick and usually prevents a person from developing a disease from the antigen. Memory cells carry out the secondary immune response.

A person is born with very few immunities but normally develops them as long as the person's immune system is healthy. The four types of immunities a person can acquire are: (1) natural acquired active immunity, (2) artificially acquired active immunity, (3) naturally acquired passive immunity, and (4) artificially acquired passive immunity.

Naturally Acquired Active Immunity

A person develops this immunity by being naturally exposed to an antigen and subsequently making antibodies and memory cells against the antigen. Having an infectious disease caused by pathogens leads to the development of this type of immunity. This immunity is usually long lasting.

Artificially Acquired Active Immunity

A person develops this immunity by being injected with a pathogen and then subsequently making antibodies and memory cells against the pathogen. Immunizations or vaccines cause this type of immunity. This type is usually long lasting.

Naturally Acquired Passive Immunity

A person is given this immunity through his mother. When a mother breast-feeds, she passes antibodies to her baby through breast milk. A mother also passes antibodies to her baby across the placenta. This type of immunity is short lived.

Artificially Acquired Passive Immunity

A person is given this immunity when she is injected with antibodies. If a snake bites a person, a physician will inject the patient with antibodies (antivenom) to neutralize the venom. This type of immunity is short lived.

Major Immune System Disorders

A number of diseases and disorders can challenge the immune system. Among them, HIV infection, AIDS, cancer, and allergies are the most significant.

Human Immunodeficiency Virus

Human immunodeficiency virus (HIV) is a viral infection that seriously damages an individual's immunity, primarily by destroying lymphocytes. It causes **acquired immunodeficiency syndrome (AIDS)** and can leave the immune system weak and susceptible to other diseases.

Routes of Transmission. HIV can be located in many body fluids including saliva, tears, blood, semen, vaginal secretions, and breast milk. The most common routes of transmission are through sexual contact, through blood, or from mother to child during pregnancy or breastfeeding. Less common routes of transmission are through accidental needlesticks, artificial insemination, and organ transplants. HIV is not transmitted through casual contact such as holding hands, hugging, and touching objects previously touched by HIV-infected persons. Statistically, persons most likely to get HIV infection are homosexual men, bisexual men, intravenous drug users who share needles, and infants born to HIV-infected mothers.

HIV Testing. A person can have an HIV infection for years before developing any symptoms of this disease. Fortunately, a few tests are available to determine if a person has been infected with HIV. The most sensitive test—but one that is very costly—is polymerase chain reaction (PCR). This test can determine the number of HIV particles in a sample of blood, even if the number is less than 25 viral particles per cubic centimeter of plasma. For this reason, this test is useful for the early diagnosis of HIV infection.

Acquired Immunodeficiency Syndrome

AIDS is the development of severe signs and symptoms caused by HIV. In the United States, AIDS is the fifth leading cause of death in individuals between the ages of 25 and 44. This disease severely suppresses a person's immune system so that what would be minor infections in healthy individuals end up being fatal in patients with AIDS.

AIDS Testing. The most commonly used test to determine the presence of the AIDS virus is called ELISA. This test is considerably less expensive than PCR but is also less reliable. ELISA cannot detect early HIV infections. For this reason, it is preferable to test a high-risk patient three times with ELISA or alternate tests to ensure an accurate diagnosis.

Counts of CD4 cells are used to diagnose the stage of HIV infection. Once CD4 counts fall below 200, a person is diagnosed with AIDS. CD4 cells are types of T cells and are important for the functions of other components of the immune system.

Signs and Symptoms. The signs and symptoms of people who have developed AIDS include low T cell counts, fever, profuse sweating, weakness, weight loss, swollen glands, frequent infections, and some rare types of cancers. Common infections include ulcers of the mouth, skin, or genitals caused by herpes viruses; tuberculosis; yeast infections within the mouth, esophagus, or vagina; pneumonia; meningitis; and encephalitis. Cytomegalovirus (CMV), which is a type of infection caused by the herpes virus, can infect the eyes and other organs. A cancer that commonly appears in AIDS patients is Kaposi's sarcoma. It forms lesions on the skin—usually on the hands and feet first.

Treatment. There is no cure for AIDS, but in the United States, treatments are available that significantly delay the progression of the disease for many patients. Treatments include the use of various antiviral drugs, but many of these drugs have serious side effects. Antibiotics are also used to treat infections.

Cancer

Cancer is defined as the uncontrolled growth of abnormal cells. Healthy cells normally know when to stop reproducing, but cancer cells have lost this ability. Cancer cells often form growths called **malignant** tumors, which are often fatal. In many cases, these cancerous cells or tumors damage normal cells of tissues and organs, which cause organ systems to fail.

At least 200 different types of cancers are known. In the United States, the three most common cancer types in men are prostate, lung, and colon cancer. The three most common types in women are breast, lung, and colon cancer. Lung cancer is the leading killer of all types of cancer for all people.

Causes. The causes of cancer are mostly unknown but certain risk factors have been identified. These factors include a suppressed immune system, radiation, tobacco, and some viruses. Many other factors are suspected. One of the best ways to prevent cancer is to not smoke and to avoid other known risk factors. A factor that is known to cause the formation of cancer is called a **carcinogen.**

Diagnosis. Most cancers are diagnosed with a **biopsy,** which is a removal of tissues for examination. CT scans are also used to help diagnose most cancer types. Other diagnostic tests include blood counts, an analysis of blood chemistry, and x-rays.

Signs and Symptoms. The symptoms of different types of cancer vary but the following are usually observed in most types: fever, chills, unintended weight loss, fatigue, and a general sense of not feeling well.

Treatment. The treatment of cancer differs depending on the type and stage of cancer. The stage of cancer refers to how large a tumor is and how far cancer cells have spread throughout the body. Table 11-1 provides a summary of cancer staging.

If tumors are localized and have not spread, the cancer can often be successfully treated by surgically removing the tumor. Other treatment options are chemotherapy and radiation therapy. Even if a cancer cannot be cured, its progression can sometimes be slowed, allowing patients to live additional years.

Allergies

An allergic reaction is an immune response to a substance, such as pollen, that is not normally harmful to the body. An allergy can also be an excessive immune response. Substances that trigger allergic responses are called **allergens.**

Allergic reactions involve IgE antibodies and mast cells. When IgE antibodies bind to allergens, they cause mast cells to release histamine and heparin. These chemicals trigger allergic reactions. A patient receiving allergy shots is being injected with tiny amounts of the allergen. This causes the body to produce IgG antibodies that will prevent IgE antibodies from binding to the allergen. IgG antibodies do not trigger immune responses because they do not activate mast cells.

Most allergies do not cause life-threatening conditions, but some do. One life-threatening condition that can result is **anaphylaxis.** In this condition, blood vessels dilate so quickly that blood pressure drops too quickly for organs to adjust.

TABLE 11-1 Cancer Staging	
Stage	**Description**
Stage 0	Very early cancer. Cancer cells are localized in a few cell layers.
Stage I	Cancer cells have spread to deeper cell layers, or some may have spread to surrounding tissues.
Stage II	Cancer cells have spread to surrounding tissues but are considered contained in the primary cancer site.
Stage III	Cancer cells have spread beyond the primary cancer site to nearby areas.
Stage IV	Cancer cells have spread to other organs of the body.
Recurrent	Cancer cells have reappeared after treatment.

Signs and Symptoms. The signs and symptoms of allergies vary depending on what part of the body is exposed to allergens. Allergens that are inhaled often cause a runny nose, sneezing, coughing, or wheezing. An allergen that is ingested causes nausea, diarrhea, or vomiting. Allergens that are contacted by skin cause rashes. Allergens in the blood, such as penicillin for people who are allergic to it, are often the most life-threatening because they can affect many organ systems.

Treatment. Many allergies are effectively treated with over-the-counter medications called **antihistamines.** Prescription-strength antihistamines are also available. Various types of nasal sprays and decongestants can also reduce the symptoms of allergies. When a person experiences anaphylaxis, an injection of **epinephrine** is usually an effective treatment. Epinephrine causes vasoconstriction, which increases blood pressure.

Pathophysiology

Common Diseases and Disorders of the Immune System

Chronic fatigue syndrome is a condition in which a person feels severe tiredness that cannot be relieved by rest and is not related to other illness.

- **Causes.** The causes are primarily unknown, although the herpes virus is suspected as a possible cause. This condition may also be caused by an autoimmune response against the nervous system.
- **Signs and symptoms.** The most common symptom is severe fatigue. Other signs and symptoms include mild fever, sore throat, tender lymph nodes in the neck or armpit, general body aches, joint pain, sleep disturbances, and depression.
- **Treatment.** Treatment includes antiviral drugs, medications to treat depression, and pain medications.

Lupus erythematosus, commonly referred to as lupus, is an autoimmune disorder that affects few or many organ systems of the body. In this condition, people produce antibodies that target their own cells and tissues. Lupus affects women more often than men.

- **Causes.** This disorder may be caused by some drugs or by bacterial infections.
- **Signs and symptoms.** The list of signs and symptoms is extensive and includes all of the following:
  - Fatigue
  - General body aches
  - Fever
  - Weight loss
  - Hair loss
  - Arthritis
  - Numbness of the fingers and toes
  - "Butterfly" rash on the face
  - Sensitivity to sunlight
  - Vision problems
  - Nausea
  - Nosebleeds
  - Headaches
  - Mental disorders
  - Seizures
  - Abnormal blood clots
  - Chest pains
  - Inflammation of heart tissues
  - Anemia
  - Shortness of breath

continued ⟶

Common Diseases and Disorders of the Immune System *(continued)*

- Fluid accumulation around the lungs
- Renal failure
- Blood in the urine

- **Treatment.** Treatment options include anti-inflammatory medications as well as protective clothing and creams to prevent damage from sunlight. Dialysis, medications to suppress the immune system, and kidney transplants may be necessary for more serious cases.

Lymphedema is the blockage of lymphatic vessels. These vessels typically drain excess fluids from various areas of the body.

- **Causes.** This condition may be caused by parasitic infections, trauma to the vessels, tumors, radiation therapy, cellulitis (a skin infection), and surgeries in which lymph tissues have been removed.
- **Signs and symptoms.** Common symptoms are swelling that lasts longer than a few days or increases over time.
- **Treatment.** Treatment options include compression stockings for swelling in the legs or arms, elevation of the affected limb, or surgery to remove abnormal lymphatic tissue.

Rheumatoid arthritis is an autoimmune disorder in which a person's immune system attacks the joints of the body. Women are more likely to be affected than men.

- **Causes.** This disorder may be caused by some bacterial infections. In addition, it can be caused by immune cells that attack the structures associated with joints.
- **Signs and symptoms.** There are a number of signs and symptoms associated with this disorder. They include fatigue, joint pain and swelling (especially in the hands and feet), body aches, cartilage and bone destruction, anemia, nodules that appear under the skin, lung tissue scarring, shortness of breath, and stomach and skin ulcers. Patients may also present with inflammation of blood vessels, heart muscle, and the eyes.
- **Treatment.** This disorder may be treated with physical therapy, pain medications, and anti-inflammatory medicines. More serious treatments include medications to suppress the immune system, the removal of antibodies from the blood through a process called apheresis, surgery to remove inflamed joint membranes, and knee and hip replacement surgeries.

Summary

The body's major line of defense is the immune system. It protects the body against infection, toxins, and cancer. These defenses can be either nonspecific or specific. Lymphocytes are the major types of cells in the immune system and are classified as either B cells or T cells.

When the body is first exposed to an antigen, a primary immune response occurs. This response is less specific and slower than a secondary immune response, which occurs the next time the body is exposed to the same antigen. An intact immune system is important because the body is attacked by numerous invaders every day. In order to effectively perform aseptic technique and infection control, the medical assistant must have a working knowledge of the immune system.

REVIEW

CHAPTER 11

CASE STUDY QUESTIONS

Now that you have completed this chapter, review the case study at the beginning of the chapter and answer the following questions:

1. Why is the 17-year-old female not likely to have AIDS?
2. What test can be done to assure the patient that she does not have AIDS?
3. What other diseases can cause the signs and symptoms of AIDS?
4. Based on her symptoms, what disease—beside AIDS—is this patient least likely to have?

Discussion Questions

1. List four types of antibodies and give their locations and functions.
2. What are nonspecific body defenses? Give examples.
3. How do secondary immune responses occur?
4. Discuss how B cells and T cells are activated.

Critical Thinking Questions

1. Why are passively acquired immunities temporary and short lasting compared to actively acquired immunities?
2. How does AIDS destroy the immune system?
3. How do vaccines produce favorable effects?

Application Activities

1. Give an example of each of the following nonspecific defense mechanisms:
   a. Mechanical barrier
   b. Chemical barrier
   c. Phagocytic cell
2. Describe what produces the following signs of inflammation:
   a. Redness
   b. Swelling
   c. Heat
   d. Pain
3. Give the functions of each of the following defensive proteins or cells:
   a. Complement proteins
   b. Macrophages
   c. Helper T cells
   d. Memory cells
   e. Plasma cells
4. What are disease-causing agents in the body called?

Internet Activity

Find a Web site that provides information on lymphedema. Research the types of patients who are most likely to develop this disorder. How can these people prevent the development of this condition?

CHAPTER 12

The Respiratory System

CHAPTER OUTLINE

- Organs of the Respiratory System
- The Mechanisms of Breathing
- Respiratory Volumes
- The Transport of Oxygen and Carbon Dioxide in the Blood

OBJECTIVES

After completing Chapter 12, you will be able to:

12.1 Explain the functions of the respiratory system.
12.2 Explain the difference between internal respiration and external respiration.
12.3 Describe how the larynx produces voice sounds.
12.4 List the structures contained within the lungs.
12.5 Describe the coverings of the lungs and chest cavity.
12.6 Describe the events that lead to the inspiration and expiration of air.
12.7 Explain how the brain controls breathing and how normal breathing patterns can be disrupted.
12.8 List and explain various respiratory volumes and tell how they are used to diagnose respiratory problems.
12.9 Describe how oxygen is transported from the lungs to body cells.
12.10 Describe how carbon dioxide is transported from body cells to the lungs.
12.11 Describe the signs, symptoms, causes, and treatments of various respiratory disorders and diseases.

KEY TERMS

alveoli
bicarbonate ions
bronchi
bronchial tree
bronchioles
chronic obstructive pulmonary disease (COPD)
cricoid cartilage
epiglottic cartilage
epiglottis
expiration
glottis
hyperventilation
inspiration
larynx
nasal conchae
nasal septum
paranasal sinuses
pharynx
pleuritis
pneumothorax
pleura
respiratory volume
sinusitis
thyroid cartilage
trachea
ventilation

Introduction

The respiratory system functions to move air in and out of the lungs. This process is called ventilation, or breathing. This system also functions to deliver oxygen (O_2) via the bloodstream. It also removes a waste product—carbon dioxide (CO_2)—from the blood. This exchange of oxygen and carbon dioxide is called external respiration.

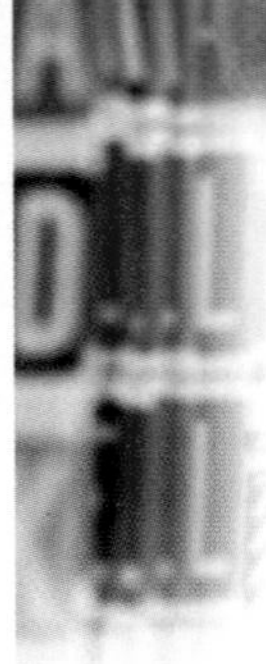

CASE STUDY

A 5-year-old boy is brought to the pediatrician's office. He has been coughing at night for the past week. Today he presents with shortness of breath, tightness in his chest, and wheezing. The doctor recognizes the child's symptoms as those of asthma and orders a bronchodilator—a drug that relaxes the muscles around the airway—to be delivered using a nebulizer. He also refers the child for allergy testing.

As you read this chapter, consider the following questions:

1. Why is the patient wheezing?
2. Is asthma a life-threatening condition?
3. What is the advantage of using a nebulizer to deliver the bronchodilator?
4. Why did the doctor refer the patient for allergy testing?

Organs of the Respiratory System

The organs of the respiratory system are the nose, pharynx, larynx, trachea, bronchial tree (including the bronchi and bronchioles), and the lungs (Figure 12-1). The nose is made of bones and cartilage and the skin covering them. The openings of the nose are called nostrils. The hairs of the nostrils prevent large particles from entering the nose through air.

The Nasal Cavity and Paranasal Sinuses

The nasal cavity is simply the hollow space behind the nose. The nasal cavity is divided into a left and right portion by the **nasal septum.** There are structures called **nasal conchae** that extend from the lateral walls of the nasal cavity. Most of the nasal cavity is lined with a mucous membrane that acts to warm and moisten air as it passes through the nasal cavity.

The nasal cavity is also lined with cells that possess cilia. As mucus traps dust and other particles in the nasal cavity, the cilia push the mucus toward the throat where it is swallowed. The enzymes of the stomach then destroy the particles in the dust.

The **paranasal sinuses** are air-filled spaces within the skull bones that open into the nasal cavity. The paranasal sinuses reduce the weight of the skull and also give your voice a certain tone. When your paranasal sinuses are "stopped up," the tone of your voice changes. The bones of the skull that contain the sinuses include the frontal, sphenoid, ethmoid, and maxillae bones.

The Pharynx

The **pharynx** is an organ of the respiratory system as well as the digestive system. During inspiration, air flows from the nasal or oral cavity into the pharynx. From the pharynx, air flows into the larynx.

The Larynx and Vocal Cords

The **larynx** is more commonly called the voice box. It sits superior to and is continuous with the trachea. It functions to move air in and out of the trachea and to produce the sounds of a person's voice. The larynx is mostly made of cartilage and muscle tissue. There are three cartilages in the larynx (Figure 12-2). The largest cartilage is called the **thyroid cartilage,** and it forms the anterior wall of the larynx. During the puberty of a male, testosterone causes the thyroid cartilage to enlarge to produce the "Adam's apple." A smaller cartilage called the **epiglottic cartilage** forms the framework of the epiglottis. The **epiglottis** is the flap-like structure that closes off the larynx during swallowing. The third cartilage of the larynx is called the **cricoid cartilage.** It forms most of the posterior wall of the larynx and a small part of the anterior wall.

The vocal cords stretch between the thyroid cartilage and the cricoid cartilage. The opening between the vocal cords is called the **glottis** (see Figure 12-2, part C). The upper vocal cords are referred to as false vocal cords because they do not produce sound. The lower vocal cords are called true vocal cords because muscles stretch and relax them to produce different types of sounds. If the true vocal cords are stretched, the voice becomes higher in pitch. When the true vocal cords are relaxed, the voice becomes lower in pitch. Men have thicker vocal cords, which is why their voices are deeper than female voices.

The Trachea, Bronchi, and Bronchioles

The **trachea** is more commonly referred to as the *windpipe*. It is a tubular organ made of rings of cartilage and smooth muscle. It extends from the larynx to the bronchi. The trachea is lined with cells that possess cilia that constantly

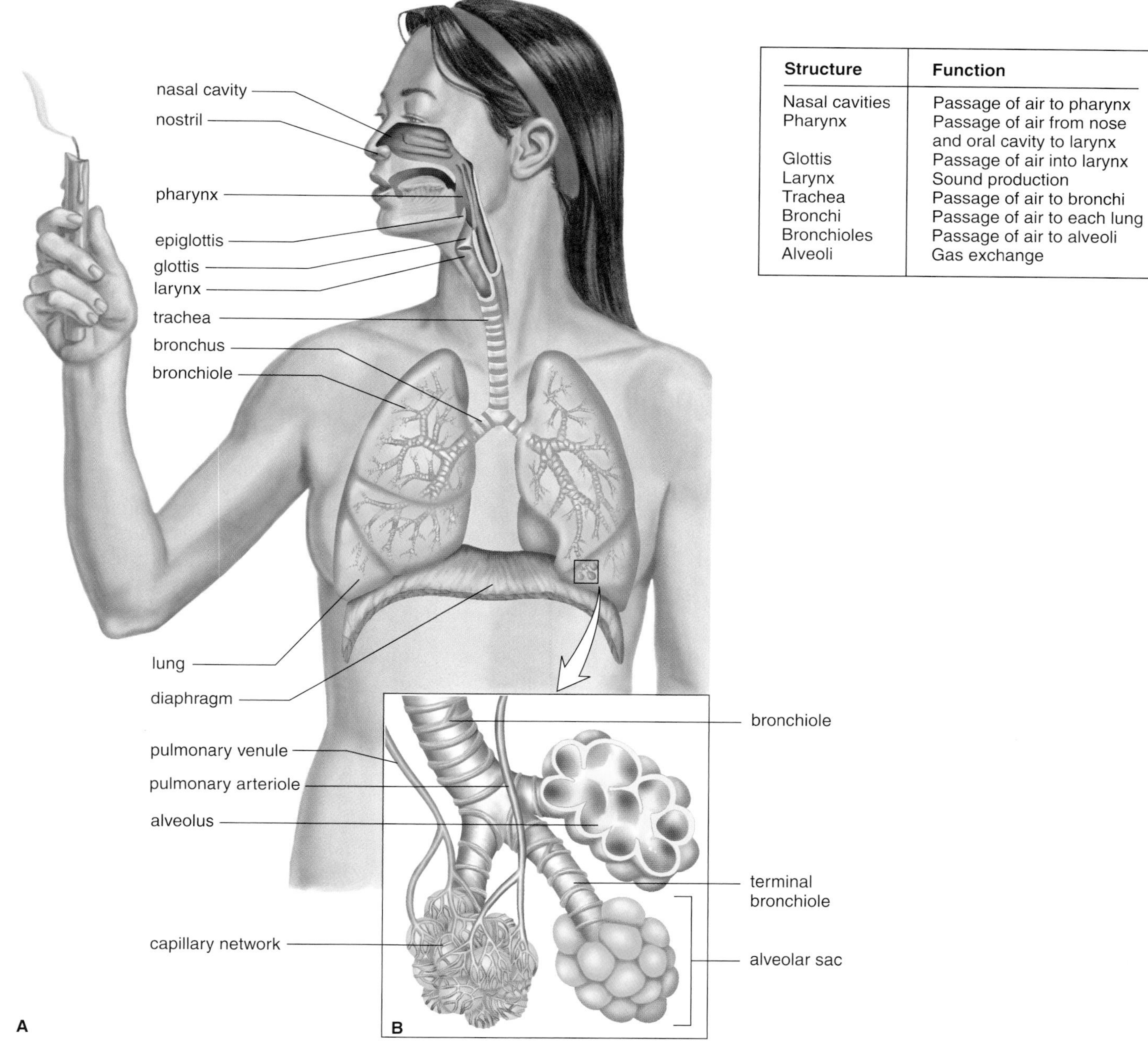

Structure	Function
Nasal cavities	Passage of air to pharynx
Pharynx	Passage of air from nose and oral cavity to larynx
Glottis	Passage of air into larynx
Larynx	Sound production
Trachea	Passage of air to bronchi
Bronchi	Passage of air to each lung
Bronchioles	Passage of air to alveoli
Alveoli	Gas exchange

Figure 12-1. (a) Organs of the respiratory system and (b) the flow of air through respiratory organs.

move mucus up to the throat where it is swallowed. Mucus traps bacteria, viruses, and any other harmful substances a person inhales—as in the process that occurs in the nasal cavity. The digestive juices of the stomach then destroy the harmful substances. Smoking destroys cilia so the only way a smoker can get mucus out of his trachea is to cough. Smokers often feel the urgency to cough more frequently than nonsmokers.

The distal end of the trachea branches and starts a series of tubes called the **bronchial tree.** The first branches off the trachea are called primary, or main stem, **bronchi.** The branches of the primary bronchi are called secondary bronchi. The secondary bronchi branch into tertiary bronchi. Tertiary bronchi branch into **bronchioles.** At the ends of the bronchioles are air sacs called alveoli.

Alveoli are very thin sacs made of simple squamous epithelial cells and are surrounded by capillaries. They are considered the "working tissue" of the lung because in the alveoli is where gaseous exchanges take place. Many physicians refer to the alveoli as the *pulmonary parenchyma* (parenchymal means "working tissue" of any organ or organ system). Blood in the capillaries releases carbon dioxide into the alveoli, and air in the alveoli releases oxygen into the blood of the capillaries. This is the process by which oxygen moves into the blood and carbon dioxide is removed.

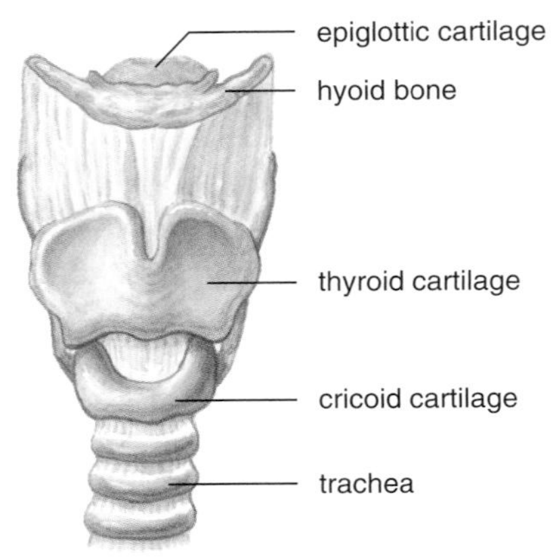

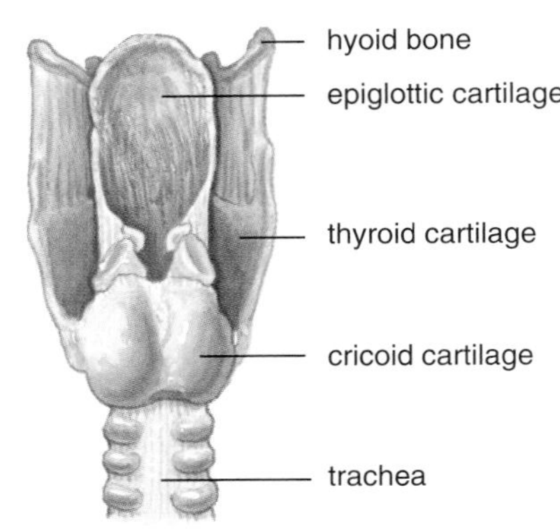

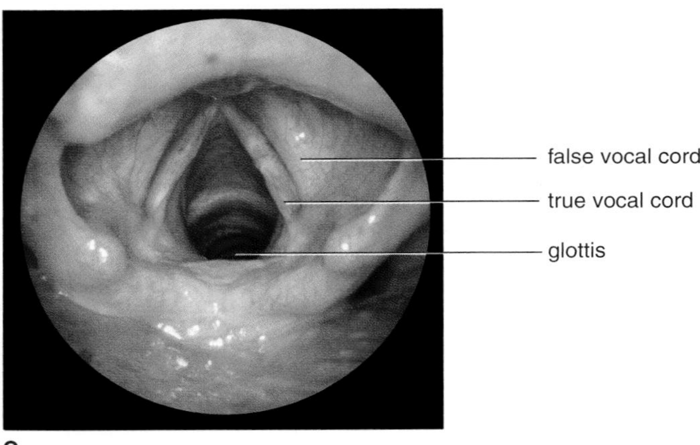

Figure 12-2. (a) Anterior view of larynx. (b) Posterior view of larynx. (c) Photograph of the vocal cords and glottis.

The Lungs

The lungs are cone-shaped organs that contain connective tissue, the bronchial tree, nerves, lymphatic vessels, and many blood vessels. The right lung is larger than the left; the right lung is divided into three lobes and the left into two. The membranes that surround the lungs are called **pleura.** Pleura produce a slippery fluid called serous fluid that helps the lungs slide easily along the thoracic wall during breathing.

The Mechanisms of Breathing

Breathing, or pulmonary **ventilation,** consists of two events—**inspiration** and **expiration.** During inspiration, or inhalation, oxygen-rich air eventually flows into the alveoli of the lungs. Air flows into the airways during inspiration because the thoracic cavity enlarges. When the thoracic cavity enlarges, pressure decreases in the cavity. The atmospheric pressure outside the body is greater than the pressure inside the cavity, and air passively flows from an area of high pressure to an area of low pressure. The events that enlarge the thoracic cavity and therefore lead to inspiration are as follows (Figure 12-3):

- The diaphragm contracts. When the diaphragm contracts, it becomes flat, which increases the amount of space in the thoracic cavity.
- The intercostal muscles raise the ribs; this further enlarges the thoracic cavity.

During expiration, or exhalation, air rich with carbon dioxide flows out of the airways. Air flows out because the thoracic cavity becomes smaller, which increases the pressure inside the cavity. When the pressure inside the cavity becomes greater than the atmospheric pressure, air flows out. The events that lead to expiration are as follows (Figure 12-3):

- The diaphragm relaxes. When the diaphragm relaxes, it domes up into the thoracic cavity, which decreases the space in the cavity.
- The intercostal muscles lower the ribs; this further decreases the size of the thoracic cavity.

Breathing is controlled by the respiratory center, which is a group of neurons in the pons and medulla oblongata. The medulla oblongata controls both the rhythm and the depth of breathing. The pons controls the rate of breathing.

Other factors that affect breathing are the carbon dioxide levels in the blood and the pH of the blood. When carbon dioxide levels rise in the blood, the rate and depth of breathing increase. The rate and depth of breathing also increase when the blood pH drops. Fear and pain also increase the breathing rate. Breathing rapidly and deeply is called **hyperventilation.** Hyperventilation decreases the amount of carbon dioxide in the blood.

The inflation reflex also helps to regulate the depth of breathing. Stretch receptors in pleural membranes are activated when the lungs are stretched past a certain point. This triggers the depth of breathing to decrease to prevent overinflation of the lungs.

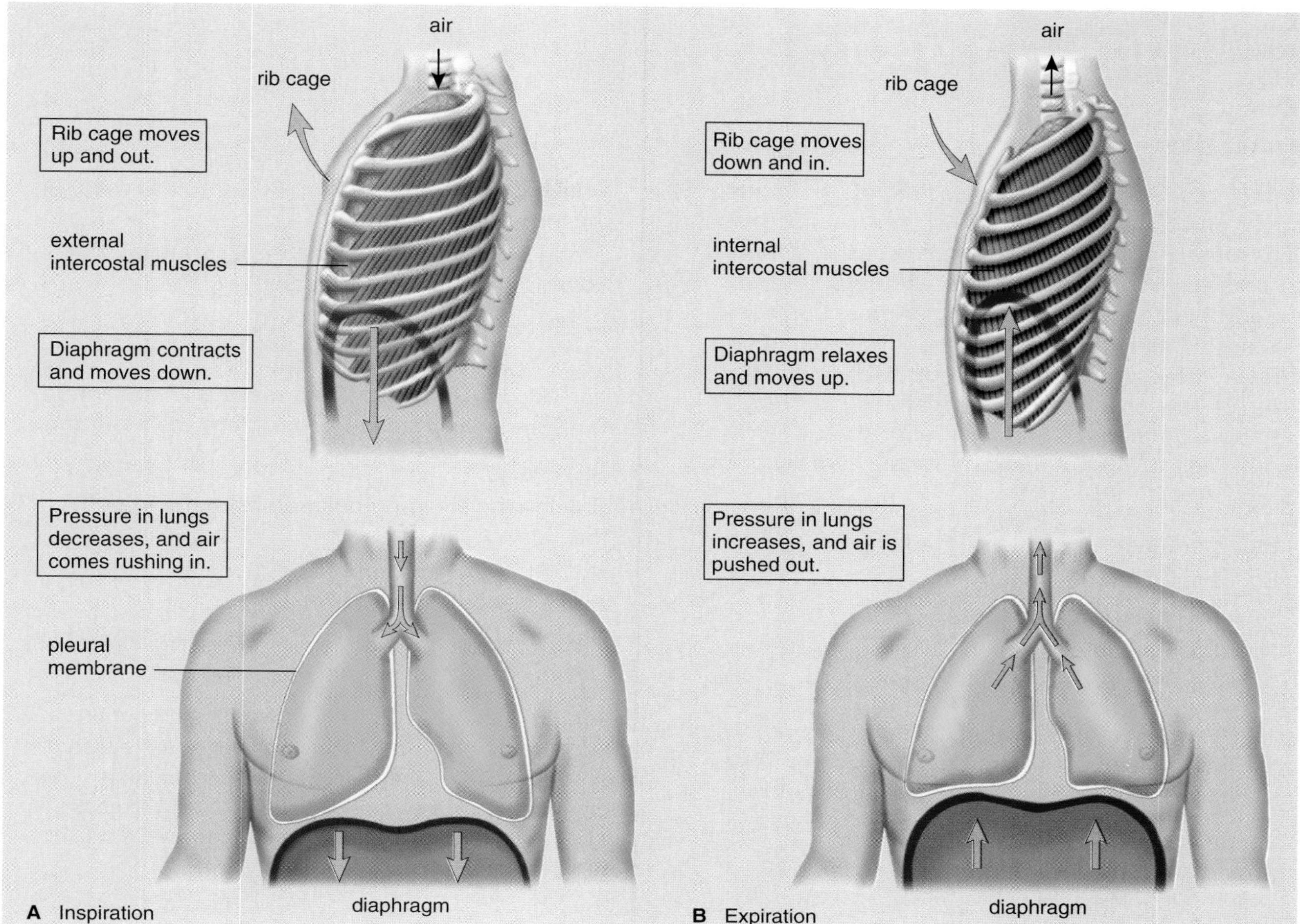

Figure 12-3. (a) Events of inspiration and (b) events of expiration.

Respiratory Volumes

During different intensities of breathing, different volumes of air move in and out of the lungs. These volumes are called **respiratory volumes** and can be measured to assess the healthiness of the respiratory system. Respiratory capacities can be calculated by adding certain respiratory volumes together. The following are the different types of volumes and capacities:

- Tidal volume: the amount of air that moves in or out of the lungs during a normal breath.
- Inspiratory reserve volume: the amount of air that can be forcefully inhaled following a normal inhalation.
- Expiratory reserve volume: the amount of air that can be forcefully exhaled following a normal exhalation.
- Residual volume: the volume of air that always remains in the lungs, even after a forceful expiration.
- Vital capacity: the total amount of air that can be forcefully exhaled after the deepest inhalation possible.
- Total lung capacity: the total amount of air the lungs can hold.

The Transport of Oxygen and Carbon Dioxide in the Blood

Once oxygen gets into the bloodstream, about 97% of it binds to **hemoglobin** in red blood cells. Hemoglobin bound to oxygen is call **oxyhemoglobin** and is bright red in color. Some oxygen stays dissolved in plasma and does not bind to hemoglobin.

Carbon dioxide in the bloodstream reacts with water to form **bicarbonate ions**; most carbon dioxide is actually carried in the blood as bicarbonate ions. When bicarbonate ions reach the respiratory membranes of the lungs, an enzyme changes them back to carbon dioxide and water. Then the carbon dioxide diffuses out of the blood and into the air of the lungs so it can be exhaled. Some carbon dioxide binds to hemoglobin or dissolves in plasma to be transported to the lungs.

Not to be confused with carbon dioxide, carbon monoxide is an odorless, clear gas that is poisonous to humans. Carbon monoxide binds to the hemoglobin at the same site that oxygen binds to it. Thus, when someone is exposed to carbon monoxide, it attaches to hemoglobin instead of oxygen causing the person to suffocate.

Educating the Patient

Snoring

Snoring occurs when the muscles of the palate, tongue, and throat relax. Airflow then causes these soft tissues to vibrate. These vibrating tissues produce the harsh sounds characteristic of snoring.

Snoring causes daytime sleepiness and is sometimes associated with sleep apnea. In this condition, the relaxed throat tissues cause airways to collapse, which prevent a person from breathing. Snoring affects approximately 50% of men and 25% of women over the age of 40. The common causes of snoring include:

- Enlargement of the tonsils or adenoids
- Being overweight
- Alcohol consumption
- Nasal congestion
- A deviated (crooked) nasal septum

The severity of snoring varies among people. The Mayo Clinic's Sleep Disorders Center uses the following scale to determine the severity of snoring:

- Grade 1: Snoring can be heard from close proximity to the face of the snoring person.
- Grade 2: Snoring can be heard from anywhere in the bedroom.
- Grade 3: Snoring can be heard just outside the bedroom with the door open.
- Grade 4: Snoring can be heard outside the bedroom with the door closed.

You can educate patients about making lifestyle modifications and using aids to help reduce their snoring:

- Lose weight
- Change the sleeping position from the back to the side
- Avoid the use of alcohol and medications that cause sleepiness
- Use nasal strips to widen the nasal passageways
- Use dental devices to keep airways open

In addition, patients may benefit from using a mask attached to a pump that forces air into their passageways while they sleep. If these therapies are not effective, patients may need surgery to trim excess tissues in the throat or laser surgery to remove a portion of the soft palate.

Pathophysiology

Common Diseases and Disorders of the Respiratory System

Asthma is a condition in which the tubes of the bronchial tree become obstructed due to inflammation.

- **Causes.** The causes can include allergens (pollen, pets, dust mites, etc.), cigarette smoke, pollutants, perfumes, cleaning agents, cold temperatures, and exercise (in susceptible individuals).
- **Signs and symptoms.** Symptoms include difficulty breathing, a tight feeling in the chest, wheezing, and coughing.
- **Treatment.** Treatment includes avoiding allergens, using a steroid inhaler to reduce inflammation, using a bronchodilator, and stopping smoking.

Bronchitis is inflammation of the bronchi and often follows a cold. Bronchitis that occurs frequently often indicates more serious conditions such as asthma or emphysema. Smokers are much more likely to develop bronchitis than are nonsmokers. Repeated episodes of bronchitis increase a person's chance of eventually developing lung cancer.

- **Causes.** This condition can be caused by viruses and gastroesophageal reflux (acids that move from the stomach into the esophagus). Exposure to cigarette smoke, pollutants, and the fumes of household cleaners can also contribute to the development of bronchitis.
- **Signs and symptoms.** The signs and symptoms include chills, fever, coughing up yellow-gray or green mucus, tightness in the chest, wheezing, and difficulty breathing.
- **Treatment.** This condition can be treated with rest, fluids, nonprescription and prescription cough medicines, and the use of a humidifier. Antibiotics are usually prescribed only for smokers. Patients who also have asthma may need to use inhalers. They should also wear masks if they may be exposed to lung irritants.

continued ⟶

Common Diseases and Disorders of the Respiratory System *(continued)*

Chronic obstructive pulmonary disease (COPD) is group of lung disorders that limit airflow to lungs and usually cause enlargement of the air sacs in lungs. Emphysema and chronic bronchitis are the most common types of COPD.

- **Causes.** The primary causes are smoking and air pollution.
- **Signs and symptoms.** Common signs and symptoms include difficulty breathing, fatigue, and frequent coughing.
- **Treatment.** Treatment should first be focused on lifestyle changes, especially stopping smoking. Other treatment options include respiratory therapy and the use of inhalers. In more serious cases, a lung transplant may be necessary.

Emphysema is a chronic condition that damages the alveoli of the lungs. It is heavily associated with smoking.

- **Causes.** The most common causes are exposure to cigarette smoke, pollutants, and the dust from grains, cotton, wood, or coal.
- **Signs and symptoms.** Symptoms include shortness of breath that progresses over time, chronic cough, unintended weight loss, and fatigue.
- **Treatment.** Stopping smoking and preventing exposure to cold environments and pollutants should be the first treatment measures. Vaccinations to prevent the flu and pneumonia as well as antibiotics to control the respiratory infections associated with emphysema may also be administered. In addition, patients can be treated with bronchodilators, supplemental oxygen, inhaled steroids, and respiratory therapy. The most serious cases may require either surgery to remove damaged lung tissue or a lung transplant.

Influenza is more commonly called the flu. Babies, the elderly, and people with suppressed immune systems are at the highest risk of developing influenza. The flu normally lasts between 5 and 10 days.

- **Causes.** This disease is caused by a number of different viruses that attack the respiratory system. It can be prevented through a flu vaccination.
- **Signs and symptoms.** Common symptoms include a runny nose, sore throat, sneezing, fever or chills, a dry cough, muscle pain, fatigue, loss of appetite, and diarrhea.
- **Treatment.** Over-the-counter pain medications can alleviate the aches and pains associated with the flu. Other treatment options include bed rest, fluids, and antiviral medications.

Laryngitis is an inflammation of the larynx. Chronic laryngitis is associated with lung cancer.

- **Causes.** The causes of this condition are varied and include the following: viruses; bacteria; polyp formation in the larynx; excessive talking, shouting, or singing; allergies; smoking; frequent heartburn; the frequent use of alcohol; damage to nerves that supply the larynx; and a stroke that paralyzes vocal cord muscles.
- **Signs and symptoms.** Signs and symptoms include a hoarse voice, sore throat, a dry cough and throat, and tickling sensations in the throat.
- **Treatment.** The most common treatment options are antibiotics, the management of heartburn, and the avoidance of cigarettes and alcohol. The treatment of more serious cases includes removing polyps in the larynx and surgery to tighten the vocal cords.

Legionnaire's disease is a type of pneumonia.

- **Causes.** This disease is caused by bacteria that usually grow in air conditioning systems.
- **Signs and symptoms.** The symptoms include fever, fatigue, difficulty breathing, frequent coughing, chest pain, muscle aches, and headache.
- **Treatment.** Antibiotics, respiratory therapy, and supportive therapy such as IV fluids are the primary treatment options.

Lung cancer is closely associated with smoking and kills more people in the United States than any other type of cancer. Smoking accounts for approximately 85% of all lung cancer cases.

- **Causes.** The primary causes are smoking and exposure to radon, asbestos, and industrial carcinogens.
- **Signs and symptoms.** The respiratory symptoms include a cough that worsens over time, coughing up blood, difficult breathing, wheezing, and recurring bronchitis. Other symptoms are chest pain, chronic hoarseness, unintended weight loss, and bone pain if the cancer spreads.
- **Classification.** Lung cancer is classified by the following types:
  - *Small cell lung cancer*. This type occurs almost exclusively in smokers. It is the most aggressive type and spreads readily to other organs. Small cell lung cancer that spreads to other organs is termed *extensive*.
  - *Squamous cell lung cancer*. This type of lung cancer arises from the epithelial cells that line the tubes of the lungs. It occurs most commonly in men.
  - *Adenocarcinoma*. This type arises from the mucous-producing cells of the lungs. It develops most commonly in women and nonsmokers.
  - *Large cell carcinoma*. This type of lung cancer arises from the peripheral parts of the lungs.
- **Stages.** Squamous cell lung cancer, adenocarcinoma, and large cell carcinoma are staged as follows:
  - Stage 0: Cancer is found only in the lining of the tubes of the lungs.
  - Stage 1: Cancer has spread from the lining of the tubes to lung tissues.

continued ⟶

- Stage 2: Cancer has spread to the lymph nodes or the chest wall.
- Stage 3: Cancer has spread to the lymph nodes and to other organs within the chest.
- Stage 4: Cancer has spread to organs outside the chest.

- **Treatment.** Treatment will vary depending on the type of cancer and the stage. Stopping smoking should be the first treatment consideration. Common treatment options include chemotherapy and radiation therapy. More serious cases may require the surgical removal of tumors (if they are confined), a lobectomy (the removal of a lung lobe or lobes), or a pneumonectomy (the removal of an entire lung).

Pleuritis is a condition in which the membranes that cover the lungs, known as pleura, become inflamed. This often causes the membranes to stick together or can cause an excess amount of fluid to form between the membranes.

- **Causes.** Causes include viruses, pneumonia, autoimmune diseases such as lupus or rheumatoid arthritis, tuberculosis, a pulmonary embolism, inflammation of the pancreas, and trauma to the chest.
- **Signs and symptoms.** Symptoms include fever or chills, a dry cough, shortness of breath, and chest pain during inhalation or exhalation.
- **Treatment.** Pain medications may be prescribed to relieve chest pain. Anti-inflammatory drugs, antibiotics, and the removal of fluid around the lungs are the primary treatment options.

Pneumonia is characterized by an inflammation of the lungs that is most often caused by a bacterial or viral infection of the lungs. There are at least 50 different types of pneumonia, and they range from mild to very serious. Double pneumonia refers to inflammation of both lungs.

- **Causes.** Pneumonia can be caused by bacteria, viruses, fungi, and parasites. It can also be caused by foreign matter that enters the lungs (for example, stomach contents that enter the lungs after vomiting). This disorder may be prevented by not smoking and, for some types of pneumonia, by vaccinations.
- **Signs and symptoms.** Common signs and symptoms include fever or chills, headache, chest or muscle pain, fatigue, difficulty breathing, and coughing up rust-colored, green, or yellowish mucus.
- **Treatment.** Rest, fluids, over-the-counter pain medications, and antibiotics are the most common treatments.

Pneumothorax is a collection of air in the chest around the lungs.

- **Causes.** Some causes of this disorder are unknown. Various respiratory diseases and trauma to the chest, such as a stabbing wound, can also contribute to the development of pneumothorax.
- **Signs and symptoms.** The primary symptoms include tightness in the chest or a sharp chest pain, shortness of breath, and a rapid heart rate.
- **Treatment.** The insertion of a chest tube to remove air from the chest and surgery to repair chest wounds are the primary treatments.

Pulmonary edema is a condition in which fluids fill spaces within the lungs. This disorder makes it very difficult for the lungs to oxygenate the blood. It most commonly occurs when the heart cannot pump all the blood it receives from the lungs. Blood then backs up in the lungs, causing fluids to seep into lung spaces.

- **Causes.** The causes of this condition are many and include the following: congestive heart failure, heart attack, cardiomyopathy, heart valve disorders, lung infections, allergic reactions, smoke inhalation, drowning, various drugs such as narcotics and heroin, chest injuries, and high altitudes. This disorder may be prevented by avoiding high altitudes and smoking. Preventing heart disease may also reduce the chance of developing this disorder.
- **Signs and symptoms.** The symptoms of pulmonary edema are shortness of breath, difficulty breathing (especially when lying down), a feeling of suffocating, wheezing, a cough that produces pink mucus, rapid weight gain, pale skin, and profuse sweating.
- **Treatment.** Treatment includes oxygen therapy, diuretics to eliminate excess fluids, and morphine to reduce anxiety and shortness of breath.

A *pulmonary embolism* is a blocked artery in the lungs. Usually the artery is blocked by a blood clot that has traveled from a vein in the legs. If an artery in the lungs is completely blocked, death can occur quickly.

- **Causes.** People at the highest risk of developing this condition are those who have had previous heart attacks, cancer, a fractured hip, or chronic lung diseases. Women who use birth control pills and individuals who have a pacemaker may be at risk for developing a pulmonary embolism. In addition, long periods of inactivity, increased levels of clotting factors in the blood (usually caused by certain cancers), injury to veins, and a stroke that causes paralysis of the arms or legs may also cause this condition. A sedentary lifestyle as well as auto or airplane travel—or any activity that requires prolonged sitting or standing—are also major risk factors for developing a pulmonary embolism. A baby aspirin taken daily, as well as plenty of fluids and frequent movement of the arms and legs, may help prevent the development of a pulmonary embolism.

continued ⟶

Common Diseases and Disorders of the Respiratory System *(continued)*

- **Signs and symptoms.** Symptoms include fainting, a sudden shortness of breath, coughing up blood, wheezing, a rapid heartbeat, profuse sweating, and chest pain that may spread to a shoulder, arm, or the face.
- **Treatment.** Support stockings can be used to promote circulation. The patient should rest until the blood clot has dissolved and may be prescribed clot-dissolving medications. Anticoagulants may be used to prevent new blood clots from forming in the deep veins of the body. Finally, surgery may be used to place a filter in the vena cava to prevent blood clots from reaching the lungs.

Severe acute respiratory syndrome (SARS) is a relatively new respiratory disease that is sometimes fatal and contagious.

- **Causes.** SARS is caused by viruses associated with the common cold as well as by unknown viruses. It can be prevented by thoroughly washing the hands, wearing a mask, and avoiding exposure to individuals with this disease.
- **Signs and symptoms.** Signs and symptoms include fever or chills, headache, a dry cough, and muscle aches.
- **Treatment.** Rest and antiviral drugs are the primary treatments.

Sinusitis is an inflammation of the membranes lining the sinuses of the skull.

- **Causes.** Bacteria, excess mucus production in the sinuses, the blockage of sinus openings, and the destruction of cilia that move mucus out of sinuses can cause this disorder.
- **Signs and symptoms.** Fever, cough, headache, a sore throat, facial pain, and nasal congestion are the common signs and symptoms.
- **Treatment.** Treatment options include the use of nasal decongestants, nasal steroid sprays, a humidifier, and antibiotics. Surgery to clear the sinuses or unblock sinus openings may be required.

Sudden infant death syndrome (SIDS) claims the life of more than 7000 babies a year in the United States. There are no characteristic signs or symptoms. Usually a baby with this disorder simply goes to sleep and never wakes up. The causes of SIDS are unknown but certain risk factors have been identified:

- Babies who are male are more likely to die of SIDS.
- Babies are most susceptible between the ages of 2 weeks and 6 months.
- Premature or low birth weight babies are more likely to have SIDS.
- A baby with a sibling who died of SIDS is more likely to also die of this disorder.
- Babies who are African American or Native American are more likely to die of SIDS.
- Babies who were prenatally exposed to alcohol, cocaine, heroine, or nicotine are at a higher risk of developing SIDS.
- Babies who sleep on their stomachs are approximately three times more likely to die of SIDS.

Tuberculosis (TB) is a disease that kills more than 2 million people worldwide each year. Although it primarily affects the lungs, it can spread to other parts of the body.

- **Causes.** This disease is caused by various strains of the bacterium *Mycobacterium tuberculosis*. Widespread tuberculosis may be complicated by the following factors:
  - HIV infection. HIV infection makes a person more vulnerable to TB.
  - Crowded living conditions. This factor allows TB to spread easily; this disease, therefore, is found in some prisons and homeless shelters.
  - Poverty. Poverty prevents some patients with TB from seeking or completing therapy.
  - Drug-resistant bacterium. Drug-resistant strains of the bacterium that causes TB have increased.
  - Long-term therapy. Current treatments require antibiotic therapy for many months, which some patients with TB do not complete.
- **Signs and symptoms.** The symptoms include a cough that lasts more than 3 weeks, unintended weight loss, fever or chills, fatigue, night sweats, pain when breathing or difficulty breathing, and pain in other affected areas.
- **Treatment.** The first step should be TB testing to detect carriers of this disease, who should then be treated. Drug-resistant cases of TB may require years of drug therapy to treat; this therapy normally lasts 6 months to a year.

Summary

The major function of the respiratory system is the exchange of oxygen and carbon dioxide between the blood and the atmosphere. In addition to this gas exchange, the respiratory system also regulates blood pH.

The organs of this system include the nose, pharynx, larynx, trachea, bronchial tree, and the lungs. Each of these structures has a role in ventilation (bringing air in and out of the body) and external respiration (the gas exchange of oxygen and carbon dioxide). Understanding this system is important in assisting with patients and instructing them in the use of an inhaler.

REVIEW

CHAPTER 12

CASE STUDY QUESTIONS

Now that you have completed this chapter, review the case study at the beginning of the chapter and answer the following questions:

1. Why is the patient wheezing?
2. Is asthma a life-threatening condition?
3. What is the advantage of using a nebulizer to deliver the bronchodilator?
4. Why did the doctor refer the patient for allergy testing?

Discussion Questions

1. Describe the actions of the diaphragm and the rib cage during inspiration and expiration.
2. List the various respiratory volumes that are commonly measured in the clinical setting. What does each volume represent?
3. Describe how the larynx varies the loudness and pitch of the voice. Besides producing sound, what is another function of the larynx?

Critical Thinking Questions

1. Smoking destroys cilia in the respiratory tract. Describe how smoking damages the lungs.
2. What effect would breathing in a paper bag have on oxygen concentrations in the blood? Would this be helpful for a person who is hyperventilating? Why or why not?

Application Activities

1. Describe the locations and functions of the following structures:
   a. pharynx
   b. larynx
   c. primary bronchi
   d. alveoli
   e. epiglottis
2. What carries most oxygen in the blood?
3. How many lobes does the left lung have? The right lung?

CHAPTER 13

The Digestive System

CHAPTER OUTLINE

- Characteristics of the Alimentary Canal
- The Mouth
- The Pharynx
- The Esophagus
- The Stomach
- The Small Intestine
- The Liver
- The Gallbladder
- The Pancreas
- The Large Intestine
- The Rectum and Anal Canal
- The Absorption of Nutrients

OBJECTIVES

After completing Chapter 13, you will be able to:

13.1 List the functions of the digestive system.
13.2 Trace the pathway of food through the alimentary canal.
13.3 Describe the structure and functions of the mouth, teeth, tongue, and salivary glands.
13.4 Describe the structure and function of the pharynx.
13.5 Describe the swallowing process.
13.6 Describe the structure of the esophagus and tell how it propels food into the stomach.
13.7 Describe the structure and functions of the stomach.
13.8 List the substances secreted by the stomach and give their functions.
13.9 Describe the structure and functions of the small intestine.
13.10 List the substances secreted by the small intestine and describe the importance of each.
13.11 Explain the structures and functions of the liver, gallbladder, and pancreas.
13.12 List the substances released by the liver, gallbladder, and pancreas into the small intestine and give the function of each secretion.
13.13 Describe the structure and functions of the large intestine.
13.14 Tell what types of nutrients are absorbed by the digestive system and where they are absorbed.
13.15 Describe the signs, symptoms, causes, and treatments of various disorders and diseases of the digestive system.

KEY TERMS

acinar cells
adenoids
alimentary canal
anal canal
appendicitis
ascending colon
bicuspids
bile
carboxypeptidase
cecum
cellulose
chief cells
chyme
chymotrypsin
cirrhosis
colitis
common bile duct
cuspids
cystic duct
defecation reflex
descending colon
disaccharide
diverticulitis
duodenum
esophageal hiatus
feces
gastric juice
gastritis
gastroesophageal reflux disease (GERD)
glycogen
hemorrhoids
hepatic duct
hepatic lobule
hepatic portal vein

KEY TERMS *(Continued)*

hepatitis
hepatocytes
hernia
ileocecal sphincter
ileum
incisors
intestinal lipase
intrinsic factor
jejunum
lactase
laryngopharynx
lingual frenulum
lingual tonsil
linoleic acid
maltase
microvilli
molars
monosaccharide
mucosa
mucous cells
nasopharynx
nucleases
oropharynx
palate
palatine tonsils
pancreatic amylase
pancreatic lipase
parietal cells
parotid glands
pepsin
pepsinogen
peptidases
pharyngeal tonsils
polysaccharide
rectum
serosa
serous cells
sigmoid colon
sublingual gland
submandibular gland
submucosa
sucrase
transverse colon
triglyceride
trypsin
uvula
vermiform appendix

Introduction

Digestion is the mechanical and chemical breakdown of foods into forms that your body cells can absorb. The organs of the digestive system carry out digestion and can be divided into two categories—those of the alimentary canal and accessory organs. Organs of the alimentary canal extend from the mouth to the anus. They are the mouth, pharynx, esophagus, stomach, small intestine, large intestine, and anal canal. The accessory organs include the teeth, tongue, salivary glands, liver, gallbladder, and pancreas (Figure 13-1).

CASE STUDY

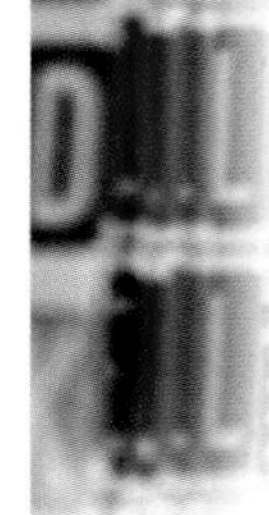

Yesterday afternoon, a 55-year-old female came to the gastroenterologist's office complaining of severe pain in her upper right abdomen. She was nauseated and stated that for several months—and especially following meals—she had been having periodic abdominal pain. After several tests, she was diagnosed as having gallstones and was scheduled for the surgical removal of her gallbladder.

As you read this chapter, consider the following questions:

1. What is the function of the gallbladder?
2. How does the gallbladder empty bile into the small intestine?
3. What conditions can result if gallstones are not removed?
4. Will this patient need to change her diet once her gallbladder is removed?

Characteristics of the Alimentary Canal

The wall of the **alimentary canal** consists of four layers:

1. Mucosa. The **mucosa** is the innermost layer of the wall and is mostly made of epithelial tissue that secretes enzymes and mucus into the lumen, or passageway, of the canal. This layer also is very active in absorbing nutrients.
2. Submucosa. The **submucosa** is the layer just deep to the mucosa. It contains loose connective tissue, blood vessels, glands, and nerves. The blood vessels in this layer carry away absorbed nutrients.
3. Muscular layer. This layer is just outside the submucosa. It is made of layers of smooth muscle tissue and contracts to move materials through the canal.
4. Serosa. The **serosa** is the outermost layer of canal and is also known as the visceral peritoneum. It secretes serous fluid to keep the outside of the canal moist and to prevent it from sticking to other organs.

Smooth muscle in the wall of the canal can contract to produce two basic types of movements—churning and

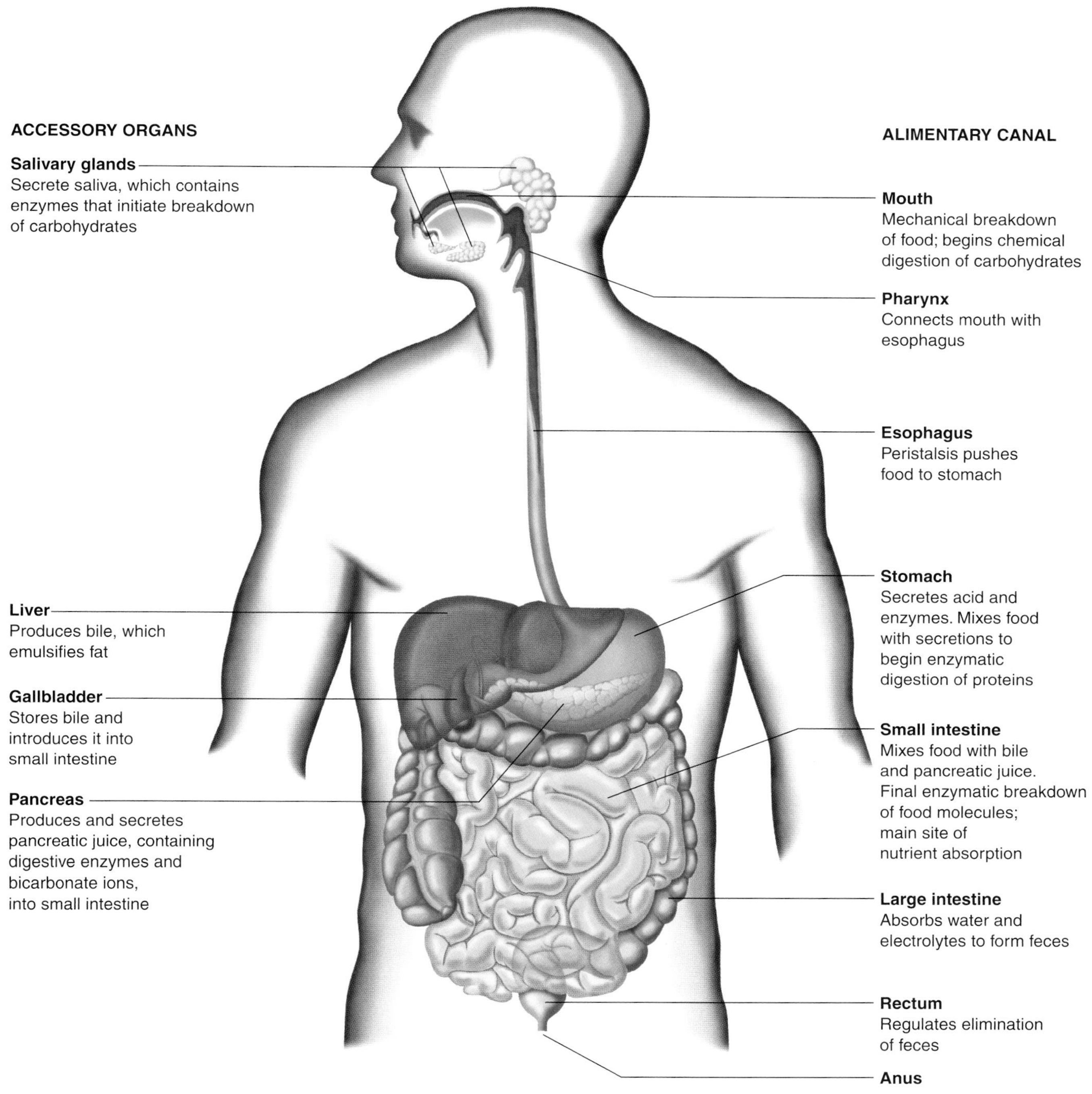
ACCESSORY ORGANS
Salivary glands
Secrete saliva, which contains enzymes that initiate breakdown of carbohydrates
Liver
Produces bile, which emulsifies fat
Gallbladder
Stores bile and introduces it into small intestine
Pancreas
Produces and secretes pancreatic juice, containing digestive enzymes and bicarbonate ions, into small intestine
ALIMENTARY CANAL
Mouth
Mechanical breakdown of food; begins chemical digestion of carbohydrates
Pharynx
Connects mouth with esophagus
Esophagus
Peristalsis pushes food to stomach
Stomach
Secretes acid and enzymes. Mixes food with secretions to begin enzymatic digestion of proteins
Small intestine
Mixes food with bile and pancreatic juice. Final enzymatic breakdown of food molecules; main site of nutrient absorption
Large intestine
Absorbs water and electrolytes to form feces
Rectum
Regulates elimination of feces
Anus

Figure 13-1. Major organs of the digestive system.

peristalsis. Churning mixes substances in the canal. Peristalsis propels substances through the tract (Figure 13-2).

The Mouth

The mouth takes in food and reduces its size through chewing. The mouth also starts to chemically digest food because saliva (spit) contains an enzyme that breaks down carbohydrates.

The cheeks consist of skin, adipose tissue, skeletal muscles, and an inner lining of moist stratified squamous epithelium. The cheeks act to hold food in the mouth. The lips contain a lot of sensory nerve fibers that can judge the temperature of food before it enters the mouth.

The tongue is mostly made of skeletal muscles and is covered by a mucous membrane. The body of the tongue is held to the floor of the oral cavity by a flap of mucous membrane called the **lingual frenulum.** The tongue acts to mix food in the mouth and to hold the food between

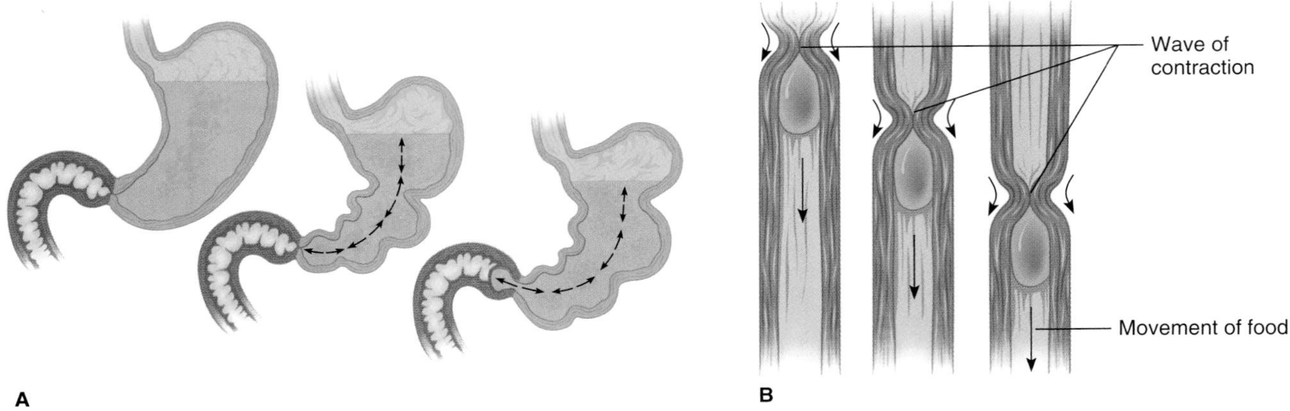

Figure 13-2. Movements through the alimentary canal. (a) Churning movements move substances back and forth to mix them. (b) Peristalsis moves contents along the canal.

teeth. It also contains taste buds. The back of the tongue contains two lumps of lymphatic tissue called **lingual tonsils.** Lingual tonsils act to destroy bacteria and viruses on the back of the tongue.

The **palate** is the roof of the mouth. It functions to separate the oral cavity from the nasal cavity. The front of the palate, the hard palate, is rigid because it has bony plates in it. The back of the palate, soft palate, lacks bony material and therefore is not rigid. The back of the soft palate hangs down into the throat, and this portion of the soft palate is called the **uvula.** The uvula acts to prevent food and liquids from entering the nose during swallowing.

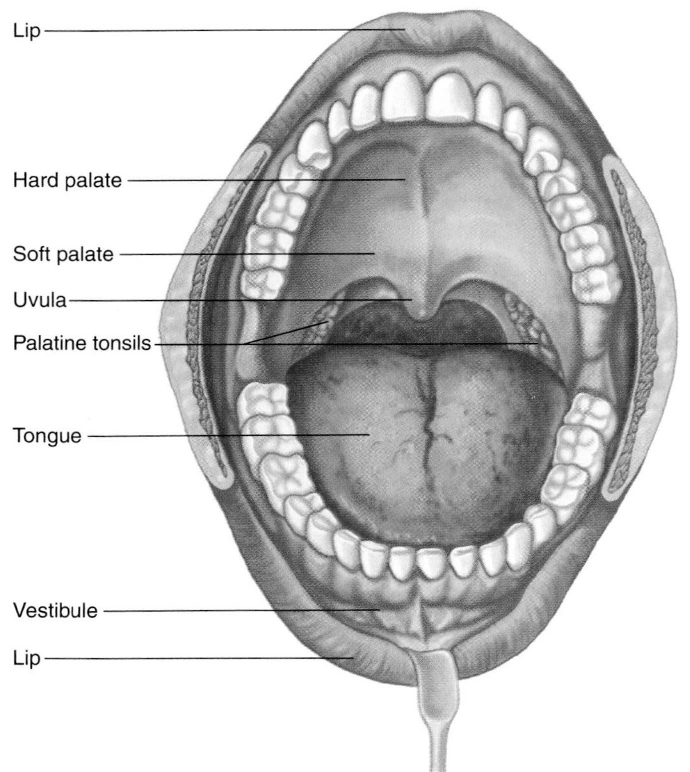

Figure 13-3. Structures of the mouth.

At the back of the mouth are two masses of lymphatic tissue called **palatine tonsils.** Just above the palatine tonsils are two more masses of lymphatic tissue called the **pharyngeal tonsils (adenoids).** These masses of lymphatic tissue act to protect the area from bacteria and viruses (Figure 13-3).

Teeth act to decrease the size of food particles, and different types of teeth are adapted to handle food in different ways. The most medial teeth, called **incisors,** act as chisels to bite off food pieces. Teeth called **cuspids** are the sharpest teeth and they act to tear tough food (Figure 13-4). The back teeth, called **bicuspids** and **molars,** are flat. They are designed to grind food (Figure 13-5).

Salivary glands secrete saliva, which is a mixture of water, enzymes, and mucus. Salivary glands are made of two types of cells—**serous cells** and **mucous cells.** Serous cells secrete a fluid made mostly of water but the fluid also contains an enzyme called amylase that digests carbohydrates. Mucous cells secrete mucus.

All major salivary glands are paired (Figure 13-6):

- **Parotid glands:** the largest of the salivary glands, located beneath the skin just in front of the ears
- **Submandibular glands:** located in the floor of the mouth just inside the surface of the mandibles (jaws)
- **Sublingual glands:** the smallest of the salivary glands, located in the floor of the mouth beneath the tongue

The Pharynx

The **pharynx** is more commonly called the throat. It is a long, muscular structure that extends from the area behind the nose to the esophagus. It acts to connect the nasal cavity with the oral cavity for breathing through the nose. It

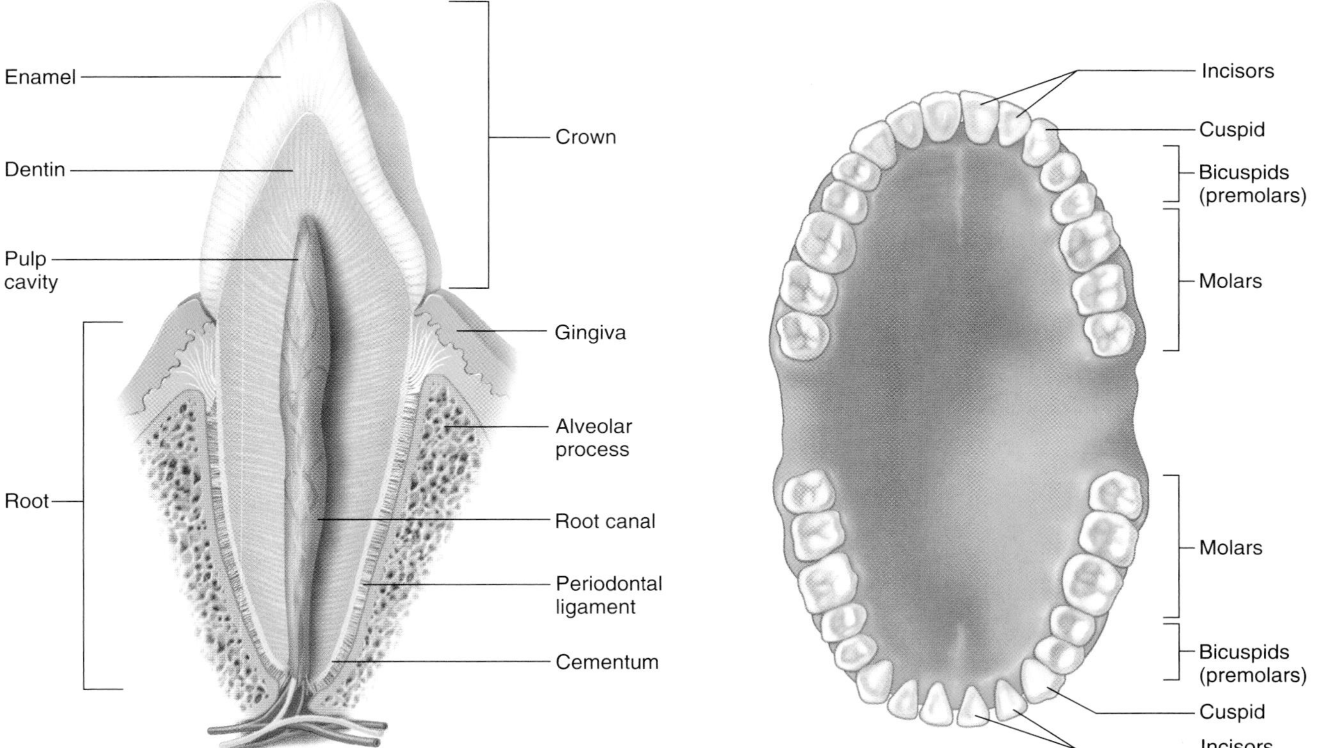

Figure 13-4. Structure of a cuspid tooth.

Figure 13-5. Types of teeth.

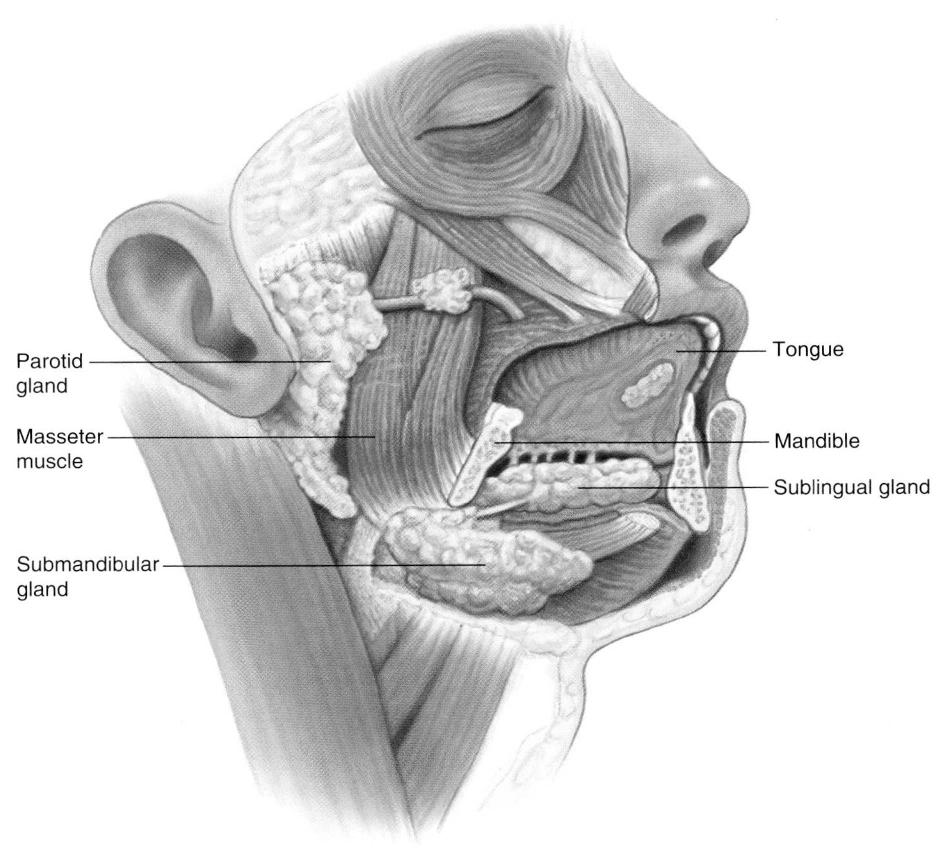

Figure 13-6. Major salivary glands.

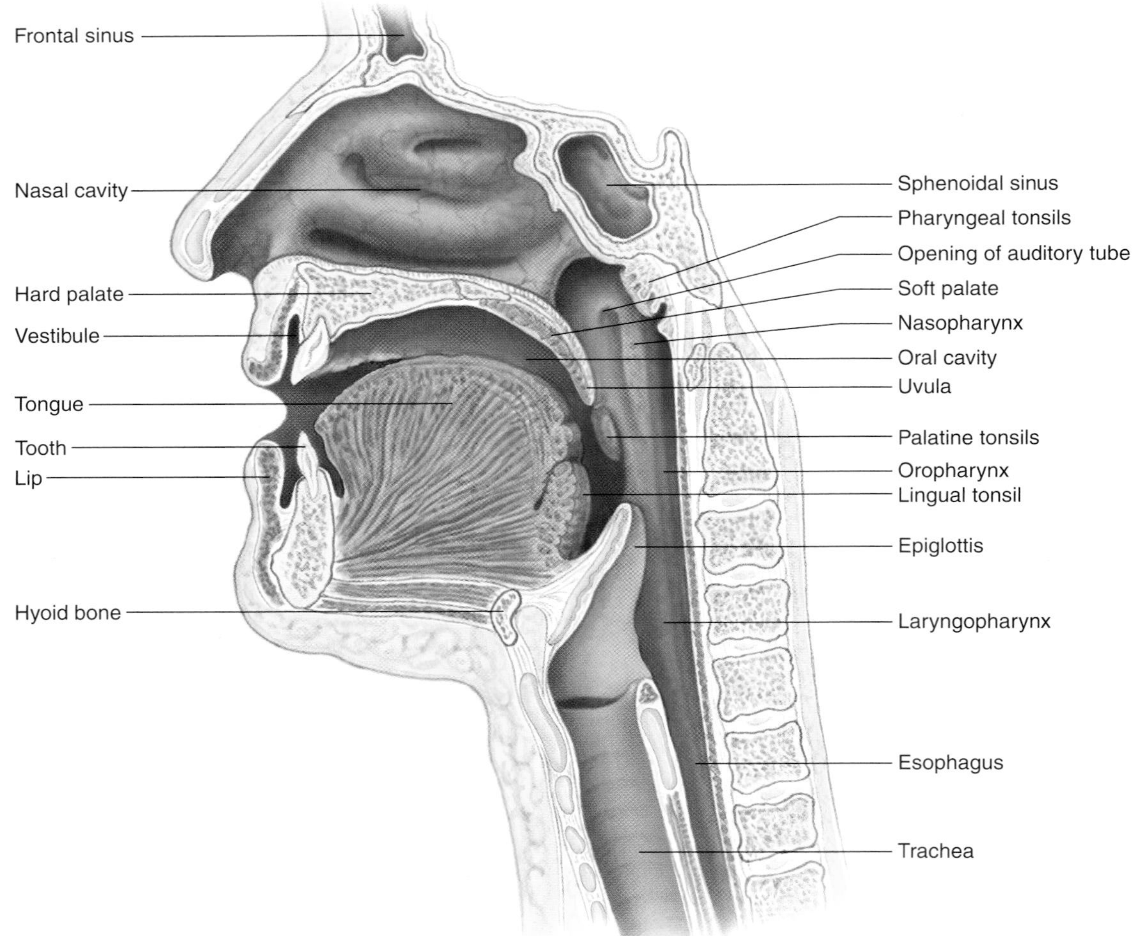

Figure 13-7. Sagittal section of the mouth, nasal cavity, and pharynx.

also acts to push food into the esophagus (Figure 13-7). The divisions of the pharynx are:

- **Nasopharynx:** the portion behind the nasal cavity.
- **Oropharynx:** the portion behind the oral cavity.
- **Laryngopharynx:** the portion behind the larynx. The laryngopharynx continues as the esophagus.

Swallowing is largely a reflex. In other words, it is an automatic response that does not require much thought. The following events occur during swallowing:

1. The soft palate rises,causing the uvula to cover the opening between the nasal cavity and the oral cavity.
2. The **epiglottis** covers the opening of the larynx so that food does not enter it (see Figure 13-7).
3. The tongue presses against the roof of the mouth, forcing food into the oropharynx.
4. The muscles in the pharynx contract, forcing food toward the esophagus.
5. The esophagus opens.
6. Food is pushed into the esophagus by the muscles of the pharynx.

The Esophagus

The esophagus is a muscular tube that connects the pharynx to the stomach (Figures 13-7 and 13-8). It descends through the thoracic cavity, through the diaphragm, and into the abdominal cavity where it joins the stomach. The hole in the diaphragm that the esophagus goes through is called the **esophageal hiatus.** This hiatus is a common place for hernias to occur. A **hernia** develops when the stomach gets pushed up into the thoracic cavity through the esophageal hiatus. The esophageal sphincter, also known as the cardiac sphincter, controls the movement of food into the stomach. **Sphincters** are circular bands of muscle located at the openings of many tubes in the body. They open and close to allow or prevent the movement of substances out of a tube.

The Stomach

The stomach lies below the diaphragm in the upper left region of the abdominal cavity. It functions to receive food from the esophagus, mix food with **gastric juice** (secretions

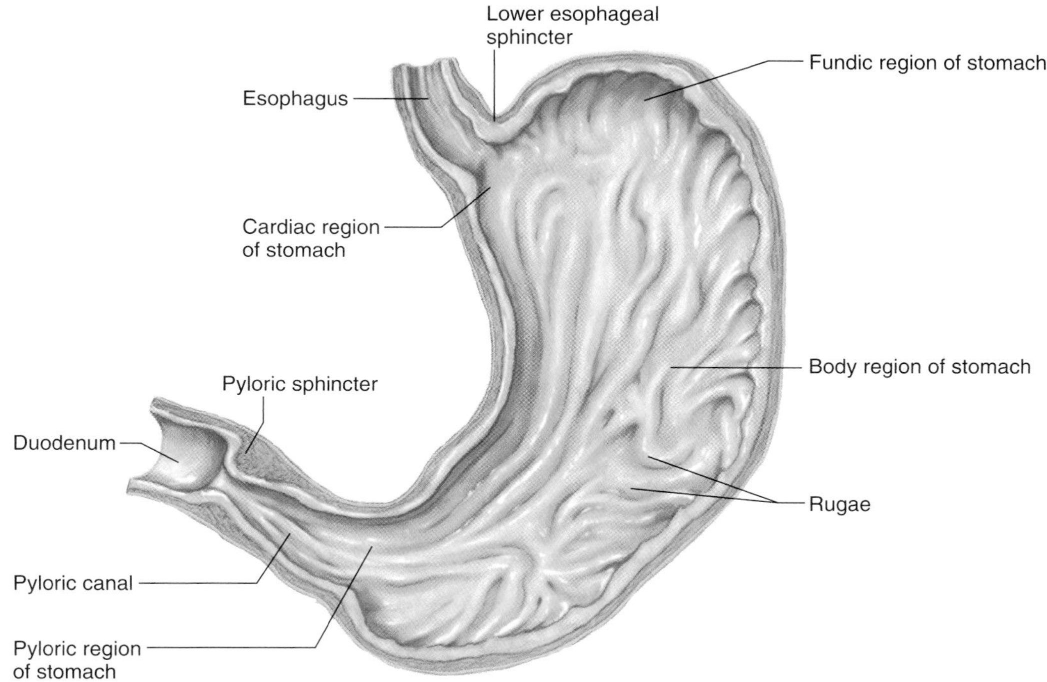

Figure 13-8. Regions of the stomach.

of the stomach lining), start protein digestion, and move food into the small intestine.

The beginning portion of the stomach that is attached to the esophagus is called the cardiac region. The portion of the stomach that balloons over the cardiac portion is called the fundic region, or fundus. The main part of the stomach is called the body, and the narrow portion that is connected to the small intestine is called the pyloric region or pylorus. A sphincter called the pyloric sphincter controls the movement of substances from the pyloric region of the stomach into the small intestine (Figure 13-8).

The lining of the stomach contains gastric glands. These glands are made of the following cell types:

- **Mucous cells.** These cells secrete mucus to protect the lining of the stomach.
- **Chief cells.** These cells secrete **pepsinogen,** which becomes **pepsin** in the presence of acid. Pepsin digests proteins.
- **Parietal cells.** These cells secrete hydrochloric acid, which is necessary to convert pepsinogen to pepsin. They also secrete **intrinsic factor,** which is necessary for vitamin B_{12} absorption.

When a person smells, tastes, or sees appetizing food, the parasympathetic nervous system stimulates the gastric glands to secrete their products. A hormone called gastrin, made by the stomach, also stimulates the gastric glands to become active. A hormone called cholecystokinin (CCK) made by the small intestine inhibits gastric glands. The stomach does not absorb many substances but it can absorb alcohol, water, and some fat-soluble drugs. The mixture of food and gastric juice is called **chyme.** Once chyme is well mixed, stomach contractions push it into the small intestine a little at a time. It takes 4 to 8 hours for the stomach to empty following a meal.

The Small Intestine

The small intestine is a tubular organ that extends from the stomach to the large intestine. It fills most of the abdominal cavity and is coiled. The small intestine carries out most of the digestion in the body and is responsible for absorbing most of the nutrients into the bloodstream.

The beginning of the small intestine is called the **duodenum.** It is C-shaped and relatively short. The middle portion of the small intestine is called the **jejunum.** It is coiled and forms the majority of the small intestine. The last portion of the small intestine is called the **ileum,** and it is directly attached to the large intestine (Figure 13-9).

The lining of the small intestine contains cells that have **microvilli.** Microvilli greatly increase the surface area of the small intestine so that it can absorb many nutrients. The lining of the small intestine also contains intestinal glands that secrete various substances. The secretions of the small intestine include mucus and water. Water aids in digestion but some toxins cause the secretion of too much water, and this leads to diarrhea—which in turn aids the body in eliminating the toxins. Mucus protects the lining of the small intestine. The following are the major enzymes secreted by the small intestine:

- **Peptidases.** These enzymes digest proteins.
- **Sucrase, maltase,** and **lactase.** These enzymes digest sugars. A person who cannot produce lactase will not be

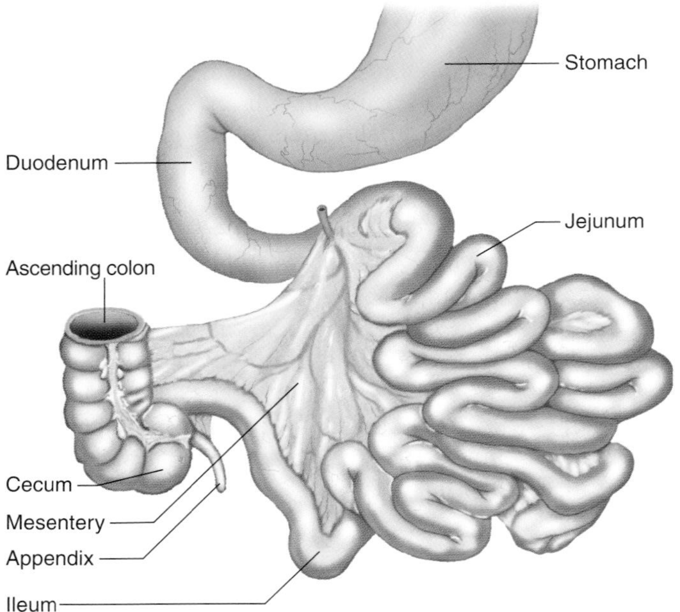

Figure 13-9. Parts of the small intestine.

able to digest lactose, which is the sugar in dairy products. This causes a condition called lactose intolerance.

- **Intestinal lipase.** This enzyme digests fats.

The parasympathetic nervous system and the stretching of the small intestine wall are the primary factors that trigger the small intestine to secrete its products. Almost all nutrients (water, glucose, amino acids, fatty acids, glycerol, and electrolytes) are absorbed by the small intestine. The wall of the small intestine contracts to mix chyme and to propel it toward the large intestine. If chyme moves too quickly through the small intestine, nutrients are not absorbed and diarrhea results. The **ileocecal sphincter** controls the movement of chyme from the ileum to the **cecum,** which is the beginning of the large intestine.

The Liver

The liver is quite large and fills most of the upper right abdominal quadrant. Part of its function is to store vitamins and iron. It is reddish-brown in color and is enclosed by a tough capsule. This capsule divides the liver into a large right lobe and a small left lobe (Figure 13-10). Each lobe is separated into smaller divisions called **hepatic lobules.** Branches of the **hepatic portal vein** carry blood from the digestive organs to the hepatic lobules. The hepatic lobules contain macrophages that destroy bacteria and viruses in the blood. Each lobule contains many cells called **hepatocytes.** Hepatocytes process the nutrients in blood and make **bile,** which is used in the digestion of fats. Bile leaves the liver through the **hepatic duct.** The hepatic duct merges with the **cystic duct** (the duct from the gallbladder) to form the **common bile duct.** This duct delivers bile to the duodenum.

The Gallbladder

The gallbladder is a small, sac-like structure located beneath the liver (Figure 13-10). Its only function is to store bile. Bile leaves the gallbladder through the cystic duct. The hormone cholecystokinin causes the gallbladder to release bile. The salts in bile break large fat globules into smaller ones so that they can be more quickly digested by the digestive enzymes. Bile salts also increase the absorption of fatty acids, cholesterol, and fat-soluble vitamins into the bloodstream.

The Pancreas

The pancreas is located behind the stomach. Pancreatic **acinar cells** produce pancreatic juice, which ultimately flows through the pancreatic duct to the duodenum (Figure 13-11). Pancreatic juice contains the following enzymes:

- **Pancreatic amylase.** This enzyme digests carbohydrates.

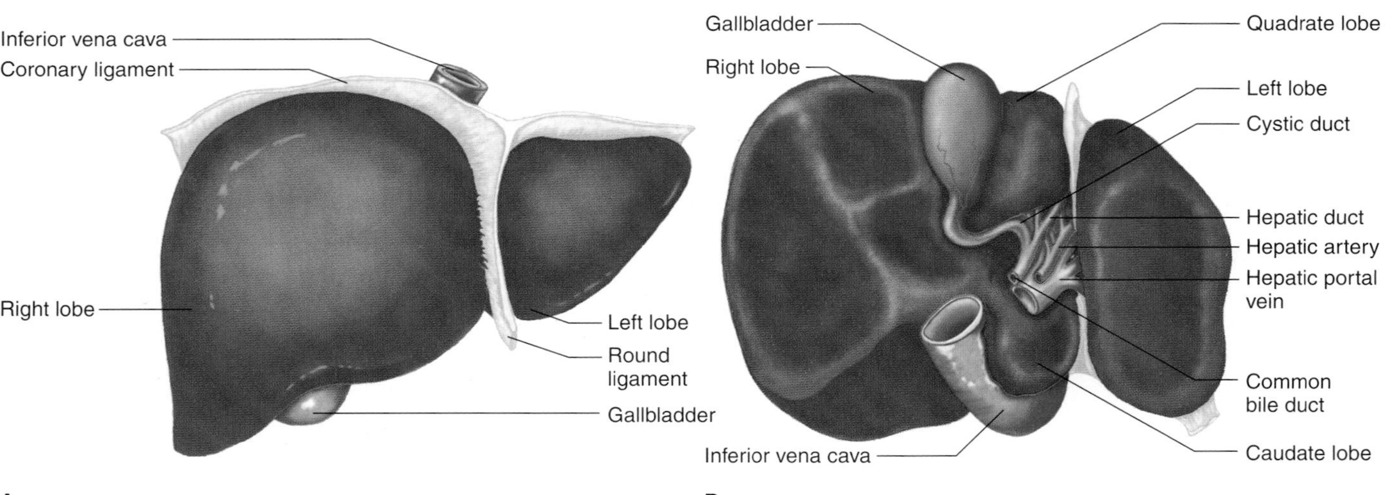

Figure 13-10. Liver and gallbladder: (a) anterior view and (b) inferior view.

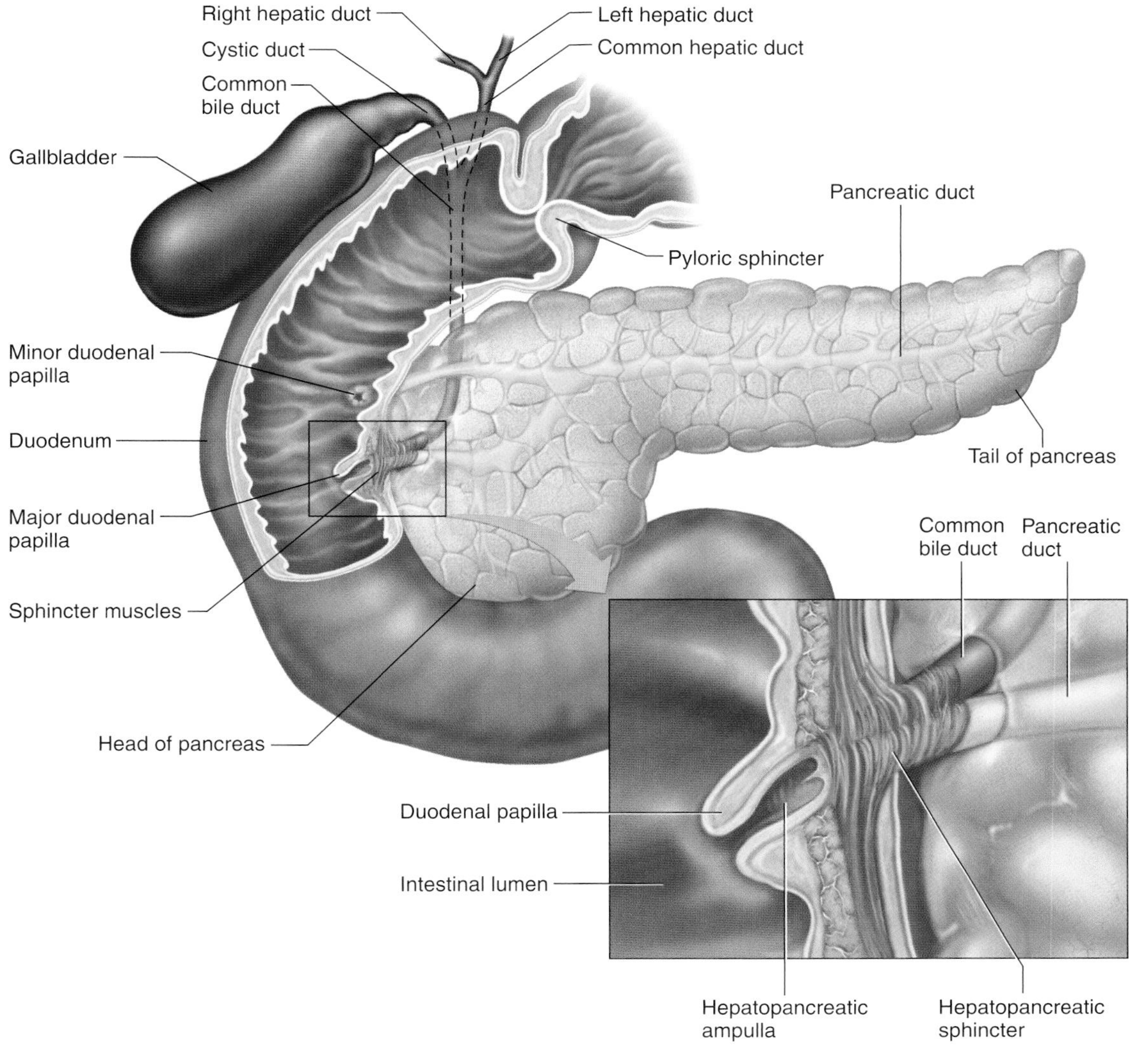

Figure 13-11. Pancreas and its connections to the gallbladder and duodenum.

- **Pancreatic lipase.** This enzyme digests lipids.
- **Nucleases.** These enzymes digest nucleic acids.
- **Trypsin, chymotrypsin,** and **carboxypeptidase.** These enzymes digest proteins.

The pancreas also secretes bicarbonate ions into the duodenum. These ions neutralize the acidic chyme arriving from the stomach. The parasympathetic nervous system stimulates the pancreas to release its enzymes. The hormones secretin and cholecystokinin also stimulate the pancreas to release digestive enzymes. Secretin and cholecystokinin come from the small intestine.

The Large Intestine

The large intestine extends from the ileum of the small intestine to where it opens to the outside world as the anus. The beginning of the large intestine is the cecum. Projecting off the cecum is the **vermiform appendix.** The appendix is mostly made of lymphoid tissue and has no significant function in humans. The cecum eventually gives rise to the **ascending colon,** which is the portion of the large intestine that runs up the right side of the abdominal cavity. The ascending colon becomes the **transverse colon** as it crosses the abdominal cavity; from there it becomes the **descending colon** as it descends the left side of the abdominal cavity. In the pelvic cavity, the descending colon then forms an S-shaped tube called the **sigmoid colon.**

The Rectum and Anal Canal

Eventually the sigmoid colon straightens out to become the **rectum.** The last few centimeters of the rectum is called the **anal canal,** and the opening of the anal canal to the outside world is called the anus (Figure 13-12).

The lining of the large intestine only secretes mucus to aid in the movement of substances. As chyme leaves the small intestine and enters the large intestine, the proximal portion of the large intestine absorbs water and a few electrolytes from it. The leftover chyme is then called **feces.**

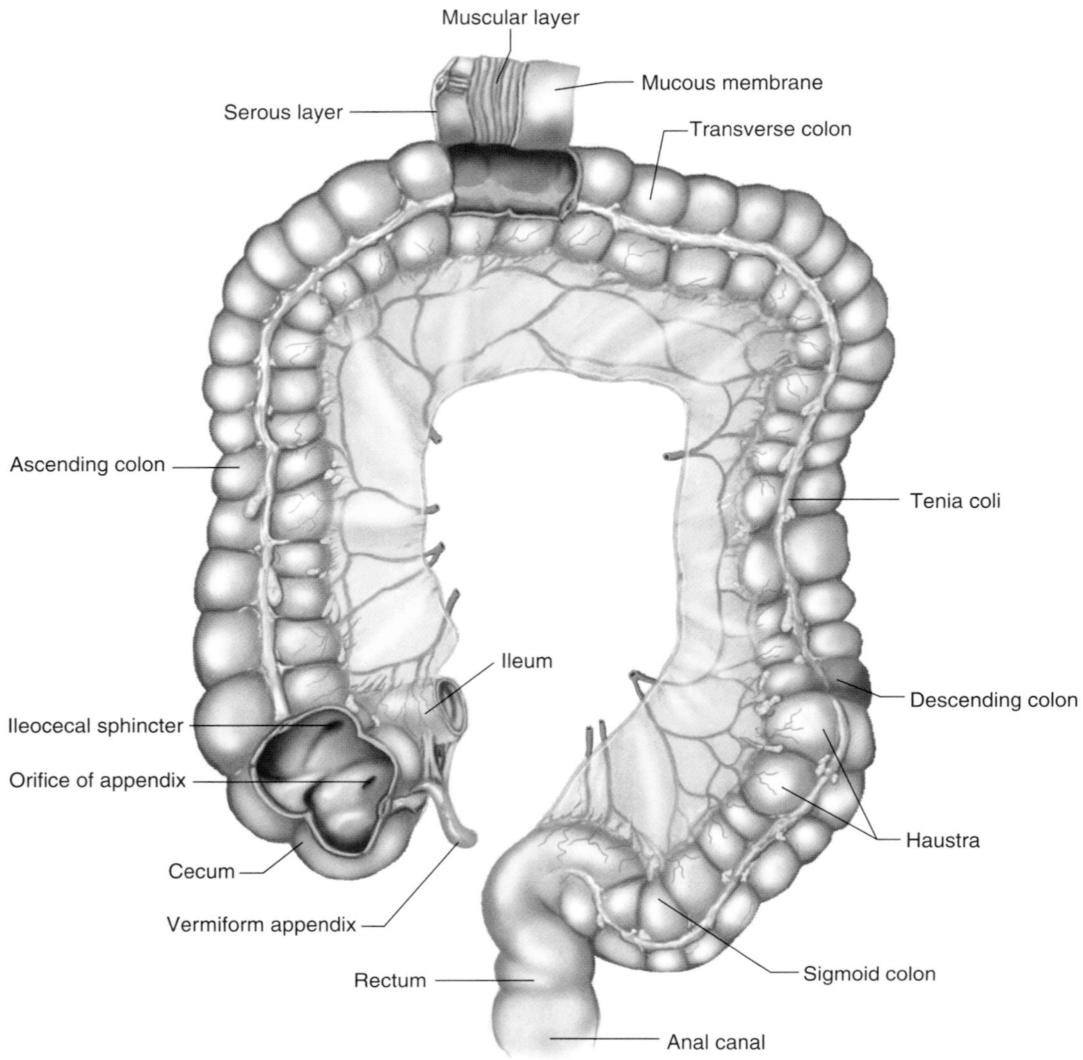

Figure 13-12. Parts of the large intestine.

Feces are made of undigested solid materials, a little water, ions, mucus, cells of the intestinal lining, and bacteria.

The contractions of the large intestine propel feces forward but these contractions normally occur periodically and as mass movements. Mass movements trigger the **defecation reflex,** which allows anal sphincters to relax and feces to move through the anus in the process of elimination. The squeezing actions of the abdominal wall muscles also aid in the emptying of the large intestine.

The Absorption of Nutrients

Nutrients are defined as necessary food substances. They include carbohydrates, proteins, lipids, vitamins, minerals, and water.

Three types of carbohydrates that humans ingest are starches **(polysaccharides),** simple sugars **(monosaccharides** and **disaccharides),** and **cellulose.** Starches come from foods such as pasta, potatoes, rice, and breads. Monosaccharides and disaccharides are obtained from sweet foods and fruits. Cellulose is a type of carbohydrate found in many vegetables that cannot be digested by humans. Therefore, cellulose provides fiber or bulk for the large intestine. This fiber helps the large intestine empty more regularly.

Most body cells use the monosaccharide glucose to make ATP. When a person has an excess of glucose, it can be stored in the liver and skeletal muscle cells as **glycogen.**

Lipids (fats) are obtained through various foods. The most abundant dietary lipids are **triglycerides.** They are found in meats, eggs, milk, and butter. Cholesterol is another common dietary lipid and is found in eggs, whole milk, butter, and cheeses. Lipids are used by the body primarily to make energy when glucose levels are low. Excess triglycerides are stored in adipose tissue. Cholesterol is essential to cell growth and function; cells use it to

TABLE 13-1 Common Vitamins and Their Importance in the Body

Vitamin	Function
Vitamin A	Needed for the production of visual receptors, mucus, the normal growth for bones and teeth, and the repair of epithelial tissues
Vitamin B_1 (thiamine)	Needed for the metabolism of carbohydrates
Vitamin B_2 (riboflavin)	Needed for carbohydrate and fat metabolism and for the growth of cells
Vitamin B_6	Needed for the synthesis of protein, antibodies, and nucleic acid
Vitamin B_{12} (cyanocobalamin)	Needed for myelin production and the metabolism of carbohydrates and nucleic acids
Biotin	Needed for the metabolism of proteins, fats, and nucleic acids
Folic acid	Needed for the production of amino acids, DNA, and red blood cells
Pantothenic acid	Needed for carbohydrate and fat metabolism
Niacin	Needed for the metabolism of carbohydrates, proteins, fats, and nucleic acids
Vitamin C (ascorbic acid)	Needed for the production of collagen, amino acids, and hormones and for the absorption of iron
Vitamin D	Needed for the absorption of calcium
Vitamin E	Antioxidant that prevents the breakdown of certain tissues
Vitamin K	Needed for blood clotting

make cell membranes and some hormones. People should have the essential fatty acid **linoleic acid** in their diet since the body cannot make it. This fatty acid is found in corn and sunflower oils. People also need a certain amount of fat to absorb fat-soluble vitamins.

Foods rich in protein include meats, eggs, milk, fish, chicken, turkey, nuts, cheese, and beans. Protein requirements vary from individual to individual, but all people must take in proteins that contain certain amino acids (called essential amino acids) because the body cannot make them. Proteins are used by the body for growth and the repair of tissues.

The fat-soluble vitamins are vitamins A, D, E, and K, and the water-soluble vitamins are all the B vitamins and vitamin C. Vitamins have many functions; they are summarized in Table 13-1.

Minerals make up about 4% of total body weight. They are primarily found in bones and teeth. Cells use minerals to make enzymes, cell membranes, and various proteins such as hemoglobin. The most important minerals to the human body are calcium, phosphorus, sulfur, sodium, chlorine, and magnesium. Trace elements are elements needed in very small amounts by the body. They include iron, manganese, copper, iodine, and zinc.

Pathophysiology

Common Diseases and Disorders of the Digestive System

Appendicitis is an inflammation of the appendix. If not treated promptly, it can be life-threatening.

- **Causes.** This disorder is caused by blockage of the appendix with feces or a tumor.
- **Signs and symptoms.** The signs and symptoms include lack of appetite, pain in or around the navel area or in the abdomen, nausea, slight fever, pain in the right leg, and an increased white blood cell count.

continued ⟶

- **Treatment.** The primary treatments are antibiotics to prevent infection or surgery to remove the appendix.

Cirrhosis is a long-lasting liver disease in which normal liver tissue is replaced with nonfunctional scar tissue.

- **Causes.** This disease is often an autoimmune disease. It may be caused by some medications and alcohol consumption. Hepatitis B and C infections can also contribute to the development of cirrhosis.
- **Signs and symptoms.** There are many symptoms to this disease. They include anemia, fatigue, mental confusion, fever, vomiting, blood in the vomit, an enlarged liver, jaundice, unintended weight loss, swelling of the legs or abdomen, abdominal pain, a decreased urine output, and pale feces.
- **Treatment.** Alcohol consumption should be discontinued. A patient with cirrhosis may be given various medications, including antibiotics and diuretics. A liver transplant may be needed for the most seriously ill patients.

Colitis is defined as inflammation of the large intestine. This condition can be chronic or short-lived, depending on the cause.

- **Causes.** Colitis can be caused by a viral or bacterial infection or the use of antibiotics. Ulcers in the large intestine, Crohn's disease, various other diseases, and stress may also contribute to the development of this disorder.
- **Signs and symptoms.** The primary symptoms are abdominal pain, bloating, and diarrhea.
- **Treatment.** The first goal of therapy is to treat the underlying causes. Changing antibiotics, treating existing ulcers, and drinking plenty of fluids are other treatment options.

Colorectal cancer usually comes from the lining of the rectum or colon. This type of cancer is curable if treated early.

- **Causes.** The causes are mostly unknown. Polyps in the colon or rectum can become cancerous, leading to this disease. Colorectal cancer may be prevented through regular screenings for polyps.
- **Signs and symptoms.** Anemia, unintended weight loss, abdominal pain, blood in the feces, narrow feces, or changes in bowel movement are all common symptoms.
- **Treatment.** Chemotherapy is the first line of treatment. Surgery to remove a cancerous tumor or the affected portions of colon or rectum may be needed in more serious cases.

Constipation is the condition of difficult defecation, which is the elimination of feces.

- **Causes.** The primary causes are a lack of physical activity, a lack of fiber in the diet, the use of certain medications, and thyroid and colon disorders.
- **Signs and symptoms.** Common signs and symptoms include infrequent bowel movements (for example, no bowel movement for 3 days), bloating, abdominal pain and pain during bowel movements, hard feces, and blood on the surface of feces.
- **Treatment.** Treatment includes an increase in fiber intake, regular exercise, and the use of stool softeners, laxatives, and enemas.

Crohn's disease is a common type of disorder called inflammatory bowel disease. It typically affects the end of the small intestine.

- **Causes.** This disease is an autoimmune disorder.
- **Signs and symptoms.** The signs and systems of Crohn's disease include fever, tender gums, joint pain, ulcers, abdominal pain and gas, constipation or diarrhea, abnormal abdominal sounds, weight loss, intestinal bleeding, and blood in the feces.
- **Treatment.** The first treatment is to change the patient's diet. Other treatments include medications to reduce inflammation and antibiotics. For the most serious cases, surgery to remove the affected part of the intestine may be needed.

Diarrhea is the condition of watery and frequent feces. Many cases of diarrhea do not require treatment because they usually stop within a day or two.

- **Causes.** The causes of diarrhea include bacterial, viral, or parasitic infections of the digestive system. It may also be caused by the ingestion of toxins; food allergies, including lactose intolerance; ulcers; Crohn's disease; laxatives; antibiotics; chemotherapy; and radiation therapy. Diarrhea may be prevented by thoroughly washing hands and cooking food properly.
- **Signs and symptoms.** The symptoms include abdominal cramps, watery feces, and the frequent passage of feces.
- **Treatment.** Patients should drink fluids to prevent dehydration. The underlying causes should be treated. Medications and dietary changes are the primary treatment options.

Diverticulitis is inflammation of diverticuli in the intestine. Diverticuli are abnormal dilations in the intestinal wall.

- **Causes.** The causes are mostly unknown. Lack of fiber in the diet and a bacterial infection of the diverticuli can cause this disorder.
- **Signs and symptoms.** Signs and symptoms include fever, nausea, abdominal pain, constipation or diarrhea, blood in the feces, and a high white blood cell count.
- **Treatment.** Treatments include a diet high in fiber, antibiotics, and surgery to remove the affected portion of the intestine.

continued ⟶

Gastritis is an inflammation of the stomach lining. It is often referred to as an "upset stomach."

- **Causes.** Gastritis can be caused by bacteria or viruses, some medications, the use of alcohol, spicy foods, excessive eating, poisons, and stress. Cooking food properly to kill harmful bacteria and viruses can help to prevent this condition.
- **Signs and symptoms.** Symptoms include nausea, lack of appetite, heartburn, vomiting, and abdominal cramps.
- **Treatment.** Lifestyle changes should be implemented to avoid foods or medications that irritate the stomach lining. Treatment with various medications to reduce the production of stomach acids can provide relief from the symptoms of this disorder.

Heartburn is also called **gastroesophageal reflux disease (GERD).** It occurs when stomach acids are pushed into the esophagus.

- **Causes.** Alcohol, some foods, a defective esophageal sphincter, pregnancy, obesity, a hiatal hernia, and repeated vomiting can contribute to the development of this disease.
- **Signs and symptoms.** Common symptoms include frequent burping, difficulty swallowing, a sore throat, a burning sensation in the chest following meals, nausea, and blood in the vomit.
- **Treatment.** Treatment includes losing weight, making dietary changes, reducing the consumption of alcohol, taking medications, and not lying down after meals.

Hemorrhoids are varicose veins of the rectum or anus.

- **Causes.** Hemorrhoids are caused by constipation, excessive straining during bowel movements, liver disease, pregnancy, and obesity.
- **Signs and symptoms.** Signs and symptoms include itching in the anal area, painful bowel movements, bright red blood on feces, and veins that protrude from the anus.
- **Treatment.** Constipation can be avoided or improved by eating a high-fiber diet. Other treatments include stool softeners, medications to reduce the inflammation of hemorrhoids, and the surgical removal of hemorrhoids.

Hepatitis is defined as inflammation of the liver. There are many different types of hepatitis.

- **Causes.** Causes include bacteria, viruses, parasites, immune disorders, the use of alcohol and drugs, and an overdose of acetaminophen. Preventive measures include getting vaccinations, practicing safe sex, avoiding undercooked food (especially seafood), and using prescription or over-the-counter drugs at their recommended dosages.
- **Signs and symptoms.** Symptoms include mild fever, bloating, lack of appetite, nausea, vomiting, abdominal pain, weakness, jaundice, the itching of various body parts, an enlarged liver, dark urine, and breast development in males.
- **Treatment.** Patients should avoid using alcohol and drugs. Various medications may be prescribed.

A *hiatal hernia* occurs when a portion of the stomach protrudes into the chest through an opening in the diaphragm.

- **Causes.** The causes are mostly unknown, although obesity and smoking are considered risk factors. Eating small meals can be an effective preventive measure.
- **Signs and symptoms.** Signs and symptoms include excessive burping, difficulty swallowing, chest pain, and heartburn.
- **Treatment.** Treatments are weight reduction, medications to reduce the production of stomach acid, and surgical repair of the hernia.

Inguinal hernias occur when a portion of the large intestine protrudes into the inguinal canal, which is located where the thigh and the body trunk meet. In males, the hernia can also protrude into the scrotum.

- **Causes.** The causes are mostly unknown, although these hernias may be caused by weak muscles in the abdominal walls.
- **Signs and symptoms.** A lump in the groin or scrotum, or pain in the groin area that gets worse when bending or straining are the common symptoms.
- **Treatment.** Pain medications may be prescribed. Surgery to repair the hernia is needed when the large intestine is pushed back into the abdominal cavity.

Oral cancer usually involves the lips or tongue but can occur anywhere in the mouth. This type of cancer tends to spread rapidly to other organs.

- **Causes.** The causes are mostly unknown, although the use of tobacco products and alcohol are known risk factors. Poor oral hygiene and ulcers in the mouth can also cause oral cancer.
- **Signs and symptoms.** Signs and symptoms include difficulty tasting, problems swallowing, and ulcers on the tongue, lip, or other mouth structures.
- **Treatment.** Radiation therapy, chemotherapy, and surgical removal of the tumor are the treatment options.

Pancreatic cancer is the fourth leading cause of cancer death in the United States.

- **Causes.** Causes are mostly unknown, although smoking is considered a risk factor.
- **Signs and symptoms.** Common signs and symptoms include depression, fatigue, lack of appetite, nausea or

continued ⟶

Common Diseases and Disorders of the Digestive System *(continued)*

vomiting, abdominal pain, constipation or diarrhea, jaundice, and unintended weight loss.

- **Treatment.** Treatment includes radiation therapy, chemotherapy, and surgical removal of the tumor.

Stomach cancer most commonly occurs in the uppermost portion of the stomach, which is called the cardiac portion. It occurs much more frequently in Japan, Chile, and Iceland than in the United States.

- **Causes.** The causes are mostly unknown, although stomach ulcers may contribute to the development of stomach cancer.
- **Signs and symptoms.** Signs and symptoms include frequent bloating, lack of appetite, feeling full after eating small amounts, nausea, vomiting (with or without blood), abdominal cramps, excessive gas, and blood in the feces.
- **Treatment.** Treatment includes radiation therapy, chemotherapy, and surgical removal of the tumor.

Stomach ulcers occur when the lining of the stomach breaks down.

- **Causes.** Stomach ulcers can be caused by bacteria, smoking, alcohol, aspirin, and excess acid secretions in the stomach. They may be prevented by stopping smoking and avoiding aspirin, certain foods, and alcohol.
- **Signs and symptoms.** Symptoms include nausea, abdominal pain, vomiting (with or without blood), and weight loss.
- **Treatment.** Treatment options include antibiotics, medications to reduce stomach acid production, surgery to remove the affected portion of the stomach, and a vagotomy (cutting the vagus nerve) in order to reduce the production of stomach acid.

Summary

The purpose of the digestive system is to provide nutrients to the body. This is accomplished by taking in food, breaking it down, and absorbing the digested molecules. The organs responsible for this process are the mouth, teeth, salivary glands, pharynx, esophagus, stomach, small intestine, pancreas, liver, gallbladder, and large intestine. An additional function of this system is to eliminate the waste products of digestion. A healthy digestive system is important for the health of all other body systems. Understanding this system is essential when assisting with procedures such as endoscopic exams and when teaching a patient about diet and nutrition.

REVIEW

CHAPTER 13

CASE STUDY QUESTIONS

Now that you have completed this chapter, review the case study at the beginning of the chapter and answer the following questions:

1. What is the function of the gallbladder?
2. How does the gallbladder empty bile into the small intestine?
3. What conditions can result if gallstones are not removed?
4. Will this patient need to change her diet once her gallbladder is removed?

Discussion Questions

1. Describe the location of the liver. What is the digestive function of the liver?
2. What substances are normally digested in the small intestine? What substances are normally absorbed through the wall of the small intestine?
3. Discuss the functions of the mouth.
4. Describe the location of the appendix and its function. Why can a person live without an appendix?

Critical Thinking Questions

1. Describe how the digestive system processes a piece of pepperoni pizza so the body can use it.
2. What complications might a person encounter after the removal of his gallbladder?
3. How does a person mechanically digest food? Why is mechanical digestion important for proper chemical digestion?

Application Activities

1. Give the locations of each of the following digestive organs:
   a. Salivary glands
   b. Gallbladder
   c. Pharynx
   d. Esophagus
   e. Small intestine
   f. Large intestine
   g. Pancreas
2. Give the functions of the following enzymes or chemicals:
   a. Amylase
   b. Lipase
   c. Lactase
   d. Pepsin
   e. Hydrochloric acid
3. Minerals make up about what percentage of total body weight? Where are minerals primarily found?

Internet Activity

Find a Web site that provides information about the health risks associated with smoking. List the effects that smoking has on the digestive system.

CHAPTER 14

The Endocrine System

KEY TERMS

acromegaly
adrenocorticotropic hormone (ACTH)
aldosterone
antidiuretic hormone (ADH)
atrial natriuretic peptide
calcitonin
cortisol
Cushing's disease
diabetes mellitus
dwarfism
estrogen
follicle-stimulating hormone (FSH)
gigantism
glucagon
gonads
G-protein
Graves' disease
growth hormone (GH)
hormone
insulin
islets of Langerhans
luteinizing hormone (LH)
melatonin
myxedema
nonsteroid hormone
optic chiasm
oxytocin (OT)
pineal body
progesterone
prolactin (PRL)
prostaglandin
steroid hormone
stressor
testosterone
thymosin
thymus gland
thyroid hormone
thyroid-stimulating hormone (TSH)

CHAPTER OUTLINE

- Hormones
- The Pituitary Gland
- The Thyroid Gland and Parathyroid Glands
- The Adrenal Glands
- The Pancreas
- Other Hormone-Producing Organs
- The Stress Response

OBJECTIVES

After completing Chapter 14, you will be able to:

14.1 Describe the general functions of the endocrine system.
14.2 Compare the endocrine and exocrine glands.
14.3 Define the term *hormone*.
14.4 Describe the locations of the pituitary gland, thyroid gland, parathyroid glands, adrenal glands, pancreas, thymus, and gonads.
14.5 List the hormones released by the pituitary gland and give the functions of each.
14.6 List the hormones released by the thyroid gland and parathyroid glands and give the functions of each.
14.7 List the hormones released by the adrenal glands and give the functions of each.
14.8 List the hormones released by the pancreas and give the functions of each.
14.9 List the hormones released by the thymus and gonads and give the function of each.
14.10 Describe the signs, symptoms, causes, and treatments of various endocrine disorders.

Introduction

The endocrine system includes the organs of the body that secrete hormones directly into body fluids such as blood. Hormones help to regulate the chemical reactions within cells. They therefore control the functions of the organs, tissues, and other cells that comprise these cells. In this chapter you will learn about the processes and organs of the endocrine system. See Figure 14-1 for an illustration of the major organs.

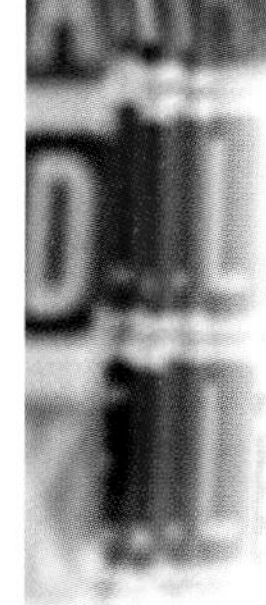

CASE STUDY

Six months ago, a 32-year-old female patient was diagnosed with a nonfunctioning tumor of her pituitary gland. This is a noncancerous tumor that does not produce any hormones. However, if it continues to grow, it can compress the pituitary gland and surrounding structures. Unfortunately, this patient's tumor has grown and now must be surgically removed.

As you read this chapter, consider the following questions:

1. Where is the pituitary gland located?
2. What structures are likely to be compressed by a tumor of the pituitary gland?
3. What hormones are normally produced by the pituitary gland?
4. What signs and symptoms would this patient have if she did not take supplemental hormones following the removal of her pituitary gland?

Hormones

Hormones can be defined as chemicals secreted by a cell that affect the functions of other cells. Once released, most hormones enter the bloodstream where they are carried to their target cells. The target cells of a hormone are the cells that contain the receptors for the hormone. A hormone cannot affect a cell unless the cell has receptors for it.

Many hormones in the body are derived from steroids. Steroids are soluble in lipids and can therefore cross cell membranes very easily. Once a **steroid hormone** is inside a cell, it binds to its receptor, which is commonly in the nucleus of the cell. The hormone-receptor complex turns a gene on or off. When new genes are turned on or off, the cell begins to carry out new functions, and this is ultimately how steroid hormones affect their target cells. Examples of steroid hormones are **estrogen, progesterone, testosterone,** and **cortisol.**

Nonsteroid hormones are those that are made of amino acids or proteins. Proteins cannot cross the cell membrane easily. Therefore, these hormones bind to receptors on the surface of the cell. The hormone-receptor complex in the membrane usually activates a **G-protein.** The G-protein causes enzymes inside the cell to be turned on. Different chemical reactions then begin inside the cell. The cell now takes on new functions.

Prostaglandins are local hormones. They are derived from lipid molecules and typically do not travel in the bloodstream to find their target cells. Instead, their target cells are located close by. They have the same effects as other hormones and are produced by many body organs, including the kidneys, stomach, uterus, heart, and brain.

The Pituitary Gland

The pituitary gland is located at the base of the brain and is controlled by the hypothalamus. This gland is well protected by a bony structure called the **sella turcica.** Just superior to the gland is the **optic chiasm,** which carries visual information to the brain for interpretation. The pituitary is divided into two lobes—the anterior and the posterior (Figures 14-1 and 14-2).

The Anterior Lobe of the Pituitary Gland

The anterior lobe of the pituitary gland secretes the following hormones:

- **Growth hormone (GH).** As its name suggests, this hormone stimulates an increase in the size of the muscles

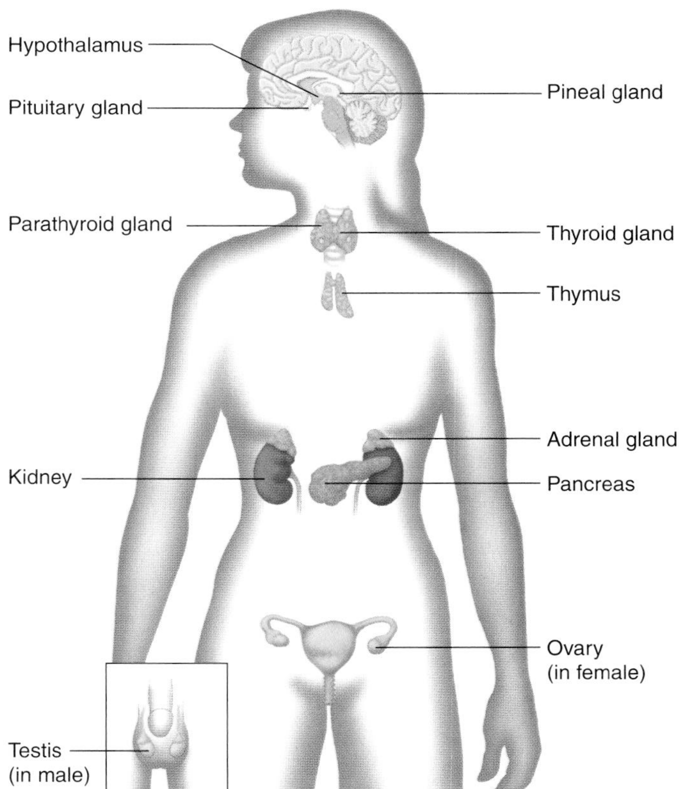

Figure 14-1. Major organs of the endocrine system.

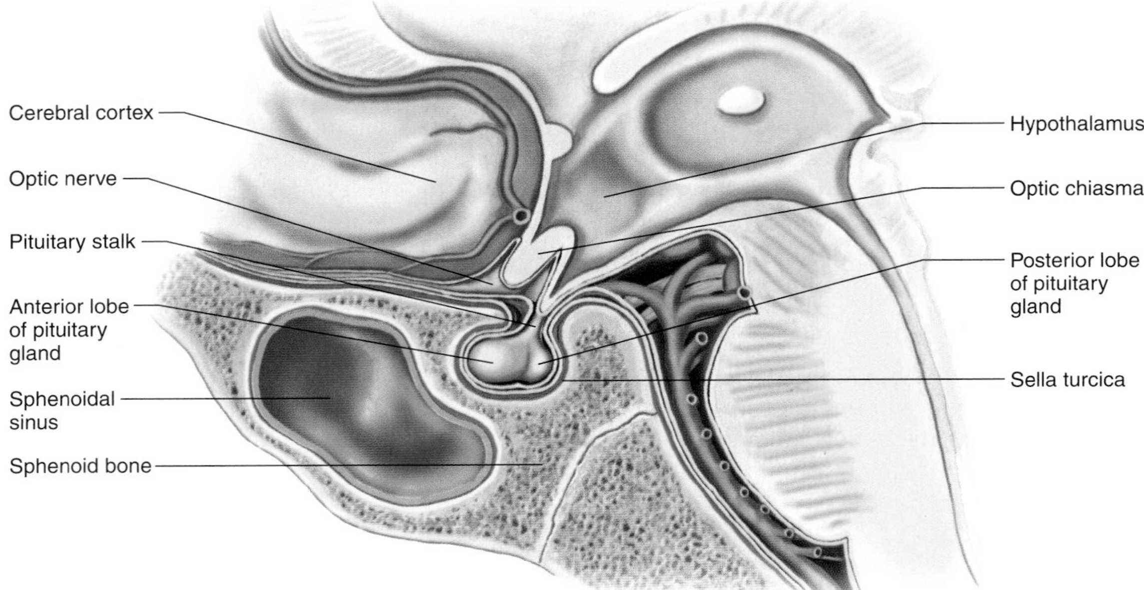

Figure 14-2. Location of the pituitary gland.

and bones in the body. It is very important in childhood for growth. It also stimulates the repair of tissues.

- **Prolactin (PRL).** This hormone stimulates milk production by mammary glands. Its function in males is not clear.
- **Adrenocorticotropic hormone (ACTH).** This hormone stimulates the adrenal cortex to release its hormones.
- **Thyroid-stimulating hormone (TSH).** This hormone stimulates the thyroid gland to release its hormones.
- **Follicle-stimulating hormone (FSH).** In females, this hormone stimulates the production of estrogen by the ovaries. More significantly, FSH stimulates maturation of the ova (eggs) before ovulation. In males, it stimulates sperm production.
- **Luteinizing hormone (LH).** In females, this hormone stimulates ovulation (the release of an egg from the ovaries) and the production of estrogen. In males, it stimulates the production of testosterone.

The Posterior Lobe of the Pituitary Gland

The posterior lobe of the pituitary gland secretes the following hormones:

- **Antidiuretic hormone (ADH).** This hormone stimulates the kidneys to conserve water. It therefore decreases urine output and helps to maintain blood pressure.
- **Oxytocin (OT).** In females, this hormone causes contractions of the uterus during childbirth. It also causes the ejection of milk from mammary glands during breast-feeding. Its function in males in not clear.

The Thyroid Gland and Parathyroid Glands

The thyroid gland consists of two lobes and sits below the larynx (voice box). It is covered by a capsule and is divided into follicles. The follicles store some of the hormones produced by the thyroid gland. Two major hormones produced by the thyroid gland are **thyroid hormones** and **calcitonin.** There are two main types of thyroid hormones—triiodothyronine (T_3) and thyronxine (T_4). The *T* stands for thyroid, and the numeral refers to the number of iodine atoms that are needed for each of these hormones to work properly.

Thyroid hormones increase energy production by cells, stimulate protein synthesis, and speed up the repair of damaged tissues. In children, they are important for normal growth and the development of the nervous system. Calcitonin lowers blood calcium levels by activating osteoblasts. Osteoblasts use excess blood calcium to build new bone tissue.

Most people have four parathyroid glands. They are small glands that are embedded into the posterior surface of the thyroid gland. The only hormone secreted by the parathyroid glands is called parathyroid hormone (PTH). This hormone acts to raise blood calcium levels by activating osteoclasts. Osteoclasts are bone-dissolving cells. When they dissolve bone, calcium is released into the bloodstream.

The Adrenal Glands

An adrenal gland sits on top of each kidney. It is divided into two portions—the adrenal medulla and the adrenal cortex. The adrenal medulla is the central portion of the gland and secretes **epinephrine** and **norepinephrine.** These hormones produce the same effects that the sympathetic nervous system produces. They increase heart rate, breathing rate, blood pressure, and all the other actions that prepare the body for stressful situations.

The adrenal cortex is the outermost portion of the adrenal gland. It secretes many hormones but the two major ones are aldosterone and cortisol. **Aldosterone** stimulates the body to retain sodium, which helps it to retain water. It is important for maintaining blood pressure. Cortisol is released when a person is stressed. It decreases protein synthesis, so it slows down the repair of tissues. Its advantage is that is also decreases inflammation, which decreases pain.

The Pancreas

The pancreas is located behind the stomach. It is an endocrine gland as well as an exocrine gland. It is considered an exocrine gland because it secretes digestive enzymes into a duct that leads to the small intestine. It is considered an endocrine gland because it contains structures known as **islets of Langerhans** that secrete hormones into the bloodstream. The islets of Langerhans secrete two hormones—**insulin** and **glucagon.**

Insulin promotes the uptake of glucose by cells. It therefore reduces glucose concentrations in the bloodstream. It also promotes the transport of amino acids into cells and increases protein synthesis. Glucagon increases glucose concentrations in the bloodstream and slows down protein synthesis.

Other Hormone-Producing Organs

The **pineal body** is a small gland located between the cerebral hemispheres. It secretes a hormone called **melatonin.** Melatonin helps to regulate your circadian rhythms, which is your biological clock. Your biological clock helps you decide when you should be awake or asleep. Melatonin is also thought to play a role in the onset of puberty.

The **thymus gland** lies between the lungs. It secretes a hormone called **thymosin.** Thymosin promotes the production of certain lymphocytes.

Sometimes referred to as the **gonads,** the ovaries and testes are reproductive organs that secrete hormones. The ovaries release estrogen and progesterone, and the testes produce testosterone. The functions of these hormones are provided in Chapter 17.

The stomach and small intestines also secrete hormones. The stomach produces gastrin, and the small intestine releases secretin and cholecystokinin. These hormones are discussed in Chapter 13.

The heart secretes a hormone called **atrial natriuretic peptide,** which regulates blood pressure. The kidneys secrete a hormone called **erythropoietin,** which stimulates blood cell production.

The Stress Response

Any stimulus that produces stress is termed a **stressor.** Stressors include physical factors such as extreme heat or cold, infections, injuries, heavy exercise, and loud sounds. Stressors can also include psychological factors such as personal loss, grief, anxiety, depression, and guilt. Even positive stimuli such as sexual arousal, joy, and happiness can be stressors.

The body's physiologic response to stress consists of a group of reactions called the general stress syndrome, which is primarily caused by the release of hormones. This syndrome results in an increase in the heart rate, breathing rate, and blood pressure. Glucose and fatty acid concentrations also increase in the blood, which leads to weight loss. Prolonged stress causes the release of cortisol. Cortisol slows down body repair because it prevents protein synthesis and inhibits immune responses, which is why a person under stress becomes more susceptible to being sick.

Pathophysiology

Common Diseases and Disorders of the Endocrine System

Acromegaly is a disorder in which too much growth hormone is produced in adults.

- **Causes.** This disorder is caused by an increased production of growth hormone or by a tumor of the pituitary gland.
- **Signs and symptoms.** The primary signs and symptoms include enlargement of the bones in the entire skull as well as in the hands and feet, and thickening of the skin. Other symptoms include headache, fatigue, profuse sweating, pain (especially in the arms and legs), gaps between the teeth, weight gain, excessive hair production, cardiovascular diseases, arthritis, and vision problems.
- **Treatment.** Treatment includes medications to lower the production of growth hormone, radiation therapy to reduce the size of a pituitary tumor, or surgery to remove a pituitary tumor.

continued ⟶

Common Diseases and Disorders of the Endocrine System *(continued)*

Addison's disease is a condition in which the adrenal glands fail to produce enough corticosteroids. It affects about 1 in every 25,000 people.

- **Causes.** The cause of this disease is most often unknown. It may be caused by an autoimmune dysfunction. It can be caused by cancer and other serious diseases that damage the adrenal glands.
- **Signs and symptoms.** The signs and symptoms may begin long before a diagnosis is made. They include weakness, fatigue, and dizziness after rising from a sitting or reclining position. Other symptoms include weight loss, muscle pain, lack of appetite, nausea, vomiting, diarrhea, and dehydration.
- **Treatment.** Because this disease can be life-threatening, the first treatment is to administer corticosteroids. Medications or other hormones may be prescribed to help balance the levels of sodium and potassium.

Cushing's disease is also known as hypercortisolism. In this condition, a person produces too much cortisol.

- **Causes.** This disease is caused by an excessive production of ACTH (a hormone that increases the production of cortisol), a tumor of the adrenal gland (the source of cortisol), a tumor of the pituitary gland (the source of ACTH), or the long-term use of steroid hormones.
- **Signs and symptoms.** Common symptoms include a round or full face, a hump of fat between the shoulders, thin arms and legs with a large abdomen, fatigue, thin skin, acne, frequent thirst, frequent urination, mental disabilities, a loss of menstrual cycle in females, high blood pressure, high glucose blood levels, and body aches in the muscles, back, or head.
- **Treatment.** The first treatment is lifestyle changes, especially stopping the use of steroid hormones. Radiation therapy or surgery may be needed to treat any tumors.

Diabetes mellitus is a chronic disease that is characterized by high glucose levels in the blood. There are at least three different types of diabetes mellitus. Type 1 is referred to as early-onset diabetes and usually develops during childhood. Type 2 is the most common type and is often called late-onset diabetes because it is primarily diagnosed in adults. Gestational diabetes occurs only in pregnant women and is usually temporary. African Americans, Hispanics, and Native Americans are more likely to develop diabetes than any other ethnic groups.

- **Causes.** This disease is caused by the production of too little or no insulin by the pancreas. Other causes include body cells having too few insulin receptors, obesity, high blood pressure, pregnancy, and high cholesterol levels in the blood.
- **Signs and symptoms.** There are many signs and symptoms of this disease. They include high levels of glucose in the blood, excessive thirst, frequent urination, fatigue, increased appetite, unexplained weight loss, blurry vision, impotence in men, nausea, skin wounds that heal slowly, high ketone levels in the urine, and foot problems (due to poor circulation).
- **Treatment.** Treatment includes daily injections of insulin, oral medications to increase insulin production, oral medications to increase the body's sensitivity to insulin, frequent monitoring of glucose levels in the blood, and frequent monitoring of ketone levels in the urine. Lifestyle changes are important and should include reducing weight (especially if obese), changing eating habits, and getting regular exercise. Lifestyle changes to prevent injury to legs or feet may also be needed.
- **Complications.** Left untreated, diabetes can result in long-term and life-threatening complications. Blood vessels become thickened, which can damage vital organs including the kidneys, eyes, heart, and brain. Long-term damage can result in kidney disease, blindness, and atherosclerosis (the buildup of fatty deposits in blood vessels). Circulation worsens, which not only affects organs but may result in slower overall healing and ulcers that develop in the feet. Because of the body's decreased ability to heal, these ulcers may require the amputation of the affected foot and possibly part of the leg.

Dwarfism is a condition in which too little growth hormone is produced.

- **Causes.** This condition can be caused by an underproduction of the growth hormone during childhood, trauma to the pituitary gland, or a pituitary tumor.
- **Signs and symptoms.** Symptoms include short height, abnormal facial features, cleft lip or palate, delayed puberty, headaches, frequent urination, and excessive thirst.
- **Treatment.** Treatment is the administration of supplemental growth hormone.

Gigantism is a condition in which too much growth hormone is produced during childhood.

- **Causes.** This condition is caused by overproduction of the growth hormone during childhood. It can also be caused by a tumor in the pituitary gland.
- **Signs and symptoms.** Very tall height, delayed sexual maturity, thick facial bones, thick skin, weakness, and vision problems are common symptoms.
- **Treatment.** Treatment includes medications to reduce growth hormone levels, radiation therapy, and surgery to remove the tumor.

Graves' disease is a disorder in which a person develops antibodies that attack the thyroid gland. This attack causes the thyroid to produce too many thyroid hormones.

continued ⟶

Common Diseases and Disorders of the Endocrine System *(continued)*

Graves' disease is the most common type of hyperthyroidism in the United States.

- **Causes.** This disease is caused by an overproduction of thyroid hormones. It is also considered an autoimmune disorder.
- **Signs and symptoms.** The most common signs and symptoms include protrusion of the eyes (exophthalmos) and thyroid enlargement (goiter). Other symptoms include insomnia, unexplained weight loss, anxiety, muscle weakness, increased appetite, excessive sweating, vision problems, thyroid enlargement, and an increased heart rate.
- **Treatment.** Treatment includes medications to reduce heart rate, sweating, and nervousness; radiation to destroy the thyroid gland; surgery to remove the thyroid gland; and supplemental thyroid hormones if the gland is destroyed or removed.

Myxedema is a disorder in which the thyroid gland does not produce adequate amounts of thyroid hormone. It is a severe type of hypothyroidism that is most common in females over age 50.

- **Causes.** Causes include the removal of the thyroid, radiation treatments to the neck area, and obesity. This disorder may be congenital.
- **Signs and symptoms.** Signs and symptoms include weakness, fatigue, weight gain, depression, general body aches, dry skin and hair, hair loss, puffy hands or feet, a decreased ability to taste food, abnormal menstrual periods, pale or yellow skin, a slow heart rate, low blood pressure, anemia, an enlarged heart, high cholesterol levels, or coma.
- **Treatment.** Treatment consists of giving supplemental thyroid hormones intravenously or orally and closely monitoring the levels of thyroid hormones.

Summary

The endocrine system regulates all chemical reactions in cells. The substances responsible for this regulation are known as hormones. Hormones are produced by endocrine glands. The major endocrine glands are the pituitary, thyroid, parathyroid, adrenal, and pancreas. Once a hormone is released into the bloodstream, it travels to its target tissue and produces a response. An awareness of this system can help medical assistants be more effective when teaching a patient about the advantages and disadvantages of hormone replacement therapy.

REVIEW

CHAPTER 14

CASE STUDY QUESTIONS

Now that you have completed this chapter, review the case study at the beginning of the chapter and answer the following questions:

1. Where is the pituitary gland located?
2. What structures are likely to be compressed by a tumor of the pituitary gland?
3. What hormones are normally produced by the pituitary gland?
4. What signs and symptoms would this patient have if she did not take supplemental hormones following the removal of her pituitary gland?

Discussion Questions

1. Explain the difference between an endocrine gland and an exocrine gland.
2. Name the major endocrine organs of the body and give their locations.
3. Explain how the body responds to stress.
4. Explain why the testes and ovaries are described as both endocrine organs and reproductive organs.

Critical Thinking Questions

1. If a patient had his pituitary gland removed, what hormone supplements would he need?
2. What is the danger of a diabetic injecting too much insulin?
3. Why is hyposecretion (insufficient secretion) of thyroid hormone in newborns more serious than hyposecretion in adults?

Application Activities

1. Tell which endocrine gland secretes the following hormones:
   a. Insulin
   b. ADH
   c. Testosterone
   d. Prolactin
   e. Growth hormone
2. Describe the effects the following hormones produce:
   a. Oxytocin
   b. Cortisol
   c. LH and FSH
   d. Glucagon
   e. Estrogen
3. For each of the following diseases, name the hormone that is involved:
   a. Acromegaly
   b. Myxedema
   c. Dwarfism
   d. Diabetes
   e. Cushing's disease
4. Define what a stressor is and give an example.

Internet Activity

Find a Web site that discusses endocrinology. Research the roles of an endocrinologist and how weight management and endocrinology are related.

CHAPTER 15

Special Senses

CHAPTER OUTLINE

- The Nose and the Sense of Smell
- The Tongue and the Sense of Taste
- The Eye and the Sense of Sight
- The Ear and the Senses of Hearing and Equilibrium

OBJECTIVES

After completing Chapter 15, you will be able to:

15.1 Describe the anatomy of the nose and the function of each part.
15.2 Describe how smell sensations are created and interpreted.
15.3 Describe the anatomy of the tongue and the function of each part.
15.4 Describe how taste sensations are created and interpreted.
15.5 Name the four primary taste sensations.
15.6 Describe the anatomy of the eye and the function of each part.
15.7 Describe various disorders of the eye.
15.8 Trace the path of a visual image through the eye and to the brain for interpretation.
15.9 Describe the anatomy of the ear and the function of each part.
15.10 Describe various disorders of the ear.
15.11 Explain how sounds travel through the ear and are interpreted in the brain.
15.12 Explain the role of the ear in maintaining equilibrium.

KEY TERMS

amblyopia
aqueous humor
astigmatism
auditory tube
auricle
cataracts
chemoreceptor
choroid
ciliary body
cochlea
conductive hearing loss
cones
conjunctiva
conjunctivitis
cornea
endolymph
external auditory canal
extrinsic eye muscles
glaucoma
gustatory receptors
hyperopia
iris
lacrimal apparatus
lacrimal gland
macular degeneration
myopia
nasolacrimal duct
olfactory
orbicularis oculi
oval window
papillae
perilymph
presbyopia
pupil

KEY TERMS *(Continued)*

retina
rods
sclera
semicircular canals
sensorineural hearing loss
sensory adaptation
strabismus
taste bud
tinnitus
tympanic membrane
vestibule
vitreous humor

Introduction

The special senses are smell, taste, vision, hearing, and equilibrium. They are called special senses because their sensory receptors are located within relatively large sensory organs in the head—the nose, tongue, eyes, and ears. This chapter introduces the structure and function of these sense organs and focuses on common diseases of the eyes and ears.

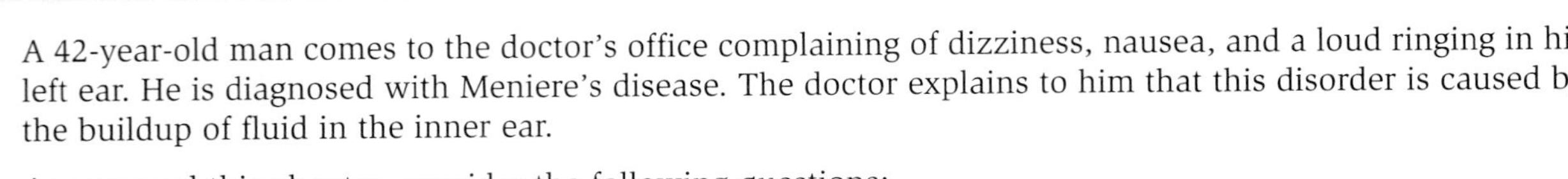

A 42-year-old man comes to the doctor's office complaining of dizziness, nausea, and a loud ringing in his left ear. He is diagnosed with Meniere's disease. The doctor explains to him that this disorder is caused by the buildup of fluid in the inner ear.

As you read this chapter, consider the following questions:

1. Why is the patient experiencing dizziness and difficulty hearing?
2. What is the clinical term for ringing in the ear?
3. What precautions should this patient take because of his dizziness?
4. A diuretic is a drug that decreases fluids in the body. Why might the doctor prescribe a diuretic?

The Nose and the Sense of Smell

Smell receptors are also called **olfactory** receptors and are **chemoreceptors.** This means that they respond to changes in chemical concentrations. Chemicals that activate smell receptors must be dissolved in the mucus of the nose. Therefore, a person who has a "dry nose" has trouble smelling.

Smell receptors are located in the olfactory organ, which is in the upper part of the nasal cavity. Humans have a relatively poor sense of smell compared to animals because chemicals must diffuse all the way up the nasal cavity in order to activate smell receptors.

Once smell receptors are activated, they send their information to the olfactory nerves. The olfactory nerves send the information along olfactory bulbs and tracts to different areas of the cerebrum. The cerebrum interprets the information as a particular type of smell (Figure 15-1).

An interesting fact about smell is that it undergoes **sensory adaptation,** which means that the same chemical can stimulate smell receptors for only a limited amount of time. Eventually, the smell receptors no longer respond to the chemical, and it can no longer be smelled. Sensory adaptation explains why you smell perfume when you first encounter it, but after a few minutes you cannot smell it or may be less aware of it.

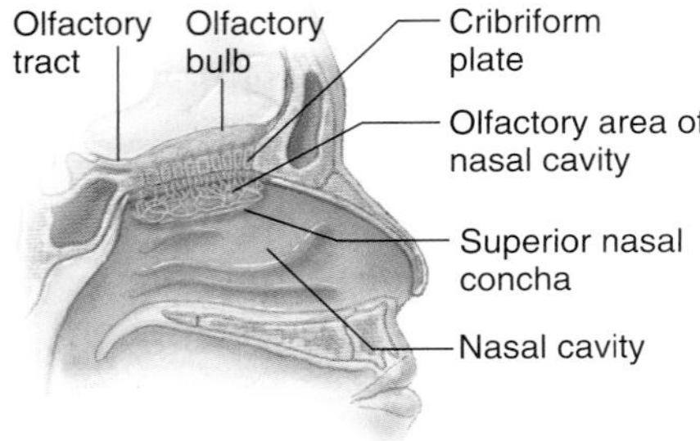

Figure 15-1. The olfactory area (organ) is located in the superior part of the nasal cavity.

The Tongue and the Sense of Taste

Taste, or **gustatory,** receptors are located on taste buds. **Taste buds** are found on the "bumps" of the tongue. These bumps are called **papillae,** which many people incorrectly think are the actual taste buds. Taste buds are microscopic and cannot be seen with the naked eye. Some taste buds are also scattered on the roof of the mouth and in the walls of the throat.

Each taste bud is made of taste cells and supporting cells. The taste cells function as taste receptors, and the supporting cells simply fill in the spaces between the taste cells. Taste cells are types of chemoreceptors because they are activated by chemicals that must be dissolved in saliva (Figure 15-2).

There are four types of taste cells, and each type is activated by a particular group of chemicals. Therefore, the following four primary taste sensations are produced:

1. Sweet. Taste cells that respond to "sweet" chemicals are concentrated at the tip of the tongue.
2. Sour. Taste cells that respond to "sour" chemicals are concentrated on the sides of the tongue.
3. Salty. Taste cells that respond to "salty" chemicals are concentrated on the tip and sides of the tongue.
4. Bitter. Taste cells that respond to "bitter" chemicals are concentrated at the back of the tongue.

Eating spicy foods activates pain receptors on the tongue. Once taste cells are activated, they send their information to several cranial nerves. The information eventually reaches the gustatory cortex in the parietal lobe of the cerebrum. The gustatory cortex interprets the information as a particular taste.

The Eye and the Sense of Sight

The sense of sight comes from the eyes and is also supported by visual accessory organs.

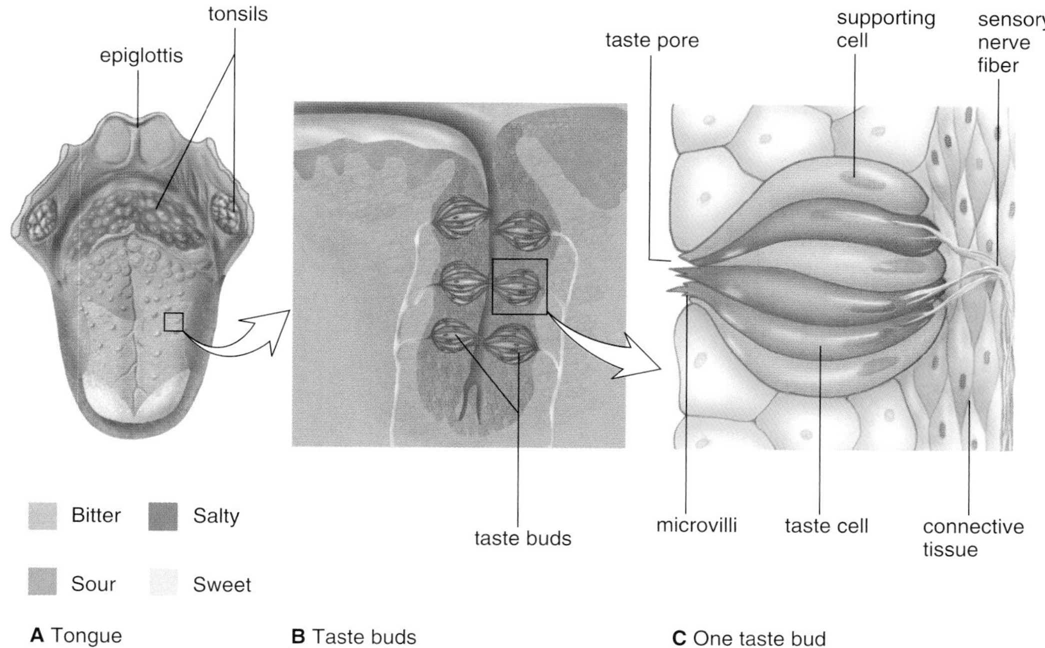

Figure 15-2. Tongue and taste buds. (a) Areas of the tongue are sensitive to different tastes, as indicated. (b) Taste buds are on and in papillae. (c) Taste buds are composed of taste cells and supporting cells.

Structure of the Eye

The eye is hollow and spherical shaped. It consists of cavities, wall layers, and other structures.

The Cavities of the Eye. Each eyeball is divided into two cavities—the anterior and the posterior.

The Anterior Cavity. The anterior cavity is in front of the lens and is filled with a watery fluid called **aqueous humor.** Aqueous humor provides nutrients to structures in the anterior cavity of the eyeball. When too much aqueous humor is produced, a person develops **glaucoma.**

The Posterior Cavity. The posterior cavity of the eyeball is behind the lens and is filled with a very thick fluid called **vitreous humor.** Vitreous humor keeps the retina flat and helps to maintain the shape of the eye.

The Wall of the Eye. In addition to the cavities of the eye, the eye is composed of a wall that has three layers: the outer, middle, and inner (Figure 15-3).

Outer Layer. The outer layer is also called the fibrous layer because it is composed of tough, dense connective tissue. The two divisions of the outer layer are the sclera and cornea. The **sclera** is the "white of the eye" and does not allow light to enter the eye. The **cornea** is anterior to the sclera and allows light to enter the eye. It is often called the "window of the eye." The entire outer layer contains no blood vessels but is supplied with many sensory receptors that can detect even the smallest of particles on the surface of the eyeball.

Middle Layer. The middle layer is also called the vascular and pigmented layer because it is richly supplied with blood vessels and pigments. The middle layer consists of the **choroid, ciliary body,** and **iris.** The choroid lines the sclera and functions to absorb extra light that has entered the eye. The ciliary body functions to hold and move the lens. The lens is moved back and forth to allow the eye to focus on images. The lens is usually transparent but "cloudy" areas called **cataracts** can form, which prevent light from reaching visual receptors. The iris, which is the most anterior structure of this layer, controls the amount of light that enters the eye. The iris also contains the color of a person's eyes. The hole in the iris is called the **pupil.**

Inner Layer. The inner layer is also called the **retina.** This layer contains visual receptors called **rods** and **cones.** Rods allow a person to see images in dim light as well as the general outlines of structures. Rods also detect black, white, and gray shades. A person who suffers from night blindness has defective rods. Cones allow a person to see images in bright light and to see details of structures. Cones also detect colors other than white, black, and gray. A person who has red-green color blindness lacks the cones needed to see reds and greens.

Visual Accessory Organs

Visual accessory organs assist and protect the eyeball. They include eyelids, conjunctivas, the lacrimal apparatus, and extrinsic eye muscles.

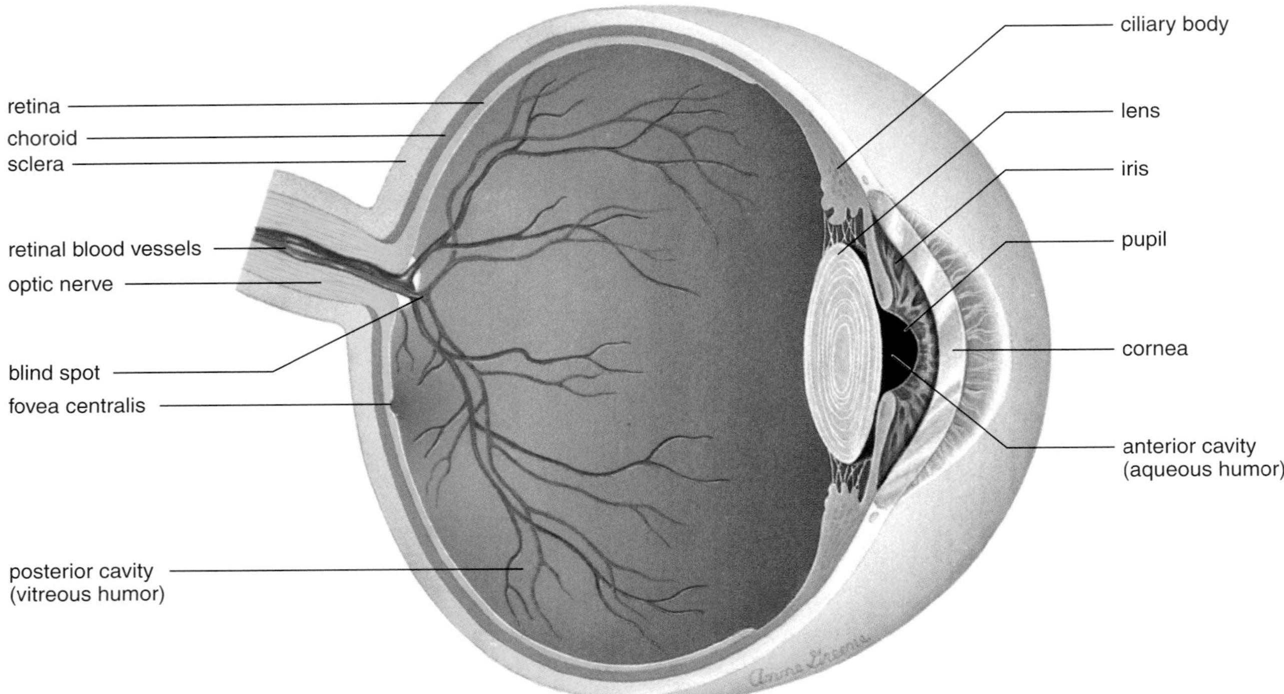

Figure 15-3. Sectioned eyeball.

Eyelids. Each eyelid is composed of skin, muscle, and dense connective tissue. The muscle in the eyelid is called the **orbicularis oculi** and is responsible for blinking. Blinking the eyelids prevents the eyeball surface from drying and also protects the eyes. A moist eyeball surface is much less likely to grow bacteria than a dry one is.

Conjunctivas. **Conjunctivas** are mucous membranes that line the inner surfaces of the eyelids; they fold back onto the anterior surface of each eyeball. They are called mucous membranes because they produce mucus that keeps the surface of the eyeballs moist.

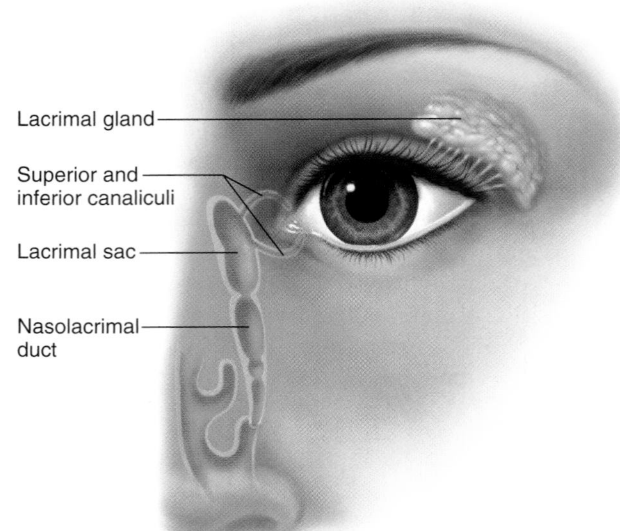

Figure 15-4. Lacrimal apparatus.

The Lacrimal Apparatus. The **lacrimal apparatus** consists of lacrimal glands and nasolacrimal ducts. **Lacrimal glands** are located on the lateral edge of each eyeball and produce tears. Tears are mostly water, but they also contain enzymes that can destroy bacteria and viruses. Tears also have an outer oily layer that prevents them from evaporating. **Nasolacrimal ducts** are located on the medial aspect of each eyeball. They drain tears into the nose. When a person cries, the abundance of tears entering the nose produces the "runny nose" associated with crying (Figure 15-4).

Extrinsic Eye Muscles. **Extrinsic eye muscles** are skeletal muscles that move the eyeball. Each eyeball has six extrinsic eye muscles attached to it that move the eyeball superiorly, inferiorly, laterally, or medially.

Visual Pathways

When visual receptors are activated, they send their information to optic nerves. Parts of the optic nerves cross at a structure called the **optic chiasm,** which is located at the base of the brain. The visual area in the occipital lobes of the cerebrum is responsible for interpreting vision. Because visual information crosses in the optic chiasm, about half of the visual information detected in each eye is interpreted on the opposite side of the brain. Therefore, half of what a person sees in the right eye is interpreted in the left side of the brain. See Table 15-1 for a summary of the parts of the eye and their functions.

TABLE 15-1 The Functions of the Parts of the Eye	
Structure	**Function**
Aqueous humor	Nourishes structures in anterior eye cavity
Vitreous humor	Holds retina in place; maintains shape of eyeball
Sclera	Protects eye
Cornea	Allows light to enter eye; bends light as it enters eye
Choroid	Absorbs extra light in eye
Ciliary body	Holds lens; moves lens for focusing
Iris	Controls amount of light entering eye
Lens	Focuses light onto retina
Retina	Contains visual receptors
Rods	Allow vision in dim light; detect black-and-white images; detect broad outlines of images
Cones	Allow vision in bright light; detect colors; detect details
Optic nerve	Carries visual information from rods and cones toward the brain

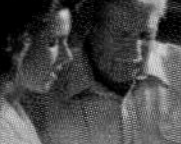

Educating the Patient

Eye Safety and Protection

Almost 90% of all eye injuries can be prevented by eye safety practices or proper protective eyewear. You can educate patients about preventing eye injuries in the home, at work, and during recreational activities.

Eye Safety in the Home

Patients should follow these suggestions to protect their eyes in the home:

- Pad or cushion the sharp corners and edges of furniture and home fixtures.
- Make sure adequate lighting and handrails are available on stairs.
- Keep personal use items (for example, cosmetics and toiletries), kitchen utensils, and desk supplies out of the reach of children.
- Keep toys with sharp edges out of the reach of children. Also, make sure toys intended for older children are kept away from younger children.
- Before mowing the lawn, remove dangerous debris.
- Wear safely goggles when operating any type of power equipment.
- Keep dangerous solvents, paints, cleaners, fertilizers, and other chemicals out of the reach of children.
- Never mix cleaning agents.

Eye Safety at Work

Approximately 15% of eye injuries in the workplace lead to temporary or permanent vision loss. Eye injuries at work can be diminished if patients take the following precautions:

- Safety eyewear should be chosen according to the type of work being performed and the type of eye protection that is needed.
- Safety eyewear should be worn whenever there is a chance of flying objects from machines.
- Safety eyewear should be worn whenever there is possible exposure to harmful chemicals or radiation.

Eye Safety During Sports and Recreational Activities

Common eye injuries that occur while playing a sport include scratched corneas, inflamed irises and retinas, bleeding in the anterior chamber of the eye, traumatic cataracts, and fractures of the eye socket. Wearing sports eye guards can prevent most sports eye injuries. These guards are recommended for baseball, basketball, soccer, football, rugby, and hockey.

Pathophysiology

Common Diseases and Disorders of the Eyes

Amblyopia is more commonly called lazy eye and occurs when a child does not use one eye regularly. A child with this disorder does not have normal depth perception and often has eyes that turn in or out.

- **Causes.** Amblyopia can be caused by any disorder of the eyes that affects normal eye development and use, including farsightedness, nearsightedness, cataracts, and astigmatism.
- **Signs and symptoms.** The most common symptoms are blurred vision and an eye that appears to turn inward.
- **Treatment.** Treating the underlying conditions and placing a patch over the normal eye are the primary treatment options.

Astigmatism means that the cornea has an abnormal shape, which causes blurred images during near or distant vision.

- **Causes.** A person with this condition is normally born with it.
- **Signs and symptoms.** There are no symptoms with this condition. However, it can be diagnosed during an ophthalmic (eye) exam.
- **Treatment.** Treatment includes corrective lenses or surgery to reshape the cornea.

Cataracts are structures in the lens that prevent light from going through the lens. Over time, images begin to look fuzzy.

- **Causes.** Aging is the most significant risk factor associated with this disorder. Cataracts can be caused by eye injuries, some medications, and certain diseases.
- **Signs and symptoms.** The primary symptom is poor or impaired vision.
- **Treatment.** Treatment includes the use of eyeglasses, medications to dilate the pupils, or surgery to remove the cataracts.

Conjunctivitis is commonly called pink eye and is highly contagious.

- **Causes.** This disease is caused by bacteria, viruses, or allergies.
- **Signs and symptoms.** The signs and symptoms are red eyes, itchy eyes, swollen eyelids, a watery discharge (in the types caused by viruses and allergies), and a stringy discharge (in the type caused by bacteria). The allergic type usually affects both eyes, whereas viral and bacterial conjunctivitis begins in one eye and then spreads to the other.
- **Treatment.** Cool compresses and anti-inflammatory drugs are used to treat conjunctivitis caused by viruses and allergies. Antihistamines are used for the type caused by allergies. The bacterial type is best treated with antibiotics.

Dry eye syndrome is one of the most common eye problems treated by physicians. This syndrome results from a decreased production of the oil within tears, which normally occurs with age.

- **Causes.** Dry eye can be caused by cigarette smoke; air conditioning; long hours at a computer; some medications; contact lenses; hormonal changes associated with menopause; and hot, dry, or windy climates.
- **Signs and symptoms.** The common eye symptoms include burning, irritation, redness, itching, and excessive tearing.
- **Treatment.** Artificial tears can provide relief to many patients. People with this condition should drink 8 to 10 glasses of water a day and make a conscious effort to blink more frequently and avoid rubbing their eyes. In addition, punctual plugs can be inserted to trap tears on the eyes, which prevents the tears from entering the nasolacrimal duct.

Glaucoma is a condition in which too much pressure is created in the eye by excessive aqueous humor. If untreated, this excess pressure can lead to permanent damage of the optic nerves, resulting in blindness.

- **Causes.** *Open-angle glaucoma* progresses relatively slowly; it can be caused by the slow drainage of aqueous humor from the anterior segment of the eye, which is the space between the cornea and the iris. *Acute-angle closure glaucoma* is a more serious type of glaucoma; it results when the space between the iris and the cornea is more narrow than normal. Certain medications, trauma, and tumors may all cause secondary glaucoma.
- **Signs and symptoms.** There are usually no symptoms of open-angle glaucoma. Common symptoms of acute-angle closure glaucoma include nausea, vomiting, extreme eye pain, headache, and a sudden loss of vision.
- **Treatment.** Treatments include medications to control pressure in the anterior segment of the eye, and surgery.

Hyperopia is commonly called farsightedness. It occurs when light entering the eye is focused behind the retina. Common causes include flat corneas or short eyes. Treatments include corrective lenses or surgery to alter the shape of the cornea.

Macular degeneration is a progressive disease that usually affects people over the age of 50. It occurs when the

continued ⟶

retina no longer receives an adequate blood supply. It is the most common cause of vision loss in the United States.

- **Causes.** Genetics, age, smoking, and exposure to ultraviolet radiation (from sunlight) are known risk factors. Nutrition plays an important role in preventing this disease—diets high in fruits and vegetables are associated with the prevention of macular degeneration.
- **Signs and symptoms.** Common symptoms include loss of central vision (may be gradual or sudden), distortions in vision (straight lines begin to look wavy, for example), and difficulty seeing details.
- **Treatment.** In most cases, there are no treatments. Laser treatments may repair the damaged blood vessels of the retina.

Myopia is commonly called nearsightedness. It occurs when light entering the eye is focused in front of the retina. Treatments include corrective lenses or surgery to alter the shape of the cornea.

Presbyopia is a common eye disorder that results in the loss of lens elasticity. It develops with age and causes a person to have difficulty seeing objects close up. Treatments include contact lenses, eyeglasses, and eye surgeries.

Retinal detachment occurs when the layers of the retina separate. It is considered a medical emergency and, if not treated right away, leads to permanent vision loss.

- **Causes.** This disorder is sometimes caused by fluids that seep between layers of the retina; this occurs most commonly in nearsighted people. In diabetics, vitreous body or scar tissue pulls the retina loose. Other causes include eye trauma that causes fluid to collect underneath the layers of the retina.
- **Signs and symptoms.** Signs and symptoms include light flashes, wavy vision, a sudden loss of vision, and a larger amount of floaters.
- **Treatment.** The treatment measures include the following:
  - Pneumatic retinopexy, which involves injecting a gas bubble into the posterior segment of the eye. The pressure flattens the retina, and the retina is later fixed in place with a laser.
  - Scleral buckle, which involves using a silicone band to hold the retina in place.
  - Replacing the vitreous body with silicone oil to reattach the retina.

Strabismus is more commonly referred to as crossed eyes. In this condition, the eyes do not focus on the same image.

- **Causes.** The causes are mostly unknown, although some known causes include eye and brain injuries, cerebral palsy, and various disorders of the retina.
- **Signs and symptoms.** Blurred vision and depth perception are the most common symptoms.
- **Treatment.** Treatment includes eyeglasses, eye exercises, a patch over the stronger eye, and surgery to realign the eyes.

The Ear and the Senses of Hearing and Equilibrium

The organ of hearing is the ear. In addition to providing the sense of hearing, the ear aids the body in maintaining balance, or equilibrium.

Structure of the Ear

The ear is divided into three parts—external ear, middle ear, and inner ear (Figure 15-5).

External Ear. The external ear is composed of the **auricle** and the **external auditory canal.** The auricle is the flap of skin and cartilage that hangs off the side of the head. It is also called the pinna and functions to collect sound waves. The external auditory canal is more commonly called the ear canal. When you stick your finger in your ear, you are sticking it in your external auditory canal. This canal carries sound waves to the **tympanic membrane** (eardrum).

Middle Ear. The middle ear begins with the tympanic membrane. This membrane is relatively thin and vibrates when sound waves hit it. On the other side of the tympanic membrane are three tiny bones called **ear ossicles**—the malleus, incus, and stapes. When the tympanic membrane vibrates, it causes the ossicles to vibrate and hit a membrane called the oval window. The **oval window** is the beginning of the inner ear.

The middle ear is connected to the throat by a tube called the **auditory tube,** which is also known as the Eustachian tube. This tube helps maintain equal pressure on both sides of the eardrum, which is important for normal hearing. Because the middle ear is connected to the throat by this tube, any throat infection can easily spread to the ear.

Inner Ear. The inner ear is a very complex system of communicating chambers and tubes. It is divided into three portions—**semicircular canals,** a **vestibule,** and a **cochlea.** There are three semicircular canals per ear, and they function to detect the balance of the body. The cochlea is shaped like a snail's shell and contains hearing receptors. The vestibule is the area between the semicircular canals and the cochlea. Like the semicircular canals, it also functions in equilibrium. When the head moves, fluids in the semicircular canals and vestibule move, which

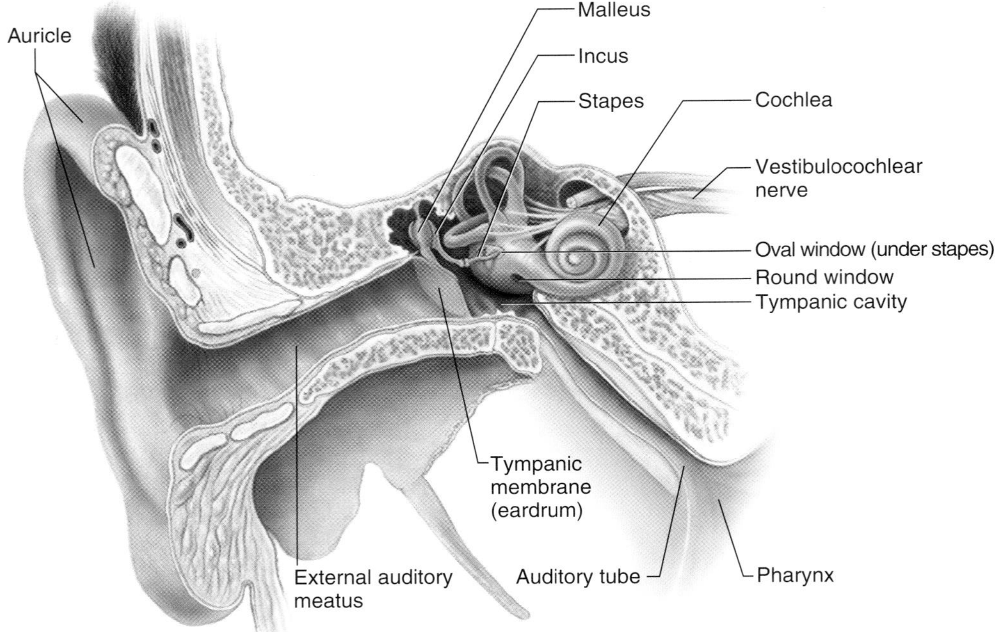

Figure 15-5. Major parts of the ear.

activates equilibrium receptors. The receptors send the information along vestibular nerves to the cerebrum for interpretation. The cerebrum can then advise the body if it needs to make any adjustments to prevent a fall.

There are two types of fluid in the inner ear—**perilymph** and **endolymph.** When these fluids move, they activate hearing and equilibrium receptors.

When sound waves reach the inner ear, fluids move and activate the hearing receptors in the cochlea. Sounds of different volumes and frequencies activate various types of hearing receptors. Once hearing receptors are activated, they send their information to auditory nerves. Auditory nerves (vestibulocochlear nerves) eventually deliver the information to the auditory cortex in the temporal lobe of

Educating the Patient

How to Recognize Hearing Problems in Infants

Hearing problems in infants are not easy to recognize. The following general guidelines can be used to teach parents how to identify normal hearing in infants. Any deviations from these guidelines may indicate a hearing loss.

- Infants up to 4 months old:
  - They should be startled by loud noises (barking dog, hand clap, etc.).
  - When sleeping in a quiet room, they should wake up at the sound of voices.
  - Around the fourth month of age, they should turn their head or move their eyes to follow a sound.
  - They should recognize the mother's or primary caregiver's voice better than other voices.
- Infants 4 to 8 months of age:
  - They should regularly turn their heads or move their eyes to follow sounds.
  - Their facial expressions should change at the sound of familiar voices or loud noises.
  - They should begin to enjoy certain sounds such as rattles or ringing bells.
  - They should begin to babble at people who talk to them.
- Babies 8 to 12 months of age:
  - They should turn quickly to the sound of their name.
  - They should begin to vary the pitch of the sounds they produce in their babbling.
  - They should begin to respond to music.
  - They should respond to the instruction "no."

the cerebrum. The auditory cortex interprets the information as sounds.

Hearing Loss

The two most common types of hearing loss are **conductive** and **sensorineural.**

Conductive Hearing Loss. Conductive hearing loss develops when sound waves cannot be conducted through the ear. For example, inserting an earplug can temporarily cause conductive hearing loss. The causes of conductive hearing loss include a buildup of earwax and damage to the tympanic membrane. Most types of conductive hearing loss are temporary.

Sensorineural Hearing Loss. Sensorineural hearing loss develops when neural structures associated with the ear are damaged. Neural structures include hearing receptors and the auditory nerve. **Tinnitus,** which is an abnormal ringing in the ear, suggests damage to the auditory nerve. Most types of sensorineural hearing loss are permanent.

Summary

The ability to detect changes in the environment is critical to survival. The human body has various organs for this purpose. The nose senses odors in the environment, the tongue senses tastes, and the eyes are important for visual sense. The ears serve two functions—hearing and equilibrium.

Each of these special senses works in concert with the nervous system to assist the body in coping with environmental changes experienced throughout the day. A medical assistant should understand the special senses in order to test distance and near visual acuity, color vision, and hearing. Knowledge of the anatomy of the eye and ear is essential when performing irrigation or instillation of these structures.

REVIEW

CHAPTER 15

CASE STUDY QUESTIONS

Now that you have completed this chapter, review the case study at the beginning of the chapter and answer the following questions:

1. Why is the patient experiencing dizziness and difficulty hearing?
2. What is the clinical term for ringing in the ear?
3. What precautions should this patient take because of his dizziness?
4. A diuretic is a drug that decreases fluids in the body. Why might the doctor prescribe a diuretic?

Discussion Questions

1. Describe how sound waves travel through the ear from the auricle to hearing receptors. Where is sound interpreted?
2. Describe the structures that light must pass through in order to reach the retina. Where is vision interpreted?
3. Identify the four primary taste sensations and tell what part of the tongue is associated with each.
4. Describe how smell receptors are activated.

Critical Thinking Questions

1. Why does a sewage treatment plant have a strong, offensive odor to visitors of the plant but not to regular workers at the plant?
2. How are the signs and symptoms of cataracts, glaucoma, and macular degeneration different?
3. Sudden loud sounds can damage the eardrums. What type of hearing loss will these sounds produce? Chronic loud sounds damage hearing receptors. What type of hearing loss do these sounds produce?

Application Activities

1. Give the functions of the following:
   a. Iris
   b. Cornea
   c. Lens
   d. Retina
   e. Ciliary body
2. State if the following structures are part of the outer, middle, or inner ear. Also give the function of each.
   a. Vestibule
   b. Cochlea
   c. External auditory canal
   e. Ear ossicles
   e. Tympanic membrane
3. What are the two kinds of cells in taste buds?
4. Where is the olfactory organ located?

Internet Activity

Find a Web site that provides information on hearing and balance. Research ways to prevent ear damage that could cause problems with balance.

CHAPTER 16

The Urinary System

CHAPTER OUTLINE

- The Kidneys
- Urine Formation
- The Ureters, Urinary Bladder, and Urethra

OBJECTIVES

After completing Chapter 16, you will be able to:

16.1 Describe the structure, location, and functions of the kidney.
16.2 Define the term *nephron* and describe its structure.
16.3 Explain how nephrons filter blood and form urine.
16.4 List substances normally found in urine.
16.5 Describe the locations, structures, and functions of the ureters, bladder, and urethra.
16.6 Explain how urination is controlled.
16.7 Describe the signs, symptoms, causes, and treatments of various diseases and disorders of the urinary system.

KEY TERMS

afferent arterioles
angiotensin II
calyces
cystitis
detrusor muscle
distal convoluted tubule
efferent arterioles
glomerular capsule
glomerular filtrate
glomerular filtration
glomerulonephritis
glomerulus
incontinence
juxtaglomerular apparatus
juxtaglomerular cells
loop of Henle
macula densa
micturition
nephrons
proximal convoluted tubule
pyelonephritis
renal calculi
renal column
renal corpuscle
renal cortex
renal medulla
renal pelvis
renal pyramids
renal sinus
renal tubule

KEY TERMS *(Continued)*

renin
retroperitoneal
trigone
tubular reabsorption
tubular secretion
urea
ureters
urethra
uric acid

Introduction

The organs of the urinary system are the kidneys, ureters, urinary bladder, and urethra (Figure 16-1). This system functions to remove waste products from the bloodstream. These waste products are excreted from the body in the form of urine. Nephrons are microscopic structures in the kidneys that filter blood and form urine.

CASE STUDY

Last week at his yearly physical, a 53-year-old male patient was diagnosed with high blood pressure. After many tests, the patient was diagnosed as having atherosclerosis of the left renal artery. All routine lab test results were normal, and the patient did not have any endocrine organ disorders.

As you read this chapter, consider the following questions:

1. How does atherosclerosis affect blood flow?
2. How does atherosclerosis of a renal artery produce high blood pressure?
3. What lifestyle changes should this patient make?
4. What can happen to the patient's kidney if his atherosclerosis is not treated?

The Kidneys

The kidneys are responsible for removing metabolic waste products from the blood. These metabolic wastes are combined with water and ions to form urine, which is excreted from the body. The kidneys also secrete the hormone erythropoietin, which helps to regulate red blood cell production, and the hormone **renin,** which helps to regulate blood pressure.

The kidneys are bean-shaped organs that are reddish brown in color. Tough, fibrous capsules cover them. The kidneys are **retroperitoneal** in position, which means that they lie behind the peritoneal cavity. They lie on either side of the vertebral column at about the level of the lumbar vertebrae.

The medial depression of a kidney is called a **renal sinus.** The entrance of the sinus is called the hilum and contains the renal artery, renal vein, and ureter. The **ureter** is a tube that carries urine out of a kidney to the urinary bladder. Inside the kidney, the ureter expands as the **renal pelvis.** The renal pelvis divides into small tubes inside the kidney called **calyces.**

The outermost layer of the kidney is called the **renal cortex,** and the middle portion is called the **renal medulla.** The renal medulla is divided into triangular-shaped areas called **renal pyramids.** The renal cortex covers the pyramids and also dips down between the pyramids. The portion of the cortex between pyramids is called a **renal column** (Figure 16-2.)

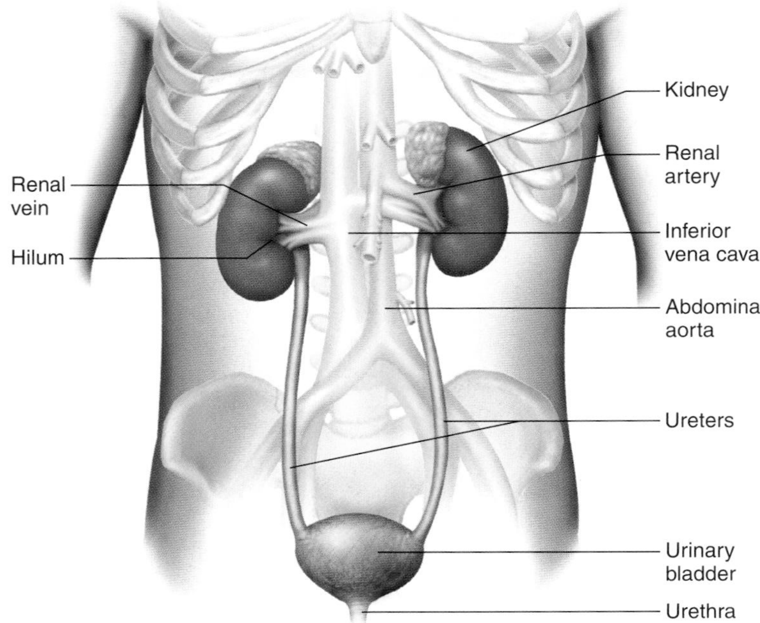

Figure 16-1. Organs of the urinary system.

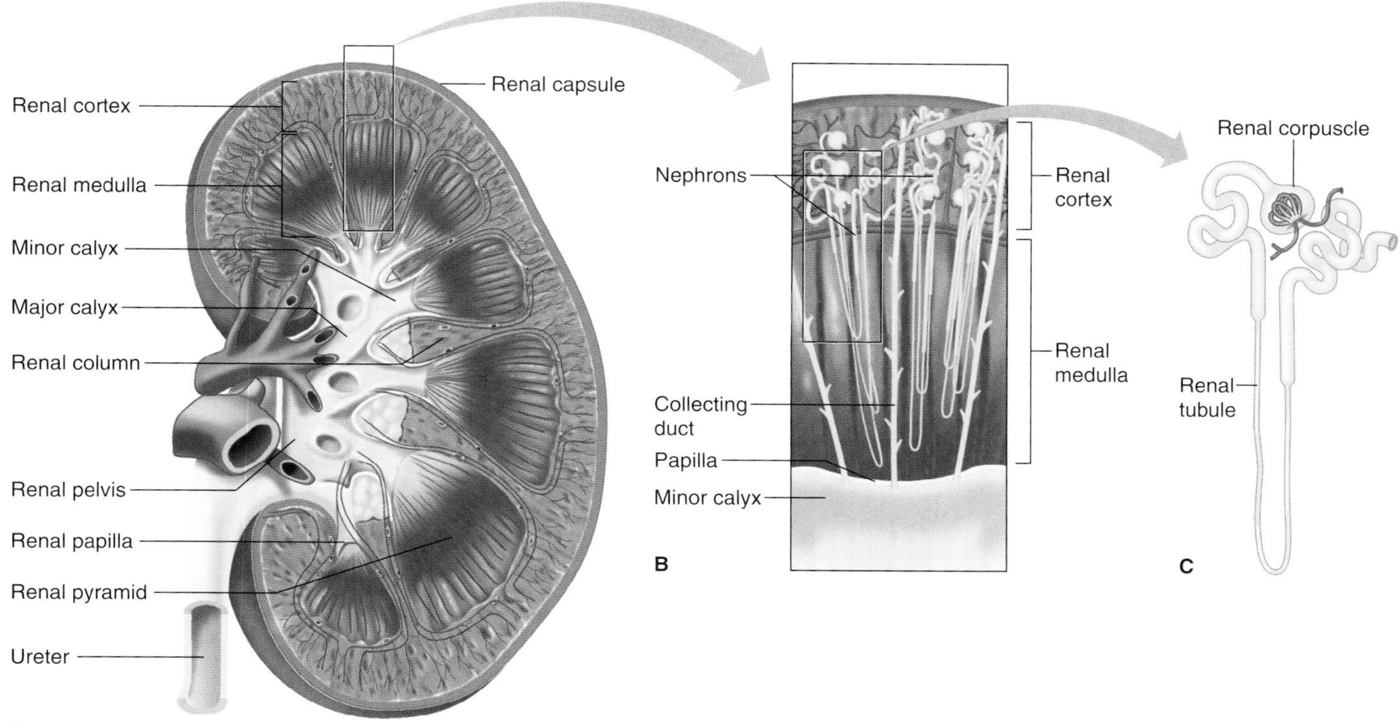

Figure 16-2. (a) Longitudinal section of a kidney, (b) the location of nephrons, and (c) a single nephron.

Blood flows through a kidney by the following pathway:

renal artery → interlobar arteries → arcuate arteries → interlobular arteries → afferent arterioles → nephrons

Blood eventually leaves the kidney through a renal vein.

Nephrons

Waste products are removed from the blood through **nephrons.** Each kidney contains about one million nephrons. Nephrons are made of a **renal corpuscle** and a **renal tubule** (Figure 16-2). A renal corpuscle is composed of a group of capillaries called a **glomerulus,** and the capsule that surrounds the glomerulus is called a **glomerular capsule.** The renal corpuscle is where blood filtration occurs.

Renal tubules extend from the glomerular capsule of a nephron. The three parts of a renal tubule are the **proximal convoluted tubule,** the **loop of Henle,** and the **distal convoluted tubule.** The proximal convoluted tubule is directly attached to the glomerular capsule and eventually straightens out to become the loop of Henle. The loop of Henle curves back toward the renal corpuscle and starts to twist again, becoming the distal convoluted tubule. Distal convoluted tubules from several nephrons merge together to form collecting ducts. These ducts collect urine and deliver it to the renal pelvis, which in turn empties urine into the ureters (Figures 16-2 and 16-3).

Afferent arterioles deliver blood to the glomeruli, and **efferent arterioles** carry blood away from them. Efferent arterioles deliver blood to peritubular capillaries, which are wrapped around the renal tubules of the nephron. Blood leaves the peritubular capillaries through the veins of the kidneys. By the time the blood leaves the peritubular capillaries, it has been cleansed of waste products. Blood flows through a nephron in the following pathway:

afferent arteriole → glomerulus → efferent arteriole → peritubular capillaries → the veins of the kidney

Juxtaglomerular Apparatus. Most nephrons contain a **juxtaglomerular apparatus,** which is made up of two structures—the **macula densa** and **juxtaglomerular cells.** The macula densa is an area of the distal convoluted tubule that touches afferent and efferent arterioles. Juxtaglomerular cells are simply enlarged smooth muscle cells in the walls of either the afferent or efferent arteriole. The juxtaglomerular apparatus secretes the hormone renin, which regulates blood pressure.

Urine Formation

The three processes of urine formation are **glomerular filtration, tubular reabsorption,** and **tubular secretion.**

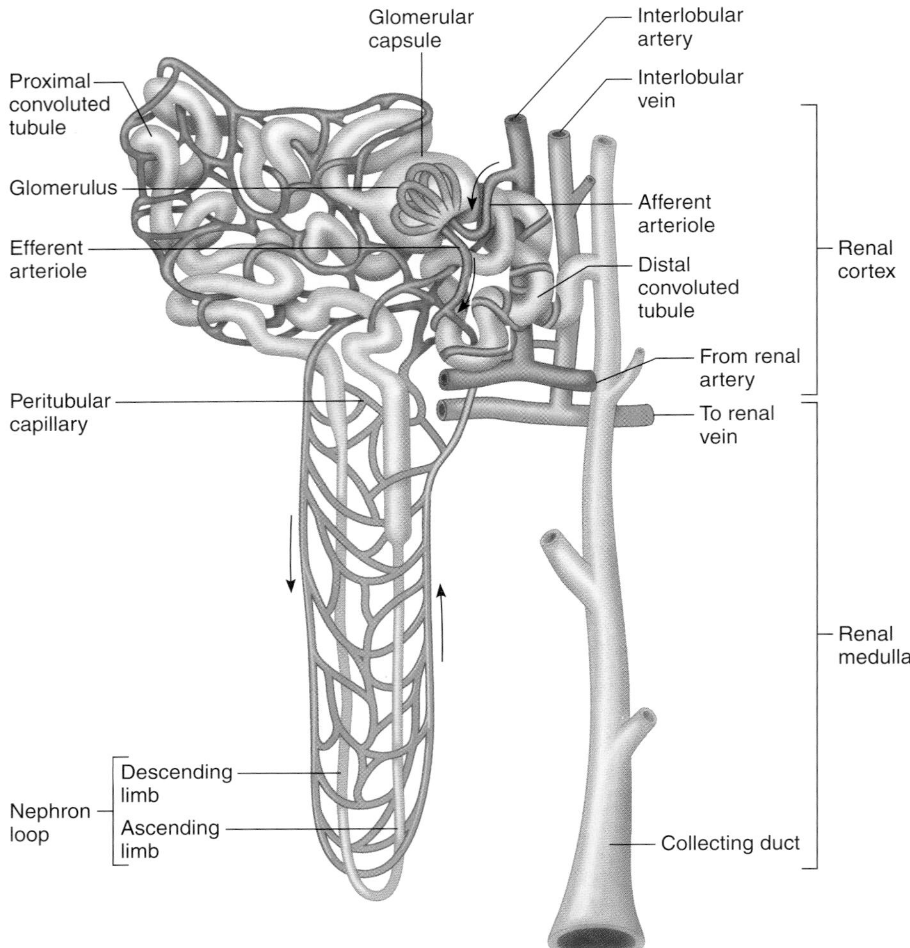

Figure 16-3. Structure of a nephron and its associated blood vessels.

Glomerular Filtration

Glomerular filtration takes place in the renal corpuscles of nephrons. In this process, the fluid part of blood is forced from the glomerulus (the capillaries) into the glomerular capsule (Figure 16-4). The fluid in the glomerular capsule is called the **glomerular filtrate.**

Glomerular filtration depends on filtration pressure, which is the amount of pressure that forces substances out of the glomerulus into the glomerular capsule. It is largely determined by blood pressure. If a person's blood pressure is too low, glomerular filtrate will not form. If filtration pressure increases, the rate of filtration and the amount of glomerular filtrate also increase.

The sympathetic nervous system largely controls the rate of filtration. If blood pressure or blood volume drops, the sympathetic nervous system causes the afferent arterioles in the kidneys to constrict. When afferent arterioles constrict, glomerular filtration pressure decreases and less glomerular filtrate is formed. When less glomerular filtrate is formed, less urine is ultimately formed. This allows the body to retain fluids that are needed to raise blood pressure and blood volume.

The juxtaglomerular apparatus also helps to regulate the filtration rate. When blood pressure drops, juxtaglomerular cells secrete renin. Renin causes the formation of **angiotensin II,** which raises blood pressure and causes the secretion of a hormone called aldosterone. Aldosterone causes the body to retain the fluids needed to maintain blood volume and pressure.

Tubular Reabsorption

Tubular reabsorption is the second process in urine formation. In this process, the glomerular filtrate flows into the proximal convoluted tubule (Figure 16-5a). The body needs to keep many of the substances (nutrients, water, and ions) that are found in glomerular filtrate. In tubular reabsorption, all the necessary substances in the glomerular filtrate pass through the wall of the renal tubule into the blood of the peritubular capillaries.

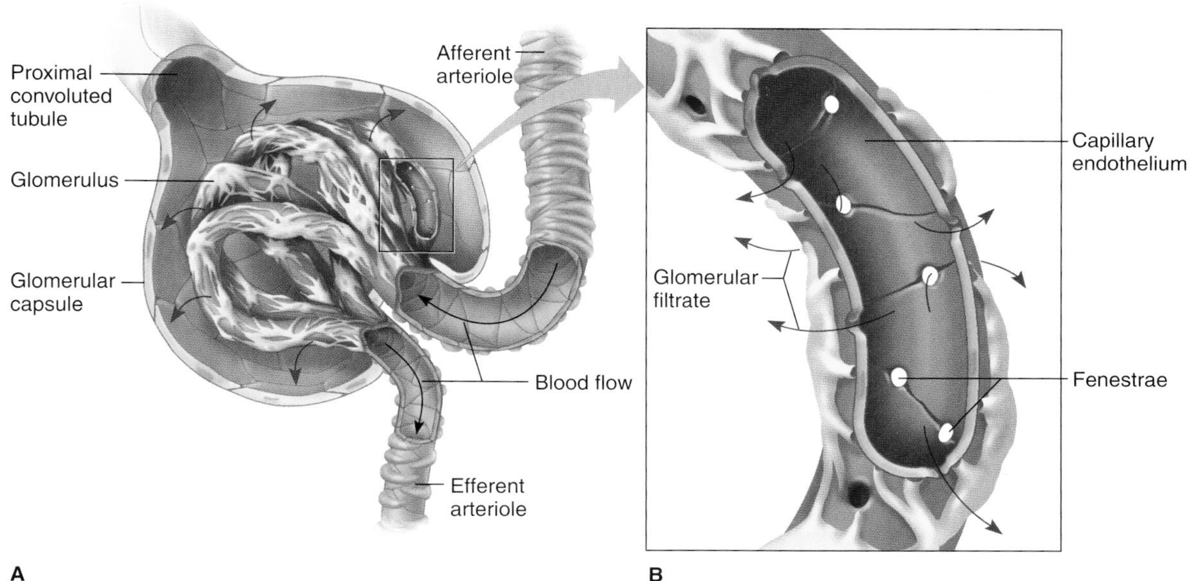

Figure 16-4. Glomerular filtration. (a) Substances move out of glomerular capillaries and into the glomerular capsule. (b) Glomerular capillaries have large holes called fenestrae that allow substances to move out of them and into a glomerular capsule.

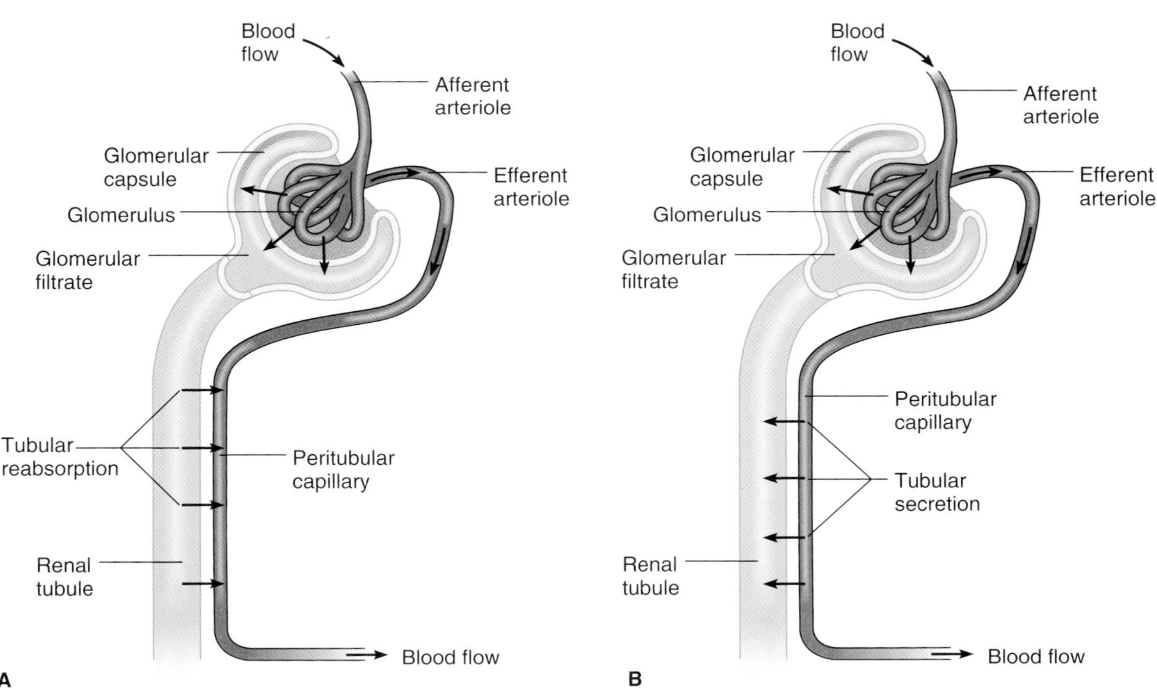

Figure 16-5. (a) Tubular reabsorption. Substances move from the glomerular filtrate into the blood of peritubular capillaries. (b) Tubular secretion. Substances move out of the blood of the peritubular capillaries into the renal tubule.

Water reabsorption varies depending on the presence of two hormones—antidiuretic hormone and aldosterone. Both of these hormones increase water reabsorption, which decreases urine production.

Tubular Secretion

Tubular secretion is the third process of urine formation. In tubular secretion, substances move out of the blood in the peritubular capillaries and into the renal tubules (Figure 16-5b). Substances that are secreted include drugs, hydrogen ions, and waste products. All of these secreted substances will be excreted in the urine.

Urine Composition

The final solution that reaches the collecting ducts of the kidneys is urine. Urine is mostly made of water but also normally contains **urea, uric acid,** trace amounts of amino acids, and various ions. Urea and uric acid are waste products formed by the breakdown of proteins and nucleic acids.

The Ureters, Urinary Bladder, and Urethra

The Ureters

Ureters are long, muscular tubes that carry urine from the kidneys to the urinary bladder. They propel urine toward the bladder through peristalsis.

Urinary Bladder

The urinary bladder is a distensible (expandable) organ that is located in the pelvic cavity. Its function is to store urine until it is eliminated from the body. The internal floor of the bladder contains three openings—one for the urethra and two for the ureters. These three openings form a triangle called the **trigone** of the bladder. The wall of the bladder contains smooth muscle, called the **detrusor muscle.** This muscle contracts to push urine from the bladder into the urethra (Figure 16-6).

The process of urination is called **micturition.** The stretching of the bladder triggers this process. The major events of micturition are the following:

1. The detrusor muscle contracts.
2. The internal urethral sphincter opens. This sphincter is located just above the opening of the urethra. When this sphincter opens, a person feels the urgency to urinate.
3. The external urethral sphincter opens. This sphincter is located below the internal urethral sphincter. A person can voluntarily keep this sphincter closed.
4. When the external urethral sphincter opens, urine flows out of the bladder through the urethra.

The Urethra

The **urethra** is a tube that moves urine from the bladder to the outside world. In females, the urethra is much shorter than in males. For this reason, females are much more susceptible to urinary tract infections.

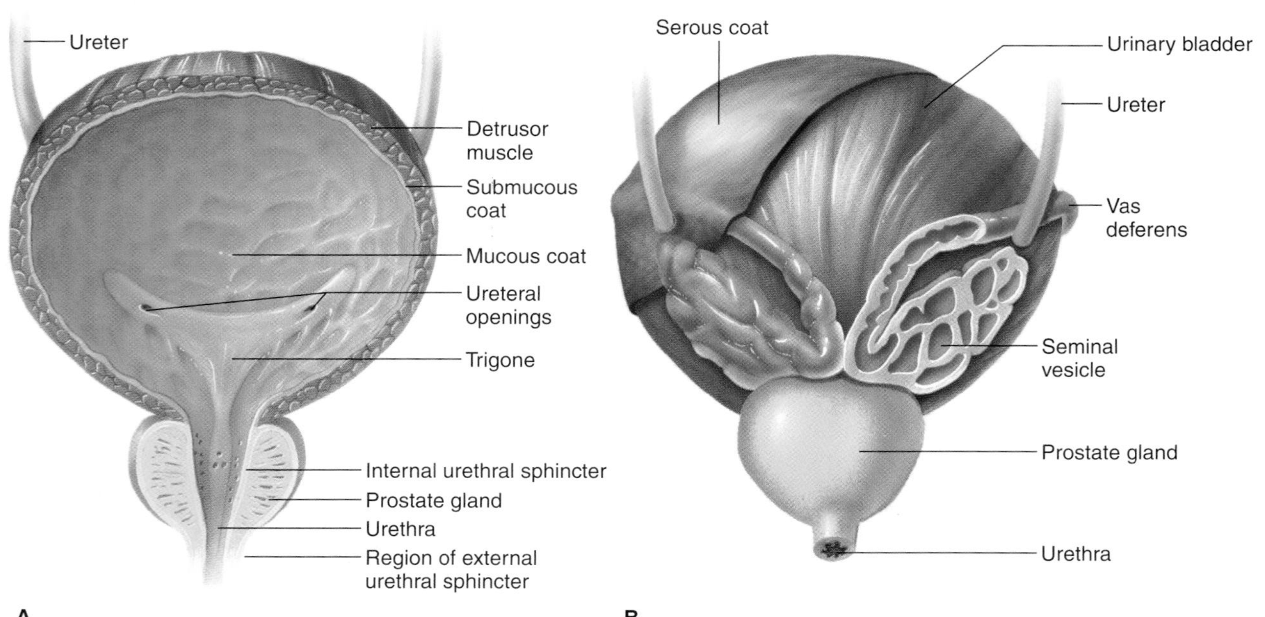

Figure 16-6. Male urinary bladder: (a) anterior view and (b) posterior view.

Pathophysiology

Common Diseases and Disorders of the Urinary System

Acute kidney failure is a sudden loss of kidney function.

- **Causes.** There are many causes and risk factors of kidney failure, including burns, dehydration, low blood pressure, hemorrhaging, allergic reactions, obstruction of the renal artery, various poisons, alcohol abuse, trauma to the kidneys and skeletal muscles, blood disorders, blood transfusion reactions, kidney stones, urinary tract infections, enlarged prostate, childbirth and immune system disorders, and food poisoning involving the bacteria *E. coli*.
- **Signs and symptoms.** The signs and symptoms include decreased urine production or no urine production, excessive urination, swelling of the arms or legs, bloating, mental confusion, coma, seizures, hand tremors, nosebleeds, easy bruising, pain in the back or abdomen, high blood pressure, abnormal heart or lung sounds, abnormal urinalysis, and an increase in potassium levels.
- **Treatment.** The first treatment measure is modifying the diet to decrease the amount of protein consumed. Controlling fluid intake and potassium levels is also recommended. Antibiotics and dialysis may also be needed.

Chronic kidney failure is a condition in which the kidneys slowly lose their ability to function. Sometimes symptoms do not appear until the kidneys have lost about 90% of their function.

- **Causes.** This disorder results from diabetes, high blood pressure, glomerulonephritis, polycystic kidney disease, kidney stones, obstruction of the ureters, and acute kidney failure.
- **Signs and symptoms.** The list of signs and symptoms is extensive and includes headache, mental confusion, coma, seizures, fatigue, frequent hiccups, itching, easy bruising, abnormal bleeding, anemia, excessive thirst, fluid retention, nausea, high blood pressure, abnormal heart or lung sounds, weight loss, white spots on the skin or increased pigmentation, high potassium levels, an increased or decreased urine output, urinary tract infections, and abnormal urinalysis results.
- **Treatment.** This disorder can be treated with antibiotics; blood transfusions; medications to control anemia; restricting the intake of fluids, electrolytes, and protein; controlling high blood pressure; and dialysis. The most serious cases may require surgery to repair an obstruction of the ureters or a kidney transplant.

Cystitis is a urinary bladder infection. Women are much more likely to develop this disorder than men because of the short length of their urethras. The urethral opening in women is also close to the anal opening, allowing bacteria from this area to be more easily introduced into the urinary tract.

- **Causes.** This infection is caused by different types of bacteria (especially those that are found in the rectum) and the placement of a catheter in the bladder. Good hygiene, urinating frequently, and wiping from front to back (for females) can help to prevent this infection.
- **Signs and symptoms.** Common symptoms include fatigue, chills, fever, painful urination, a frequent need to urinate, cloudy urine, and blood in the urine.
- **Treatment.** This infection is treated with antibiotics.

Glomerulonephritis is an inflammation of the glomeruli of the kidney.

- **Causes.** This disorder is caused by renal diseases, immune disorders, and bacterial infections.
- **Signs and symptoms.** The signs and symptoms are hiccups, drowsiness, coma, seizures, nausea, anemia, high blood pressure, increased skin pigmentation, abnormal heart sounds, abnormal urinalysis results, blood in the urine, and a decreased or increased urine output.
- **Treatment.** Treatment begins with a low-sodium, low-protein diet. Medications to control high blood pressure, corticosteroids to reduce inflammation, and dialysis are other treatment options.

Incontinence is a condition in which a person (other than a child) cannot control urination. This condition can be either temporary or long lasting. Women are more likely to develop incontinence than men are.

- **Causes.** This condition can be caused by various medications, excessive coughing (for example, in smokers), urinary tract infections, nervous system disorders, and bladder cancer. In men, prostate problems can lead to the development of this disorder. The weakness of the urinary sphincters from surgery, trauma, or pregnancy can also cause incontinence. It may be prevented by avoiding urinary bladder irritants such as coffee, cigarettes, diuretics, and various medications.
- **Signs and symptoms.** The primary symptom is the involuntary leakage of urine.
- **Treatment.** Treatment includes various medications, incontinence pads, removal of the prostate, Kegel exercises to increase the control of urinary sphincters, and surgery to repair damaged bladders or urethral sphincters.

continued ⟶

Common Diseases and Disorders of the Urinary System *(continued)*

Polycystic kidney disease is a disorder in which the kidneys enlarge because of the presence of many cysts within them. The disease develops relatively slowly, with symptoms worsening over time.

- **Causes.** The causes are hereditary (via an inherited dominant gene from a parent).
- **Signs and symptoms.** Fatigue, high blood pressure, anemia, pain in the back or abdomen, joint pain, heart murmurs, the formation of kidney stones, kidney failure, blood in the urine, and liver disease are the symptoms of this disorder.
- **Treatment.** Treatment includes medications to control anemia and high blood pressure, blood transfusions, draining of the cysts, dialysis, and surgery to remove one or both kidneys.

Pyelonephritis is a type of complicated urinary tract infection. It begins as a bladder infection and spreads to one or both kidneys. This condition can develop suddenly, or it may be long lasting.

- **Causes.** This disorder is caused by bacteria, a bladder infection, kidney stones, or an obstruction of the urinary system ducts.
- **Signs and symptoms.** Signs and symptoms include fatigue, mental confusion, fever, nausea, pain in the back or abdomen, enlarged kidneys, painful urination, and cloudy or bloody urine.
- **Treatment.** Treatment includes intravenous fluids, pain medication, and antibiotics.

Renal calculi are more commonly called kidney stones. These stones can become lodged in the ducts within the kidneys or ureters.

- **Causes.** This condition is caused by gouty arthritis, defects of the ureters, overly concentrated urine, and urinary tract infections.
- **Signs and symptoms.** The signs and symptoms include fever, nausea, severe back or abdominal pain, a frequent urge to urinate, blood in the urine, and abnormal urinalysis results.
- **Treatment.** Treatment includes pain medication, intravenous fluids, medications to decrease stone formation, surgery to remove kidney stones, and lithotripsy (a procedure that uses shock waves to break up stones).

Summary

The kidneys, ureters, bladder, and urethra work together to remove waste products from the blood. The nephrons of the kidneys are involved in urine formation. The ureters, bladder, and urethra are responsible for eliminating urine from the body. The kidneys also play an important role in regulating blood cell production and blood pressure. Knowledge of the anatomy and physiology of the urinary system is important when collecting urine specimens, performing urinary testing, and assisting with cystoscopy.

REVIEW

CHAPTER 16

CASE STUDY QUESTIONS

Now that you have completed this chapter, review the case study at the beginning of the chapter and answer the following questions:

1. How does atherosclerosis affect blood flow?
2. How does atherosclerosis of a renal artery produce high blood pressure?
3. What lifestyle changes should this patient make?
4. What can happen to the patient's kidney if his atherosclerosis is not treated?

Discussion Questions

1. Describe the three steps in the formation of urine.
2. Describe the composition of normal urine.
3. What are the differences between a renal corpuscle and a renal tubule?
4. Explain the functions of the kidneys.

Critical Thinking Questions

1. Why are females more likely than males to develop urinary tract infections?
2. What is the significance of proteins in urine?
3. The position of the kidneys is retroperitoneal. What would be the easiest way for a surgeon to reach a kidney?
4. What effect would vascular shock have on urine production?

Application Activities

1. Define the following parts of a kidney:
   a. Renal pyramid
   b. Renal cortex
   c. Renal medulla
   d. Renal pelvis
2. Name the three openings of the urinary bladder.
3. What is the name of the tubes that carry urine from the kidneys to the bladder?
4. What is the name of the tube that carries urine from the bladder to the outside world?

CHAPTER 17

The Reproductive System

KEY TERMS

acrosome
alveolar glands
amnion
areola
blastocyst
bulbourethral glands
cervical orifice
cervicitis
cervix
cleavage
clitoris
corpus luteum
ductus arteriosus
ductus venosus
dysmenorrhea
ectoderm
embryonic period
endoderm
endometriosis
endometrium
epididymis
epididymitis
erectile tissue
fallopian tubes
fertilization
fetal period
fibroid
fimbriae
follicular cells
foramen ovale
glans penis
gonadotropin-releasing hormone (GnRH)
human chorionic gonadotropin (HCG)

CHAPTER OUTLINE

- The Male Reproductive System
- The Female Reproductive System
- Sexually Transmitted Diseases
- Pregnancy
- The Birth Process
- Contraception
- Infertility

OBJECTIVES

After completing Chapter 17, you will be able to:

17.1 List the organs of the male reproductive system and give the locations, structures, and functions of each.
17.2 Describe how sperm cells are formed.
17.3 List the actions of testosterone.
17.4 Describe the substances found in semen.
17.5 Describe the processes of erection and ejaculation.
17.6 Describe the causes, signs and symptoms, and treatment of various disorders of the male reproductive system.
17.7 List the organs of the female reproductive system and give the locations, structures, and functions of each.
17.8 Explain how eggs develop.
17.9 List the actions of estrogen and progesterone.
17.10 Explain how and when ovulation occurs.
17.11 Describe what happens to an egg after ovulation occurs.
17.12 List the purpose and events of the menstrual cycle.
17.13 Define menopause and explain what causes it.
17.14 List the most common sexually transmitted diseases and give the signs, symptoms, causes, and treatments of each.
17.15 Explain how and where fertilization occurs.
17.16 Describe the process of implantation.
17.17 Explain the difference between an embryo and a fetus.
17.18 Describe the changes that occur in a woman during pregnancy.
17.19 List several birth control methods and explain why they are effective.
17.20 List the causes and treatment of infertility.
17.21 Describe the causes, signs and symptoms, and treatment of various disorders of the female reproductive system.

KEY TERMS *(Continued)*

hysterectomy
impotence
infundibulum
inner cell mass
interstitial cell
labia majora
labia minora
lactogen
mammary glands
menopause
menses
menstrual cycle
mesoderm
mons pubis
morula
myometrium
neonatal period
neonate
oocyte
oogenesis
ovulation
parathyroid hormone
perimetrium
placenta
polar body
postnatal period
premenstrual syndrome (PMS)
prenatal period
prepuce
primary germ layer
primordial follicle
prostate gland
prostatitis
relaxin
scrotum
semen
seminal vesicles
seminiferous tubules
spermatids
spermatocytes
spermatogenesis
spermatogenic cells
spermatogonia
testes
umbilical cord
uterus
vagina
vaginitis
vas deferens
vasectomy
vestibular glands
yolk sac
zona pellucida
zygote

Introduction

The male and female reproductive systems function together to produce offspring. The female reproductive system nurtures a developing offspring. If a female breast-feeds, her reproductive system is also used to nurture a newborn baby. The male and female reproductive systems also produce a number of important hormones.

CASE STUDY

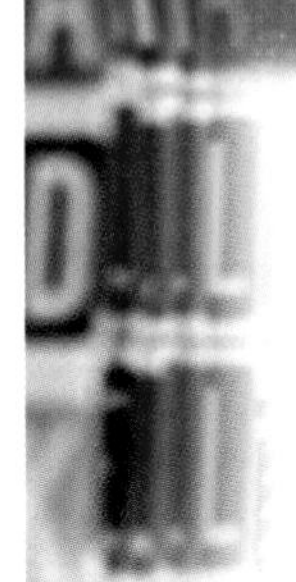

Last week, a 27-year-old female came to the doctor's office complaining of abnormal vaginal discharge, pain during urination, and pain in her abdominopelvic area. Her symptoms have been occurring for a couple of weeks but have recently started to get worse. She says that her sexual partner also has abnormal discharge coming from his penis but is not experiencing any pain. The doctor diagnoses her with a urinary tract infection and a sexually transmitted disease caused by bacteria. The doctor also tells the patient that she has peritonitis, which is inflammation in the abdominopelvic cavity. The patient is treated with antibiotics and pain medication. The doctor tells her that her sexual partner must also be treated with antibiotics.

As you read this chapter, consider the following questions:

1. What sexually transmitted diseases are caused by bacteria?
2. How did the infection spread to the patient's abdominopelvic cavity?
3. Why is her sexual partner not experiencing pain in his abdominopelvic cavity?
4. Why is it important for her sexual partner to be treated with antibiotics?
5. Why is it common for women with sexually transmitted diseases to also have urinary tract infections?

The Male Reproductive System

Testes

Testes are the primary organs of the male reproductive system because they produce the sex cells (sperm) of the male (Figure 17-1). They also make the male hormone **testosterone.** Most males have two testes that are held just below the pelvic cavity in the **scrotum.** A fibrous capsule encloses each testis and invades the testis to divide it into lobules. Each lobule is filled with **seminiferous tubules,** which are filled with **spermatogenic cells.** These cells give rise to sperm cells. Between the seminiferous tubules are cells called **interstitial cells** that make testosterone.

Sperm Cell Formation. Spermatogenic cells of the seminiferous tubules begin the process of making sperm

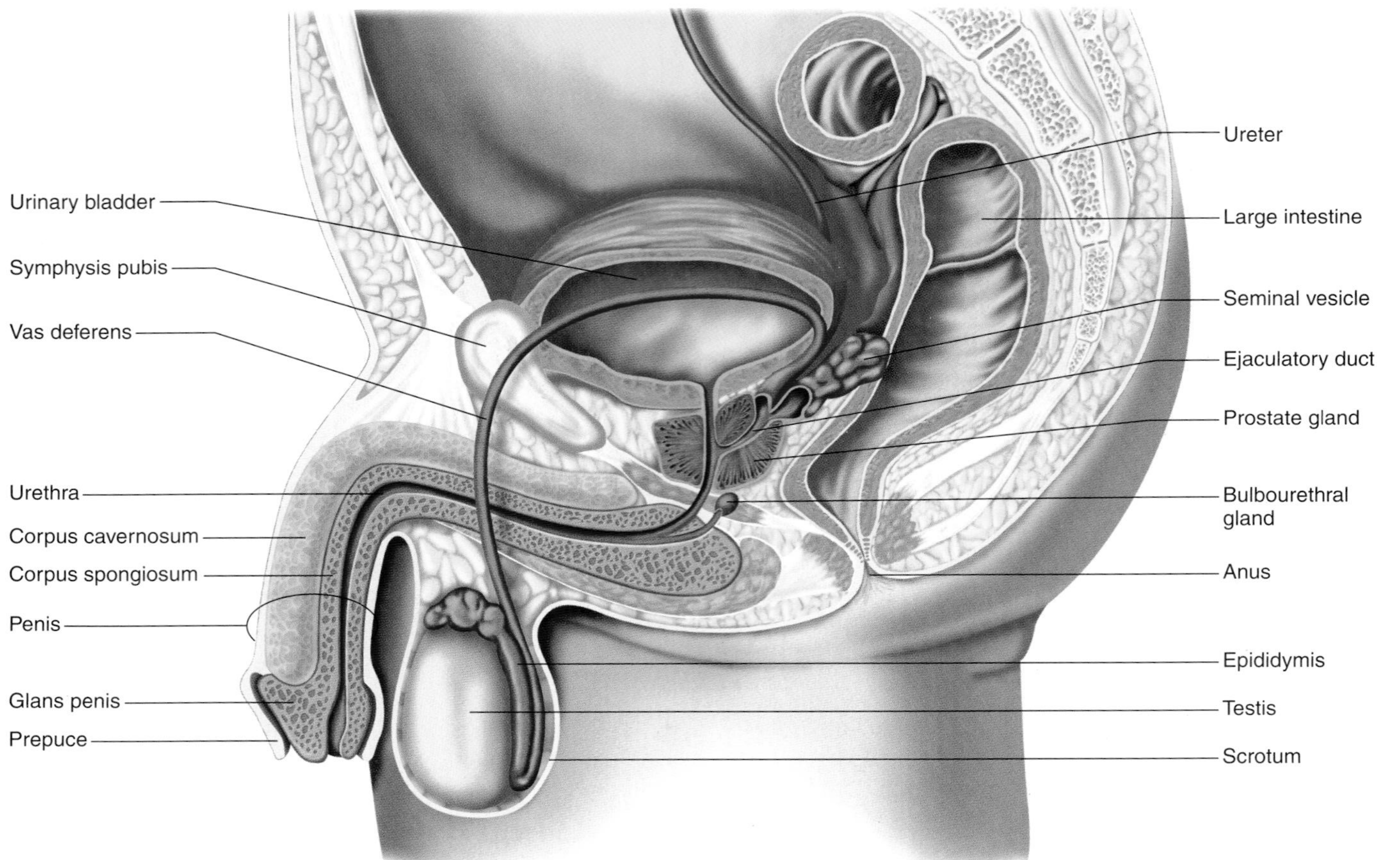

Figure 17-1. Sagittal view of male reproductive organs. The male reproductive system produces sperm and delivers them in a form that keeps them viable long enough to fertilize an egg.

cells, but the sperm cells do not mature until they go to the **epididymis. Spermatogenesis** is the process of sperm cell formation. At the beginning of spermatogenesis, spermatogenic cells are called **spermatogonia.** Spermatogonia contain 46 chromosomes. These cells undergo mitosis, and the resulting cells are called primary **spermatocytes.** Primary spermatocytes also contain 46 chromosomes, which is the normal number of chromosomes. At about the time of puberty, primary spermatocytes undergo a process called **meiosis.** In meiosis, each primary spermatocyte divides to make two secondary spermatocytes. Each secondary spermatocyte divides to make two **spermatids.** Therefore, from one primary spermatocyte, four spermatids are formed. Spermatids develop flagella to become mature sperm cells. They contain only 23 chromosomes (Figure 17-2).

Structure of Sperm Cells. A mature sperm (Figure 17-3) has following three parts: the head, the midpiece, and the tail.

The Head. The head is oval in structure and holds a nucleus with 23 chromosomes. The head is covered with an enzyme-filled sac called an **acrosome,** which helps the sperm penetrate an egg at the time of fertilization.

The Midpiece. This portion of the sperm is between the head and tail. It is filled with mitochondria that generate the energy needed by the cell to move.

The Tail. The tail is a flagellum that moves in such a way as to propel the sperm forward in the female reproductive tract.

Internal Accessory Organs of the Male Reproductive System

The internal accessory organs of the male reproductive system are the epididymis, **vas deferens, seminal vesicles, prostate gland,** and **bulbourethral glands.**

Epididymis. An epididymis sits on top of each testis. It is a highly coiled tube that receives spermatids from seminiferous tubules as these cells are formed. Inside the epididymis, spermatids mature to become sperm cells.

Vas Deferens. A tube called a vas deferens is connected to each epididymis. These tubes carry sperm cells from an epididymis to the urethra in the pelvic cavity of the male. When a male has a **vasectomy,** this is the tube that is cut and tied.

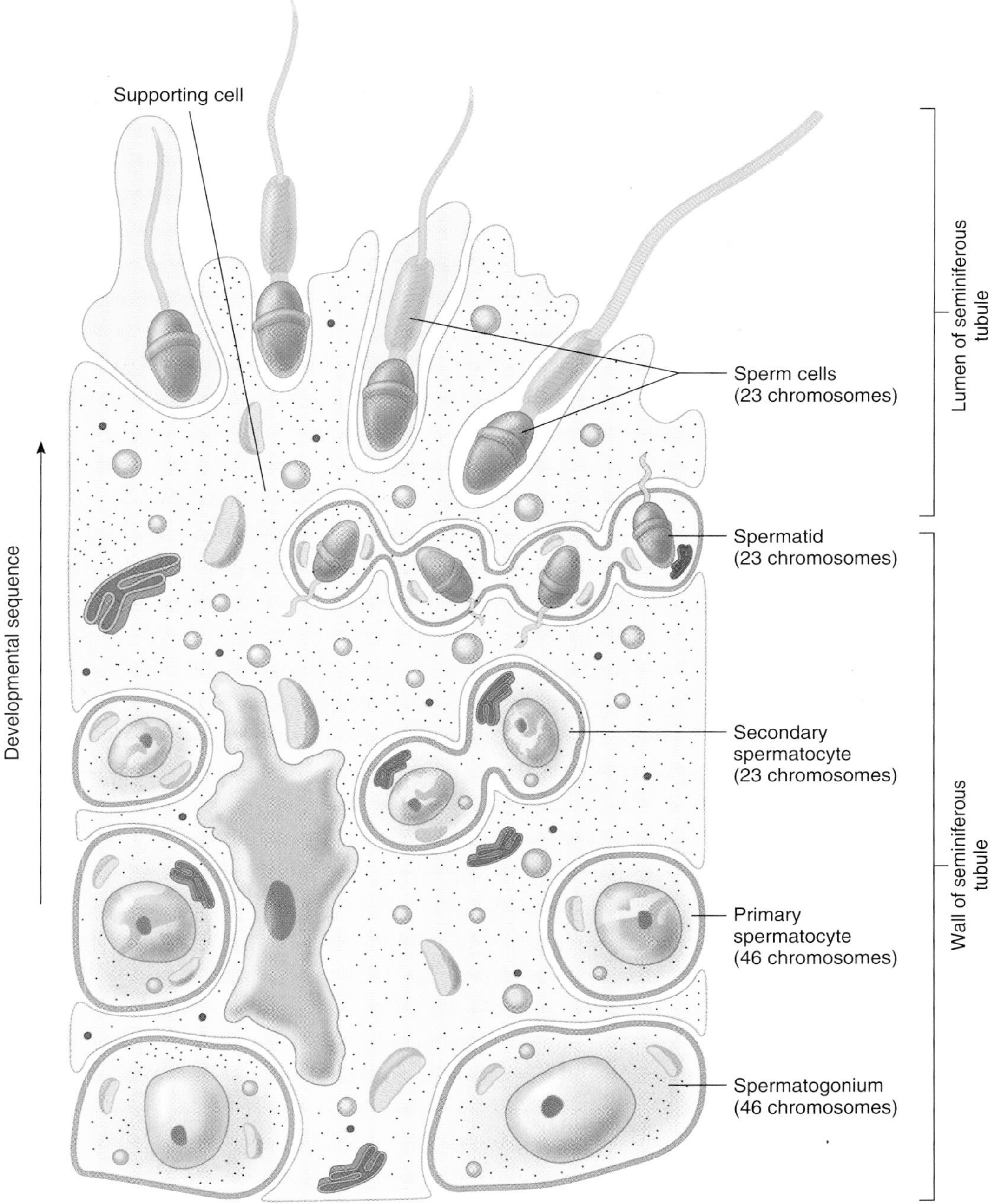

Figure 17-2. The process of spermatogenesis.

Seminal Vesicle. Seminal vesicles are sac-like organs that secrete an alkaline fluid rich in sugars and **prostaglandins.** The sugars are used by sperm cells to make energy, and the prostaglandins stimulate muscular contractions in the female reproductive system. These muscular contractions help to propel sperm forward in the female reproductive tract. Seminal vesicles release their product into the vas deferens just before ejaculation.

Prostate Gland. The prostate gland surrounds the proximal portion of the urethra. It makes a milky, alkaline fluid and secretes this fluid into the urethra just before ejaculation. This fluid helps to protect the sperm when they enter the female reproductive system.

Bulbourethral Glands. Bulbourethral glands are inferior to the prostate gland. They make a mucus-like fluid that is secreted before ejaculation into the urethra. This fluid lubricates the end of the penis in preparation for sexual intercourse.

Semen. **Semen** is a mixture of sperm cells and fluids from the seminal vesicles, prostate gland, and bulbourethral glands. This mixture is alkaline and contains

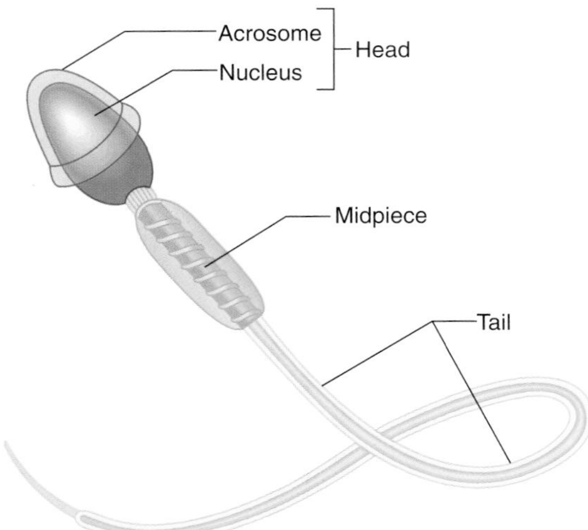

Figure 17-3. Parts of a mature sperm cell.

nutrients and prostaglandins. One milliliter of semen usually contains about 120 million sperm cells.

External Organs of the Male Reproductive System

The two male external reproductive organs are the scrotum and the penis (Figure 17-1).

Scrotum. The scrotum is a pouch of skin that holds the testes. It is lined with a serous membrane that secretes serous fluid to ensure that the testes move freely within it.

Penis. The penis is a cylindrical organ that moves urine and semen to the outside world. The body, or shaft, of the penis contains specialized tissue called **erectile tissue.** The urethra runs the length of the penis. The end of the penis is enlarged into a cone-shaped structure called the **glans penis.** If a male has not been circumcised, a piece of skin, called the **prepuce,** covers the glans penis. The function of the penis is to deliver sperm to the female reproductive tract. The penis also functions in urination because it contains the urethra.

Erection, Orgasm, and Ejaculation

During sexual arousal, the parasympathetic nervous system causes erectile tissue of the penis to become engorged with blood, which produces erection of the penis. During orgasm, sperm cells are propelled out of the testes toward the urethra. The secretions of the prostate, seminal vesicles, and bulbourethral glands are also released into the urethra. The movement of the sperm and secretions into the urethra is called emission. The process of ejaculation occurs when semen is forced out of the urethra. After ejaculation, sympathetic nerve fibers cause the erectile tissue to release blood, and the penis gradually returns to a nonerect state.

Male Reproductive Hormones

The hypothalamus, anterior pituitary gland, and the testes secrete hormones that regulate male reproductive functions. At the onset of puberty, the hypothalamus releases a hormone called **gonadotropin-releasing hormone (GnRH).** GnRH stimulates the anterior pituitary gland to release **follicle-stimulating hormone (FSH)** and **luteinizing hormone (LH).** FSH causes spermatogenesis to begin, and LH stimulates interstitial cells to produce testosterone.

Testosterone stimulates the development of male secondary sex characteristics, which are defined as characteristics that are typically unique to males. Examples of these characteristics are chest hair, thick facial hair, enlarged muscles, enlarged bones, and thickening of vocal cords that produces a deep voice. Testosterone also stimulates the maturation of male reproductive organs.

Testosterone levels in the male are regulated by a negative feedback mechanism. When testosterone levels in the blood increase above normal, the hypothalamus no longer releases GnRH. Therefore, the anterior pituitary gland no longer secretes LH and FSH, which causes testosterone levels to fall. When testosterone levels fall below normal, the hypothalamus begins to secrete GnRH again, which causes the anterior pituitary gland to release LH and FSH again. Testosterone levels begin to rise again, and the cycle repeats itself.

Pathophysiology

Common Diseases and Disorders of the Male Reproductive System

Epididymitis is inflammation of an epididymis. Most cases start out as an infection of the urinary tract that spreads to an epididymis.

- **Causes.** The causes include the use of certain medications, placement of a catheter in the urethra, and bacteria—especially those that cause gonorrhea and chlamydia.
- **Signs and symptoms.** Signs and symptoms include fever, pain in the testes, a lump in the testes, swelling of the scrotum, painful ejaculation, blood in the semen, pain during urination, discharge from the urethra, and enlarged lymph nodes in the pelvic area.
- **Treatment.** Treatment includes pain medication, antibiotics for both the patient and his sexual partner,

continued ⟶

Common Diseases and Disorders of the Male Reproductive System *(continued)*

elevation of the scrotum, and ice packs applied to the scrotum.

Erectile dysfunction is more commonly called **impotence.** It is a disorder in which a male cannot maintain an erect penis to complete sexual intercourse. It is estimated that half of all men between the ages of 40 and 70 have some degree of impotence. Most causes are physical and not psychological.

- **Causes.** Anxiety and depression can cause erectile dysfunction. Common causes include diabetes, high blood pressure, anemia, coronary artery disease, peripheral vascular problems, low testosterone production, various medications, smoking, excessive alcohol consumption, and drugs such as cocaine, marijuana, and heroin.
- **Signs and symptoms.** Signs and symptoms are an inability to achieve an erection and an inability to maintain an erection long enough to complete sexual intercourse.
- **Treatment.** The first treatment step should be lifestyle changes to quit smoking and stop using alcohol or drugs. Counseling to reduce anxiety and depression may also be helpful. Other treatment options include various medications, penile implants, and penile injections of medications if oral medications do not work.

Prostate cancer is the third most common cause of cancer death in men of all ages, although it most frequently occurs in men over the age of 40. In the United States, most cases of prostate cancer are diagnosed before they cause signs or symptoms because most men over age 40 are screened regularly.

- **Causes.** The causes are mostly unknown, although decreased testosterone production may contribute to the development of this disease.
- **Signs and symptoms.** Common symptoms include anemia, weight loss, incontinence, difficult urination, painful urination, pain in the lower back or abdomen, pain during bowel movements, high levels of PSA (a specific type of antigen) in the blood, blood in the urine, and bone pain in advanced cases.
- **Treatment.** Treatments are hormone therapy, chemotherapy, radiation therapy to destroy the tumor, and surgery to remove the prostate.

Prostatitis is an inflammation of the prostate gland. If it develops suddenly, it is called *acute prostatitis.* The slow development of this condition is termed *chronic prostatitis.*

- **Causes.** This condition can be caused by excessive alcohol consumption, a bacterial infection, a catheter in the urethra, trauma to the urethra or urinary bladder, and scarring of the urethra or prostate due to frequent infections. Urinating frequently can help to prevent infection.
- **Signs and symptoms.** Signs and symptoms include fever; pain in the scrotum, pelvic area, or abdomen; difficult urination; frequent urination; painful urination; blood in the urine; painful ejaculation; blood in the semen; discharge from the urethra; a low sperm count; and white blood cells in urine or semen.
- **Treatment.** This condition is treated with antibiotics and may also be treated with surgery to repair damage to the urethra.

The Female Reproductive System

Ovaries and Egg Cell Formation

The ovaries are the primary sex organs of the female because they produce the sex cells (eggs) of the female (Figures 17-4 and 17-5). They also produce **estrogen** and **progesterone.** Most females have two ovaries. They are oval in shape and are located in the pelvic cavity. Each ovary is divided into an inner area called the medulla and an outer area called the cortex. The medulla contains nerves, lymphatic vessels, and many blood vessels. The cortex contains small masses of cells called ovarian follicles. Epithelial tissue and dense connective tissue cover each ovary.

Before a female child is born, **primordial follicles** develop in her ovarian cortex. Each primordial follicle contains a large cell called a primary **oocyte** (immature egg) and smaller cells called **follicular cells.** Unlike males, who make sperm cells throughout their entire life, a female is born with the maximum number of primary oocytes she will ever produce.

Oogenesis is the process of egg cell formation. At the onset of puberty, some primary oocytes are stimulated to continue meiosis. When a primary oocyte divides, it becomes one **polar body** (a nonfunctional cell) and a secondary oocyte. It is the secondary oocyte that is released from an ovary each month during a process called **ovulation.** When the secondary oocyte is fertilized, it divides to form a mature, fertilized egg cell. Therefore, the process of meiosis begins before a female is born and is completed only if a secondary oocyte is fertilized. The mature egg cell contains 23 chromosomes; when it combines with a sperm cell, the resulting cell contains 46 chromosomes.

Internal Accessory Organs of the Female Reproductive System

The female reproductive internal accessory organs are the **fallopian tubes, uterus,** and **vagina.**

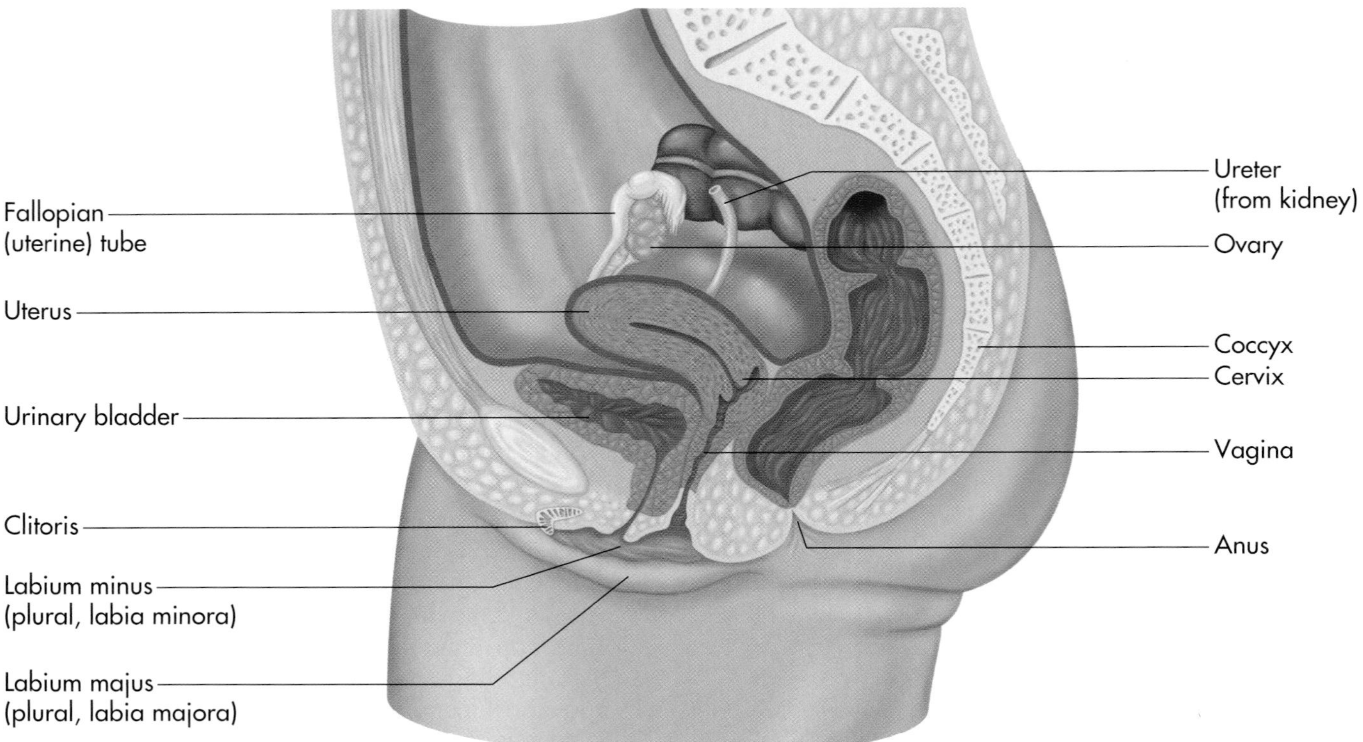

Figure 17-4. Sagittal view of female reproductive organs. The female reproductive system produces eggs for fertilization and provides the place and means for a fertilized egg to develop.

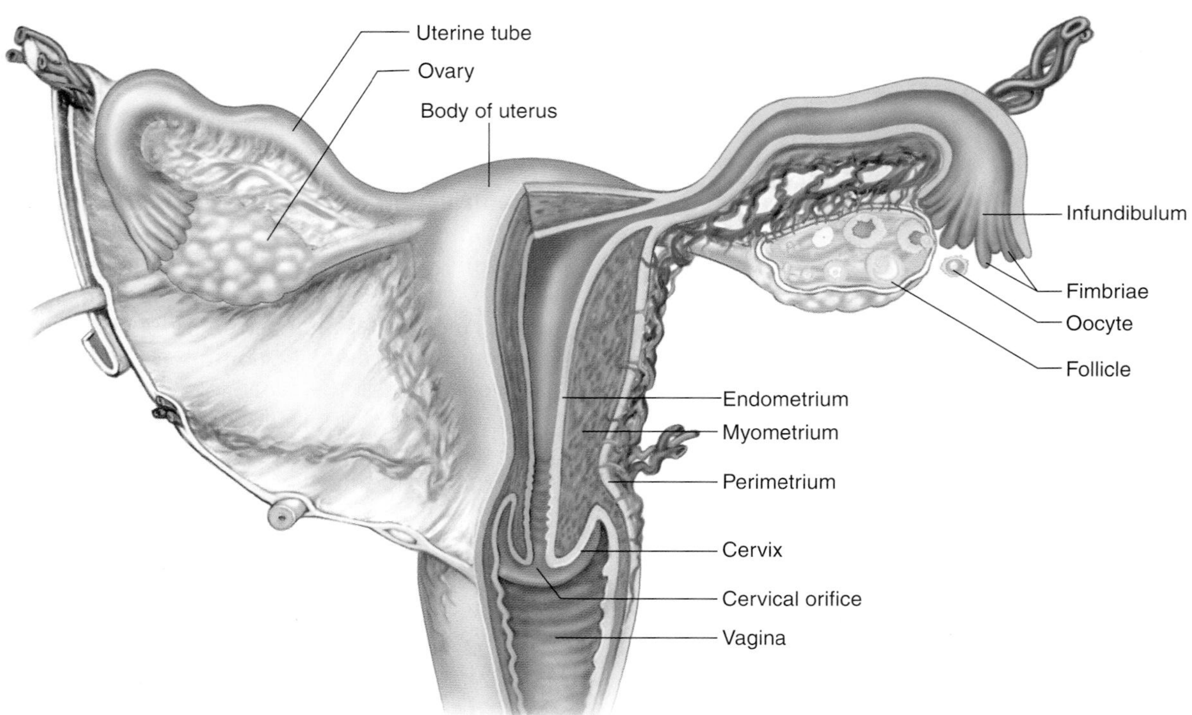

Figure 17-5. Anterior view of internal female reproductive organs. Ovulation of an oocyte is also demonstrated.

Fallopian Tubes. A fallopian tube opens near each ovary and into the uterus. The end of a fallopian tube near an ovary is expanded and is called an **infundibulum** and **fimbriae.** The infundibulum and its fimbriae function to "catch" a secondary oocyte as it leaves an ovary. Fallopian tubes are lined with ciliated cells that sweep the oocyte toward the uterus.

Uterus. The uterus is a hollow, muscular organ that functions to receive an embryo and sustain its development. The upper two-thirds of the uterus is called the body of the uterus, and the narrow, lower portion of the uterus, that extends into the vagina is called the **cervix.** The opening of the cervix is called the **cervical orifice.**

The wall of the uterus has three layers—the **endometrium, myometrium,** and **perimetrium.** The endometrium is the innermost lining of the uterus and contains numerous tubular glands that secrete mucus. The myometrium is the middle, thick, muscular layer. The perimetrium is a thin layer that covers the myometrium. It secretes serous fluid that coats the uterus.

Vagina. The vagina is a tubular organ that extends from the uterus to the outside of the body. It functions to receive an erect penis during sexual intercourse, and it provides an open passageway for uterine secretions and offspring. The opening of the vagina is posterior to the urinary opening and anterior to the anal opening. The wall of the vagina has three layers—an innermost mucosal layer that secretes mucus, a middle muscular layer, and an outermost fibrous layer.

External Accessory Organs of the Female Reproductive System

Mammary glands are the accessory organs of the female reproductive system (Figure 17-6). They secrete milk after pregnancy.

Mammary glands are located beneath the skin in the breast area. A nipple is located near the center of each breast. The pigmented area that surrounds the nipple is called the **areola.** Each gland is made of 15 to 20 lobes and contains **alveolar glands** that make milk under the influence of the hormone prolactin. The hormone oxytocin induces alveolar ducts to deliver milk through openings in the nipples. Therefore, if a woman wants to breast-feed, she must produce adequate amounts of prolactin and oxytocin.

External Organs of the Female Reproductive System

The female external reproductive organs are the **labia majora, labia minora,** and **clitoris**.

Labia Majora. The labia majora are rounded folds of adipose tissue and skin that serve to protect the other external female reproductive organs. At their anterior ends, the labia majora form the **mons pubis,** which is a fatty area that overlies the pubic bones. The labia majora and mons pubis are typically covered in pubic hair in post-pubescent females.

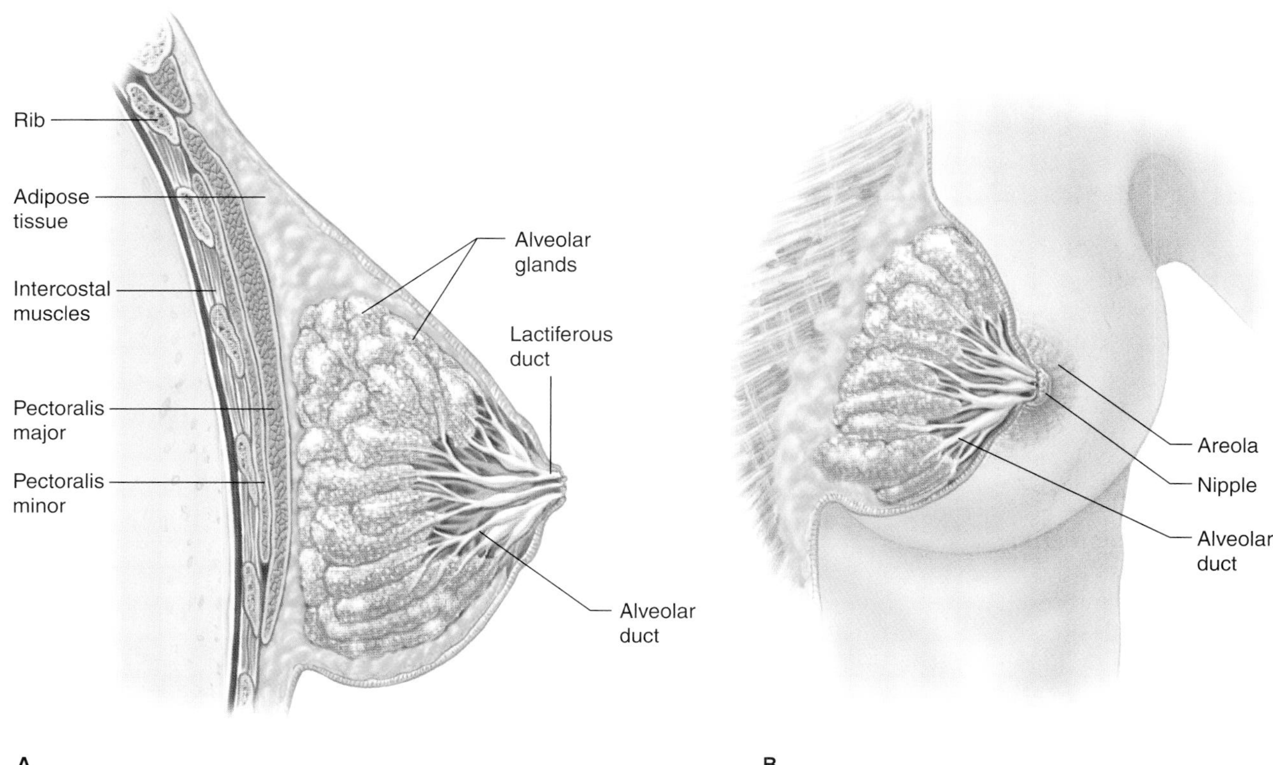

Figure 17-6. Mammary glands: (a) sagittal view and (b) anterior view.

Labia Minora. The labia minora are folds of skin between the labia majora. They are pinkish in color because of their high degree of vascularity. They merge together anteriorly to form a hood over the clitoris.

The space enclosed by the labia minora is called the vestibule. **Vestibular glands** secrete mucus into this area during sexual arousal. This mucus facilitates insertion of the penis into the vagina.

Clitoris. The clitoris is anterior to the urethral opening. It contains erectile tissue and is rich in sensory nerves.

Erection, Lubrication, and Orgasm

During sexual arousal, nervous stimulation causes the clitoris to become erect and the vestibular glands to become active. At the same time, the vagina elongates. If the clitoris is sufficiently stimulated, an orgasm occurs. During orgasm, the walls of the uterus and fallopian tubes contract to help propel sperm toward the upper ends of the fallopian tubes.

Female Reproductive Hormones

At the onset of puberty, the hypothalamus secretes increasing amounts of GnRH. GnRH causes the anterior pituitary gland to release FSH and LH. FSH and LH then stimulate the ovary to produce estrogen, progesterone, and mature follicles. Estrogen and progesterone also stimulate enlargement of the reproductive organs and the production of female secondary sex characteristics, which are characteristics that are typically unique to females. They include breast development, increased vascularization of the skin, and increased fat deposits in the breasts, thighs, and hips.

Female Reproductive Cycle

The female reproductive cycle is also called the **menstrual cycle.** It consists of regular changes in the uterine lining that leads to a monthly "period," or bleeding. **Menopause** is the termination of the menstrual cycle because of normal aging of the ovaries. The following steps are the major hormonal changes that occur during one reproductive cycle:

1. The anterior pituitary gland releases FSH. FSH stimulates an ovarian follicle to mature.
2. The maturing follicle secretes estrogen. Estrogen causes the uterine lining to thicken.
3. The anterior pituitary gland releases a sudden surge of LH. The LH surge triggers ovulation.
4. Following ovulation, follicular cells of the follicle become a **corpus luteum.**
5. The corpus luteum secretes progesterone, which causes the uterine lining to become more vascular and glandular.
6. If the released oocyte is not fertilized, the corpus luteum degenerates.
7. The degenerating corpus luteum causes estrogen and progesterone levels to fall. The decline in estrogen and progesterone levels causes the uterine lining to break down, and bleeding **(menses)** starts.
8. When the anterior pituitary releases FSH, the reproductive cycle begins again.

Pathophysiology

Common Diseases and Disorders of the Female Reproductive System

Breast cancer affects approximately one in eight women. Depending on tumor size and how far cancer cells have spread, breast cancer is classified in stages from 0 to 4, with stage 4 cancer being the most serious. Early diagnosis through regular mammograms and self-breast examinations greatly increases the success of treatment.

- **Causes.** The causes are largely unknown, although breast cancer may be related to hormonal changes or the presence of certain genes.
- **Signs and symptoms.** Signs and symptoms include a lump in the breast that is usually painless and firm, a lump in the armpit, discharge from the nipples, dimpled skin on the breast or nipple, and breast pain. Swelling of the arm and bone pain may be present in advanced cases.
- **Treatment.** Nonsurgical treatment methods include hormone therapy, radiation therapy, and chemotherapy. Surgical options include surgery to remove affected lymph nodes, lumpectomy (surgery to remove a lump), and mastectomy (surgery to remove a breast).

Cervical cancer develops slowly and most of the time is treatable without removing the uterus. Early screening for cervical cancer is successful with a yearly Pap smear, which is a test that looks for abnormal cells in the cervix.

- **Causes.** A weak immune system may be a factor in the development of this cancer. It can also be caused by sexual intercourse early in life, multiple sexual partners, and infection with the human papilloma virus.
- **Signs and symptoms.** Primary symptoms include frequent vaginal discharge, sporadic vaginal bleeding, vaginal bleeding after sexual intercourse, and abnormal cells in the cervix. Patients who are in later stages of this disease may experience pain in the pelvic area or legs, or bone fractures.

continued ⟶

Common Diseases and Disorders of the Female Reproductive System *(continued)*

- **Treatment.** Radiation therapy, chemotherapy, the removal of diseased tissue, and the removal of the uterus **(hysterectomy)** are the treatments for this disease.

Cervicitis is defined as an inflammation of the cervix, which is usually caused by an infection.

- **Causes.** Causes include bacterial or viral infections and allergic reactions to spermicidal creams and latex condoms.
- **Signs and symptoms.** Frequent vaginal discharge, pain during intercourse, and vaginal bleeding after intercourse are common signs and symptoms.
- **Treatment.** This condition is treated with antibiotics and by changing the method of contraception.

Dysmenorrhea is the condition of experiencing severe menstrual cramps that limit normal daily activities. It is a common cause of lost time from work for women.

- **Causes.** Causes include anxiety, endometriosis, pelvic inflammatory disease, fibroid tumors in the uterus, ovarian cysts, abnormally high levels of prostaglandins, and multiple sexual partners.
- **Signs and symptoms.** Common symptoms are abdominal pains, including sharp or dull pain in the pelvic area.
- **Treatment.** Nonsurgical treatments include pain medication, anti-inflammatory drugs, medications that inhibit prostaglandin formation, oral contraceptives, and antibiotics in the case of pelvic inflammatory disease. Surgical treatments include hysterectomy and surgery to remove cysts or fibroids.

Endometriosis is a condition in which tissues that make up the lining of the uterus grow outside the uterus.

- **Causes.** The cause of this disorder is unknown; it may be inherited.
- **Signs and symptoms.** Signs and symptoms include infertility, heavy bleeding from the uterus, pain in the abdomen or pelvis, painful periods, spotting between periods, and pain during sexual intercourse.
- **Treatment.** Oral contraceptives, pain medications, and various hormone therapies may be prescribed. Surgical treatments include laser surgery to remove endometrial tissue outside the uterus, and hysterectomy.

Fibrocystic breast disease is the presence of abnormal tissue in the breasts. It is a common disorder and occurs in more than 60% of women in the United States between the ages of 30 and 50. It is rare in women who have gone through menopause.

- **Causes.** This disorder is caused by hormonal changes associated with the menstrual cycle and various dietary substances (for example, caffeine).
- **Signs and symptoms.** Common symptoms include breasts that feel "bumpy," breast tenderness or pain, itchy nipples, and dense tissues as seen in a mammogram.
- **Treatment.** Treatments are changing one's diet, taking oral contraceptives, and preventing pain by wearing support bras.

Fibroids are benign (noncancerous) tumors that grow in the uterine wall. They are most common in African American women.

- **Causes.** The causes are mostly unknown, although it has been found that tumors enlarge as estrogen levels increase.
- **Signs and symptoms.** The signs and symptoms are pressure in the abdomen, severe menstrual cramps, abdominal gas, heavy menstrual bleeding, and an enlarged uterus.
- **Treatment.** Treatment includes pain medications, hormone treatments to shrink tumors, surgery to remove tumors, hysterectomy, and surgery to decrease the blood supply to the uterus.

Ovarian cancer is more deadly than other types of cancer because its signs and symptoms are usually mild until the disease has spread to other organs. It is the fifth leading cause of cancer death in women.

- **Causes.** The causes are unknown, although the presence of certain genes has been indicated as a risk factor. Some oral contraceptives may lower the risk of developing this disease.
- **Signs and symptoms.** Abdominal and pelvic discomfort, unusual menstrual cycles, indigestion, bloating, nausea, and excessive hair growth are signs and symptoms.
- **Treatment.** Treatments are radiation therapy, chemotherapy, and surgery to remove the ovaries.

Premenstrual syndrome (PMS) is a collection of symptoms that occur just before a menstrual period.

- **Causes.** The causes are mostly unknown.
- **Signs and symptoms.** The signs and symptoms include anxiety, depression, irritability, acne, fatigue, food cravings, bloating, aches in the head or back, abdominal pain, breast tenderness, muscle spasms, diarrhea, weight gain, and loss of sex drive.
- **Treatment.** PMS is commonly treated with pain medications, diuretics, medications to treat depression or anxiety, and oral contraceptives.

Vaginitis is the condition of having abnormal vaginal discharge. Some vaginal discharge is normal for all women,

continued ⟶

Common Diseases and Disorders of the Female Reproductive System *(continued)*

and it varies throughout the menstrual cycle. Normal vaginal discharge is clear, whitish, or yellowish in color.

- **Causes.** This condition can be caused by yeast infections, tampon use, poor hygiene, bacteria, antibiotics, and sexually transmitted diseases. Vaginitis may be prevented through good hygiene.
- **Signs and symptoms.** Common symptoms include fever, vaginal itching, abnormal increases in the amount of vaginal discharge, decreases in the amount of vaginal discharge, an abnormal color of vaginal discharge (brown or pinkish), and vaginal discharge that has an abnormal odor.
- **Treatment.** The patient may be given medications for fungal or bacterial infections, or the patient and her sexual partner may be treated for sexually transmitted diseases.

Uterine cancer is most common in women between the ages of 60 and 70. In the United States, it occurs in about 1% of women.

- **Causes.** The causes are mostly unknown, although it may be related to increased levels of estrogen.
- **Signs and symptoms.** Signs and symptoms include abdominal pain, abnormal bleeding from the uterus, pelvic pain, and a thin, white vaginal discharge in postmenopausal women.
- **Treatment.** Treatment includes radiation therapy, chemotherapy, and surgery to remove the uterus, fallopian tubes, and ovaries.

Sexually Transmitted Diseases

Sexually transmitted diseases (STDs) can be caused by bacteria, viruses, or parasites.

Bacterial Causes of STDs

STDs caused by bacteria are chlamydia, syphilis, and gonorrhea. The symptoms of STDs caused by bacterial infections are often absent or too mild to be noticed in both men and women. These symptoms include:

- Discharge from the vagina or penis
- Burning sensations during urination
- Pelvic pain
- Pain in the testes

STDs caused by bacteria are easily and effectively treated with antibiotics. However, both partners must take antibiotics to prevent reinfection. These STDs can lead to complications if left untreated. The most common complication of an untreated bacterial STD is *pelvic inflammatory disease (PID)*. PID is a leading cause of infertility in women because it leads to scarring of the fallopian tubes.

Viral Causes of STDs

STDs caused by viruses are herpes and AIDS. *Herpes simplex 1* usually infects the mouth and causes fever blisters, or cold sores. *Herpes simplex 2* affects the genital area. This virus usually causes only genital ulcers, but it can also infect the eyes, lungs, skin, brain, and a developing fetus. There is no cure for any type of herpes but medication is available to prevent outbreaks. *AIDS* is discussed in Chapter 11.

Parasitic Causes of STDs

Parasites can cause STDs. *Crabs* is an STD caused by bloodsucking insects called lice. Lice that invade hair in the genital region are called pubic lice. They typically attach to pubic hair to lay their eggs. They produce severe itching and can be seen with a magnifying glass and sometimes with the naked eye. They are usually treated with insecticides. It is also important to wash all clothing and linens during treatment.

Trichimonas is caused by a parasitic protozoan. It most often does not produce noticeable symptoms in males. In females, it usually produces a large amount of foul-smelling vaginal discharge. This disease also causes itching and swollen labia. It is easily treated with specific antibiotics.

Pregnancy

Fertilization

Pregnancy is defined as the condition of having a developing offspring in the uterus. Pregnancy results when a sperm cell unites with an egg in a process called **fertilization** (Figure 17-7).

Prior to fertilization, an egg is released from an ovary, and it travels through a fallopian tube. During sexual intercourse, the male deposits semen into the vagina. Sperm cells must travel up through the uterus to the fallopian tubes to fertilize the egg.

Prostaglandins in semen stimulate the flagella of sperm cells to undulate, causing the swimming action of sperm. Prostaglandins also stimulate muscles in the uterus and fallopian tubes to contract. These contractions help the sperm reach the egg. Normally about 10 to 14 days after ovulation, high estrogen levels stimulate the uterus and

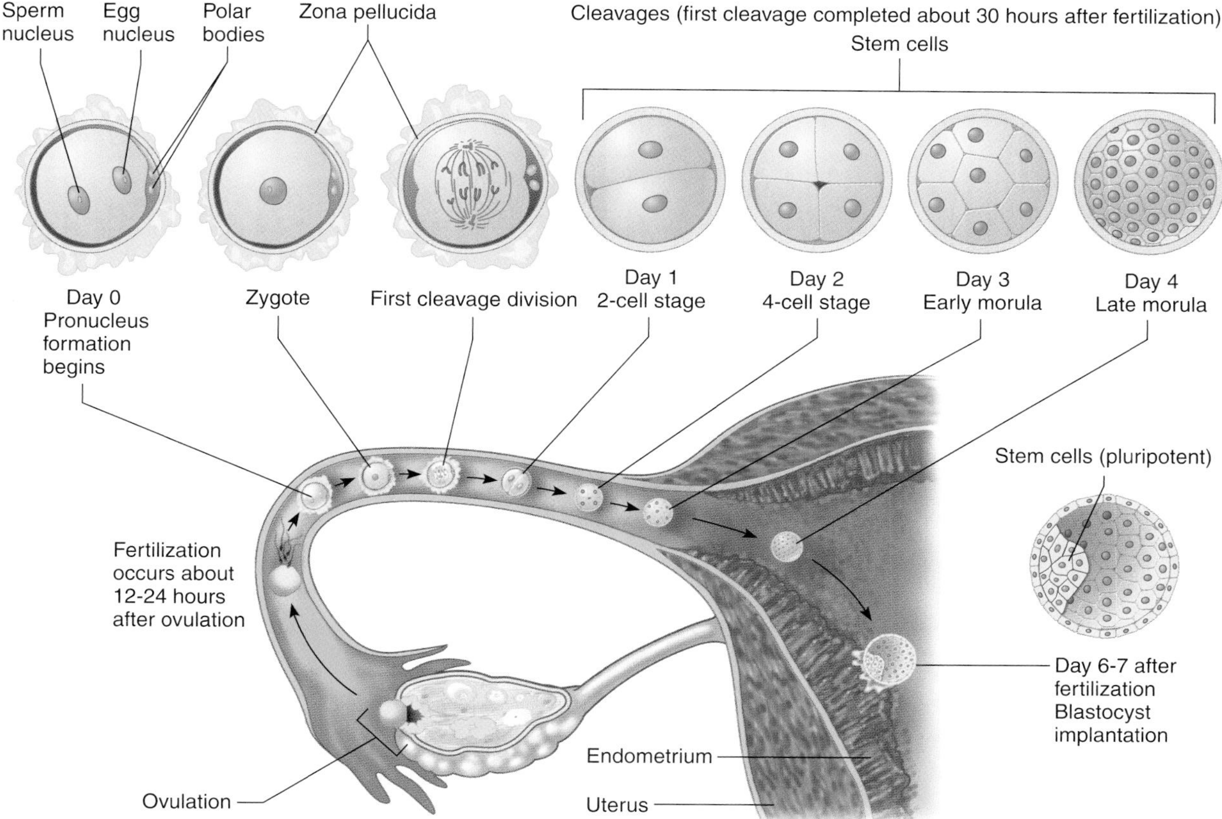

Figure 17-7. Stages of early embryo development.

cervix to secrete a thin watery fluid that also promotes the movement of sperm toward the egg.

Although many sperm cells normally reach an egg, only one unites with the egg to fertilize it. The sperm cell that unites with the egg penetrates the follicular cells and a layer called the **zona pellucida,** which surround the cell membrane of the egg. The acrosome of the sperm releases enzymes to help the sperm penetrate the membrane of the egg. Once a sperm unites with an egg, the egg releases enzymes that prevent other sperm from invading it. The enzymes cause the zona pellucida to become hard and therefore impenetrable to other sperm.

The nucleus of the egg (with 23 chromosomes) and the nucleus of the sperm (with 23 chromosomes) eventually fuse together to make one nucleus that contains 46 chromosomes. The cell that is formed by this union is called a **zygote.**

The Prenatal Period

The **prenatal period** is the time before the offspring is born. The prenatal period is divided into an **embryonic period** (weeks 2 through 8 of pregnancy) and a **fetal period** (week 9 to the delivery of the offspring).

About one day after the zygote forms, it begins to undergo mitosis at a relatively rapid rate. This rapid cell division is called **cleavage.** The resulting ball of cells is called a **morula.** The morula travels down the fallopian tube to the uterus. Fluid then invades the morula, and this organism is called a **blastocyst.** The blastocyst implants in the wall of the uterus. The process of moving from zygote formation to implantation of the blastocyst takes about one week. Once the blastocyst implants, a group of cells in the blastocyst, called the **inner cell mass,** gives rise to an embryo. Other cells in the blastocyst, along with cells of the uterus, eventually form the **placenta.**

The Embryonic Period. The embryonic period extends from the second week of pregnancy to the end of the eighth week of development. During this stage, the placenta, **amnion, umbilical cord,** and **yolk sac** form along with most of the internal organs and external structures of the embryo (Figure 17-8). The cells of the inner cell mass organize into layers called **primary germ layers.** All organs are formed from the primary germ layers, which include the ectoderm, mesoderm, and endoderm.

- The **ectoderm** gives rise to nervous tissue and some epithelial tissue.
- The **mesoderm,** the middle layer, gives rise to connective tissues and some epithelial tissue.
- The **endoderm** gives rise to epithelial tissues only.

The placenta allows nutrients and oxygen from maternal blood to pass to embryonic blood. It also allows waste

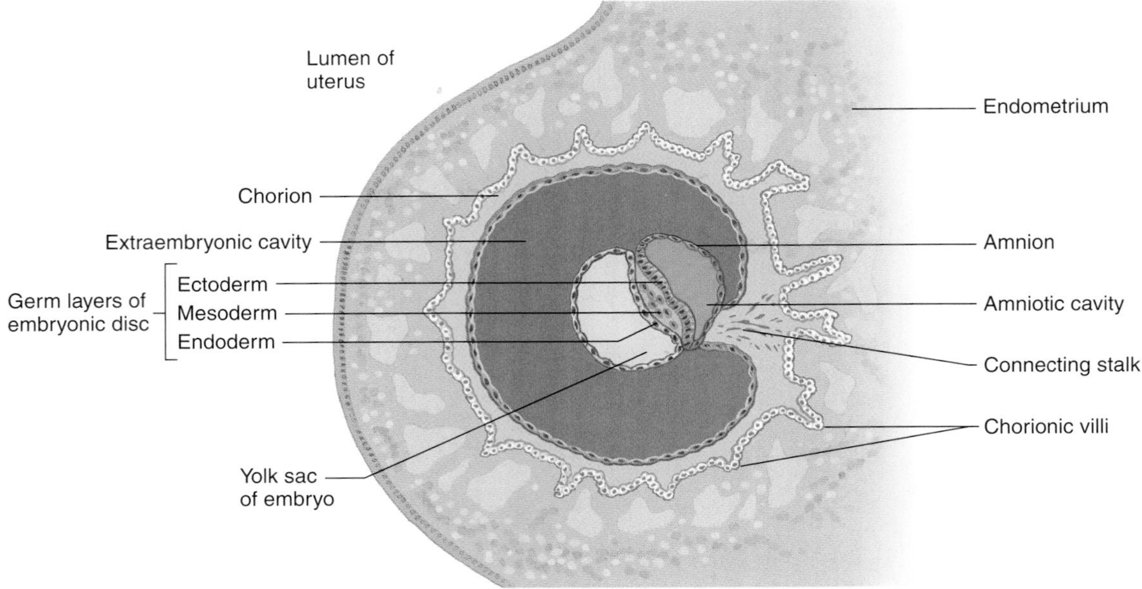

Figure 17-8. Primary germ layers and membranes associated with an embryo.

products from the fetal blood to pass into maternal blood. The amnion is a protective, fluid-filled sac that surrounds the embryo. The umbilical cord contains three blood vessels—one umbilical vein and two umbilical arteries. These blood vessels transport blood between the fetus and the placenta.

The yolk sac makes new blood cells for the fetus as well as cells that eventually become sex cells of the baby. By the end of the embryonic stage, the baby closely resembles a human because all external structures (arms, hands, legs, feet, etc.) have formed.

The Fetal Period. The fetal period begins at the end of the eighth week of development and ends at birth. During this period, the growth of the offspring, which is now called a fetus, is rapid. By the twelfth week bones have begun to harden and the external reproductive organs can be distinguishable as male or female.

The growth rate of the fetus slows down in the fifth month but skeletal muscles become active. In the sixth month, the fetus starts to gain substantial weight. In the seventh month, the eyelids open. In the last three months of pregnancy, fetal brain cells divide rapidly and organs continue to grow. The testes of the male descend into the scrotum. The last organ systems to completely develop are the digestive and respiratory systems. By the end of the ninth month, the fetus is usually positioned upside down in the uterus.

Fetal Circulation

Throughout prenatal development, the placenta and umbilical blood vessels carry out the exchange of nutrients, oxygen, and waste products between maternal and fetal blood. Therefore, the fetus does not need to send blood to the lungs to pick up oxygen nor does it need to send blood to the liver to process nutrients.

Fetal circulation has some important differences from normal circulation, which are illustrated in Figure 17-9. In the fetal heart, a hole called the **foramen ovale** is located between the right atrium and the left atrium. Therefore, in the fetal heart, most blood flows from the right atrium into the left atrium. In the adult heart, blood flows from the right atrium into the right ventricle so it can be pumped to the lungs. However, some fetal blood does flow from the right atrium into the right ventricle, and the right ventricle then delivers the blood to the pulmonary trunk.

In the fetus, there is a connection between the pulmonary trunk and the aorta called the **ductus arteriosus.** This connection allows blood to flow from the pulmonary trunk into the aorta. In the adult, this connection does not exist and blood flows from the pulmonary trunk to the lungs.

The fetus also contains a blood vessel that allows most of the blood to bypass the liver. This vessel is called the **ductus venosus.** After a baby is born, the foramen ovale, ductus arteriosus, and ductus venosus close.

Hemoglobin within the fetus has a much higher affinity for oxygen than does the normal hemoglobin that is found after birth and growth. Therefore, the fetus's blood is adapted to carry more oxygen.

Hormonal Changes During Pregnancy

Many hormonal changes take place when a woman is pregnant. Following implantation of the embryo, the cells of the embryo begin to secrete **human chorionic gonadotropin (HCG).** HCG maintains the corpus luteum in the ovary so it will continue to secrete estrogen and progesterone. The

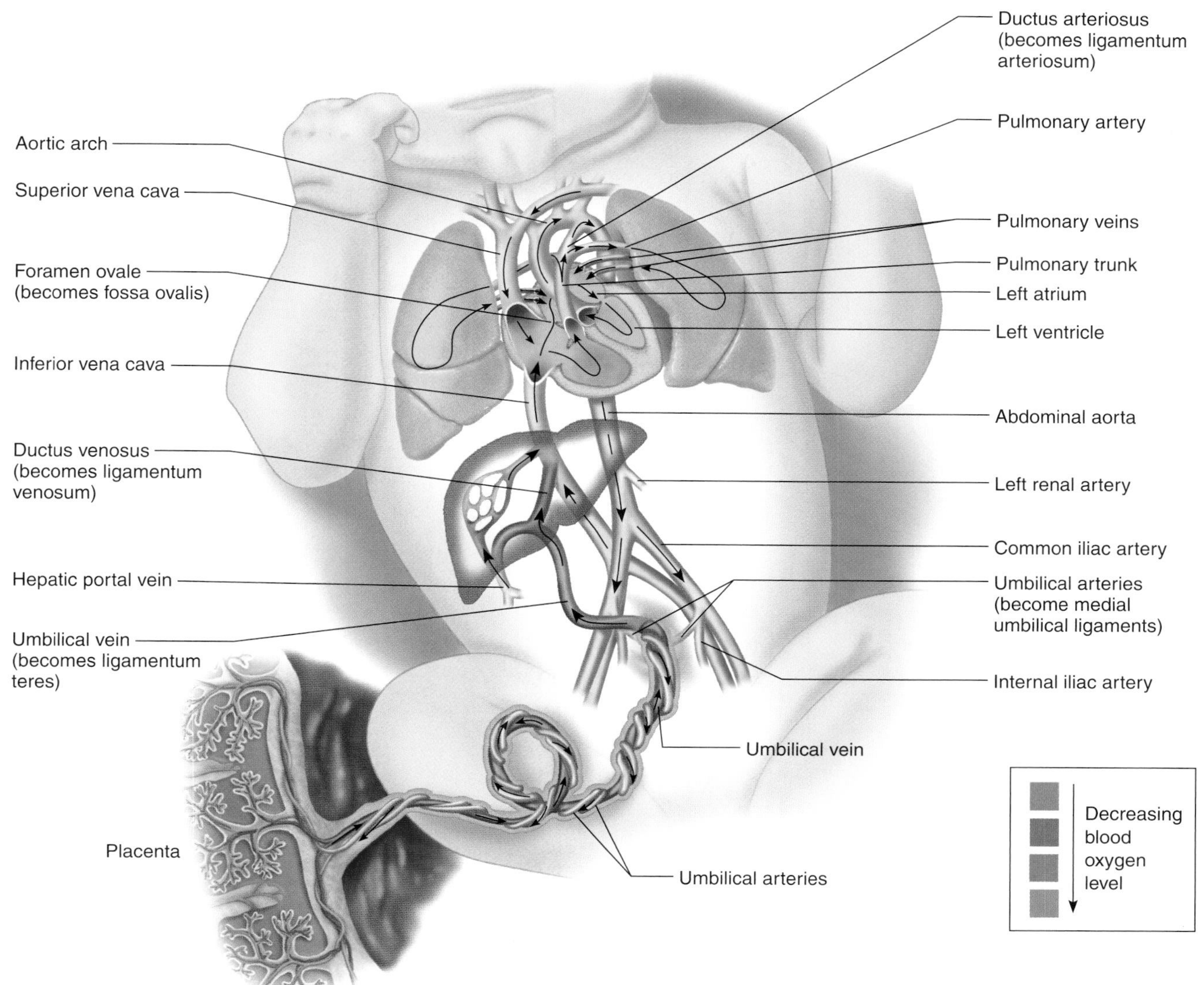

Figure 17-9. Fetal circulation.

placenta also secretes large amounts of progesterone and estrogen.

Progesterone and estrogen stimulate the uterine lining to thicken. They also inhibit the anterior pituitary gland from secreting FSH and LH to prevent ovulation during pregnancy. Estrogen and progesterone also stimulate the development of the mammary glands, inhibit uterine contractions, and stimulate the enlargement of female reproductive organs.

Another hormone called **relaxin,** which comes from the corpus luteum, inhibits uterine contractions and relaxes the ligaments of the pelvis in preparation for childbirth. The placenta also secretes **lactogen,** a hormone that stimulates the enlargement of mammary glands. **Aldosterone,** which is secreted from the adrenal gland, increases sodium and water retention. The secretion of **parathyroid hormone** (PTH) increases, helping to maintain high calcium levels in the blood.

The Birth Process

The birth process ends pregnancy. This process begins when progesterone levels fall. When progesterone levels fall, uterine contractions are no longer inhibited and the uterus secretes prostaglandins. Prostaglandins stimulate uterine contractions, which cause the posterior pituitary gland to release **oxytocin.** Oxytocin stimulates strong uterine contractions until the birth process ends. Following the birth of a baby, the placenta is expelled from the uterus (Figure 17-10).

The Postnatal Period

The **postnatal period** is the period following birth. The first four weeks of the postnatal period is called the **neonatal period** and the offspring is called a **neonate.** The neonatal period is marked by adjustment to life outside the uterus. The lungs of the neonate must expand, which

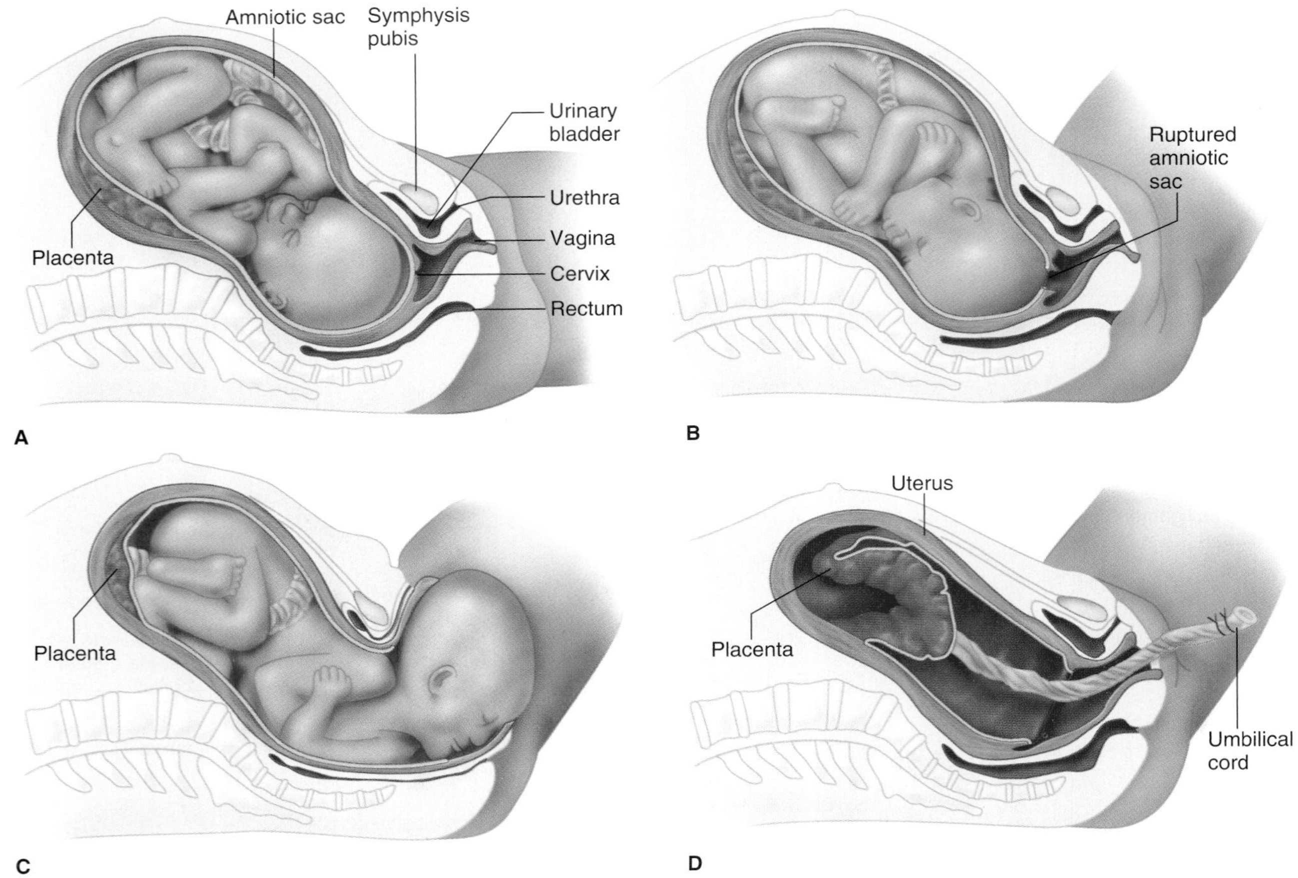

Figure 17-10. Stages of the birth process: (a) the fetal position before birth; (b) dilation of the cervix; (c) delivery of the fetus; and (d) delivery of the placenta.

is why the first breath of a baby is forceful. The liver of the newborn is immature, so the baby must obtain most of its glucose from fat stores in the skin. The newborn urinates a lot because the kidneys are too immature to concentrate urine well. In addition, body temperature tends to be unstable. The umbilical vessels of the newborn must constrict, and the foramen ovale, ductus arteriosus, and ductus venosus must close.

Milk Production and Secretion

During pregnancy, hormones stimulate the breasts to enlarge. After childbirth, prolactin causes the mammary glands to produce milk. The hormone oxytocin stimulates the ejection of milk from mammary gland ducts. As long as milk is removed from the mammary glands, milk production will continue. Once a female stops breast-feeding, the hypothalamus will inhibit the release of prolactin and oxytocin so that milk production will stop.

Contraception

Birth control methods, also referred to as contraception, reduce the risk of pregnancy. Although many methods of birth control are available, some are more reliable than others. The following are the most commonly used birth control methods:

- Coitus interruptus. The penis is withdrawn from the vagina before ejaculation. This method is not very reliable because small amounts of semen may enter the vagina before ejaculation.
- Rhythm method. The rhythm method requires abstinence from sexual intercourse at about the time a female is ovulating. However, predicting ovulation can be difficult; therefore, this type of contraception can be unreliable.
- Mechanical barriers. Mechanical barriers prevent sperm from entering the female reproductive tract. They include condoms, diaphragms, and cervical caps.
- Chemical barriers. Chemical barriers destroy sperm in the female reproductive tract. They primarily include spermicides.
- Oral contraceptives. Birth control pills are oral contraceptives. These pills normally include low doses of estrogen or progesterone that prevent the LH surge necessary for ovulation. These pills therefore prevent ovulation.
- Injectable contraceptives. Depo-Provera is one brand of injectable contraceptive. It prevents ovulation and

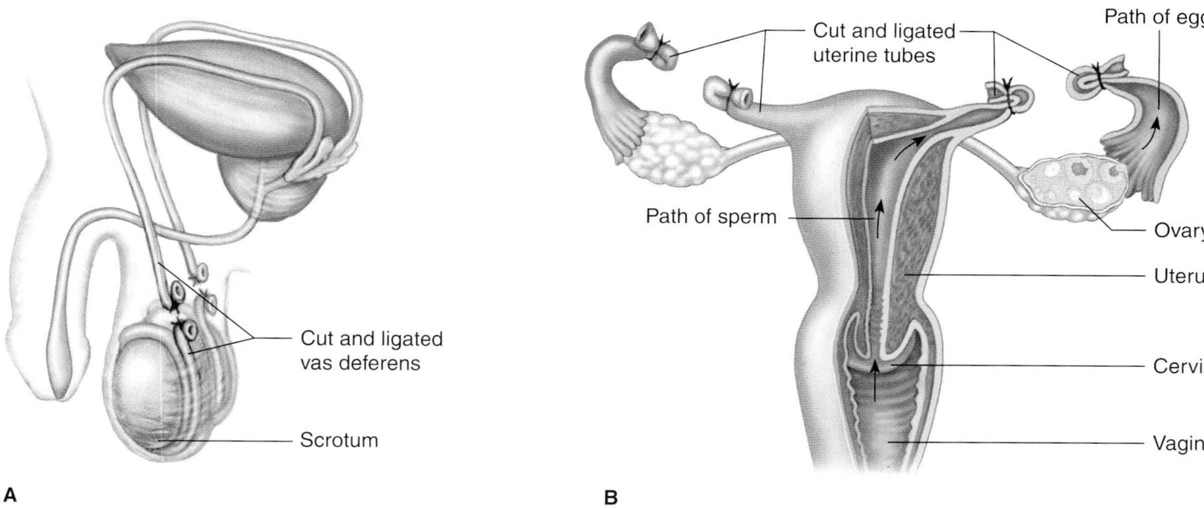

Figure 17-11. (a) Vasectomy involves cutting and ligating the vas deferens. (b) Tubal ligation involves cutting and ligating each fallopian tube.

alters the lining of the uterus so that implantation of a blastocyst is not likely.

- Contraceptive implants. Contraceptive implants are small rods of progesterone that are implanted beneath the skin. They also prevent ovulation.
- Intrauterine devices. An intrauterine device (IUD) is a small, solid device that a physician places in the uterus. It prevents the implantation of a blastocyst.
- Surgical methods. *Tubal ligation* is a surgical method used in females to prevent pregnancy. In this process, each fallopian tube is cut and tied to prevent sperm from reaching the oocyte. *Vasectomy* is a surgical method used in males to prevent pregnancy. In this process, each vas deferens is cut and tied to prevent sperm from being ejaculated. Figure 17-11 illustrates these methods.

Infertility

Infertility is the inability to conceive a child. If a couple has never been pregnant and has tried for 12 months to achieve pregnancy, they are said to have primary infertility. If a couple has had at least one pregnancy but has not been able to get pregnant after one year, they are said to have secondary infertility.

In the United States, about 15% of infertility causes are unknown, about 35% are due to problems in the male, and about 50% are due to problems in the female. Common causes of infertility due to male factors include the following:

- Impotence
- Retrograde ejaculation
- Low or absent sperm count
- Use of various medications or drugs
- Decreased testosterone production
- Scarring of the male reproductive tract from sexually transmitted diseases
- Mumps that infect the testes
- Inflammation of the epididymis or testes

Infertility due to female factors includes these common causes:

- Scarring of fallopian tubes from sexually transmitted diseases
- Pelvic inflammatory disease
- Inadequate diet
- Lack of ovulation
- Lack of menstrual cycles
- Endometriosis
- Abnormal shape of the uterus or cervix
- Hormone imbalances
- Cysts in ovaries
- Being over the age of 40

Women are most likely to get pregnant in their early 20s. By the time a woman reaches the age of 40, her chance of conceiving a child is less than 10% each month. In general, infertility in men is not age related.

Infertility Tests

A number of tests are used to diagnose infertility. They include the following:

- Semen analysis. This test determines the thickness of semen and how many normal sperm cells are in a sample.
- Monitoring of morning body temperature. If a woman's body temperature does not rise slightly once a month, which is best determined by taking her temperature first thing in the morning, a woman may not be ovulating.

- Blood hormone measurements. In females, various hormone levels can be monitored to predict ovulation and the general health of ovaries. In males, testosterone levels are primarily measured.
- Endometrial biopsy. This test determines the health of the uterine lining.
- Urinary analysis for luteinizing hormone. The absence of this hormone in urine may indicate a lack of ovulation.
- Hysterosalpingogram. This type of x-ray uses dye to visualize the shape of the uterus and the fallopian tubes. If a woman has excess scar tissue in her fallopian tubes, the dye cannot run through them.
- Laparoscopy. Laparoscopy is a procedure that is used to visualize pelvic organs.

Treatment of Infertility

Many treatments are available for infertility, but often there is no cure for this condition. Common treatments include surgery to repair abnormal fallopian tubes, fertility drugs to increase ovulation, and hormone therapies. In cases where infertility cannot be cured, procedures such as artificial insemination or in vitro fertilization may help a couple to conceive.

Summary

The ability to reproduce is one of the basic characteristics of life. The male and female reproductive systems work together to produce offspring. The male produces sperm and delivers them to the female. The female produces ova and once fertilization occurs, she nurtures the fetus until birth. The medical assistant must understand the anatomy and physiology of the reproductive systems in order to assist with exams and procedures such as colposcopy and vasectomy. Knowledge of the system is also important when teaching patients about breast and testicular self-examination and sexually transmitted diseases.

REVIEW

CHAPTER 17

CASE STUDY QUESTIONS

Now that you have completed this chapter, review the case study at the beginning of the chapter and answer the following questions:

1. What sexually transmitted diseases are caused by bacteria?
2. How did the infection spread to the patient's abdominopelvic cavity?
3. Why is her sexual partner not experiencing pain in his abdominopelvic cavity?
4. Why is it important for her sexual partner to be treated with antibiotics?
5. Why is it common for women with sexually transmitted diseases to also have urinary tract infections?

Discussion Questions

1. Describe the components of semen. What is the function of each component?
2. What are male and female secondary sex characteristics? Give examples of each.
3. Explain the difference between the embryonic period and the fetal period.

Critical Thinking Questions

1. Why is coitus interruptus not a reliable birth control method?
2. Why do condoms prevent the spread of sexually transmitted diseases while most other methods of birth control do not?
3. What changes occur as a result of a tubal ligation?

Application Activities

1. Describe the functions of the following parts of a sperm:
   a. Head
   b. Midpiece
   c. Tail
2. List the primary sex organs of the male. List the primary sex organs of the female.
3. List the structures that are derived from the following embryonic germ layers:
   a. Endoderm
   b. Mesoderm
   c. Ectoderm

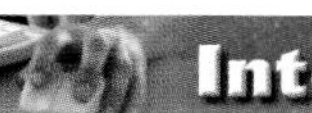

Internet Activity

Find a Web site that discusses AIDS, and answer the following questions:

a. How can AIDS be prevented?
b. What are the current treatments of AIDS?
c. Is an AIDS vaccine currently available?

SECTION 3

ASSISTING WITH PATIENTS

CHAPTER 18

Interviewing the Patient, Taking a History, Documentation

AREAS OF COMPETENCE

2003 Role Delineation Study

CLINICAL

Patient Care

- Obtain patient history and vital signs

GENERAL

Communication Skills

- Adapt communications to individual's ability to understand
- Recognize and respond effectively to verbal, nonverbal, and written communications

Legal Concepts

- Perform within legal and ethical boundaries
- Prepare and maintain medical records
- Document accurately

KEY TERMS

addiction
chief complaint
mirroring
substance abuse
verbalizing

CHAPTER OUTLINE

- The Patient Interview and History
- Your Role as an Observer
- Documenting Patient Information
- Recording the Patient's Medical History

OBJECTIVES

After completing Chapter 18, you will be able to:

18.1 Name the skills necessary to conduct a patient interview.
18.2 Explain the procedure for conducting a patient interview.
18.3 Recognize the signs of anxiety; depression; and physical, mental, or substance abuse.
18.4 State the six Cs for writing an accurate patient history.
18.5 Document on the patient's chart accurately.
18.6 Identify parts of the health history form.

Introduction

As a medical assistant, it is your job to prepare the patient and the patient's chart before the physician enters the examination room to examine the patient. You are the first contact with the patient in the examination room. How you conduct yourself during those first few moments can make a major difference in the patient's attitude. The patient must cooperate fully to provide the information the physician needs to diagnose and treat the patient successfully. Conducting the patient interview and recording the necessary medical history are essential to the practitioner's examination process.

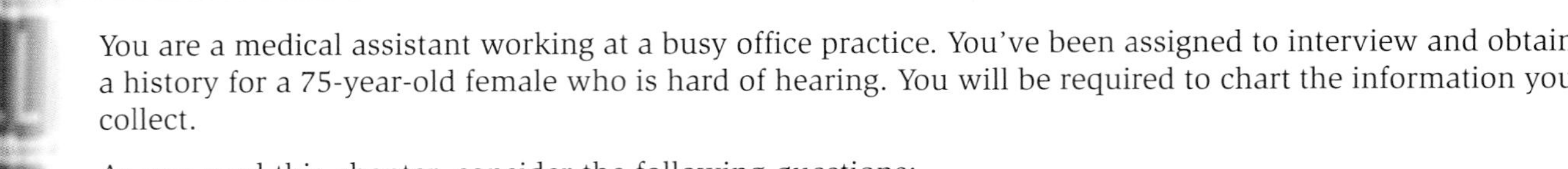

You are a medical assistant working at a busy office practice. You've been assigned to interview and obtain a history for a 75-year-old female who is hard of hearing. You will be required to chart the information you collect.

As you read this chapter, consider the following questions:

1. How can you ensure that the interview process goes smoothly?
2. Why is it important that you maintain a positive relationship with this patient?
3. What steps will you take to make sure all the documentation is completed correctly and accurately?

The Patient Interview and History

The first step in the examination process is the patient interview. A well-conducted interview helps establish a beneficial relationship between you and the patient (Figure 18-1).

When a patient makes an office visit for a medical problem, you will ask the patient (or an attending family member) for specific pieces of information called data. These data include symptoms and the **chief complaint** (a subjective statement made by a patient describing the patient's most significant symptoms or signs of illness). Medicare and most insurers require this information. When a patient makes an office visit for a routine checkup, you will ask the patient about general health and lifestyle and about any changes in health status since the last visit.

The initial interview with the patient in the examining room is more than the process of filling out a standard form. It is an important communication tool that allows an exchange of information. The interview provides far more pertinent information than you and the physician could obtain from the standardized form alone.

A patient's medical and health history is the basis for all treatment rendered by the practitioner. The history provides information for research, reportable diseases, and insurance claims. The information contained on the chart becomes a legal record of the treatment rendered to the patient. It must be complete and accurate to be a good defense in case of legal action. All information regarding the patient should be documented precisely and accurately.

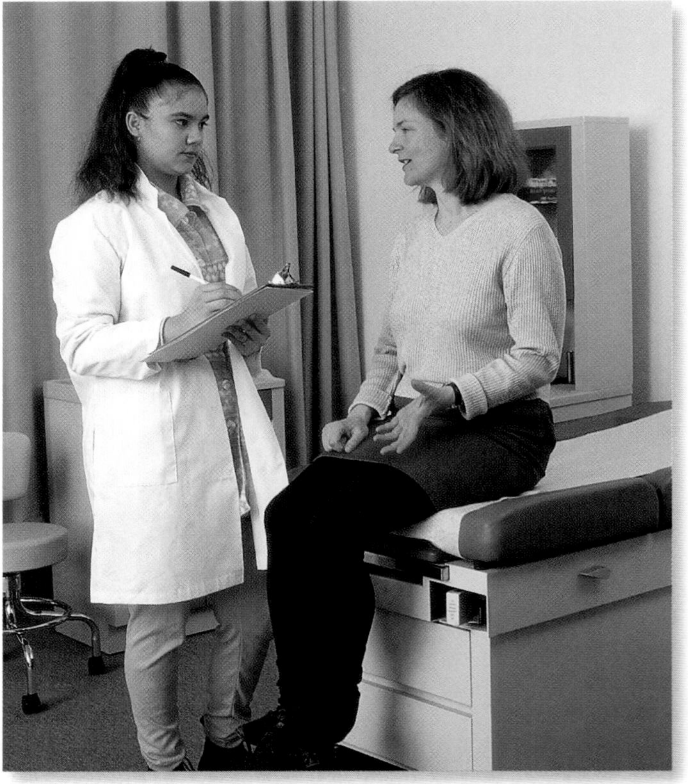

Figure 18-1. Encourage the patient to verbalize her concerns.

Patient Rights, Responsibilities, and Privacy

It is important to remember that all the data you obtain are subject to legal and ethical considerations. Most states have adopted a version of the American Hospital Association's Patient's Bill of Rights, written in 1973 and revised in 1992. Each state encourages health-care workers to be aware of and follow this document when caring for patients. The statement guarantees the patient's right to:

- Receive considerate and respectful care
- Receive complete and current information concerning his or her diagnosis, treatment, and prognosis
- Know the identity of physicians, nurses, and others involved with his or her care as well as know when those involved are students, residents, or trainees
- Know the immediate and long-term costs of treatment choices
- Receive information necessary to give informed consent prior to the start of any procedure or treatment
- Have an advance directive concerning treatment or be able to choose a representative to make decisions
- Refuse treatment to the extent permitted by law
- Receive every consideration of his or her privacy
- Be assured of confidentiality
- Obtain reasonable responses to requests for services
- Obtain information about his or her health care, be allowed to review his or her medical record, and to have any information explained or interpreted
- Know whether treatment is experimental and be able to consent or decline to participate in proposed research studies or human experimentation
- Expect reasonable continuity of care
- Ask about and be informed of the existence of business relationships between the hospital and others that may influence the patient's treatment and care
- Know which hospital policies and practices relate to patient care, treatment, and responsibilities
- Be informed of available resources for resolving disputes, grievances, and conflicts, such as ethics committees or patient representatives
- Examine his or her bill and have it explained, and be informed of available payment methods

Medical assistants should also know that patients have certain responsibilities when they seek medical care. Patients are responsible for:

- Providing information about past illnesses, hospitalizations, medications, and other matters related to their health status. If an incorrect diagnosis is made because a patient fails to give the physician the proper information, the physician is not liable.
- Participating in decision making by asking for additional information about their health status or treatment when they do not fully understand information and instructions.
- Providing health-care agencies with a copy of their written advance directive if they have one.
- Informing physicians and other caregivers if they anticipate problems in following a prescribed treatment.
- Following the physician's orders for treatment. If a patient willfully or negligently fails to follow the physician's instructions, that patient has little legal recourse.
- Providing health-care agencies with necessary information for insurance claims and working with the health-care facility to make arrangements to pay fees when necessary.

Additionally, in April of 2003, the enforcement of the Health Insurance Portability and Accountability Act (HIPAA) began. If this act is not followed, individual health-care workers can be subject to fines up to $250,000 and 10 years in jail. The privacy standards of this act ensure the following:

- Health-care facilities must provide patients with a written notice of their practices regarding the use and disclosure of all individually identifiable health information
- Health-care facilities may not use or disclose protected health information for any purpose that is not in the privacy notice
- Patient consent is required when protected information is used or disclosed for purposes of treatment, payment, or health operations
- Written authorization is required for other types of disclosures
- Hospitals must make the privacy notice available either prior to, or at the time of, the delivery of care
- A privacy notice must be posted in a clear and prominent location within the hospital facility

Interviewing Skills

To conduct a successful patient interview and obtain a history and health information, you will need to apply a variety of skills, including the following:

- Effective listening
- Being aware of nonverbal clues and body language
- Using a broad knowledge base
- Summarizing to form a general picture

Effective Listening. Listening attentively is one of the most important skills you will need for a successful interview. When you listen to what the patient is saying, you not only listen for details but also try to get an overall view of the patient's situation. As you become more experienced in conducting patient interviews, these skills will improve.

One way to be a good listener is to hear, think about, and respond to what the patient has said. This technique is called active listening. Passive listeners simply sit back and hear. When you are an active listener, you pay attention and provide feedback. For example, you might repeat what the patient says in your own words or ask questions so that you understand details.

Being Aware of Nonverbal Clues and Body Language. Verbal communication is the asking and answering of questions. To conduct a successful interview, you must also be aware of nonverbal communication. The patient's tone of voice, facial expression, and body language are examples of nonverbal communication. These signs often communicate more than words could ever say. For example, a patient who has difficulty making eye contact may be embarrassed by some symptoms and may need your extra patience and encouragement to report symptoms fully. A child or adolescent may deny or exaggerate pain. Pay attention to the patient's facial expression and how much the patient guards the area in question.

Using a Broad Knowledge Base. To conduct a successful interview, you must have a broad knowledge base so that you can ask questions that will elicit the most meaningful information about the patient. You must take every opportunity to expand your knowledge base by learning more about medical terminology, symptoms, and diseases.

Summarizing to Form a General Picture. You will gather a variety of subjective and objective data as you conduct a patient interview. You must consider the relative importance of each piece of information so that you can summarize the data to formulate a general picture of the patient.

Interviewing Successfully

One of the main goals of the patient interview is to give the patient an opportunity to fully explain in her own words the reason for the current office visit. These eight steps will help you conduct a successful interview.

1. Do your research before the patient interview
2. Plan the interview
3. Approach the patient and request the interview
4. Make the patient feel at ease
5. Conduct the interview in private without interruptions
6. Deal with sensitive topics with respect
7. Do not diagnose or give a diagnostic opinion
8. Formulate the general picture

Doing Research Before the Patient Interview. Before the interview review the patient's medical record for history, medications, and chronic problems (for example, diabetes or high blood pressure). Note whether the patient has family problems that might have an impact on health issues.

Planning the Interview. Develop a plan for the interview. Have a general idea of the questions you will ask. For example, if a client is being treated for high blood pressure, you might ask about headaches or tinnitis (ringing in the ears), which are common signs of high blood pressure. Planning the interview helps you maintain your focus and ensures that you will obtain all the necessary information.

Approaching the Patient and Requesting the Interview. Ask the patient whether you may pose some questions about the reason for the visit and the patient's current health situation. You may need to explain that the questions are necessary to plan the most effective care. It is more courteous to seek permission to ask questions than to say that you "need to take a history." Asking permission helps the patient feel more comfortable and emphasizes the importance of the interview process. It also makes the patient feel more like a participant in the medical care being provided.

Making the Patient Feel at Ease. Using certain words or phrases known as icebreakers can help set the stage for the interview. Icebreakers put the patient at ease and create a relaxed atmosphere. Examples of icebreakers include acknowledging the patient's reason for the visit, introducing yourself, or commenting about the weather. Icebreakers that also convey a sincere and sensitive interest in the patient are asking the patient how she prefers to be addressed or clarifying the pronunciation of a difficult name.

Another way to convey an image of a professional who is sensitive to the patient's needs is to sit with the patient and appear relaxed. By appearing relaxed, you help the patient relax and encourage a more open and comfortable interview.

Conducting the Interview in Private Without Interruptions. After setting the stage for the interview, ensure privacy by showing the patient to a private room or area or by closing the door if the patient is already in a private room. You can then begin to ask relevant questions. Some approaches are more effective than others, as shown in Table 18-1. Listening carefully to the patient's responses may lead you to ask questions other than those in your interview plan.

Developing a rapport with the patient is essential. Keep the atmosphere relaxed, do not rush, maintain eye contact, and use the patient's name in conversation. Avoid interruptions, such as taking phone calls and letting people walk in and out of the room.

Dealing With Sensitive Topics With Respect. Sometimes you will have to ask patients questions about sensitive topics. Such topics may be related to sexuality, lifestyle, or behaviors that put a person at risk for diseases, such as those that are sexually transmitted. You must approach these topics gently so that the patient does not feel threatened by the questioning. You can show respect for the patient's rights and privacy by knowing when to stop. Both verbal and nonverbal clues can guide you in this area.

TABLE 18-1 Methods of Collecting Patient Data	
Effective Methods	**Characteristics**
Asking open-ended questions	Requires more than a yes or no answer; allows the patient to more fully explain the situation, resulting in more relevant data. Instead of asking, "Do you have a cough?" ask, "Can you tell me about your symptoms?"
Asking hypothetical questions	Allows you to determine the patient's knowledge of the situation and whether it is accurate. For example, ask a patient who has been prescribed nitroglycerin for chest pain, "What would you do if you have chest pain?"
Mirroring patient's responses and verbalizing the implied	Allows nonthreatening ways for the patient to discuss the situation further and to provide underlying meaning. *Mirroring* means restating what the patient says in your own words. *Verbalizing* the implied means stating what you believe the patient is suggesting by his response. You might say, "So the pain started about three days ago and has been getting worse each day, and today it has not let up at all."
Focusing on patient	Shows the patient that you are really listening to what he is saying. You maintain eye contact (as culturally appropriate), assume a relaxed and open body posture, and use the proper responses.
Encouraging patient to take the lead	Motivates the patient to discuss or describe the situation in his own way. Ask a question such as "Where would you like to begin?"
Encouraging patient to provide additional information	Conveys sincere interest in the patient by continuing to explore topics in more detail when appropriate. You might ask the patient if he has experienced a symptom before or if he associates it with a change in routine.
Encouraging patient to evaluate his situation	Provides an idea of the patient's point of view about the situation; allows you to determine the patient's knowledge of the situation and possible fears. Ask the patient, "What do you think is going on here?"
Ineffective Methods	**Characteristics**
Asking closed-ended questions	Provides little information because closed-ended questions offer the patient little freedom to explain his answers. Closed-ended questions require only yes or no answers.
Asking leading questions	Leading questions suggest a desired response instead of the patient's true response. The patient tends to agree with such statements instead of elaborating on them. An example of a leading question is "You seem to be making progress, don't you agree?" This type of question limits the patient's response.
Challenging patient	The patient may feel you are disagreeing with what he is saying if you ask an emotional question or use a certain tone of voice. The patient may become defensive, which might block further communication.
Probing	Continuing to question a patient after he appears to have finished giving information can make him feel that you are invading his privacy. The patient may become defensive and withhold information.
Agreeing or disagreeing with patient	When you agree or disagree with a patient, it implies that the patient is either "right" or "wrong." This action can block further communication.

Avoiding Making a Diagnosis or Giving a Diagnostic Opinion. Only the physician can make a diagnosis, based on the patient's symptoms and complaints. If the patient asks for your opinion about a diagnosis, explain that the physician should be asked about diagnoses. If pressed, you may need to say that it is not your place to give opinions about a diagnosis. Never go beyond the scope of your knowledge or job description.

Formulating the General Picture. Summarize the key points of the interview. Ask the patient whether he has questions or other information to add. You will be most successful with the interview process if you remain alert and organized but flexible. Procedure 18-1 demonstrates the proper approach to an interview.

Your Role as an Observer

During the preexamination stage of the office visit, you will gather most of your information through verbal and nonverbal communication. The nonverbal communication that occurs during the interview and history taking, however, sometimes reveals more about a patient than the patient's words. Listening attentively and observing the patient closely may help you detect a problem that might otherwise go unnoted.

Anxiety

Anxiety is a common emotional response in patients. Some patients respond with anxiety to a specific fear, such as fear of pain. Others simply feel anxious when they are in an unfamiliar situation. For example, many patients have what is called "white coat syndrome," which is anxiety related to seeing a physician.

To recognize anxiety, you must understand that its levels vary from mild to severe. A patient with mild anxiety may have a heightened ability to observe and to make connections. A patient with severe anxiety has difficulty focusing on details, feels panicky, and is virtually helpless. A heightened focus or a lack of focus in a patient can hinder your ability to get the information and cooperation you need.

When you observe signs of anxiety in a patient, make every effort to help her relax and release or reduce the anxious feelings. You may be able to help by allowing the patient to describe her feelings. If a patient becomes agitated while discussing a physical complaint, you may need to postpone talking about the matter until the patient is calmer. In either situation, give support in nonverbal ways by trying to make the patient as comfortable as possible. Give the patient time to respond and then wait quietly, provide privacy, make eye contact, and communicate at the level of the patient.

Depression

Some symptoms of depression are the same as those of many common illnesses. Many patients with major depression develop great skill in hiding depression or are unaware they are suffering from it. Thus, depression may be difficult to recognize. Many patients, especially the elderly, have undiagnosed depression.

To recognize depression, you must be aware of common symptoms associated with the condition. Classic symptoms of depression are profound sadness and fatigue. In addition, a depressed person may have difficulty falling asleep at night or getting up in the morning. The depressed patient may suffer from loss of appetite, loss of energy, or both.

Depression seems to occur most frequently during late adolescence, in middle age, and after retirement. It is common in the elderly but is often mistaken for senility. If you observe any signs of depression, indicate them in the patient's chart and alert the physician.

PROCEDURE 18.1

Using Critical Thinking Skills During an Interview

Objective: To be able to use verbal and nonverbal clues to optimize the process of obtaining data for the patient's chart

OSHA Guidelines: This procedure does not involve exposure to blood, body fluids, or tissues.

Materials: Patient chart, pen with black ink

Method

Example 1: Getting at an Underlying Meaning

1. You are interviewing a female patient with type 2 diabetes who has recently started insulin injections. She is in the office for a follow-up visit.
2. You ask her how she is managing her diabetes. (This open-ended questioning allows the patient to explain the situation in her own words and often provides more information than closed-ended questioning.)
3. The patient states that she "just can't get used to the whole idea of injections."
4. To encourage her to verbalize her concerns more clearly, you can **mirror** her response, or restate her comments in your own words. For example, you might say, "You seem to be having some difficulty giving yourself injections." (Your response should encourage her to verbalize the specific area in which she is having problems [for example, loading the syringe, injecting herself, finding the time for the injections, and so on].) Another method you can use is to **verbalize** the implied, which means that you state what

continued →

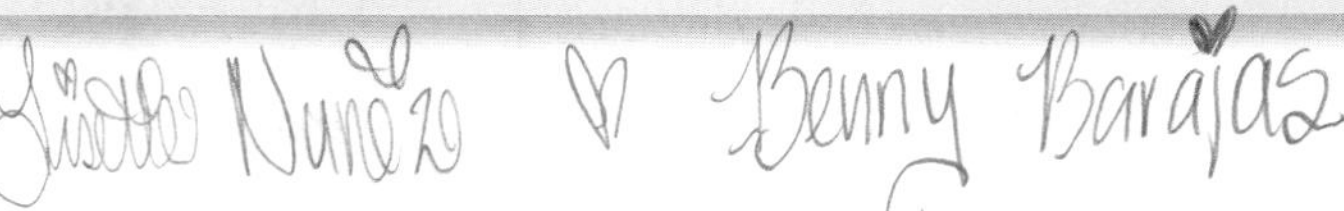

PROCEDURE 18.1

Using Critical Thinking Skills During an Interview *(continued)*

you think the patient is suggesting by her response.

5. After you determine the specific problem, you will be able to address it in the interview or note it in the patient's chart for the doctor's attention.

Example 2: Dealing With a Potentially Violent Patient

1. You are interviewing a 24-year-old male patient who is new to the office. He appears agitated. You ask his reason for seeing the doctor today.
2. The patient explains that he does not want to talk to "some assistant" about his problem. He just wants to see the doctor.
3. You say that you respect his wish not to discuss his symptoms but explain that you need to ask him a few questions so that the doctor can provide the proper medical care. (The patient has the right to refuse to answer a question, even if it is a reasonable one.)
4. The patient begins to yell at you, saying he wants to see the doctor and doesn't "want to answer stupid questions" (Figure 18-2).
5. The fact that the patient appears agitated and begins to raise his voice in anger should be a warning to you that he may become violent. It would be best not to handle this patient by yourself.
6. If you are alone with the patient, leave the room and request assistance from another staff member.

Example 3: Gathering Symptom Information About a Child

1. A parent brings a 6-year-old boy to the office because the child is complaining about stomach pain.
2. To gather the pertinent symptom information, ask the child various types of questions. (Talking to the child first allows him to feel that his view of the problem is important.)
   a. Can he tell you about the pain? (Open-ended questioning allows him to tell you about his problem in his own words.)
   b. Can he tell you exactly where it hurts (Figure 18-3)?
   c. Is there anything else that hurts?
3. To confirm the child's answers, ask the parent to answer similar questions.
4. You should then ask the parent additional questions. Begin with an open-ended question, as above. Follow up with specific questions such as these.
   a. How long has he had the pain?
   b. Is the pain related to any specific event (such as going to school)?
5. Ask the child to confirm the parent's answers. He may be able to provide additional information at this time.

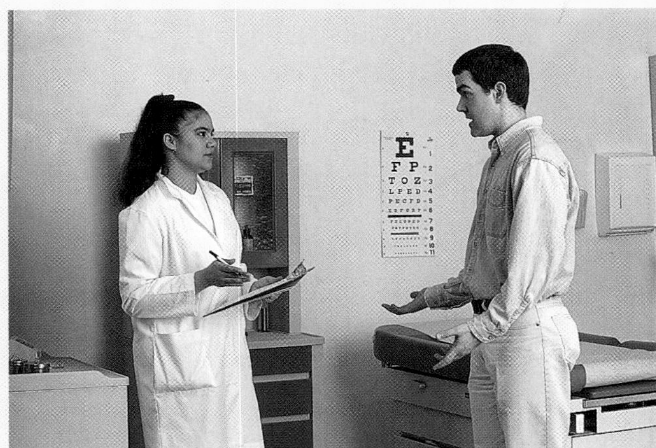

Figure 18-2. Do not try to handle a patient who may become violent by yourself. Ask for help from other staff members.

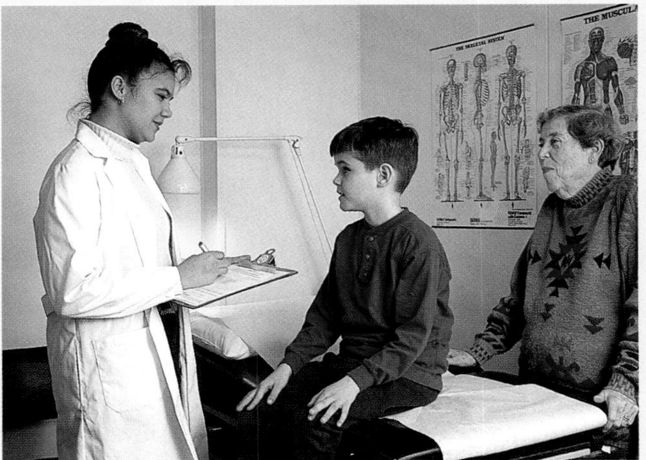

Figure 18-3. Gather any symptom information you can from a child. Then ask the parent or caregiver similar questions.

CAUTION *Handle With Care*

Signs of Depression, Substance Abuse, and Addiction in Adolescents

Signs of depression, substance abuse, and addiction are often hard to distinguish in adolescents. Part of the difficulty is that adolescents are particularly skilled at hiding signs of all three disorders.

Various signs may indicate depression in an adolescent. One teenager may lose interest in or be unable to enjoy everyday activities. Another may sleep for long periods and have difficulty getting up in the morning, whereas yet another may sleep very little. Chronic fatigue or aches and pains may signal depression, as may trouble with concentration or school absenteeism. These signs may also indicate substance abuse or addiction.

It is important to know the difference between substance abuse and addiction. **Substance abuse** refers to the use of a substance, even an over-the-counter drug, in a way that is not medically approved. Inappropriate use includes such practices as using diet pills to stay awake or consuming large quantities of cough syrup that contains codeine. It also includes taking larger-than-prescribed doses of a medication. Substance abusers are not necessarily addicts, however.

Addiction refers to a physical or psychological dependence on a substance. Addiction usually involves a pattern of behavior that includes an obsessive or compulsive preoccupation with a substance and the security of its supply as well as a high rate of relapse after withdrawal.

As a medical assistant, you should not try to make a diagnosis. Quite probably an adolescent with one or more of these disorders will be uncooperative and refuse to answer relevant questions. You must be aware, however, of physical signs or behaviors that may be associated with depression, substance abuse, or addiction in an adolescent patient. The following signs or behaviors are important clues that you should report immediately to the doctor.

- The patient complains of altered eating habits or disturbed sleep patterns (either too much or too little sleep).
- The patient's weight has changed drastically (either up or down) since the previous office visit.
- The patient appears lethargic or sullen or exhibits radical mood changes.
- The patient has slurred speech.
- The patient appears to have illogical thought patterns.
- The patient appears to have needle tracks (anywhere on the body, especially on the arms or legs).
- The patient has pinpoint (highly constricted) pupils.

Signs of depression, addiction, and substance abuse in adolescents can be difficult to distinguish. Signs of substance abuse or addiction can be mistaken for depression. The reverse is also true. Sometimes all three conditions exist simultaneously. If you have any clues that point to one of these conditions in an adolescent patient, notify the physician immediately. For symptoms that may be signs of these disorders, see the Caution: Handle With Care section.

Physical and Psychological Abuse

Abuse can involve people from all walks of life and of all ages. Abuse can be physical, psychological, or both. As a medical assistant, you are in a unique position to detect abuse in the patients you see. (See Chapter 22 for additional information related to child abuse, domestic violence, and elder abuse.)

Although you must not make hasty judgments, you may suspect abuse when a patient speaks in a guarded way. An unlikely explanation for an injury may also be a sign of abuse. There may be no history of the injury, or the history may be suspicious. In either case the following injuries may be signs of physical abuse:

- Head injuries and skull fractures
- Burns (especially those that appear to be deliberate, such as from a cigarette or an iron)
- Broken bones
- Bruises (especially multiple bruises, those that are clearly in the shape of an object, and those in various stages of healing)

Although a patient can recover physically from abuse, the emotional and psychological scars may last a lifetime. Other signs of physical abuse (including sexual abuse and neglect) and signs of psychological abuse include the following:

- A child's failure to thrive
- Severe dehydration or underweight
- Delayed medical attention
- Hair loss

- Drug use
- Genital injuries

Battered Women. Women who are abused by their partners may come to the medical office with bruises or other injuries. Often they are afraid to discuss the problem. A woman may fear that her partner will "get even" if she tells anyone about what happened. The woman may not feel strong enough emotionally to leave an abusing partner. If you suspect abuse, bring it to the physician's attention immediately. You or the physician, or the two of you together, may be able to convince the patient to seek help. Obtain the battered-woman hotline number for your area, and have it available for quick reference.

Abused Children. Children are often the targets of violence, much of which occurs in the home. In addition to being physically, emotionally, or sexually abused, children can be abused by being neglected. If you suspect child abuse, you must report it to the proper authorities. Keep the child abuse hotline number for your area on file.

The Abused Elderly. Physical or mental disabilities can make elderly people dependent on others for care. When such care is perceived as a burden by the caregiver, elder abuse may occur. The disabilities that make an elderly person dependent can also leave him defenseless against abuse. Such a patient may have suspicious injuries or show signs of neglect. Find out whether there is an elder abuse hotline number for your area, and if so keep it available for quick reference.

Drug and Alcohol Abuse

Substance abuse and addiction to drugs or alcohol are serious social problems. Symptoms of substance abuse or addiction differ from drug to drug, as indicated in Table 18-2. Addiction, however, typically causes a gradual decline in

TABLE 18-2 Symptoms Associated With Commonly Abused Drugs

Drug Names/Type	Trade or Other Name	Symptoms, Effects
Amphetamines/stimulants	Benzedrine, Dexedrine, methamphetamine, black beauty, speed, uppers	Altered mental status, from confusion to paranoia; hyperactivity, then exhaustion; insomnia; loss of appetite
Anabolic steroids	Anadrol, Dianabol, Deca-durabotin, Depo-testosterone	Irritability, aggression, nervousness, male-pattern baldness
Barbiturates/sedatives	Amobarbital, phenobarbital, Butisol, secobarbital, yellow jackets, red birds	Slowed thinking, slowed reflexes, slowed respiration, loss of anxiety
Benzodiazepines/sedatives	Ativan, diazepam, Librium, Valium, downers, candy	Poor coordination, drowsiness, increased self-confidence
Cocaine/stimulant	Coke, snow, crack	Alternating euphoria and apprehension, intense craving for more of the drug
Ecstasy/psychoactive	Adam, XTC, MDMA	Confusion, depression, anxiety, paranoia, increase in heart rate and blood pressure
GHB/depressants	G, liquid ecstasy, georgia homeboy	Slow pulse and breathing, lowered blood pressure, drowsiness, poor concentration
Inhalants	Solvents: paint thinner; gases: aerosol, butane or propane	Stimulation, intoxication, hearing loss, arm or leg spasms
LSD (lysergic acid diethylamine)/hallucinogen	Acid, microdot	Heightened sense of awareness, grandiose hallucinations, mystical experiences, flashbacks
Marijuana/cannabinoids/ Hashish	Pot, grass, joint, reefer, weed, bone, buds, hash, boom	Altered thought processes, distorted sense of time and self, impaired short-term memory
Opium, morphine, codeine/ opiate narcotics	Monkey, white stuff	Decreased level of consciousness, detachment, drowsiness, impaired judgment
PCP (phencyclidine)/ hallucinogen	Angel dust	Decreased awareness of surroundings, hallucinations, poor perception of time and distance, possible overdose and death

the quality of someone's work or relationships. The patient may behave erratically, have frequent mood changes, suffer from loss of appetite, and be constantly tired.

Someone who is abusing alcohol may have no apparent signs or symptoms at first. As time goes on, however, that person may suffer from blackouts (failure to remember what happened while drinking) or may become secretive and guilty about drinking and deny that there is a problem. She may suffer from bruises, trembling hands, or chronic stomach problems.

Even though the patient may feel she does not have a problem of substance abuse or addiction, members of the health-care team may recognize a problem. Then their job is to try to persuade the patient to seek help.

Documenting Patient Information

Whenever you interview a patient, keep in mind that the patient chart is a legal document. The chart can be used as evidence in a court of law. Therefore, you must meet certain guidelines when recording data.

The Six Cs of Charting

To help ensure that you record patient data accurately, you must follow the six Cs of charting. These guidelines are as follows.

1. *Client's words* must be recorded exactly. The doctor may uncover clues to use in diagnosing the patient's condition. Place quotation marks to indicate what the patient said.
2. *Clarity* is essential when you describe the patient's condition. You must use medical terminology and precise descriptions.
3. *Completeness* is required on all the forms used in the patient record.
4. *Conciseness* can save time and space when you are recording information.
5. *Chronological order* and dates on all entries in patient records are critical in the documentation of patient care. This information can also be used for legal questions regarding medical services. Most charts are arranged with the most recent information on top. This type of charting is known as *reverse chronological order.*
6. *Confidentiality* is essential to protect the patient's privacy. You cannot discuss a patient's records, forward them to another office, fax them, or show them to anyone except the doctor unless the patient gives you written permission to do so.

Contents of Patient Charts

Each physician's office has its own forms and medical charts. All records, however, must contain the following standard information.

- The patient registration form carries the date of the patient's current visit and generally lists the patient's age, address, Social Security number, medical insurance, occupation, education, racial or ethnic background, marital status, number of children, and nearest relative.
- Patient medical history usually includes the chief complaint, history of the present illness, past medical history (including medical treatment, surgeries, known allergies, and current medications), family history, and social and occupational history (including diet, exercise, smoking, and use of alcohol or drugs). This section may also be used to record the results of a general physical examination. See Figure 18-4 for one example.
- Test results include those performed in the office and those received from other physicians, hospitals, or independent laboratories. Physicians may have tests run on a patient's blood, urine, or tissue samples to aid in their diagnoses. Figure 18-5 shows an example of a laboratory report of a panel of chemical tests on blood performed by an outside laboratory.
- Records from other physicians or hospitals are accompanied by a copy of the patient's written authorization to release the records.
- The physician's diagnosis and treatment plan are specific and detailed.
- Operative reports include a record of all procedures, surgeries, follow-up care, and additional notes the physician makes regarding the patient's case. Continuation forms can be used for additional information. Some medical offices also keep a separate log of telephone calls to and from the patient.
- Informed consent forms verify that the patient has understood the treatment offered and the possible outcomes or side effects of it. The patient signs the consent form but may withdraw consent if she decides to change or discontinue treatment.
- A discharge summary form is used when a patient is hospitalized. This form includes information that summarizes the reason the patient entered the hospital; tests, procedures, or operations performed in the hospital; medications administered; and the disposition, or outcome, of the case.
- Correspondence with or about the patient is marked or stamped with the date the document was received in the physician's office.

When recording information in the patient chart, be sure to date and initial every item. This documentation makes it easy to tell which items you entered into the chart and which items others entered. The physician usually initials reports before they are filed to prove that she saw them.

Methods of Charting

Various methods of charting are used on the medical record. Most methods are based on a series of steps to document the information. These steps are referred to as

The Medical Center at Springfield
Medical History

Name Age Sex S M W D
Address Phone Date
Occupation Ref. by
Chief Complaint
Present Illness
History —Military
—Social
—Family
—Marital
—Menstrual Menarche Para. LMP
—Illness Measles Pert. Var. Pneu. Pleur. Typh. Mal. Rh. Fev. Sc. Fev. Diphth. Other
—Surgery
—Allergies
—Current Medications

Physical Examination

Temp. Pulse Resp. BP Ht. Wt.
General Appearance Skin Mucous Membrane
Eyes: Vision Pupil Fundus
Ears:
Nose:

Figure 18-4. Your office may have its own patient history form. This is a sample form.

the SOAP method of documentation (Figure 18-6). Understanding the parts of SOAP will help you document information in a logical manner.

1. **Subjective** data. You obtain subjective data from conversation with the patient or an attending family member. Subjective data include thoughts, feelings, and perceptions, including the chief complaint.
2. **Objective** data. Objective data are readily apparent and measurable; for example, vital signs or test results and the physician's examination.
3. Assessment. Assessment is the physician's diagnosis or impression of the patient's problem.
4. Plan of action. Options for treatment, the type of treatment chosen, medications, tests, consultations, patient education, and follow-up are included in a plan of action.

Three common methods for maintaining notes on a patient chart include:

1. Conventional or source-oriented medical records (SOMR). Information is arranged according to who supplied that data—the patient, the doctor, a specialist, or someone else. The medical form may have a space for patient remarks followed by a section for the doctor's comment.
2. Problem-oriented medical records (POMR). This method is used more extensively and includes the database; the problem list; an educational, diagnostic, and treatment plan; and the progress notes.
3. Computerized medical records. This method uses a combination of SOMR and POMR but provides accessibility by the physician or other health-care workers at any time from a computer terminal.

Recording the Patient's Medical History

A patient's medical history includes pertinent information about the patient and the patient's family. Age, previous illnesses, surgical history, allergies, medication history, and family medical history are key items.

When recording a patient history, you must do more than fill out the form (Figure 18-7). You must review the pieces of information, organize them, determine their importance, and document the facts. When you write your first histories, you may find it to be a lengthy process. When you become more experienced, however, you will be able to write histories more quickly.

Whenever you write information on the chart you must consider its completeness and accuracy. For example,

Morris A. Turner, MD

MEDLAB

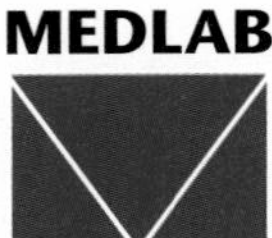

266 Line Road
Montclair, Delaware 00956
800-555-4567

C.L.I.A. #21-1862

WELLS, KARLA	09/12/04	09/12/04	09/13/04
Patient Name	Date Drawn	Date Received	Date of Report

F (Sex) 43 (Age)

Lisa W. Clark, MD
22 Landover Lane
Newark, Delaware 00964

23341 — ID Number

67294 — Account Number

166241809 — Patient ID/Soc. Sec. Number

897211 — Specimen Number

TEST NAME	RESULT ABNORMAL	RESULT NORMAL	UNITS	REFERENCE RANGE
CHEM-SCREEN PANEL				
GLUCOSE		76.0	MG/DL	65.0–115
SODIUM		139.0	MMOL/L	134–143
POTASSIUM		4.00	MMOL/L	3.60–5.10
CHLORIDE		107.0	MMOL/L	96.0–107
BUN		17.0	MG/DL	6.00–19.0
BUN/CREATININE RATIO		14.2		
URIC ACID		4.30	MG/DL	2.20–6.20
PHOSPHATE		2.40	MG/DL	2.40–4.50
CALCIUM		9.50	MG/DL	8.60–10.0
MAGNESIUM		1.75	MEG/L	1.40–2.00
CHOLESTEROL	237.0		MG/DL	130–200
CHOL. PERCENTILE	90.0		PERCENTILE	1.00–75.0
HDL CHOLESTEROL	41.0		MG/DL	48.0–89.0
CHOL./HDL RATIO		5.80		
LDL CHOL., CALCULATED	175.0		MG/DL	65.5–130
TRIGLYCERIDES		104.0	MG/DL	00.0–200
TOTAL PROTEIN		6.60	GM/DL	6.40–8.00
ALBUMIN		4.10	GM/DL	3.70–4.80
GLOBULIN		2.50	GM/DL	2.20–3.60
ALB/GLOB RATIO		1.64		1.10–2.10
TOTAL BILIRUBIN		0.80	MG/DL	0.20–1.30
DIRECT BILIRUBIN		0.15	MG/DL	0.00–0.20
ALK. PHOSPHATASE		44.0	UNITS/L	25.0–125
G-GLUTAMYL TRANSPEP.		8.00	UNITS/L	1.00–63.0
AST (SGOT)		21.0	IU/L	1.00–40.0
ALT (SGPT)		14.0	IU/L	1.00–50.0
LD		134.0	IU/L	90.0–250
IRON		130.0	MCG/DL	35.0–180

Figure 18-5. Laboratory reports provide physicians with valuable information about patients' health. Test results are accompanied by normal ranges appropriate for the laboratory's testing procedures.

OUTLINE FORMAT PROGRESS NOTES

Patient Name Hansen (LAST) Christopher (FIRST) M. (MIDDLE) Date of Birth 3 / 1 / 65 Chart # H234

Prob. No. or Letter	DATE	S Subjective	O Objective	A Assess	P Plans	Page 1
	6/16/04	Patient complaining of pain in lower right quadrant. Has been running fever of between 100.5° F and 101.3° F since Sunday morning. Has queasy feeling in stomach and has been unable to eat since yesterday morning.				
			BP 125/75. Temperature 101.2° F. Abdominal exam revealed rebound tenderness and distension in lower right quadrant.			
				Appendicitis		
					1. Admit to hospital 2. Surgically remove appendix.	

Start each Progress Note (Subjective, Objective, Assessment, and Plans) at the appropriate shaded column to create an outline form. Write through the intervening columns to the right margin of the page.

PROGRESS NOTES

TO REORDER CALL TOLL FREE: (800)BIBBERO (800 242-2376)
FORM # 26-7215-01

Figure 18-6. When you use the SOAP approach to documenting patient information, start each progress note at the appropriate shaded column to create an outline form. Write through the intervening columns to the right margin of the page.

if a patient's chief complaint is pain in the left shoulder, you should probe the patient for some pertinent information:

- When did the pain start, and how long have you had the pain? (For example, the type of accident or injury, or the number of days or weeks, etc.)
- When does the pain occur? (For example, on movement, in the morning or evening, etc.)
- Can you describe the pain? (For example, dull, aching, burning, sharp, etc.)
- Rate the pain on a scale of 1 to 10, with 10 being the worst. (A diagram is frequently used for this rating, as shown in Figure 18-8.)

Providing this detailed information is important to the patient's care and treatment. In addition, you will need to chart other information prior to the physician visit. Figure 18-9 shows two types of forms used by the medical assistant and the practitioner when seeing a patient. All information should all be charted completely and accurately. Pay special attention to spelling. If you do not know how to spell a word, look it up or ask someone. Use only approved and recognized abbreviations. Many facilities have a written document identifying these abbreviations. Remember that the chart is a legal document; therefore, special attention to detail is required when charting.

The Health History Form

The medical office usually has a standard medical history form that is used for all patients. The specific arrangement and wording of items vary from office to office. The following sections contain brief descriptions of each of the parts of this form.

Personal Data. This information is obtained from the administrative sheet and includes the patient's name, Social Security number, birth date, and other basic data.

Chief Complaint. Abbreviated as CC, the chief complaint is the reason the patient came to visit the practitioner. It should be short and specific and should cover subjective and objective data.

History of Present Illness. This history includes detailed information about the chief complaint, including when the problem started and what the patient has done to treat the problem (including any medications taken). For example, a chief complaint might be "sore throat" and the history of the present illness would include when the sore throat started (e.g., 3 days ago), how severe the pain is on a scale of 1 to 10 (e.g., pain scale rating of 6 out of 10), and what treatments have been used (e.g., throat lozenges and 4 to 6 aspirin daily).

Past Medical History. The past medical history includes any and all health problems both present and past, including major illnesses and surgery. The past medical history would also include important information about medications and allergies. It should list any medications taken by the patient, including their dosages and the reasons for taking them. Over-the-counter and herbal medications should be considered as well. Known or suspected

HEALTH HISTORY
(Confidential)

Name__________ Today's Date__________

Age_____ Birthdate__________ Date of last physical examination__________

What is your reason for visit?__________

SYMPTOMS Check (✓) symptoms you currently have or have had in the past year.

GENERAL
☐ Chills
☐ Depression
☐ Dizziness
☐ Fainting
☐ Fever
☐ Forgetfulness
☐ Headache
☐ Loss of sleep
☐ Loss of weight
☐ Nervousness
☐ Numbness
☐ Sweats

MUSCLE/JOINT/BONE
Pain, weakness, numbness in:
☐ Arms ☐ Hips
☐ Back ☐ Legs
☐ Feet ☐ Neck
☐ Hands ☐ Shoulders

GENITO-URINARY
☐ Blood in urine
☐ Frequent urination
☐ Lack of bladder control
☐ Painful urination

GASTROINTESTINAL
☐ Appetite poor
☐ Bloating
☐ Bowel changes
☐ Constipation
☐ Diarrhea
☐ Excessive hunger
☐ Excessive thirst
☐ Gas
☐ Hemorrhoids
☐ Indigestion
☐ Nausea
☐ Rectal bleeding
☐ Stomach pain
☐ Vomiting
☐ Vomiting blood

CARDIOVASCULAR
☐ Chest pain
☐ High blood pressure
☐ Irregular heart beat
☐ Low blood pressure
☐ Poor circulation
☐ Rapid heart beat
☐ Swelling of ankles
☐ Varicose veins

EYE, EAR, NOSE, THROAT
☐ Bleeding gums
☐ Blurred vision
☐ Crossed eyes
☐ Difficulty swallowing
☐ Double vision
☐ Earache
☐ Ear discharge
☐ Hay fever
☐ Hoarseness
☐ Loss of hearing
☐ Nosebleeds
☐ Persistent cough
☐ Ringing in ears
☐ Sinus problems
☐ Vision – Flashes
☐ Vision – Halos

SKIN
☐ Bruise easily
☐ Hives
☐ Itching
☐ Change in moles
☐ Rash
☐ Scars
☐ Sore that won't heal

MEN only
☐ Breast lump
☐ Erection difficulties
☐ Lump in testicles
☐ Penis discharge
☐ Sore on penis
☐ Other

WOMEN only
☐ Abnormal Pap smear
☐ Bleeding between periods
☐ Breast lump
☐ Extreme menstrual pain
☐ Hot flashes
☐ Nipple discharge
☐ Painful intercourse
☐ Vaginal discharge
☐ Other

Date of last menstrual period__________
Date of last Pap smear__________
Have you had a mammogram?__________
Are you pregnant?__________
Number of children__________

CONDITIONS Check (✓) conditions you have or have had in the past.

☐ AIDS
☐ Alcoholism
☐ Anemia
☐ Anorexia
☐ Appendicitis
☐ Arthritis
☐ Asthma
☐ Bleeding Disorders
☐ Breast Lump
☐ Bronchitis
☐ Bulimia
☐ Cancer
☐ Cataracts

☐ Chemical Dependency
☐ Chicken Pox
☐ Diabetes
☐ Emphysema
☐ Epilepsy
☐ Glaucoma
☐ Goiter
☐ Gonorrhea
☐ Gout
☐ Heart Disease
☐ Hepatitis
☐ Hernia
☐ Herpes

☐ High Cholesterol
☐ HIV Positive
☐ Kidney Disease
☐ Liver Disease
☐ Measles
☐ Migraine Headaches
☐ Miscarriage
☐ Mononucleosis
☐ Multiple Sclerosis
☐ Mumps
☐ Pacemaker
☐ Pneumonia
☐ Polio

☐ Prostate Problem
☐ Psychiatric Care
☐ Rheumatic Fever
☐ Scarlet Fever
☐ Stroke
☐ Suicide Attempt
☐ Thyroid Problems
☐ Tonsillitis
☐ Tuberculosis
☐ Typhoid Fever
☐ Ulcers
☐ Vaginal Infections
☐ Venereal Disease

MEDICATIONS List medications you are currently taking	**ALLERGIES** To medications or substances
Pharmacy Name__________ Phone__________	

(All information is strictly confidential)

FAMILY HISTORY Fill in health information about your family.

Relation	Age	State of Health	Age at Death	Cause of Death	Check (✓) if, your blood relatives had any of the following:	Disease	Relationship to you
Father						Arthritis, Gout	
Mother						Asthma, Hay Fever	
Brothers						Cancer	
						Chemical Dependency	
						Diabetes	
						Heart Disease, Strokes	
Sisters						High Blood Pressure	
						Kidney Disease	
						Tuberculosis	
						Other	

HOSPITALIZATIONS

Year	Hospital	Reason for Hospitalization and Outcome

PREGNANCY HISTORY

Year of Birth	Sex of Birth	Complications if any

Have you ever had a blood transfusion? ☐ Yes ☐ No
If yes, please give approximate dates.__________

SERIOUS ILLNESS/INJURIES	DATE	OUTCOME

HEALTH HABITS Check (✓) which substances you use and describe how much you use.

	Caffeine	
	Tobacco	
	Drugs	
	Other	

OCCUPATIONAL CONCERNS
Check (✓) if your work exposes you to the following:

	Stress	
	Hazardous Substances	
	Heavy Lifting	
	Other	

Your occupation:

I certify that the above information is correct to the best of my knowledge. I will not hold my doctor or any members of his/her staff responsible for any errors or omissions that I may have made in the completion of this form.

__________ Signature __________ Date

__________ Reviewed By __________ Date

Figure 18-7. The health history form must be complete and accurate. This sample form is started by the patient, then checked and completed by the medical assistant.

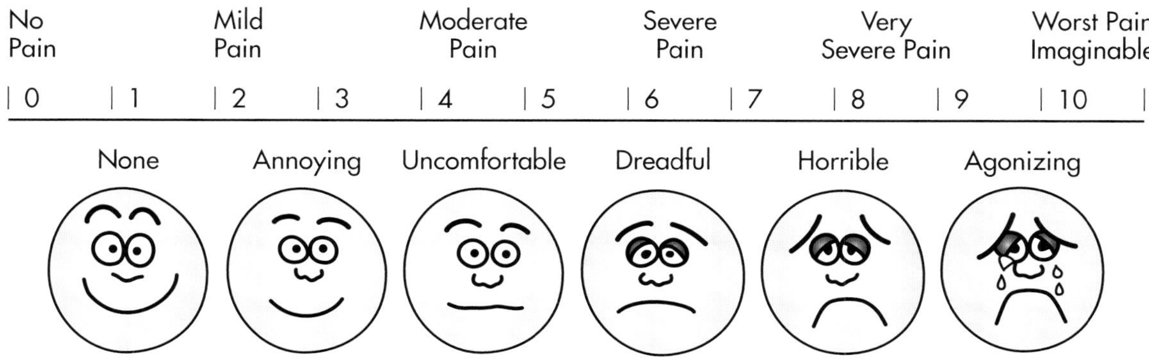

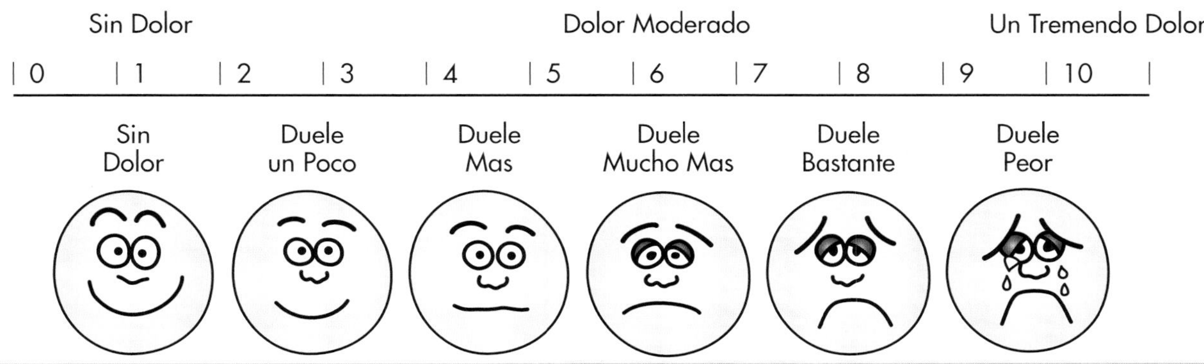

Figure 18-8. Assessing a patient's pain is part of the interview and history-taking process. This common chart is used to make the process easier for the patient and the medical assistant.

allergies to medications or other substances should be listed and clearly visible. Some facilities use a red sticker or other means on charts to identify allergies immediately.

Family History. This section includes information about the health of the patient's family members. Many times the family history can help lead a practitioner to the cause of a current medical problem. Obtain specific information about family members' current ages and medical conditions or, if deceased, their age at death and the cause. Ask open-ended questions about the siblings, parents, and grandparents. Because the death of a parent or sibling or the limited knowledge of an adopted child can be difficult to discuss, use great care and sensitivity when asking these questions.

Social and Occupational History. Information such as marital status, sexual behaviors and orientation, occupations, hobbies, and the use of chemical substances help determine a patient's risk for disease. Patients should be asked about their use of alcohol, tobacco, recreational drugs, or other chemical substances. Be aware that patients may feel uncomfortable or may refuse to provide certain information. Depending on the circumstances, you may ask the question later in the interview. For example, an adolescent child may not want to answer questions about his sexual behaviors in front of his parents. Occupational information regarding the patient's level of stress, exposure to hazardous substances, and heavy lifting may also be included here.

Review of Systems. Some of this information may be started by the patient but is completed by the practitioner. This systematic review of each of the systems of the body includes questions and an examination by the practitioner. The information is obtained in an orderly fashion but may vary depending on the physician or practitioner.

Wildwood Medical Clinic
Progress Notes

Name: Carrie Shaw Chart #: 01769

DATE	
10/12/04	Patient c/o headache and cough X 3 days. HA is dull ache,
	pain scale 7/10 cough—non-productive. — H. Walton CMA

Name Jennifer Haddix DOB 12/05/80 Date 08/28/04

ALLERGIES: Bee Stings, Penicillin

Review of Systems

Systems	NL	Note	Systems	NL	Note
Constitutional			Musculoskeletal		
Eyes			Skin/breasts		
ENT/mouth			Neurologic		
Cardiovascular			Psychiatric		
Respiratory			Endocrine		
GI			Hem/lymph		
GU			Allergy/immun		

Current Medicines	Date	Current Diagnosis
ClaritinD prN MVI T qd Ortho Novum 7/7/7 T qd		

Note

H: 5'7" W: 140 T: 97.8 P: 88 R: 20

B/P Sitting 122/78 or Standing ______ Supine ______

Last Tetantus 06/12/99

L.M.P. 08/20/04

O2 Sat: 98% Pain Scale: 6/10

Social Habits	Yes	No
Tobacco		✓
Alcohol	✓	occ
Rec. Drugs		✓

CC: (L) Shoulder pain X 3 days due to fall. "Sharp pain that hurts when I move"

HPI:

Figure 18-9. These example forms are completed by the medical assistant prior to the physician visit. All information must be complete and accurate as shown.

Summary

As a medical assistant, you will play a key role in a patient's visit to the physician's office. Because you will begin the examination by interviewing the patient, you will set the tone of the visit. Keep in mind that some patients may be nervous or uncomfortable. It is important to make them feel at ease. Using interviewing skills effectively will help make the interview productive as well as comfortable for the patient. Taking a thorough history and using proper documentation methods will also allow you to ensure that patient records are complete and accurate. They will also help the practitioner to diagnose and treat the patient successfully.

REVIEW

CHAPTER 18

CASE STUDY QUESTIONS

Now that you have completed this chapter, review the case study at the beginning of the chapter and answer the following questions:

1. How can you ensure that the interview process goes smoothly?
2. Why is it important that you maintain a positive relationship with this patient?
3. What steps will you take to make sure all the documentation is completed correctly and accurately?

Discussion Questions

1. Explain the difference between subjective and objective data. Give examples of each type.
2. Describe the technique you would use to obtain accurate information from a pediatric patient.
3. What is the significance of each of the parts of the health history form?

Critical Thinking Questions

1. A patient comes into the office with abdominal pain. On her chart is a notation that she is coming in with symptoms of appendicitis. What questions might you ask her to assist the doctor in determining whether her condition is appendicitis?
2. A parent brings in her 3-year-old son, who has chronic diarrhea. You note that the child has a large bruise on the side of his face. He appears very thin and pale. You suspect he may have been abused. What questions might you ask to obtain the information necessary to rule out or confirm abuse?
3. A 31-year-old male patient comes to the clinic after a fall that occurred at work. During the interview, he complains of pain in his left leg and right elbow. He is unable to describe what happened and says he just blacked out. What observations should you make, and what questions should you ask this patient?
4. While interviewing and recording the health history of a patient, you are required to list all the medications the patient is taking. The patient names several medications and provides the dosages; however, you cannot spell one of them and you are not sure about how to write the abbreviations for the dosages. What should you do?

Application Activities

1. Have a partner assume the role of a patient who has come into the office with what appears to be the flu. Conduct an interview and take a patient history.
2. With a partner, practice role-playing both effective and ineffective methods of collecting patient data. Create situations and questions that encourage and discourage communication. Compare and contrast the differences. Use Table 18-1 as a guideline.

Internet Activity

1. Explore the Internet to find resources for charting medical and health information. Find sites for medical abbreviations, medical terminology, and medications, and then create favorites or quick links from the browser on your computer for handy reference when writing in the patient's chart.
2. Research the Internet for a commonly abused drug, and create a brief oral or written report. Include the following information:
   - **a.** The drug's trade and common names
   - **b.** How it affects the body both physically and psychologically
   - **c.** The signs and symptoms of abuse
   - **d.** How you would notice if a patient is abusing this drug

Visit the National Institute of Drug Abuse at **www.nida.nih.gov** to begin your research.

CHAPTER 19

Obtaining Vital Signs and Measurements

KEY TERMS

afebrile
antecubital space
apex
apical
auscultated blood pressure
axilla
brachial artery
calibrate
Celsius (centigrade)
dyspnea
Fahrenheit
febrile
hyperpnea
hypotension
meniscus
palpatory method
radial artery
sphygmomanometer
stethoscope
tachypnea
tympanic thermometer

AREAS OF COMPETENCE

2003 Role Delineation Study

CLINICAL

Patient Care

- Obtain patient history and vital signs

GENERAL

Communication Skills

- Adapt communications to individual's ability to understand
- Recognize and respond effectively to verbal, nonverbal, and written communications
- Utilize electronic technology to receive, organize, prioritize, and transmit information

CHAPTER OUTLINE

- Vital Signs
- Body Measurements

OBJECTIVES

After completing Chapter 19, you will be able to:

19.1 Recognize common terminology and abbreviations used in documenting and discussing vital signs.
19.2 Describe the instruments used to measure vital signs and body measurements.
19.3 Explain the procedure used to measure vital signs and body measurements.
19.4 Demonstrate the procedures for measuring vital signs and body measurements.

Introduction

Vital signs are one of the most important assessments you can make when preparing the patient to be examined by the practitioner. Temperature, pulse, respirations, and blood pressure give information about how a patient will adjust to changes within the body and in the environment. Changes in the vital signs can indicate an abnormality.

Measurements such as height, weight, and head circumference can indicate physical growth and development, especially in infants and children. These measurements are also used to evaluate health problems, such as obesity. You must be accurate when performing and recording vital signs and measurements. The practitioner uses your results when making a diagnosis.

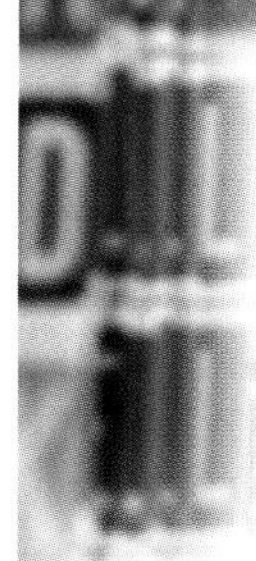

CASE STUDY

A 68-year-old female has been a patient for two years at the clinic where you work as a medical assistant. She suffers from both hypertension and obesity and is taking a diuretic medication (HCTZ, or hydrochlorothiazide) daily.

As you read this chapter, consider the following questions:

1. Why is it essential for you to take accurate measurements of this patient?
2. How can you help ensure the accuracy of these measurements?

Vital Signs

As a medical assistant, you will usually take the vital signs before the doctor examines the patient. Temperature, pulse, respiration, and blood pressure (vital signs) provide the doctor with information about the patient's overall condition.

Preexamination procedures in some offices are performed in a general area outside the patient examination room. In other offices and in most pediatric offices, these measurements are taken in the examination room. In either case you will usually take the measurements before the patient disrobes. Follow the standard procedure used in your office. Also be certain to follow the HIPAA regulations and provide for the privacy of your results.

General Considerations

Vital signs are the primary indicators of a patient's overall general condition. The four vital signs are as follows:

1. Temperature
2. Pulse
3. Respiration
4. Blood pressure

Vital signs are usually measured at every office visit. There is a standard range of values for each measurement, as shown in Table 19-1. Each patient has an individual baseline value that is normal for that patient, however. The difference between a patient's current values and normal values can help the physician in making a diagnosis.

TABLE 19-1 Normal Ranges for Vital Signs

	Age				
Vital Sign	**0–1 year**	**1–6 years**	**6–11 years**	**11–16 years**	**Adult**
Temperature					
Oral (°F)	96–99.5 (less than 4 weeks)	98.5–99.5	97.5–99.6	97.6–99.6	97.6–99.6
Rectal (°F)	99.0–100.0	99.0–100.0	98.5–99.6	98.6–100.6	98.6–100.6
Pulse (beats per minute)	80–160	75–130	70–115	55–110	60–100
Respirations (per minute)	26–40	20–30	18–24	16–24	12–20
Blood Pressure (mm Hg)					
Systolic*	74–100	80–112	80–120	88–120	90–120
Diastolic*	50–70	50–80	50–80	58–80	60–80

*According to the American Heart Association, patients with systolic readings from 120 to 139 mm Hg and diastolic readings from 80 to 89 mm Hg are considered prehypertensive.

TABLE 19-2 OSHA Guidelines for Taking Measurements of Vital Signs	
Situation	**OSHA Guidelines**
Before and after all patient contact	Examination area cleaned according to OSHA standards Aseptic hand washing (Procedure 1-1 in Chapter 1)
Temperature by oral or rectal route Contact with patient with lesions Contact with patient suspect for infectious disease	Gloves worn Biohazard bags used for disposal of used thermometer sheaths, otoscope tips, alcohol swabs, dressings, and bandages
In presence of patient suspect for airborne infectious disease (particularly sneezing)	Mask worn Patient weighed, measured, and examined in room away from staff and other patients Protective clothing (laboratory coat, gown, or apron) worn Biohazard bags used as above

You must follow closely the guidelines from the Department of Labor's Occupational Safety and Health Administration (OSHA) for taking measurements of vital signs (Table 19-2). These guidelines are intended to prevent transmission of disease from the patient. They help protect you and keep the workplace safe.

Temperature

When you take a patient's temperature, you will determine whether the patient is **febrile** (has a body temperature above the patient's normal range) or whether the patient is **afebrile** (has a body temperature at about the patient's normal range). A fever is usually a sign of inflammation or infection. You can take a temperature in one of four locations:

1. Mouth (oral)
2. Ear (tympanic)
3. Rectum (rectal)
4. Armpit, or **axilla** (axillary)

Temperature can be measured in degrees **Fahrenheit** (°F) or degrees **Celsius** (**centigrade;** °C). Figure 19-1, gives equivalent values for the two temperature scales. Normal adult oral temperature is considered to be about 98.6°F or 37.0°C. Rectal and tympanic temperatures are normally 1° higher than an oral temperature. The rectal method usually provides the most accurate body temperature; however, the oral method is more commonly used and is accurate when performed properly. Axillary temperatures are normally 1° lower than oral temperatures because the area is outside the body and exposed to air.

Temperature is measured with a thermometer. Thermometers may be one of three types: electronic digital, tympanic, or disposable.

Electronic Digital Thermometers. Electronic digital thermometers are used frequently in medical offices. These thermometers provide a digital readout of the patient's temperature (Figure 19-2). They are accurate, fast, easy to read, and comfortable for the patient.

Fahrenheit and Celsius Equivalents for Temperature

°F	°C	°F	°C	°F	°C	°F	°C
95.0	35.0	98.4	36.9	101.8	38.8	105.2	40.7
95.2	35.1	98.6	37.0	102.0	38.9	105.4	40.8
95.4	35.2	98.8	37.1	102.2	39.0	105.6	40.9
95.6	35.3	99.0	37.2	102.4	39.1	105.8	41.0
95.8	35.4	99.2	37.3	102.6	39.2	106.0	41.1
96.0	35.6	99.4	37.4	102.8	39.3	106.2	41.2
96.2	35.7	99.6	37.6	103.0	39.4	106.4	41.3
96.4	35.8	99.8	37.7	103.2	39.6	106.6	41.4
96.6	35.9	100.0	37.8	103.4	39.7	106.8	41.6
96.8	36.0	100.2	37.9	103.6	39.8	107.0	41.7
97.0	36.1	100.4	38.0	103.8	39.9	107.2	41.8
97.2	36.2	100.6	38.1	104.0	40.0	107.4	41.9
97.4	36.3	100.8	38.2	104.2	40.1	107.6	42.0
97.6	36.4	101.0	38.3	104.4	40.2	107.8	42.1
97.8	36.6	101.2	38.4	104.6	40.3	108.0	42.2
98.0	36.7	101.4	38.6	104.8	40.4		
98.2	36.8	101.6	38.7	105.0	40.6		

Note: °F = (°C × ⁹⁄₅) + 32; °C = (°F − 32) × ⁵⁄₉. Conversions are rounded to nearest tenth.

Figure 19-1. Use this chart to convert Fahrenheit temperature readings to Celsius and vice versa.

One type of electronic thermometer is designed for oral, rectal, or axillary use. This type of thermometer has a battery-powered display unit, a wire cord, and a temperature-sensitive probe covered by a disposable plastic tip. Separate probes and tips are available for oral or rectal use. Most units have an audible indicator, such as a beep, to let you know when the temperature has registered and is displayed.

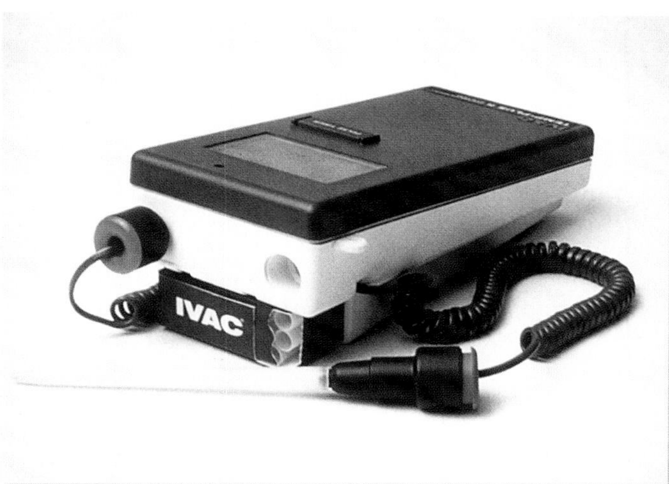

Figure 19-2. The electronic digital thermometer provides a digital readout of the patient's temperature.

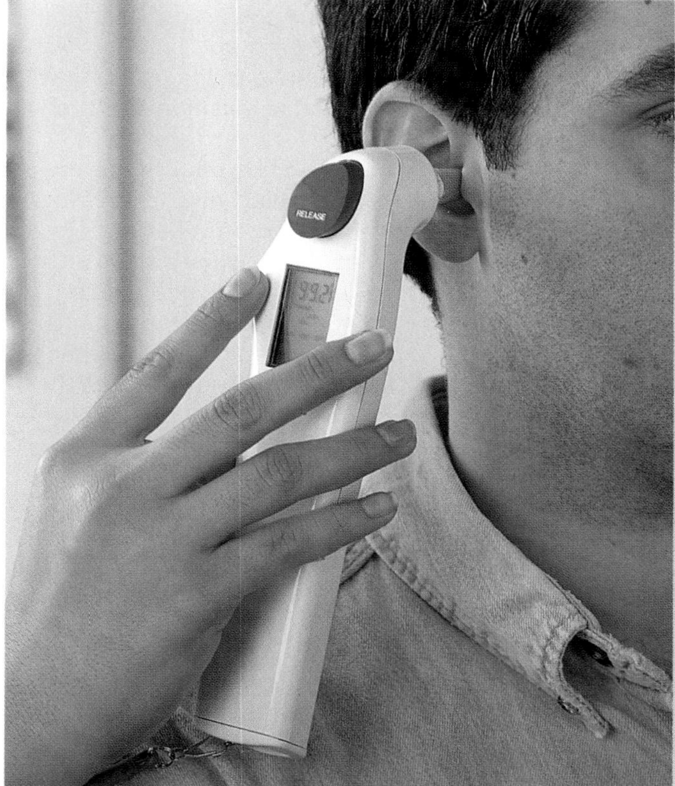

Figure 19-3. The tympanic thermometer measures infrared energy emitted from the tympanic membrane. The result, converted to body temperature, is displayed within seconds of insertion of the shielded tip into the ear.

Tympanic Thermometers. Another type of electronic thermometer, the **tympanic thermometer,** is designed for use in the ear, as shown in Figure 19-3. This thermometer measures infrared energy emitted from the tympanic membrane (eardrum). This energy is converted into a temperature reading. Because of its speed, ease of use, and comfort for the patient, the tymp ter is popular in pediatric offices. The tip is disposable sheath to prevent cross-contamina

Disposable Thermometers. Disposable, use thermometers are usually made of thin strips tic with specially treated dot or strip indicators. indicators change color according to the temperature. T type of thermometer is used most commonly for oral and axillary temperature measurements, particularly in children. Typically, it does not give as accurate a reading as other types of thermometers do. However, disposable thermometers are useful for patients in their homes.

Taking Temperatures

Using the proper instrument and technique provides the most accurate temperature readings. Temperatures can vary according to the location used. Thus, you must be sure to indicate the site (oral, rectal, axillary, tympanic) of the temperature measurement when you enter the reading in the patient's chart. If no site is specified, it is presumed to be oral. All temperature measurements should be recorded to the nearest one-tenth of a degree.

Using Tympanic Thermometers. Although accurate when used correctly, tympanic thermometers can give incorrect readings if you do not follow the proper technique exactly. For a description of tympanic thermometers and potential problems with their use, see the Caution: Handle With Care section.

Although you must follow manufacturers' instructions precisely, these thermometers are easy to use. First remove the thermometer from its recharging cradle, then wait for the indicator light to show that the unit is ready. Attach a disposable sheath, and place the thermometer in the opening of the ear so that the fit is snug. Pull the ear up and back for adults and down and back for children. Press the button, and the result will be displayed within seconds. Be certain to press the correct button to read the temperature. Another button on the thermometer releases the sheath. You do not want to release the sheath into the patient's ear.

Measuring Oral Temperatures. To take an oral temperature, make sure the patient is able to hold the thermometer in the mouth. The patient must also be able to breathe through the nose. Place the thermometer under the tongue in either pocket just off-center in the lower jaw. The patient should hold the thermometer with lips closed. Wait at least 15 minutes after a patient has been eating, drinking, or smoking before taking an oral temperature; otherwise, you may obtain an inaccurate result.

Measuring Rectal Temperatures. Temperatures are sometimes measured rectally in infants or adults in whom an oral temperature cannot be taken. When taking rectal temperatures, you must wear gloves to prevent contamination from microorganisms present in the stool.

To take a rectal temperature, use an electronic thermometer with a rectal probe and disposable rectal tip. The

…TION *Handle With Care*

…rmometers: What You Need to Know

…rs are popular in medical of- …tric offices, because they are fast …n used correctly. They are also par- …y useful with uncooperative patients and with patients who have been eating, drinking, or smoking, because tympanic temperature readings are not affected by these activities.

If you do not use the proper technique, however, you can get inaccurate temperature readings with a tympanic thermometer. Here is a summary of what you need to know.

Why the Eardrum?

The idea of using the tympanic membrane as a site for temperature measurement originated in the 1960s as a means of measuring temperature in astronauts. The eardrum is an ideal place to measure temperature because it shares the same blood supply with the hypothalamus, the organ that controls body temperature.

How Do Tympanic Thermometers Work?

Tympanic thermometers work by measuring infrared energy, a type of heat energy, emitted from the tympanic membrane (eardrum). The thermometer converts this information into a temperature reading, usually within seconds. Most tympanic thermometers run on a rechargeable battery that must be recharged between uses.

Where Problems Can Occur

The technique for taking a tympanic temperature may vary slightly, depending on which brand of thermometer you use. You must follow the manufacturer's instructions for your instrument to get accurate results.

Most units have an indicator to let you know when the thermometer is ready for use. Some units require taking the temperature within a certain period after removing the thermometer from its charging base. Read the manufacturer's instructions for specific information.

There can be problems with most units if the outer opening of the ear is not sealed completely when the probe is placed at the ear canal. An improper seal may also mean that the thermometer is not aimed at the eardrum and will give an inaccurate reading. You may need to tug gently on the ear to position the thermometer properly and aim it at the eardrum.

If the thermometer has been charging for several hours before use, the initial reading may be inaccurately high. Therefore, some experts believe you should take two measurements on the first patient after charging the unit and record only the second reading.

Even with good technique, errors can sometimes occur. If you do obtain a reading that does not appear to match the patient's general condition, repeat the temperature measurement to be sure.

patient should be positioned on one side or on the stomach with the anus exposed. The left side is the preferred position. The bulb of the thermometer should be inserted slowly and gently until it is covered or until you feel resistance, at approximately 1 inch for adults and ½ inch for infants and small children. Hold the thermometer in place while taking the temperature.

Measuring Axillary Temperatures. To take an axillary temperature, first have the patient sit or lie down. Place the tip of the thermometer in the middle of the axilla, with the shaft facing forward. The patient's upper arm should be pressed against his side, and his lower arm should be crossed over the stomach to hold the thermometer in place. Make sure the tip of the thermometer touches skin on all sides of the probe.

Special Considerations in Children. Taking a child's or an infant's temperature can be a challenge. If the infant or child is likely to cry or become agitated, take the temperature last. Measure pulse, respiration, and blood pressure (if ordered) before you take the temperature to avoid having these measurements elevated because of the child's agitation.

Oral thermometers are not appropriate for children under 5 years of age because these children are too young to safely hold the thermometer in their mouths. Instead, take axillary, rectal, or tympanic temperatures. If you use a rectal thermometer, hold it in place until the temperature registers, because the thermometer can be expelled easily. Furthermore, children, especially infants, can injure themselves if they move while having a rectal temperature taken. Tympanic thermometers are especially useful in pediatric offices because of their speed and safety.

Pulse and Respiration

Pulse and respiration are related because the circulatory and respiratory systems work together. Pulse is measured as the number of times the heart beats in 1 minute. Respiration is the number of times a patient breathes in 1 minute.

One breath, or respiration, equals one inhalation and one exhalation. Usually if either the pulse or respiration rate is high or low, the other is also. The usual ratio of the pulse rate to the respiration rate is about 4:1 (for example, a pulse of 80 and a respiration of 20).

Pulse. A pulse rate gives information about the patient's cardiovascular system. It is an indirect measurement of the patient's cardiac output. If the pulse is abnormally fast, slow, weak, or irregular, the patient may have a medical problem.

Measure the pulse of adults at the **radial artery,** where it can be felt in the groove on the thumb side of the inner wrist. Press lightly on this pulse point with your fingers and not your thumb (a pulse is located in your thumb, and you may feel it instead of the patient's pulse), and count the number of beats you feel in 1 minute. Office policy may direct that you count the pulse for 30 seconds and multiply the results by 2 to obtain the beats per minute. If you take a pulse for less than 1 minute and notice irregularities, you must count for 1 full minute and document the irregularities.

In young children the radial artery may be hard to feel. You may instead take the pulse at the **brachial artery,** which is in the bend of the elbow (the **antecubital space**).

You may not be able to feel the brachial artery in an infant. If you cannot, then take the pulse over the **apex** (the left lower corner) of the heart, where the strongest heart sounds can be heard. Count the **apical** pulse while you listen with a **stethoscope,** an instrument that amplifies body sounds. The apex is located in the fifth intercostal space between the ribs on the left side of the chest, directly below the center of the clavicle. Consult Figure 19-4 for placement of the stethoscope.

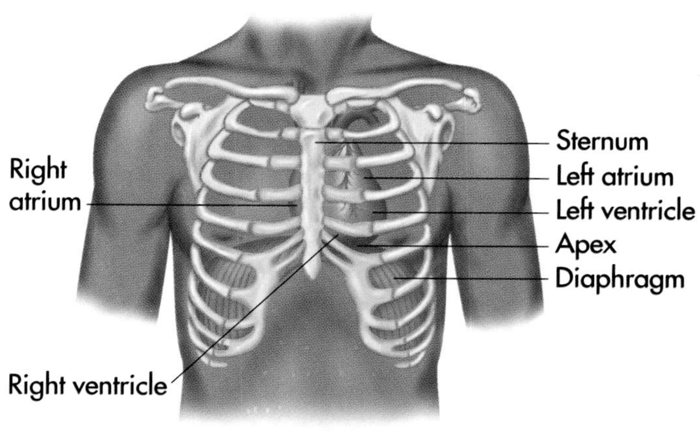

Figure 19-4. A stethoscope is used over the apex of the heart to listen for the pulse in patients in whom pulse is not otherwise detectable.

You may also use other locations to take a pulse. Figure 19-5 shows the location of common pulse points.

Electronic Pulse. The pulse may also be measured electronically using a device attached to the finger or sometimes the earlobe. Figure 19-6 shows one type of device used as part of an electronic blood pressure machine. A pulse oximeter machine, which measures the oxygen level of the blood, can also be used (Figure 19-7). When using these devices, be certain to attach the clip firmly to the finger or lobe. The clip uses an infrared light to measure the pulse and

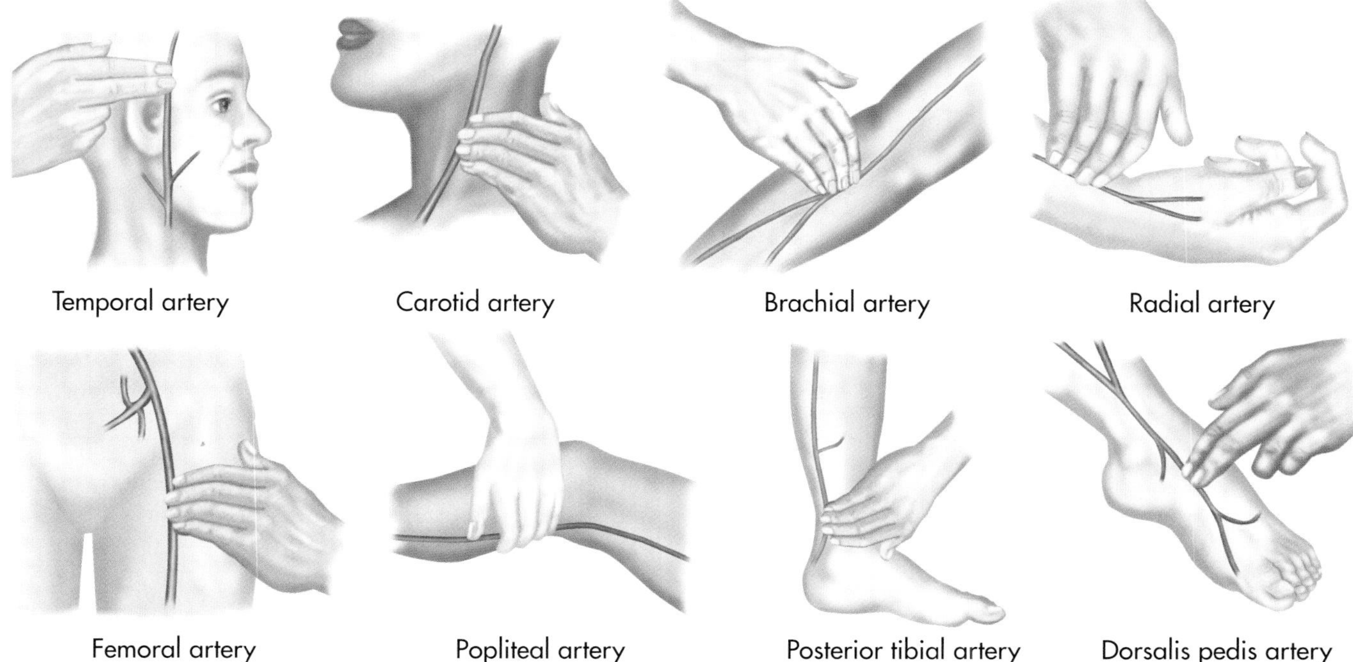

Figure 19-5. There are many locations on the body where major arteries are close enough to the surface to allow a pulse to be felt and counted.

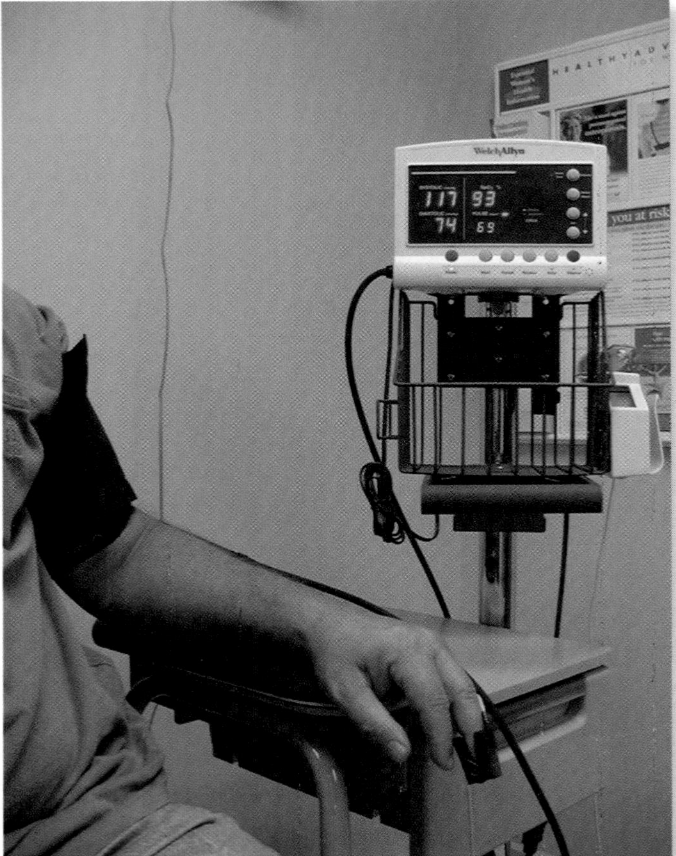

Figure 19-6. Pulse, blood pressure, and oxygen saturation can all be measured with this electronic blood pressure device.
Photo courtesy of Total Care Programming.

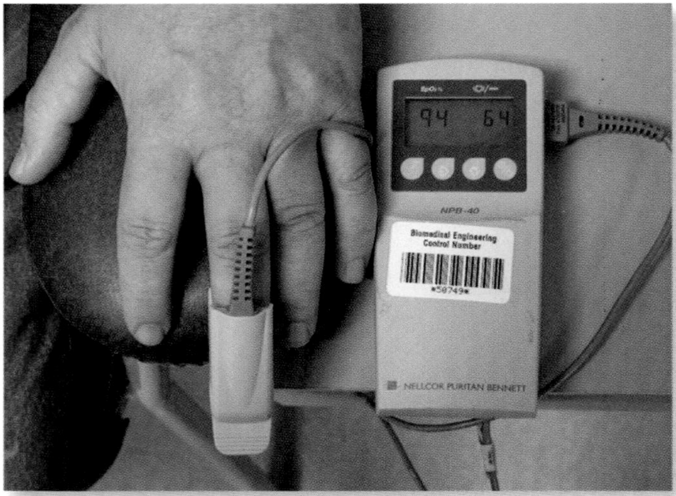

Figure 19-7. A pulse oximeter measures the pulse and oxygen saturation of the blood.
Photo courtesy of Total Care Programming.

oxygen levels, so it works best when no nail polish is present on the patient's finger. The pulse reading and the oxygen saturation of the blood will display on the screen. If the pulse is outside the normal range (see Table 19-1), it should be taken again or performed manually. If the oxygen level is less than 92%, the patient should be asked to take deep breaths during the procedure to increase her oxygen level.

Respiration. Respiration rate indicates how well a patient's body is providing oxygen to tissues. The best way to check respiration is by watching, listening, or feeling the movement at the patient's chest, stomach, back, or shoulders. If you cannot see the chest movement, then place your hand over the patient's chest, shoulder, or abdomen and listen for the movement of air. You may not be able to see or hear the breathing of some patients. Many times the most reliable method for measuring respiration is with a stethoscope. Place the stethoscope on one side of the spine in the middle of the back to count respirations. You need to do this subtly, however, because once the patient is aware that respiration is being measured, he may unintentionally alter his breathing. You may tell the patient that you want to listen to his lungs.

Counting respirations for less than 1 full minute may cause you to miss certain breathing abnormalities. Irregularities such as **dyspnea** (difficult or painful breathing), **tachypnea** (rapid breathing), or **hyperpnea** (deep, rapid breathing) are important indications of possible infection or disease.

Respiration rates are higher in infants and children than in adults. Become familiar with the normal ranges of respiration for each age group, as presented in Table 19-1.

Blood Pressure

Blood pressure (also known as arterial blood pressure) is the force at which blood is pumped against the walls of the arteries. The standard unit for measuring blood pressure is millimeters of mercury (mm Hg). The pressure measured when the left ventricle of the heart contracts is known as the **systolic pressure.** The pressure measured when the heart relaxes is known as the **diastolic pressure.** The diastolic pressure indicates the minimum amount of pressure exerted against the vessel walls at all times.

Expected adult systolic readings range from 100 to 120 mm Hg. Expected adult diastolic readings range from 60 to 80 mm Hg. These values may increase with advancing age. Readings that are higher than these values are considered prehypertensive.

Certain disease states may cause blood pressure to rise above or fall below these ranges. Thus, it is important to recognize these abnormalities. **Hypertension,** or high blood pressure, is a major contributor to heart attack and stroke. The doctor may ask a patient whose blood pressure is elevated to return in 2 months or less for a checkup or blood pressure check. If the blood pressure remains elevated, the patient may be diagnosed with hypertension. **Hypotension,** or low blood pressure, is not generally a chronic health problem. Slightly low blood pressure may be normal for some patients and does not usually require treatment. Severe hypotension may be present with shock, heart failure, severe burns, and excessive bleeding.

Blood Pressure Measuring Equipment. Blood pressure is measured with an instrument called a **sphygmomanometer.** A sphygmomanometer consists of an inflatable cuff, a pressure bulb or automatic device for inflating the cuff, and a manometer to read the pressure. The three basic types of sphygmomanometers differ in how the pressure is displayed.

Aneroid Sphygmomanometers. Aneroid sphygmomanometers have a circular gauge for registering pressure. The needle on the gauge rotates as pressure rises. This type of sphygmomanometer is very accurate. Each measurement line indicates 2 mm Hg (Figure 19-8).

Electronic Sphygmomanometers. Electronic sphygmomanometers provide a digital readout of blood pressure on a lit display (Figure 19-9). Unlike mercury and aneroid sphygmomanometers, these devices do not require use of a stethoscope to determine blood pressure. Although they are easy to use, electronic sphygmomanometers are very costly and may give you an inaccurate reading. However, electronic sphygmomanometers are often used, and newer models have improved accuracy. If you question the results of an electronic blood pressure measurement, take it again with an aneroid cuff.

Mercury Sphygmomanometers. Mercury sphygmomanometers contain a column of mercury. The mercury column rises with an increase in pressure as the cuff is inflated. Mercury sphygmomanometers may be wall-mounted units, tabletop units, or freestanding units on wheels. Mercury instruments are used less frequently because the government has restricted the use of mercury due to its affects on the environment. Consequently, no new mercury sphygmomanometers are being manufactured.

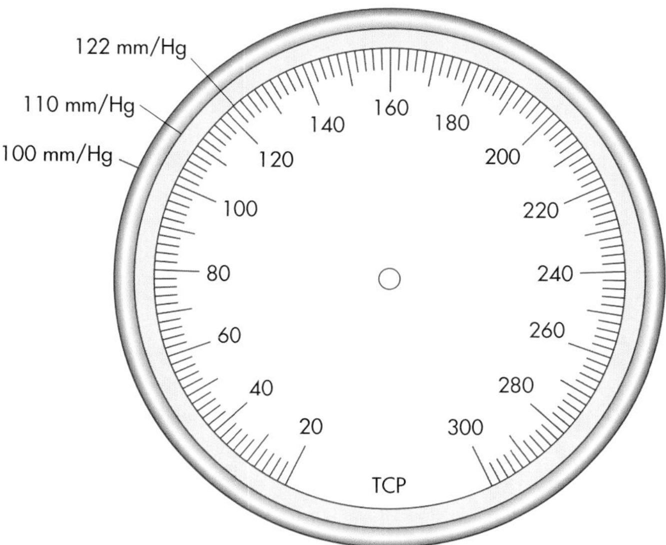

Figure 19-8. Each line on the aneroid gauge indicates 2 mm Hg. To prevent inaccuracies, look directly at this gauge when performing a blood pressure test.

Borrowed from Kathryn Booth, *Health Care Science Technology: Career Technology, 1st ed.,* Peoria, IL: Glencoe/McGraw-Hill, 2004.

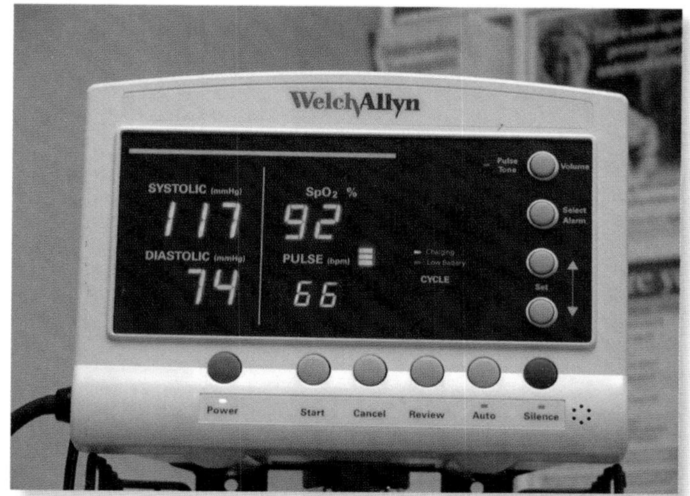

Figure 19-9. This electronic sphygmomanometer displays the patient's blood pressure, pulse, and oxygen saturation. If you question any of the results, repeat the test using a manual method.

Calibrating the Sphygmomanometer. To ensure that sphygmomanometers are working properly, you or a medical supply dealer must calibrate them regularly. To **calibrate** means to standardize a measuring instrument. Mercury sphygmomanometers must be checked for faults, serviced, and calibrated every 6 to 12 months. Aneroid sphygmomanometers must be checked, serviced, and calibrated every 3 to 6 months. Follow the manufacturer's instructions for an electronic sphygmomanometer.

Each time you use a mercury or aneroid sphygmomanometer, you need to ensure that it is correctly calibrated. To do so, follow these steps.

- For a mercury sphygmomanometer, check that the **meniscus** (curve in the air-to-liquid surface of the specimen in the cylinder) of mercury on the mercury column rests at zero when you view it at eye level.
- For an aneroid sphygmomanometer, check that the recording needle on the dial rests within the small square at the bottom of the dial. To calibrate the dial, use a Y connector to attach the dial to a pressure bulb and a calibrated mercury manometer. Use the pressure bulb to elevate both manometer readings to 250 mm Hg. As you let the pressure fall, record both readings at four different points. The difference between paired readings should not exceed 3 mm Hg.

Do not use a sphygmomanometer that is not correctly calibrated. The patient's blood pressure reading will not be accurate.

The Stethoscope. A stethoscope amplifies body sounds, making them louder. It consists of earpieces, binaurals, rubber or plastic tubing, and a chestpiece (Figure 19-10). For best results the earpieces should fit snugly and comfortably in your ears. When placing them in your

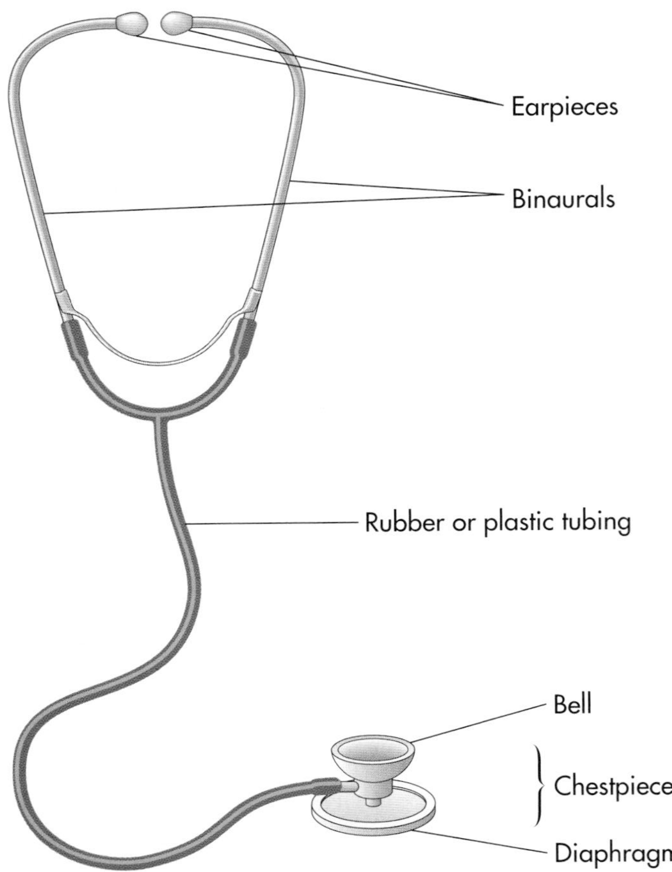

Figure 19-10. The stethoscope amplifies body sounds.

ears, face the angle of the earpiece up and forward for the best fit.

The chestpiece consists of two parts: the diaphragm and the bell. The diaphragm is the larger, flat side of the chestpiece. It is covered by a thin, plastic disk. The diaphragm must be placed firmly against the skin for proper amplification of sound. The diaphragm is best at amplifying high-pitched sounds, such as bowel and lung sounds.

The bell is the cone-shaped side of the stethoscope chestpiece. It must be held lightly against the skin to amplify sound. The bell is best at amplifying low-pitched sounds, such as vascular and heart sounds. With practice you may find you prefer to use one side rather than the other for various purposes.

Measuring Blood Pressure. To measure blood pressure, wrap the rubber cuff of the sphygmomanometer around the patient's upper arm, just above the pulse point of the brachial artery. This pulse point is located in the bend of the elbow, or the **antecubital space.** If the patient has an injury to one arm, or has had a mastectomy (breast removal), then place the cuff on the other arm. Otherwise, palpate the pulse in both arms, and use the one with the stronger pulse. Inflate the cuff, then while you release the air in the cuff, listen with the stethoscope. The cuff is usually inflated to 30 mm Hg above the palpatory result, or approximately 180 to 200 mm Hg. You will hear vascular sounds that will change. These sounds are also called Korotkoff sounds. They are produced by the obstruction and release of the arterial blood flow.

The first heartbeat you hear is the systolic pressure. As the pressure in the cuff is released, this strong heartbeat changes to a softer, muffled sound. The point at which the sound disappears is the diastolic pressure. The patient's blood pressure reading is recorded as the numbers registered for the first and last sounds separated by a slash mark, as in BP 120/76. Although only the systolic and diastolic readings are usually recorded for adults, a third number may be included at times. For example, if there is a pressure difference greater than 10 mm Hg between the muffled sound and its disappearance, the blood pressure is recorded with all three sounds noted, such as 120/80/60. The process of taking blood pressure is described in Procedure 19-1.

Special Considerations in Adults. Blood pressure is elevated during and just after exercise. If a patient has engaged in strenuous activity before the examination, you should wait 15 minutes before taking blood pressure measurements. This waiting period also applies to patients with ambulatory disabilities, to those who are obese, and to those who have a known blood pressure problem. If you ensure that patients have relaxed for 15 minutes before you measure their blood pressure, you will get an accurate reading.

Blood pressure may also be elevated when a patient is anxious or under extreme stress. If the patient seems stressed, allow him to rest for about 5 minutes before measuring his blood pressure. To help the patient relax, try to engage the person in conversation rather than calling attention to the fact that you are waiting to take his blood pressure. If the patient still appears anxious or under stress, take his blood pressure anyway, and make a notation for the physician (who may want to repeat the measurement later in the visit).

There are certain instances when you should not take a blood pressure measurement on a particular arm. Blood pressure should not be taken on an arm that is on the same side as a mastectomy or on an arm that has an injury, a blocked artery, or a device under the skin (implant) at the site. In such cases use the other arm or the upper leg. Note the measurements and their locations in the patient's chart.

Be sure you use the proper size cuff when taking blood pressure. The bladder inside the cuff should encircle 80% to 100% the distance around the arm or leg. Although the standard adult cuff can be used for most adults, some may require the larger size. Using an improper size may result in an inaccurate reading.

Sometimes a patient is aware that a blood pressure reading is abnormally high or low. If the patient is upset about a reading, tell her that the physician may take another reading later, perhaps on the other arm.

Special Considerations in Children. Blood pressure in children or infants is not routinely measured at

PROCEDURE 19.1

Taking the Blood Pressure of Adults and Older Children

Objective: To accurately measure blood pressure in adults and older children

OSHA Guidelines

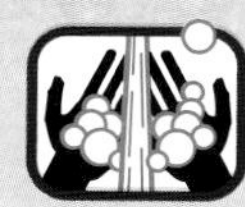

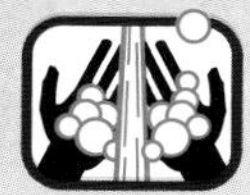

Materials: Aneroid or mercury sphygmomanometer, stethoscope, alcohol gauze squares, patient's chart, and black pen.

Method

1. Gather the equipment and make sure the sphygmomanometer is in working order and is correctly calibrated.
2. Identify the patient and introduce yourself.
3. Wash your hands and explain the procedure to the patient.
4. Have the patient sit in a quiet area. If she is wearing long-sleeved clothing, have her loosely roll up one sleeve. If she cannot, have her change into a gown. (A sleeve that is tightly rolled up may restrict the blood flow and give inaccurate readings. The cuff should not be placed over clothing for the same reason.)
5. Have the patient rest her bared arm on a flat surface so that the midpoint of the upper arm is at the same level as the heart.
6. Select a cuff that is the appropriate size for the patient. The bladder inside the cuff should encircle 80% of the arm in adults and 100% of the arm in children under the age of 13. If you are not sure about the size, use a larger cuff.
7. Locate the brachial artery in the antecubital space.
8. Position the cuff so that the midline of the bladder is above the arterial pulsation. Then wrap and secure the cuff snugly around the patient's bare upper arm. The lower edge of the cuff should be 1 inch above the antecubital space, where the head of the stethoscope is to be placed.
9. Place the manometer so that the center of the aneroid dial or mercury column is at eye level and easily visible and so that the tubing from the cuff is unobstructed.
10. Close the valve of the pressure bulb until it is finger-tight.
11. Inflate the cuff rapidly to 70 mm Hg with one hand, and increase this pressure by 10 mm Hg increments while palpating the radial pulse with your other hand. Note the level of pressure at which the pulse disappears and subsequently reappears during deflation. This procedure, the **palpatory method,** provides a necessary preliminary approximation of the systolic blood pressure to ensure an adequate level of inflation when the actual auscultatory measurement is made.
12. Open the valve to release the pressure, deflate the cuff completely, and wait 30 seconds. (If you do not deflate the cuff completely and wait, blood may pool in the artery and give a falsely high reading.)
13. Place the earpieces of the stethoscope in your ear canals, and adjust them to fit snugly and comfortably. When placed in the ears, they should point up or toward the nose. Switch the stethoscope head to the diaphragm position. Confirm the setting by listening as you tap the stethoscope head gently.
14. Place the head of the stethoscope over the brachial artery pulsation, just above and medial to the antecubital space but below the lower edge of the cuff. Hold the stethoscope firmly in place between the index and middle fingers, making sure the head is in contact with the skin around its entire circumference. (Do not hold the stethoscope with the thumb, because the pulse of your thumb can interfere with the reading.)
15. Inflate the bladder rapidly and steadily to a pressure 20 to 30 mm Hg above the level previously determined by palpation. Then partially open (unscrew) the valve, and deflate the bladder at 2 mm per second while you listen for the appearance of the Korotkoff sounds.
16. As the pressure in the bladder falls, note the level of pressure on the manometer at the first appearance of repetitive sounds. This reading is the systolic pressure.
17. Continue to deflate the cuff gradually, noting the point at which the sound changes from strong to muffled.
18. Continue to deflate the cuff, and note when the sound disappears. This reading is the diastolic pressure.

continued ⟶

PROCEDURE 19.1

Taking the Blood Pressure of Adults and Older Children *(continued)*

19. Deflate the cuff completely, and remove it from the patient's arm.
20. Record the three numbers, separated by slashes, in the patient's chart. (This value is an exact measurement of the **auscultated blood pressure,** meaning that it was determined by listening with a stethoscope.) Remember to indicate the date and time of the measurement, the arm on which the measurement was made, the subject's position, and the cuff size when a nonstandard size is used.
21. Fold the cuff and replace it in the holder.
22. Inform the patient that you have completed the procedure.
23. Disinfect the earpieces and diaphragm of the stethoscope with gauze squares moistened with alcohol.
24. Properly dispose of the used gauze squares and wash your hands.

each visit. Instead, the measurement is taken on the order of the doctor. The procedure is the same as that for taking blood pressure in adults, except for these modifications.

1. Ideally, take the patient's blood pressure before performing other tests or procedures that may cause anxiety. In this way you can avoid a falsely high result.
2. Be sure to use the correct cuff size for the child or infant. The bladder width should not exceed two-thirds the length of the upper or lower arm. The bladder should cover three-fourths the circumference of the extremity.
3. Do not attempt to estimate an infant's blood pressure in the manner described in Procedure 19-1—the palpatory method usually cannot be used on an infant.
4. Inflate the pressure cuff to 20 mm Hg above the point at which the radial pulse disappears.
5. Deflate the cuff at a rate of 2 mm Hg per second.
6. You may continue to hear a heartbeat on a child or infant until the pressure reaches zero, so note when the strong heartbeat becomes muffled.

Body Measurements

Certain measurements are obtained prior to the patient's being seen by the practitioner. These include height and weight for adults and older children, and weight, length, and head circumference for infants. Usually these measurements are taken before or after the vital signs, depending on the office policy. Depending on the patient, you may choose to take the patient's vital signs first. For example, if a patient may become upset about her weight, you should take her vital signs first so that the patient's vital signs will not be affected by the weight results. Follow the policy at your facility.

At the first visit these measurements provide baseline values for a patient's current condition. Any extreme or abnormal changes may indicate a disease or disorders of metabolism. Metabolism includes the processes that break down food and convert it into energy or build it into body tissue. Abnormal changes in weight, height, and body proportions may indicate a metabolic problem.

Weight and height measurements of children and adolescents, taken at each office visit, allow the physician to follow growth and development. Many physicians use growth charts to compare a child's growth with that of other children the same age (Figure 19-11). These charts help physicians recognize possible growth and nutritional problems.

Measurements are also important in determining certain treatment regimens. For example, dosages of certain medications are based on patient weight. These measurements may also be necessary for correct interpretation of certain diagnostic tests, such as electrocardiography. Metric conversions for weight and height measurements are given in Figures 19-12 and 19-13.

Measuring the Weight of Adults

An adult's weight is taken at each office visit. Weight should be listed in the patient's chart to the nearest quarter of a pound. The steps for weighing an adult are described in Procedure 19-2.

Measuring the Height of Adults

The height of an adult should be measured at the patient's initial visit and whenever a complete physical examination is performed or at least yearly. Height should be measured to the nearest quarter of an inch.

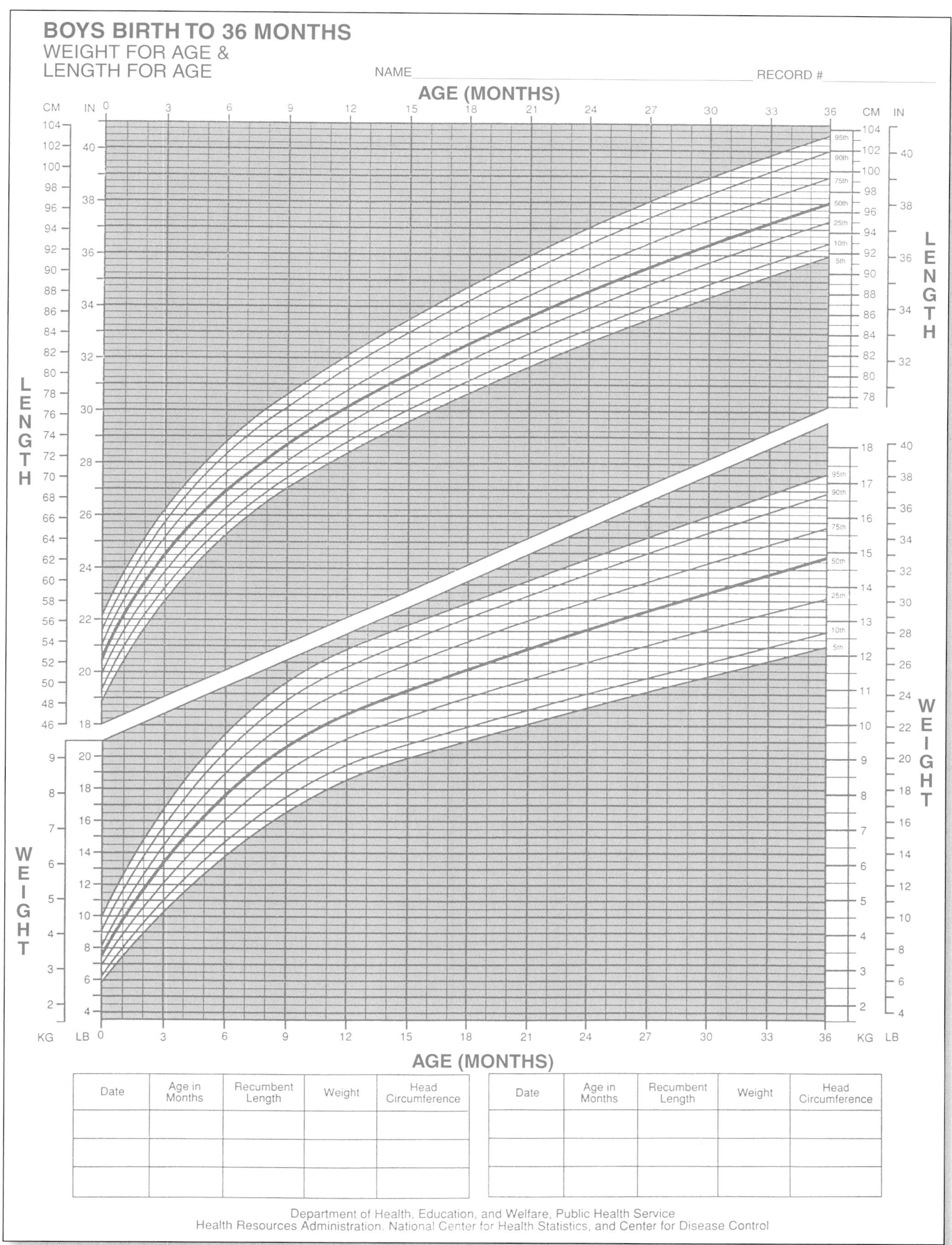

Figure 19-11. The curved lines on this growth chart show the normal range of growth for boys from birth to age 36 months.

Metric Conversions for Weight

lb	kg	lb	kg	lb	kg
10	4.5	95	43.1	180	81.7
15	6.8	100	45.4	185	84.0
20	9.1	105	47.7	190	86.3
25	11.4	110	49.9	195	88.5
30	13.6	115	52.2	200	90.8
35	15.9	120	54.5	205	93.1
40	18.2	125	56.8	210	95.3
45	20.4	130	59.0	215	97.6
50	22.7	135	61.3	220	99.9
55	25.0	140	63.6	225	102.2
60	27.2	145	65.8	230	104.4
65	29.5	150	68.1	235	106.7
70	31.8	155	70.4	240	109.0
75	34.1	160	72.6	245	111.2
80	36.3	165	74.9	250	113.5
85	38.6	170	77.2		
90	40.9	175	79.5		

Note: kg = lb × 0.454; lb = kg × 2.205. Conversions are rounded to nearest tenth.

Figure 19-12. Use this chart to convert pounds to kilograms and vice versa.

Metric Conversions for Height

in	cm	in	cm	in	cm
20	51	42	107	62	157
22	56	44	112	64	163
24	61	46	117	66	168
26	66	48	122	68	173
28	71	50	127	70	178
30	76	52	132	72	183
32	81	54	137	74	188
34	86	56	142	76	193
36	91	58	147	78	198
38	97	60	152	80	203
40	102				

Note: cm = in × 2.54; in = cm × 0.394. Conversions are rounded to nearest whole number.

Figure 19-13. Use this chart to convert inches to centimeters and vice versa.

Measure the patient's height after weighing the patient. Most office scales have a height bar located in the center of the scale. This bar is calibrated in inches and quarter inches (Figure 19-14). The steps for measuring the height of an adult are described in Procedure 19-2.

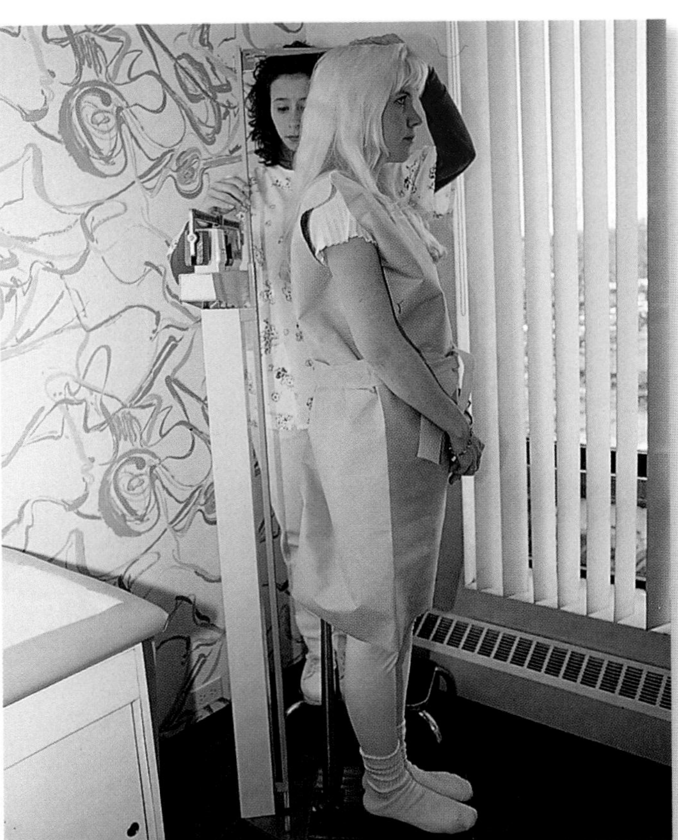

Figure 19-14. The scale with attached height bar is used for measuring the height and weight of children and adults.

Measuring the Weight of Children and Infants

Children and infants are weighed at each office visit. Children who can stand may be weighed on an adult scale. If toddlers cannot remain still on an adult scale, weight may be determined by weighing an adult holding the toddler, then subtracting the weight of the adult.

Infants are weighed on infant scales, which typically measure pounds and ounces. Infant scales are sometimes built into a pediatric examination table. The steps for weighing children and infants are described in Procedure 19-3.

Measuring the Height of Children and Infants

The height of children and length of infants is measured at each office visit. Measure children in the same manner as you measure an adult. Some offices are equipped with height bars or wall charts that are separate from a scale. Use these devices in the same way as those that are attached to a scale.

Measure infants while they are lying down. In this instance you are measuring length instead of height. Some pediatric examination tables have a built-in bar for

PROCEDURE 19.2

Measuring Adults and Children

Objective: To accurately measure weight and height of adults and children

OSHA Guidelines

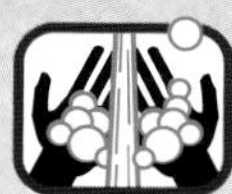
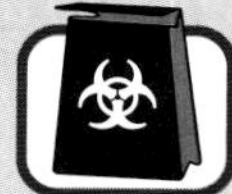
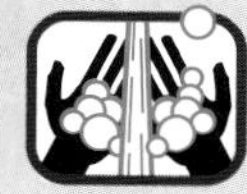

Materials: For an adult or older child, adult scale with height bar, disposable towel; for toddler, adult scale with height bar or height chart, disposable towel

Method

Adult or Older Child: Weight

1. Identify the patient and introduce yourself.
2. Wash your hands and explain the procedure to the patient.
3. Check to see whether the scale is in balance by moving all the weights to the left side. The indicator should be level with the middle mark. If not, check the manufacturer's directions and adjust it to ensure a zero balance. If you are using a scale equipped to measure either kilograms or pounds, check to see that it is set on the desired units and that the upper and lower weights show the same units.
4. Place a disposable towel on the scale.
5. Ask the patient to remove her shoes, if that is the standard office policy. (Use the same procedure for all visits for consistency.)
6. Ask the patient to step on the center of the scale, facing forward. Assist as necessary.
7. Place the lower weight at the highest number that does not cause the balance indicator to drop to the bottom.
8. Move the upper weight slowly to the right until the balance bar is centered at the middle mark, adjusting as necessary.
9. Add the two weights together to get the patient's weight.
10. Record the patient's weight in the chart to the nearest quarter of a pound or tenth of a kilogram.
11. Return the weights to their starting positions on the left side.

Adult or Older Child: Height

12. With the patient off the scale, raise the height bar well above the patient's head and swing out the extension.
13. Ask the patient to step on the center of the scale and to stand up straight and look forward.
14. Gently lower the height bar until the extension rests on the patient's head.
15. Have the patient step off the scale before reading the measurement.
16. If the patient is fewer than 50 inches tall, read the height on the bottom part of the ruler; if the patient is more than 50 inches tall, read the height on the top movable part of the ruler at the point at which it meets the bottom part of the ruler. Note that the numbers increase on the bottom part of the bar and decrease on the top, moveable part of the bar. Read the height in the right direction.
17. Record the patient's height.
18. Have the patient put her shoes back on, if necessary.
19. Properly dispose of the used towel and wash your hands.

Toddler: Weight

1. Identify the patient and obtain permission from the parent to weigh the toddler.
2. Wash your hands and explain the procedure to the parent.
3. Check to see whether the scale is in balance, and place a disposable towel on the scale.
4. Ask the parent to hold the patient and to step on the scale. Follow the procedure for obtaining the weight of an adult.
5. Have the parent put the child down or hand the child to another staff member.
6. Obtain the parent's weight.
7. Subtract the parent's weight from the combined weight to determine the weight of the child.
8. Record the patient's weight in the chart to the nearest quarter of a pound or tenth of a kilogram.

Toddler: Height

9. Measure the child's height in the same manner as you measure adult height, or have the child stand with his back against the height chart. Measure height at the crown of the head.
10. Record the height in the patient's chart.
11. Properly dispose of the used towel and wash your hands.

PROCEDURE 19.3

Measuring Infants

Objective: To accurately measure weight and length of infants and infant head circumference.

OSHA Guidelines

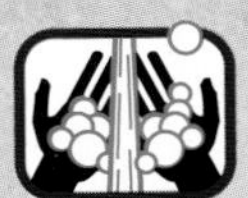

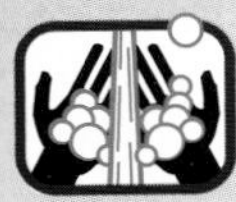

Materials: Pediatric examination table or infant scale, cardboard, pencil, yardstick, tape measure, disposable towel

Method

Weight

1. Identify the patient and obtain permission from the parent to weigh the infant.
2. Wash your hands and explain the procedure to the parent.
3. Ask the parent to undress the infant. (The infant's clothing and diaper can affect the results.)
4. Check to see whether the infant scale is in balance, and place a disposable towel on it.
5. Have the parent place the child face up on the scale (or on the examination table if the scale is built into it). Keep one hand over the infant at all times to prevent a fall. (When weighing a male infant, it is a good idea to hold a diaper over his penis to catch any urine the infant might void.)
6. Place the lower weight at the highest number that does not cause the balance indicator to drop to the bottom.
7. Move the upper weight slowly to the right until the balance bar is centered at the middle mark, adjusting as necessary.
8. Add the two weights together to get the infant's weight.
9. Record the infant's weight in the chart in pounds and ounces or to the nearest tenth of a kilogram.
10. Return the weights to their starting positions on the left side.

Length: Scale With Length (Height) Bar

11. If the scale has a height bar, move the infant toward the head of the scale or examination table until her head touches the bar.
12. Have the parent hold the infant by the shoulders in this position.
13. Holding the infant's ankles, gently extend the legs and slide the bottom bar to touch the soles of the feet.
14. Note the length and release the infant's ankles.
15. Record the length in the patient's chart.

Length: Scale or Examination Table Without Length (Height) Bar

11. If neither the scale nor the examination table has a height bar, have the parent position the infant close to the head of the examination table and hold the infant by the shoulders in this position.
12. Place a stiff piece of cardboard against the crown of the infant's head, and mark a line on the towel or paper, or hold a yardstick against the cardboard.
13. Holding the infant's ankles, gently extend the legs and draw a line on the towel or paper to mark the heel, or note the measure on the yardstick.
14. Release the infant's ankles and measure the distance between the two markings on the towel or paper using the yardstick or a tape measure.
15. Record the length in the patient's chart.

Head Circumference

Measurement of head circumference may be performed at the same time as weight and length, or it may be part of the general physical examination.

16. With the infant in a sitting or supine position, place the tape measure around the infant's head at the forehead.
17. Adjust the tape so that it surrounds the infant's head at its largest circumference.
18. Overlap the ends of the tape, and read the measure at the point of overlap.
19. Remove the tape, and record the circumference in the patient's chart.
20. Properly dispose of the used towel and wash your hands.

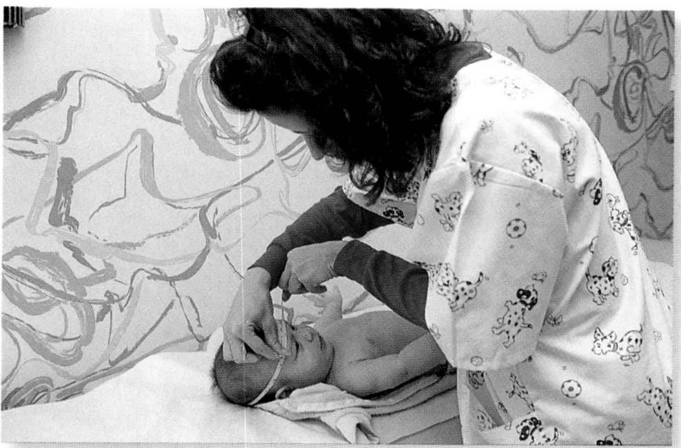

Figure 19-15. The medical assistant uses a flexible tape to measure the circumference of an infant's head.

measuring length. You can also use a tape measure or yardstick. The steps for measuring the height of a child or the length of an infant are described in Procedure 19-3.

Measuring the Head Circumference of Infants

The circumference of an infant's head is an important measure of growth and development. You may be asked to perform this measurement (Figure 19-15) when you measure the infant's length. In some offices you will be asked to assist the doctor with this measurement during the general physical examination. The steps for measuring the circumference of an infant's head are described in Procedure 19-3.

Summary

One of your duties as a medical assistant will be to measure and record the patient's vital signs, weight, and height. Gathering this information is crucial to the outcome of the patient's visit. Remember that the physician relies on these data as they appear on the chart from visit to visit and when making a diagnosis. Using the proper techniques and the same equipment each and every time you measure a patient's weight, height, and vital signs will help you to provide information that is precise and accurate.

REVIEW

CHAPTER 19

CASE STUDY QUESTIONS

Now that you have completed this chapter, review the case study at the beginning of the chapter and answer the following questions:

1. Why is it essential for you to take accurate measurements of this patient?
2. How can you help ensure the accuracy of these measurements?
3. Describe how you would perform vital signs and measurements on an uncooperative child or crying infant.
4. Describe how you might obtain height and weight measurements of a patient who is deaf.

Discussion Questions

1. What are the pros and cons of using growth charts when charting children's growth?
2. Compare and contrast the different types of sphygmomanometers.

Critical Thinking Questions

1. A 45-year-old patient comes to the clinic for a follow-up appointment regarding her elevated blood pressure. Prior to seeing the patient, you note on her chart that her last blood pressure reading was 152/90 and her weight was 295 pounds. Which of these measurements should you first take for this patient and why?
2. You take the pulse and blood pressure of a 68-year-old male with an electronic sphygmomanometer and note the following results: BP 169/98, P 104. Are these within normal limits for this patient? If not, what should you do?

Application Activities

1. Pair up with a classmate and practice measuring each other's weight and height.
2. Practice measuring vital signs of several classmates. Compare your measurements with others to verify accuracy.

Internet Activity

1. Take a virtual field trip to one of the following organizations using the Web links provided here. Research the site to determine methods of preventing and treating high blood pressure (hypertension). Use the information to develop a teaching plan for a patient with hypertension.

   National Heart, Lung, and Blood Institute
   www.nhlbi.nih.gov

   American Health Association
   www.americanheart.org

CHAPTER 20

Assisting With a General Physical Examination

AREAS OF COMPETENCE

2003 Role Delineation Study

CLINICAL

Fundamental Principles

- Comply with quality assurance practices

Patient Care

- Prepare patient for examinations, procedures, and treatments
- Assist with examinations, procedures, and treatments

GENERAL

Professionalism

- Display a professional manner and image
- Treat all patients with compassion and empathy

Communication Skills

- Recognize and respect cultural diversity

Instruction

- Instruct individuals according to their needs

KEY TERMS

auscultation
cerumen
clinical diagnosis
culture
differential diagnosis
digital examination
fenestrated drape
inspection
kyphosis
manipulation
mensuration
nasal mucosa
palpation
patient compliance
percussion
prognosis
quadrant
SARS (severe acute respiratory syndrome)
symmetry

CHAPTER OUTLINE

- The Purpose of a General Physical Examination
- The Role of the Medical Assistant
- Safety Precautions
- Preparing the Patient for an Examination
- Examination Methods
- Components of a General Physical Examination
- Completing the Examination

OBJECTIVES

After completing Chapter 20, you will be able to:

20.1 State the purpose of a general physical examination.
20.2 Describe the role of the medical assistant in a general physical examination.
20.3 Explain safety precautions used during a general physical examination.
20.4 Outline the steps necessary to prepare the patient for an examination.

OBJECTIVES *(Continued)*

20.5 Describe how to position and drape a patient in each of the ten common examination positions.

20.6 Explain ways to assist patients from different cultures, patients with disabilities, children, and pregnant women.

20.7 Identify and describe the six examination methods used in a general physical examination.

20.8 List the components of a general physical examination.

20.9 Explain the special needs of the elderly for patient education.

20.10 Identify ways to help a patient follow up on a doctor's recommendations.

Introduction

Whether a patient comes for a regular checkup or to have a problem diagnosed and treated, the physical examination is the first step in the process for the physician or practitioner. During the physical examination, the medical assistant must make the client comfortable and assist the physician as necessary. A skilled medical assistant who is sensitive to patient needs plus proficient in performing these skills can create an atmosphere that results in a positive outcome for the patient during the physical examination.

CASE STUDY

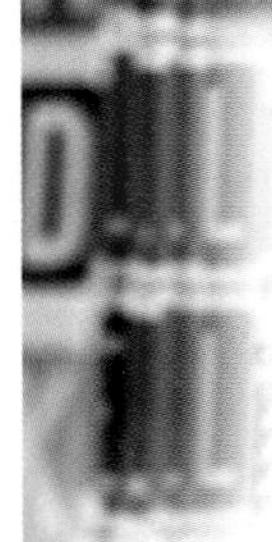

A 50-year-old male patient who cannot speak English comes for a general physical examination. You must prepare the patient for the examination, including proper positioning, explain each component of the exam, and assist the physician as necessary.

As you read this chapter, consider the following questions:

1. English is the only language you speak. How can you provide adequate explanation?
2. How can you prevent embarrassment when preparing the patient for the examination?
3. During what parts of the examination do you expect to provide assistance for the physician?

The Purpose of a General Physical Examination

Physicians perform general physical examinations for two purposes. The first is to examine a healthy patient to confirm an overall state of health and to provide baseline values for vital signs and measurements. The second is to examine a patient to diagnose a medical problem.

To confirm a patient's health status, physicians usually perform examinations on a routine basis, such as once a year. Some examinations are done to fulfill a requirement before an individual starts school, begins a new job, or starts an exercise program.

To diagnose medical problems, physicians usually focus on a particular organ system, as indicated by the patient's chief complaint. Because organ systems are so interdependent, however, physicians generally perform an overall physical examination even when a specific medical problem exists.

During a general physical examination, physicians check all the major organs and body systems. They can determine much about a patient's general condition of health from the examination. If appropriate, they also try to make a **clinical diagnosis,** a diagnosis based on the signs and symptoms of a disease.

After forming an initial diagnosis of a patient's problem, physicians may order laboratory or other diagnostic tests. These tests are done to confirm a clinical diagnosis or to rule out other possible disorders. These additional steps are necessary when a patient has symptoms that may indicate more than one condition. Determining the correct diagnosis when two or more diagnoses are possible is called making a **differential diagnosis.**

Laboratory and diagnostic tests may also aid physicians in developing a **prognosis,** or a forecast of the probable course and outcome of the disorder and the prospects of recovery. In addition, such tests help physicians formulate a treatment plan or appropriate drug therapy. Physicians may ask to have these tests repeated as part of the follow-up evaluation of a patient's progress.

The Role of the Medical Assistant

Your job as a medical assistant is to assist both the doctor and the patient during the general physical examination. Your presence enables the doctor to perform his examination as efficiently and professionally as possible. Patients benefit from your positive and caring attention; you contribute to their confidence in the care they receive.

As described in Chapters 18 and 19, the process begins when you first have contact with the patient. You interview the patient, write an accurate history, determine vital signs, and measure weight and height. You then assist the doctor during the examination.

Generally, your responsibilities include ensuring that all instruments and supplies are readily available to the doctor during the examination. You also ensure that the patient is physically and emotionally comfortable during the examination. It is important to observe the patient for signs that indicate distress or the need for assistance. Elderly patients, who may have physical limitations or special needs, often require extra time and attention.

Safety Precautions

As you prepare for and assist with a general physical examination, you will use a variety of safety measures. Some of these are outlined by the Department of Labor's Occupational Safety and Health Administration (OSHA). OSHA standards and guidelines (detailed in Chapter 1) are designed to protect employees and make the workplace safe. The Department of Health and Human Services' Centers for Disease Control and Prevention (CDC) establishes the guidelines intended to protect both patients and health-care professionals in the medical office and the hospital setting. (These guidelines are also discussed in Chapter 1.) Taken together, these safety measures help protect you, the physician, and the patient from disease transmission.

Safety measures that you must take before, during, and after a general physical examination include the following.

1. Perform a thorough hand washing before and after contact with each patient and before and after each procedure. Procedure 1-1 in Chapter 1 describes how to perform aseptic hand washing. Additionally, according to OSHA standards, you can use an approved waterless, alcohol-based hand cleaner between patients if no gross contamination or visible soilage is on your hands.
2. Wear gloves whenever there is a possibility that you may come in contact with blood, body fluids, nonintact skin, or moist surfaces (during the examination of the patient or when handling specimens). Refer to Chapter 1 for details on personal protective equipment.
3. Wear a mask in the presence of a patient suspected of having an infectious disease that is transmitted by airborne droplets, such as **severe acute respiratory syndrome (SARS)** or tuberculosis (TB) (Table 20-1).
4. Patients with highly contagious infectious diseases, such as diphtheria or chickenpox, must be examined under isolation precautions, such as in a private room. Wear personal protective equipment during contact. For more information on isolation guidelines, see Chapter 2. (Because infectious diseases are common in children, you are most likely to deal with them in a pediatrician's office.)

TABLE 20-1 Infectious Diseases Transmitted by Airborne Droplets

Viral Infections	Bacterial Infections
Chickenpox	Epiglottitis (caused by *Haemophilus influenzae* type B)
Diphtheria	Meningitis
Herpes zoster (shingles)	Pertussis (whooping cough)
Meningitis	Pneumonia
Mumps	Tuberculosis
Pneumonia	
Rabies	
Rubella (German measles)	
Rubeola (measles)	
Severe acute respiratory syndrome (SARS)	

Note: Health-care professionals should use masks when coming in contact with patients suspected of having any of these diseases.

5. Discard in biohazardous waste containers all disposable equipment and supplies that come in contact with a patient's blood or body fluids. See Chapter 1 for guidelines on the proper disposal of biohazardous waste.
6. Clean and disinfect the examination room following the examination of each patient. Refer to Chapter 4 for information on cleanliness in the examination room.
7. Sanitize, disinfect, and sterilize equipment, as appropriate, after the examination of each patient. Chapter 2 describes these procedures in detail.

Preparing the Patient for an Examination

You can help prepare patients for examinations by making sure that they are comfortable and know what to expect. It is easier for the doctor to obtain an accurate assessment of a patient's condition when the patient is emotionally and physically prepared.

Emotional Preparation

To prepare patients, begin by explaining exactly what will occur during the examination. Use simple, direct language that patients can understand. Describe what patients can expect to feel and how their cooperation can contribute to the success of the procedure.

Emotional preparedness is particularly important when dealing with children. They deserve to have the same sort of information and reassurance as adults. To involve children in the examination process, you might allow them to inspect the blunt instruments. Speak to them calmly during the procedure, and praise them when they are cooperative.

Infants and toddlers are likely to be afraid of you because you are a stranger. Approach these children slowly, smile, and use a gentle voice. Children of preschool age are sometimes uncooperative and challenging. In such cases remain calm, perform the procedures quickly, and restrain the child (with assistance from the parent) when appropriate. To prevent children from getting injured, watch them at all times.

If you are a male medical assistant, a female doctor may ask you to remain in the room when she examines a male patient. Likewise, if you are a female medical assistant, a male doctor may ask you to remain in the room when he examines a woman. These measures are for the protection of both the patient and the doctor. Such policies depend on the standard procedures in each medical practice or facility.

Physical Preparation

To ensure that the patient is physically prepared before the doctor enters the examination room, give the patient an opportunity to empty his bladder or bowels. If a urine specimen is needed, it should be collected at this time. That way the patient will be more comfortable during the examination.

When the patient is ready, ask him to disrobe and put on an examination gown or cover himself with a drape. The extent of disrobing depends on the type of examination and the doctor's preference. If the doctor requests a gown for the patient, show the patient how to put on the gown. Include specific instructions on whether the gown should open in the back or front and whether it should be left open or tied. Leave the examination room while the patient disrobes to give him privacy, unless he needs and requests assistance.

Positioning and Draping

During the examination, the patient may need to assume a variety of positions. These positions facilitate the physician's examination of certain areas of the body. The physician will indicate which positions are needed for specific examinations. You will help the patient assume these positions. Some positions are embarrassing or physically uncomfortable for some patients. If you perceive embarrassment, explain the need for the position, and help the patient assume the position when necessary. Help minimize the time a patient spends in any embarrassing or uncomfortable position.

If a patient is physically uncomfortable in a position, you may be able to ease the discomfort by using a small pillow to support part of the body. You may have to help the patient maintain a position during the examination. Always try to make the patient as comfortable as possible.

When you need to make changes in the patient's position, do so gradually. If your office is equipped with an examination table that can be adjusted automatically, learn to use the controls efficiently to maximize patient comfort. Always tell the patient what movement to expect.

When patients have assumed the correct position, cover them with an appropriate drape. Drapes vary in size. Make sure you choose one that will help keep the patient warm and maintain privacy. You will position drapes differently depending on the examination position and the parts of the patient's body that the physician examines.

Examination Positions

The positions commonly used during a medical examination include the following:

- Sitting
- Supine (recumbent)
- Dorsal recumbent
- Lithotomy
- Trendelenburg's
- Fowler's
- Prone

- Sims'
- Knee-chest
- Proctologic

Sitting. In the sitting position, the patient sits at the edge of the examination table without back support (see Figure 20-1a). The physician examines the patient's head, neck, chest, heart, back, and arms. While the patient is in the sitting position, the physician evaluates the patient's ability to fully expand the lungs. She then checks the upper body parts for **symmetry,** the degree to which one side is the same as the other. In this position the drape is placed across the patient's lap for men or across the patient's chest and lap for women.

If a patient is too weak to sit unsupported, another position is necessary. One possible alternative is the supine position.

Supine (Recumbent). In the supine, or recumbent, position, the patient lies flat on the back (Figure 20-1b). (*Supine* means "lying down faceup"; *recumbent* means "lying down." Either term is used to describe this position.) This is the most relaxed position for many patients. A doctor can examine the head, neck, chest, heart, abdomen, arms, and legs when a patient is in the supine position. The patient is normally draped from the neck or underarms down to the feet.

The supine position may not be comfortable for patients who become short of breath easily. Also, patients with a back injury or lower-back pain may find it uncomfortable. You can make these patients more comfortable by placing a pillow under their heads and under their knees. Some patients, however, may need to be placed in the dorsal recumbent position.

Dorsal Recumbent. In the dorsal recumbent position, the patient lies faceup, with his back supporting all his weight. (The term *dorsal* refers to the back.) This position is the same as the supine position, except that the patient's knees are drawn up and the feet are flat on the table, as shown in Figure 20-1c. The physician may examine the head, neck, chest, and heart while a patient is in this position. The patient is normally draped from the neck or underarms down to the feet.

Patients who have leg disabilities may find the dorsal recumbent position uncomfortable or even impossible. On the other hand, patients who are elderly or have painful disorders such as arthritis or back pain may find the dorsal recumbent position more comfortable than the supine position because the knees are bent. This position is sometimes used as an alternative to the lithotomy position when patients have severe arthritis or joint deformities.

Lithotomy. The lithotomy position is used during examination of the female genitalia. In this position, the patient lies on her back with her knees bent and her feet in stirrups attached to the end of the examination table. You may need to help the patient place her feet in the stirrups. She should then slide forward to position her buttocks near the edge of the table, as shown in Figure 20-1d.

Many women are embarrassed and physically uncomfortable in this position, so you should not ask a patient to remain in this position any longer than necessary. Use a large drape that covers the patient from the breasts to the ankles. Placing the drape with one point or corner between the legs will make the examination easier in this position.

A patient with severe arthritis or joint deformities in the hips or knees may have difficulty assuming the lithotomy position. She may be able to place only one leg in the stirrup, or she may need your assistance in separating her thighs. An alternative position for such a patient is the dorsal recumbent position. Other patients who may have difficulty with the lithotomy position are those who are obese or in the late stages of pregnancy.

Trendelenburg's. In Trendelenburg's position, the patient is supine on a tilted table with the head lower than the legs. Some tables have flexible positioning so that the patient's legs can be bent with the feet lower than the knees, as shown in Figure 20-1e. Although physicians do not generally use this position for physical examinations, they use it in certain surgical procedures or emergencies. If this position is necessary on a standard examination table, you can place the patient with the feet at the head of the table and then raise the head. This position may be used for a patient with low blood pressure or a patient experiencing shock. It cannot be used for patients who have a head injury, however. The drape is typically positioned from the neck or underarms down to the knees.

Fowler's. In Fowler's position, the patient lies back on an examination table on which the head is elevated, as shown in Figure 20-1f. Although the head of the table can be raised to a 90° angle, the most common position is a 45° angle. The doctor may examine the head, neck, and chest areas while the patient is in this position. The patient is usually draped from the neck or underarms down to the feet.

Fowler's position is one of the best positions for examining patients who are experiencing shortness of breath or individuals with a lower-back injury.

Prone. In the prone position, the patient is lying flat on the table, facedown. The patient's head is turned to one side, and his arms are placed at his sides or bent at the elbows, as shown in Figure 20-1g. The patient is normally draped from the upper back to the feet.

With the patient in this position, the physician can examine the back, feet, or musculoskeletal system. The prone position is unsuitable for women in advanced stages of pregnancy, obese patients, patients with respiratory difficulties, or the elderly.

Sims'. In Sims' position, the patient lies on the left side. The patient's left leg is slightly bent, and the left arm is placed behind the back so that the patient's weight is resting primarily on the chest. The right knee is bent and raised toward the chest, and the right arm is bent toward

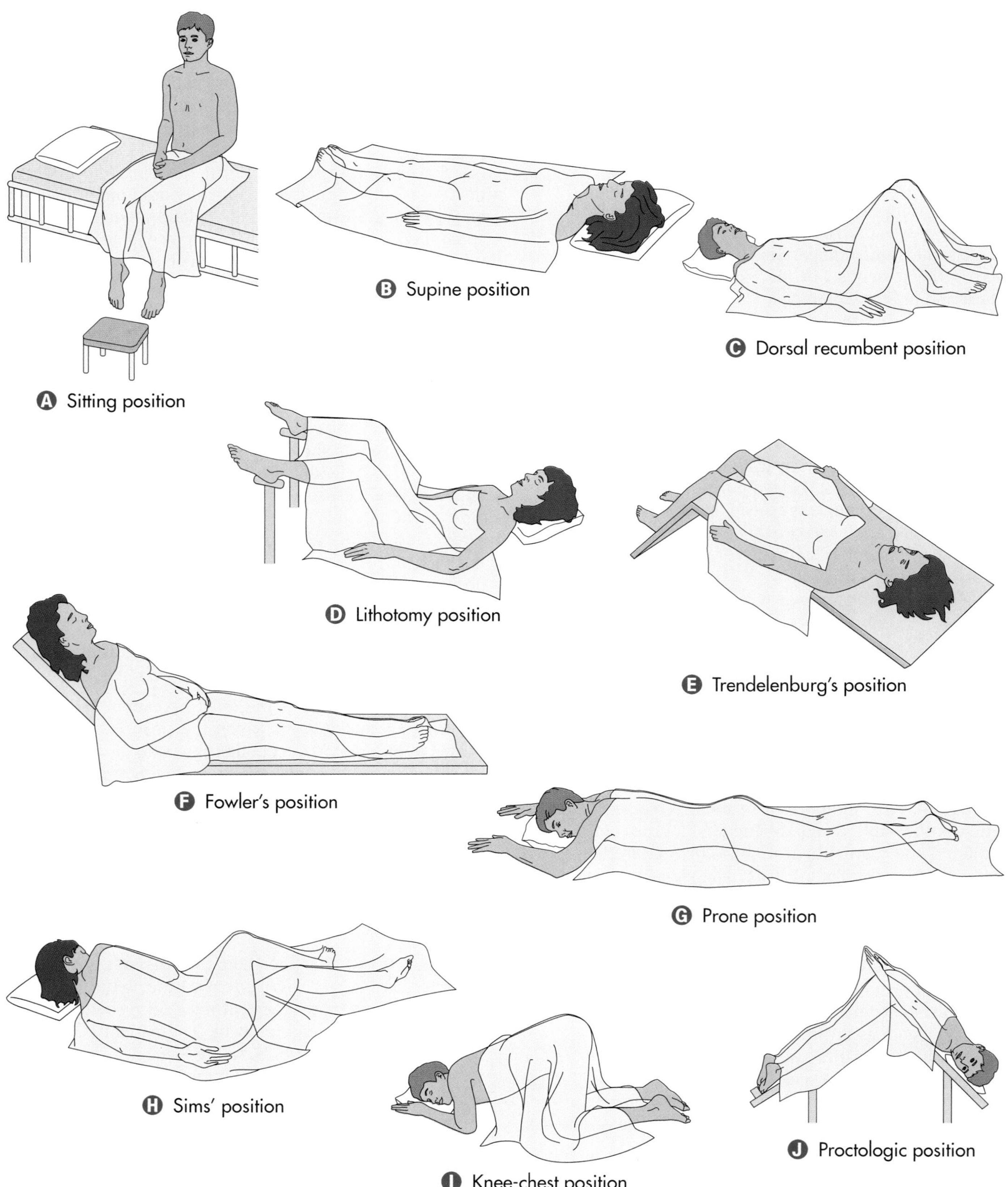

Figure 20-1. These positions may be used during the general physical examination.

the head for support, as shown in Figure 20-1h. The patient is draped from the upper back to the feet.

Sims' position is used during anal or rectal examinations and may also be used for perineal and certain pelvic examinations. Patients with joint deformities of the hips and knees may have difficulty assuming this position.

Knee-Chest. In the knee-chest position, the patient is lying on the table facedown, supporting the body with the knees and chest. The patient should have the thighs at a 90° angle to the table and slightly separated. The head is turned to one side, and the arms are placed to the side or above the head, as shown in Figure 20-1i. The patient may need your assistance to assume this position correctly and to maintain it during the examination.

The knee-chest position is used during examinations of the anal and perineal areas and during certain proctologic procedures. Some patients—those who are pregnant, obese, or elderly—have difficulty assuming this position. An alternative that puts less strain on the patient and is easier to maintain is the knee-elbow position. This position is the same as the knee-chest position except that the patient supports body weight with the knees and elbows rather than the knees and chest. In either of these two positions, the patient is commonly covered with a **fenestrated drape,** in which a special opening provides access to the area to be examined.

Proctologic. The proctologic position may be used as an alternative to the Sims' or knee-chest position. In the proctologic position, also called the jackknife position, the patient is bent at the hips at a 90° angle. The patient can assume this position by standing next to the examination table and bending at the waist until the chest rests on the table. If an adjustable examination table is available, the patient can assume the position by lying prone on the table, which is then raised in the middle with both ends pointing down. This places the patient at the correct 90° angle, as shown in Figure 20-1j. In either variation of this position, the patient is draped with a fenestrated drape, as in the knee-chest position.

The steps for placing patients into these positions are described in Procedure 20-1.

PROCEDURE 20.1

Positioning the Patient for an Examination

Objective: To effectively assist a patient in assuming the various positions used in a general physical examination

OSHA Guidelines

Materials: Adjustable examination table or gynecologic table, step stool, examination gown, drape

Method

1. Identify the patient and introduce yourself.
2. Wash your hands.
3. Explain the procedure to the patient.
4. Provide a gown or drape if the physician has requested one, and instruct the patient in the proper way to wear it after disrobing. Allow the patient privacy while disrobing, and assist only if the patient requests help.
5. Explain to the patient the necessary examination and the position required.
6. Ask the patient to step on the stool or the pullout step of the examination table. If necessary, assist the patient onto the examination table.
7. Assist the patient into the required position:
   a. Sitting. Do not use this position for patients who cannot sit unsupported.
   b. Supine (Recumbent). Do not use this position for patients with back injuries, low back pain, or difficulty breathing. Place a pillow or other support under the head and knees for comfort, if needed.
   c. Dorsal Recumbent. This position may be difficult for someone with leg disabilities. It may be used for patients when lithotomy is difficult.
   d. Lithotomy. This position is used to examine the female genitalia, with the patient's feet placed in stirrups. Assist as necessary. The patient's buttocks should be near the edge of the table. Drape the client with a large drape to help prevent embarrassment.
   e. Trendelenburg. This position is a supine position with the patient's head lower than her feet. It is used infrequently in the physician's office but may be necessary for low blood pressure or shock.

continued →

PROCEDURE 20.1

Positioning the Patient for an Examination *(continued)*

f. Fowler's. Adjust the head of the table to the desired angle. Help the patient move toward the head of the table until the patient's buttocks meet the point at which the head of the table begins to incline upward (Figures 20-2 and 20-3).

g. Prone. This position is when the patient lies face down. It is not used for later stages of pregnancy, obese patients, patients with respiratory difficulty, or certain elderly patients.

h. Sims'. In this position, the patient lies on her left side with her left leg slightly bent and her left arm behind her back. Her right knee is bent and raised toward her chest and her right arm is bent toward her head. This position may be difficult for patients with joint deformities.

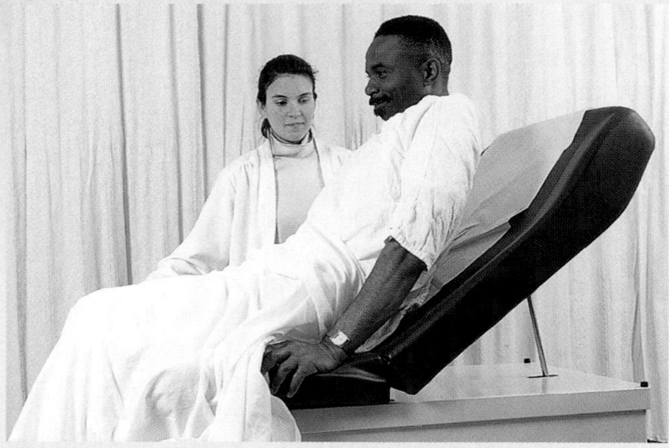

Figure 20-3. Encourage the patient to slide back until the buttocks meet the point at which the head of the table begins to incline upward.

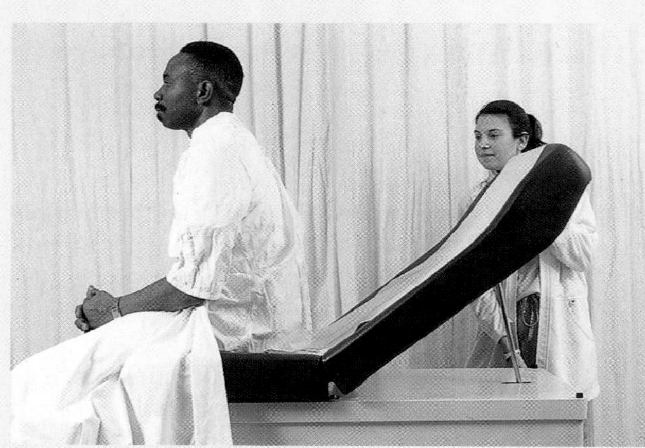

Figure 20-2. Adjust the head of the examination table to a 45° angle.

i. Knee-Chest. This position is difficult for patients to assume. The patient is face down, supporting his weight on his knees and chest or an alternative knee-elbow position. This position is used for rectal and perineal exams. Keep the patient in this position for the shortest amount of time as possible.

j. Proctologic. This position is also used for rectal and perineal exams. In this position, the patient bends over the exam table with his chest resting on the table.

8. Drape the client to prevent exposure and avoid embarrassment. Place pillows for comfort as needed.

9. Adjust the drapes during the examination.

10. On completion of the examination, assist the client as necessary out of the position and provide privacy as the client dresses.

Special Considerations: Patients From Different Cultures

During your career you will come in contact with patients from many different cultures. A **culture,** in this sociological sense, is defined as a pattern of assumptions, beliefs, and practices that shape the way people think and act. Avoid the temptation to stereotype an individual or group on the basis of a single patient's behavior. Stereotyping can lead to incorrect judgments, which may influence the care you provide to patients. Avoid making judgments about patients or cultural groups on the basis of your experience with other patients or with your own family and friends.

Patients from different cultures may never have had a medical examination by a physician and may not know what to expect. These patients may be more modest than other patients and may have a greater need for privacy. They may not want the physician to examine certain areas of their bodies. Procedure 20-2 describes techniques you can use to ensure effective communication with patients from other cultures while meeting their privacy needs.

PROCEDURE 20.2

Communicating Effectively With Patients From Other Cultures and Meeting Their Needs for Privacy

Objective: To ensure effective communication with patients from other cultures while meeting their needs for privacy

OSHA Guidelines: This procedure does not involve exposure to blood, body fluids, or tissues.

Materials: Examination gown, drapes

Method

Effective Communication

1. When it is necessary to use a translator, direct conversation or instruction to the translator.
2. Direct demonstrations of what to do, such as putting on an examination gown, to the patient.
3. Confirm with the translator that the patient has understood the instruction or demonstration.
4. Allow the translator to be present during the examination if that is the patient's preference.
5. If the patient understands some English, speak slowly, use simple language, and demonstrate instructions whenever possible.

Meeting the Need for Privacy

1. Before the procedure, thoroughly explain to the patient or translator the reason for disrobing. Indicate that you will allow the patient privacy and ample time to undress.
2. If the patient is reluctant, reassure him that the physician respects the need for privacy and will look at only what is necessary for the examination.
3. Provide extra drapes if you think doing so will make the patient feel more comfortable.
4. If the patient is still reluctant, discuss the problem with the physician; the physician may be able to negotiate a compromise with the patient.
5. During the procedure, ensure that the patient is undraped only as much as necessary.
6. Whenever possible, minimize the amount of time the patient remains undraped.

Special Considerations: Patients With Disabilities

As a medical assistant, you will come in contact with patients with physical disabilities. These patients will have different strengths and weaknesses. They will also vary in their ability to ambulate (move from place to place). Many patients with physical disabilities require the use of devices such as wheelchairs, canes, or walkers or other special equipment that permits or enhances mobility.

Depending on the extent of their disability, these patients may require extra assistance in preparing for a general physical examination. You may need to help them disrobe, move from a mobility device to the examination table, and assume certain positions on or off the examination table. At all times you should ask another staff member for assistance if you are not sure whether you can safely move or lift a patient on your own. Procedure 20-3 describes the steps you would take to transfer a patient from a wheelchair to the examination table.

Special Considerations: Children

No matter what type of office you work in, you will probably deal with children at times. You will base your choice of an examination position for children on each child's age and ability to cooperate. Although young infants are usually examined on an examination table, older infants and toddlers may need to be examined while held on a parent's lap. Some toddlers may cooperate while standing on the examination table with a parent nearby. Preschool children can usually be placed on the examination table if a parent is nearby. Regardless of their position, watch children at all times to prevent injury.

When examining young children, doctors typically perform percussion and auscultation first, because children are more likely to be calm and quiet at the outset. Doctors always examine painful areas last. Doctors may examine older children's genitalia last, because after a certain age children tend to find such an examination embarrassing.

Special Considerations: Pregnant Women

When a pregnant patient needs a general physical examination, remember that she has several special needs. Some positions (such as the prone or lithotomy positions) are not recommended for a pregnant patient, especially during late stages of pregnancy. Other positions may be

PROCEDURE 20.3

Transferring a Patient in a Wheelchair and Preparing for an Examination

Objective: To assist a patient in transferring from a wheelchair to the examination table safely and efficiently

OSHA Guidelines

Materials: Adjustable examination table or gynecologic table, step stool (optional), examination gown, drape

Method

Never risk injuring yourself; call for assistance when in doubt. As a rule you should not attempt to lift more than 35% of your body weight.

Preparation Before Transfer

1. Identify the patient and introduce yourself.
2. Wash your hands.
3. Explain the procedure in detail.
4. Position the wheelchair at a right angle to the end of the examination table. This position reduces the distance between the wheelchair and the end of the examination table across which the patient must move.
5. Lock the wheels of the wheelchair to prevent the wheelchair from moving during the transfer.
6. Lift the patient's feet and fold back the foot and leg supports of the wheelchair.
7. Place the patient's feet on the floor, and ensure that the patient will not slip on the floor. (The patient should have shoes or slippers with nonskid soles.) Place your feet in front of the patient's feet to prevent further slipping.
8. If needed, place a step stool in front of the table, and place the patient's feet flat on the stool.

Transferring Patient by Yourself

9. Face the patient, spread your feet apart, align your knees with the patient's knees, and bend your knees slightly. (If you lift while bending at the waist instead of bending your knees, you can cause serious injury to your back.)
10. Have the patient hold on to your shoulders.
11. Place your arms around the patient, under the patient's arms (Figure 20-4).
12. Tell the patient that you will lift on the count of 3, and ask the patient to support as much of his own weight as possible (if he is able).
13. At the count of 3, lift the patient.

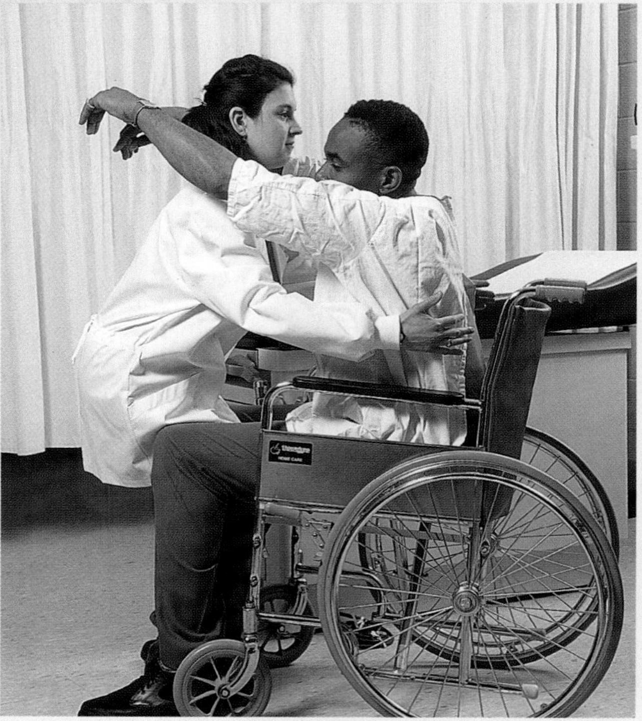

Figure 20-4. Align your knees, slightly bent, with the patient's knees. Have the patient hold on to your shoulders while you place your arms around the patient, under the patient's arms.

14. Pivot the patient to bring the back of the patient's knees against the table.
15. Gently lower the patient into a sitting position on the table. If the patient cannot sit unassisted, help him move into a supine position (Figure 20-5).
16. Move the wheelchair out of the way.
17. Assist the patient with disrobing as necessary, providing a gown and drape.

Transferring Patient With Assistance

9. Working with your partner, you both face the patient, spread your feet apart, position yourselves so that one of each of your knees is aligned with the patient's knees, and bend your knees slightly. (If you lift while bending at your waist instead of bending your knees, you can cause serious injury to your back.)
10. Have the patient place one hand on each of your shoulders and hold on.

continued ⟶

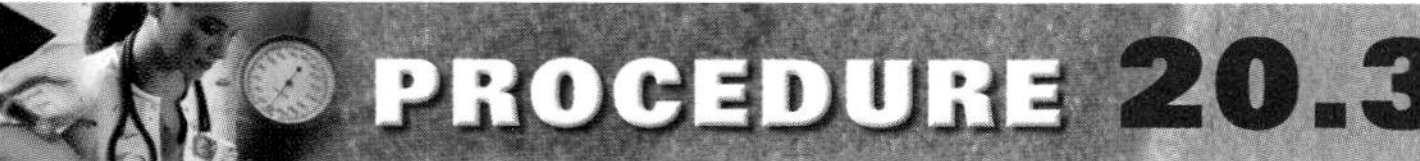

PROCEDURE 20.3

Transferring a Patient in a Wheelchair and Preparing for an Examination *(continued)*

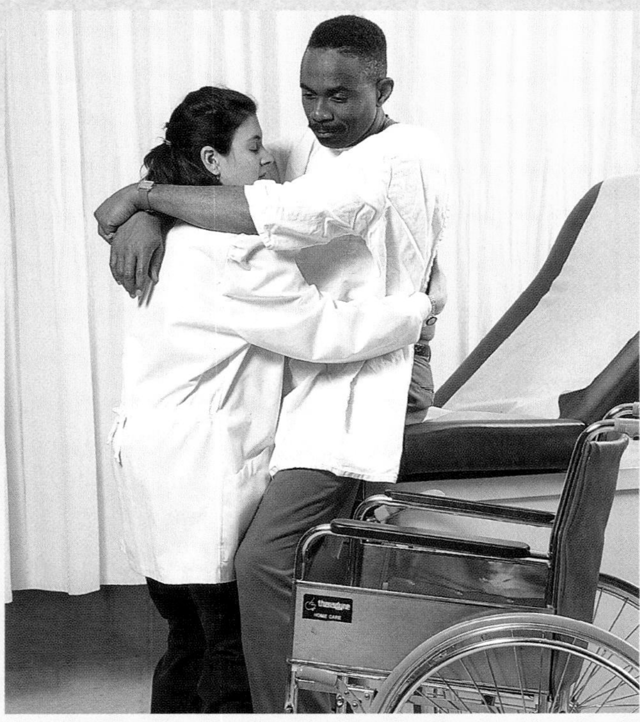

Figure 20-5. When you have lifted the patient, pivot him to bring the back of the knees against the table. Gently lower the patient into a sitting position, or into a supine position if the patient cannot sit unassisted.

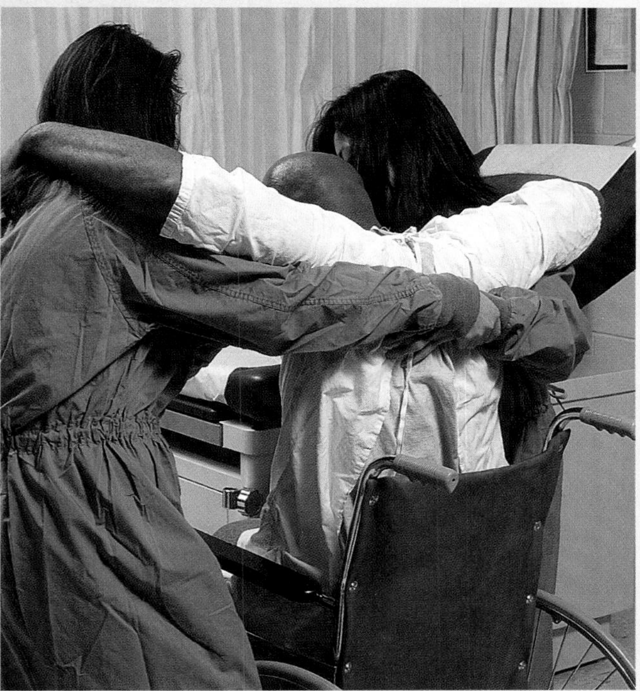

Figure 20-6. If you have an assistant, have the patient place one hand on each of your shoulders. Each of you should place your outermost arm around the patient, under one of the patient's arms. Interlock your wrists and, together, lift the patient.

11. Each of you places your outermost arm around the patient, one under each of the patient's arms. Then interlock your wrists (Figure 20-6).
12. Tell the patient that you will lift on the count of 3, and ask the patient to support as much of his own weight as possible (if he is able).
13. At the count of 3, you should lift the patient together.
14. The stronger of the two of you should pivot the patient to bring the back of the patient's knees against the table.
15. Working together, gently lower the patient into a sitting position on the table. If the patient cannot sit unassisted, help him move into a supine position (Figure 20-7).
16. Move the wheelchair out of the way.
17. Assist the patient with disrobing as necessary, providing a gown and drape.

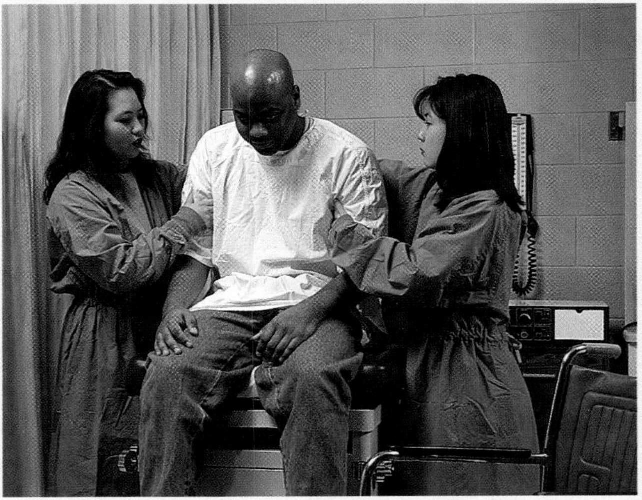

Figure 20-7. The stronger of the two of you should pivot the patient to bring the back of the patient's knees against the table. Gently lower the patient into a sitting position, or a supine position if the patient cannot sit unassisted.

PROCEDURE 20.4

Meeting the Needs of the Pregnant Patient During an Examination

Objective: To meet the special needs of the pregnant woman during the general physical examination

OSHA Guidelines 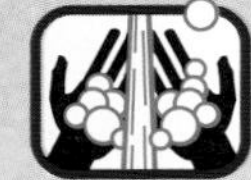

Materials: Patient education materials, examination table, examination gown, drape

Method

Providing Patient Information

1. Identify the patient and introduce yourself.
2. Assess the patient's need for education by asking appropriate questions.
3. Provide any appropriate instructions or materials.
4. Ask the patient whether she has any special concerns or questions about her pregnancy that she might want to discuss with the physician.
5. Communicate the patient's concerns or questions to the physician; include all pertinent background information on the patient.

Ensuring Comfort During the Examination

1. Identify the patient and introduce yourself.
2. Wash your hands.
3. Explain the procedure to the patient.
4. Provide a gown or drape, and instruct the patient in the proper way to wear it after disrobing. (Allow the patient privacy while disrobing, and assist only if she requests help.)
5. Ask the patient to step on the stool or the pullout step of the examination table.
6. Assist the patient onto the examination table.
7. Keeping position restrictions in mind, help the patient into the position requested by the physician.
8. Provide and adjust additional drapes as needed.
9. Keep in mind any difficulties the patient may have in achieving a certain position; suggest alternative positions whenever possible.
10. Minimize the time the patient must spend in uncomfortable positions.
11. If the patient appears to be uncomfortable during the procedure, ask whether she would like to reposition herself or take a break; assist as necessary.
12. To prevent pelvic pooling of blood and subsequent dizziness or hyperventilation, allow the patient time to adjust to sitting before standing after she has been lying on the examination table.

difficult or impossible for a pregnant woman to achieve. Procedure 20-4 outlines steps you can take to ensure that a pregnant woman's needs are addressed during an examination.

Examination Methods

There are six methods for examining a patient during a general physical examination. These methods enable the physician to gather important information about the patient's condition, and they are normally performed in the following sequence:

1. Inspection
2. Palpation
3. Percussion
4. Auscultation
5. Mensuration
6. Manipulation

Inspection

Inspection is the visual examination of the patient's entire body and overall appearance. During inspection the physician assesses posture, mannerisms, and hygiene. The physician also inspects parts of the body for size, shape, color, position, symmetry, and the presence of abnormalities such as rashes or growths. You can help the physician perform the inspection by making sure that good lighting is available and that the patient's body parts are properly exposed.

Palpation

The doctor uses **palpation** (touch) extensively in the general physical examination. During palpation the doctor assesses characteristics such as texture, temperature, shape, and the presence of vibrations or movements. The doctor may palpate superficially (on the skin surface), or she may palpate with additional pressure. She uses extra pressure when assessing characteristics of underlying tissues and organs. Depending on the characteristic the doctor is measuring, she may perform palpation using the fingertips, one hand, two hands (bimanual), or the palm of the hand.

Percussion

Percussion involves tapping or striking the body to hear sounds or feel vibrations. Physicians use percussion to determine the location, size, or density of a body structure or organ under the skin. For example, physicians use percussion to determine whether the lungs contain air or fluid.

The physician may perform percussion by striking the body directly with one or two fingers. More commonly, however, he performs indirect percussion by placing one finger of one hand on the area and striking it with a finger from the other hand.

Auscultation

Auscultation is the process of listening to body sounds. Doctors use auscultation to detect the flow of blood through an artery. Doctors perform auscultation extensively in the general examination to assess sounds from the heart, lungs, and abdominal organs. They use a stethoscope to hear most of these sounds.

Mensuration

Mensuration is the process of measuring. In addition to the measurements you take before the examination—weight and height—you may need to take other measurements during the examination. For example, measurements may be done to monitor the growth of the uterus during pregnancy or to note the length and diameter of an extremity. You will usually use a tape measure or small ruler to take measurements.

Manipulation

Manipulation is the systematic moving of a patient's body parts. Physicians may palpate an area of the body while manipulating it to check for abnormalities that affect movement. Physicians often use manipulation to determine the range of motion of a joint.

Components of a General Physical Examination

Each physician performs the general physical examination in a certain order. Most physicians begin by assessing the patient's overall appearance and the condition of the patient's skin, nails, and hair. They usually then proceed with the examination in the following order, using the examination methods described in the previous section:

1. Head
2. Neck
3. Eyes
4. Ears
5. Nose and sinuses
6. Mouth and throat
7. Chest and lungs
8. Heart
9. Breasts
10. Abdomen
11. Genitalia
12. Rectum
13. Musculoskeletal system
14. Neurological system

Learn the standard order that the physicians in your facility follow when performing the general examination. You should also be familiar with the components of the examination and the instruments and supplies needed for each component (see Table 20-2 and Figure 20-8). Instruments and supplies are discussed in detail in Chapter 4 and should include the following basic items:

- Penlight
- Otoscope/ophthalmoscope
- Vision chart
- Color vision chart
- Audiometer
- Nasal speculum
- Gloves
- Tongue depressor
- Stethoscope
- Vaginal speculum
- Lubricant
- Tape measure

Certain parts of the examination are your responsibility, and you should know how to perform them. You should also understand the physician's responsibilities.

Part of the medical assistant's role in the general examination is to ensure that the patient is as comfortable as possible. You can do this by helping to protect the patient's modesty as much as you can. For example, when the physician removes a drape or gown to expose an area for inspection, watch the patient for signs of embarrassment. If you notice any such signs, do your best to keep the patient covered without hindering the physician's examination.

General Appearance

The physician usually begins the examination by reviewing the patient's general appearance and noting whether the patient appears to be in good health and of an acceptable weight. The physician also notes whether the patient appears to be distressed or in pain and assesses the level of the patient's alertness. Then the physician examines the patient's skin, nails, and hair.

Skin. The physician may prefer to examine all of the patient's skin at one time or to look at certain areas of skin

TABLE 20-2 Components and Materials of a General Physical Examination

Component	Materials Required*
General appearance (skin, nails, hair)	No special materials needed
Head	No special materials needed
Neck	No special materials needed
Eyes and vision**	Penlight, ophthalmoscope, vision and color vision charts
Ears and hearing**	Otoscope, audiometer
Nose and sinuses	Penlight, nasal speculum
Mouth and throat	Gloves, tongue depressor
Chest and lungs	Stethoscope
Heart	Stethoscope
Breasts	No special materials needed
Abdomen	Stethoscope
Genitalia (women)	Gloves, vaginal speculum, lubricant
Genitalia (men)	Gloves
Rectum	Gloves, lubricant
Musculoskeletal system	Tape measure
Neurological system	Reflex hammer, penlight

*Gloves should always be worn if your hands will come in contact with the patient's nonintact skin, blood, body fluids, or moist surfaces or if the patient is suspected of having an infectious disease.

**Procedures performed alone by the medical assistant are described in Chapter 21; all other listed procedures are performed by a physician with help from a medical assistant.

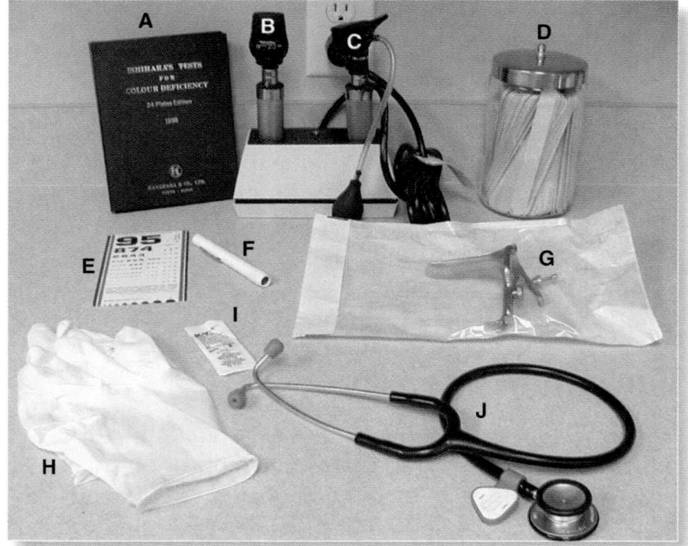

Figure 20-8. Some common instruments and supplies for the general physical examination are (a) color vision chart, (b) ophthalmoscope, (c) otoscope, (d) tongue blades, (e) near vision chart, (f) penlight, (g) vaginal speculum, (h) gloves, (i) lubricant, and (j) stethoscope.

while examining specific body parts. The physician notes the color, texture, moisture level, temperature, and elasticity of the skin. The condition of the skin is a good indicator of overall health. If the physician notices any lesions, she wears gloves to prevent possible transmission of microorganisms. The physician may also request that a specimen be taken from a lesion or wound for later examination to determine the infecting microorganism.

Nails. When the physician examines the patient's nails, he looks at both the nails and the nail beds. The condition of the nails may indicate poor nutrition, disease, infection, or injury. If applicable, remind the patient to remove nail cosmetics prior to the appointment.

Hair. The physician notes the patient's pattern of hair growth and the texture of the hair on the patient's scalp and on the rest of the body. Sudden hair loss or changes in hair growth may be indicators of an underlying disease.

Head

After reviewing the patient's general appearance, the doctor examines the patient's head. He looks for any abnormal condition of the scalp or skin, puffiness around the eyes or lips or in other areas of the face, or any abnormal growths.

Neck

To check the neck, the doctor palpates the patient's lymph nodes, thyroid gland, and major blood vessels. Enlarged lymph nodes may be a sign of infection or a blood cancer. An enlarged thyroid gland may indicate thyroid disease. The doctor also checks the neck for symmetry and range of motion.

Eyes

The physician examines the patient's eyes—particularly the eyelids and conjunctiva—for the presence of disease or abnormalities. She checks eye muscles by observing the patient's ability to follow the movement of a finger. She checks the pupils for their response to light (the pupils should contract—become smaller—when a penlight is directed toward them). Then she uses an ophthalmoscope to examine the patient's retinas and other internal structures of the eyes.

You may be required to perform various vision tests either before or after the general physical examination. (The tests are described in Chapter 21.)

Ears

The doctor checks the patient's outer ears for size, symmetry, and the presence of lesions, redness, or swelling. Using an otoscope, he then examines the inner structures of the patient's ears. The doctor may ask you to assist in keeping the patient's head still during the otoscopic examination, particularly when the patient is a young child. Although this procedure is usually painless, patients with an ear infection may find it uncomfortable or painful.

The doctor checks the patient's ear canals for redness, drainage, lesions, foreign objects, or the presence of excessive **cerumen** (a waxy secretion from the ear, also known as earwax). During the most important part of the examination of the ears, the doctor assesses the color, shape, and reflectiveness of the eardrums. If an eardrum bulges outward or reflects light abnormally, the middle ear could be infected.

One of your responsibilities may be to perform various hearing tests either before or after the general physical examination. (These tests are described in Chapter 21.)

Nose and Sinuses

When examining the nose, the physician checks for the presence of infection or allergy. She uses a penlight to view the color of the **nasal mucosa** (lining of the nose) and notes any discharge, lesions, obstructions, swelling, or inflammation. A mucosa that is red or swollen and is accompanied by a yellowish discharge usually indicates an infection. A pale, swollen mucosa accompanied by a clear discharge indicates an allergy. When examining adults, the physician uses the nasal speculum to view the structures of the nose.

The physician may use palpation to check for tenderness in a patient's sinuses. Tenderness is an indication of inflammation or swelling.

Mouth and Throat

The doctor checks the condition of the patient's mouth to get a general impression of overall health and hygiene. Using a tongue depressor to draw back the patient's cheeks, the doctor examines the lining of the cheeks, the underside of the tongue, and the floor of the mouth. Changes in color or any lesions in these areas may indicate possible infection or oral cancer. The doctor also assesses the condition of the teeth and gums. When examining children, she counts the number of teeth. Most doctors leave this part of the examination of infants and toddlers until last, because children of this age tend to resist opening their mouths.

The doctor examines the patient's throat carefully because it is a common site of infection. She uses a tongue depressor to press the patient's tongue down and out of the way while asking the patient to say "ah." This procedure allows the doctor to view the throat and tonsils more clearly while checking them for redness or swelling, which can indicate the presence of infection.

Chest and Lungs

The physician usually assesses the patient's chest and lungs while the patient sits at the end of the examination table. When the patient is examined in this position, the chest can expand to its maximum capacity. Typically, the physician removes the patient's gown or lowers the drape from the waist up. Then he asks the patient to breathe normally or to take deep breaths. A patient who becomes dizzy during deep breathing may be hyperventilating. **Hyperventilation** is overly deep breathing that leads to a loss of carbon dioxide in the blood. You can help by having the patient breathe into a paper bag. If no bag is available, the patient can breath into cupped hands. With your help the patient should recover quickly.

The physician inspects the patient's chest from the back, side, and front. He checks its shape, symmetry, and postural position and looks for the presence of any type of deformity. Postural abnormalities such as **kyphosis** often occur in the elderly. Frequently, especially in elderly women, these abnormalities are caused by osteoporosis, the loss of bone density. This bone density loss causes the patient to have a rounded back, or "humpback."

The physician also palpates the chest and performs percussion to check for the presence of fluid or a foreign mass in the lungs. The physician then uses a stethoscope to auscultate the chest from the back, side, and front. He listens to the lung sounds during both normal and deep breathing. The stethoscope allows him to hear abnormal breathing that may result from such disorders as bronchitis, asthma, or pneumonia.

Heart

The doctor usually examines the patient's heart and vascular system at the same time as, or immediately after, the lung examination. He may palpate the area first to locate the correct anatomical landmarks for placing the stethoscope. He may use percussion to check the size of the heart. The patient should not speak while the physician auscultates the heart sounds with the stethoscope. The physician notes the rate, rhythm, intensity, and pitch of the heart.

Breasts

During a general physical examination, every woman should have a complete breast examination. Breast cancer is the most common cancer in women. Because growths are also possible in men's breasts, doctors should perform a breast examination on all patients.

The doctor begins the examination with the patient in a sitting position. The doctor asks the patient to hold her arms at her sides while he inspects the breasts for symmetry, contour, masses, and retracted areas. The doctor then asks the patient to raise her arms above her head while he palpates the lymph nodes under her arms.

Next, the doctor asks the patient to lie down and place her hand under her head on the first side to be examined. The doctor may ask you to place a small pillow or folded towel under the patient's shoulder blade on the same side. This procedure allows the breast tissue to flatten evenly against the chest wall, permitting easier palpation. The doctor then palpates the breast in a circular, systematic manner to check for lumps, examines the areola and nipple, and then repeats the procedure on the other side.

When examining male patients, the doctor palpates the patient's breasts and lymph nodes in the same manner that he does with his female patients. The doctor also checks the breasts of his male patients for lesions or swelling.

Abdomen

The physician examines the patient's abdomen while the patient is in a supine position with arms down at the sides. The abdominal muscles should be completely relaxed for this part of the examination. The physician may ask you to place a small pillow under the patient's head or knees (or both) to keep the abdomen relaxed. If the patient is wearing a gown, it is raised to just under the breasts. If the patient is draped, the drape must be lowered to just above the genitalia to allow a complete view of the area. A separate drape should be placed to cover a female patient's breasts.

The order of examination methods for the abdomen is different from the order for other areas. The physician begins with inspection and auscultation, followed by percussion and palpation. Following this order allows the physician to listen to bowel sounds before palpating the abdominal organs. Palpation of this area can change bowel sounds in such a way that the physician could misdiagnose a patient's condition.

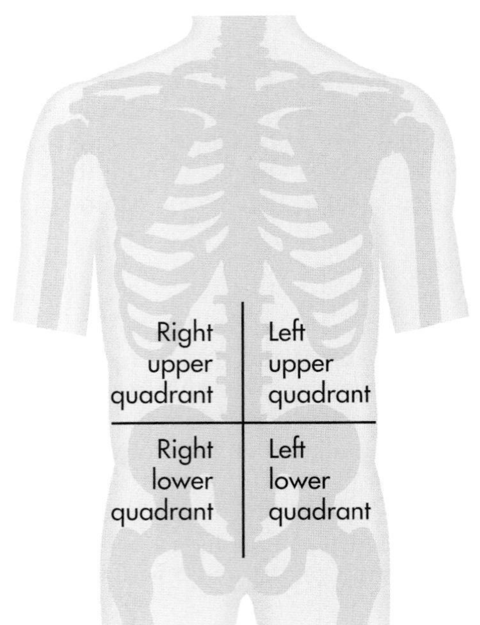

Figure 20-9. The abdomen is typically divided into four equal sections, or quadrants.

The physician must assess the abdomen thoroughly, because there are many organs in the abdominal cavity. The physician describes observations based on a system of landmarks that map out the abdominal region. The abdomen is typically divided into four equal sections, or **quadrants,** as shown in Figure 20-9. Some physicians divide the abdomen into nine sections, similar to a tick-tack-toe board, as shown in Figure 20-10.

If the physician has not assessed the skin in this area already, she begins with an inspection of the abdominal skin's color and surface and follows with an inspection of the shape and symmetry of the abdomen. She then uses auscultation to check bowel and vascular sounds and uses percussion to note the size and position of the organs. Lastly, she uses palpation to check muscle tone and to determine the presence of any tenderness or masses.

Female Genitalia

Female patients may feel self-conscious or anxious in the lithotomy position—which is most commonly used during examination of the genitalia. The medical assistant may help the patient relax during this procedure and may assist patients in maintaining the position.

If the doctor who performs the examination is male, a female medical assistant should always be in the room to protect both the patient and doctor from potential lawsuits. This type of examination may be performed by a specialist or by a primary care physician. The procedure for a gynecologic examination is described in detail in Chapter 22.

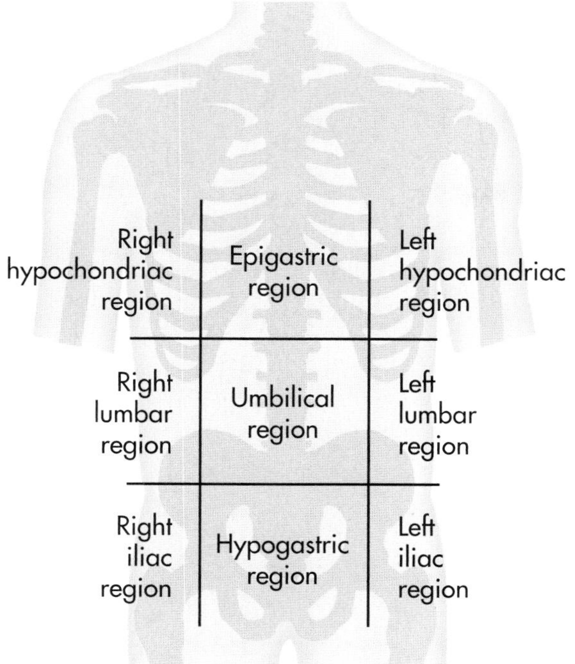

Figure 20-10. Some physicians divide the abdomen into nine sections, similar to a tick-tack-toe board.

Male Genitalia

During the examination of the genitalia, men may be just as embarrassed or uncomfortable as women may be. If the physician who is performing the assessment is female, a male medical assistant should be in the room to protect both the patient and physician from potential lawsuits.

The procedure begins with the patient in the supine position. The physician puts on gloves and visually inspects the patient's penis for signs of infection or structural abnormalities, palpating any lesions. The physician then examines the scrotum in the same manner, palpating the testicles for lumps. The patient is asked to stand while the physician checks for any bulges in the groin that may indicate a hernia. At the same time, the physician palpates the local lymph nodes to check for any abnormality.

Rectum

The doctor usually examines the rectum after examining the genitalia. You may need to assist an adult patient into a dorsal recumbent or Sims' position. The doctor normally examines a child when the child is in the prone position and inspects only the external areas of the rectum.

In adults the doctor uses **digital examination** to palpate the rectum for lesions or irregularities. Doctors recommend that patients older than age 40 have a yearly digital examination for early detection of colorectal cancer. For this examination the doctor puts on a clean pair of gloves. You assist by applying lubricant to the doctor's gloved index finger before the examination begins. As with examination of the genitalia, patients often find digital examination of the rectum embarrassing and uncomfortable.

After performing the procedure, the doctor may request that any stool found on the glove be tested for the presence of occult blood. The presence of occult blood in the stool is a possible indication of colorectal cancer or gastrointestinal bleeding. This test—often called by its brand name, Hemoccult or Seracult test—involves placing a sample of stool on a special cardboard slide. You assist by presenting the slide to the doctor. To produce an accurate test, three consecutive bowel movements are tested; this sample is usually the first. After the examination you may be responsible for instructing the patient on how to collect the additional two samples. The procedure is outlined on the package of the occult blood-testing kit.

After the rectal examination, offer the patient the opportunity to clean the anal area before you adjust the drape. Dispose of gloves and soiled materials in a biohazardous waste container.

Musculoskeletal System

If the physician did not examine the patient's back during the chest examination, he does so during the musculoskeletal assessment. The physician checks for good posture from the back and side. He may ask the patient to walk so that he can assess her gait. The physician always asks a child to bend at the waist so that he can check for the presence of **scoliosis,** a lateral curvature of the spine. This procedure is discussed further in Chapter 22, Procedure 22-2.

During the musculoskeletal assessment the physician determines range of motion, the strength of various muscle groups, and body measurements. The physician also examines the arms, hands, legs, and feet for any lesions, deformities, or circulatory problems.

The physician checks a patient's range of motion to detect joint deformities and to learn whether the patient has any limitations in movement caused by an injury or other conditions, such as arthritis. Checking a patient's range of motion also allows the physician to follow a patient's progress during recovery from an injury or surgery.

As part of the assessment of a child's health, the physician asks the child to perform certain tasks, such as walking a straight line and balancing or hopping on one foot. The physician uses these tasks to evaluate the child's development and coordination and to provide the physician with information about the functioning of the child's neurological system.

Neurological System

The doctor's neurological assessment includes an evaluation of the patient's reflexes, mental and emotional status (including intelligence, speech, and behavior), and sensory and motor functions. The doctor often performs the neurological assessment at the same time as the musculoskeletal assessment because both systems are involved in movement and coordination.

The doctor may incorporate certain aspects of the neurological assessment into other parts of the examination. For example, testing how a patient's pupils react to light is part of an eye examination, but because this test also examines the patient's light reflex, the test includes a neurological assessment as well.

The doctor checks the patient's reflexes to assess both sensory and motor nerve pathways at different areas of the spinal cord. To check reflexes, the doctor uses a reflex hammer to tap tendons in different areas of the patient's body.

Most examinations of children also include an intellectual assessment, in which the doctor asks the child general questions appropriate to the child's age. Doctors may also test the mental status and memory of older adults to detect disorders such as senility and Alzheimer's disease in patients who show signs of confusion or complain of memory loss.

Completing the Examination

After the physician completes the examination, you should help the patient into a sitting position. Then allow the patient to perform any necessary self-hygiene measures.

Additional Tests or Procedures

Before the patient dresses, check to see whether the physician has ordered any additional tests or procedures that are more conveniently performed while the patient is undressed. These tests might include taking body fat measurements or blood samples or preparing the patient for a diagnostic or therapeutic procedure, such as an x-ray or physical therapy session. The physician may also ask you to perform other procedures. Some of these procedures, which are covered in other chapters, include the following:

- Cold or heat therapy (Chapter 25)
- Applying a bandage (Chapter 26)

CAUTION ***Handle With Care***

Helping Patients With Suspected Breast Cancer

If the physician detects a suspicious lump in a patient's breast during the general physical examination, your main concern is to help the patient remain calm. Although most suspicious lumps are not cancerous, the patient is likely to be anxious and upset about the finding. The best thing you can do for her is to schedule her for a mammogram as soon as possible.

Preparing the Patient for a Mammogram

To alleviate some of the patient's fears, explain exactly what a mammogram is. Give the patient the following information.

1. A mammogram is a special type of x-ray of the breast that is used to detect cancer and other abnormalities of the breast.
2. A technician specially trained in performing mammography will position the patient's breast along a flat plastic plate. A second plate will be brought into position and pressure will be applied for about 20 to 30 seconds to flatten the breast (to obtain a clearer x-ray) while the x-ray is taken. This will be done in two directions (planes) for each breast.
3. Mammography is generally not a painful procedure, but some women may find it uncomfortable. Many professionals suggest that patients avoid scheduling a mammogram during the week prior to a menstrual period to reduce potential discomfort.
4. The mammography appointment normally takes ½ to 1 hour. The actual mammography takes only about 15 minutes.
5. Because the patient will have to undress from the waist up, she should wear a separate top and slacks or a skirt rather than a dress.
6. The patient should have no creams, powders, or deodorants on her breasts or underarms when the mammography is performed because chemicals in these preparations can produce misleading images in the mammogram.

Answer any questions the patient has, and provide patient education materials related to mammography and breast disease. Reassure her that most lumps are not cancerous.

If your office refers patients to a particular facility that you are familiar with, give the patient an idea of how long she can expect to wait for the results. Ensure her that she will be notified as soon as the physician receives the report. You may want to schedule a follow-up visit at this time, based on when results are expected.

Because this is a difficult time for a patient, you should be as supportive as possible. You can help the patient cope by showing your concern and giving her prompt attention. Tell the patient that if she has any questions at all, she should call the physician.

- Collecting culture specimens (Chapters 28, 29, and 30)
- Administering an injection (Chapter 33)
- Applying a topical medication (Chapter 33)

If the physician has not ordered any additional procedures—or if wearing clothing does not interfere with the procedures ordered—the patient may dress. Help the patient get off the examination table, and allow her to dress in privacy. Make sure she knows you are available to assist if she needs help dressing.

The physician may ask you to perform other tests and procedures that can be done after the patient has dressed, including these procedures, which are discussed in detail where noted:

- Vision and hearing tests (Chapter 21)
- Otic or ophthalmic irrigation (Chapter 21)
- Administration of certain medications (Chapter 33)
- Pulmonary function tests (Chapter 34)

Patient Education

The general physical examination provides you with the opportunity to assess the patient's educational needs. Basing your findings on the patient's interview, history, and examination, you can identify areas in which the patient may benefit from additional education.

Pay special attention to educating patients about risk factors for disease. For example, women are often instructed about the risk factors for breast cancer. The risk factors include being older than 50 (many physicians recommend that women older than 40 have a mammogram every 2 years and that women older than 50 have one every year), having a family history of breast cancer, having the first child after age 30, never being pregnant, and beginning to menstruate at an early age.

The physician may also request that you teach patients how to administer certain medications or how to perform self-help or diagnostic techniques, such as a breast

Educating the Patient

How to Perform a Breast Self-Examination

You may be responsible for reinforcing patient education about monthly breast self-examination (BSE), which can be instrumental in the early detection of breast cancer. Figure 20-11 shows the steps suggested by the National Cancer Institute for performing this procedure.

Check the office policy to see which of several methods it recommends for teaching BSE. One approach uses the following steps.

1. Explain the purpose of BSE.
2. Assist the patient to the standing position, and instruct her to use a large mirror to view the breasts during this part of the procedure.
3. Explain to the patient what she should look for when inspecting her breasts while standing.
4. Demonstrate the positioning of arms and hands for this visual inspection: first, her arms at her sides; then, her arms raised and her hands clasped behind her head; finally, her arms lowered with her hands on her hips.
5. Demonstrate, on the patient's breast, how to perform the small rotary motions with the flat pads of the fingers from the outer rim (including the armpit and collarbone area) toward the nipple. (Synthetic breast models are available that may be helpful in teaching the proper technique.)
6. Demonstrate how to inspect the nipples.
7. Ask the patient to practice the procedure.
8. Observe the patient's self-examination technique. (If the patient is reluctant to examine herself in front of you, have her repeat the highlights of the procedure.)
9. Assist the patient to lie down, with a small pillow or folded towel under the shoulder on the side to be examined.
10. Repeat steps 5 through 8.
11. Suggest that the patient mark her calendar for a monthly reminder to perform the examination 1 week after the onset of menses.
12. Give the patient educational materials that explain how to perform BSE.

Make sure the patient knows that she should perform BSE around the same date of each month—after her period ends, if she is still menstruating. (At this time the breasts are most normal and least swollen and lumpy.) You must also emphasize that BSE is not a substitute for mammograms or regular breast examination by a doctor. Early cancer detection depends on the performance of all three types of breast examination.

continued ⟶

Educating the Patient

How to Perform a Breast Self-Examination *(continued)*

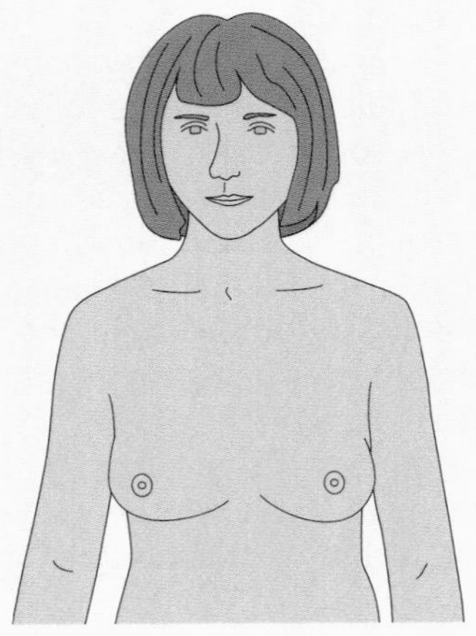

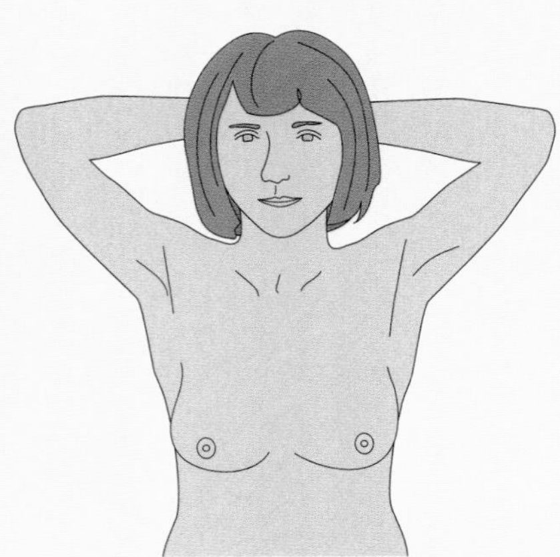

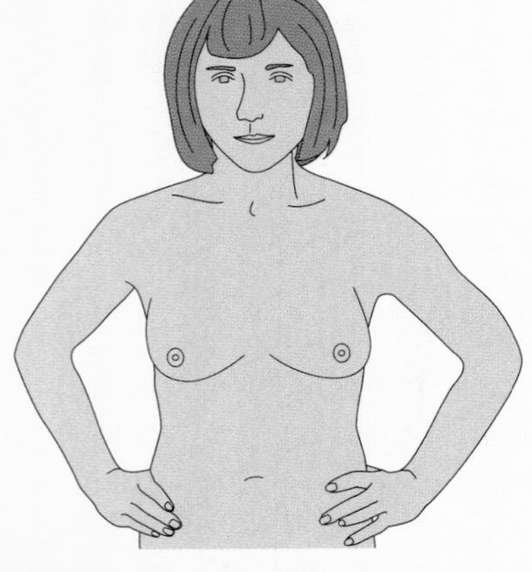

❶ Stand before a mirror. Inspect both breasts for anything unusual such as any discharge from the nipples or puckering, dimpling, or scaling of the skin.

The next two steps are designed to emphasize any change in the shape or contour of your breasts. As you do them, you should be able to feel your chest muscles tighten.

❷ Watching closely in the mirror, clasp your hands behind your head, and press your hands forward.

❸ Next, press your hands firmly on your hips, and bow slightly toward your mirror as you pull your shoulders and elbows forward.

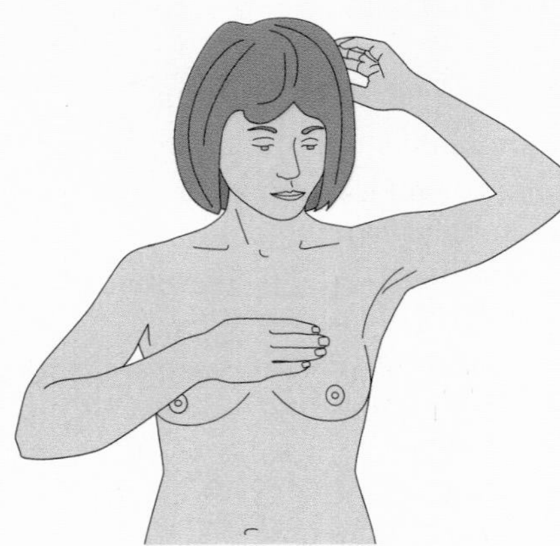

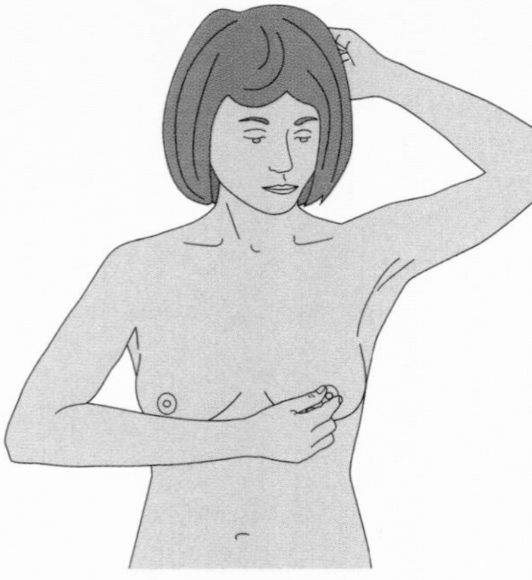

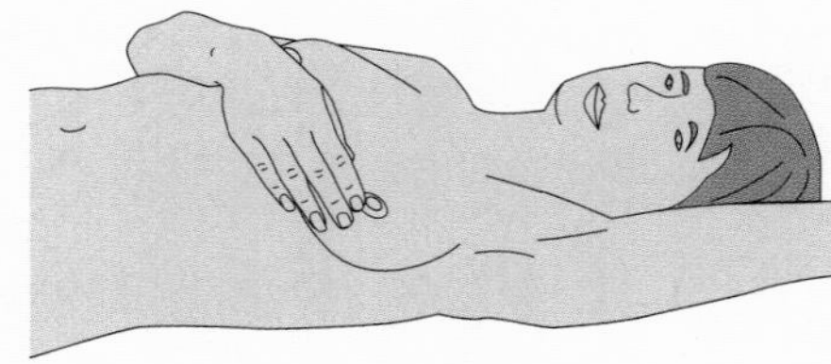

Some women do the next part of the exam in the shower because fingers glide over soapy skin, making it easy to concentrate on the texture underneath.

❹ Raise your left arm. Use three or four fingers of your right hand to explore your left breast firmly, carefully, and thoroughly. Beginning at the outer edge, press the flat part of your fingers in small circles, moving the circles slowly around the breast. and the underarm, including the underarm itself. Feel for any unusual lump or mass under the skin.

❺ Gently squeeze the nipple and look for a discharge. (If you have any discharge during the month—whether or not it is during BSE—see your doctor.) Repeat steps 4 and 5 on your right breast.

❻ Steps 4 and 5 should be repeated lying down. Lie flat on your back with your left arm over your head and a pillow or folded towel under your left shoulder. This position flattens the breast and makes it easier to examine. Use the same circular motion described earlier. Repeat the examination on your right breast.

Figure 20-11. The National Cancer Institute includes these instructions and illustrations in the brochure *Breast Exams: What You Should Know* (NIH Publication No. 90-2000).

self-exam, at home (see the Educating the Patient section). These procedures may involve collecting samples for occult blood testing or urine testing, applying cold or hot packs, or instilling eyedrops. It is important to teach the patient the correct way to perform a diagnostic test. If a specimen is incorrectly obtained, the test results will be inaccurate.

Regardless of the type of instruction, be sure that you address patients at a language level they can understand without talking down to them. To ensure that they understand fully, ask patients to repeat each instruction and to perform each demonstration as you give it to them. (For additional patient education tips related to specialty examinations, refer to Chapters 22 and 23.) Give patients written instructions that they can refer to at home.

Special Problems of the Elderly

The elderly often have a greater need for patient education than do younger patients because certain diseases are common in older patients. Moreover, the elderly frequently are

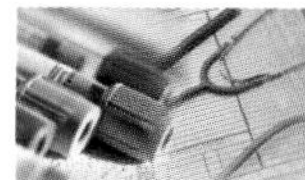

Diseases and Disorders

Helping Elderly Patients With Depression

Depression is a common problem among elderly people. Studies published by the National Institutes of Health (NIH) indicate that at least 5% of elderly people attending primary care clinics suffer from depression. For elderly people in nursing homes, that percentage rises to between 15% and 25%. The NIH also indicates that only about 10% of elderly people who need treatment for depression ever receive it. Additionally, the NIH considers depression in people age 65 and older to be a major public health concern. Suicide is more common among the elderly than any other age group.

One reason for this low rate of treatment is that many older people—and their families—believe that depression is a normal consequence of growing old. Older people may experience the deaths of a spouse and siblings; they have to adjust to retirement and, possibly, loneliness. They may have to deal with a relocation. They may suffer economic hardship and are likely to experience a variety of physical ailments. Because of these circumstances, doctors and family may miss the signs of depression.

Recognizing the Symptoms

There is, unfortunately, no specific diagnostic test for depression, so a diagnosis must be made on the basis of symptoms. The symptoms of depression in the elderly are similar to those in other age groups and include the following:

- Decreased ability to enjoy life or to show an interest in activities or people
- Slow thinking, indecisiveness, or difficulty in concentrating
- Increased or decreased appetite
- Increased or decreased time spent sleeping
- Recurrent feelings of worthlessness
- Loss of energy and motivation
- Exaggerated feelings of sadness, hopelessness, or anxiety
- Recurrent thoughts of death or suicide

The failure to realize that symptoms such as these indicate an illness prevents many older people from seeking help. Yet there is evidence that treatment for depression in the elderly can be highly effective.

Treatment for Depression

Treatment for depression generally combines a course of antidepressant drugs with psychotherapy. Older people generally respond to antidepressants more slowly than younger people do, so older people may not experience relief until more than 6 weeks after starting treatment. For this and other reasons, compliance in taking medications for depression is a problem with elderly people. Many of them do not understand depression and the importance of taking medications as prescribed. They may also be frightened by the idea of taking medication for a mental problem.

Psychotherapy aims to help older people talk through their anxieties, develop coping skills, and improve the quality of their lives. Again, compliance is a problem. Many older people are unwilling to admit that they have a mental-health problem and refuse to follow up on referrals to mental-health professionals.

Benefits of Treatment

Elderly people who follow a course of treatment for depression benefit in a number of ways. They gain:

- Relief from many of the symptoms associated with depression
- Relief from some of the pain and suffering associated with physical ailments
- Improved physical, mental, and social well-being

Health-care providers can play a significant role in recognizing symptoms of depression in the elderly and in encouraging them to get the treatment they need.

not aware of these diseases or of advances in their treatment. Here are some common problems of the elderly:

- Incontinence
- Depression
- Lack of information on preventive medicine
- Lack of compliance when taking medications

Incontinence. Physicians estimate that most patients who suffer from incontinence (involuntary leakage of urine) can be helped. Because most people are too embarrassed to ask for help or are unaware of possible solutions, however, only 1 out of 12 persons actually seeks help for the condition.

Depression. Depression is common in the elderly, but many of the symptoms of depression mimic those of other conditions. You can help elderly patients—and their families—recognize the signs of depression. Knowing what to look for may help patients seek help sooner than they otherwise would and receive prompt diagnosis and treatment. See the Diseases and Disorders section for a discussion of symptoms and treatment of depression in the elderly.

Lack of Information on Preventive Medicine. Many of the elderly are still not aware of the concept of preventive medicine (measures taken to prevent illness). Many come from environments in which people went to a doctor only when they were very ill. Thus, they do not realize the importance of preventive measures such as regular checkups and yearly digital rectal examinations to detect colorectal cancer. Older women often do not recognize the need for regular mammograms and Pap smears to detect cancers of the breast and cervix.

Use any educational tools available to you to make elderly patients more aware of these disorders and the importance of preventive measures. If you reinforce the doctor's recommendations with education, you increase the chance that patients will heed the advice they are given.

Lack of Compliance When Taking Medications. Some elderly people need several medications, and many of them find it difficult to keep track and take the right medication at the right time. You can help by telling elderly patients about available medication reminder boxes, timers, or medication organizers (Figure 20-12). These devices can help ensure **patient compliance** (obedience in following the physician's orders). Patient compliance helps patients remain healthier and get well faster.

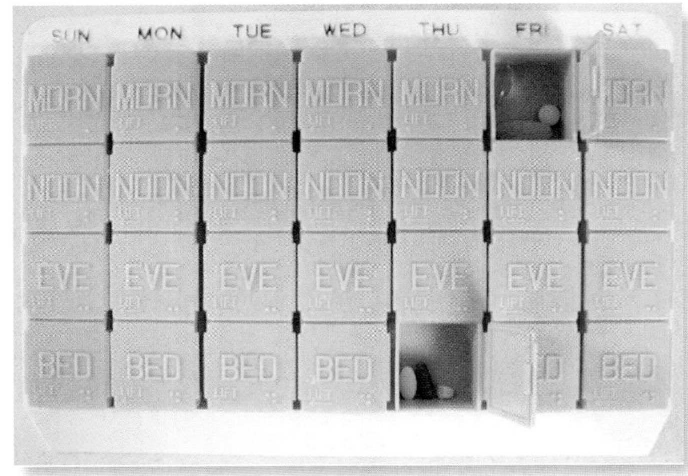

Figure 20-12. This pill case allows the elderly patient to keep weekly track of medications to be taken at different times of the day.

Follow-up

After the examination, you must help the patient follow up on all of the doctor's recommendations. Follow-up may include these actions:

1. Scheduling the patient for future visits at the office
2. Making outside appointments for certain diagnostic tests, such as mammograms or other radiologic procedures, or for therapeutic procedures, such as physical therapy
3. Helping the patient and the patient's family plan for home nursing care after an illness or a surgical procedure
4. Helping the patient obtain help from community or social service organizations, such as adult day care, counseling, or meal programs

Patient follow-up is particularly crucial for patients suspected of having breast cancer. You have an important responsibility to track patients who have suspicious findings on a breast examination. See the Caution: Handle With Care section for an explanation of the steps you can take to help such patients. Patients may file medical malpractice suits if doctors fail to diagnose breast cancer. In fact, this is currently the most frequent cause of malpractice suits.

Summary

The general physical examination provides substantial information about a patient's overall health status and assists the physician in making a diagnosis, prognosis, and treatment plan. The general physical examination is the cornerstone of medical care.

The physician uses a number of assessment methods to gather information during the examination. Although one common order of examination is presented in this chapter, you should learn the order preferred by the physician(s) you assist. Be aware, too, that a physician may change the order of an examination to accommodate the needs of a particular patient.

During the examination, your first priority as a medical assistant is to address the comfort, privacy, and educational needs of the patient. You must also anticipate the needs of the physician throughout the procedure. In addition, you must be aware of the special needs of children, pregnant women, and the elderly and the areas in which patient education is likely to be needed.

REVIEW

CHAPTER 20

CASE STUDY QUESTIONS

Now that you have completed this chapter, review the case study at the beginning of the chapter and answer the following questions:

1. English is the only language you speak. How can you provide adequate explanation?
2. How can you prevent embarrassment when preparing the patient for the examination?
3. During what parts of the examination do you expect to provide assistance for the physician?

Discussion Questions

1. How can a medical assistant help prepare a patient emotionally and physically for a general physical examination?
2. In what ways do children and the elderly present special problems during or after a general physical examination?
3. Discuss how you would care for a patient who has just found out from the practitioner that she has a breast lump.

Critical Thinking Questions

1. How might the physician change the typical order of the general physical examination for an infant who is suffering from an ear infection and appears agitated?
2. What steps can you take to help ensure that an elderly patient takes her medicine properly?
3. How can you help a patient who is in a wheelchair prepare for an examination?
4. An elderly patient arrives at the clinic for a physical examination. She is using a walker, has weakness and arthritis in her legs, and is hard of hearing. You need to place her in position for an examination of the head, neck, chest, and heart. What should you do?
5. A Spanish-speaking 5-year-old child arrives at your clinic for a physical in preparation for school. The mother is with the child and speaks and understands very little English. You must prepare the child for the examination, and no interpreter is available. What should you do?

Application Activities

1. With a partner, practice assisting each other in assuming the various examination positions and in placing drapes properly.
2. Interview a physician to find out what order of components she follows when performing a general physical examination. Present your findings to the class.
3. With a partner, role-play a situation in which a patient has just found out that she has a breast lump. As the medical assistant, you will need to discuss the mammogram and interact with the patient appropriately. Change places, and role-play a situation in which a patient needs to be taught how to perform a breast self-examination.

Internet Activity

1. Mammography is an essential screening procedure for female clients. The screening procedure is done at health-care facilities all over the United States. To ensure quality, the FDA certifies facilities. Search the FDA Internet site, and find out the names of facilities in your area that are certified to perform mammography. Try the Food and Drug Administration at **www.fda.gov**.
2. Research elderly depression on any of the following association Web sites. Choose one aspect of the disease to research, such as incidence, diagnosis, symptoms, treatment, or suicide. Write a brief summary or report to share with your class.

   National Alliance for the Mentally Ill (NAMI) at **www.nami.org**
   Depression and Bipolar Support Alliance (DBSA) at **www.DBSAlliance.org**
   National Institute of Mental Health (NIMH) at **www.nimh.nih.gov**
   National Mental Health Association (NMHA) at **www.nmha.org**
   National Institute on Aging at **www.nia.nih.gov**

CHAPTER 21

Providing Eye and Ear Care

KEY TERMS

audiologist
audiometer
bone conduction
decibel
eustachian tube
frequency
incus
labyrinth
lens
malleus
ophthalmologist
optometrist
orbit
otologist
stapes

AREAS OF COMPETENCE

2003 Role Delineation Study

CLINICAL

Diagnostic Orders

- Perform diagnostic tests

Patient Care

- Prepare patient for examinations, procedures, and treatments
- Assist with examinations, procedures, and treatments
- Prepare and administer medications and immunizations
- Maintain medication and immunization records

GENERAL

Communication Skills

- Adapt communications to individual's ability to understand

Instruction

- Instruct individuals according to their needs
- Explain office policies and procedures
- Teach methods of health promotion and disease prevention

CHAPTER OUTLINE

- Vision
- The Aging Eye
- Vision Testing
- Treating Eye Problems
- Hearing
- The Aging Ear
- Hearing Loss
- Hearing and Diagnostic Tests
- Treating Ear and Hearing Problems

OBJECTIVES

After completing Chapter 21, you will be able to:

21.1 Describe the anatomy and physiology of the eye.
21.2 State ways that vision changes with age.
21.3 Describe ways to detect vision problems.
21.4 List treatments for eye disorders.
21.5 Identify ways that patients can practice preventive eye care.
21.6 Describe the anatomy and physiology of the ear.

OBJECTIVES *(Continued)*

21.7 State ways that hearing changes with age.
21.8 List the types of hearing loss.
21.9 Explain the procedures for screening and diagnosing ear problems.
21.10 Describe treatments for ear and hearing disorders.
21.11 Explain how patients can be educated about preventive ear care.

Introduction

Part of your clinical assisting duties for a general medical practice may involve performing basic tests for vision and hearing. You may also assist the doctor in providing treatment related to the eyes and ears. You will be expected to know the basic structure and function of these organs and to advise patients about general eye and ear care and concerns. Specialized examinations and treatments for the eye and the ear are discussed in Chapter 23 under ophthalmology and otology, respectively.

CASE STUDY

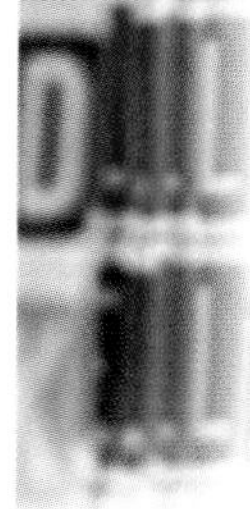

A 6-year-old is brought into the office today where you work as a medical assistant. His mother states that he has not been responding to her when she speaks to him. She also notes that he has been turning up the television volume for the last week. The boy complains of a feeling of fullness in his ears. He is afebrile. The physician determines that the patient has bilateral cerumen plugs and orders ear irrigation with 200 cc of room-temperature water. She also orders a hearing test.

As you read this chapter, consider the following questions:

1. What is cerumen?
2. Why is it important to use room-temperature water when irrigating a patient's ear?
3. What other factors might contribute to the patient's hearing loss?
4. Why is it important to test the patient's hearing after cerumen removal?
5. What device is used to perform a hearing test?

Vision

A person's visual system consists of the eyes; the optic nerve, which connects the eye to the vision center of the brain; and several accessory structures. If these parts of the system are healthy and normal, the individual is able to see normally.

The Eye

The eye is a complex organ that processes light to produce images. It is made up of three main layers and a number of specialized parts, as shown in Figure 21-1.

The Outer Layer. The white of the eye, called the **sclera,** is the tough, outermost layer of the eye. This layer, through which light cannot pass, covers all except the front of the eye. Here the sclera gives way to the cornea. The **cornea** is a transparent area on the front of the eye that acts as a window to let light into the eye.

The Middle Layer. The **choroid** is the middle layer of the eye, which contains most of the eye's blood vessels. In the anterior part of the choroid are the iris and the ciliary body. The **iris** is the colored part of the eye. It is made of muscular tissue. As this tissue contracts and relaxes, an opening at its center grows larger or smaller. This opening is the **pupil.** The size of the pupil regulates the amount of light that enters the eye. In bright light the pupil becomes smaller. In dim light it becomes larger.

The **ciliary body** is a wedge-shaped thickening in the middle layer of the eyeball. Muscles in the ciliary body control the shape of the lens—making the lens more or less curved for viewing either near or distant objects. The **lens** is a clear, circular disk located just posterior to the iris. Because the lens can change shape, it helps the eye focus images of objects that are near or far away.

The space between the cornea and the lens contains a liquid called **aqueous humor,** which is produced by capillaries in the ciliary body. The part of the eye behind the lens is filled with a jellylike substance called **vitreous humor,** which helps the eye hold its shape.

The Inner Layer. The inner layer of the eye consists of the **retina.** Nerve cells at the posterior of the retina

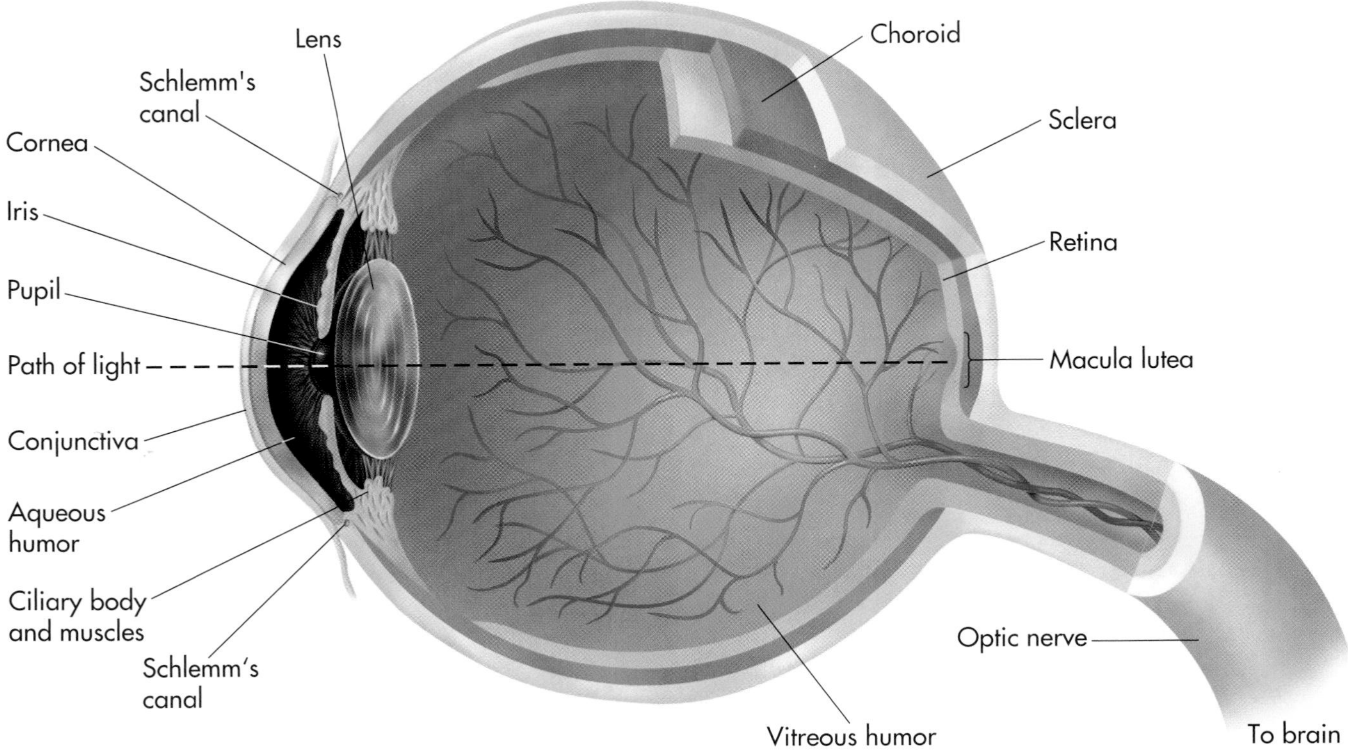

Figure 21-1. The eye is composed of a number of structures that work in harmony to produce vision.

sense light. There are two types of nerve cells, each named for its shape. **Rods** are highly sensitive to light. They function in dim light but do not provide a sharp image or detect color. **Cones** function only in bright light. They are sensitive to color and provide sharp images.

There are three types of cones—one each for detecting red, green, or blue light. A person who completely lacks cones cannot see colors and is said to be color-blind. Someone who lacks one type of cone is partially color-blind and has difficulty telling two or more colors apart.

The Process of Seeing

The eye works much like a camera. Light reflected from an object, or produced by one, enters the eye from the outside and passes through the cornea, pupil, lens, and fluids in the eye. The cornea, lens, and fluids help focus the light onto the retina by bending, or refracting, the light. As in a camera, an image of an object is carried by light patterns. The image is projected upside down—on film in a camera and on the retina in an eye. The retina converts the light into nerve impulses. These impulses are transmitted along the optic nerve to the brain. This nerve, which consists of about a million fibers, serves as a flexible cable connecting the eyeball to the brain. The brain interprets these impulses, turns the image right-side up, and "develops" a picture of the object from which the light originally came.

Accessory Structures

Several structures protect, lubricate, and move the eye, all of which contribute to healthy vision. These structures include the following:

- Eye sockets
- Eyebrows and eyelashes
- Eyelids
- Conjunctiva
- Lacrimal apparatus
- Eye muscles

The eye sockets, or **orbits,** form a protective shell around the eyes. Eyebrows and eyelashes also serve to protect the eyes by reducing the chances that sweat and direct sunlight will enter the eyes. The eyelids are a part of the blinking reflex, which protects the eyes from foreign materials such as dust. Blinking also helps lubricate the eyes by spreading tears over their surface. The protective membrane that lines the eyelids and covers the anterior of the sclera is the **conjunctiva.**

The lacrimal apparatus consists of the **lacrimal gland** (the source of tears) and a drainage system. Tears moisten and lubricate the eye and wash away foreign materials. They also inhibit the growth of bacteria. Excess tears drain from the eye through ducts located in the inner corner of the eye. The ducts empty into the nose.

In addition to the muscles inside the eye, there are six muscles that attach to the outside of each eyeball. These muscles control the movement of the eyes and normally allow both eyes to move in harmony.

The Aging Eye

With age, a number of changes occur in the structure and function of the eye.

- The amount of fat tissue diminishes; this loss may cause the eyelids to droop
- The quality and quantity of tears decrease
- The conjunctiva becomes thinner and may be drier because of a decrease in tear production
- The cornea begins to appear yellow, and a ring of fat deposits appears around it
- The sclera may develop brown spots
- Changes in the iris cause the pupil to become smaller, limiting the amount of light entering the eye
- The lens becomes denser and more rigid; this trend reduces the amount of light that reaches the retina and makes focusing more difficult
- Yellowing of the lens causes problems in distinguishing colors
- Changes in the retina may make vision fuzzy
- The ability of the eye to adapt to changes in light intensities may be reduced; glare can become painful as this ability diminishes
- Night vision may be impaired
- Peripheral vision is reduced, limiting the area a person can see and reducing depth perception
- The vitreous humor breaks down, producing tiny clumps of gel or cellular material that cause floaters—dark spots or lines—that appear in a person's field of vision
- Rubbing of the vitreous humor on the retina produces flashes of light or "sparks"

Because of changes that impair vision—such as reductions in the field of vision, in depth perception, and in visual clarity—elderly people may fall more often than younger people. See the Educating the Patient section for some tips for preventing such falls.

Vision Testing

When doctors perform complete physical examinations, they usually screen patients for vision problems and for the general health of the eyes. An **ophthalmologist** (a medical doctor who is an eye specialist) usually performs

Educating the Patient

Preventing Falls in the Elderly

Falls can occur at any age, but in the elderly they can have especially serious consequences. Bones become brittle with age, and falls can cause breaks in major bones, such as the hip. Complications from falls and bone fractures can lead to death in individuals in this age group.

The elderly are prone to falling because of vision problems, possible poor health, slowing reflexes, and changes in the ear that cause equilibrium problems. In addition, medications can increase the risk of falls because they may make the patient less alert. Discuss a safety checklist with elderly patients and their families. Point out that by taking the precautions listed, elderly patients can reduce the risk of falling. Make sure patients and their families understand these instructions.

- Remove reading glasses before getting up and walking around.
- Make sure that potentially hazardous areas, such as stairs and doorway entrances, are well lit.
- Use night-lights in the bedroom and bathroom to help prevent falls at night.
- When getting up from a reclining or recumbent position, sit at the edge of the bed for a few minutes before trying to stand to allow blood flow to adjust.
- Wear well-fitting shoes with low heels and slippers with nonslip soles.
- Use a cane or walker if you are unsteady on your feet.
- Secure rugs and floor coverings to the floor to prevent slippage.
- Attach all electrical cords to the walls or floor moldings.
- Place sturdy banisters along all stairs inside and outside the home.
- Install secure handrails near the bathtub and toilet.
- Use nonslip mats in the bathtub and shower.
- Minimize clutter in the home.
- Store frequently used items within easy reach.

Career Opportunities

Ophthalmic Assistant

To gain medical assistant credentials, you must fulfill the requirements of either the American Association of Medical Assistants (for a Certified Medical Assistant) or the American Medical Technologists (for a Registered Medical Assistant). After obtaining your medical assistant certification or registration, you may wish to acquire additional skills in specialty areas through course work or on-the-job training. Although this course work or training may not lead to an additional certification or degree, it will enable you to expand your role in the medical office and advance your career as the demand for skilled health professionals increases.

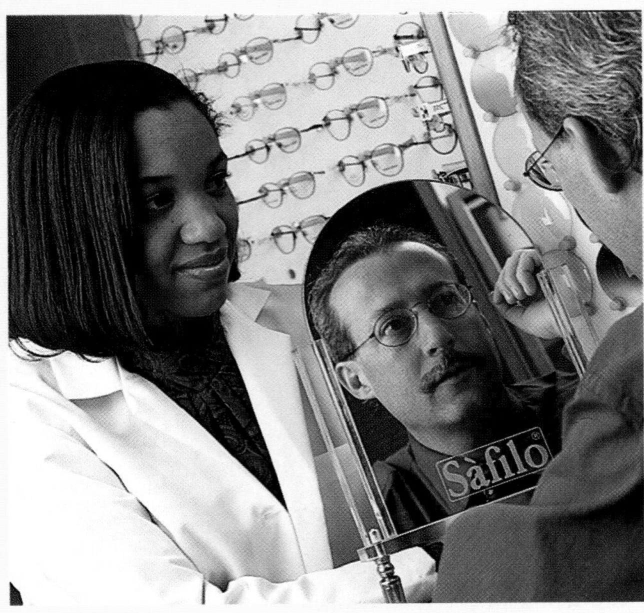

Skills and Duties

An ophthalmic assistant provides administrative and clinical support for an ophthalmologist. The assistant works with patients, assists with surgery, and keeps instruments and equipment in proper working order.

The ophthalmic assistant works with patients in a number of ways. Taking the medical history is basic to the ophthalmic assistant's job. She must gather information about the patient's ocular history, family medical history, past and present systemic illnesses, medications, and allergies. She needs to preserve patient confidentiality and use proper recording techniques.

An ophthalmic assistant may conduct tests that evaluate aspects of vision, such as distance acuity, near acuity, and color perception. She must understand how these tests work and how to run them and be prepared to help patients with special needs as she conducts the tests. Tonometry, the measurement of fluid pressure in the eyeball with a machine called a tonometer, may also be the responsibility of an ophthalmic assistant.

When patients need help with their eyeglasses, the ophthalmic assistant is often the person who records prescriptions, adjusts and repairs damaged frames and lenses, and instructs patients in the care of their eyeglasses. The assistant is trained to administer eye medications to patients in the form of drops, ointments, and irrigating solutions.

The ophthalmic assistant may also assist the ophthalmologist with minor surgery. She prepares the room and instruments, instructs the patient before and after the procedure, and assists the doctor during the surgical procedure.

The operation and care of specialized ophthalmologic instruments, such as ophthalmoscopes, retinoscopes, tonometers, and slitlamps, are often the responsibility of an ophthalmic assistant. She must maintain infection control in the office or operating room, including sanitization, disinfection, and sterilization of instruments and surfaces.

Workplace Settings

The ophthalmic assistant always works under the supervision of an ophthalmologist. She may work in a private office or in a hospital setting.

Education

Certification as an ophthalmic assistant requires a high school diploma or equivalency, followed by a clinical program approved by the Joint Review Committee for Ophthalmic Medical Personnel (JRCOMP). After completing the program, the student must pass an examination that tests seven basic content areas: history taking, basic skills and lensometry, patient services, basic tonometry, instrument maintenance, general medical knowledge, and special studies. She must also provide a current CPR card (such as those issued by the Red Cross or the American Heart Association) and an

continued ⟶

Career Opportunities

Ophthalmic Assistant *(continued)*

endorsement from her supervising ophthalmologist. After passing the examination, the student gains the title of Certified Ophthalmic Assistant (COA). Certification must be renewed every 3 years.

Where to Go for More Information

American Academy of Ophthalmology
655 Beach Street
San Francisco, CA 94109
(415) 561-8500

Association of Technical Personnel
in Ophthalmology
50 Lee Road
Chestnut Hill, MA 02167
(617) 232-4433

Joint Commission on Allied Health Personnel
in Ophthalmology
2025 Woodlane Drive
St. Paul, MN 55125-2995
(800) 284-3937

a thorough eye examination (described in Chapter 23). She tests the external as well as internal structures of the eyes, along with eye movement and coordination. The kinds of testing you will perform or help perform will depend on where you work. You will, however, be expected to assist the doctor and ensure that the patient is comfortable.

Types of Vision Screening Tests

Screening tests are used to detect a number of common visual problems. Some problems may involve the ability to see clearly. Others may involve the ability to distinguish shades of gray or colors. When you record the results of vision tests, you will use the following abbreviations:

- O.D. (right eye)
- O.S. (left eye)
- O.U. (both eyes)
- $\overline{cc}$ (with correction)

Distance Vision. To test the distance vision of adults, the Snellen letter chart (Figure 21-2) is commonly used. This chart has several rows of letters of the alphabet. Within each row, letter size is the same, but from row to row, letter size decreases from top to bottom. Patients are asked to read the letters from larger to smaller. A chart such as the Snellen E chart (Figure 21-3a), the Landolt C chart (similar to Snellen E, using the letter C), or a pictorial chart (Figure 21-3b), is used for children and adults who do not know the alphabet.

When distance vision is tested, normal vision is referred to as 20/20. This number means that at the standard testing distance of 20 feet (first number), a patient can see what a person with normal vision can see at 20 feet (second number). A patient who has 20/80 vision can see at 20 feet what a person with normal vision sees at 80 feet. The first number (20) always stays the same because a patient always stands 20 feet away from the chart. The second number, however, changes with a patient's visual acuity. If a patient misses only one or two letters on a line during vision testing, record the results with a minus sign. For example, one letter missed with the right eye would be O.D. 20/30 −1. Two letters would be O.D. 20/30 −2.

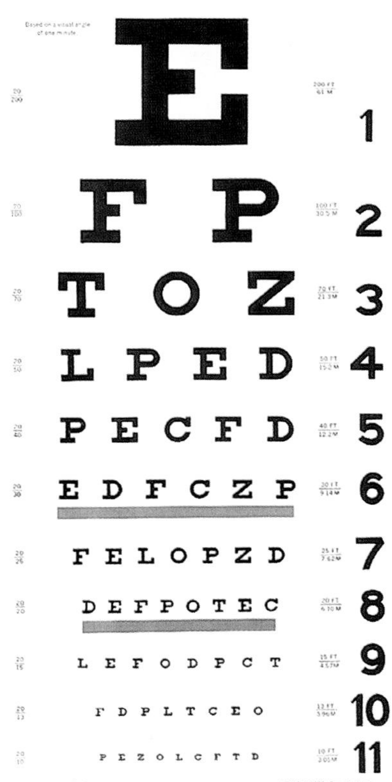

Figure 21-2. The Snellen letter chart is used to test the ability to see objects that are relatively far away.

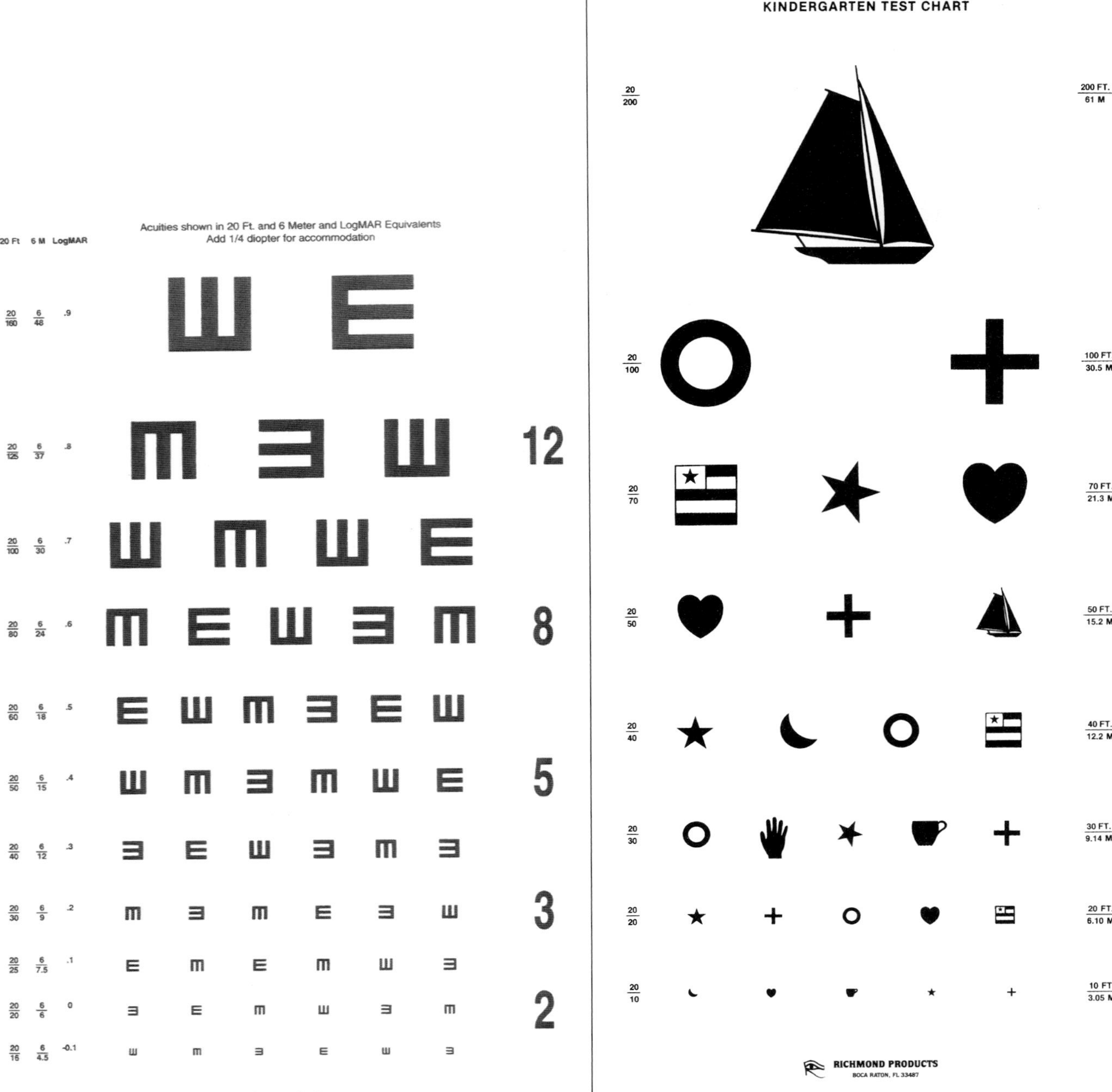

Figure 21-3. The Snellen E eye chart (left) or a pictorial (right) eye chart is used to test the vision of children and nonreading adults. (Courtesy Richmond Products, Inc.)

Near Vision. To test for near vision, special handheld charts are used. These cards contain letters, numbers, or paragraphs in various sizes of print (Figures 21-4 and 21-5). They may be held and read at a normal reading distance or mounted in a plastic and metal frame and read through optical lenses.

Contrast Sensitivity. To test for the ability to distinguish shades of gray (contrast sensitivity), the Pelli-Robson contrast sensitivity chart, the Vistech Consultants vision contrast test system (Figure 21-6), or another testing system is used. Newer systems use special equipment to provide contrast variations in a projected image. These tests can detect cataracts or problems of the retina even before the sharpness of the patient's vision is impaired.

Color Vision. To test color vision, illustrations such as those of the Ishihara color system or the Richmond pseudoisochromatic color test (Figure 21-7) are used. These illustrations contain numbers or symbols made up of colored dots that appear among other colored dots. The

V = .50 D.

The fourteenth of August was the day fixed upon for the sailing of the brig Pilgrim, on her voyage from Boston round Cape Horn, to the western coast of North America. As she was to get under way early in the afternoon, I made my appearance on board at twelve o'clock in full sea-rig, and with my chest, containing an outfit for a two or three years voyage, which I had undertaken from a determination to cure, if possible, by an entire change of life, and by a long absence from books and study, a weakness of the eyes which had obliged me to give up my pursuits, and which no medical aid seemed likely to cure. The change from the tight dress coat, silk cap and kid gloves of an undergraduate at Cambridge, to the

V = .75 D.

loose duck trousers, checked shirt and tarpaulin hat of a sailor, though somewhat of a transformation, was soon made, and I supposed that I should pass very well for a Jack tar. But it is impossible to deceive the practiced eye in these matters; and while I supposed myself to be looking as salt as Neptune himself, I was, no doubt, known for a landsman by every one on board, as soon as I hove in sight. A sailor has a peculiar cut to his clothes, and a way of wear-

V = 1. D.

ing them which a green hand can never get. The trousers, tight around the hips, and thence hanging long and loose around the feet, a superabundance of checked shirt, a low-crowned, well-varnished black hat, worn on the back of the head, with half a fathom of black ribbon hanging over the left eye, and a peculiar tie to the black silk neckerchief, with sundry other *details*, are signs the want of which betray the beginner at once.

V = 1.25 D.

Beside the points in my dress which were out of the way, doubtless my complexion and hands would distinguish me from the regular *salt*, who, with a sun-browned cheek, wide step and rolling gait, swings his bronzed and toughened hands athwartships half open, as though just to ready to grasp a rope. "With all my imperfections

V = 1.50 D.

on my head," I joined the crew, and we hauled out into the stream and came to anchor for the night. The next day we were employed in preparation for sea, reeving and studding-sail gear, crossing royal yards, putting on chafing gear, and taking on board our powder. On the

V = 1.75 D.

following night I stood my first watch. I remained awake nearly all the first part of the night, from fear that I might not hear when I was called; and when I went on deck, so great were my ideas of the importance of my trust, that I

V = 2. D.

walked regularly fore and aft the whole length of the vessel, looking out over the bows and taffrail at each turn, and was not a little surprised at the unconcerned manner in which the billows turned up their

Your glasses are of value to you only as they accurately interpret your prescription and this only as they are fitted and serviced in accordance with these needs. They are a therapeutic device.

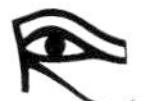

RICHMOND PRODUCTS
BOCA RATON, FL 33487

No. 11974 R

Figure 21-4. This near-vision chart is used to test the ability to see objects at a normal reading distance. (Courtesy Richmond Products, Inc.)

patient is asked to identify what he sees. A patient who is color-blind will not be able to report seeing the numbers or symbols. Color blindness may be inherited; it occurs more commonly in males. Changes in one's ability to see colors, however, may indicate a disease of the retina or optic nerve. For details on how to perform color vision and other vision tests, see Procedure 21-1.

Special Considerations. Certain patients may need special attention when having vision tests. For example, children may be uncooperative or unable to follow directions. To encourage cooperation, show a child the chart you will be using before you begin the test. Point to the symbols and read them aloud once so the child knows the proper term for each symbol. Most physicians use pictorial charts

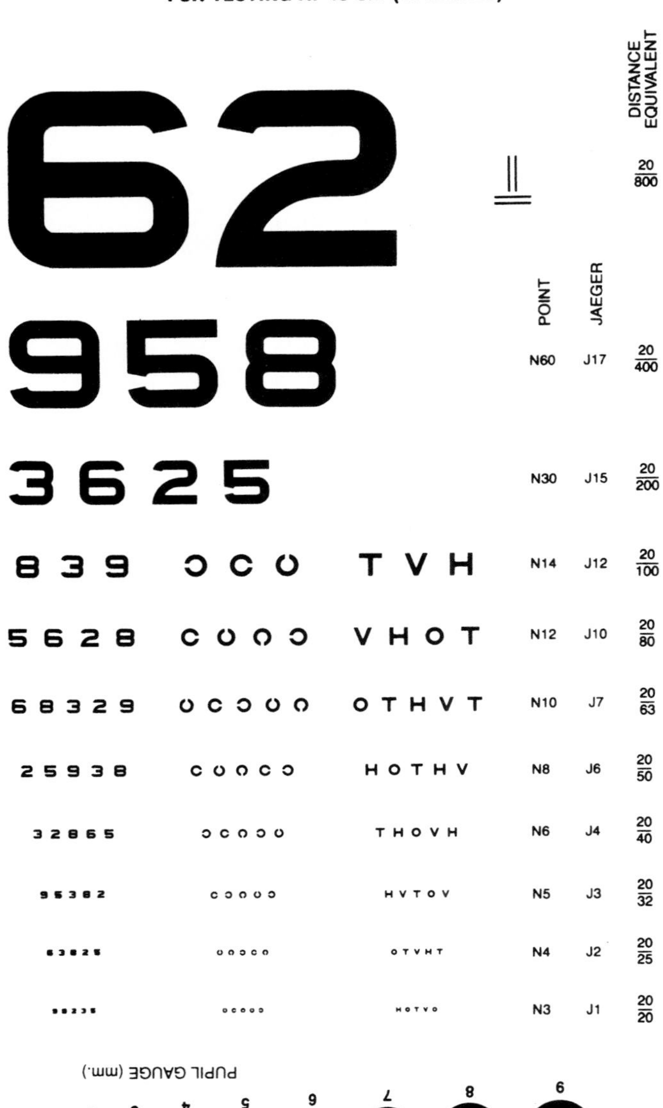

Figure 21-5. The Richmond pocket vision screener is also used to test the ability to see close objects. (Courtesy Richmond Products, Inc.)

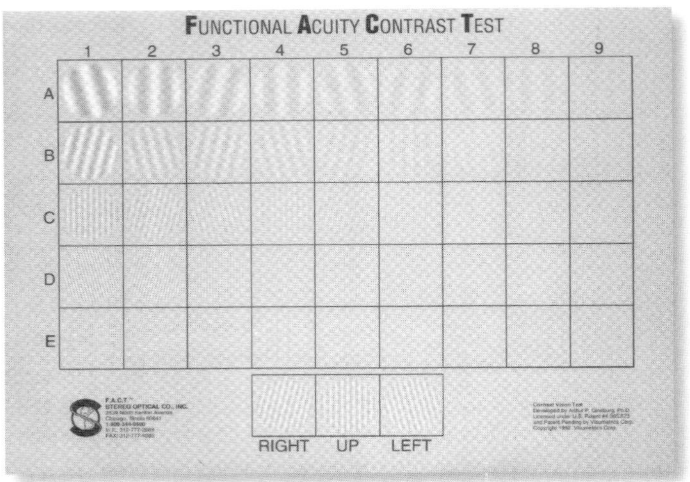

Figure 21-6. The Functional Acuity Contrast Test (FACT™) is used to test the ability to differentiate various shades of gray. (Stereo Optical Co., Inc., Chicago, IL. Copyright Vision Sciences Research Corporation, San Ramon, CA. Developed by Dr. Arthur P. Ginsburg)

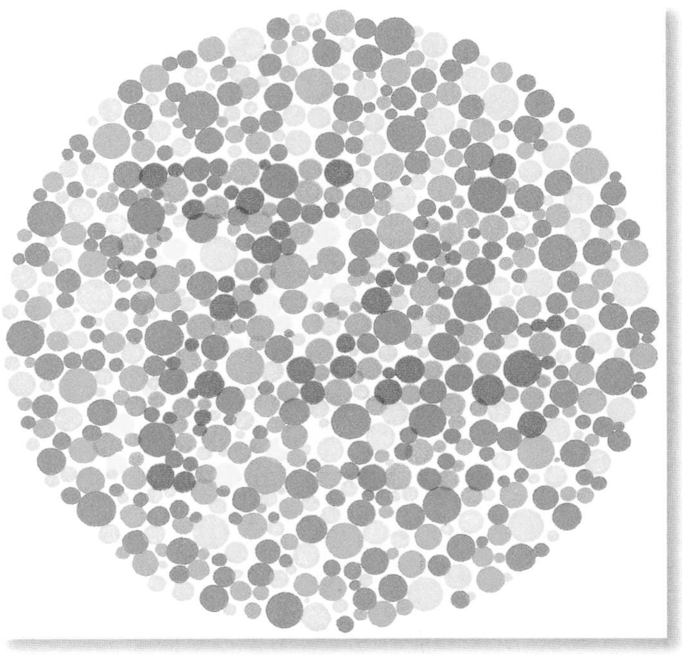

Figure 21-7. The Richmond pseudoisochromatic color chart is used to test a person's ability to see colors. (Courtesy Richmond Products, Inc.)

when they start screening a child's vision at the 4-year or 5-year checkup. You can provide assistance during the test by guiding the child through each step in the procedure or by covering the child's eye. Watch the child closely for signs that she is having difficulty seeing the chart. Examples of signs include straining, blinking or watering of the eyes, and puckering of the face.

If a child has difficulty following directions, enlist the parent's or guardian's help. He may be able to explain or interpret information for the child more effectively than you can. Ask the parent if he has ever observed signs of vision problems in his child. For example, does the child rub her eyes frequently, blink a great deal, or hold books very close to her face? Be sure to note the answers in the child's chart so the physician is aware of them.

A patient with Alzheimer's disease may also require special attention during a vision test. Before the test, encourage a family member to stay with the patient so he is more comfortable. During the test use simple language to explain the procedure and demonstrate whenever possible. Proceed through the examination slowly, one step at a time. Because the patient's memory and language skills may be impaired, you may need to repeat directions many times and help him name a particular object. If he appears to have trouble with one part of the examination, proceed to another part and return later to the part that was difficult for him.

PROCEDURE 21.1

Performing Vision Screening Tests

Objectives: To screen a patient's ability to see distant or close objects, to determine contrast sensitivity, or to detect color blindness

OSHA Guidelines

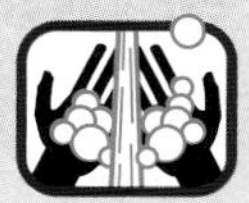
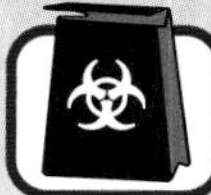
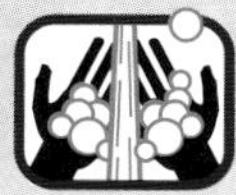

Materials: Occluder or card, alcohol, gauze squares, appropriate vision charts to test for distance vision, near vision, contrast sensitivity, and color blindness

Method

Distance Vision

1. Wash your hands, identify the patient, introduce yourself, and explain the procedure.
2. Mount one of the following eye charts at eye level: Snellen letter or similar chart (for patients who can read); Snellen E, Landolt C, pictorial, or similar chart (for patients who cannot read). If using the Snellen letter chart, verify that the patient knows the letters of the alphabet. With children or nonreading adults, use demonstration cards to verify that they can identify the pictures or direction of the letters.
3. Make a mark on the floor 20 feet away from the chart.
4. Have the patient stand with the heels at the 20-foot mark or sit with the back of the chair at the mark.
5. Instruct the patient to keep both eyes open and not to squint or lean forward during the test.
6. Test both eyes first, then the right eye, and then the left eye. (Different offices may test in a different order. Follow your office policy.) Refer to Figure 21-8.
7. Have the patient read the lines on the chart (or identify the picture/direction), beginning with the 20-foot line. If the patient cannot read this line, begin with the smallest line the patient can read. (Some offices use a pointer to select one symbol at a time in random order to prevent patients from memorizing the order. It is common to start with children at the 40- or 30-foot line, or larger if low vision is suspected, and proceed to the 20-foot line.)

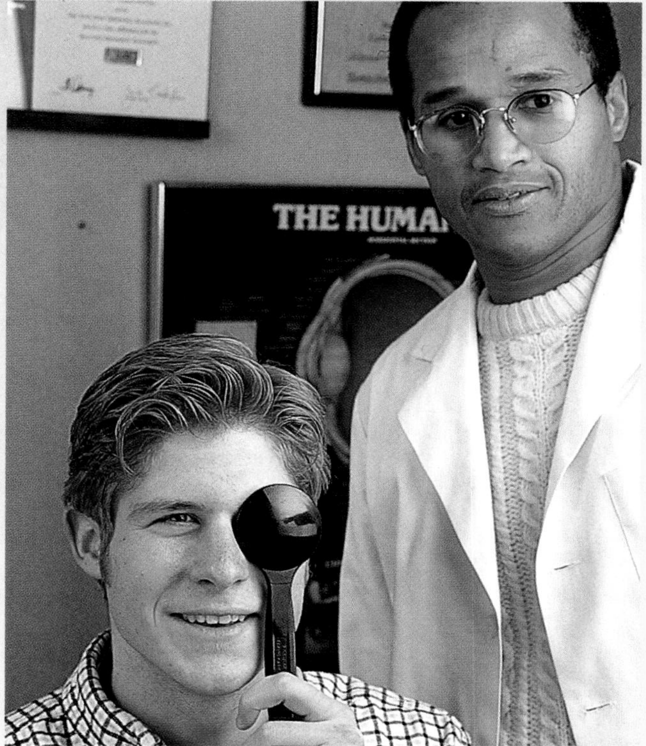

Figure 21-8. Have the patient cover the left eye with the occluder. The patient should keep both eyes open and not squint.

8. Note the smallest line the patient can read or identify. (When testing children, note the smallest line on which they can identify three out of four or four out of six symbols correctly.)
9. Record the results as a fraction (for example, O.U. 20/40 –1 if the patient misses one letter on a line or O.U. 20/40 –2 if the patient misses two letters on a line).
10. Show the patient how to cover the left eye with the occluder or card. Again, instruct the patient to keep both eyes open and not to squint or lean forward during the test.
11. Have the patient read the lines on the chart.
12. Record the results of the right eye (for example, O.D. 20/30).
13. Have the patient cover the right eye and read the lines on the chart.

continued ⟶

PROCEDURE 21.1

Performing Vision Screening Tests *(continued)*

14. Record the results of the left eye (for example, O.S. 20/20).
15. If the patient wears corrective lenses, record the results using $\overline{cc}$ (if your office uses this abbreviation for "with correction") in front of the abbreviation (for example, $\overline{cc}$ O.U. 20/20).
16. Note and record any observations of squinting, head tilting, or excessive blinking or tearing.
17. Ask the patient to keep both eyes open and to identify the two colored bars, and record the results in the patient's chart.
18. Clean the occluder with a gauze square dampened with alcohol.
19. Properly dispose of the gauze square and wash your hands.

Near Vision

1. Wash your hands, identify the patient, introduce yourself, and explain the procedure.
2. Have the patient hold one of the following at normal reading distance (approximately 14 to 16 inches): Jaeger, Richmond pocket, or similar chart or card.
3. Ask the patient to keep both eyes open and to read or identify the letters, symbols, or paragraphs.
4. Record the smallest line read without error.
5. If the card is laminated, clean it with a gauze square dampened with alcohol.
6. Properly dispose of the gauze square and wash your hands.

Contrast Sensitivity

1. Wash your hands, identify the patient, introduce yourself, and explain the procedure.
2. Mount a contrast sensitivity chart at eye level. (The following steps apply to use of the Vistech Consultants vision contrast test system. The procedures for using other contrast sensitivity charts vary slightly.)
3. Make a mark on the floor 10 feet from the chart.
4. Have the patient stand with the heels at the mark or sit with the back of the chair at the mark.
5. Test both eyes first.
6. Beginning with circle A1, have the patient identify the direction of the stripes in each circle in row A—left, right, up and down, or blank.
7. In column A on the answer grid that accompanies the chart, mark the point for the last circle for which the patient can correctly identify the direction of the stripes. (If the point falls within the shaded area, the patient's vision is within the normal range.)
8. Repeat steps 6 and 7 for rows B through E.
9. Have the patient cover his left eye with an occluder or card, and repeat steps 6 through 8 for the right eye.
10. Have the patient cover his right eye, and repeat steps 6 through 8 for the left eye.
11. Clean the occluder or card with a gauze square dipped in alcohol.
12. Properly dispose of the used gauze square and wash your hands.

Color Vision

1. Wash your hands, identify the patient, introduce yourself, and explain the procedure.
2. Hold one of the following color charts or books at the patient's normal reading distance (approximately 14 to 16 inches): Ishihara, Richmond pseudoisochromatic, or similar color-testing system.
3. Ask the patient to tell you the number or symbol within the colored dots on each chart or page.
4. Proceed through all the charts or pages.
5. Record the number correctly identified and failed with a slash between them (for example, 13 passed/1 failed).
6. If the charts are laminated, clean them with a gauze square dampened with alcohol.
7. Properly dispose of the gauze square and wash your hands.

Treating Eye Problems

Some common eye problems include conjunctivitis (inflammation of the conjunctiva), blepharitis (inflammation of the eyelid), and corneal abrasions (scratching of the cornea). The eye is an extremely delicate organ. Even what seems to be a minor injury or infection can have lasting consequences. Therefore, you must use the greatest caution as well as proper techniques when treating a patient's eyes. You should also provide patients with information on how

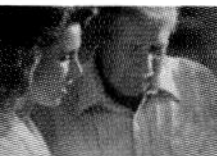

Educating the Patient

Preventive Eye-Care Tips

You can help patients take care of their eyes and protect their vision by providing them with guidelines to follow. Go over each item slowly and carefully. Ask whether the patient has questions before moving on to the next item. Answer all the patient's questions, and make sure the patient understands the answers. Eye-care tips include the following.

1. Get regular health checkups. Patients may not appreciate the connection between their general health and their eyes. Point out that high blood pressure and diabetes can cause eye problems.
2. Get regular eye examinations. Most people need eye examinations every 1 to 2 years. Patients with diabetes should see their eye-care specialists more frequently.
3. Be alert for the warning signs of eye disease. Tell patients to call their eye-care specialist immediately if they experience any of these signs:
   - Eye pain
   - Loss of vision
   - Double or blurred vision
   - Headache with blurred vision
   - Redness of the eye or eyelid
   - A gritty or sticky feeling around the eye
   - Excessive tearing
   - Difficulty seeing in the dark
   - Flashes of light
   - Halos around lights
   - Sensitivity to light
   - Loss of color perception
4. Wear sunglasses with ultraviolet protection to shield the eyes from bright sunlight, even in the winter. Recommend that patients ask to have ultraviolet protection added when purchasing new distance prescription glasses. Explain to patients that the cornea can get sunburned, which can be painful and damaging. Also tell patients that excessive exposure to the sun is a contributing factor in malignant melanoma of the eye—a dangerous type of skin cancer that may spread through the bloodstream or lymphatic system.
5. Wear protective eye equipment to prevent eye injury. Indicate to patients that they should wear protective eyewear every time they participate in sports, work with chemicals, or encounter a situation in which they may be exposed to flying debris.
6. Use nonprescription eye medications properly. Show patients how to use eyedrops; emphasize that the tip of the dropper should never touch the eye. Explain to patients that medications should be used only as indicated on the label and discarded after the condition has cleared up.

to routinely care for their eyes. See the Educating the Patient section for specific guidelines to follow when presenting preventive eye-care information.

Administration of Medications to the Eye

Your responsibilities as a medical assistant include dispensing medications and explaining their use. Some medications are used to diagnose conditions, whereas others are used to treat conditions. Only medications for ophthalmic use should be used in the eye. You should teach patients to check medication labels carefully before administering them at home. *Optic* medications for use in the eye could easily be confused with *otic* medications for the ear. Medications other than optic medications may be too concentrated or may contain substances that will injure sensitive eye tissue.

If you administer eye medications as part of your job, avoid touching a dropper or ointment tube tip to the eye. Such touching can injure the eye, cause an infection, and contaminate the medication. Procedure 21-2 describes the proper technique for administering eye medications.

Eye Irrigation

When foreign materials enter the eye, they must be flushed out. Flushing (or irrigation) should be done with a sterile solution especially formulated for this purpose. Someone's eye may also need to be irrigated to relieve discomfort from irritating substances, such as smog, pollen, chemicals, or chlorinated water. The steps involved in irrigating the eye are outlined in Procedure 21-3.

Vision Aids

Vision screening tests may indicate that a patient has a vision problem. Common refractive disorders, such as myopia, hyperopia, presbyopia, and astigmatism, are discussed in detail in Chapter 23. Most of these vision prob-

PROCEDURE 21.2

Administering Eye Medications

Objective: To instill medication into the eye for treatment of certain eye disorders

OSHA Guidelines

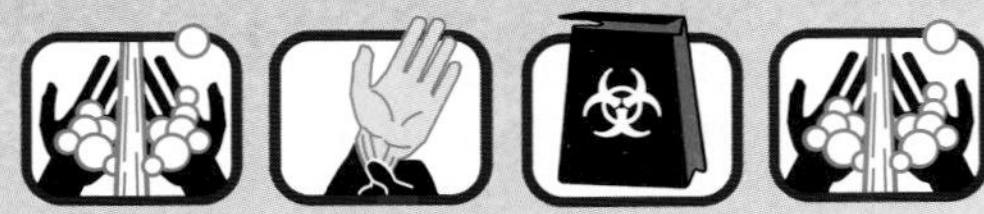

Materials: Medication (drops, cream, or ointment), tissues, eye patch (if applicable)

Method

1. Identify the patient, introduce yourself, and explain the procedure.
2. Review the doctor's medication order. This should include the patient's name, drug name, concentration, number of drops (if a liquid), into which eye(s) the medication is to be administered, and the frequency of administration.
3. Compare the drug with the medication order three times.
4. Ask whether the patient has any known allergies to eye medications.
5. Wash your hands and put on gloves.
6. Assemble supplies.
7. Ask the patient to lie down or to sit back in a chair with the head tilted back.
8. Give the patient a tissue to blot excess medication as needed.
9. Remove an eye patch, if present.

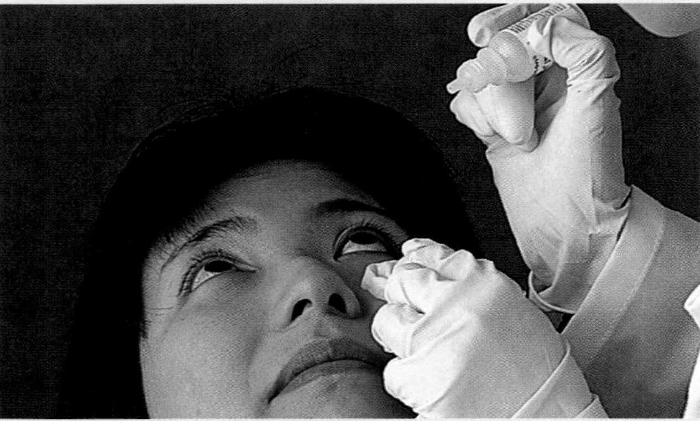

Figure 21-9. Use a tissue to press down on the patient's cheekbone just below the eyelid, opening up a pocket of space between the eyelid and the eye.

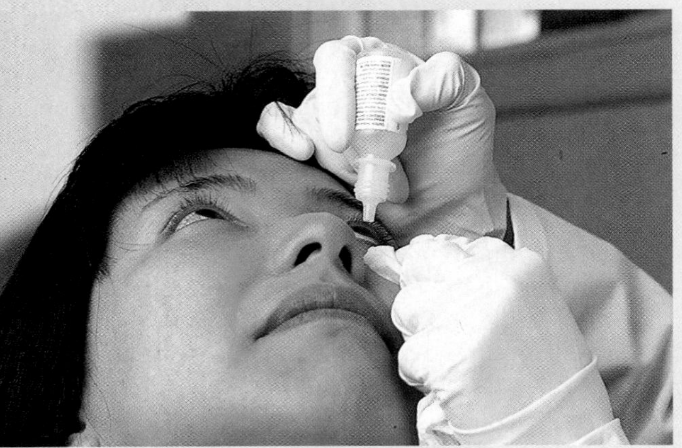

Figure 21-10. The bottle should be approximately ½ inch from the conjunctiva as you prepare to instill drops in the patient's eye.

10. Ask the patient to look at the ceiling. Instruct the patient to keep both eyes open during the procedure.
11. With a tissue, gently pull the lower eyelid down by pressing downward on the patient's cheekbone just below the eyelid with your nondominant hand. This pressure will open a pocket of space between the eyelid and the eye (Figure 21-9).

Eyedrops

12. Resting your dominant hand on the patient's forehead, hold the filled eyedropper or bottle approximately ½ inch from the conjunctiva (Figure 21-10).
13. Drop the prescribed number of drops into the pocket. If any drops land outside the eye, repeat instilling the drops that missed the eye.

Creams or Ointments

12. Rest your dominant hand on the patient's forehead, and hold the tube or applicator above the conjunctiva.
13. Evenly apply a thin ribbon of cream or ointment along the inside edge of the lower eyelid on the conjunctiva, working from the medial (inner) to the lateral (outer) side (Figure 21-11).

All Medications

14. Release the lower lid and instruct the patient to gently close the eyes.

continued ⟶

PROCEDURE 21.2

Administering Eye Medications *(continued)*

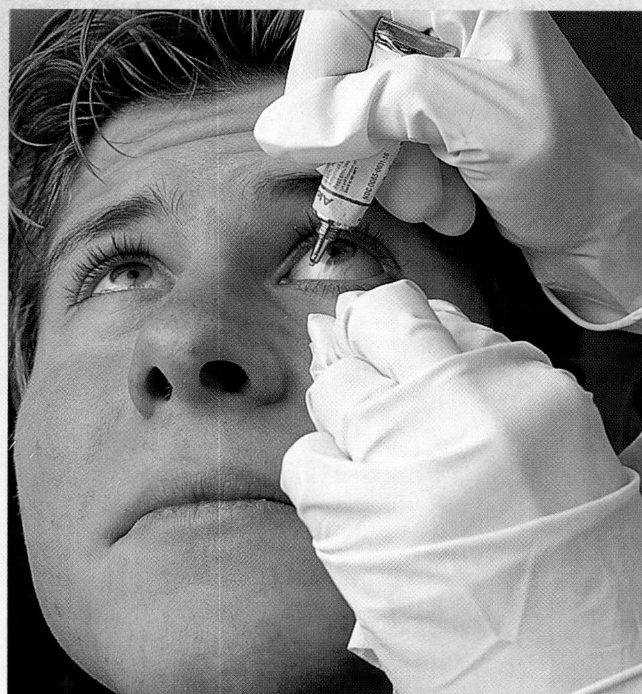

Figure 21-11. Apply a thin ribbon of cream or ointment along the inside of the lower eyelid on the conjunctiva.

15. Repeat the procedure for the other eye as necessary.
16. Remove any excess medication by wiping each eyelid gently with a fresh tissue from the medial to the lateral side (Figure 21-12).
17. Apply a clean eye patch to cover the entire eye as necessary.
18. Ask whether the patient felt any discomfort, and observe for any adverse reactions. Notify the doctor as necessary.
19. Instruct the patient on self-administration of medication and patch application as necessary.
20. Ask the patient to repeat the instructions.
21. Provide written instructions.
22. Properly dispose of used disposable materials.
23. Remove gloves and wash your hands.
24. Document administration in the patient's chart. Include the drug, concentration, number of drops, time of administration, and which eye(s) received the medication.

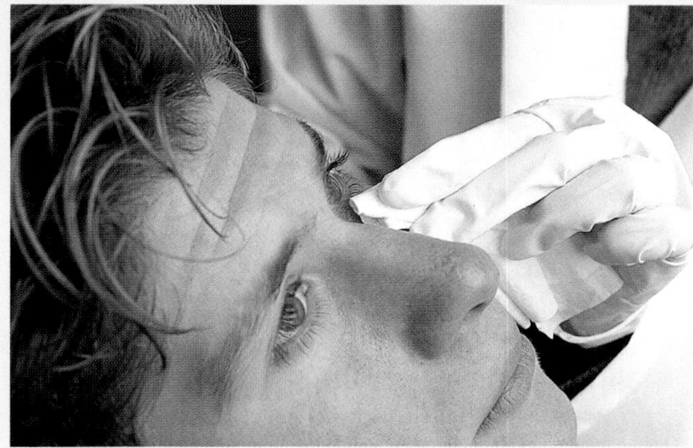

Figure 21-12. Use a tissue to remove excess medication from the eyelid.

lems are corrected with eyeglasses or contact lenses. These corrective aids are usually prescribed by an ophthalmologist or an **optometrist** (a trained and licensed vision specialist who is not a physician). You may be asked to assist patients who have vision problems by providing them with information on vision and eye-care specialists or by making appointments for them.

Hearing

The ability to hear depends on the normal functioning of a number of structures in the ear. It also depends on the normal transmission of nerve impulses from the ear to the brain.

The Ear

The ear is the organ that enables people to hear. It also helps people maintain balance. As shown in Figure 21-13, the ear is divided into three parts:

1. External ear
2. Middle ear
3. Inner ear

The External Ear. The external, or outer, ear is made up of the outer part of the ear, or **auricle,** and the ear canal. The auricle is made of cartilage and is covered with skin. The ear canal is lined with skin that contains hairs and glands that produce **cerumen,** a waxlike

PROCEDURE 21.3

Performing Eye Irrigation

Objective: To flush the eye to remove foreign particles or relieve eye irritation

OSHA Guidelines

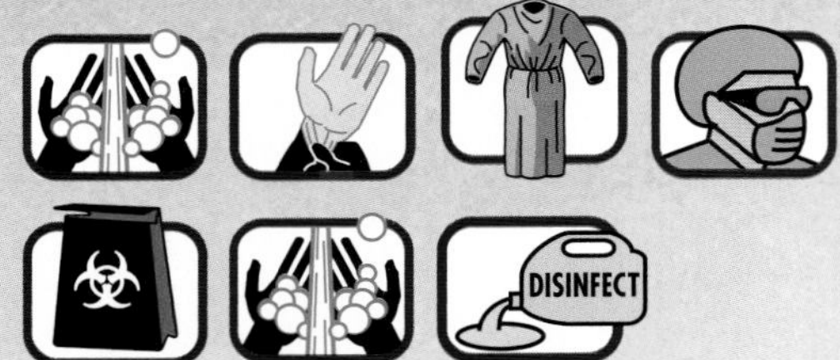

Materials: Sterile irrigating solution, sterile basin, sterile irrigating syringe and kidney-shaped basin, tissues

Method

1. Identify the patient, introduce yourself, and explain the procedure.
2. Review the physician's order. This should include the patient's name, irrigating solution, volume of solution, and for which eye(s) the irrigation is to be performed.
3. Compare the solution with the instructions three times.
4. Wash your hands and put on gloves, a gown, and a face shield (splashing is possible when a syringe is used).
5. Assemble supplies.
6. Ask the patient to lie down or to sit with the head tilted back and to the side that is being irrigated. The solution should not spill over into the other eye.
7. Place a towel over the patient's shoulder (or under the head and shoulder, if the patient is lying down). Have the patient hold the kidney-shaped basin at the side of the head next to the eye to be irrigated.
8. Pour the solution into the sterile basin.
9. Fill the irrigating syringe with solution (approximately 50 mL).
10. Hold a tissue on the patient's cheekbone below the lower eyelid with your nondominant hand, and press downward to expose the eye socket.
11. Holding the tip of the syringe ½ inch away from the eye, direct the solution onto the lower conjunctiva from the inner to the outer aspect of the eye. (Avoid directing the solution against the cornea because it is sensitive; do not use excessive force.)
12. Refill the syringe and continue irrigation until the prescribed volume of solution is used or until the solution is used up.
13. Dry the area around the eye with tissues.
14. Properly dispose of used disposable materials.
15. Remove gloves, gown, and face shield, and wash your hands.
16. Record in the patient's chart the procedure, the amount of solution used, time of administration, and eye(s) irrigated.
17. Put on gloves and clean the equipment and room according to OSHA guidelines.

substance also called earwax. The eardrum, or **tympanic membrane,** is a fibrous partition located at the inner end of the canal. The eardrum separates the external ear from the middle ear.

The Middle Ear. The middle ear is a small, air-filled cavity between the eardrum and the inner ear. It contains three small bones: the hammer, the anvil, and the stirrup. The **malleus,** or hammer, is attached to the eardrum, and the **stapes,** or stirrup, is attached to the inner ear. The **incus,** or anvil, lies between them. An opening in the middle ear, the **eustachian tube,** leads to the back of the throat. The eustachian tube helps equalize air pressure on both sides of the eardrum.

The Inner Ear. The inner ear, or **labyrinth,** contains a number of important structures. Among these are the **cochlea,** a spiral-shaped canal that contains the hearing receptors, and three **semicircular canals,** which help a person maintain balance.

The Hearing Process

A sound consists of waves of different frequencies that move through the air. The external ear initiates sound conduction when it collects these waves and channels them to the eardrum. There the waves make the eardrum vibrate. The vibrations, in turn, are amplified by the bones

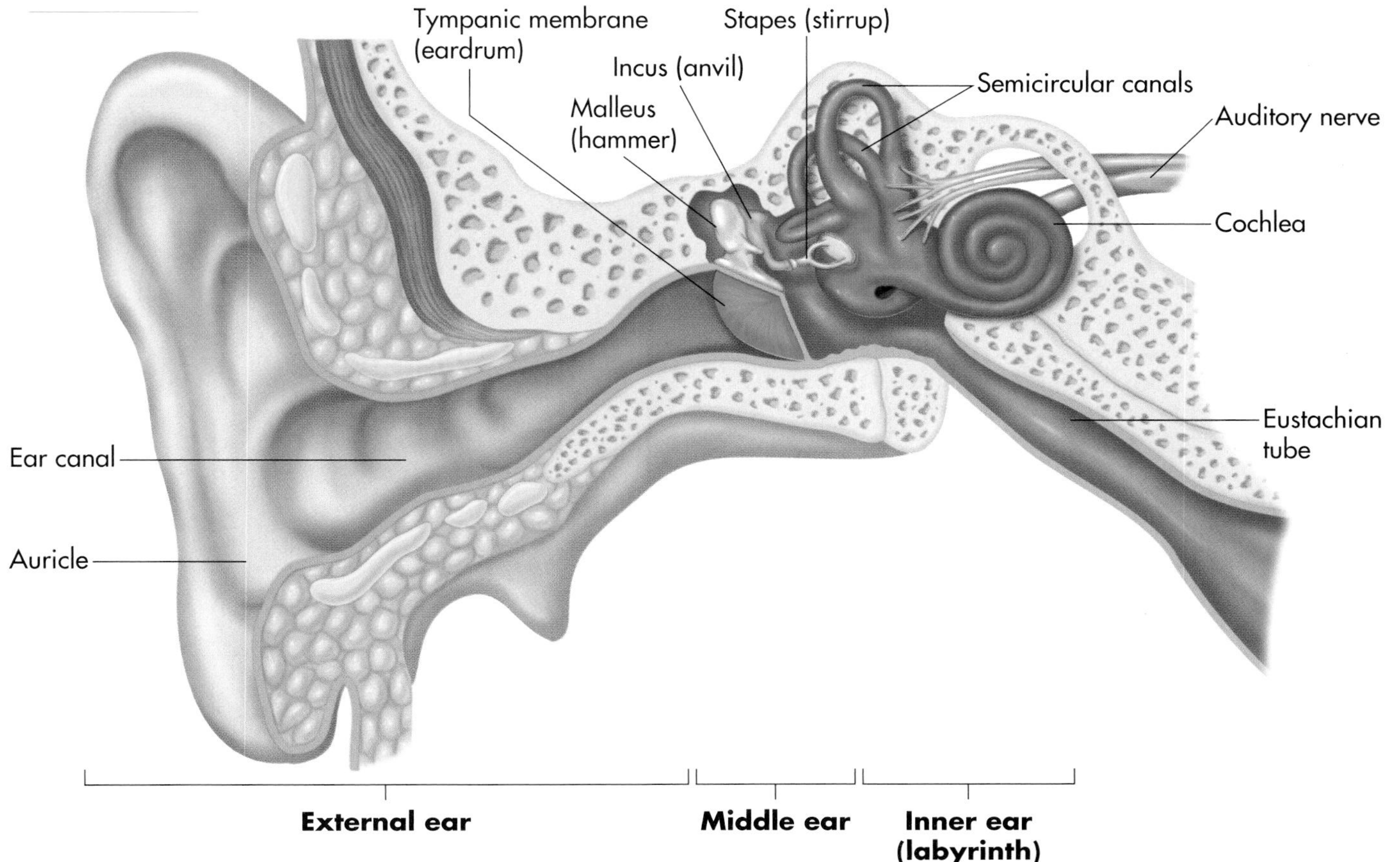

Figure 21-13. The ear is composed of a number of structures that work in harmony to produce hearing and a sense of balance.

of the middle ear. The amplified waves enter the inner ear and the cochlea. These waves cause tiny hairs that line the cochlea to bend. Movements of the hairs trigger nerve impulses. The impulses are transmitted by the auditory nerve to the brain, where they are perceived as sound.

Sound waves are also conducted through the bones of the skull directly to the inner ear, a process called **bone conduction.** This alternative pathway for sound bypasses the external and middle ears. When you hear your own voice, the sound has reached your inner ear mainly through bone conduction. By comparing a person's ability to sense sounds by bone conduction and through the entire ear, doctors can often identify what part of the ear is causing a hearing problem. For example, if bone conduction is normal, a hearing problem likely involves the middle or external ear rather than the inner ear.

The Ear and Balance

The brain constantly monitors the position of one's body on the basis of information it receives from the semicircular canals, eyes, and muscles. Each canal is at a right angle to the other two. In other words, each is oriented in a different dimension or plane: height, depth, and width. Together they detect any change in the position of the body. Such information is passed on to the brain along with data from the eyes and muscles. The brain then uses the information to maintain balance.

The Aging Ear

As a person grows older, a number of changes occur in the ear. The external ear appears larger because of continued growth of cartilage and the loss of skin elasticity. The ear lobe gets longer and may have a wrinkled appearance. The glands that produce cerumen become less efficient, producing earwax that is much drier. The ear canal also becomes narrower.

In the middle ear, changes in the eardrum cause it to shrink and appear dull and gray. The joints between the bones of the middle ear degenerate, so they do not move as freely. In the inner ear, the semicircular canals become less sensitive to changes in position, and this reduced sensitivity affects balance.

Problems with equilibrium make the elderly prone to falls. Some ear disorders are also more common in older individuals.

Hearing Loss

Hearing loss is actually a symptom of a disease, not a disease in itself. Contrary to what most people believe, hearing loss is not a normal part of the aging process and should always be evaluated for proper treatment.

Types of Hearing Loss

There are two types of hearing loss, conductive and sensorineural. The two types differ in the point at which the hearing process is interrupted.

A conductive hearing loss is caused by an interruption in the transmission of sound waves to the inner ear. Conditions that can cause conductive hearing loss include obstruction of the ear canal, infection of the middle ear, and reduced movement of the stirrup.

A sensorineural hearing loss occurs when there is damage to the inner ear, to the nerve that leads from the ear to the brain, or to the brain itself. In this kind of loss, sound waves reach the inner ear, but the brain does not perceive them as sound. This type of hearing loss can be hereditary, can be caused by loud noises or viral infections, or can occur as a side effect of medications.

Sensorineural hearing loss can be differentiated from conductive hearing loss by hearing tests. It is possible for both types of hearing loss to occur together.

Noise Pollution

Prolonged exposure to loud noises is a common cause of hearing loss because of damage to the sensitive cells in the cochlea. People who work around noisy equipment, including construction workers, aircraft personnel, and machine operators, are likely to suffer from this type of hearing loss unless they protect their ears (see Figure 21-14). Repeatedly listening to loud music from a personal stereo set at too high a volume can also damage the ears.

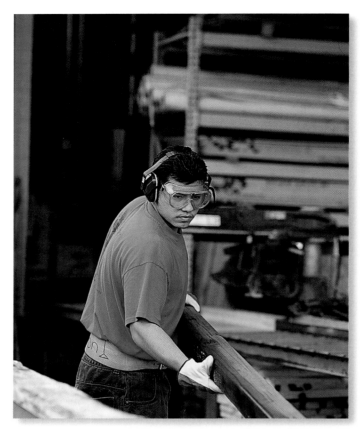

Figure 21-14. Loud noises, such as those produced by a jet engine, can damage hearing unless appropriate ear protectors are worn.

Working With Patients With a Hearing Impairment

You may come in contact with patients of all ages who have hearing impairments. Many patients wear hearing aids to amplify normal speech. Some patients, however, may not admit they have a problem—out of fear, vanity, or misinformation. It is estimated that one-third of patients between the ages of 65 and 74 and one-half of those between the ages of 75 and 79 suffer from some loss of hearing.

To improve communication with a patient whose hearing is impaired, you can do the following:

- Speak at a reasonable volume. Do not shout. Shouting can actually make your words harder to understand. A hearing aid filters out loud sounds, so the patient may not hear everything you say if you shout.
- Speak in clear, low-pitched tones. Elderly patients lose the ability to hear high-pitched sounds first.
- Avoid speaking directly into the patient's ear. Stand 3 to 6 feet away, and face the patient so she can see your lip movements and facial expressions. Avoid covering your mouth with your hands. Speak at a normal rate.
- Avoid overemphasizing your lip movements, which makes lipreading difficult.
- Avoid hand gestures unless they are appropriate.
- If the patient does not understand what you say, restate the message in short, simple sentences. Have the patient repeat the message to verify that your words were understood.
- Treat patients who have a hearing impairment with patience and respect.

Hearing and Diagnostic Tests

Various tests are performed to find out whether a person hears normally. If the tests reveal a problem, follow-up tests are performed to determine the cause of the problem.

Hearing Tests

As part of a general examination, physicians may perform a simple hearing test with one or more tuning forks. Physicians use the tuning forks to determine whether there is a

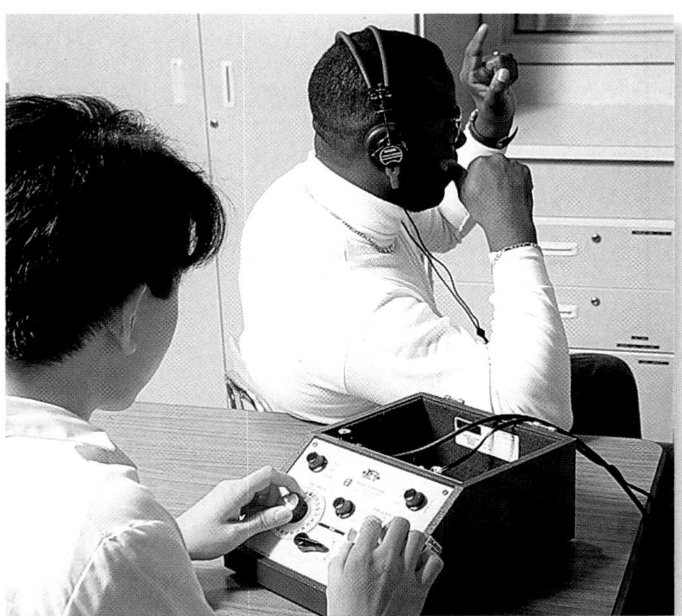

Figure 21-15. An audiometer is used to test hearing.

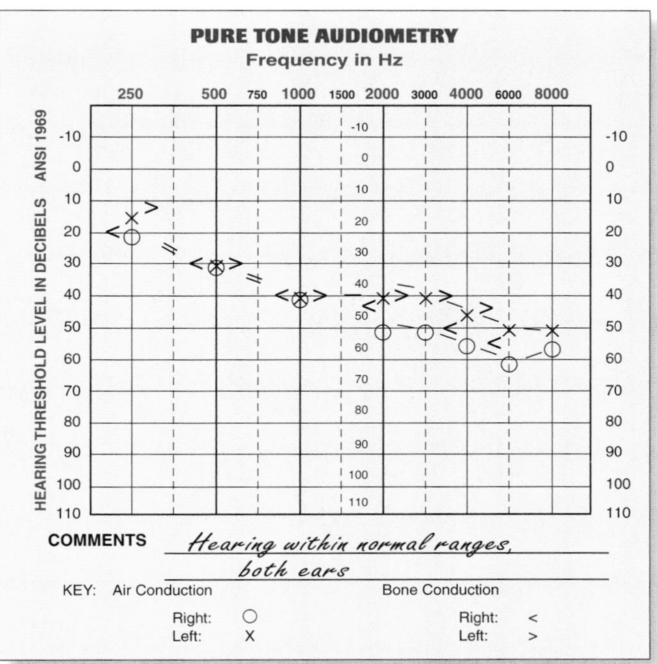

Figure 21-16. The results of an audiometer test are displayed on a graph that indicates the response of each ear to various sounds conducted through air and bone.

hearing loss. Tuning forks can also be helpful in differentiating conductive from sensorineural hearing loss.

If you have the necessary training, you may help perform a test that uses an audiometer, as shown in Figure 21-15. An **audiometer** is an electronic device that measures hearing acuity by producing sounds in specific frequencies and intensities. A **frequency** is the number of complete fluctuations of energy per second in the form of waves. Frequency is best described as the pitch of sound. High frequency is high-pitched, and low frequency is low-pitched. The audiometer allows a physician or other health practitioner to test a person's hearing and to determine the nature and extent of a person's hearing loss.

Many types of audiometers are available. Some machines automatically generate the various tones at different **decibels** (units for measuring the relative intensity of sounds on a scale from 0 to 130) and print out the patient's responses. Others must be manually adjusted and the results charted by hand, as shown in Figure 21-16.

During the test the patient wears a headset to hear the sounds produced by the audiometer. Depending on the particular unit, the patient indicates hearing a sound by raising a finger or by pushing a button. In the former case the person administering the test records the response. In the latter case the response may be recorded automatically or by the test giver.

Adults and children who can understand directions and respond appropriately can be screened in this manner. If you work in a pediatrician's office, you may also help check an infant's response to sounds. These tests require special techniques because infants cannot understand directions. The general steps involved in performing hearing tests on different age groups are outlined in Procedure 21-4.

Diagnostic Testing

A diagnostic test called tympanometry measures the eardrum's ability to move and thus gauges pressure in the middle ear. Tympanometry is used to detect diseases and abnormalities of the middle ear.

To perform the test, a small, soft-rubber cuff is placed over the external ear canal, producing an airtight seal. The tympanometer then automatically measures air pressure and prints out a graph of the results.

Treating Ear and Hearing Problems

Some common ear problems that you may encounter in the physician's office include cerumen impaction (a buildup of earwax in the ear canal), rupture of the eardrum, otitis media (inflammation of the middle ear), and otitis externa (inflammation of the outer ear). Physicians use various approaches and techniques with each problem to restore the health of a patient's ears. For a detailed description of the techniques used for patients with otitis media, see the Diseases and Disorders section.

Physicians also employ special techniques and devices to improve patients' hearing and maintain the health of their ears. As a medical assistant, you can provide patients with information on preventive ear-care techniques, as described in the Educating the Patient section.

PROCEDURE 21.4

Measuring Auditory Acuity

Objective: To determine how well a patient hears

OSHA Guidelines

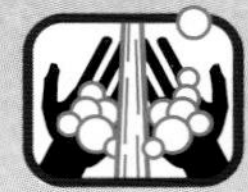

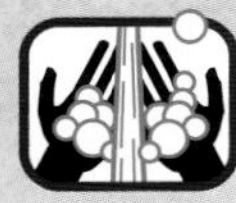

Materials: Audiometer, headset, graph pad (if applicable), alcohol, gauze squares

Method

Adults and Children

1. Wash your hands, identify the patient, introduce yourself, and explain the procedure.
2. Clean the earpieces of the headset with a gauze square dampened with alcohol.
3. Have the patient sit with his back to you.
4. Assist the patient in putting on the headset, and adjust it until it is comfortable.
5. Tell the patient he will hear tones in the right ear.
6. Tell the patient to raise his finger or press the indicator button when he hears a tone.
7. Set the audiometer for the right ear.
8. Set the audiometer for the lowest range of frequencies and the first degree of loudness (usually 15 decibels). (When using automated audiometers, follow the instructions printed in the user's manual.)
9. Press the tone button or switch and observe the patient.
10. If the patient does not hear the first degree of loudness, raise it two or three times to greater degrees, up to 50 or 60 decibels.
11. If the patient indicates that he has heard the tone, record the setting on the graph.
12. Change the setting to the next frequency. Repeat steps 9, 10, and 11.
13. Proceed to the mid-range frequencies. Repeat steps 9, 10, and 11.
14. Proceed to the high-range frequencies. Repeat steps 9, 10, and 11.
15. Set the audiometer for the left ear.
16. Tell the patient that he will hear tones in the left ear, and ask him to raise his finger or press the indicator button when he hears a tone.
17. Repeat steps 8 through 14.
18. Set the audiometer for both ears.
19. Ask the patient to listen with both ears and to raise his finger or press the indicator button when he hears a tone.
20. Repeat steps 8 through 14.
21. Have the patient remove the headset.
22. Clean the earpieces with a gauze square dampened with alcohol.
23. Properly dispose of the used gauze square and wash your hands.

Infants and Toddlers

1. Identify the patient and introduce yourself.
2. Wash your hands.
3. Pick a quiet location.
4. The patient can be sitting, lying down, or held by the parent.
5. Instruct the parent to be silent during the procedure.
6. Position yourself so your hands are behind the child's right ear and out of sight.
7. Clap your hands loudly. Observe the child's response. (Never clap directly in front of the ear because this can damage the eardrum. As an alternative to clapping, use special devices, such as rattles or clickers, that may be available in the office to generate sounds of varying loudness.)
8. Record the child's response as positive or negative for loud noise.
9. Position one hand behind the child's right ear, as before.
10. Snap your fingers. Observe the child's response.
11. Record the response as positive or negative for moderate noise.
12. Repeat steps 6 through 11 for the left ear.

Ear Medications and Irrigation

Part of your job may be to administer ear medications to patients. You may also teach patients how to administer ear medications at home. The proper procedure for administering eardrops is described in Procedure 21-5.

Irrigating the ear may relieve inflammation or irritation of the ear canal and may help loosen and remove impacted cerumen (earwax) or a foreign body. This procedure is performed in the physician's office. The steps used to irrigate the ear are described in Procedure 21-6.

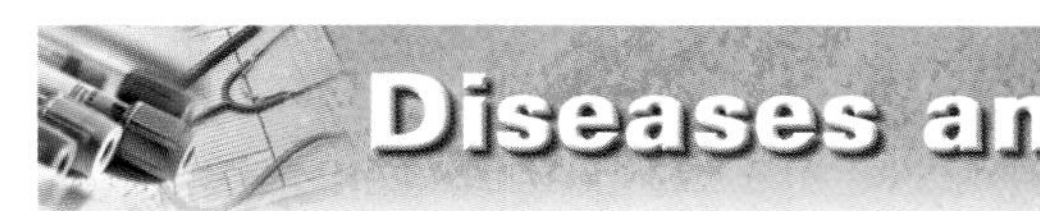

Diseases and Disorders

Otitis Media: The Common Ear Infection

Otitis media, commonly referred to as an ear infection, affects almost all children by age 6. This inflammation of the middle ear accounts for 24.5 million doctor visits each year—second only to upper respiratory infections.

Ear infections typically start when fluid becomes trapped in the middle ear. The lining of the middle ear and eustachian tube is blanketed with a layer of fluid similar to that found in the nose. The normal flow of this fluid from the ear into the back of the nose helps keep the middle ear and the eustachian tube free of bacteria. When a child gets a cold or flu, the lining of the eustachian tube and middle ear can become inflamed and can trap the fluid. The child can develop one of the following four types of otitis media.

1. Acute otitis media typically refers to a bacterial infection of the middle ear that comes on suddenly. This type is common in children and typically follows an upper respiratory tract infection. The symptoms include pain, a feeling of fullness in the ear, some loss of hearing, and possible fever. In severe cases the eardrum may rupture because of the fluid pressure. Acute infections are usually treated with oral antibiotics. If not treated, this type of otitis media can cause permanent hearing loss.
2. Recurrent otitis media is diagnosed when a child contracts acute otitis media again and again, perhaps once or twice every month.
3. Otitis media with effusion, also known as OME, involves an accumulation of fluid in the middle ear. Children with OME do not exhibit any symptoms, and they may not experience any discomfort.
4. Chronic otitis media is diagnosed when fluid is present in the ear and fails to clear up after 3 months or more. Infection may or may not be present. Without treatment the undrained fluid thickens, resulting in possible changes in the shape of the eardrum. These changes may cause temporary hearing loss. Antibiotics and reconstructive surgery may be used to treat chronic otitis media.

If a child suffers from recurrent or chronic otitis media, myringotomy, or the surgical insertion of tubes, may be recommended to keep the fluid draining continuously. This procedure usually removes enough fluid so the infection clears up. Depending on the type of tube, it falls out on its own within 3 to 18 months of insertion.

Ear infections may be difficult to identify, especially in a young child who cannot talk. The following symptoms may be indications of a possible ear infection, particularly if more than one is present:

- Tugging or rubbing the ear
- Fever ranging from 100° to 104°F
- Difficulty balancing
- Excessive crankiness
- Difficulty hearing or speaking
- An unwillingness to lie down (The pain may become more severe in a reclining position because of increased pressure against the eardrum.)

Hearing Aids

Hearing aids may be worn inside or outside the ear. If worn outside, they may be located behind the ear, mounted on eyeglasses, or worn on the body. Hearing aids consist of the following parts:

- A tiny microphone to pick up sounds
- An amplifier to increase the volume of sounds
- A tiny speaker to transmit sounds to the ear

You may need to teach patients how to obtain a hearing aid. You can also pass along tips to patients to help them take proper care of their hearing aids and to troubleshoot problems.

Obtaining a Hearing Aid. A patient with signs of hearing loss should be referred to an **otologist,** a medical doctor specializing in the health of the ear, or an **audiologist,** a specialist who focuses on evaluating and correcting hearing problems. Audiologists are not medical doctors and do not treat diseases of the ear. Instead, they evaluate the patient's hearing, fit hearing aids, give instruction in the use of hearing aids, and provide service for hearing aids if necessary. It is important for hearing aids to fit properly. If they do not, sounds may not be transmitted well into the ear.

Care and Use of Hearing Aids. Hearing aids run on batteries that typically last about 2 weeks. Therefore, the patient must keep a fresh supply of batteries on hand. The hearing aid itself must be routinely cleaned, or the microphone, switches, or dials may not work properly. Moisture can damage the aid, so it must not get wet. Hair sprays can clog hearing aid openings or interfere with the operation of moving parts. For these reasons spray should

Educating the Patient

Preventive Ear-Care Tips

You can help patients protect their ears and take care of their hearing by providing them with guidelines to follow. As with any patient education, go over items slowly, ask patients whether they have questions before moving on, and answer questions completely. Ear-care tips include the following.

1. Get routine hearing examinations. Screening for hearing problems is often part of a comprehensive physical examination. Encourage patients who have not had their hearing screened or who suspect they have hearing problems to arrange for testing by their doctor. Older patients, who may not admit they have a problem, may need special encouragement.
2. Avoid injury when cleaning the ears. Instruct patients in proper ear care. Point out that they should not put objects in the ear that might injure the eardrum or ear canal.
3. Avoid injury from nonprescription ear-care products. Tell patients to check with a doctor before using nonprescription products for softening earwax.
4. Use proper ear protection. Urge patients to wear ear protectors around loud work equipment and to avoid listening to loud music. It is especially important to keep the volume at a reasonable level when listening through earphones.
5. Use all medications properly. Show patients how to use eardrops; emphasize that they must follow instructions precisely. Explain to patients that following instructions applies to all medications because many, including aspirin and some antibiotics, may cause hearing loss if used improperly.
6. Be alert for warning signs. Tell patients to call their doctor immediately if they experience any of these signs of ear problems:
   - Ear pain
   - Stuffiness
   - Discharge from the ear
   - Vertigo (dizziness)

   Also have patients notify the doctor if they have any of these signs of hearing problems:
   - Tinnitus (ringing)
   - Hearing others' speech as mumbled sounds
   - Speaking in a very loud voice without being aware of it

PROCEDURE 21.5

Administering Eardrops

Objective: To instill medication into the ear to treat certain ear disorders

OSHA Guidelines

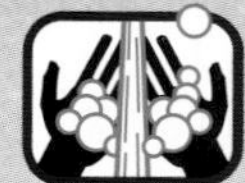 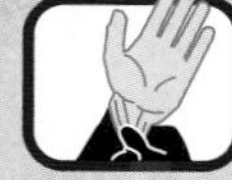 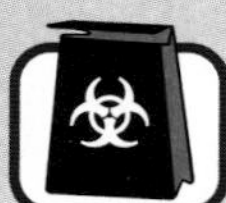 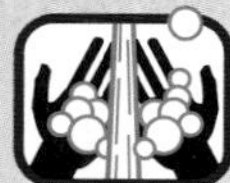

Materials: Liquid medication, cotton balls

Method

1. Identify the patient, introduce yourself, and explain the procedure.
2. Check the physician's medication order. It should include the patient's name, drug name, concentration, number of drops, into which ear(s) the medication is to be administered, and the frequency of administration.
3. Compare the drug with the instructions three times.
4. Ask whether the patient has any allergies to ear medications.
5. Wash your hands and put on gloves.
6. Assemble supplies.
7. If the medication is cold, warm it to room temperature with your hands or by placing the bottle in a pan of warm water. *Warning:* Internal ear structures are very sensitive to extreme heat or cold. Administration of cold medications can result in vertigo (dizziness) or nausea.
8. Have the patient lie on the side with the ear to be treated facing up.
9. Straighten the ear canal by pulling the auricle upward and outward for adults (Figure 21-17),

continued ⟶

PROCEDURE 21.5

Administering Eardrops *(continued)*

down and back for infants and children (Figure 21-18).

10. Hold the dropper ½ inch above the ear canal.
11. Gently squeeze the bottle or dropper bulb to administer the correct number of drops (Figure 21-19).
12. Have the patient remain in this position for 10 minutes.
13. If ordered, loosely place a small wad of cotton in the outermost part of the ear canal.
14. Note any adverse reaction, notifying the physician as necessary.
15. Repeat the procedure for the other ear if ordered.
16. Instruct the patient on how to administer the drops at home.
17. Ask the patient to repeat the instructions.
18. Provide written instructions.
19. Remove the cotton after 15 minutes.
20. Properly dispose of used disposable materials.
21. Remove gloves and wash your hands.
22. Record in the patient's chart the medication, concentration, number of drops, time of administration, and which ear(s) received the medication.

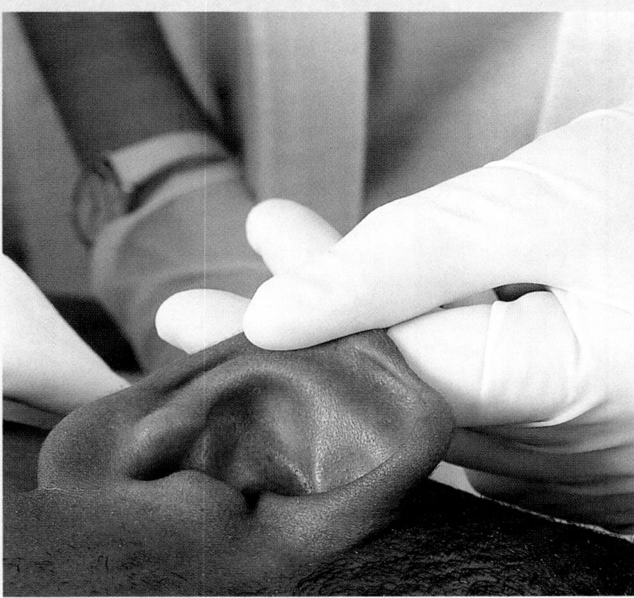

Figure 21-17. Straighten an adult's ear canal by pulling the auricle upward and outward.

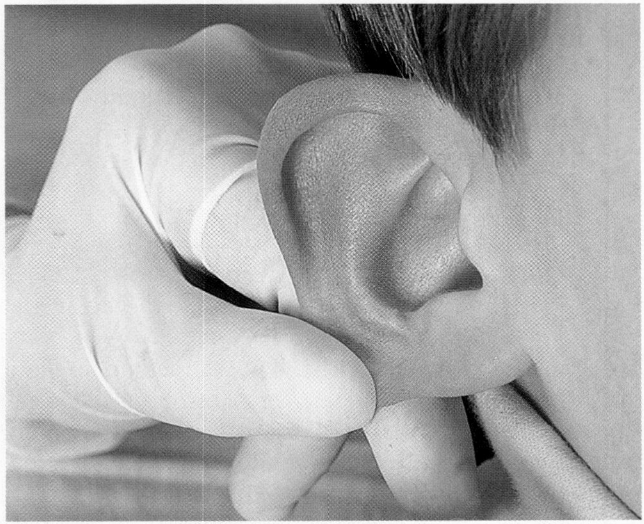

Figure 21-18. Straighten an infant's or a child's ear canal by pulling the auricle downward and back.

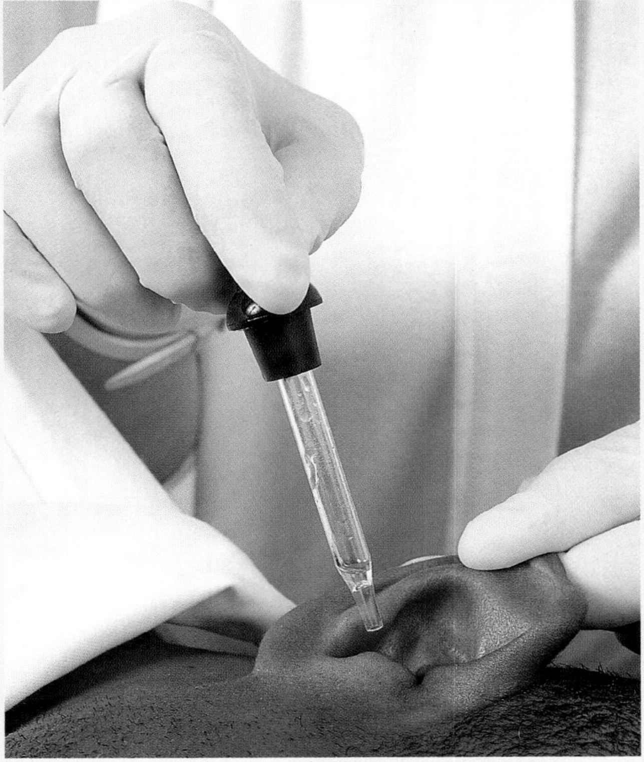

Figure 21-19. Apply slow, gentle pressure to the dropper bulb so you can count the drops and administer the prescribed number.

PROCEDURE 21.6

Performing Ear Irrigation

Objective: To wash out the ear canal to remove impacted cerumen, relieve inflammation, or remove a foreign body

OSHA Guidelines

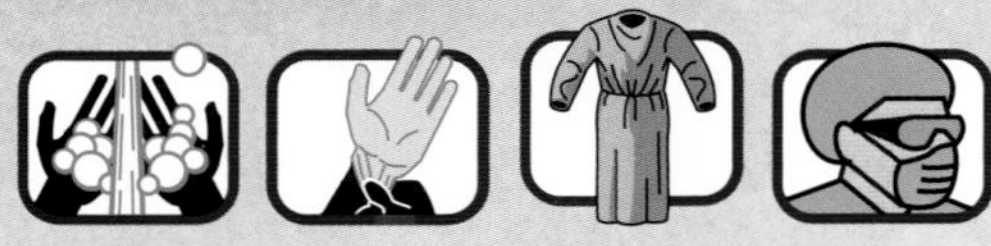

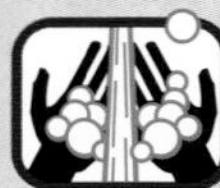
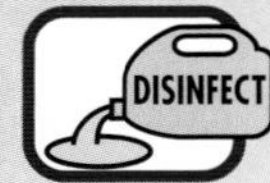

Materials: Fresh irrigating solution, clean basin, clean irrigating syringe, towel or absorbent pad, kidney-shaped basin, cotton balls

Method

1. Identify the patient, introduce yourself, and explain the procedure.
2. Check the doctor's order. It should include the patient's name, irrigating solution, volume of solution, and for which ear(s) the irrigation is to be performed. If the doctor has not specified the volume of solution, use the amount needed to remove the wax.
3. Compare the solution with the instructions three times.
4. Wash your hands and put on gloves, a gown, and a face shield (splashing is possible when a syringe is used).
5. Look into the patient's ear if cerumen or a foreign body needs to be removed so you will know when you have completed the irrigation.
6. Assemble the supplies.
7. If the solution is cold, warm it to room temperature by placing the bottle in a pan of warm water. *Warning:* Internal ear structures are very sensitive to extreme heat or cold. Administration of cold liquids can result in vertigo or nausea.
8. Have the patient sit or lie on her back with the ear to be treated facing you.
9. Place a towel over the patient's shoulder (or under the head and shoulder if she is lying down), and have her hold the kidney-shaped basin under her ear.
10. Pour the solution into the other basin.
11. If necessary, gently clean the external ear with cotton moistened with the solution.
12. Fill the irrigating syringe with solution (approximately 50 mL).
13. Straighten the ear canal by pulling the auricle upward and outward for adults, down and back for infants and children.
14. Holding the tip of the syringe ½ inch above the opening of the ear, slowly instill the solution into the ear. Allow the fluid to drain out during the process.
15. Refill the syringe and continue irrigation until the canal is cleaned or the solution is used up.
16. Dry the external ear with a cotton ball, and leave a clean cotton ball loosely in place for 5 to 10 minutes.
17. If the patient becomes dizzy or nauseated, allow her time to regain balance before standing up. Then assist her as needed.
18. Properly dispose of used disposable materials.
19. Remove gloves, gown, and face shield, and wash your hands.
20. Record in the patient's chart the procedure and result, amount of solution used, time of administration, and ear(s) irrigated.
21. Put on gloves and clean the equipment and room according to OSHA guidelines.

be applied before a hearing aid is inserted. Cerumen often builds up behind hearing aids that are worn in the ear. Wax buildup reduces sound transmission. If buildup occurs, the earwax plug can be removed by ear irrigation.

Other Devices and Strategies

People whose hearing cannot be substantially improved by hearing aids may need to use other devices or strategies to overcome the problem. These devices include appliances that light up as well as ring, such as telephones, doorbells, smoke detectors, alarm clocks, and burglar alarms. Patients can purchase amplifiers for the telephone, television set, and radio. Many closed-captioned television programs are also available. To benefit from closed captioning, the patient must have a television set with a decoder that translates the captioning and displays the captions on the screen.

Summary

You can help prevent, detect, and treat eye and ear problems in your work as a medical assistant. Because conditions that affect the eyes and ears can have an impact on vision, hearing, and balance, these conditions affect a patient's quality of life. Vision and hearing provide people with information about the world around them; balance allows people to move securely and effectively through their environment.

A basic understanding of the anatomy and physiology of the eyes and ears will help you provide good eye and ear care to patients. You must also become familiar with many health, medication, safety, and hygiene concerns to teach patients to care for their own eyes and ears properly. Take time to comprehend and master the various tests of vision and hearing so you can provide accurate information to the physician about each patient's performance on each test.

Be sensitive to the needs of individual patients as you care for their eyes and ears. Learn all you can about how to meet the special needs of children, elderly patients, and patients with conditions that make preventing, detecting, and treating eye and ear problems a challenge. Practice the administration of eye and ear medications until it becomes second nature to provide the prescribed treatment calmly, accurately, and with the least discomfort to the patient.

The more knowledgeable and proficient you become, the better the eye and ear care you will provide. Knowing just what you are doing and why will make your assistance to the patient and the physician a valuable asset to the office.

REVIEW

CHAPTER 21

CASE STUDY QUESTIONS

Now that you have completed this chapter, review the case study at the beginning of the chapter and answer the following questions:

1. What is cerumen?
2. Why is it important to use room-temperature water when irrigating a patient's ear?
3. What other factors might contribute to the patient's hearing loss?
4. Why is it important to test the patient's hearing after cerumen removal?
5. What device is used to perform a hearing test?

Discussion Questions

1. How can you help elderly patients cope with the changes that occur in the eyes and ears as a result of aging?
2. Which common warning signs of eye problems and of ear problems might people tend to ignore and why?
3. Discuss the difference between sensorineural and conductive hearing loss, and give an example of how each might be caused.

Critical Thinking Questions

1. What questions might you ask as you interview an 80-year-old patient who comes to the office for an eye examination?
2. What questions might you ask as you interview a patient who comes into the office complaining of poor hearing?
3. What questions would you ask, in order, of a patient who comes into the office complaining that her hearing aid does not seem to be working properly?

Application Activities

1. Research a procedure, such as radial keratotomy, used to help restore people's vision. Present an oral report to the class in which you describe the procedure, its results, and the characteristics of good candidates for the procedure.
2. Practice conducting vision tests with your classmates.
3. Shop around for a hearing aid. Find out how much aids cost, what sizes are available, the cost of a fitting, and how to change batteries and clean a hearing aid properly. Present your findings in a written report. Remark on the service you received and whether you would recommend the place or places where you shopped.

SECTION 4

SPECIALTY PRACTICES AND MEDICAL EMERGENCIES

CHAPTER 22

Assisting With Examinations in the Basic Specialties

KEY TERMS

acute
arterial blood gases
chronic
colposcopy
embolism
fixative
medical practice act
puberty
speculum

AREAS OF COMPETENCE

2003 Role Delineation Study

CLINICAL

Fundamental Principles

- Apply principles of aseptic technique and infection control

Patient Care

- Obtain patient history and vital signs
- Prepare patient for examinations, procedures, and treatments
- Assist with examinations, procedures, and treatments

GENERAL

Communication Skills

- Recognize and respect cultural diversity
- Adapt communications to individual's ability to understand

Legal Concepts

- Perform within legal and ethical boundaries

Instruction

- Instruct individuals according to their needs
- Teach methods of health promotion and disease prevention

CHAPTER OUTLINE

- The Medical Assistant's Role in Specialty Examinations
- Internal Medicine
- Pediatrics
- Obstetrics and Gynecology

OBJECTIVES

After completing Chapter 22, you will be able to:

22.1 Briefly describe the medical specialties of internal medicine, pediatrics, and obstetrics and gynecology.

22.2 Describe the types of examinations and diagnostic tests performed in each of these specialties and the medical assistant's role in them.

OBJECTIVES *(Continued)*

22.3 List and describe some common diseases and disorders seen in these medical specialties and typical treatments for them.

22.4 Explain the medical assistant's duties in assessing for chronic fatigue syndrome.

22.5 Identify common signs of domestic violence and child abuse.

22.6 Describe the medical assistant's responsibilities in performing a scoliosis examination.

22.7 Describe the medical assistant's role in assisting with a cervical biopsy.

Introduction

Specialty examinations are usually performed by specialists. Specialists are physicians, such as pediatricians and gynecologists, who have taken additional training beyond medical school and their required residencies to become board-certified in their respective specialties. Physicians who wish to become board-certified must pass rigorous examinations in their chosen specialty and be elected by the board for that specialty.

As a medical assistant, you may be employed to assist with examinations in the basic specialties. This chapter introduces you to the basic specialties of internal medicine, pediatrics, and obstetrics and gynecology. You will learn about the types of examinations and diagnostic tests used in these specialties and about the common diseases and disorders seen in these specialities. You will also learn to watch for the signs of domestic violence and child abuse.

CASE STUDY

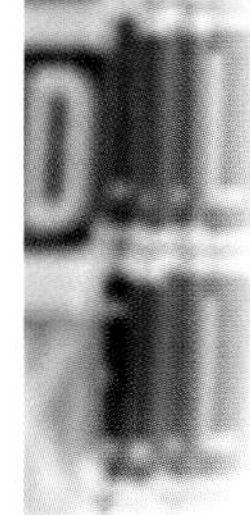

After working for a year in the office of a general practice physician, you want a chance to increase your knowledge and skills. There are three opportunities available to you: an internal medicine practice, a pediatrician's office, and an obstetrics and gynecology clinic. Because you are looking for change, you must first learn about the types of patients and procedures you might encounter in these facilities.

As you read this chapter, consider the following questions:

1. What kind of patients would you see in each of these offices?
2. What additional duties and procedures would you perform?

The Medical Assistant's Role in Specialty Examinations

Different and additional duties may be required of the medical assistant working in basic specialties. These duties and procedures are based on your education, training, and certification. They are also based on your state's medical practice act. A **medical practice act** is a law that defines the exact duties that physicians and other health-care personnel may perform. It determines the ways that you can assist in examinations, procedures, and diagnostic tests. It also determines which of these tasks you can perform alone. For example, many states have acts that give physicians the right to delegate certain clinical procedures to medical assistants and other qualified health professionals. A medical assistant is allowed to perform clinical procedures only under the supervision of the physician or other licensed health-care professional who is granted the right and who delegates the specific clinical procedures to the medical assistant. Because state laws vary, you will need to know the scope of practice for medical assistants in the state where you work.

If you work for a specialist, she may have her own rules regarding examinations, procedures, and diagnostic tests with which she permits assistance. The physician may want to perform some procedures alone, with only minimal assistance from you. She may need more assistance with other procedures. She may ask you to perform some procedures on your own.

You must have a thorough understanding of basic anatomy and physiology of various body systems (see Chapters 5–17) to perform procedures alone and to communicate effectively with patients. You must also be familiar with the specific examinations and steps for the procedures in the specialty in which you are employed. Acquiring this knowledge will help you become a valuable member of your practice.

Providing Emotional Support

You will often deal with a variety of diseases and disorders in a specialty setting. Patients' illnesses may be acute, chronic, or both. **Acute** means that a disease's onset and progress is rapid, as in acute appendicitis. An illness that lasts a long time or recurs frequently is referred to as **chronic,** such as chronic osteoarthritis. Patients may have strong reactions to acute or chronic illness, including fear, defensive behavior, and frustration with physical limitations. Your empathy and support will help patients identify and cope with their feelings and behaviors.

Providing Patient Education

Patients do not generally visit specialists as frequently as they do a general practitioner, and they may have more questions than during a general physical examination. Consequently, communicating effectively with patients and providing educational materials will be one of your primary responsibilities. You will explain the functioning of the appropriate body system and the purpose of and preparation for specific examination procedures and tests. You will also teach patients how to perform prescribed home-care regimens. Remember that just giving patients a brochure may not be enough. Make sure the patient knows what is necessary and has an opportunity to ask questions. Sometimes you can ask patients to tell you what they already know before you begin your patient education.

Internal Medicine

Internal medicine is the specialty of an internist, who diagnoses and treats disorders and diseases of the body's internal organs. The internist is often the first doctor to see a patient with a complaint. Internists treat medical problems with medicine, either alone or in combination with other modalities (therapeutic agents). In some cases an internist refers the patient to a doctor in one of the internal medicine subspecialties.

Assisting With the Physical Examination

An internist's physical examination is usually conducted in the same way as is the general physical examination described in Chapter 20. As you gather information and prepare a patient for a physical examination, you may be expected to assess for chronic fatigue syndrome. You may also use this opportunity to detect possible substance abuse, domestic violence, or elder abuse. These topics were introduced in Chapter 18.

Assessing for Chronic Fatigue Syndrome. Chronic fatigue syndrome (CFS) is an accumulation of at least four or more of the following symptoms:

- Impairment in short-term memory or concentration
- Sore throat
- Tender lymph nodes
- Muscle pain
- Multijoint pain without swelling or redness
- Headaches of a new type, pattern, or severity
- Unrefreshing sleep
- Postexertional malaise lasting more than 24 hours

There is no test for CFS, so physicians diagnose it by ruling out other diseases with similar symptoms, such as acquired immunodeficiency syndrome (AIDS), thyroid problems, anemia, and hepatitis. When diagnosing CFS, the physician must realize that fatigue caused by stress or depression is one of the most common reasons for a patient's visit.

Symptoms of CFS can begin suddenly but may continue for 3 to 4 years. The cause of CFS is unknown. However, it may be triggered by viral infections, transient traumatic conditions, stress, or toxins. Patients with CFS are treated for the symptoms as needed. Treatments may include physical activity, education, antidepressants, nonsteroidal anti-inflammatory agents such as naproxen (Aleve) or ibuprofen (Motrin), antimicrobials, and dietary supplements.

Because you check vital signs, take history, and chart, you are in a position to notice the symptoms for this disorder. Procedure 22-1 explains how to assess for CFS.

Detecting Substance Abuse. You should be alert for signs of substance abuse when you assist with an examination. Signs of substance abuse vary, depending on the type of drug and the individual's response to it. In general, signs you can observe are as follows:

- Alcohol: depressed pulse rate, respiration, and blood pressure; slurred speech; odor of alcohol on breath; reduced coordination and reflexes; poor vision and depth perception
- Cocaine and amphetamines: excitation, increased pulse rate and blood pressure, increased respiration and body temperature, dilated pupils, loss of appetite
- Hallucinogens such as LSD and angel dust: hallucinations, poor perception of time and distance, severe panic, violent and bizarre behavior
- Inhalants such as nitrous oxide and household solvents: muscle weakness, hearing loss, changes in heart rate, nausea, dizziness
- Marijuana: reddening of the eyes, increased heart rate, heightened appetite, muscular weakness
- Narcotics such as codeine and morphine: drowsiness, depressed respiration, constricted pupils, nausea, vomiting, constipation
- Sedatives such as barbiturates: nausea, slurred speech, drunken behavior without odor of alcohol

If you see any of these signs of substance abuse in a patient, inform the physician. Also inform the physician if you find such indications in someone who works in your office. If your state requires reporting suspected substance abuse by health-care workers, be sure you know the procedure for doing so.

PROCEDURE 22.1

Performing an Assessment for Chronic Fatigue Syndrome

Objective: To assess a patient for possible chronic fatigue syndrome

OSHA Guidelines: This procedure does not involve exposure to blood, body fluids, or tissues.

Materials: Patient chart, pen

Method

When a patient makes an office visit for fatigue, be alert to the possibility that the patient may have chronic fatigue syndrome. You can give a more accurate report to the physician if you work from a checklist of symptoms.

1. Identify the patient and introduce yourself.
2. Question the patient (Figure 22-1) about the following:
   - Persistent, overwhelming fatigue (that does not go away even with rest) for at least 6 months
   - Lingering fatigue after levels of exercise that would normally be easily tolerated
   - Frequent headaches
   - Sore throat and swollen lymph nodes in neck or armpits
   - Low-grade fever
   - Unexplainable muscle weakness or pains
   - Pain in joints without swelling
   - Forgetfulness or confusion
   - Irritability

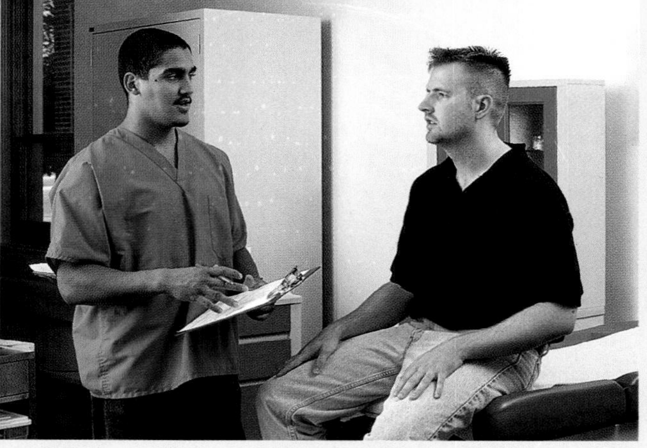

Figure 22-1. During the patient interview you can use your interviewing skills to help determine whether CFS may be the cause of fatigue.

   - Depression
   - Sensitivity to light
   - Impaired vision
   - Sleep disturbances
   - Inability to concentrate or perform mental tasks such as arithmetic
   - Numbness or tingling sensations
3. Document any of these symptoms in the patient's chart, and report them to the internist, who will follow up with appropriate diagnostic tests.

Detecting Domestic Violence. During a physical examination, you and the internist are in a position to detect signs of domestic violence. It is crucial that you bring to the doctor's attention any clues you notice during the initial interview. The doctor can then use your observations to examine and question the patient for possible internal injuries. See the Caution: Handle With Care section for guidelines on dealing with this issue.

Detecting Elder Abuse. It is difficult to detect elder abuse. There is no uniform and comprehensive definition of this type of abuse, and bruises from falls and other accidents can be mistaken for abuse. Also, the signs of neglect can be similar to the signs of some chronic medical conditions.

There are three basic categories of elder abuse: domestic elder abuse, institutional elder abuse, and self-neglect, or self-abuse. Elders can be abused physically, sexually, or psychologically. Elders may also be neglected, abandoned, or exploited materially or financially. Elders may even choose to neglect or abuse themselves. More than one type of abuse can occur simultaneously. Elder abuse occurs in all racial, socioeconomic, and religious groups. However, most victims are older women with chronic illness or disabilities. Risk factors or situations that increase the possibility of elder abuse include

- History of alcoholism, drug abuse, or violence in the family
- History of mental illness in the abuser or victim
- Isolation of the victim from family members and friends other than the abuser
- Recent stressful events affecting the abuser or victim

You can assist the doctor by taking a careful history. Ask the patient about living arrangements, social contact,

CAUTION *Handle With Care*

Domestic Violence Detection

Physicians and medical assistants are in a position to detect signs of domestic violence. These signs can be seen in unusual bruising or injuries that the patient may try to hide or excuse. You may hear signs in a patient's tone of voice or choice of words during a conversation in the office or over the telephone. Many times patients who are abused blame themselves.

You play an important role in noticing these signs, and you must inform the physician of any signs that you detect. You must also create a supportive office environment where the patient can seek help. Encourage the physician to join the American Medical Association's National Coalition of Physicians Against Family Violence, if she is not already a member. This organization provides posters—which often help patients feel encouraged to discuss domestic violence—in addition to pamphlets and other information.

Reporting suspected domestic violence is mandatory in some states. You should have a folder that contains lists of the phone numbers for domestic violence hotlines, women's shelters, and other helpful resources. You can offer the following general guidelines to women.

- Ignoring the problem never works—silence does not help anyone.
- Understand that abusive family members may not be able to help themselves.
- Call for help if a physical threat exists.

and emotional stress. Try to note the interaction between caregiver and patient. If you suspect abuse, inform the doctor. He will then be able to direct the physical examination toward possible internal injuries, malnutrition, or lack of cognitive ability. Signs of neglect include the following:

- Foul odor from the patient's body
- Poor skin color
- Inappropriate clothing for the season
- Soiled clothing
- Extreme concern about money

You can increase your awareness by consulting the guidelines for diagnosis and treatment of elder abuse and neglect published by the American Medical Association (AMA). Most states require doctors who suspect elder abuse or neglect to report their concerns to a designated office. Early intervention usually results in better living arrangements for both the patient and the caregiver.

Diagnostic Testing

Based on a patient's physical examination, an internist may order a number of diagnostic tests. As a medical assistant in an internist's office, you must be familiar with commonly ordered tests. They include urine and blood tests, radiologic tests, bacterial cultures, electrocardiograms (ECGs), and pulmonary function tests, all of which are discussed in later chapters. Descriptions of a few specific diagnostic tests follow.

Measurement of Arterial Blood Gases. The internist may order measurement of **arterial blood gases** to determine the exchange of oxygen and carbon dioxide in the lungs and to monitor blood chemistry. Blood is drawn from an artery (instead of a vein) for this test, which is usually performed by a respiratory therapist. The oxygen measurement for arterial blood (partial pressure of oxygen) indicates how well the lungs are providing oxygen to body tissues. The carbon dioxide measurement for arterial blood (partial pressure of carbon dioxide) evaluates how well the lungs are eliminating carbon dioxide. These measurements help the physician diagnose and monitor conditions such as central nervous system (CNS) depression, pulmonary disorders, and kidney diseases.

Radiologic Tests. The physician orders a radiologic test to confirm or rule out a diagnosis. The choice of radiologic procedure depends on the suspected problem. Internists order plain films (roentgenograms or x-rays), computed tomography (CT) scans, magnetic resonance imaging (MRI), ultrasound, and radionuclide imaging (also known as nuclear imaging). Radiologic procedures are discussed in detail in Chapter 35.

Although you will not perform radiologic procedures, the physician will expect you to set up appointments and explain procedures to the patient. You may need to explain what kinds of preparations the patient must make prior to the test. Be sure to ask the radiologic facility about the requirements for the specific type of test.

Chest X-Ray. Internists may order a chest x-ray, which can reveal respiratory and cardiac disorders such as pneumonia, tuberculosis, or cardiomegaly (enlarged heart). It may also reveal abnormal masses in the upper thoracic region.

Venography and Venous Ultrasonography. Venography and venous ultrasonography are tests used to rule out deep-vein thrombosis (DVT). A patient has DVT when there is a thrombus, or blood clot, in the veins. If the thrombus becomes dislodged and travels in the bloodstream, it is known as an embolus. This moving blood clot can obstruct a blood vessel, causing an **embolism.** An embolism can be fatal, depending on its location. Risk factors for DVTs are poor circulation, vein injury, prolonged bed rest, recent surgery or childbirth, irregular blood coagulation, and use of oral contraceptives.

For a venogram, a contrast medium is injected into a vein, and x-rays are taken of the veins. Venous ultrasonography uses inaudible sound waves that bounce off liquid (in this case, blood) to form a two-dimensional image. Internists generally prefer venous ultrasonography to venography because it is noninvasive.

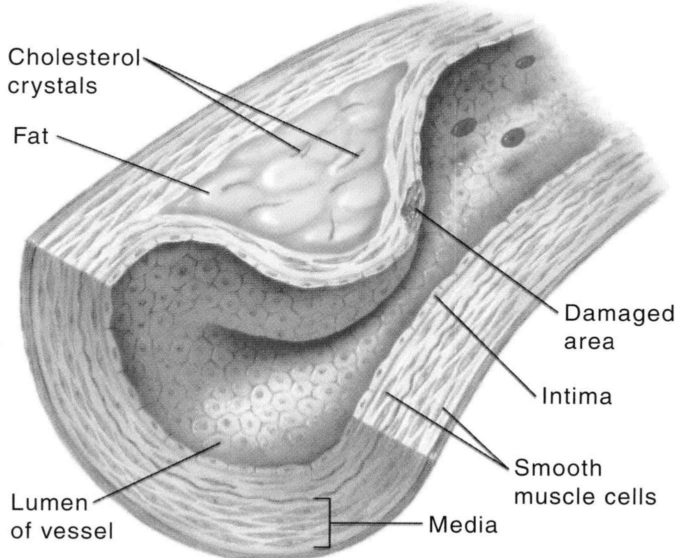

Figure 22-2. High cholesterol can lead to atherosclerosis. Help patients reduce their cholesterol through proper diet and exercise, along with medication, if prescribed.

Source: McGraw-Hill's Digital Asset Library.

Diseases and Disorders

Internists treat a variety of diseases and disorders. Some of the most common include diseases of aging, infectious diseases, and sexually transmitted diseases.

Diseases of Aging. The elderly constitute a large percentage of patients in an internal medicine practice. Many of the serious disorders frequently seen in the elderly are discussed in Chapter 23. They include hypertension, coronary artery disease, and diabetes mellitus. Other disorders, such as constipation, diarrhea, and osteoporosis—while not serious for young and middle-aged adults—can create major problems for the elderly.

Constipation-Diarrhea Cycle. The cycle of constipation followed by diarrhea occurs when people's diets lack the fiber and liquids to maintain healthy bowel function and they use harsh laxatives to treat their constipation. The patient then complains of diarrhea and asks for antidiarrheal medication, which in turn causes constipation again. Encourage elderly patients to eat more high-fiber foods, such as cereals, fruits, and vegetables, and to increase their fluid intake.

Hyperlipidemia. Hyperlipidemia is a condition in which cholesterol levels are above normal. It is not just a disease of the elderly, but it can cause serious problems for older people. High cholesterol levels can lead to atherosclerosis, the accumulation of fatty deposits along the inner walls of arteries (Figure 22-2). These deposits, along with other substances in the blood, can form an atherosclerotic plaque. This plaque can narrow the opening in an artery to the point of obstructing blood flow. Atherosclerosis is a primary cause of cardiovascular disease, including stroke.

Your role as a patient educator is vital to helping people with high cholesterol levels. Take every opportunity to teach patients about eating foods with lower amounts of cholesterol (see Chapter 31). Provide patients with printed materials on cholesterol, available from the AMA and other sources. The doctor may also prescribe medication to lower cholesterol in patients when diet modification and exercise are not adequate.

Osteoporosis. Osteoporosis is an endocrine and metabolic disorder of the musculoskeletal system. The condition is prevalent in the elderly and is more common in women than men. It is characterized by hunched-over posture (Figure 22-3). The disorder may be caused by inadequate calcium consumption, estrogen deficiency, or alcoholism. Prevention methods include regular exercise, a diet high in calcium (perhaps including supplemental calcium), and hormone replacement therapy in women who are menopausal or postmenopausal.

Alzheimer's Disease. Alzheimer's disease is a severely debilitating brain disorder. Warning signs include changes in personality, mood, or behavior; recent memory loss and an increase in forgetfulness; decreased ability to perform familiar tasks; difficulty with use of language and abstract thinking; decreased powers of judgment; and disorientation to time or place. Because there is no cure, the primary role of caregivers is to provide comfort and safety to the patient.

Infectious Diseases. An internist is usually the primary physician for treating infectious diseases. Most of the infectious diseases discussed in Chapters 2 and 3 are treated by either an internist or a pediatrician. Descriptions of other common infectious diseases follow.

Infectious Mononucleosis. Infectious mononucleosis (mono) is caused by either the cytomegalovirus (CMV) or the Epstein-Barr virus (EBV). Unexplained fever, fatigue, and sore throat are usually the dominant symptoms. If patients have these symptoms without any apparent cause, the doctor orders blood tests to rule out mononucleosis.

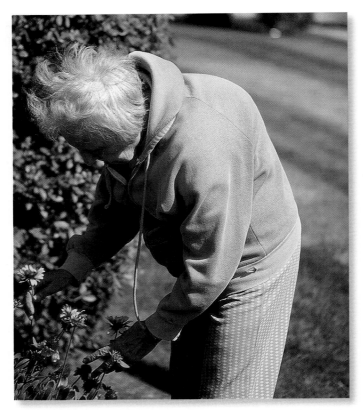

Figure 22-3. Osteoporosis is most prevalent in elderly women.

Other symptoms may include weakness, headache, and swollen lymph nodes. With proper rest, nutrition, and antibiotics to prevent secondary infections, patients usually recover from acute symptoms in 7 to 10 days. Complete recovery may take as long as a month or more. The virus that causes mono is contagious. It is transmitted through the saliva of an infected patient by coughing, sneezing, or kissing. Precautions should be taken to prevent the spread, especially to highly susceptible patients.

Lyme Disease. Lyme disease is a serious infection caused by a spirochete bacterium carried by the deer tick. When the condition is diagnosed early, treatment with antibiotics is effective. Diagnosis is difficult, however, because symptoms can occur in any order or overlap.

The first symptom of Lyme disease is often the appearance of a raised, red dot at the site of the tick bite. A circular rash may surround the bite (Figure 22-4). In many cases, however, the bite goes unnoticed. Headache, fever, and fatigue develop, followed by muscle aches and inflammation of the joints. Left untreated, the disease can progress to arthritis and heart and neurological problems.

When a tick bite is reported, tell the patient to save the tick and place it in a plastic bag. It should be taken to a U.S. Department of Agriculture Extension Office for identification. A tick identified as a deer tick will be tested for the presence of the spirochete bacterium. Even if the tick tests positive for Lyme disease bacteria, the risk of the patient contracting the disease is not great if the tick was removed from the patient within 24 hours. Your main role in dealing with Lyme disease is patient education. Many doctors' offices display pamphlets or posters to show patients how to prevent and recognize symptoms of Lyme disease.

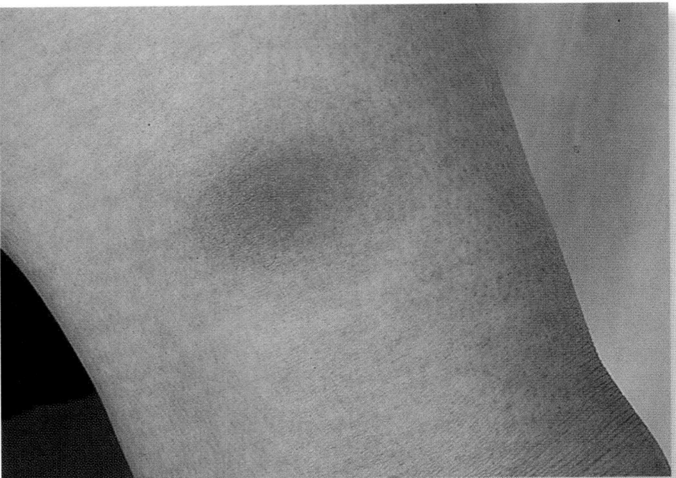

Figure 22-4. A bull's-eye rash is a symptom of the first stage of Lyme disease.

Pneumonia. Pneumonia is an acute infection of the lung tissue caused by bacteria or viruses. It often occurs in conjunction with a chronic weakening illness. Symptoms range from coughing, sputum production, and chest pain to chills and fever. It is treated with bed rest, antibiotics, adequate fluids, respiratory support measures, and pain medication.

Rabies. Rabies is a virus transmitted to humans by a bite from a mammal, such as a dog, rat, or bat. A patient who has been bitten by an animal that may be rabid should receive a rabies vaccination, which is a series of injections. Dogs, cats, and people who are at risk for exposure to the virus should have the vaccination at regular intervals. Patients must be vaccinated during the incubation period, before symptoms appear. Symptoms are nonspecific at onset and include malaise, fatigue, anxiety, or insomnia. Later there are neurological symptoms. After symptoms have occurred, nearly 100% of people who are infected with rabies die.

Staphylococcal and Streptococcal Infections (Staph and Strep). Staphylococci and streptococci are common bacteria, with many species occurring naturally in the body. When the body's resistance is low, however, these bacteria can cause infections, such as strep throat, skin abscess, impetigo, and pneumonia. Antibiotics are the standard treatment for staphylococcal and streptococcal infections. Because these organisms become resistant to antibiotics, however, researchers are constantly working to develop effective new drugs. Always stress to patients the importance of finishing the entire course of prescribed medication. Otherwise the patient will not receive enough of the

Educating the Patient

Teaching Patients About Sexually Transmitted Diseases

You must provide complete and detailed information with a nonjudgmental and supportive attitude when you teach patients about sexually transmitted diseases. Begin with the principle that all STDs are preventable. The key to prevention is avoiding sexual activities in which blood, semen, or vaginal secretions pass from one person to another.

There are various levels of protection in connection with STDs. The only absolute methods of "safe sex" are abstinence (no sex) and masturbation (self-stimulation). The next level is mutual monogamy, in which partners have sex only with each other. Emphasize that monogamy provides protection from STDs only if neither partner has an STD when the relationship begins. A final level of prevention applies to people who do not practice abstinence or mutual monogamy but wish to protect themselves and others from STDs. The following measures provide some protection.

- Use a latex condom and spermicide for every act of intercourse. (Use a latex condom during oral sex.)
- Know all your sexual partners, and discuss STD prevention with them.
- Have a physician regularly screen you for STDs because many people, especially men, have no signs when they are infected.
- Consult a physician if any signs of STDs develop, such as a blister, sore, discharge, rash, or abdominal pain.

Encourage patients to ask questions and discuss any concerns they have. Explain the need to make follow-up appointments with a physician if appropriate.

Teaching a patient who has been diagnosed with an STD how to treat or manage the disease is especially important. Make sure the patient understands all directions and the necessity for treatment. Bacterial infections such as chlamydia, gonorrhea, and syphilis can be cured with antibiotics as long as the patient takes all the medication in the prescribed manner. Viral infections such as AIDS, genital herpes, and genital warts cannot be cured, although they can be treated and managed to differing degrees.

Emphasize to patients with an STD that they should avoid all sexual contact until the infection has been treated completely. Many STDs can be spread through any type of genital contact, including vaginal intercourse, anal sex, and oral sex. Herpes can be spread through kissing if there are herpes sores in the mouth. Encourage patients to inform each person with whom they had sexual contact that they have contracted an STD. Explain that unless all sexual partners are treated successfully, the disease will pass back and forth indefinitely.

You can reinforce your education efforts by providing patients with materials on the prevention and treatment of STDs. Keep a variety of pamphlets, books, and other resources in your office to help patients cope with and manage STDs.

drug to kill the organism, and the organism will build up a tolerance to the antibiotic.

Sexually Transmitted Diseases. Sexually transmitted diseases (STDs)—diseases acquired through sexual contact with an infected person—are also infectious diseases. The number and severity of these diseases, their high incidence, and the great amount of misinformation about them warrant a discussion apart from other infectious diseases. (AIDS is discussed in Chapter 3.) Internists, infectious disease specialists, pediatricians, urologists, and gynecologists are all involved in the diagnosis and treatment of STDs.

Patient Education About STDs. Your role as an educator is vital in dealing with patients who have STDs. Some patients may be hesitant to ask for information. Providing educational materials in the examination room will help answer their questions and put them at ease. These materials deal with sensitive or embarrassing topics, and the patient's privacy must be maintained. Printed materials are available from several medical agencies and should be provided to your patients. In addition, you must educate patients about prevention and treatment of STDs. The Educating the Patient section provides more information on this topic.

Common Types of STDs. Your role in assisting the doctor in the treatment of STDs will involve emphasizing to the patient the importance of completing the course of therapy and avoiding sexual contact while the infection is still active. Sexual partners must also be treated to avoid reinfection. Several types of STDs are fairly common.

Candidiasis is a yeast infection. It is not a true STD but is included with the STDs because the infection can be transmitted between sexual partners. Symptoms include severe genital itching, redness and swelling of the vaginal or vulval tissue, light yellow or white patches (usually cheesy or curdlike) on the vagina, and vaginal discharge. The infection is treated with an antimycotic (antifungal) drug.

Chlamydia usually produces symptoms of discharge and uncomfortable urination, although it may be asymptomatic, particularly in women. Untreated, the disease can cause scarring of the fallopian tubes and eventual infertility. Diagnosis is made by aspirating pus from the urethra of men, the endocervix of women, or other infected tissue and having it examined in a laboratory. Chlamydia is treated with antibiotics.

Genital herpes is a type of herpes virus. Symptoms include blisterlike sores on the genitalia, difficult urination, swelling of the legs, fatigue, and a general ill feeling. Because this disease is cyclical, symptoms disappear and reappear periodically. Although there is no cure for genital herpes, an antiviral drug can reduce or suppress the symptoms. Herpes may be transmitted to the fetus during pregnancy or delivery. It is often fatal to an infant.

Genital warts and human papilloma virus (HPV) are found on or in men and women. Patients may generally be asymptomatic, but some have burning and itching in the genital area. There appears to be an increased risk of cancer of the vulva, vagina, and cervix in women with genital warts. There is no treatment for the virus. Its symptoms usually disappear within 6 to 18 months in a person with a normal immune system. However, even though the symptoms subside, the virus remains present in the patient.

Gonorrhea causes inflammation of the genitalia, with a greenish yellow discharge from the cervix, sore throat, anal discharge, swollen glands, and lower abdominal pain. Treatment is with antibiotics such as penicillin or tetracycline.

Trichomoniasis symptoms in women include inflammation of the genital area and an abundant white or yellow vaginal discharge with a foul odor. (It is usually asymptomatic in men.) The infection is diagnosed by inspecting a specimen of the discharge under the microscope. The condition is usually treated with a course of antibiotics.

Other Diseases and Disorders. Internists may diagnose and treat other diseases and disorders, including anemia, appendicitis, arthritis, gout, and peptic ulcer (Table 22-1). They may also refer patients to a physician in one of the highly specialized areas.

TABLE 22-1 Common Diseases and Disorders Treated by Internists

Condition	Description	Treatment
Anemia	Results from deficiency of iron or vitamins, such as folic acid and vitamin B_{12}; can also result from loss of blood (acute blood loss anemia); body's cells do not get enough oxygen, resulting in fatigue, listlessness, pallor, inability to concentrate, difficulty breathing on exertion	Oral supplements of appropriate vitamin or iron; if caused by acute blood loss, blood transfusion
Appendicitis	Acute inflammation of appendix as result of serious infection, blood clotting, or tissue destruction; inflammation may lead to rupture or perforation of the appendix, which can be fatal; symptoms include general abdominal pain and tenderness often starting at the umbilical area and radiating to lower right quadrant, fever, loss of appetite, gastrointestinal (GI) distress	Surgical removal of appendix
Arthritis	Chronic inflammatory disease of tissues of joints; symptoms include pain and stiffness in joints	Medication to reduce inflammation and pain; surgery in severe cases
Gout	Metabolic disease involving acute joint pain, most commonly in the big toe at night; caused by overproduction or retention of uric acid	Medication and diet restrictions to decrease production of uric acid and promote its excretion
Peptic ulcer	Lesion of mucous membrane of esophagus, stomach, or duodenum (first section of small intestine); symptoms include heartburn, vomiting, and dull, gnawing pain or burning sensation in area	Medication and diet restrictions to reduce amount and acidity of gastric juices; stress reduction; surgery in severe cases

Pediatrics

A pediatrician specializes in the health care of children, monitoring their development and diagnosing and treating their illnesses. Just as with internal medicine, there are subspecialties of pediatrics, such as surgery and oncology. To be a good pediatric medical assistant, you must first like children of all ages. If you do, you will be better able to relate to them and to communicate with them effectively.

Parent or caregiver education, adherence to immunization schedules (see Chapter 2), and child abuse detection are primary areas of responsibility for medical assistants who work in pediatrics. You will also assist with the physical examination and treatment of the pediatric patient. Your role as liaison in these areas between caregiver and physician will be an important one.

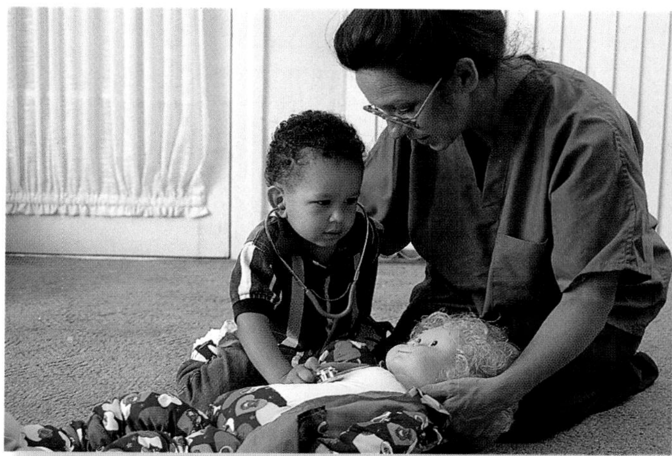

Figure 22-5. Providing a pediatric patient with a diversion may help alleviate the child's fear.

Assisting With a Pediatric Physical Examination

Many of the examination procedures for a pediatric patient are the same as those for an adult. While you prepare the child or adolescent for examination, you might discuss with the parent, caregiver, or child such topics as eating habits, sleep patterns, daily activities, immunization schedules, and toilet training. This discussion will provide important clues to possible abnormal mental, physical, emotional, or social development. Topics such as STDs and drugs and alcohol may be appropriate for you to discuss with an adolescent. Point out potential problems to the doctor.

Be mindful of adolescents' sensitivity toward rapid growth and physical, sexual, and social development when you prepare them for examination. Adolescents and preadolescents often feel awkward and self-conscious about being examined. They may also prefer to dress alone and to be alone with the doctor.

Some children are afraid of going to the doctor's office. You can help relieve a child's fear by calmly explaining procedures before they occur, giving the reason for each procedure, and being cheerful and mindful of a child's feelings. Allowing a child to examine some of the instruments may also alleviate fear (Figure 22-5). If a patient is physically resistant to examination, you may need to call for assistance from the doctor or caregiver, or the child may need to be restrained.

Try to speak in terms aimed at the child's age level, and kneel if necessary to make eye contact with the child. Treat the child with respect and provide positive reinforcement when a child is cooperative. Avoid making light of crying or pain. Make a game out of some aspect of a procedure, and provide a small token reward at the end of a visit. For infants a gentle approach, such as talking quietly and holding them comfortingly, is helpful.

Examining the Well Child. Parents should bring their infants and children to the pediatrician for regular checkups and growth monitoring. The American Academy of Pediatrics recommends the following frequency.

- Infants need seven well-baby examinations during their first year, at these intervals: 2 weeks, 1 month, 2 months, 4 months, 6 months, 9 months, 1 year.
- Children in the second year of life should have checkups at 15 and 18 months.
- From the age of 2, children should have checkups every year.

Follow Universal Precautions and prepare for the physical examination the same way you would for an adult, except for draping and positioning. Ask the parent of an infant or toddler to remove all the child's clothing except the diaper because the child should be nude for the examination. Then keep the child covered until the physician enters the examining room.

An infant or toddler may be crying during the examination. To assist the physician in hearing chest sounds with a stethoscope, ask the parent to allow the child to suck on a pacifier to quiet the crying. Feeding the child during the examination is not encouraged because stomach sounds interfere with clear auscultation.

Parents play a more active role during the examination of infants and toddlers than they play during the examination of older children. You or the parent may assist the child into position during the examination, or the physician may allow the parent to hold the child. Distracting infants and toddlers with mobiles, shiny surfaces, or toys may help the examination go more smoothly.

Examining for Scoliosis. One examination performed frequently in the pediatric office is that for scoliosis, an abnormal lateral curving of the spine into an S curve. It can appear in a child of any age but is more common in adolescent girls during their growth spurt. This condition is undetectable when the child is young. As she grows, however, it can be detected in an examination. Procedure 22-2 explains how to perform a scoliosis examination.

Report any symptoms that you notice during your examination to the pediatrician. If the pediatrician confirms

PROCEDURE 22.2

Performing a Scoliosis Examination

Objective: To assess a patient for possible scoliosis

OSHA Guidelines: This procedure does not involve exposure to blood, body fluids, or tissues.

Materials: Patient chart, pen

Method

Scoliosis is an abnormal, lateral curving of the spine into an S shape (Figure 22-6). It results from rotation of the spinal column, with the thorax usually curving to the right and the lumbar spine to the left. The two forms of scoliosis are functional, caused by poor posture or uneven leg lengths, and structural, resulting from vertebral deformities.

Genetic scoliosis, a type of structural scoliosis, is seldom apparent before the age of 10. It is most noticeable at the beginning of the preadolescent growth spurt. It is seven times more common in girls than in boys. Screening for scoliosis by school nurses is routine in most schools. It can be detected in an examination. You can perform a scoliosis examination on a child as follows.

1. Identify the patient and introduce yourself.
2. Explain the procedure.
3. Have the child remove his shirt and stand up straight. Look to see whether one shoulder is higher than the other or one shoulder blade is more prominent.
4. With the child's arms hanging loosely at his sides, check whether one arm swings away from the body more than the other, whether one hip is higher or more prominent than the other, and whether the child seems to tilt to one side.

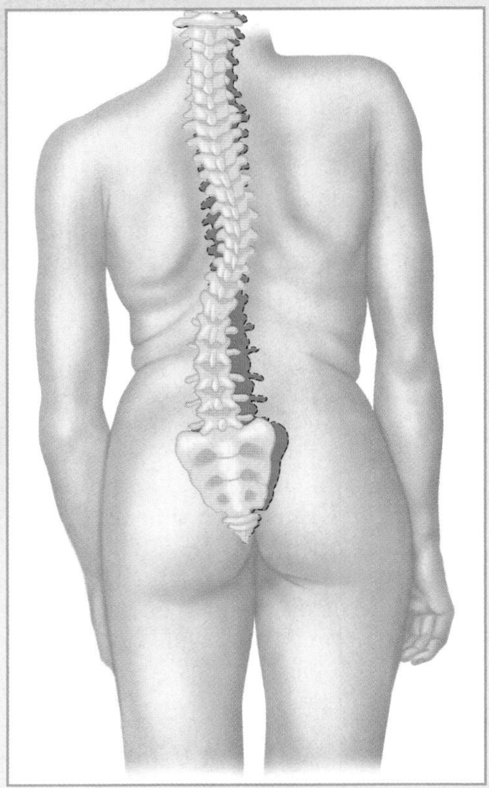

Figure 22-6. Scoliosis causes the spine to curve into an S shape.

5. Have the child bend forward, with arms hanging down and palms together at knee level. Check to see whether there is a hump on the back at the ribs or near the waist.
6. Document your findings in the patient's chart, and report them to the doctor.

scoliosis, she may recommend exercises, a Milwaukee brace (Figure 22-7), surgical rod implantation, or a combination of therapies.

Your role as educator in regard to scoliosis is important. Untreated scoliosis can cause debilitating symptoms as the patient matures to adulthood. Encourage parents to bring older children and adolescents to the office annually for routine screening. If the Milwaukee brace is prescribed, the adolescent may need encouragement from you and the physician to wear the brace as directed.

Detecting Child Abuse or Neglect. Child abuse is an all-too-common and potentially fatal problem. Whenever a child comes to the office, you should watch for any signs of serious problems in the relationship between the parent or caregiver and the child. Also notice any signs of physical injury, such as unexplained bruises or burns. Any suspicious lesion on a child's genitalia should prompt an investigation of sexual abuse. Possible signs of neglect include dirty or neglected appearance, hunger, extreme sadness or fear, and an inability to communicate. Note any suspicions in the chart, and report them to the doctor before he sees the patient. The doctor will respond to your information by examining the child for clues to indicate the following:

- Internal injuries: tenderness when palpated or auscultated

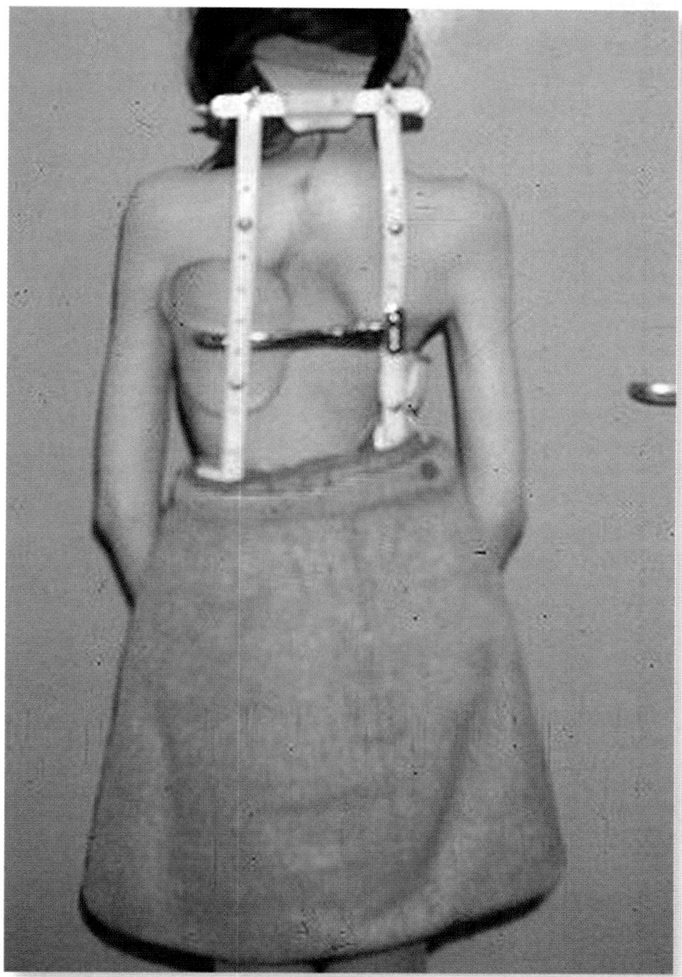

Figure 22-7. A spinal brace like this one may be used for scoliosis, which is an abnormal curvature of the spine.

- Malnutrition: tooth discoloration, unhealthy gums or skin color
- Lack of cognitive ability: dulled neurological responses

Studies show that certain risk factors are usually present in parents who abuse their children. Some risk factors are stress, single parenthood, inadequate knowledge of normal developmental expectations, lack of family support, family hostility, financial problems, and mental health problems. Other risk factors include prolonged separation of parent and child, ambivalent feelings toward the child, and a mother younger than 16 years. Additional risk factors include an unhealthy or unsafe home environment, inappropriate supervision, substance abuse, a parental crime record, a negative attitude toward pregnancy, and a history of parents having been abused.

Intervention, such as home visits by nurses, can significantly lower the rate of child abuse. Managed care systems may provide this service as part of their postpartum program. These nurses provide information on normal child growth and development and routine health needs, serve as informational support persons, and refer families to appropriate services when they require assistance.

You are legally responsible for reporting suspected child abuse or neglect. Contact the child protection agency in your community. Post the appropriate telephone number in your office.

Examining for Growth Abnormalities. Pediatricians look for any sign of growth abnormality during routine well-child visits. Physicians compare a child's physical, intellectual, and social signs to charts showing national averages. In general, physicians look for signs that the child is in the appropriate stage of growth for her age. Growth can be divided into five stages.

Stages One and Two: The First and Second Years. Infancy, the first year of life, is marked by the development of strength and coordination of the trunk, head, and limbs. Intellectual growth primarily involves receiving information through the senses and performing motor (physical) functions in response to the environment. In the second year of life, the child develops fine motor skills (involving control of smaller muscles, such as those in the fingers) and manual dexterity. Sociologically, the child develops some independence and begins to test parental limits.

Stage Three: Ages 3 to 5 Years. During ages 3 to 5 years, the child develops physical skills of muscle coordination and both large motor skills (involving control of larger muscles, such as those in the arms and legs) and fine motor skills. Intellectually, the child observes and copies older children and adults without fully understanding them. The child also learns to initiate play with others and begins to make requests of family members.

Stage Four: Age 6 Years to Puberty. The fourth stage occurs from approximately age 6 to **puberty,** the period of adolescence when a person begins to develop sexual traits. Muscle coordination and fine and large motor skills develop further. The child begins to get involved in scholastic and extracurricular activities. The child also develops an identity, based partially on both intellectual and physical skills, and learns how to achieve goals in the environment.

Stage Five: Adolescence. Physical growth and development in the teenage years are centered on normal sexual change. Girls usually begin puberty between 8 and 14 years of age; boys begin between 9½ and 16, on average. Menarche, the onset of menstruation, usually occurs about 2½ years after the onset of puberty. The beginning of nocturnal emissions of seminal fluid signals sexual maturation in boys. This awareness of sexuality is accompanied by concern with body image. Intellectually, adolescents are able to understand abstract concepts and think about themselves in terms of the past and future. The process of developing independence, a personal identity, and future plans is also important during this time of life.

General Eye Examination. As part of the general examination, the pediatrician examines the interior of the child's eyes with an ophthalmoscope. You will probably

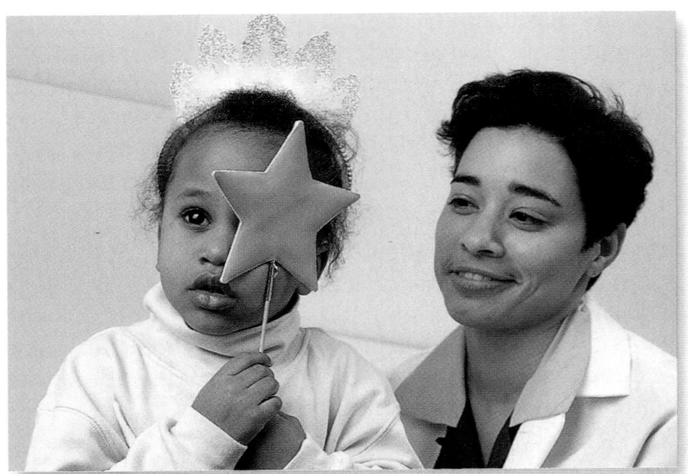

Figure 22-8. Making a game out of the visual acuity test helps put a child at ease.

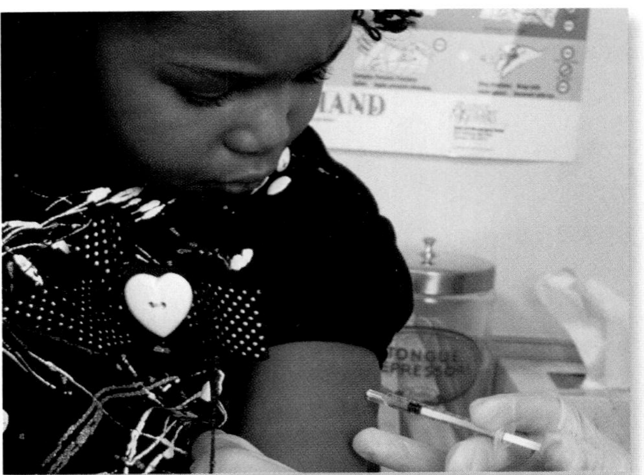

Figure 22-9. Immunizations are part of routine well-child visits in a pediatric practice.

perform the visual acuity test (Figure 22-8). Make a game of covering the child's eye if the child resists this part of the procedure. Watch for signs of visual difficulty during the test, such as tilting the head in a certain direction, blinking, squinting, or frowning. If the caregiver brought the child in specifically for a vision test, record in the child's chart whatever symptoms the caregiver mentions.

General Ear Examination. A pediatric ear examination is important because so many children have ear infections or upper respiratory infections involving the ear. Because children's eustachian tubes are more horizontal than those of adults, fluid collects more easily in the tubes and can promote bacterial growth. The tubes are also short and connected to the throat. Any upper respiratory infections can easily travel to the ear. (The ear examination is described in Chapter 21.)

Diagnostic Testing

Many adult diagnostic procedures are also used for children. The pediatrician uses the same laboratory tests and radiologic tests. He performs some diagnostic tests in the office.

Because streptococcal infection can be especially serious in a child, some pediatricians perform a rapid test for the presence of streptococcal bacteria so they can immediately start the appropriate medical treatment. If the test is positive, the physician begins treatment with antibiotics specifically for this type of bacteria.

Some physicians believe the rapid strep test is not always reliable. To confirm a negative test result, these physicians also do a throat culture. A throat culture can determine which of the streptococcal bacteria is present or whether other organisms are causing the symptoms. The results can indicate a possible change in medication. The method for obtaining a throat culture is outlined in Chapter 28. You may also be required to collect a pediatric urine specimen. This process is described in Procedure 29-2 in Chapter 29. Additionally, collecting blood may be part of your responsibility. This procedure is discussed in Chapter 30.

Immunizations

Immunizations are usually given during routine office visits (Figure 22-9). Public health authorities recommend a schedule (see Chapter 2) for immunizing children against diseases such as hepatitis B, diphtheria, tetanus, pertussis (whooping cough), poliomyelitis, measles, mumps, rubella (German measles), chickenpox, and *Haemophilus influenzae* type B (Hib). Many vaccines have largely eliminated the threat of these once-prevalent, life-threatening diseases.

The first vaccine, for hepatitis B, is given to a newborn the day after birth. Some vaccines require a series of doses to give immunity. Booster doses may be required for a particular vaccine at a later age. The patient must not have an illness or fever at the time of immunization. If these conditions exist, reschedule the appointment.

Pediatric Diseases and Disorders

If you work in a pediatric office, you should know the signs and symptoms of common childhood diseases. Some diseases, including chickenpox, influenza, measles, mumps, rubella, scarlet fever, and tetanus, are described in Chapter 2. Other common diseases are outlined in Table 22-2. Many common disorders found in children are not specific diseases. Upper respiratory infections, including colds and viral influenza, occur frequently among children.

It is important not to make assumptions regarding diagnosis or treatment. When reported symptoms include fever, sore throat, runny nose, and earache, any number of conditions could be the cause. Encourage the parent to bring the child to the office. You should, however, tell the doctor as soon as possible when a child has an extremely high fever. The doctor may want the child to go to an emergency room. Do not recommend aspirin for fever in

TABLE 22-2 Common Pediatric Diseases and Disorders		
Condition	**Description**	**Treatment**
Head lice	Small insects easily spread among children by head-to-head contact and by sharing objects such as combs and hairbrushes; lice live on scalp and lay eggs strongly attached to hair shafts; symptoms include itchy scalp; identify by locating crawling lice or nits (eggs) attached to hair; examine parted hair carefully at scalp and bottom of hair strands	Antilice shampoo or 1% permethrin cream rinse; removal of eggs with fine-tooth comb; disinfection of clothing, bedding, and washable toys by machine washing and drying in hot cycles or by dry cleaning; tight bagging for 30 days of items that cannot be washed; disinfection of combs and brushes (used for hair) by washing in shampoo
Herpes simplex virus (HSV)	In children virus causes cold-sore blisters on or near mouth; diagnosis made by inspecting lesions; first stage (2–12 days before appearance of blister) involves tingling and itching sensations; later blister ruptures and forms yellow crust; outbreak takes about 3 weeks to heal completely	Application of ice cube to blister, which may promote faster healing; ointments to alleviate cracking and discomfort; avoidance of sun exposure because it may trigger outbreak
Impetigo	Highly contagious dermatologic disease caused by staphylococcal, sometimes streptococcal, bacteria; transmitted by direct contact; causes inflammation and pustules, which are small lymph-filled bumps that rupture and become encrusted before healing; frequently seen around mouth and nostrils	Avoidance of scratching lesions and sharing utensils, towels, bed linens, or bath or pool water that could cause further transmission; careful washing of affected areas two to three times per day to keep lesions clean and dry; topical antibacterial cream
Infectious conjunctivitis ("pink eye")	Highly contagious streptococcal or staphylococcal bacterial infection of conjunctiva of eye; transmitted by direct contact; causes redness, pain, swelling, discharge; usually begins in one eye and spreads to other	Avoidance of scratching eyes and sharing utensils, towels, or bed linens that could cause further transmission; warm compresses to relieve discomfort; antibiotic drops or ointment
Pinworms	Parasites transmitted by swallowing worm eggs, by touching something that infected person has touched, or by putting infested sand or dirt into mouth; when eggs hatch in body, worms attach to intestinal lining; mature females travel to areas just outside rectum to lay eggs, which causes itching	Medication usually given to whole family to treat and prevent further infestation
Ringworm	Contagious fungal infection involving scalp, groin, feet, or other areas of body, causing flat, dry, and scaly or moist and crusty lesions; lesions develop into clear center with outer ring; when scalp is affected, may cause bald patches	Oral and topical antifungal medication; isolation to prevent spreading; frequent changing of towels, bedding, with no sharing with others in family; caution that child not use others' combs or brushes
Streptococcal sore throat ("strep throat")	Contagious disease caused by streptococcal bacteria and spread by droplet; complications include progression to rheumatic fever (with arthritis, nephritis, and inflammation of endocardium, or inner lining of heart); symptoms include headache, high fever, vomiting, and extremely painful, swollen, and red or white sore throat; causes difficulty swallowing	Streptococci-specific antibiotics given as soon as possible; because of potential complications, therapy based on the practitioner's experience is sometimes given without confirmed diagnosis from throat culture; antibiotics are adjusted with confirmation of infecting organism; possible hospitalization in acute cases

children. The use of aspirin in children has been associated with Reye's syndrome, a potentially fatal disease of the central nervous system and liver. Acetaminophen (Tylenol) is preferred for treating fever in children.

Some less common diseases and disorders can be found in children. You need to be aware of the basic symptoms and the treatments for these disorders.

AIDS. Most childhood cases of human immunodeficiency virus (HIV) infection are transmitted from a mother to her infant. When a woman is HIV-positive, her baby has a 15% to 30% chance of being infected. All babies born to HIV-positive mothers have HIV antibodies that are detectable through testing at birth. The antibodies persist for a period of 15 to 18 months, but not all such babies remain permanently infected. AIDS has no cure, but treating the pregnant woman and newborn child with antiviral agents has been shown to lower the rate of HIV infection in the child.

Attention Deficit Hyperactivity Disorder and Learning Disabilities. Attention deficit hyperactivity disorder (ADHD) and learning disabilities (LD) are found in children, adolescents, and adults. These disorders can cause gross motor disability, inability to read or write, hyperactivity, distractibility, impulsiveness, and generally disruptive behavior. ADHD encompasses all conditions formerly identified as hyperactivity, or hyperkinesis, and attention deficit. LD encompasses a wide range of conditions that interfere with learning, including dyslexia (reading problems), dysgraphia (writing problems), and dyscalculia (math problems).

ADHD is misunderstood, misdiagnosed, and overdiagnosed in children. Some physicians fail to recognize ADHD as a cause of academic, social, and emotional problems. Others are quick to attribute too many such problems to ADHD. When ADHD is the correct diagnosis, methylphenidate hydrochloride (Ritalin) and other drugs may alleviate the symptoms but not without risk of adverse effects, such as insomnia, increased heart rate and blood pressure, and interference with growth rate. Successful treatment usually requires a combination of drug and behavioral therapies and educational, psychological, and emotional support tailored to the child.

Cerebral Palsy. Cerebral palsy, a birth-related disorder of the nerves and muscles, is the most frequent crippling disease in children. It is caused by brain damage that occurs before, during, or shortly after birth or in early childhood. Signs of spastic cerebral palsy (the most common form) include hyperactive tendon reflexes, rapid alteration between muscular contraction and relaxation, permanent muscle shortening, and underdevelopment of extremities. Among people who have this disease, 40% are mentally retarded, 25% have seizures, and 80% have impaired speech. There is no known cure, but the effects of the disorder can be alleviated with physical therapy, speech therapy, orthopedic surgery, splints, skeletal muscle relaxants, and anticonvulsant medication.

Congenital Heart Disease. Congenital heart disease is caused by a cardiovascular malformation in the fetus before birth. If the fetus survives, the newborn is usually small. The defect may be so small, however, that it may not be recognized until days, months, or even years later. Some patients have such a mild case of the disease that no treatment is necessary. Others require only low-risk surgery. In still others major high-risk surgery is necessary. Many patients diagnosed with the problem are treated with antibiotics to avoid secondary infections.

A cardiovascular defect can be caused by genetic mutations (changes in the genes), maternal infections (such as rubella or cytomegalovirus), maternal alcoholism, or maternal insulin-dependent diabetes. Blue lips and fingernails, signs of cyanosis in a newborn, are obvious indications of a cardiac defect.

Down Syndrome. Down syndrome is a genetic disorder resulting from one extra chromosome in each of the millions of cells formed during development of the fetus. It is the most common chromosomal abnormality in humans. Down syndrome is not caused by any parental behavior, such as diet or activity. The estimated risk for a Down syndrome birth increases, however, as maternal age increases. Down syndrome is characterized by low muscle tone, which can be alleviated with physical therapy. Characteristic facial features are also evident (Figure 22-10). These include broad face, flattened nasal bridge, narrow

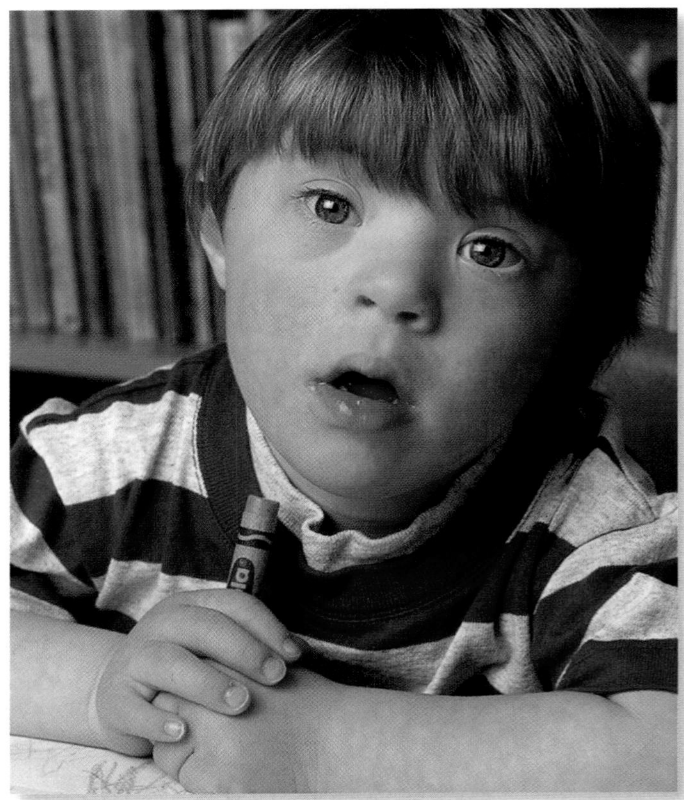

Figure 22-10. A child with Down syndrome usually has distinct facial features.

nasal passages (increasing the risk of congestion), slanting eyes (vision problems are common), and small teeth and ears. Mental retardation, which can range from mild to severe, is also a characteristic of Down syndrome.

Hepatitis B. Infection with the hepatitis B virus (HBV) can lead to a serious and chronic infection of the liver. A child can carry the virus for years and only later develop liver failure or liver cancer. The virus can be transmitted across the placenta or during birth if the mother is infected. The disease may also be transmitted sexually, by blood transfusion, or by direct contact. It is frequently seen among drug abusers who share needles. Immunization is available, and children should be immunized starting the day after birth. Children who have not been immunized should begin to receive the series of immunizations for protection from infection.

Respiratory Syncytial Virus. The respiratory syncytial virus (RSV) is a major cause of lower respiratory disease in infants and young children. RSV is seen yearly in the winter and spring outbreaks of pneumonia, bronchiolitis, and tracheobronchitis. It is highly contagious, and reinfection is common. Treatment is difficult because the infection is viral rather than bacterial. Antibiotics are thus effective for treating only the possible secondary infections that develop during or after contracting RSV.

Sudden Infant Death Syndrome. Sudden infant death syndrome (SIDS)—formerly known as crib death—is the sudden death of an infant that remains unexplained after all other possible causes have been carefully ruled out. Most SIDS cases occur before the infant is 6 months of age. Victims appear to be healthy and are more likely to be male than female. SIDS occurs during sleep. Some factors that may put babies between the ages of 1 week and 1 year at high risk have been identified:

- Being exposed to smoke in utero and to secondhand smoke after birth
- Being overheated when ill
- Being exclusively bottle-fed
- Being born prematurely
- Receiving little or no prenatal care

The National Sudden Infant Death Foundation has local chapters for parents whose babies have died of the syndrome. Counseling and information are available through local health organizations. Support groups are very helpful to the parents of a SIDS infant. Recommend and refer families when necessary.

Spina Bifida. Spina bifida is a defect of spinal development that results when tissues fail to close properly around the spinal cord during the first trimester of pregnancy. Neurological symptoms are common because the spinal cord is not fully protected by the bony and connective tissues of the spine. These symptoms may vary with the severity of the defect, ranging from foot weakness and bladder or bowel problems to paralysis of the lower extremities and mental retardation. The skin over the spinal cord often has a depression, tuft of hair, or port wine stain when the defect is not readily apparent.

The treatment and outcome of spina bifida are based on the extent of damage. Surgical closure or implants are sometimes required. Unfortunately, the neurological conditions cannot be reversed.

Viral Gastroenteritis. Gastroenteritis is an inflammation of the stomach and intestines. Gastroenteritis caused by a virus may be called the flu, traveler's diarrhea, or food poisoning. Viral gastroenteritis usually subsides within 1 to 2 days. It can be serious in young children, however, because it can cause extreme fluid loss that results in dehydration and electrolyte imbalances.

Symptoms include fever, nausea, abdominal cramping, diarrhea, and vomiting. Gastroenteritis is treated with bed rest, increased fluid intake, dietary modifications (usually only clear liquids), and medication for vomiting and diarrhea if necessary. Antibiotics may be prescribed if evidence of bacterial involvement is present.

Patient and Caregiver Education for Pediatric Patients

Patients and caregivers in a pediatrician's office usually have many questions. You will be able to answer some of the questions yourself, sparing valuable time for the pediatrician. Helpful brochures and booklets are available from the American Academy of Pediatrics. You should obtain the current list of publications and encourage your employer to order what the office needs.

Obstetrics and Gynecology

An obstetrician/gynecologist (OB/GYN) specializes in the female reproductive system. Physicians who focus on caring for women during pregnancy and childbirth are called obstetricians. Physicians who treat other conditions of the female reproductive system are called gynecologists.

As a medical assistant in an OB/GYN office, you will need to be familiar with the female reproductive system and its functions, including pregnancy, fertility, and menopause. Review the female reproductive system in Chapter 17. You need to know about the common diagnostic tests and procedures performed in this specialty. You must also be familiar with the common diseases and disorders in obstetrics and gynecology, be prepared to answer patients' questions, and provide patient education materials.

Assisting With the Gynecologic Physical Examination

An annual gynecologic examination is recommended for all women age 18 and older. The examination is intended to provide an overview of a woman's health and to provide the opportunity for important cancer-screening examinations and tests. A female medical assistant should be in the examining room during the physical examination to assist a male doctor and to provide legal protection. Your role during the examination is similar to that for the general physical examination.

Ask the patient to empty her bladder; if a urine specimen is needed, it should be collected at this time. Provide the patient with a gown before the examination, and give her privacy while she changes. When you interview her, discuss her gynecologic and general health, and inquire about any changes in appetite, weight, or emotional status. Also find out the date of her last menstrual period. Then have her sit on the examining table while you check her vital signs.

The Physician's Interview. The gynecologic physical examination is more than an internal pelvic examination. It is an evaluation of the patient's total health and a review of factors that could be an indication of possible cancer or STDs. The physician asks questions about the patient's menstrual cycle and about any abnormal discharge or discomfort during sexual intercourse. The physician also listens to the patient's heart and lungs before beginning the gynecologic examination.

Breast Examination. The physician examines the patient's breasts and underarm areas to check for abnormal lumps that could be cancerous. Your role as patient educator is crucial. Patients must understand the need for regular breast examinations. When interviewing the patient and after the examination, emphasize the breast cancer detection guidelines of the American Cancer Society and National Cancer Institute:

1. Beginning at age 40, all women should be encouraged to have a mammogram every year. Mammography should begin earlier in patients with a strong family history of breast cancer.
2. Women should have breast examinations during their annual routine checkups at least every three years for women ages 20 to 39 and yearly for women 40 and older.
3. Women should do breast self-examination (BSE) monthly.

These guidelines emphasize the importance of education and awareness of the patient.

While reviewing the patient's chart, the physician checks to see when the last mammogram was performed. He may also ask the patient whether she knows how to perform a BSE and whether she is performing it monthly. If needed, he may ask you to instruct the patient in performing the BSE. The teaching technique for the BSE is found in the Educating the Patient section on page 319 of Chapter 20.

Pelvic Examination. During the pelvic examination the doctor checks the external genitalia, cervix, vaginal wall, internal reproductive organs, and rectum. Examination methods include palpation and inspection with a **speculum,** an instrument that expands the vaginal opening to permit viewing of the vagina and cervix. The doctor wears gloves and uses a lubricant for patient comfort.

Your role is to assist the patient into position, with her feet in the stirrups of the examining table and her buttocks at the end of the table. Drape her so that only the area between the thighs is exposed. Assist the doctor by having gloves and instruments ready for use and by applying lubricant to the doctor's gloved fingers. You may also warm the speculum for the patient's comfort. Be prepared to provide reassurance and explanation to a patient who appears to be uncomfortable or nervous. Encourage her to breathe deeply to help relax the pelvic muscles and reduce discomfort. See Procedure 22-3 for further instructions on how to assist with a gynecological examination.

After checking the vagina and cervix and while the speculum is still in place, the doctor will most likely take a Pap smear (Papanicolaou smear) (Figure 22-11). The doctor then removes the speculum and begins the bimanual phase of the examination. She will ask for your assistance in removing the examining gloves, putting on new gloves, and lubricating two fingers. Placing those fingers in the vagina and using the other hand to palpate the abdomen, the doctor assesses the position of the uterus. She may then place a lubricated finger in the rectum and palpate for abnormal growths with the other hand by pressing on the lower abdomen.

When the doctor completes the examination, she usually asks the patient if she has any questions or concerns. Ask the patient whether she has additional questions after the doctor leaves the examining room. You may need to provide written information in addition to answering the patient's questions orally.

The medical assistant in many OB/GYN offices provides handouts describing female anatomy and recommended

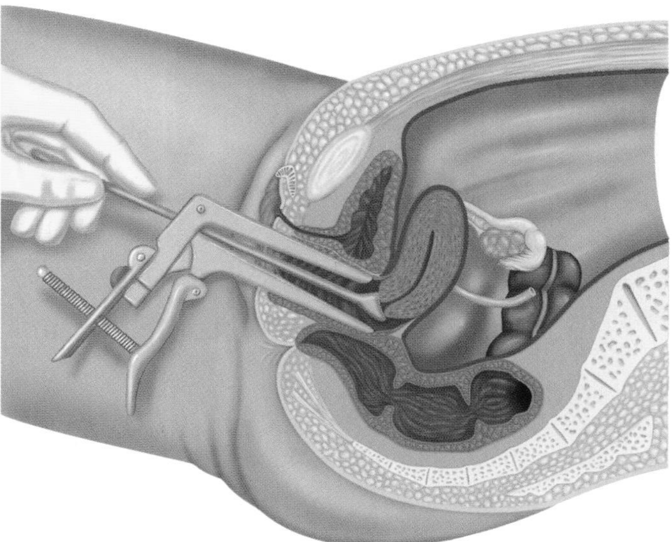

Figure 22-11. A speculum is used to expand the vaginal opening to help view the vagina and cervix.

PROCEDURE 22.3

Assisting with a Gynecological Examination

Objective: To assist the physician and maintain the client's comfort and privacy during a gynecological examination

OSHA Guidelines

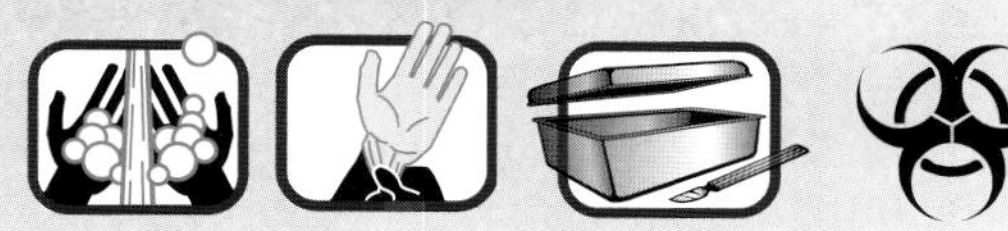

Materials: Gown and drape, vaginal speculum, cervical brush and/or scraper, cotton-tipped applicator, examination gloves, tissues, laboratory requisition, water-soluble lubricant, examination table with stirrups, examination light, microscopic slide(s), tissues, spray fixative, pen and pencil

Method

1. Gather equipment and make sure all items are in working order. Write the patient's name and date on the microscopic slide with pencil.
2. Identify the patient and explain the procedure. The patient should remove all clothing, including underwear, and put the gown on with the opening in the front.
3. Ask the patient to sit on the edge of the examination table with the drape until the physician arrives.
4. When the physician is ready, have the patient place her feet into the stirrups and move her buttocks to the edge of the table. This is the lithotomy position.
5. Provide the physician with gloves and an examination lamp as she examines the genitalia by inspection and palpation.
6. Pass the speculum to the physician. For a metal speculum, you may warm it in warm water. For a plastic speculum, a water-soluble lubricant is used. Have this available to the physician as required.
7. For the Pap (Papanicolaou) smear, be prepared to pass a cotton-tipped applicator and cervical brush or scraper for the collection of the specimen. Have the labeled slide available for the physician to place the specimen on the slide. Depending on the physician and the specimen collected, two or more slides may be necessary. They may be labeled based on where the specimen was collected: endocervical = E, vaginal = V, and cervical = C.
8. Once the specimen is on the slide, a cytology fixative must be applied immediately. The **fixative** holds the cells in place until a microscopic examination is performed. A spray fixative is common, and it should be held 6 inches from the slide and sprayed lightly with a back and forth motion. Allow the slide to dry completely.
9. After the physician removes the speculum, a digital examination is performed to check the position of the internal organs. Provide the physician with additional lubricant as needed.
10. Upon completion of the examination, help the patient switch from the lithotomy position to a supine or sitting position.
11. Provide tissues for the patient to remove the lubricant, and ask the patient to get dressed. Assist as necessary or provide for privacy. Explain the procedure for communicating the laboratory results.
12. After the patient has left, don gloves and clean the examination room and equipment. Dispose of the disposable speculum, cervical scraper, and other contaminated waste in a biohazardous waste container.
13. Store the supplies, straighten the room, and discard the used examination paper on the table.
14. Prepare the laboratory slide, and place it and the specimen in the proper place for transport to an outside laboratory.
15. Remove your gloves and wash your hands.

female screening procedures. Printed materials are available from a variety of sources, including the AMA, government agencies, and pharmaceutical companies. The Web site of the National Women's Health Information Center, www.4women.gov, is an excellent resource.

Life Cycle Changes

Women experience physical changes as a result of maturation. The two distinct changes that occur as part of the life cycle involve menstruation and menopause.

Menstruation. Menstruation is a woman's normal cycle of preparation for conception (the union of egg and sperm that initiates pregnancy). The normal age range of menarche, the beginning of menstruation, is 10 to 15 years of age. Each month (averaging every 28 days) the endometrium, which lines the uterus, is shed in vaginal bleeding. If the woman becomes pregnant, this shedding does not occur, and the woman misses her menstrual period. Note the last menstrual period (LMP) for each patient in her chart at each visit. A period lasts an average of 5 days, with durations of 3 to 7 days considered normal. Menstrual cycles are prompted by changes in hormonal (estrogen and progesterone) levels.

Menopause. Menopause is the cessation of the menstrual cycle. Menopause is a natural occurrence, not a disease or disorder. Several stages surround menopause. Premenopause is the time period before menopause, during which the menstrual periods may be irregular. The time just before and after menopause is called perimenopause. During perimenopause a woman may experience irregular periods, hot flashes, and vaginal dryness, all caused by changing levels of estrogen. Because hormonal change is occurring, the woman may experience mood swings or other psychological changes.

Menopause can also be brought on by the surgical removal of the uterus and ovaries (see the discussion of hysterectomy in this chapter). The symptoms and treatment are the same as those of naturally occurring menopause.

A woman entering menopause may feel embarrassed to discuss her symptoms with you. Reassure her not only that it is a natural occurrence but also that there are ways to make menopause more comfortable.

Diagnostic Tests and Procedures

The physician uses a number of diagnostic tests, including urine and blood tests (described in Chapters 29 and 30). Many OB/GYN offices have their own small laboratories for immediate results, especially for pregnancy-related tests.

Pregnancy Test. Pregnancy tests are done on a specimen of blood or urine (the patient's first urine of the morning). These tests detect whether or not the hormone human chorionic gonadotropin (HCG), which is produced during pregnancy, is present. A variety of testing kits are available, including over-the-counter urine self-test kits that the patient can use at home.

These tests are not foolproof; false positives and false negatives do occur. An abnormal pregnancy can result in a lower level of HCG, not detectable by the tests. Urine specimens that contain blood, protein, or drugs can also give a false positive result. False negatives may result from testing too early or from a urine specimen that is too dilute. The tests are also subject to human error. The physician confirms pregnancy after taking the patient's history, performing an examination, and ordering a pregnancy test.

Tests for STDs. The doctor diagnoses and treats STDs by taking bacterial and tissue cultures, examining lesions, ordering blood tests, and discussing the patient's history, as appropriate for the specific disease. Some facilities do not permit the release of these results, even to the parents of a minor, without the patient's written consent. Be sure you are familiar with your state's regulations regarding the reporting of STDs to the state epidemiology department.

Radiologic Tests. Several radiologic tests are used in obstetrics and gynecology. The gynecologist uses x-ray, ultrasonography, CT scan, and MRI. X-rays are avoided when a patient is pregnant. If it is crucial for a pregnant woman to have an x-ray, a lead apron must cover her abdomen, and she must be made aware that the x-ray could possibly cause an abnormality in the fetus. You will usually schedule the appointment for radiologic tests. Tell the patient when and where to go for the test, and answer her questions about the procedure. Medical assistants need further training to assist with x-ray procedures.

Hysterosalpingography. Hysterosalpingography is an x-ray examination of the fallopian, or uterine, tubes and the uterus that uses a contrast medium, such as dye or air. Because the procedure is quite uncomfortable, the physician may prescribe a sedative.

Mammogram. A mammogram is a low-dose x-ray of the breast, taken with a special mammogram camera. It can detect cancer about 2 years before it can be palpated with BSE. A first, or baseline, mammogram is taken when a woman is between the ages of 35 and 40 for later comparison.

A patient should schedule mammography for the week after her menstrual period, when the breasts are most normal and least swollen. The procedure involves compressing the breast to obtain a clear x-ray (Figure 22-12). Tell the

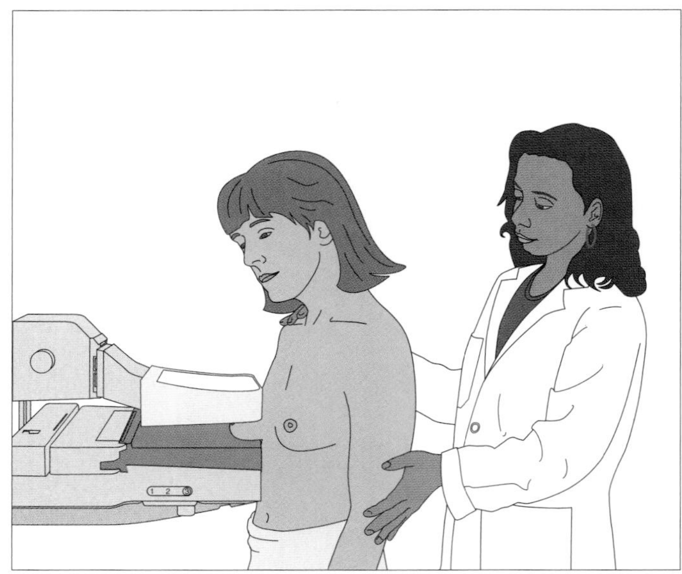

Figure 22-12. Mammography consists of two views of each breast and is achieved by compressing the breast between the radiography plates.

patient that although the procedure is uncomfortable, it is usually not painful. The patient should avoid wearing perfume, deodorant, or body powders on the day of the examination because they can cause false readings.

Fetal Screening. Tests for determining the health of an unborn child are performed on many women. Some, such as an ultrasound, may be performed routinely. Other tests are used only for women whose unborn babies are at high risk of having birth defects. Fetal screening tests can indicate the presence of several birth defects, including Down syndrome and spina bifida. The doctor will consider the patient's age and medical history and the age of the unborn baby when ordering fetal screening tests.

Alpha Fetoprotein. Alpha fetoprotein (AFP) is a protein produced by the unborn child that normally passes into the blood of the mother. A blood test determines whether the AFP level in the blood is normal. Too little or too much AFP in the blood can indicate a fetal abnormality. AFP is also measured in amniotic fluid collected by amniocentesis.

Ultrasound. Ultrasound translates the echoes of sound waves into a picture of an internal part of the body. The picture or image is called a sonogram, and it can help identify and diagnose cysts and tumors in the abdominal cavity or obstructions of the urinary tract. Ultrasound is painless and safe to use on pregnant women to determine fetal size and position. It is also used to guide a physician in performing amniocentesis.

A patient who is going to have an ultrasound examination during early pregnancy should be instructed not to urinate before the test, because a full bladder allows a better view of the uterus. The patient is asked to lie on an examining table, and a gel or lotion is applied to enhance sound wave conduction and reduce friction of the transducer on the skin (Figure 22-13).

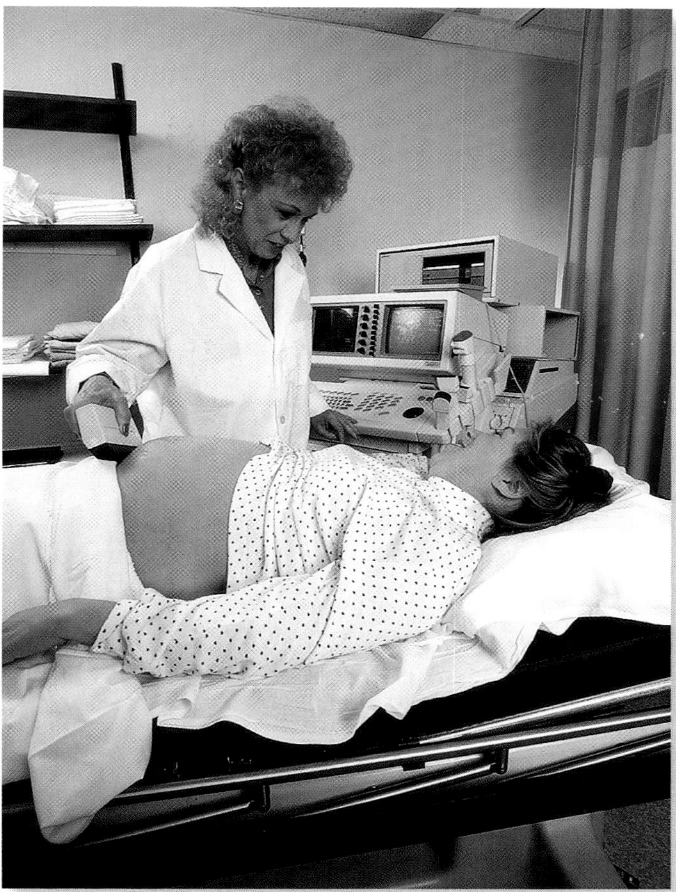

Figure 22-13. An ultrasound technician lightly rubs the transducer over a pregnant woman's abdomen to reveal the anatomy of her fetus.

Diagnostic and Therapeutic Procedures. Many surgical OB/GYN procedures require the use of needles or other instruments to obtain tissue or amniotic fluid samples. Some procedures are used for obstetric reasons only; others may be used gynecologically and obstetrically.

Amniocentesis. Amniocentesis is a procedure performed when a genetic or metabolic defect is suspected in a fetus. The test involves removing a small amount of amniotic fluid, which surrounds the fetus, from the uterus. The doctor inserts a needle, which is guided with ultrasonography, through the anesthetized lower abdominal wall. Fetal skin cells obtained from the fluid are then grown in a culture and examined for chromosomal abnormalities. The level of AFP may also be measured in amniotic fluid.

Biopsy. Biopsy is the surgical removal of tissue for later microscopic examination. It is the most accurate and, in some cases, the only way to diagnose breast and other cancers. Biopsy of the endometrium, which is the mucous membrane lining the uterus, may help the doctor diagnose uterine cancer and show whether ovulation is occurring. It may also indicate whether infection, polyps, or abnormal cells are present. If a patient's Pap smear indicates abnormal cells, a cervical or endocervical biopsy may be performed to rule out or diagnose cervical cancer. Procedure 22-4 explains how to assist with a cervical biopsy.

To assist with these biopsies, you must have knowledge of the female anatomy, the order of procedure, and the instruments used. You will also need to instruct patients about having an escort, appropriate clothing, and any special dietary restrictions. A careful medical history must be obtained to screen for problems such as possible allergic reactions. The day before the biopsy, you might call the patient to confirm the appointment and address any concerns.

A biopsy is considered minor surgery and consequently requires observance of Universal Precautions and sterile technique. Depending on the extent and site of the biopsy, the patient may be given sedation or local anesthesia. During the procedure you may be responsible for clipping excess material from sutures (stitches) and any other special assistance the doctor requests. You must place the biopsy specimen in a sterile, solution-filled container provided by the laboratory. You may assist with or perform the cleaning and bandaging of the site after the procedure.

PROCEDURE 22.4

Assisting With a Cervical Biopsy

Objective: To assist the physician in obtaining a sample of cervical tissue for analysis

OSHA Guidelines

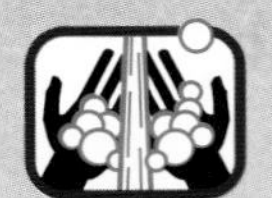
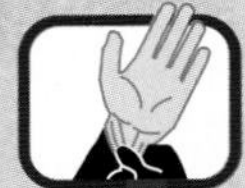
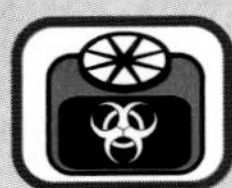
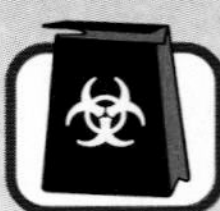
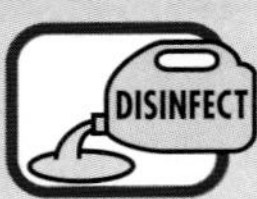

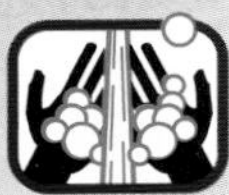

Materials: Gown and drape, tray or Mayo stand, disposable cervical biopsy kit (disposable forceps, curette, and spatula in a sterile pack), transfer forceps, vaginal speculum, biopsy specimen container, clean basin, sterile cotton balls, sterile gauze squares, sanitary napkin

Method

1. Identify the patient and introduce yourself.
2. Look at the patient's chart, and ask the patient to confirm information or explain any changes. Specific patient information you need to ask about and note in the chart includes the following:
   - Date of birth and Social Security number (verify that you have the correct chart for the correct patient)
   - Date of last menstrual period
   - Method of contraception if any
   - Previous gynecologic surgery
   - Use of hormone replacement therapy or other steroids
3. Describe the biopsy procedure to the patient, noting that a piece of tissue will be removed to diagnose the cause of her problem. Explain that it may be painful but only for the brief moment during which tissue is taken.
4. Give the patient a gown, if needed, and a drape. Direct her to undress from the waist down and to wrap the drape around herself. Tell her to sit at the end of the examining table.
5. Wash your hands and put on examination gloves.
6. Using sterile method, open the sterile pack to create a sterile field on the tray or Mayo stand, and arrange the instruments with transfer forceps. Add the vaginal speculum and sterile supplies to the sterile field.
7. When the physician arrives in the examining room, ask the patient to lie back, place her heels in the stirrups of the table, and move her buttocks to the edge of the table.
8. Assist the physician by arranging the drape so that only the genitalia are exposed, and place the light so that the genitalia are illuminated.
9. Use transfer forceps to hand instruments and supplies to the physician as he requests them. When he is ready to obtain the biopsy, tell the patient that it may hurt. If she seems particularly fearful, instruct her to take a deep breath and let it out slowly.
10. When the physician hands you the instrument with the tissue specimen, place the specimen in the specimen container and discard the instrument in the appropriate container.
11. Label the specimen container with the patient's name, the date and time, cervical or endocervical (as indicated by the physician), the physician's name, and your initials.
12. Place the container and the cytology laboratory requisition form in the envelope or bag provided by the laboratory.
13. When the physician has removed the vaginal speculum, place it in the clean basin for later sanitization, disinfection, and sterilization. Properly dispose of used supplies and disposable instruments.
14. Remove the gloves and wash your hands.
15. Tell the patient that she may get dressed. Inform her that she may have some vaginal bleeding for a couple of days, and provide her with a sanitary napkin. Instruct her not to take tub baths or have intercourse and not to use tampons for 2 days. Encourage her to call the office if she experiences problems or has questions.

Colposcopy. **Colposcopy** is the examination of the vagina and cervix with an instrument called a colposcope. Assisting with the colposcopy procedure is similar to assisting with a cervical biopsy. The physician first cleanses the cervix with saline solution. She then cleanses the cervix with acetic acid, which makes abnormal tissue appear white. The physician inserts the colposcope into the vagina and uses the attached magnifying lens to identify abnormal cells, such as cancerous or precancerous cells.

This procedure is often performed prior to a biopsy after results of a Pap smear show the presence of abnormal cells. The abnormal cells may not be cancerous but may be caused by infection or medication.

Dilation and Curettage (D and C). A D and C consists of widening the opening of the cervix (dilation) and scraping the uterine lining (curettage). Reasons for the D and C procedure include assessing the size and shape of the uterus, removing polyps and fibroids from the endometrium, obtaining endometrial specimens for biopsy, performing an abortion, and completing an incomplete miscarriage. Other diagnoses for which a D and C may be performed include abnormal uterine bleeding, abnormal menstrual bleeding, postcoital bleeding, spotting between periods, postmenopausal bleeding, and an imbedded intrauterine device (IUD).

The procedure is usually performed in a hospital or outpatient surgical facility. Tell the patient she will need to have someone take her to and from the facility. Inform the patient that she will have anesthesia before the doctor performs a routine pelvic examination. The doctor then swabs the vagina with an antiseptic and inserts a speculum. After dilating the cervix, the doctor uses a curette to remove a portion of the endometrium to assess the texture. Both cervical and endometrial tissue may be sent to a laboratory for examination. Exploration of the uterine cavity and removal of any abnormal growths complete the procedure.

Instruct the patient not to have intercourse, take tub baths, or use tampons for 1 week after the procedure. She should also avoid strenuous activity.

Fine-Needle Aspiration. During fine-needle aspiration the physician uses a fine needle to remove by vacuum a sample of tissue from a cyst, lump, or tumor of the breast. This procedure may be used instead of mammography to diagnose breast disorders in pregnant patients, thus avoiding the use of radiation. Patients with fibrocystic breast disease (involving multiple cystic lumps within the breast tissue) may have needle aspiration of a cyst followed by replacement of the cystic fluid with a steroid to prevent recurrence.

Hysterectomy. A hysterectomy is the surgical removal of the uterus. If surgery includes removal of one or both fallopian tubes, it is called a hysterosalpingectomy. Surgical removal of the uterus, the fallopian tubes, and the ovaries is called a hysterosalpingo-oophorectomy. A hysterectomy or a related surgery may be performed for the following reasons: cervical or endometrial cancer; severe endometriosis; unusual bleeding; a leiomyoma, or fibroid; defects of pelvic supports; pregnancy-related problems; and pelvic adhesions or other causes of uterine pain not controllable by other methods.

Inform the patient that a procedure of this type is major surgery that requires hospitalization. It also requires preadmission urine and blood tests, cleansing enemas, and shaving of the pelvic area. Normal activities, including sexual intercourse, can usually be resumed within a few weeks.

Premenopausal women who have hysterectomies or hysterosalpingectomies may begin menopause sooner than they otherwise would have. Premenopausal women who have hysterosalpingo-oophorectomies will experience menopause immediately after the surgery. In the past, some doctors prescribed hormone replacement therapy to help alleviate menopausal symptoms.

Laparoscopy. A laparoscope is a long tubular instrument. It contains fiber-optic threads that illuminate the organs and a lens that resembles a small telescope. A physician can use the laparoscope to view the internal female organs. Laparoscopy is used to help determine the cause of infertility, to obtain tissue samples, to remove abnormal growths, and to surgically sterilize a patient. It is also used in the treatment of ectopic pregnancies, endometriosis, and laparoscopy-assisted hysterectomy.

The patient is anesthetized before a tube is inserted into a small incision in or near the navel. Carbon dioxide or another gas is pumped into the abdomen to spread the organs apart and thereby make them easier to see. The patient's body is then tilted with her head lower than her hips to allow the intestines to move away from the lower abdomen. This positioning permits a clearer view of the ovaries, uterus, and fallopian tubes.

Pap Smear. A Pap smear is used to determine the presence of abnormal or precancerous cells. As discussed earlier, during a pelvic examination, cells from the cervix, endocervix, and vagina are smeared on a special, properly labeled slide. They are then sprayed with a fixative and sent to a laboratory for microscopic analysis. The test results are classified according to level of abnormality, using the standardized Bethesda system (Table 22-3).

Pregnancy

Pregnancy progresses in three stages. These stages are referred to as trimesters, and each lasts for 3 months. Figure 22-14 shows the developing fetus during each stage of growth.

First Trimester. After conception, the resulting cell begins to divide. This cluster of cells, the embryo, is implanted in the uterine wall about 36 hours after fertilization. Implantation initiates the embryonic period, during which most of the organ systems develop. The embryonic period lasts 8 weeks, after which the embryo is called a fetus. Week 12 marks the end of the first trimester, or one-third of the pregnancy.

Second Trimester. Fine, soft hair (lanugo) appears on the shoulders, back, and head of the fetus during the fourth month. By the twentieth week fetal movement may be felt, and the pregnant woman begins to show fullness in the abdomen. There are identifiable periods of fetal sleep and wakefulness as the second trimester ends at the completion of the sixth month.

Third Trimester. The last trimester encompasses the most noticeable period of growth, both in the fetus and in the mother. By the end of 30 weeks, the fetus has assumed a head-down position and has a 50% chance of survival if

TABLE 22-3 The Bethesda System for Classification of the Papanicolaou Smear

Classification	What It Means	Tests and Treatments That May Be Included
Negative	No intraepithelial lesion or malignancy	Continue routine Pap smears
ASC—atypical squamous cells, which may present in one of two types:	ASC— abnormalities in the squamous cells, which are the thin, flat cells on the cervix	
ASC-US—atypical squamous cells of undetermined significance	ASC-US—Considered a mild abnormality; may be related to HPV infection	Repeat the Pap smear; sometimes changes can go away without treatment
ASC-H—atypical squamous cells that cannot exclude a high-grade squamous intraepithelial lesion	ASC-H—May be at risk of being precancerous	HPV testing; repeat Pap test; colposcopy and biopsy; administer estrogen cream
AGC—atypical glandular cells (mucus-producing cells)	Glandular cells do not appear normal, but it is uncertain what the changes mean	Colposcopy and biopsy; endocervical curettage
AIS—endocervical adenocarcinoma in situ	Precancerous cells are found in the glandular tissue	Colposcopy and biopsy; endocervical curettage
LSIL—low-grade squamous intraepithelial lesion May also be called mild dysplasia or cervical intraepithelial neoplasia-1 (CIN-1)	Early changes in cells and an area of abnormal tissue; mild abnormalities caused by HPV infection	Colposcopy and biopsy
HSIL—high-grade squamous intraepithelial lesion May also be called moderate dysplasia, severe dysplasia, CIN-2, CIN-3, or carcinoma in situ (CIS)	Marked changes in the size and shape of the abnormal (precancerous) cells; a higher likelihood of progressing to invasive cancer	Colposcopy and biopsy; endocervical curettage; further treatment with cryotherapy, laser therapy, conization, or hysterectomy

it is born at this time. The fetus is said to have come full term after it is approximately 9 months (40 weeks) old.

Nägele's Rule. To estimate the delivery date for a pregnant woman, most doctors use Nägele's rule. Begin with the first day of the patient's last menstrual period, subtract 3 months, and add 7 days plus 1 year. If, for example, the first day of the last menstrual period was June 30, 2004, subtracting 3 months would give you March 30, 2004. After the addition of 7 days plus 1 year, April 6, 2005, would be the estimated delivery date.

Prenatal Care. Pregnant women need to be particularly attentive to nutrition, exercise, medical monitoring, and childbirth classes. They should avoid using tobacco, alcohol, and drugs. Normal manifestations during pregnancy include morning sickness (usually in the first trimester), weight gain, urinary frequency, fatigue, depression, constipation, and swollen hands and feet.

You may perform or assist with routine tests for pregnant women, or you may send them to an outside laboratory. These tests may include the complete blood count (CBC), Rh-antibody determination, blood typing, Pap smear, urinalysis, and hematocrit. Others may include tests for syphilis, hepatitis B antibodies, HIV, and chlamydia.

Assisting With Prenatal Care. You will play an important role in encouraging the obstetric patient to have regular checkups and to take proper care of herself. You will also help teach and support both parents throughout the pregnancy. You must document all information given to or taken from the patient.

Providing information on the effects of using drugs or alcohol during pregnancy is particularly important. Alcohol, for example, crosses the placental barrier and directly affects fetal development. Drinking alcohol during pregnancy can cause fetal alcohol syndrome (FAS). This syndrome may include fetal growth deficiencies, mental retardation or

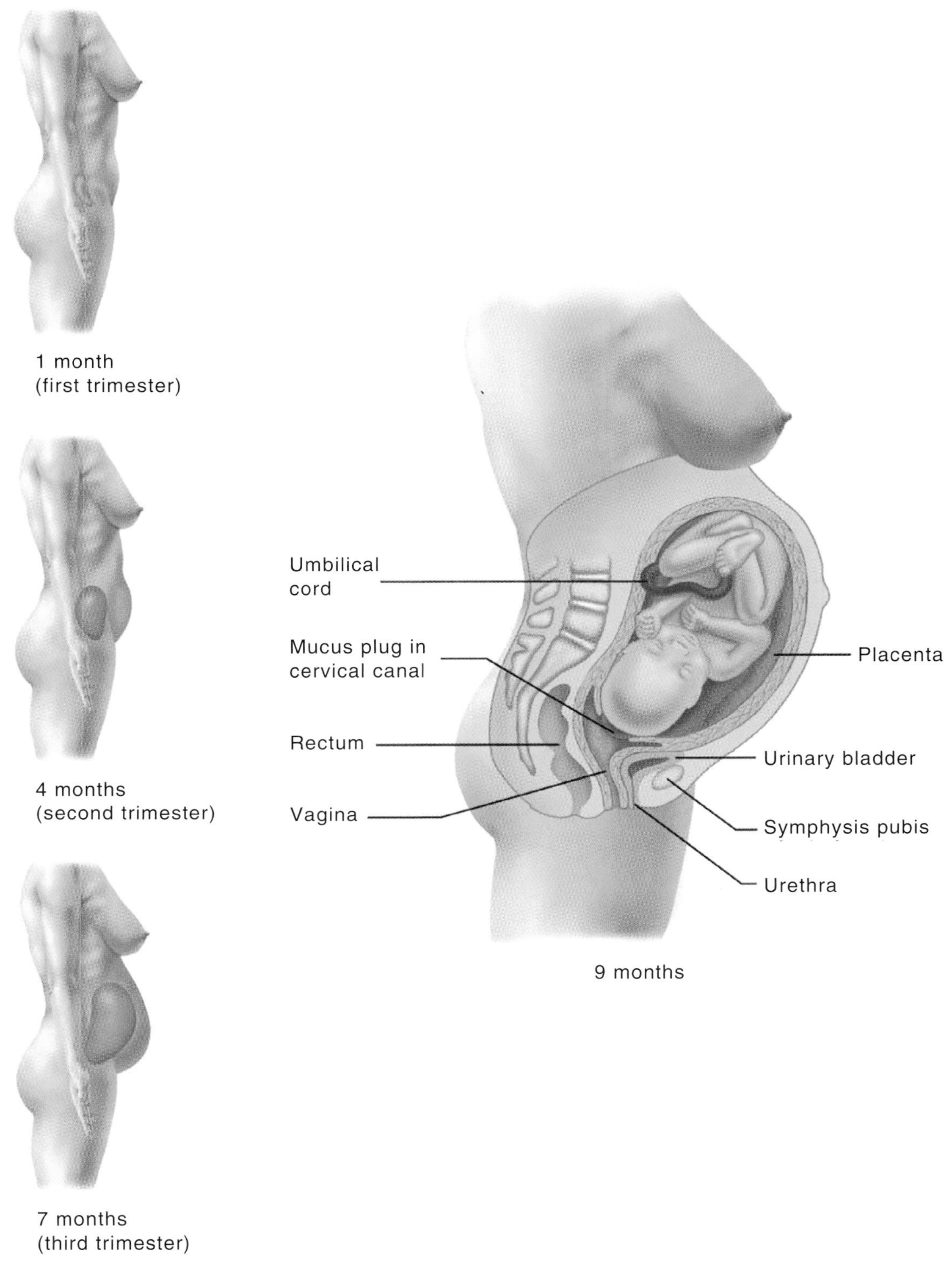

Figure 22-14. The fetus develops over the course of three trimesters.
Source: McGraw-Hill's Digital Asset Library.

learning disabilities, heart defects, cleft palate, a small head, a small brain, and deformed limbs. There is no known safe level of alcohol consumption during pregnancy. You can help prevent FAS by teaching all pregnant patients about the potential effects of alcohol on their unborn babies. If a pregnant patient who is an alcoholic expresses a desire to stop drinking, inform the physician, who may wish to discuss admission to an alcoholic rehabilitation program with her. You may also refer the patient to Alcoholics Anonymous or a similar community group for assistance. Drug use during pregnancy poses similar problems for a woman's developing fetus.

When assisting with routine prenatal patient visits, you may:

1. Ask the patient about any problems and record any symptoms she reports.
2. Ask the patient to empty her bladder and obtain a urine specimen in the cup you provide.
3. Weigh the patient and note her weight in the chart.
4. Perform the reagent urine test (chemical analysis) and note the results in her chart.
5. Give the patient a drape and ask her to undress from the waist down if the physician will be performing an internal examination.
6. Assist the patient to the examining table. Take her vital signs. Record them in her chart.
7. Assist the physician as needed with the examination. Provide the flexible centimeter tape measure and Doppler, an instrument used to listen to fetal heartbeat.
8. Assist the patient from the examining table after the examination.

Prenatal Care by the Doctor. The doctor carefully monitors the progress of a pregnancy. She watches blood pressure, weight changes, and urinalysis results for possible signs of preeclampsia. Increased blood pressure (hypertension), unusual weight gain due to edema, and protein in the urine are signs of this serious complication of pregnancy. The doctor examines urine specimens for possible urinary tract infections and occasionally asks for other laboratory tests, such as a complete blood count. She may prescribe special vitamins and iron as dietary supplements.

Labor. Changes occur in the mother's body chemistry when the fetus is ready to be born. These changes signal the release of the hormone oxytocin, which initiates labor. The first stage of labor is marked by regular contractions and cervical dilation. The second stage is characterized by complete cervical dilation and the entrance of the head (or buttocks if it is a breech birth) into the vagina. Further contractions and the mother's bearing down push the baby into the birth canal and out of the mother's body. The last contractions push out the placenta and its membranes (afterbirth), attached to the baby with the umbilical cord. This is the third and final stage of labor.

Delivery. At birth a newborn's average weight and length are 7.5 lb and 20 inches. The baby's mouth and nose are suctioned to clear them of mucus. Crying indicates that the baby is breathing on her own. The lungs inflate, and the color of the skin changes from bluish to normal. The physician clamps, ties, and cuts the umbilical cord and presents the baby to the mother.

If the pregnant woman cannot deliver the baby vaginally, the physician may deliver the baby by performing an operation known as a cesarean section. Several conditions may require a cesarean section, such as a large baby in a breech position. To perform a cesarean section, the physician makes a series of incisions. First the skin, underlying muscles, and abdomen are opened. Then the uterus is opened, and the infant is removed.

Newborn Function Testing. The newborn is assessed at 1 and 5 minutes after delivery for neurological function. This is known as the Apgar test. The tests are repeated until the infant's condition stabilizes. With the Apgar test, the baby's heart rate, respiratory effort, muscle tone, reflex irritability, and color are each evaluated with a score of 0, 1, or 2. The best possible Apgar rating is 10 (five evaluations with a score of 2). A score of 7 to 9 is adequate; 4 to 6 indicates that treatment and close observation are warranted; below 4 requires immediate treatment.

Breast-Feeding. Human milk is the preferred form of nutrition for an infant. Colostrum, the first milk the mother produces after delivery, is rich in antibodies that provide passive natural immunity to the baby as well. Breast-feeding is economical and convenient. There is no need to buy or make formula or wash bottles and nipples. Breast milk is always available to the baby at the correct temperature.

A woman's success at breast-feeding depends largely on her desire to breast-feed, her satisfaction with it, and her available support systems. You can support patients who choose to breast-feed by providing them with pamphlets and other written materials. Emphasize how essential the mother's nutritional intake is, and explain that she needs to follow a high-protein, high-calorie diet. Patients who need help may be referred to lactation consultants or support groups such as the La Leche League.

Contraception

Couples who want to prevent pregnancy practice contraception. The type of contraception chosen is based on variables such as price, convenience, effectiveness, and side effects. The only method that is 100% effective is abstinence. Contraceptive methods include the following:

- The birth control pill is a daily oral contraceptive. Synthetic hormones in the pills inhibit ovulation.
- The birth control patch is placed on the lower abdomen or buttocks. It is replaced once a week for 3 weeks, then no patch is used the 4th week.
- Subdermal implants consist of 6 capsules of synthetic hormone that are surgically implanted under the skin of the arm. They provide 5 years of contraception and are reversible.
- Injection is a method in which a synthetic hormone is administered every 3 months to inhibit ovulation.
- A condom is worn on the penis or inserted into the vagina to serve as a barrier to sperm.
- Spermicidal foam, cream, jelly, and vaginal suppositories contain spermicides (sperm-killing chemicals). They are inserted into the woman's vagina.
- A diaphragm is a dome-shaped rubber cup prescribed to fit over the patient's cervix and used with spermicide to provide a barrier to sperm.

- A vaginal contraceptive ring is inserted by the woman for 3 weeks and then removed for 1 week.
- A cervical cap is similar to a diaphragm, except that it covers a smaller area of the woman's cervix.
- An IUD is a small piece of plastic or metal that fits inside the uterus and inhibits fertilization or implantation. Insertion of an IUD is performed by a doctor.
- Sterilization is a surgical procedure. A man can have a vasectomy, in which the doctor removes a section of each tube that carries sperm from each testicle to the penis. A female can have her fallopian tubes cut or blocked.
- Periodic abstinence (sometimes called the rhythm method) involves refraining from sexual intercourse when a woman is fertile and likely to become pregnant.
- Withdrawal consists of withdrawing the penis from the vagina before ejaculation occurs.
- Postcoital pills taken to prevent implantation of the embryo in the uterus must be taken within 72 hours of having unprotected sex.

Contraception information should be obtained and provided to patients as required. The Planned Parenthood Federation, the National Library of Medicine, and the FDA are valuable resources.

Infertility

Infertility is the inability of a couple to conceive a child. Physicians usually test both the man and woman for infertility. Depending on the cause of the problem, the physician may treat the man, the woman, or both.

If you work in an OB/GYN office, the physicians may test couples for fertility and provide them with treatments or options so they can have children. In such an office you should be familiar with basic infertility tests and treatments. You may need to explain procedures to couples, assist with tests or treatments, and provide emotional support and encouragement.

Tests to determine the cause of infertility in a woman examine whether ovulation occurs, whether the fallopian tubes are clear of obstruction, whether the uterus is healthy enough to support the implantation and growth of a fetus, and whether the woman is healthy enough to maintain pregnancy. Tests to determine the cause of infertility in a man examine whether the sperm are healthy and numerous enough to fertilize an egg.

TABLE 22-4 Common Obstetric and Gynecologic Diseases and Disorders

Condition	Description	Treatment
Cancer	Common occurrence in cervix, endometrium (uterus), ovaries; cells divide uncontrollably, eventually forming tumor or other growth of abnormal tissue; most often seen in women between the ages of 50 and 60; symptoms differ for each type of cancer	Surgery (hysterectomy), radiation, chemotherapy, hormones; for ovarian cancer, surgical removal of all reproductive organs, affected lymph nodes, appendix, and some muscle tissue, followed by chemotherapy (to extend survival time)
Ectopic pregnancy	Fertilized egg unable to move out of fallopian tube into uterus for implantation; patient experiences pain within a few weeks of conception; can be fatal	Surgery to remove embryo from fallopian tube before tube ruptures
Endometriosis	Endometrial tissue present outside uterus, usually in pelvic area; not life-threatening but may cause sterility; symptoms include abnormal menstruation and pain (sometimes severe) in lower abdominal area and back	Hormone therapy, hysterectomy for severe cases, endometrial ablation (1-day surgery, alternative to hysterectomy), leuprolide acetate injection
Fibroids, or leiomyomas	Common, benign, smooth tumors of muscle cells (not fibrous tissue) grouped in uterus; symptoms include excessive menstruation and bloating; diagnosis by bimanual examination and ultrasound	Surgery for severe cases
Fibrocystic breast disease	Benign, fluid-filled cysts or nodules in breast; sometimes confused with malignant growths in breast until complete diagnostic tests performed; symptoms include pain and tenderness	Depending on severity, vitamin E supplements, hormones, compresses, analgesics, aspiration, biopsy; restricted caffeine intake

continued →

TABLE 22-4 Common Obstetric and Gynecologic Diseases and Disorders *(continued)*

Condition	Description	Treatment
Menstrual disturbances	May be (1) amenorrhea (absence of menstruation), (2) dysmenorrhea (painful menstruation), (3) menorrhagia (excessive amount of menstrual flow or prolonged period of menstruation), or (4) metrorrhagia (bleeding between menstrual periods)	Treatment according to symptoms; analgesics; possibly D and C; for severe cases, hysterectomy
Ovarian cysts	Sacs of fluid or semisolid material, usually benign and without symptoms; occur anytime between puberty and menopause; extensive ovarian cysts may cause pelvic discomfort, lower back pain, and abnormal bleeding	Analgesics and bed rest if severe pain; hormone therapy; surgery, usually reserved for cysts that rupture or are large enough to put pressure on surrounding organs
Pelvic inflammatory disease (PID)	Acute, chronic infection of reproductive tract; causes include untreated STDs, such as gonorrhea and chlamydia, and organisms such as staphylococci and streptococci; symptoms include vaginal discharge, fever, and general discomfort	Antibiotics
Pelvic support problems	Abnormal weakening of vaginal tissue, unusual increase in abdominal pressure, congenital weakening (weakness since birth); symptoms include urine leakage, pelvic heaviness ("bottom falling out"), pain or discomfort in pelvic area, pulling or aching feeling in lower back, abdomen, or groin	Kegel or perineal exercises to strengthen muscles, insertion of pessary (device to hold pelvic organs in place), surgery to repair muscles
Polyps	Red, soft, and fragile growths, with slender stem attachment, sometimes found on mucous membranes of cervix or endometrium; may cause pain	Depending on size and shape, may be removed in office or hospital
Premenstrual dysphoric disorder (PMDD)	A severe form of premenstrual syndrome that affects 5% of women; symptoms have a very disrupting effect on the patient's life; screening tests and physician evaluation are necessary for diagnosis	Medications, including antidepressants, antianxiety drugs, analgesics, hormones, and diuretics; exercise, relaxation, diet modification, vitamins, minerals, and herbal preparations are also useful
Premenstrual syndrome (PMS)	Symptoms include swelling, bloating, weight gain, breast tenderness, headaches, and mood shifts 1 week to 10 days before menstruation	Vitamins, diuretics, hormones, oral contraceptives, tranquilizers, other medications; stress-reduction methods as needed; restricted intake of dietary sodium, alcohol, and caffeine
Sexual function disorders	Interruption or lack of sexual response cycle (excitement, plateau, orgasm, and resolution); unhealthy view of one's feelings about oneself as a woman and feelings toward sex; sometimes caused by painful intercourse, abusive partner, unrealistic demands on oneself, or menopause	Counseling (for both woman and partner) to teach relaxation, effective communication, and identification of cycle stages and natural responses
Vaginitis	Inflammation of vagina caused by bacteria, viruses, yeasts, or chemicals in sprays, douches, or tampons; symptoms include itching, redness, pain, swelling	Treatment prescribed according to cause; avoiding douches, tampons, tight pants, wiping from back to front; sometimes avoiding sex during treatment

themselves locally—with a skin rash or nasal congestion—or may manifest themselves throughout the body.

The most severe kind of allergic reaction is anaphylaxis, or anaphylactic shock, which is life-threatening. Symptoms of anaphylaxis include respiratory distress, difficulty in swallowing, pallor, and a drastic drop in blood pressure that can lead to circulatory collapse. When anaphylaxis occurs, immediate medical intervention is needed to save the patient's life. Chapter 26 addresses emergency medical intervention in anaphylaxis.

Allergy Examinations

An allergy examination involves a medical history and, usually, several diagnostic tests. You may assist with these tests or perform them yourself under a physician's supervision. Skin tests, for example, involve introducing solutions containing suspected allergens onto or just below the skin. Any reaction is observed and assessed.

As an allergist's medical assistant, you will need to understand the function of the immune system and how allergies are commonly treated. Allergy treatments include allergen avoidance, medications, and desensitization to a substance by means of injections. Part of your job will be to encourage patients to make necessary lifestyle changes to avoid allergens. You will also help them adhere to regimens of injections or medication.

Allergy Testing

Three tests are commonly performed in the allergist's office. They are the scratch test, the intradermal test, and the patch test. The radioallergosorbent test is performed in a laboratory.

Scratch Test. A **scratch test** is performed to test the patient for specific allergies. Extracts of suspected allergens are applied to the patient's skin, usually on the arms or back. One site is always a negative control— a solution like the one used to carry the allergens but containing no allergen is applied. Then the skin is scratched to allow the extracts to penetrate. Procedure 23-1 describes how to

PROCEDURE 23.1

Performing a Scratch Test

Objective: To determine substances to which a patient has an allergic reaction

OSHA Guidelines

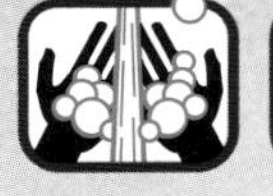
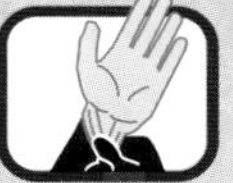
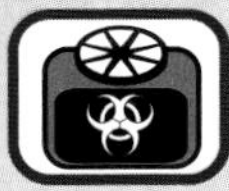

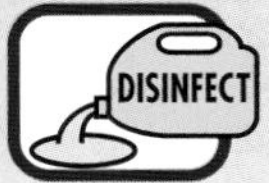

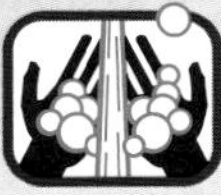

Materials: Disposable sterile needles or lancets, allergen extracts, control solution, cotton balls, alcohol, timer, adhesive tape, ruler, cold packs or ice bag

Method

1. Wash your hands and assemble the necessary materials.
2. Identify the patient and introduce yourself.
3. Show the patient into the treatment area. Explain the procedure and discuss any concerns.
4. Put on examination gloves and assist the patient into a comfortable position.
5. Swab the test site, usually the upper arm or back, with an alcohol-soaked cotton ball. Allow the test site to air-dry.

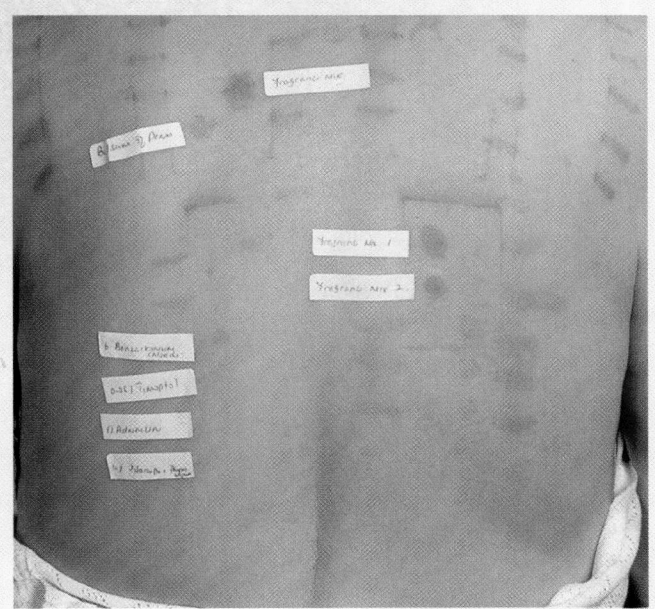

Figure 23-1. Label each site with the name of the allergen or an accepted abbreviation.

6. Apply small drops of the allergen extracts and control solution onto the test site at evenly spaced intervals, about 1½ to 2 inches apart.

continued ⟶

PROCEDURE 23.1

Performing a Scratch Test *(continued)*

7. Identify the sites (if more than one) with adhesive-tape labels (Figure 23-1).
8. Open the package containing the first needle or lancet, making sure you do not contaminate the instrument.
9. Using a new sterile needle or lancet for each site, scratch the skin beneath each drop of allergen, no more than ⅛-inch deep.
10. Start the timer for the 20-minute reaction period.
11. After the reaction time has passed, cleanse each site with an alcohol-soaked cotton ball. (Do not remove identifying labels until the doctor has checked the patient.)
12. Examine and measure the sites (Figure 23-2).
13. Apply cold packs or an ice bag to sites as needed to relieve itching.
14. Record the test results in the patient's chart, and initial your entries.
15. Properly dispose of used materials and instruments.
16. Clean and disinfect the area according to OSHA guidelines.
17. Remove the gloves and wash your hands.

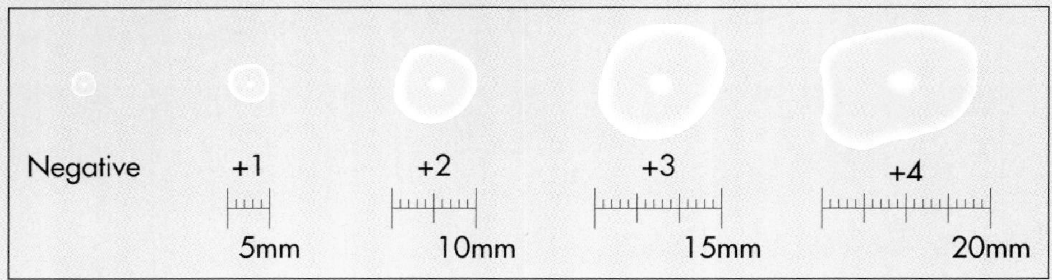

Figure 23-2. Physicians classify skin reactions as either negative (no greater than the reaction to the control) or positive. Positive reactions are rated on a scale of +1 to +4, depending on the size of the wheal.

perform a scratch test using sterile needles or lancets. Some allergists prefer to use multiple applicators that allow the tester to apply allergens to and puncture the skin in several places at once, as shown in Figure 23-3.

Be sure to let the patient know that the procedure may cause some discomfort and that itching afterward can be relieved with cold packs. The doctor interprets the test results. Because a delayed reaction is possible, the doctor may wish to recheck the scratch sites in 24 hours. When the results of the scratch test are inconclusive, another test, such as an intradermal test, may be ordered.

Intradermal Test. An allergist performs an **intradermal test** by introducing dilute solutions of allergens into the skin of the inner forearm or upper back with a fine-gauge needle. The intradermal test is more sensitive than the scratch test. A small blister, also known as a wheal, that is filled with the introduced fluid appears on the skin over the injection site. The allergic reaction time is about 15 to 30 minutes, although some substances may cause delayed reactions. If no reaction appears, the test can be repeated with a more concentrated solution to confirm the

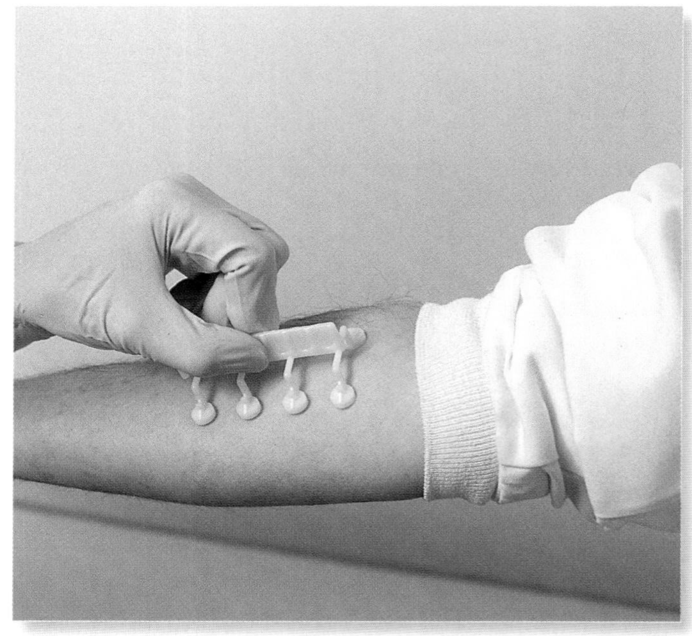

Figure 23-3. A multiple applicator allows the medical assistant to apply several allergens at one time.

result. If a severe reaction occurs, the doctor will order epinephrine to be administered.

The tuberculin test, or purified protein derivative (PPD) test, is a type of intradermal skin test. In most offices today it is administered with a needle and syringe. (In the past this test was administered using a disposable device consisting of a disk with tines and was called a tine test.) An extract from the tubercle bacillus is injected into the skin. The results are read in 48 to 72 hours. Raising and hardening of the skin around the area (induration), rather than redness alone, indicate a positive reaction.

Patch Test. You perform a **patch test** by placing a linen or paper patch on uninvolved skin and then using a dropper to soak the patch with the suspected allergen (Figure 23-4). Cellophane or another occlusive, usually covered with an adhesive patch, is then applied over the linen or paper patch. The test is used to discover the cause of contact dermatitis.

Radioallergosorbent Test (RAST). The RAST measures blood levels of antibodies to particular allergens. You obtain a blood sample from the patient and send it to a laboratory. There the blood serum is exposed to suspected allergens, and the levels of antibodies are measured. This test usually provides more information than skin testing but is more expensive.

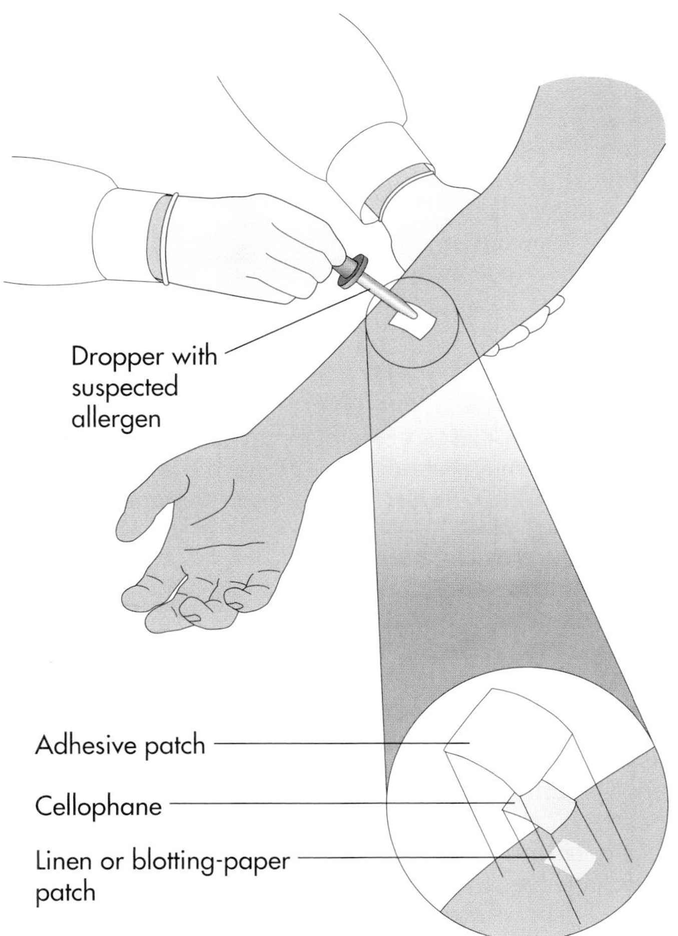

Figure 23-4. A patch test is usually done on the arm and is read in 48 hours.

Cardiology

A physician specializing in heart diseases and disorders is called a cardiologist. To assist a cardiologist, you must be familiar with the structure of the cardiovascular system and the typical examinations and measurements associated with it. You also need to know about common heart diseases and their treatments.

Many of the diagnostic tests performed in this specialty, including electrocardiography and stress testing, are described in detail in Chapter 34. Imaging techniques, such as x-rays and echocardiography, may also be employed. You will assist with or perform some of these tests. Because caring for a heart condition often involves many lifestyle changes, your role in educating the patient about topics such as diet and exercise will be especially important. You will also provide emotional support to patients with serious illnesses.

Cardiology Examinations

A general cardiovascular examination usually begins with cardiac auscultation to obtain a blood pressure reading and an evaluation of overall cardiac health. The cardiologist also palpates the heart and chest wall and the vessels in the extremities to detect abnormal vibrations, pulses, swelling, or temperature. In addition, an electrocardiogram may be obtained.

Electrocardiogram. An electrocardiogram (abbreviated ECG or EKG) provides a measurement of the electrical activity of the heart. Electrocardiography is a painless, safe diagnostic test that is a routine part of a cardiovascular examination. Electrodes are placed on the skin in particular areas of the chest and limbs. The heart's electrical activity is shown as a tracing on a strip of graph paper.

Stress Test. An ECG is usually obtained in one of two ways. A resting ECG is performed while the patient is lying down. A **stress test** involves recording an ECG while the patient is exercising on a stationary bicycle, treadmill, or stair-stepping ergometer. This test measures the patient's response to a constant or increasing workload. Part of your job may involve keeping the equipment properly maintained and calibrated. You may also be responsible for administering the test itself. A doctor should always be present, however, because of the risk of cardiac crisis.

Before the test the patient has a screening appointment with the doctor, during which you take a careful medical history and explain pretest requirements. On the day of the test, be sure the patient has followed pretest directions, such as abstaining from smoking or consuming alcohol, and has signed the proper consent form.

The patient is prepared as for an ECG by having the electrodes attached to the skin. Show the patient how to

Career Opportunities

Doppler and Stress Testing

To gain medical assistant credentials, you must fulfill the requirements of either the American Association of Medical Assistants (for a Certified Medical Assistant) or the American Medical Technologists (for a Registered Medical Assistant). After obtaining your medical assistant certification or registration, you may wish to acquire additional skills in specialty areas through course work or on-the-job training. Although this course work or training may not lead to an additional certification or degree, it will enable you to expand your role in the medical office and advance your career as the demand for skilled health professionals increases.

Skills and Duties

Doppler and stress testing are two procedures that help physicians diagnose cardiac problems. The Doppler test uses an ultrasound transducer, a device that emits and receives ultrasonic waves, to provide a sound wave image of blood flow. The stress test monitors the effect of physical activity on a person's heart. Both procedures can be performed by a medical assistant with appropriate training.

The Doppler test takes between 5 and 10 minutes. The medical assistant applies a special gel to the patient's chest. The gel facilitates the transmission of sound waves. The medical assistant then moves the transducer across the patient's chest, producing a picture on the Doppler screen. This picture can be videotaped or copied in still photographs for later viewing. The assistant records the results of the session and reports them to the physician.

To perform a stress test, the medical assistant uses an electrocardiograph, a machine that monitors the electrical activity of the heart and records the activity as an electrocardiogram (ECG) on special graph paper. The medical assistant attaches metal electrodes (sensors) from the electrocardiograph to the patient's chest, arms, and legs. A baseline ECG of the patient's heartbeat at rest is then obtained.

The patient then exercises on a treadmill or bicycle, with the level of difficulty increasing every 2 to 3 minutes. The medical assistant monitors the patient's blood pressure and ECG and stops the test as soon as the patient experiences fatigue, breathlessness, chest pain, or unusual ECG readings. (A physician is always present during a stress test to deal with cardiac emergencies.) After the test is completed, the assistant records the patient's vital signs. Medical assistants who specialize in Doppler and stress testing may also maintain the equipment, schedule appointments, type test results and physician instructions, and maintain patient files.

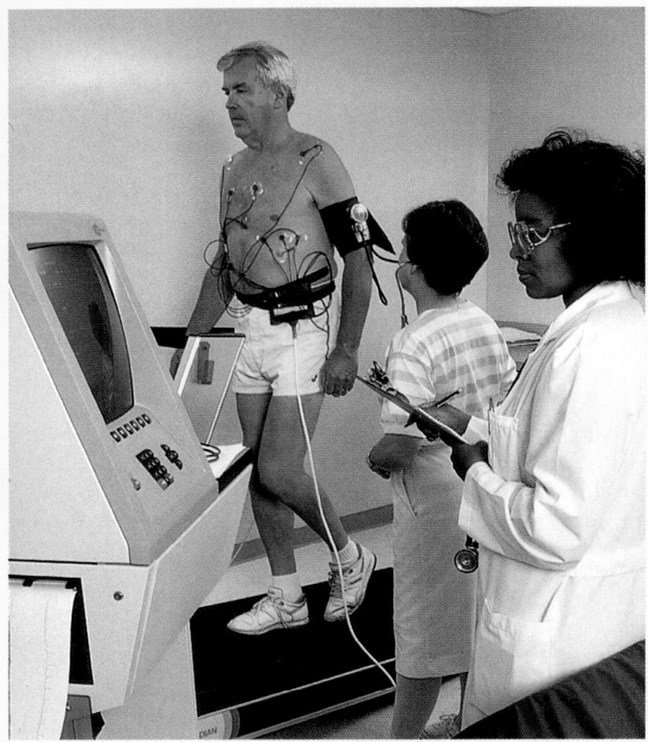

Workplace Settings

Most medical assistants who perform Doppler and stress tests work in a hospital or cardiologist's office. Some medical assistants may perform these tests in clinics, rehabilitation centers, and managed care facilities.

Education

Medical assistants interested in Doppler and stress testing must, at minimum, have a high school diploma. Many medical assistants who specialize in stress testing are trained on the job, a process that takes between 8 and 16 weeks. In addition, some colleges and hospitals offer a 1-year certificate program for stress testing.

To perform Doppler testing, medical assistants must receive additional education. Many colleges offer 2-year programs specializing in noninvasive technology, which features tests such as the Doppler.

continued ⟶

Career Opportunities

Doppler and Stress Testing *(continued)*

Although the job outlook for this area is good, the demand for a technician who performs only these tests may not be high. Health-care professionals who have other skills in addition to training in Doppler and stress testing will find the greatest demand for their services.

Where to Go for More Information

American College of Cardiology
9111 Old Georgetown Road
Bethesda, MD 20814
(301) 897-5400

American Medical Association
Division of Allied Health Education
and Accreditation
515 North State Street
Chicago, IL 60610
(312) 464-5000

American Society for Cardiovascular
Professionals
120 Falcon Drive, Unit 3
Fredericksburg, VA 22408
(540) 891-0079

use the ergometric device. If the device is a treadmill, show the patient how to step on and off it and how to use the metal railing for balance. (Exercise electrocardiography, or stress testing, is further described in Chapter 34.)

A type of stress test called the stress thallium ECG is performed by injecting the radioisotope thallium (^{201}Tl) into the patient's veins at the time of peak stress. The patient is checked several minutes later to find out how much thallium has been taken up by the heart. Damaged areas do not take up the thallium as rapidly as healthy areas do.

Holter Monitor. The Holter monitor is an ECG device that includes a small cassette recorder, allowing readings to be taken over a specific period of time. Electrodes are attached to the patient's chest wall in the physician's office. The patient wears a recording device on a belt or sling (Figure 23-5). The patient returns home, and the device monitors heart activity for 24 hours. (Ambulatory electrocardiography, or Holter monitoring, is fully described in Chapter 34.)

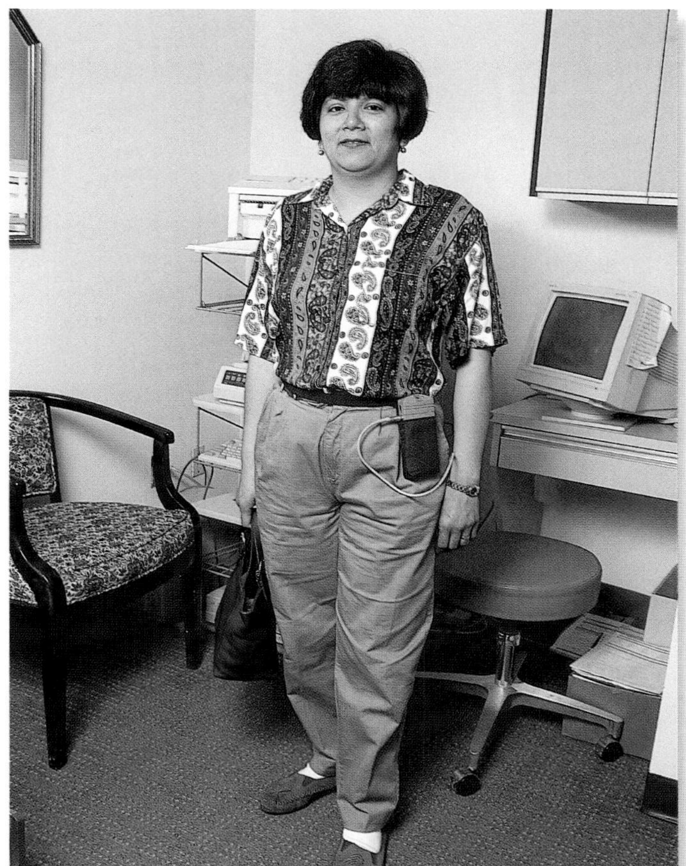

Figure 23-5. A Holter monitor allows the doctor to assess heart function during periods of normal activity.

Radiography Techniques

Various radiography techniques are used in cardiology. Chest x-rays can reveal conditions such as cardiac enlargement. In radionuclide studies, the patient ingests or is injected with a radioactive contrast medium, often referred to as a dye. X-rays are then taken. For example, fluoroscopy studies are x-ray examinations in which a contrast medium is injected and pictures of the heart in motion are projected onto a closed-circuit television screen. A venogram allows evaluation of the deep veins of the legs. **Angiography** is an x-ray examination of a blood vessel after the injection of a contrast medium. The test, performed in a hospital, usually evaluates the function and structure of one or more arteries.

Ultrasound, a noninvasive diagnostic method, is also used in cardiology. Doppler ultrasonography tests the body's main blood vessels for conditions such as weaknesses in vessel walls or blocked arteries. With the use of a handheld probe, sound waves are transmitted through the skin and are reflected by the blood cells moving through the blood vessels.

Echocardiography tests the structure and function of the heart through the use of reflected sound waves, or echoes. Sound waves of an extremely high frequency are projected through the chest wall into the heart and are reflected back through a mechanical device. The echoes, which are recorded on paper, can indicate conditions such as structural defects and fluid accumulation (Figure 23-6).

Cardiac catheterization is a diagnostic method in which a catheter (a slender, hollow tube) is inserted into a vein or artery in the right or left arm or leg and passed through the blood vessels into the heart. The cardiologist can use this method to take blood samples for analysis, measure the pressure in the heart's chambers, and view the heart's motions with the aid of fluoroscopy. The procedure is performed in the hospital and is often combined with angiography.

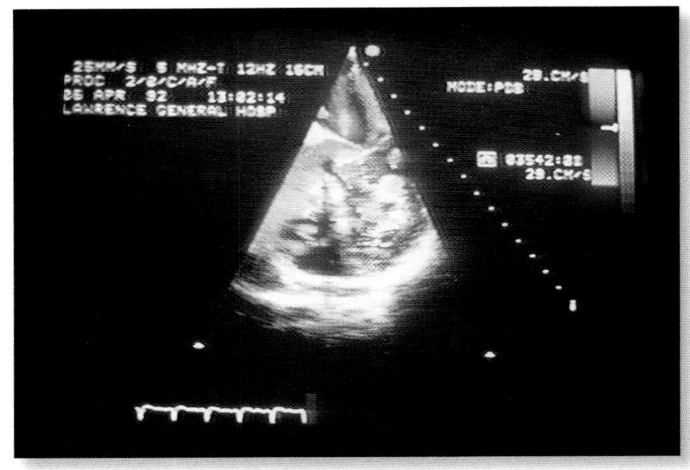

Figure 23-6. An echocardiograph shows the structures and function of the heart.

Cardiac Diseases and Disorders

All of these diagnostic tests are used to reveal heart diseases and disorders. Table 23-1 lists the types of diseases and disorders you may encounter in a cardiologist's office.

TABLE 23-1 Types of Cardiovascular Diseases and Disorders

Category of Disease/Disorder	Common Conditions	Treatment
Arterial/vascular disorders	Aneurysms: abnormal dilation of artery wall caused by area of weakness	Medication, surgery
	Arteriosclerosis: thickening or hardening of arterial wall	Medication, lifestyle and diet management, surgery
	Atherosclerosis: accumulation of deposits along inner walls of arteries, obstructing blood flow	Medication, lifestyle and diet management, surgery
	Hypertension: persistent high blood pressure; systolic pressure greater than 120 mm Hg, diastolic pressure greater than 80 mm Hg	Medication, lifestyle and diet management, stress management
	Varicose veins: distended veins in the legs caused by weakening of vein walls and failure of one-way valves inside veins	Wearing of elastic stockings, weight loss, elevation of legs, weight control, surgery
Cardiomyopathy: disease of heart muscle causing fatigue, breathing problems, and leading to heart failure	Dilated cardiomyopathy: dilated heart chambers	Medication, heart transplant surgery
	Hypertrophic cardiomyopathy: thickening of heart walls and narrowing of chambers	Medication, heart transplant surgery
	Restrictive cardiomyopathy: decrease in elasticity and narrowing of heart chambers	Medication, heart transplant surgery
Coronary artery disease: condition involving partial or complete blockage of major coronary arteries that surround heart	Angina pectoris: disorder caused by reduced blood supply to heart muscle	Medication, rest, lifestyle management
	Myocardial infarction: death of heart tissue because of oxygen deprivation	Medication, oxygen administration, rest, lifestyle management

continued →

TABLE 23-1 Types of Cardiovascular Diseases and Disorders *(continued)*

Category of Disease/Disorder	Common Conditions	Treatment
Dysrhythmias: disorders of heartbeat	Atrial fibrillation: uncoordinated atrial contractions, resulting in diminished cardiac output	Medication, cardioversion (delivery of electric shock to myocardium, or heart muscle)
	Conduction delays or blocks: problems with transmission of electrical impulses in heart	Medication, implantation of pacemaker
	Tachycardia: rapid heartbeat (more than 100 beats per minute)	Medication, diet management
Heart failure	Congestive heart failure: inability of heart to pump blood effectively, causing fluid to build up in tissues and lungs	Medication, diet management, rest
Inflammations: infections of heart tissue, often caused by systemic infections	Endocarditis: inflammation of heart lining, including valves	Medication, surgery to repair or replace valves
	Myocarditis: inflammation of myocardium, or heart muscle	Specific treatment for underlying cause, medication, rest
	Pericarditis: inflammation of pericardium (tissue sac covering heart)	Medication, rest
Valvular diseases: disorders in which heart valves do not open or close fully	Aortic stenosis: narrowing of aortic valve opening, restricting blood flow	Surgical replacement of valve
	Mitral stenosis: narrowing of mitral valve opening, restricting blood flow	Medication, rest, surgical repair or replacement of valve
	Mitral valve prolapse: condition in which a portion of mitral valve falls into left atrium during systole	Medication (usually antibiotic prophylaxis to prevent subacute bacterial endocarditis)

Dermatology

Dermatologists diagnose and treat skin diseases and disorders such as acne, eczema, and skin cancer. Some skin conditions involve only the skin itself; others are a sign of disease elsewhere in the body.

To assist in a dermatologist's office, you must understand the basic elements of dermatologic examinations and procedures. You should develop familiarity with skin disorders and their treatments. You also need to understand the terminology used to describe skin lesions, as outlined in Table 23-2.

Assisting with positioning and draping during a skin examination and taking skin scrapings or wound cultures might be among your duties in a dermatologist's office. You might also perform procedures such as administering sunlamp treatments and applying topical medications. You will also instruct patients about caring for a skin condition or wound site at home.

Dermatology Examinations

During a **whole-body skin examination,** the dermatologist examines the visible top layer of the entire surface of the skin, including the scalp, the genital area, and the areas between the toes. The physician uses a magnifying lens and a bright light to look for lesions, especially suspicious moles or precancerous growths. The physician may photograph or sketch a lesion to aid in detecting future changes.

Your role in this examination includes preparing patients and helping them into the proper position before examination of each skin area. During the examination, drape patients to protect their privacy as much as possible while exposing the area to be examined. The physician may also ask you to take photographs or make sketches of lesions.

Another type of dermatologic examination is the **Wood's light examination,** in which the physician inspects the patient's skin under an ultraviolet lamp in a darkened room. This examination highlights certain abnormal skin characteristics and aids in diagnosis. The dermatologist may also perform more limited, focused examinations to evaluate specific skin conditions or disorders.

Dermatologic Conditions and Disorders

The condition of the skin plays a large part in a person's appearance. Patients with skin disorders, therefore, may worry about their attractiveness to and acceptance by

TABLE 23-2 Skin Lesions			
Type of Lesion	**Appearance**	**Type of Lesion**	**Appearance**
Macule: flat, discolored spot on skin (less than 1 cm in diameter), such as freckle or flat mole	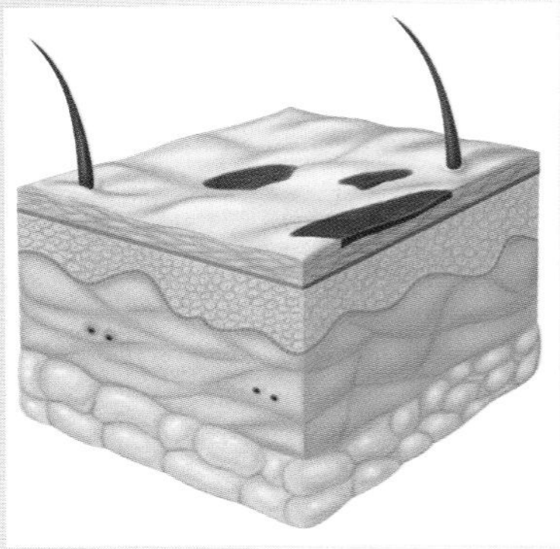	Bulla: large vesicle (more than 1 cm in diameter), such as burn blister	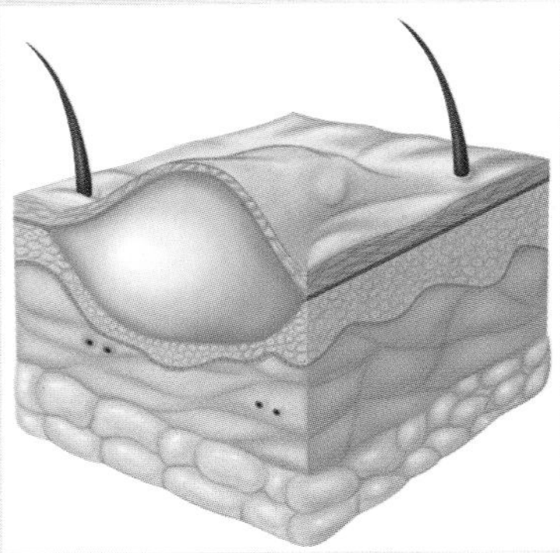
Papule: firm, raised lesion (less than 1 cm in diameter), such as wart or raised mole	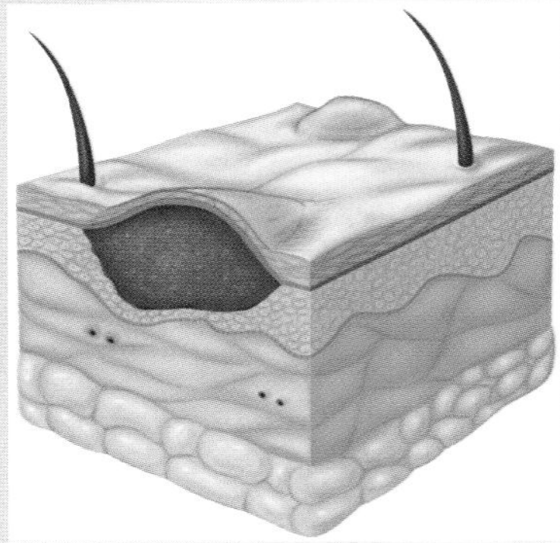	Pustule: raised lesion containing pus, such as acne or impetigo pustule	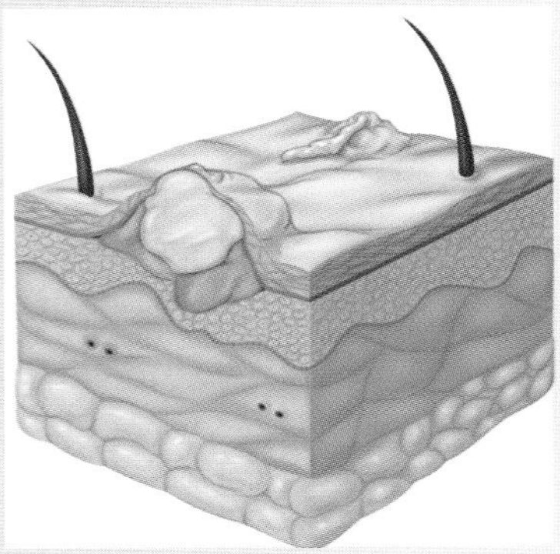
Nodule: raised, firm lesion larger and deeper than papule, such as sebaceous cyst	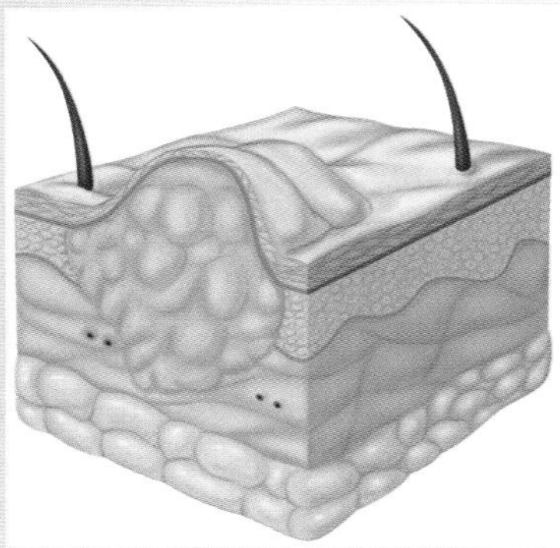	Ulcer: depression in skin formed when skin layers are destroyed, such as pressure sore	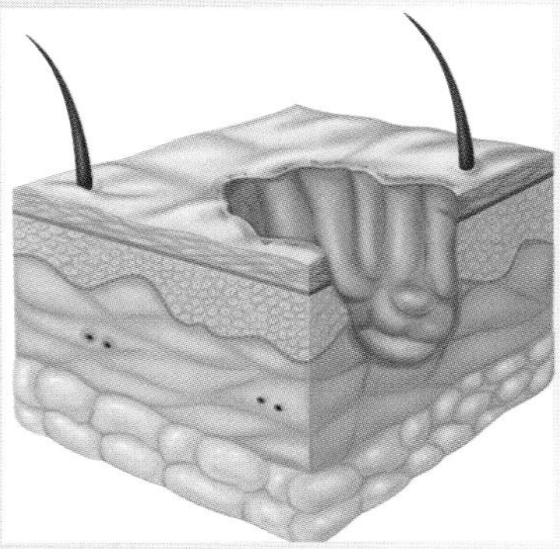
Vesicle: small skin elevation (less than 1 cm in diameter) filled with clear fluid, such as blister	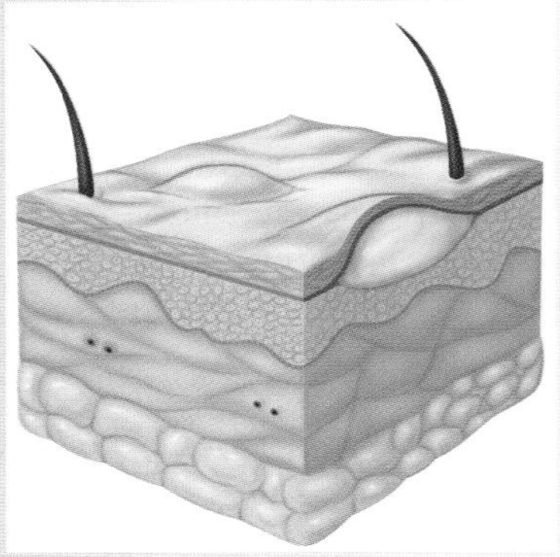	Tumor: solid abnormal mass of cells larger than 1 cm	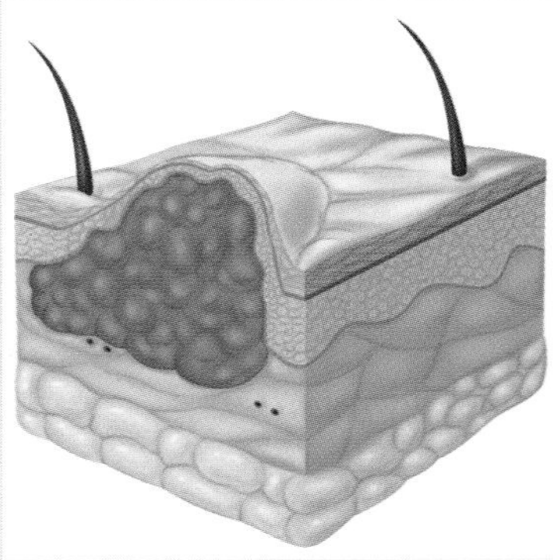

continued →

TABLE 23-2 Skin Lesions *(continued)*			
Type of Lesion	**Appearance**	**Type of Lesion**	**Appearance**
Wheal: temporary elevation of skin caused by swelling, as with hives or insect bites, or by administration of an intradermal injection		Fissure: crack in skin, such as fissure caused by athlete's foot	

others. Allow patients to express their anxieties; in return, provide encouragement about the course and outcome of their treatment.

Acne Vulgaris. Acne vulgaris, also called acne, is an inflammation of the follicles of the skin's sebaceous (oil) glands. It causes skin eruptions of pimples, blackheads, and cysts, mainly on the face but sometimes on the back or other areas. Acne occurs most frequently in adolescents but can affect adults as well. Its ultimate cause is unknown, but it is thought to involve a hormonal dysfunction that creates excess skin oil (sebum). The sebum hardens at the follicle openings, closing off the flow of skin secretions and causing eruptions.

Medications, either topical or oral, do not cure acne; rather, the treatments help to manage the outbreaks and are based on the type of acne diagnosed. Most often, medications used for treatment include those that:

- Help to unplug pores and stop them from getting plugged with oil
- Kill bacteria, such as antibiotics
- Reduce the amount of sebum produced
- Reduce the effects of hormones contributing to the acne

Retinoic acid cannot be used by patients who are pregnant or likely to become pregnant, because retinoic acid damages the fetus.

Patients need to understand the prescribed treatment regimen and its requirements, such as avoiding sun overexposure if vitamin A products are being used. You may also be asked to instruct patients in proper skin cleansing and care.

Contact Dermatitis. Contact dermatitis is a skin inflammation that can be caused by irritants as diverse as rough fabrics, cosmetics, pollen, or plants such as poison ivy or poison oak. Symptoms include redness, itching, edema, and lesions.

Treatment of contact dermatitis depends on the cause and type of lesions. Anti-inflammatory medications may be applied to the skin, or antihistamines may be taken internally. Corticosteroids are prescribed for severe inflammation. The dermatologist may wish to use a patch test to determine whether a condition is caused by a specific allergen. If such a cause is found, the patient should be taught how to avoid that substance and what to do after accidental exposure.

Ringworm. Ringworm, or tinea, is a term for various fungal infections that most often affect the feet (athlete's foot, or tinea pedis), groin (jock itch, or tinea cruris), and scalp (tinea capitis). Ringworm produces flat lesions on the body that are dry and scaly or moist and crusty. These lesions eventually develop a clear center with an outer ring, for which these infections are named. When ringworm appears on the scalp, it creates small lesions and scaly bald patches.

Ringworm is treated with topical antifungal medications and, when an infection is well established, oral medications. Ringworm is contagious, so instruct the infected individual in how to prevent contamination. The person should not share bedding, combs, towels, or other personal items with anyone until the infection is gone.

Moles. A mole (nevus) is a raised or unraised brown, black, or tan spot on the skin, with even coloring, a round or oval shape, and clear borders. It is usually less than 6 mm in diameter. It may be present at birth, but most appear during childhood or adolescence. Most moles are harmless; in fact, everyone has some. Because moles have the potential to become malignant, however, they must be monitored for bleeding, itching, or changes in color, size, shape, or texture. Some people choose to have a harmless mole removed because it is cosmetically unappealing or because it is in a place especially vulnerable to injury.

Skin Cancer. One of the most serious conditions treated in a dermatologist's office is skin cancer. Skin cancer

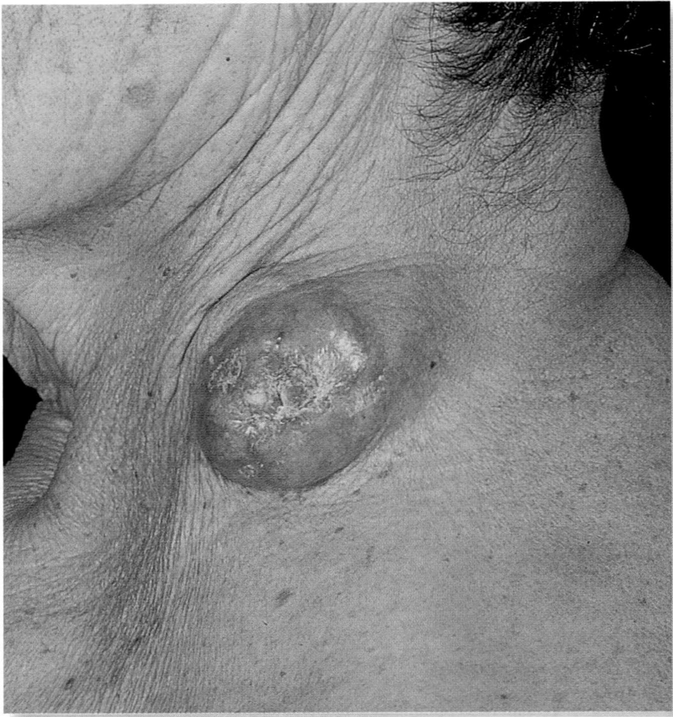

Figure 23-7. Left untreated, basal cell carcinomas can damage bones or blood vessels.

can appear in the form of basal cell carcinomas, squamous cell carcinomas, and malignant melanomas. Overexposure to the sun is a risk factor for all these types of skin cancer. Other triggers include x-rays, irritants, various chemical carcinogens, and the presence of premalignant lesions. The following people have a higher-than-average risk of developing skin cancer: those who have had severe, blistering sunburns in their teens or 20s; those who have fair skin and hair and light-colored eyes; and those who work outdoors.

Basal cell carcinomas are malignant lesions that occur most often on areas exposed to the sun, such as the face and neck. Basal cell carcinomas are the most common malignant tumor in Caucasians. The lesions look like small, waxy craters with rolled borders (Figure 23-7).

Squamous cell carcinomas also appear on sun-exposed areas. The lesions often look ulcerated or have a crust (Figure 23-8). They invade deeper into the skin and have a greater tendency to spread to other areas of the body than do basal cell carcinomas.

Malignant melanomas, which originate in cells that produce the pigment melanin, are the most dangerous type of skin cancer (Figure 23-9). Malignant cells may spread through the bloodstream or lymphatic system to the liver, lungs, and other parts of the body. A sudden or continuous change in the appearance of a mole may signal melanoma. Early diagnosis is critical for successful treatment.

Treatments for skin cancer vary with the type of cancer and its extent. Treatments include surgery, electrosurgery, cryosurgery, radiation therapy, and chemotherapy.

Warts. Warts (verrucae) are benign skin tumors that result from a viral skin infection. If a wart is scratched open, the virus may spread by contact to another part of the body or to another person. There are several kinds of warts. Common warts are raised, rounded, flesh-colored lesions that usually occur on the hands and fingers. Plantar warts appear on the soles of the feet. Venereal warts appear on the genitalia and anus and are transmitted through sexual contact.

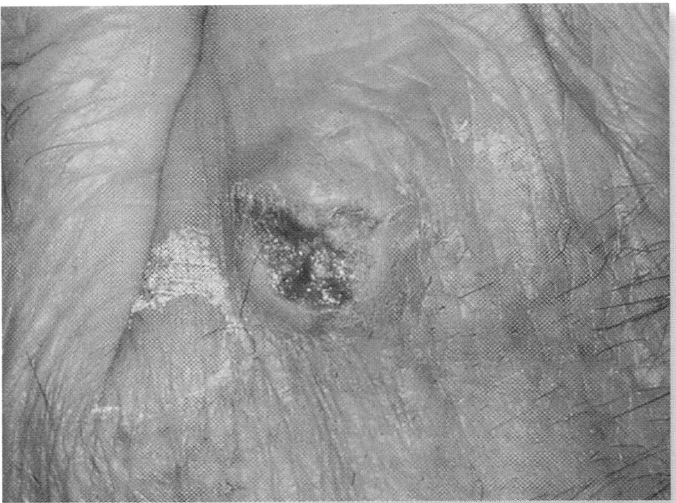

Figure 23-8. Repeated injury to an area, as well as sun exposure, is a risk factor for squamous cell carcinoma.

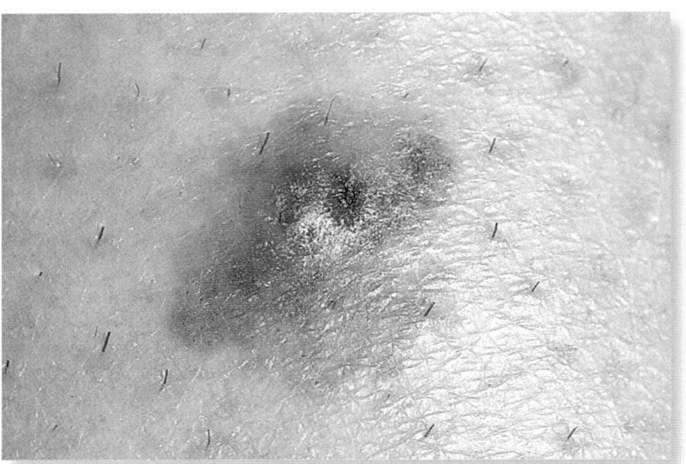

Figure 23-9. Early diagnosis is critical in successfully treating malignant melanoma.

Treatment depends on the type of wart. Some warts go away without treatment. Physicians often remove warts by burning or freezing the wart tissue. Instruct the patient to keep the wart removal site clean and dry until a scab forms or the wart falls off in a few days.

Other Conditions and Disorders. The following conditions may also be diagnosed and treated in a dermatologist's office:

- Eczema: skin inflammation that may be an allergic response to allergens, such as chemicals or foods

- Impetigo: highly contagious bacterial skin infection
- Psoriasis: chronic noninfectious disease that manifests itself in itching lesions covered with scales
- Herpes zoster: acute viral infection of nerves under the skin, often called shingles; causes painful skin eruptions
- Scabies: contagious skin disease caused by a mite; causes intense itching

Endocrinology

Endocrinologists treat diseases and disorders of the endocrine system, which includes glands that regulate and coordinate the systems of the body. Hormonal imbalances can affect the basic processes of growth, metabolism, and reproduction. In the endocrinologist's office you will assist with examinations as well as collect specimens for analysis.

Endocrine Examinations

Before an examination you will take a thorough medical history. The physician will assess the patient's skin condition, weight, and cardiac functioning for clues about illness. Most of the endocrine glands are located deep within the body; only the thyroid, the testes and, to some extent, the ovaries can be examined with palpation or auscultation. Therefore, diagnostic urine and blood tests are essential. You may be asked to collect a urine specimen or draw blood (see Chapters 29 and 30). Other diagnostic tools used in endocrinology include radiologic tests such as x-rays and iodine scans.

An endocrinologist will perform a complete physical examination, including palpation of the thyroid gland. In a thyroid scan the patient receives an oral or intravenous (IV) dose of radioactive iodine, and the thyroid is x-rayed as the material is absorbed. Ultrasound can also be employed to view glands or detect tumors. Urine and blood may be tested for the presence of glucose or hormones.

Endocrine Diseases and Disorders

An endocrine disorder commonly treated by endocrinologists is diabetes mellitus. This name is used for several related disorders characterized by hyperglycemia, an elevated level of glucose in the blood. When blood sugar is abnormally low, the condition is called hypoglycemia. Normally, the glucose level is regulated by insulin, a hormone secreted by the pancreas. A deficiency of insulin interferes with the metabolism of carbohydrates, proteins, and fats, raising the glucose level in the blood.

One form of diabetes, insulin-dependent diabetes mellitus (IDDM), may appear before age 30. Non-insulin-dependent diabetes mellitus (NIDDM) usually appears after age 40. Other forms of diabetes can occur during pregnancy (gestational diabetes) or as a result of other disorders. Symptoms include excessive thirst, hunger, excessive urination, and fatigue. Diabetes is treated through diet and weight control, oral medications, and insulin injections. Special, thorough patient education is necessary for the patient to cope successfully with the blood glucose monitoring, dietary restrictions, and self-care measures associated with this disorder (Figure 23-10). Physicians must pay special attention to certain secondary conditions, such as eye and foot problems, in patients with diabetes.

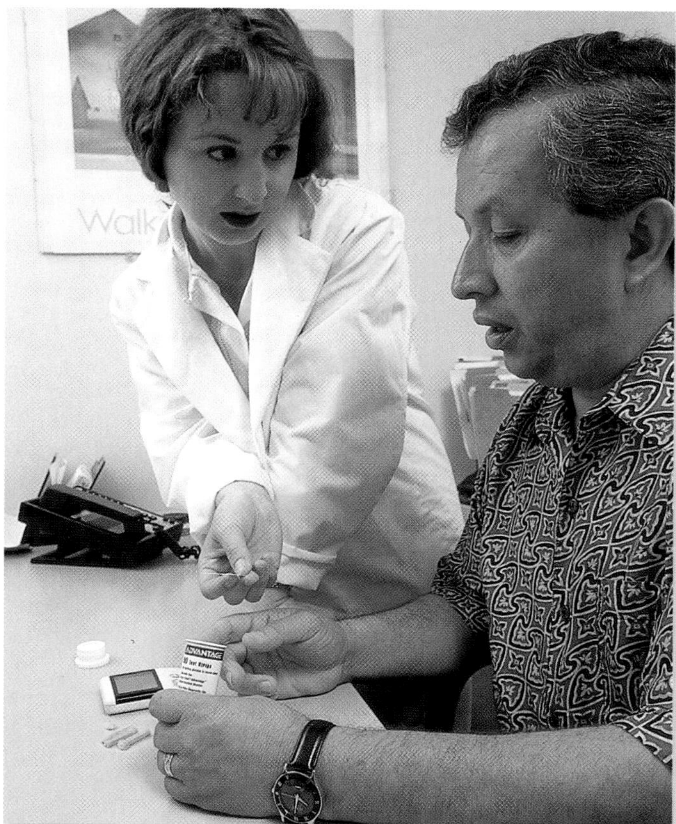

Figure 23-10. Patients with diabetes can use a glucometer to monitor their own blood glucose levels.

Thyroid Gland Dysfunctions. Several of the most common endocrine system disorders occur when there is a dysfunction of the thyroid gland. These disorders include hypothyroidism, hyperthyroidism, and goiter.

Hypothyroidism. Hypothyroidism is characterized by decreased activity of the thyroid gland and underproduction of the hormone thyroxine. This shortage can cause cretinism in children, with resulting mental and physical retardation. Underproduction of thyroxine in adults results in myxedema. Patients with this condition have fatigue, low blood pressure, dry skin and hair, facial puffiness, and goiter. Treatment for hypothyroidism consists of thyroid hormone supplements.

Hyperthyroidism. Hyperthyroidism, also called Graves' disease, is characterized by increased thyroid gland activity. Too much thyroxine is produced, and the patient has anxiety, irritability, elevated heart rate and blood pressure, tremors, and weight loss despite an increased appetite. Sometimes hyperthyroidism causes the patient's eyes to protrude, a condition known as exophthalmos. Treatment includes the administration of radioactive iodine, antithyroid drugs, or surgery to remove part or all of the thyroid gland. Many patients require supplemental thyroid hormones following treatment for a hyperactive thyroid.

Goiter. An enlarged thyroid gland, commonly called a goiter, is usually caused by a deficiency of iodine in the diet. Iodine is found in seafood, iodized salt, and vegetables grown in soil containing iodine. Without this mineral the thyroid gland enlarges in an attempt to produce more thyroid hormones. Treatment usually involves the administration of iodine.

Cushing's Syndrome. Cushing's syndrome results from overproduction of hormones by the adrenal cortex. This overproduction may be caused by a tumor of the pituitary gland or adrenal cortex. Cushing's syndrome may be a side effect of certain prescription medications. Symptoms include high blood pressure, muscle weakness, easily bruised skin with purple streaks, a rounded face, a fatty hump between the shoulders, and rapidly deposited fat that causes obesity in the trunk while the arms and legs remain slender. Some diabetic symptoms, such as hyperglycemia, may also appear. Treatments include medications to suppress adrenal function and surgical removal of tumors causing the disorder.

Gastroenterology

Gastroenterologists diagnose and treat disorders of the entire gastrointestinal (GI) tract, from the mouth to the anus, as well as the liver and pancreas. (Proctologists treat disorders of the rectum and anus only.)

A patient who sees a GI specialist has usually been referred by a family doctor, internist, or pediatrician who suspects a GI problem requiring additional expertise. You will need to understand the basic elements of GI examinations and procedures to assist in a gastroenterologist's office. You must also be familiar with common GI disorders, their treatments, and the terminology used to describe them.

In a gastroenterologist's office you will tell patients how to prepare for examinations, whether in the office, a radiology facility, or a hospital. You will order informational brochures and make them available to patients. You will also be prepared to answer patient questions.

Gastrointestinal Examinations

The gastroenterologist's examination of the patient's GI tract covers the mouth (lips, oral cavity, and tongue), the abdomen and lower thorax, the lower sigmoid colon, the rectum, and the anus. Your role as a medical assistant will be to prepare the equipment and the patient.

Depending on the patient's symptoms, the physician may perform an invasive examination procedure during the patient's first visit. Formerly, such procedures were performed only in hospitals or special medical facilities. Now many GI specialists' offices are equipped for these procedures and the management of possible resulting emergencies.

You must provide reassurance during examinations and help patients be as comfortable as possible. Your duties during the procedures will vary according to your state's scope of practice and the physician for whom you work. Instruct patients in advance to arrange for someone to drive them to and from the examination. After a procedure in which patients have had a local anesthetic at the back of the throat, caution them to avoid eating until the drug has been eliminated from the body. Otherwise, they could choke or aspirate food particles into the trachea.

Gastric Lavage. Gastric lavage involves obtaining a sample of stomach contents by inserting an orogastric tube into the mouth (or nasogastric tube through the nose) and passing it down through the esophagus into the stomach. The patient is usually sedated. You will spray the back of the throat with a local anesthetic to inhibit the gag reflex. The patient should be awake, however, to assist in swallowing the tube. The gastric sample is suctioned up through the tube and sent to a laboratory for analysis.

Endoscopy. **Endoscopy** generally refers to any procedure in which a scope is used to visually inspect a canal or cavity within the body. Several endoscopic examinations are performed with a flexible fiber-optic tube that has a lighted instrument on the end. These examinations provide direct visualization of a body cavity and provide a means for collecting tissue biopsies and removing polyps, as in the colon. Endoscopy helps diagnose tumors, ulcers, structural abnormalities, and other problems. It is particularly useful in performing procedures that formerly would have required an incision, such as removing stones from the bile duct.

Peroral Endoscopy. Peroral endoscopy involves inserting the scope by way of the mouth (Figure 23-11). The patient is sedated, and the gag reflex is inhibited with a local anesthetic. The peroral endoscopic procedures include panendoscopy (esophagus, stomach, and duodenum), esophagoscopy (esophagus only), gastroscopy (stomach only), and duodenoscopy (duodenum only).

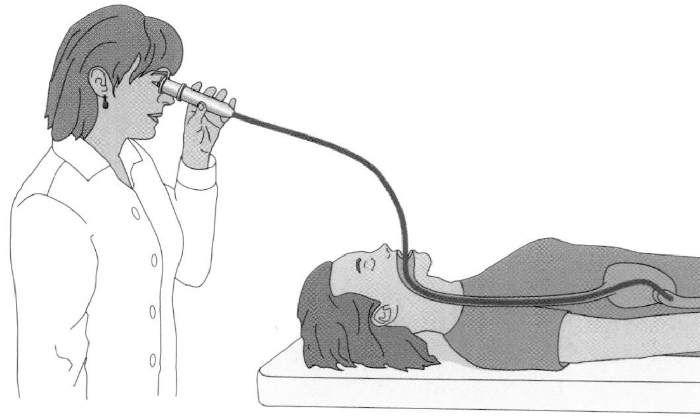

Figure 23-11. To perform peroral endoscopy, the physician inserts a scope into the patient's mouth.

Colonoscopy. **Colonoscopy,** which is performed by inserting a colonoscope through the anus, can provide direct visualization of the large intestine. The gastroenterologist uses this procedure to determine the cause of diarrhea, constipation, bleeding, or lower abdominal pain.

Patient preparation is designed to clear the colon of fecal material so that the colon can be seen clearly. Instruct patients to follow a liquid diet for 24 to 48 hours before the procedure. Patients should take a prescribed cathartic on the two evenings prior to the colonoscopy. Instruct patients to use one or more prepackaged enema preparations on the night before and the day of the procedure. (Alternatively, provide patients with 4 liters of a prepared electrolyte solution to consume over a 2- to 4-hour period. During this time patients should keep a record of their intake, output, and symptoms. Tell patients to expect diarrhea and possibly mild cramps.)

Immediately before the procedure instruct patients to empty the bladder. Patients should be given a sedative or an analgesic before undergoing the procedure. Patients lie in the Sims' position as the scope is guided through the large intestine. The doctor may manipulate the abdomen to facilitate passage of the scope.

Proctoscopy. **Proctoscopy** is an examination of the lower rectum and anal canal. After an initial digital examination, the proctoscopy is performed with a 3-inch instrument called a proctoscope. This examination can detect hemorrhoids, polyps, fissures, fistulas, and abscesses.

Sigmoidoscopy. **Sigmoidoscopy** is similar to colonoscopy, except that only the sigmoid area of the large intestine (the S-shaped segment between the descending colon and the rectum) is examined. Sigmoidoscopy is an important part of many complete physical examinations and is performed by many general practitioners and internists. It aids in diagnosing colon cancer, ulcerations, polyps, tumors, bleeding, and other lower intestinal problems.

Patient preparation involves using one or two prepackaged enemas either the night before or the morning of the procedure, depending on the doctor's instructions. The method for assisting the doctor during a sigmoidoscopy is described in Procedure 23-2. The sigmoidoscope, a lighted

PROCEDURE 23.2

Assisting With a Sigmoidoscopy

Objective: To assist the doctor during the examination of the rectum, anus, and sigmoid colon using a sigmoidoscope

OSHA Guidelines

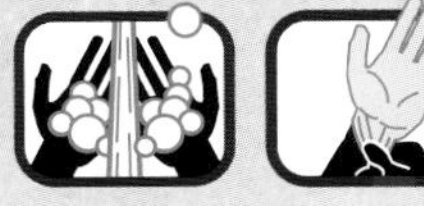
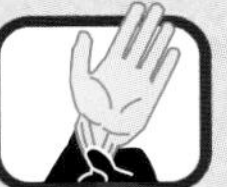
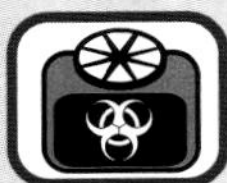
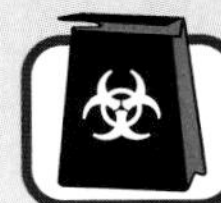
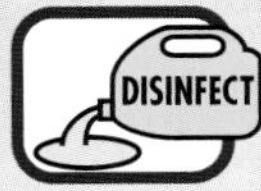

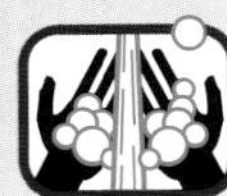

Materials: Sigmoidoscope, suction pump, lubricating jelly, drape, patient gown, tissues

Method

1. Wash your hands and assemble and position materials and equipment according to the preference of the doctor.
2. Test the suction pump.
3. Identify the patient and introduce yourself.
4. Show the patient into the treatment room. Explain the procedure and discuss any concerns the patient may have.
5. Instruct the patient to empty the bladder, take off all clothing from the waist down, and put on the gown with the opening in the back.
6. Put on examination gloves and assist the patient into the knee-chest or Sims' position. Immediately cover the patient with a drape.
7. Use warm water to bring the sigmoidoscope to slightly above body temperature; lubricate the tip.
8. Assist as needed, including handing the doctor the necessary instruments and equipment.
9. Monitor the patient's reactions during the procedure, and relay any signs of pain to the doctor.
10. Clean the anal area with tissues after the examination.
11. Properly dispose of used materials and disposable instruments.
12. Remove the gloves and wash your hands.
13. Help the patient gradually assume a comfortable position.
14. Instruct the patient to dress.
15. Put on clean gloves.
16. Sanitize reusable instruments and prepare them for disinfection and/or sterilization, as necessary.
17. Clean and disinfect the equipment and the room according to OSHA guidelines.
18. Remove the gloves and wash your hands.

instrument with a magnifying lens, allows the doctor to see and to examine the mucous membrane of the sigmoid colon.

Diagnostic Testing

Common diagnostic tests in this specialty include analysis of the contents of the stomach, analysis of a stool specimen, and urine and blood tests. Gastroenterologists sometimes use imaging techniques, such as x-rays, ultrasound, radionuclide imaging, computed tomography, and magnetic resonance imaging.

Laboratory Tests. A GI specialist may order laboratory analysis of stomach contents (obtained by gastric lavage) to determine the presence of bacteria or gastric bleeding. The physician may also request blood or urine tests. Another important test for GI specialists is the occult blood test, in which the feces are analyzed for occult, or hidden, bleeding from the intestinal tract. (This test is discussed in Chapter 20.)

Radiologic Examinations. Most GI radiologic examinations are not performed in an office, but you should know enough about them to answer patients' questions. Generally, these examinations are performed in a hospital x-ray laboratory or an outpatient facility. You may be responsible for scheduling tests at such facilities for patients. You can help prepare the patient in general terms for these examinations; however, the patient should discuss specific preparation with personnel from the radiologic facility.

Cholecystography. **Cholecystography** is a gallbladder function test performed by x-ray with a contrast agent. The patient swallows tablets of the contrast agent the night before the test. X-rays taken 12 to 14 hours later should show the contrast agent in the gallbladder. The patient then swallows a substance high in fat, which should make the gallbladder contract and empty the contrast agent into the duodenum. If the contrast agent is not taken up by the gallbladder or if the gallbladder does not contract properly, the doctor can determine whether there is bile duct obstruction or gallstones.

Ultrasound. Ultrasound is used commonly for diagnosing problems in the gallbladder, pancreas, spleen, and liver. The patient should have nothing to eat or drink after midnight of the night before and on the morning of the examination. Some gastroenterologists may perform ultrasound examinations in the office.

Barium Swallow. The barium swallow (also called an upper GI series) is used to detect abnormalities in the esophagus, stomach, and small intestine. The patient swallows a liquid containing barium, an insoluble contrast agent. This material is viewed using fluoroscopy (moving x-ray images) as the liquid is swallowed and passes into the stomach. X-ray films are taken at frequent intervals to record the diagnostic images. The patient is asked to move into various positions while the barium is tracked through the small intestine. To prepare for this test, the patient should have nothing to eat or drink after midnight of the night before and on the morning of the procedure.

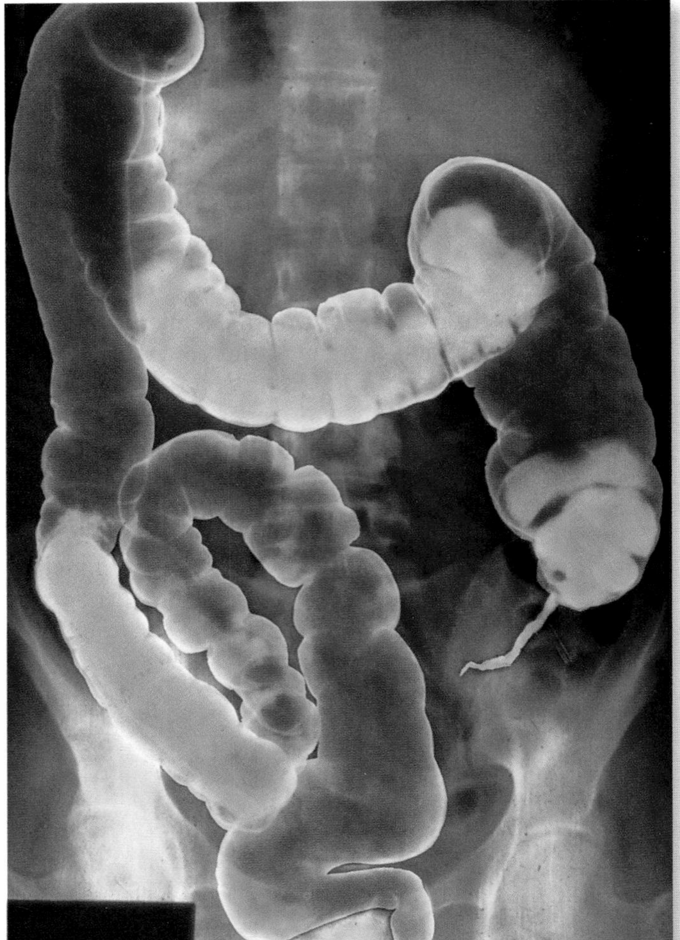

Figure 23-12. During a barium enema the barium is tracked on x-rays.

Barium Enema. A barium enema (also called a lower GI series) is used to detect abnormalities in the large intestine. Barium is given as an enema in this test. A balloon-like tube is inflated in the rectum during the x-ray, and the patient is asked to move into various positions to ensure that the barium is distributed completely (Figure 23-12).

Patients must eat no meats or vegetables for 1 to 3 days before the test to avoid incorrect indications on the x-ray. For 24 hours before the test, they must also follow a liquid diet, which includes drinking special liquid laxative preparations and more than a quart of water. The staff at the facility performing the test instructs patients about the specific steps, but the intent is to cleanse the colon completely.

Radionuclide Imaging. Radiology subspecialists who are trained in nuclear medicine perform nuclear medicine studies with radionuclide imaging. The patient is first injected with a radioactive substance, then waits a prescribed length of time for the radioactive substance to be taken up by the body part that is being imaged. The patient is scanned or photographed with a special gamma camera, which can read the radioactive areas to determine abnormalities in their composition. This technique is commonly used for liver, spleen, thyroid, and bone scans.

Gastrointestinal Diseases and Disorders

The level of discomfort from GI disorders can be misleading in relation to severity. There may be severe pain with intestinal gas, which is not serious, whereas there is virtually no pain in the initial stage of appendicitis, which is potentially life-threatening. Be sure that your notes are accurate and complete when a patient reports GI symptoms. Note the level of the patient's pain and whether over-the-counter drugs have been administered. Common diseases and disorders treated by a GI specialist are outlined in Table 23-3.

TABLE 23-3 Common Gastrointestinal Diseases and Disorders

Condition	Description	Treatment
Abdominal hernia	Weakness of abdominal wall muscle with outpouching, caused by heavy lifting; exacerbated by general lack of muscle tone; usually asymptomatic except for outpouching; severe pain may indicate complication of strangulated hernia, causing lack of blood supply	Surgery to repair muscle
Anal fissure	Ulcer in anal wall; symptoms include painful defecation with burning; may develop into fistula (abnormal duct to rectum)	Dependent on extent, may include surgery to repair
Cholecystitis	Inflammation of gallbladder; may be caused by intolerance to fatty foods, gallstones, or bacterial infection; symptoms include pain, nausea, diarrhea	Avoidance of fatty foods for intolerance; lithotripsy (noninvasive shock waves) to break up stones; antibiotic for bacterial infection
Cholelithiasis	Formation of gallstones from cholesterol in bile; symptoms include pain, nausea, diarrhea; complications include secondary bacterial infection	Lithotripsy, antibiotics to prevent secondary infection
Colitis	Inflammation of colon caused by bacteria, food intolerance, anxiety, or emotional disorder; symptoms include cramping, pain, diarrhea or bloody diarrhea with mucus or pus, fever, malaise, weight loss, nausea; complications include life-threatening infection or blood poisoning, liver damage, hemorrhoids, anemia, arthritis	Diet modification (clear liquid for acute phase), medication, psychotherapy, fluid replacement, surgery for severe cases; surgery may include insertion of elimination tube (colostomy tube) for temporary or permanent elimination of solid waste
Constipation	Hard feces or stools, decrease in frequency of or ability to have bowel movements, complication of fecal impaction	Diet modification, stool-softener medication, enemas, surgery if necessary for impaction
Diarrhea	Abnormally frequent and watery bowel movements caused by bacterial or viral infection or food poisoning, complication of dehydration with fluid-electrolyte imbalance	Diet modification, antibiotics for bacterial infection, medication to prevent dehydration
Diverticulitis	Inflammation of diverticulum, usually in colon; symptoms may be absent, may include abdominal pain	Diet modification, surgery possible for severe cases

continued ⟶

TABLE 23-3 Common Gastrointestinal Diseases and Disorders *(continued)*

Condition	Description	Treatment
Gastritis	Inflammation of stomach lining, causing excess secretion of gastric acids and bloating; numerous causes	Diet modification, drug therapy
Gastroesophageal reflux	Gastric acid rising into esophagus due to abnormal valve function; causes heartburn; symptoms may be similar to those of angina, dysphagia (inability to swallow)	Diet modification (including eating small meals), antacids, upright eating, remaining upright for several hours after eating, surgery (rarely)
Hemorrhoids	Enlargement of veins in rectal or anal area, may protrude from anus; symptoms include itching, pain, red blood with defecation	Diet modification, surgery
Hiatal hernia	Protrusion of stomach through diaphragm defect into thorax; symptoms similar to those of gastroesophageal reflux plus pain	Diet therapy with small and frequent meals, exercise, upright eating, medication
Stomatitis (canker sores)	Sore gums or other oral areas caused by herpes virus or acidic body chemistry; exacerbated by emotional distress, foods high in acid; symptoms include ulcerations (canker sores) with burning, sometimes swelling	Bland diet, avoidance of stress, medicated mouth rinses, topical anesthetic

Neurology

Neurologists diagnose and treat diseases and disorders of the central nervous system and associated systems. Nervous system injuries or diseases can result in loss of sensation, loss or impairment of voluntary movement, seizures, or mental confusion.

Your duties in a neurologist's office include assisting with examinations by readying equipment for use, positioning the patient, and handing the doctor tools and other items. You may be asked to perform parts of these examinations. You may also assist with certain diagnostic tests, such as electroencephalography. Your responsibilities will include instructing and educating patients and their families about procedures, disorders, and treatments.

Neurological Examinations

The neurologist evaluates five categories of neurological function in a complete examination:

1. Cognitive function (mental status)
2. Cranial nerves
3. Motor system
4. Reflexes
5. Sensory system

Cognitive function can be assessed by observing general appearance and grooming as well as by asking patients specific questions. The neurologist also determines the status of the cranial nerves, which affect smell and taste, eye movements, hearing, voice quality, facial expression, and facial mobility. The physician may, for example, ask patients to close their eyes and then identify familiar smells. The neurologist observes patients' faces for symmetry of movement and tests visual and auditory acuity. The physician assesses motor ability by testing coordination, observing gait, and determining muscle strength. Finally, the neurologist tests patients' reflexes and examines the function of the sensory system in areas of tactile sensation, pain and temperature sensitivity, and awareness of vibration. You are likely to assist the physician in completing these examinations, and you may perform certain components yourself.

Diagnostic Testing

Common diagnostic tests in neurology include electroencephalography and various radiologic tests. You may assist in performing these tests. Many tests are done at a site apart from the physician's office. In such cases you will need to schedule the procedures, instruct patients about pretest preparations, and educate them about the procedure and what to expect.

Electroencephalography. **Electroencephalography** records the electrical activity of the brain on a strip of graph paper. The tracing is an electroencephalogram (EEG). Electrodes are attached to the patient's scalp, and readings are taken while the patient is at rest and engaged in specific activities (Figure 23-13). An EEG can be used to detect or examine conditions such as tumors, seizure disorders, or

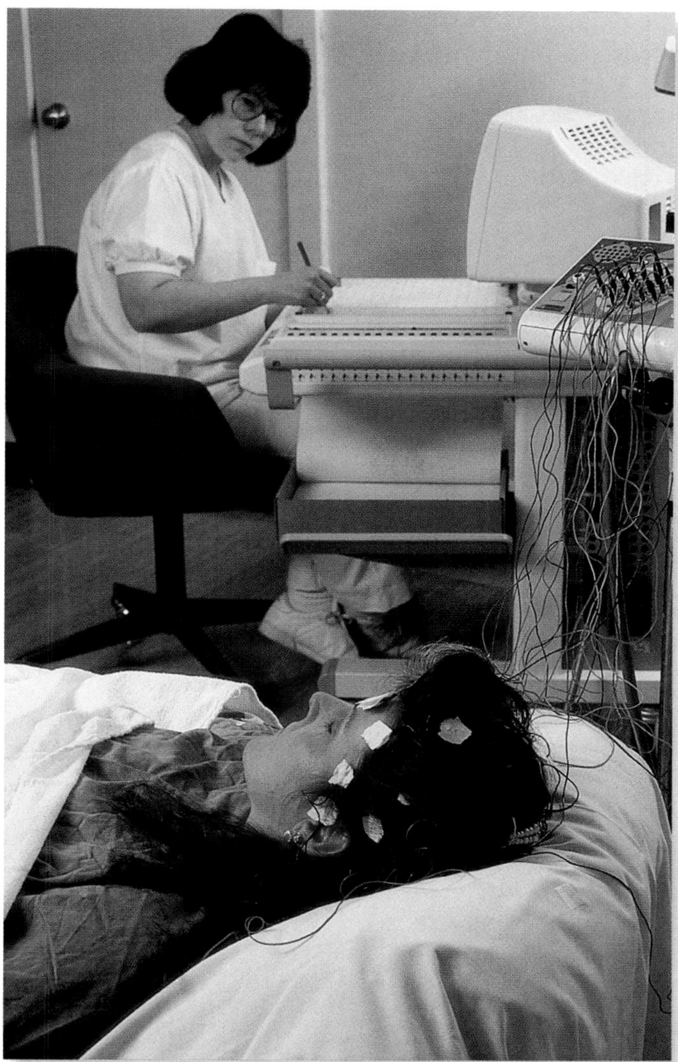

Figure 23-13. EEG readings are taken first while the patient is at rest and then while the patient is breathing deeply or observing a flashing light.

brain injury. You may assist with electrode placement or, after training, obtain the EEG on your own.

Imaging Procedures. Several imaging techniques are used as neurological diagnostic tools. Types of procedures include angiograms, brain scans, computed tomography, magnetic resonance imaging, myelography, and skull x-rays.

Cerebral Angiography. Cerebral angiography (or angiogram) is a radiologic study of the cerebral blood vessels. After a contrast medium is injected into an artery, x-rays are taken to visualize the cerebral blood vessels.

Brain Scan. A brain scan is performed by injecting the patient with radioisotopes and, after a period of time, using a scanner to detect the material. The radioisotopes tend to gather in areas of abnormality, such as tumors or abscesses.

Computed Tomography. **Computed tomography,** often called a CT scan, is a radiographic examination that produces a three-dimensional, cross-sectional view of the brain. Often one scan is done without a contrast medium. Then a contrast medium is injected for greater clarity. CT scans can help diagnose a wide range of conditions, including tumors, blood clots, and brain swelling.

Magnetic Resonance Imaging. **Magnetic resonance imaging** (MRI) is a viewing technique that enables physicians to see areas inside the body without exposing the patient to x-rays or surgery. The procedure, which takes 30 to 60 minutes, requires the patient to lie still on a padded table that is moved into a tunnellike structure (Figure 23-14). A powerful magnetic field produces an image of internal body structures.

Positron Emission Tomography. **Positron emission tomography,** often called a PET scan, studies the blood flow and metabolic activity in the brain to help physicians identify certain neurological and central nervous system disorders. These disorders include Parkinson's disease, multiple sclerosis, Alzheimer's disease, transient ischemic attack (TIA), amyotrophic lateral sclerosis (ALS), Huntington's disease, epilepsy, stroke, and schizophrenia.

Myelography. **Myelography** is an x-ray visualization of the spinal cord after the injection of a radioactive contrast

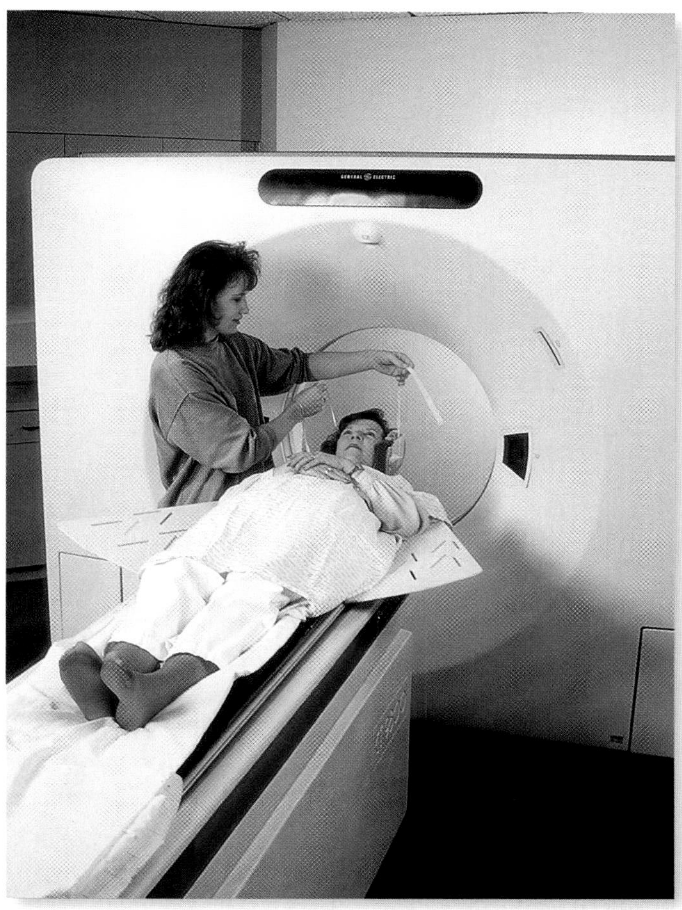

Figure 23-14. Magnetic resonance imaging is used to diagnose disorders in many specialties.

medium or air into the spinal subarachnoid space (between the second and innermost of three membranes that cover the spinal cord). This test can reveal tumors, cysts, spinal stenosis, or herniated disks.

Skull X-Ray. Skull x-rays may be used to detect breaks in the skull. They can also be used to locate tumors.

Other Tests. Other diagnostic tests do not involve imaging techniques. They include lumbar puncture and electromyography. A lumbar puncture, or spinal tap, involves collecting a sample of cerebrospinal fluid. A needle is inserted between two lumbar vertebrae and into the subarachnoid space. The collected fluid is sent to a laboratory for analysis. This test is used to diagnose infection, to measure cerebrospinal fluid pressure, and to check for blood cells and proteins in the fluid.

Electromyography is used to detect neuromuscular disorders or nerve damage. Needle electrodes are inserted into some of the patient's skeletal muscles. When the muscles contract, a monitor records the nerve impulses and measures conduction time.

Neurological Diseases and Disorders

Common diseases of the neurological system are described in Table 23-4. Trauma can also cause damage to the nervous system. Traumatic injuries can result in loss of sensation

TABLE 23-4 Common Diseases of the Neurological System

Condition	Description	Treatment
Alzheimer's disease	Disabling disease that usually affects elderly people; involves dementia and deterioration of physical function	Frequent stimulation to possibly help slow deterioration, medications that may slow progression of some symptoms
Bell's palsy	Suddenly occurring cranial nerve disease that causes weakness or paralysis on one side of face	Usually resolves without treatment in 1 to 8 weeks
Encephalitis	Inflammation of brain tissue usually caused by viral infection; symptoms include fever, headache, vomiting, stiff neck, drowsiness	Medication, rest
Epilepsy	Disease caused by misfiring of nerve groups in brain, resulting in seizures	Medication
Herpes zoster	Disease caused by virus that causes chickenpox; symptoms include painful blisters that form along path of one or more nerves	Medication to relieve pain
Meningitis	Inflammation of meninges (membranes covering brain and spinal cord) caused by bacterial or viral infection; symptoms include fever, chills, stiff neck, headache, vomiting	Medication such as antibiotics and drugs to reduce swelling
Migraine headaches	Severe headaches caused by vascular disturbance and characterized by pain, nausea, and sometimes visual disturbances	Medication
Multiple sclerosis	Degenerative disease of central nervous system that results in visual problems, muscle weakness, paralysis	Anti-inflammatory medications used during attacks
Neuritis	Inflammation of one or more nerves; symptoms include severe pain and discomfort or paralysis of affected area	Medication and rest
Parkinson's disease	Progressive neurological disease, causing symptoms of muscular rigidity and tremors	Medication to relieve symptoms
Sciatica	Inflammation of sciatic nerve causing pain in back of thigh and down leg	Medication to relieve pain, rest, heat applications

and voluntary motion. Paralysis on one side of the body, as a result of damage to the opposite side of the brain, is called hemiplegia. Paraplegia involves motor or sensory loss in the lower extremities. Paralysis of the arms, legs, and muscles below the place where the spinal cord is damaged is called quadriplegia.

Patients with acquired immunodeficiency syndrome (AIDS) may exhibit specific neurological symptoms related to their disease. These include:

- Meningitis caused by a fungal infection
- Encephalopathy (degenerative effect on the brain), resulting in headaches, difficulty concentrating, and apathy
- Peripheral neuropathies (disorders of the peripheral nerves) that result in pain or changes in gait

Oncology

An oncologist specializes in the detection and treatment of tumors and cancerous growths. The term *cancer* refers to a number of oncologic diseases that affect different body systems. All cancers are characterized by the uncontrolled growth and spread of abnormal cells.

A tumor is a lump of abnormal cells. Tumors are classified as benign or malignant. Benign tumors contain abnormal cells, but the cells do not invade and actively destroy surrounding tissue. Malignant tumors contain cells that grow uncontrollably, invading and actively destroying the tissue around them. Malignant, or cancerous, growths are capable of **metastasis,** the transfer of abnormal cells to body sites far removed from the original tumor. When cells become malignant, the process is called carcinogenesis.

You will encounter patients with a variety of medical conditions in an oncologist's office. You must be aware of the various types of cancer, what their symptoms are, and how they are treated (Table 23-5). Part of your job will involve preparing patients for the side effects of cancer treatment and helping patients deal with them. Patient and family education and support are essential.

Diagnostic Testing

Cancer is detected and diagnosed through a variety of procedures. You will schedule some of these tests and provide pretest instructions and explanations to patients. You may obtain blood specimens for some tests and assist in other diagnostic procedures, including:

- X-rays
- CT scan
- MRI
- Blood tests, especially those to detect tumor markers, such as carcinoembryonic antigen (CEA) (increased levels of CEA indicate a variety of cancers), CA125, and CA15-3

TABLE 23-5 Common Cancers by Body System

Body System	Symptoms	Treatment
Skeletal System		
Osteosarcoma: malignant lesion, usually in femur, tibia, or humerus	Pain and swelling, central hardened portion with softer edges, possible pathologic fracture	Radiation and chemotherapy to minimize tumor, surgery
Chondrosarcomas: malignant tumors of cartilage	Dull pain and swelling	Radiation and chemotherapy to minimize tumor, surgery
Nervous System		
Malignant gliomas: tumors of brain and brainstem	Headache, vomiting, changes in sensation or personality	Surgery, radiation, chemotherapy
Endocrine System		
Thyroid cancer	Nodules on thyroid gland	Surgery, radiation
Pancreatic cancer	Weight loss, abdominal pain, jaundice; very lethal form of cancer	Surgery, chemotherapy with radiation
Circulatory System		
Leukemia: several diseases involving abnormal overproduction of cells in bone marrow	Fatigue, paleness, repeated infections	Chemotherapy, bone marrow transplants

continued ⟶

TABLE 23-5 Common Cancers by Body System *(continued)*		
Body System	**Symptoms**	**Treatment**
Lymphoma: cancers of lymph system; divided into Hodgkin's lymphoma and non-Hodgkin's lymphoma	Enlarged lymph nodes, itching, fever, weight loss	Chemotherapy, radiation
Respiratory System		
Lung cancer	Often no early symptoms; later, new cough or cold that lingers; chest, shoulder, and/or back pain; wheezing and shortness of breath; hoarseness; coughing up blood; swelling in the face and neck; difficulty in swallowing; weight loss and anorexia; increased fatigue; recurrent respiratory infections	Surgery, radiation, chemotherapy
Digestive System		
Oral cancer: cancer of mouth or throat	May begin with painless sore or mass; later, difficulty chewing or swallowing	Surgery, radiation, chemotherapy
Esophageal cancer	Often no early symptoms; later, difficulty swallowing, regurgitation of food	Surgery, radiation, chemotherapy
Stomach cancer	Indigestion, weight loss, nausea	Surgery, chemotherapy
Liver cancer	Abdominal pain, fatigue, jaundice	Surgery, liver transplant
Colorectal cancer	Changes in bowel habits, blood in stools, rectal or abdominal pain	Surgery combined with radiation or chemotherapy
Urinary System		
Bladder cancer	Urinary frequency or urgency, blood in urine	Surgery, chemotherapy
Kidney cancer	Back or abdominal pain, blood in urine	Surgery, radiation, chemotherapy
Reproductive System		
Cervical cancer	Usually none, possible painless vaginal bleeding; abnormal Pap smear (Papanicolaou smear)	Surgery, radiation, chemotherapy
Endometrial cancer: cancer of uterine lining	Postmenopausal bleeding	Surgery, radiation, chemotherapy
Ovarian cancer	Usually none, possible abdominal pain	Surgery, radiation, chemotherapy
Breast cancer	Lump or thickening in breast, changed appearance, discharge	Surgery, radiation, chemotherapy
Prostate cancer	Often none; possible difficult, frequent, or painful urination	Surgery, radiation, chemotherapy
Testicular cancer	Lump in testicle	Surgery, radiation, chemotherapy

- Ultrasonography
- Biopsy, the removal of a sample of fluid or tissue from a growth (see the discussion of surgery as a medical specialty later in this chapter)

Cancer Treatment

Cancer treatments fall into three general categories: surgery, radiation therapy, and chemotherapy. Often a combination of these treatment methods is used. All methods damage healthy as well as cancerous cells. The success of treatment depends on many factors, and recovery varies greatly from patient to patient.

Surgery. Surgical removal of all or part of the tumor and some surrounding tissue is one method of cancer treatment. It is most effective when the tumor appears to be contained within a particular organ or is localized in an area of the skin. Surgery is often followed, however, by either radiation therapy or chemotherapy.

Radiation Therapy. Radiation therapy uses radiation to kill and stop the growth of tumor cells. It is often used in conjunction with surgery or chemotherapy. Radiation therapy is effective because radiation has the most damaging effect on cells that are undergoing rapid division, such as cancer cells.

Chemotherapy. Chemotherapy is also used in conjunction with other therapies. Chemotherapy uses strong anticancer drugs to kill malignant cells. As with radiation therapy, rapidly dividing cells, such as cancer cells, are most strongly affected by these medications. Although it is unlikely that you will prepare or administer anticancer drugs, you need to be aware that they are highly toxic. General protective guidelines must be followed whenever there is risk of contact with the drugs or patients' body fluids. Measures include wearing complete personal protective equipment and properly handling and disposing of materials contaminated with body fluids.

Ophthalmology

An ophthalmologist treats the eyes and related tissues. Chapters 15 and 21 cover the anatomy of the eye and the types of eye examinations and procedures that might be encountered in a general physician's office. Some of these examinations and procedures will also be performed in an ophthalmologist's office. The most common eye disorders that an ophthalmologist treats are visual defects, which are

PROCEDURE 23.3

Preparing the Ophthalmoscope for Use

Objective: To ensure that the ophthalmoscope is ready for use during an eye examination

OSHA Guidelines This procedure does not involve exposure to blood, body fluids, or tissues.

Materials: Ophthalmoscope, lens, spare bulb, spare battery

Method

1. Wash your hands.
2. Take the ophthalmoscope out of its battery charger. In a darkened room turn on the ophthalmoscope light.
3. Shine the large beam of white light on the back of your hand to check that the instrument's tiny lightbulb is providing strong enough light (Figure 23-15).
4. Replace the bulb or battery if necessary. (The battery is located in the ophthalmoscope's handle.)
5. Make sure the instrument's lens is screwed into the handle. If it is not, attach the lens.

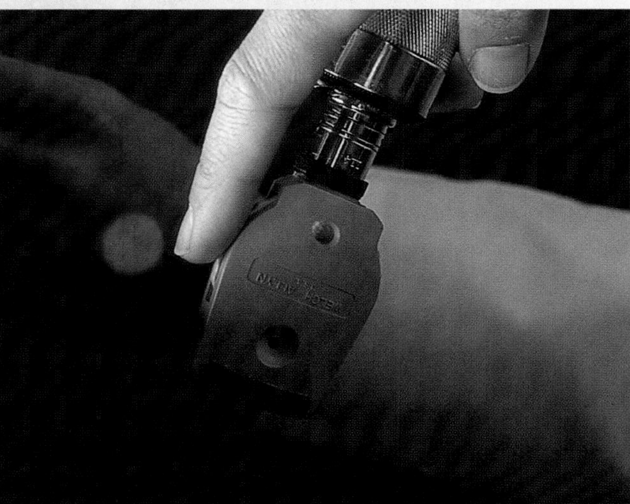

Figure 23-15. Shine the ophthalmoscope light on your hand to check the strength of the beam.

often correctable with eyeglasses or contact lenses. Ophthalmologists also treat eye injuries and remove foreign bodies from the eye. More serious disorders, such as cataracts and glaucoma, require medication or surgery. In an ophthalmologist's office you may perform some of the procedures that involve measuring various aspects and functions of the eye, such as visual acuity, color vision, and intraocular pressure.

Ophthalmic Examinations

An ophthalmologist performs an eye examination by inspecting the interior of the patient's eyes, including the retina, optic nerve, and blood vessels. The physician uses an **ophthalmoscope,** a handheld instrument with a light, to view the inner eye structures. You will maintain and prepare this instrument for the physician's use, as described in Procedure 23-3.

An ophthalmologist also tests the patient's visual fields. The visual field is the entire area visible to the eye when the patient looks at an object straight ahead. Visual fields are assessed by the confrontation method. The doctor stands or sits about 2 feet in front of the patient. The patient covers one eye, and the doctor closes her own opposite eye. (This makes the visual fields of the two individuals roughly the same.) Then the doctor moves a pencil or other object into the patient's horizontal or vertical visual field, asking the patient to say "Now" when the object comes into view. Defects in field of vision are noted. Convergence of the eyes is tested by bringing the handheld object to the patient's nose as the eyes focus on it.

The ophthalmologist also routinely tests for glaucoma with the aid of a tonometer (Figure 23-16). The tonometer measures intraocular pressure, shown by the eyeball's resistance to indentation. Your role is to explain the procedure to the patient, instill anesthetizing eyedrops into the patient's eyes when required, assist the patient into position, and hand the doctor the instruments.

The eye examination may also include a **refraction examination** to verify the need for corrective lenses. Normally, the lens and other parts of the eye work together to focus images on the retina. When errors of refraction exist, images are focused incorrectly, causing conditions such as farsightedness and nearsightedness. A refraction examination is performed with a retinoscope or a Phoroptor, the trademark name for a device that contains many different lenses. The doctor has the patient look through a succession of lens combinations to find out which one creates the clearest image (Figure 23-17).

Another instrument the ophthalmologist may use during the examination is the **slitlamp.** This instrument consists of a magnifying lens combined with a light source. It is used to provide a minute examination of the eye's anatomy. Patients rest their chin on the device's chin rest and stare straight ahead while the doctor shines a narrow beam (slit) of light into the eye and looks at the eye through the instrument's lens.

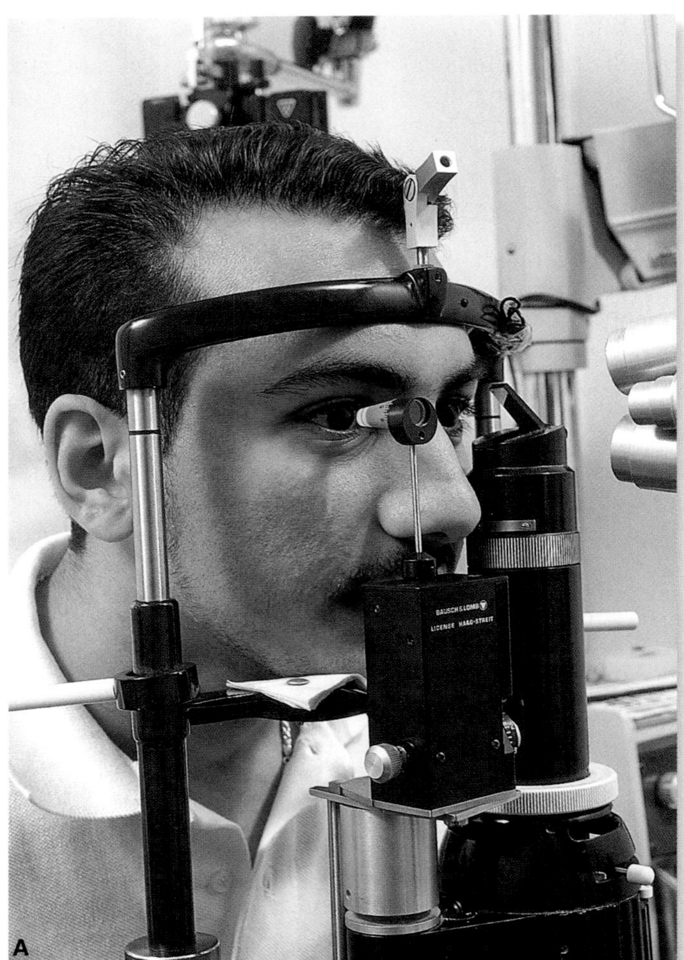

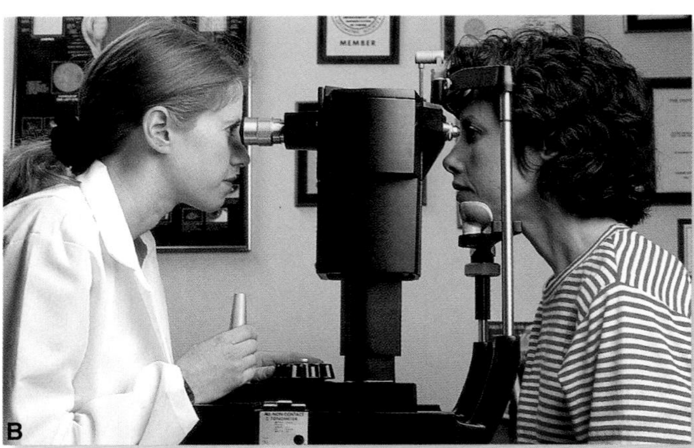

Figure 23-16. The two types of tonometers are (a) the applanation tonometer, which actually touches the eyeball during assessment, and (b) the noncontact, or air-puff, tonometer, which directs a puff of air at the cornea.

Eye Diseases and Disorders

An ophthalmologist treats a wide range of eye diseases and disorders. Some, such as a sty or conjunctivitis, do not greatly affect vision and may be treated by a general

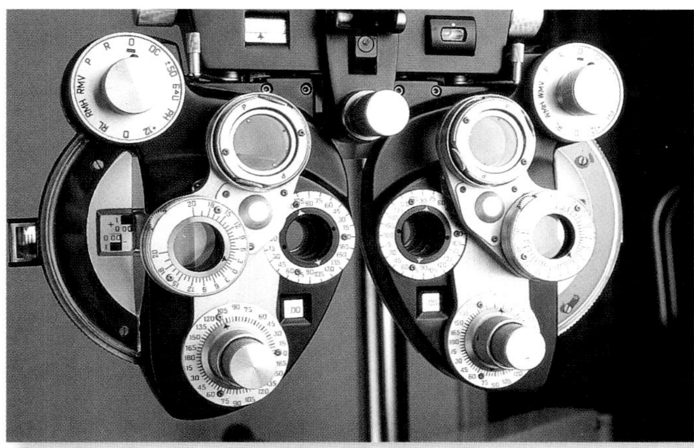

Figure 23-17. The Phoroptor helps the ophthalmologist assess errors of refraction.

practitioner. Others affect the internal workings of the eye and require the attention of a specialist.

Disorders of External Eye Structures. Some disorders affect external eye structures. These structures include the eyelid and the eyelashes.

Blepharitis. Blepharitis is a chronic inflammation of the edges of the eyelid, more common in older individuals than in younger people. It can be caused by infection or by the same skin condition that causes dandruff. Symptoms include red, swollen eyelids with scaling or crusting of skin at the edges. The patient's eyes may be irritated and itchy. Proper eye care and hygiene often clear up the condition successfully. Antibiotic creams may be necessary in severe cases.

Ptosis. Ptosis is a drooping of the upper eyelid in which the lid partially or completely covers the eye. It is caused by weakness of or damage to the muscle that raises the eyelid or by problems with the nerve that controls the muscle. Often no treatment is required, although surgery may be performed if the condition interferes with vision or if the patient is concerned about appearance.

Sty. A sty (external hordeolum) is the result of an infection of an eyelash follicle. A red, painful swelling appears on the edge of the eye and typically forms a white head of pus. The head bursts and drains before it heals in about a week. Applying warm, moist compresses to the sty may help it drain sooner.

Disorders of Structures at the Front of the Eye. Another group of disorders affects structures at the front of the eye. These structures include the conjunctiva and the cornea.

Conjunctivitis. Conjunctivitis, or pinkeye, is an inflammation of the conjunctiva caused by allergy, an irritant, or infection. It is a common disorder that is annoying but normally not serious.

Allergic conjunctivitis occurs when a person has an allergic reaction to pollen, makeup, or other substance. The symptoms are itchy, red eyes. The doctor may prescribe medication to relieve troublesome symptoms and suggest avoidance of the trigger whenever possible. Conjunctivitis may also be caused by irritants such as dust, smoke, wind, pollutants, and excessive glare.

Infectious conjunctivitis can be caused by either a bacterial or a viral infection. Both forms are easily spread and have symptoms including redness and a gritty feeling in the eye. Bacterial infections typically produce pus, which may form a crust on the eye during sleep. Viral infections usually produce a watery discharge. Although eye irrigation or saline drops may be used to soothe eyes affected by either type of infection, only bacterial infections are treated with antibiotic drops or ointment.

Because you may not know the cause of a patient's conjunctivitis (allergies, irritants, bacteria, viruses), take precautions to avoid spreading infection. As with any potentially infectious disease, use Universal Precautions in medical settings. Wear appropriate personal protective equipment when dealing with any patient who has conjunctivitis.

Corneal Ulcers and Abrasions. Ulcers (lesions) on the cornea may be the result of injury, infection, or both. An injury such as an abrasion (scratch) on the cornea can become infected with bacteria, viruses, or fungi. The symptoms of a corneal ulcer include pain or discomfort and unclear vision. Treatment consists of antibiotic eyedrops or ointments and use of an eye patch.

Disorders Involving Internal Eye Structures. Another group of disorders affects structures inside the eye. Cataracts, for example, affect the lens. Glaucoma can damage several internal eye structures.

Cataracts. Cataracts are cloudy or opaque areas in the normally clear lens of the eye. Cataracts develop gradually, blocking the passage of light through the eye. The result is a progressive loss of vision in one or both eyes. In severe cases you can actually see the cloudy lens through the pupil of the eye (Figure 23-18).

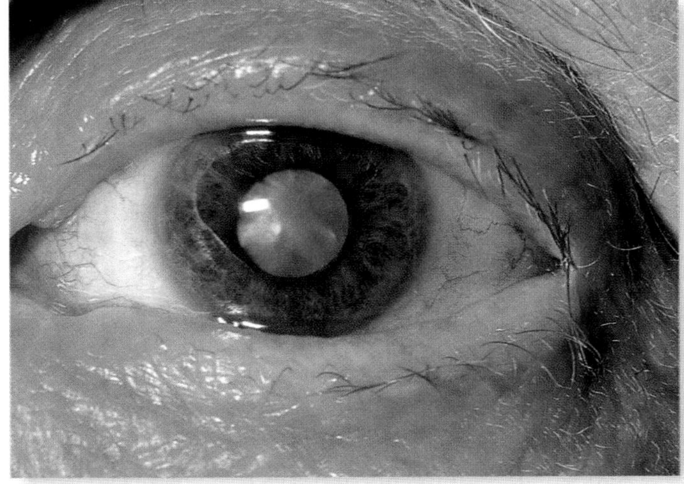

Figure 23-18. The lens of an eye with a cataract has a clouded appearance.

Cataracts are more common in the elderly than in younger people because the lens deteriorates with aging. Cataracts can also be caused by iritis, injury, ultraviolet radiation, or diabetes. Some cataracts are congenital. Cataracts are treated by surgically removing the lens and using an artificial lens in its place. The artificial lens may be in the form of special eyeglasses, special contact lenses, or an intraocular lens inserted at the time of cataract surgery.

Glaucoma. Glaucoma is a condition in which fluid pressure builds up inside the eye. This pressure damages the internal structures of the eye and gradually destroys vision. Glaucoma is the second leading cause of blindness in the United States and the first cause among African Americans.

Aqueous humor is produced by capillaries in the ciliary body. This fluid circulates between the lens and the cornea. The fluid drains out of this area through the angle formed by the iris and the cornea. The aqueous humor diffuses into a vascular channel (Schlemm's canal) that encircles the cornea where it meets the sclera (see Figure 15-3 in Chapter 15). The aqueous humor then returns to the systemic circulation (the circulation of the blood to body tissues).

In a patient with glaucoma, the fluid drains out of the eye too slowly or fails to drain at all. The result is a buildup of intraocular pressure. Retinal nerve fibers are damaged, and blood vessels are destroyed, leading to loss of vision and possible blindness.

Glaucoma is treated with medication that reduces pressure in the eye. Drops, pills, or both may be prescribed to reduce the production of aqueous humor. A procedure called an iridotomy is sometimes performed. This procedure is a type of laser surgery in which a small hole is created in the iris that allows the excess fluid to drain. If the surgery is not effective, an iridectomy (removal of part of the iris) is done to create a larger opening in the iris to allow drainage.

Iritis. Iritis, also known as uveitis, is an inflammation of the iris and sometimes the ciliary body. White blood cells from the inflamed area and protein that leaks from small blood vessels float in the aqueous humor. The symptoms of iritis are pain or discomfort in one or both eyes; pain may be worse in bright light. The eye is red, and loss of vision may occur. Left untreated, iritis can lead to other complications, such as glaucoma and cataracts. Iritis is treated with anti-inflammatory drops or ointment.

Disorders of the Retina. Several serious disorders affect the retina, the internal layer of the back of the eye. These disorders include retinal detachment, diabetic retinopathy, and macular degeneration.

Retinal Detachment. Retinal detachment occurs when the retina separates from the underlying choroid layer. When this separation occurs, vision is damaged.

Retinal detachment is rare; however, it is more common as people age. Early symptoms of detachment include flashes of light or floating black shapes, both of which can occur as the hole in the retina forms. Patients occasionally describe their field of vision as being like a window shade that has been pulled down. Peripheral vision is lost as the retina detaches. Vision becomes progressively blurred as detachment continues.

When detected early, a hole can be "sealed" so that the retina does not detach. If the retina has already detached, some vision can often be restored with new surgical and laser treatments.

Diabetic Retinopathy. Diabetic retinopathy is a complication of diabetes. People who have had diabetes for a long time or who do not keep their condition under control experience damage to small blood vessels that supply the retina. The vessels initially leak fluid, which distorts vision. As the disease progresses, fragile new blood vessels grow on the retina and bleed into the vitreous humor. Scar tissue may also form on the retina. The result is loss of vision. The damage usually cannot be repaired, but the disorder can be controlled to prevent further loss of vision.

Macular Degeneration. The macula is the area of the retina responsible for the central area of a person's visual field. For unknown reasons the macula begins to deteriorate as some individuals age. Macular degeneration causes loss of vision in the center of an image; peripheral vision remains intact. Macular degeneration is the leading cause of blindness among the elderly in the United States.

Loss of sharp vision occurs very gradually and without pain. One of the first signs is difficulty in reading. The loss of vision often appears as a dark spot in the center of the field of vision. If macular degeneration is detected early, laser surgery may restore some vision or prevent further loss.

Disorders Involving Eye Movement. Normally, both eyes move together when people look at objects. Strabismus is the name for a deviation of one eye. Strabismus in young children is caused by misaligned or unbalanced eye muscles. A condition called amblyopia may occur as the misaligned eye becomes "lazy." The brain tends to ignore what the lazy eye sees; if the condition is not treated, vision will be affected in this eye. Treatment involves putting a patch over the fully working eye to force the child to use the other eye. Eyeglasses may be used along with the patch. In some cases surgery on the eye muscle is required.

Strabismus in adults usually results from problems with the nerves connecting the brain and the eye muscles or with the muscles themselves. Conditions that can cause such problems include diabetes, high blood pressure, brain injury, muscular dystrophy, and inflammation of certain cerebral arteries. Treatment depends on the cause of the condition.

Refractive Disorders. Refraction refers to the way light from objects is focused through the eye to form an image on the retina. The normal eye focuses light exactly at the retina, producing a clear image (Figure 23-19). In some

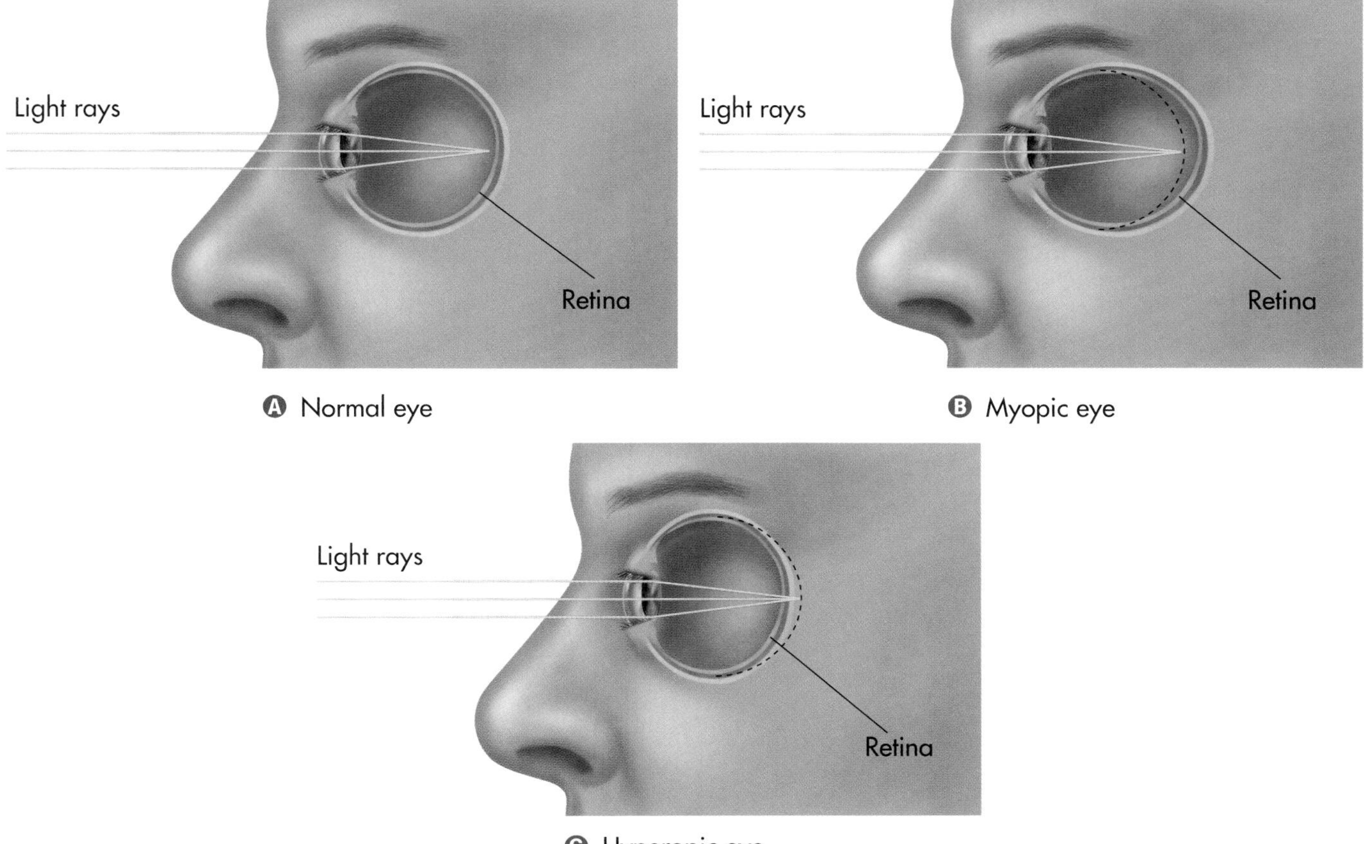

Figure 23-19. (a) In the normal eye, light rays are focused directly on the retina. (b) With myopia an elongated eyeball causes light rays to be focused in front of the retina. (c) With hyperopia a shortened eyeball causes light rays to be focused behind the retina.

people the eye focuses light either in front of or behind the retina, so the image is not clear. The problem may be due to abnormal shape of the eye or to abnormal focusing of the light by the cornea and lens. The four most common refractive disorders are nearsightedness, farsightedness, presbyopia, and astigmatism.

Myopia (Nearsightedness). Myopia is the condition in which images of distant objects come into focus in front of the retina and are blurred (Figure 23-19). This condition occurs if the eye is too long or if the cornea and lens bend light rays more than normally. Nearby objects are usually seen clearly, but objects far away are unclear.

Nearsightedness is corrected with eyeglasses or contact lenses that have inwardly curving (concave) lenses. The lenses correct the bending of light rays so that they focus on the retina. Surgical and laser techniques are also used to correct myopia by changing the shape of the cornea.

Hyperopia (Farsightedness) and Presbyopia. Hyperopia, or hypermetropia, causes images to come into focus behind the retina (Figure 23-19). The eyeball may be too short, or the cornea and lens may bend light rays less than normally. Faraway objects are usually seen clearly, but nearby objects are unclear. Young eyes can compensate for the problem by a process known as accommodation. The ciliary muscles contract during accommodation, thickening the lens and increasing its convexity. These changes allow the image to come into focus on the retina.

Patients with mild farsightedness may have no symptoms or may have blurred vision. They may have symptoms of eyestrain (an aching in the eye) because the ciliary muscles are overworked. Farsightedness is corrected with eyeglasses or contact lenses that have outwardly turning (convex) lenses. Aging usually causes the ciliary muscles to weaken, so a person may need stronger eyeglasses over time.

Presbyopia is a condition that most commonly affects people starting in their mid-40s. Older eyes tend to lose the ability to accommodate because the lens becomes more rigid. As a result images come into focus behind the retina, as they do with farsightedness. Individuals find they must hold reading materials farther away to see them clearly. Corrective lenses are used to treat this condition.

Astigmatism. Sometimes vision is distorted because the cornea is unevenly curved. This condition is called astigmatism. Astigmatism may cause vertical or horizontal lines to appear out of focus. It can occur along with either nearsightedness or farsightedness. Astigmatism is treated with lenses that correct the unevenness of the cornea.

A surgical vision-correcting treatment for myopia and astigmatism is radial keratotomy. The procedure, which is done on an outpatient basis under local anesthesia, involves making corneal incisions in a wheel-spoke configuration. The incisions allow the eye to return to a normal or almost normal shape. This procedure has been very successful for some patients. Others, however, have experienced complications, including worsening of vision. Newer techniques that use lasers to correct vision are largely replacing the radial keratotomy method.

Orthopedics

Orthopedics is the medical specialty focusing on disorders, injuries, and diseases of the muscular and skeletal systems. The two systems are so interdependent that they are sometimes referred to as the musculoskeletal system, especially by orthopedists. In the office of an orthopedist, you will be asked to assist with general examinations. Other responsibilities may include assisting with x-rays, helping with casting, applying hot or cold treatments (discussed in Chapter 25), and educating patients about therapy regimens. You must be knowledgeable about the musculoskeletal system and its common disorders and treatments.

Orthopedic Examinations

An orthopedist uses inspection, palpation, and a variety of diagnostic tests to assess the structure and function of the musculoskeletal system. The patient is asked to stand, walk, and perform several range-of-motion exercises. In these maneuvers the patient moves a joint in a variety of ways; the doctor usually measures the degree of mobility with a device called a goniometer. A complete examination takes some time, and you may need to help drape, position, or physically support the patient, especially if the patient is elderly or incapacitated. You may also be responsible for instructing the patient about care for a musculoskeletal condition, including how to perform therapeutic exercises.

Orthopedists use a variety of diagnostic tests. As in most other specialties, x-rays play a vital role in diagnosis. They are especially useful in determining the nature and extent of a bone injury. Other common radiographic examinations in the orthopedic specialty include the following:

- CT scan
- MRI
- Angiography (for affected vascular structures)
- Myelography (for spinal disorders)
- Diskography (for intervertebral disk disorders)
- Arthrography (for joint disorders)
- Bone scans

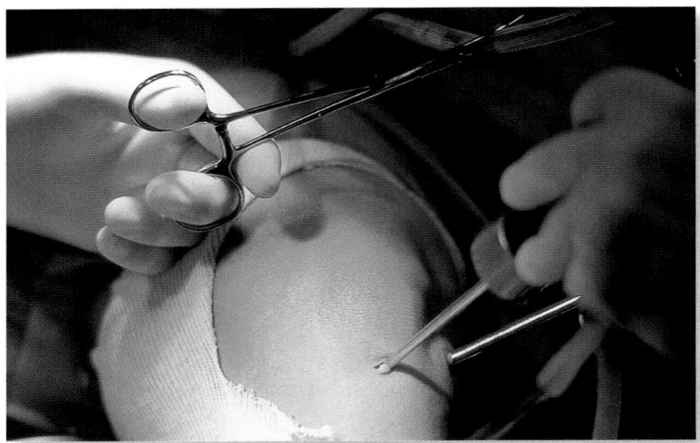

Figure 23-20. Arthroscopy can be used for diagnosis as well as biopsy and surgical repair.

Arthroscopy enables the orthopedist to see inside a joint, usually the knee or shoulder, with an arthroscope. This tubular instrument includes an optical system; when the tube is inserted into the joint, it can be visualized (Figure 23-20). Arthroscopy is used to give the physician a closer look at conditions such as injuries and degenerative joint diseases and to guide surgical procedures.

Bone and muscle biopsies may be performed to detect disorders such as bone infection and muscle atrophy. Electromyography is another diagnostic tool used in this specialty. An orthopedist may also order urine and blood tests to detect levels of substances such as calcium or phosphorus.

Orthopedic Diseases and Disorders

Table 23-6 lists many of the diseases and disorders you will encounter in an orthopedic specialty. Back pain, especially lower-back pain, is a common disorder. It can have many causes, including muscle strain, osteoarthritis, and the presence of a tumor. The orthopedist determines the nature of the problem based on the symptoms and diagnostic x-rays and CT scans. Treatments include the application of heat, administration of analgesics or muscle relaxants, exercise therapy, special braces, and traction.

Another condition that is commonly encountered in the orthopedist's office is a **fracture,** or break in a bone. Fractures and their treatment are discussed in Chapter 26.

Otology

An otologist treats diseases and disorders of the ears. Procedures common to this specialty are sometimes performed by other physicians as well, especially general practitioners, internists, and allergists. Chapters 15 and 21 cover the anatomy of the ear and the types of ear examinations and procedures that might be done in a general practitioner's office. Some of these are performed in an otologist's office too. You may assist with or perform

TABLE 23-6 Common Diseases and Disorders of the Musculoskeletal System

Condition	Description	Treatment
Arthritis	Inflammation of joints—rheumatoid or degenerative (osteoarthritis); rheumatoid arthritis causes joint stiffness and soreness, pain, and swelling and may lead to deformity; osteoarthritis produces pain, stiffness, and possible enlargement of bones, without deformity	Anti-inflammatory medications, application of heat, rest, exercise, occupational and physical therapy, surgery such as joint replacement (arthroplasty)
Bursitis	Inflammation of one or more bursae (sacs surrounding joints); symptoms include pain (especially on movement), restricted motion, and swelling	Anti-inflammatory medications
Carpal tunnel syndrome	Compression of median nerve, causing wrist pain and numbness	Rest and occupational adjustments, splinting of wrists, injection of corticosteroids, surgical decompression of nerve
Dislocation	Displacement of bones at joint so that parts that are supposed to make contact no longer come together; occurs most often to fingers, shoulder, knee, and hip	Relocation, or shifting bones back into place; anti-inflammatory medications
Herniated intervertebral disk (HID)	Protruding contents of disk compress nerve roots and cause severe pain	Rest, traction, physical therapy, muscle relaxants, surgery
Osteomyelitis	Infection of bone; principal symptom is pain	Antibiotics and analgesics, surgery
Osteoporosis	Metabolic disorder that causes decreased bone mass; bones become brittle and fracture easily	Exercise, dietary supplements, hormone therapy, drug therapy (alendronate)
Paget's disease	Chronic condition that causes bone deformities and affects 2% to 3% of people over age 50	Exercise, dietary supplements, hormone therapy, drug therapy (alendronate)
Scoliosis	Abnormal curving of spine	Back brace, surgery
Sprain	Injury to ligament caused by joint overextension; symptoms include pain, swelling, and discoloration	Rest, support, application of cold, anti-inflammatory medications
Tendonitis	Inflammation of tendon	Rest, support, anti-inflammatory medications

auditory screening, and you may help with diagnostic tests such as tympanometry. Otology specialists whose practices include problems affecting the nose and throat are called otorhinolaryngologists.

Common Disorders of the Outer Ear

Several disorders affect the external parts of the ear. These include cerumen impaction, otitis externa, and pruritus.

Cerumen Impaction. A condition called cerumen impaction occurs when the ear canal becomes blocked by a buildup of cerumen (earwax). The symptoms include a feeling that the ear is stopped up, partial hearing loss, ringing in the ear, and occasionally, pain. The wax can be softened with special eardrops, and irrigation can be performed to remove the wax.

Otitis Externa. Otitis externa is an infection of the outer ear, usually caused by bacteria or fungi. The infection can be localized, as with a boil or abscess, or the entire ear canal lining can be affected. Fungal infections are common in swimmers because of persistent moisture in the ear canal.

Symptoms of otitis externa include itching, pain, and pus in the ear. This infection is sometimes treated with a combination of an antibiotic or antifungal agent and an anti-inflammatory medication.

Pruritus. A common problem in the elderly is pruritus, or itching, of the ear canal. Because the sebaceous glands produce less wax with aging, the ear becomes dry and itchy. Dryness can be overcome by a regular routine of lubricating the ear canal with a few drops of mineral oil.

Common Disorders of the Middle Ear

Middle ear disorders involve the eardrum and the chamber behind it. They include otitis media, mastoiditis, otosclerosis, and ruptured eardrum.

Otitis Media. Otitis media is an inflammation of the middle ear characterized by a buildup of fluid. It is most commonly referred to as an ear infection. For detailed information on otitis media, see Chapter 15.

Mastoiditis. The mastoid bone is located just behind the ear. It is connected to the middle ear by air cells, or sinuses, in the bone. Sometimes, if left untreated, an infection in the middle ear can spread to the mastoid bone through these air cells. Although mastoiditis is fairly rare, it may be serious because the mastoid air cells are close to the organs of hearing, important nerves, the covering of the brain, and the jugular vein. Severe cases of mastoiditis may require removal of the affected bone.

Otosclerosis. Otosclerosis occurs when bone tissue grows abnormally around the stapes, or stirrup (the innermost of the three tiny bones that connect the eardrum and the inner ear). This overgrowth of tissue prevents the stapes from transmitting sound vibrations to the inner ear. The result is hearing loss that involves one or both ears. The condition is often hereditary.

Symptoms of otosclerosis include gradual loss of hearing and tinnitus (described in the next section). Surgery to replace the stapes can restore or improve hearing in almost 90% of patients with otosclerosis. Alternatively, a hearing aid may improve hearing for some patients.

Ruptured Eardrum. The eardrum may become ruptured in several ways: by a sharp object, an explosion, a blow to the ear, or a severe middle ear infection. Sometimes the eardrum is ruptured by a sudden change in air pressure, as might occur when flying in an airplane or diving. Symptoms include pain, partial hearing loss, and a slight discharge or bleeding. The symptoms typically last only a few hours. A ruptured eardrum usually heals on its own in 1 to 2 weeks, but the doctor may prescribe an antibiotic or the use of a temporary patch to prevent infection.

Common Disorders of the Inner Ear

Disorders of the inner ear, or labyrinth, affect the cochlea and the semicircular canals. They include labyrinthitis, Ménière's disease, presbycusis, and tinnitus.

Labyrinthitis. Labyrinthitis is an infection of the labyrinth, most commonly caused by a virus. Because the labyrinth includes the semicircular canals, which are involved in balance, this infection causes symptoms of dizziness or vertigo. The room may appear to spin, and any movement exacerbates the sensation, sometimes to the point of nausea and vomiting. Although disturbing, labyrinthitis disappears on its own within 1 to 3 weeks. The patient may need to rest in bed for a few days, and medication can be given for symptoms.

Ménière's Disease. Ménière's disease is caused by increased fluid in the labyrinth. The pressure of the fluid disturbs the sense of balance and may even rupture the labyrinth wall or damage the cochlea with its hearing receptors. One or both ears may be affected. Symptoms of this disorder include vertigo, nausea, vomiting, distorted hearing, and tinnitus. Some people may suffer hearing loss ranging from mild to severe. Medications may be used to combat vertigo, nausea, and vomiting. Other treatments that help some people include using diuretics and following a low-sodium diet.

Presbycusis. Presbycusis is a type of sensorineural hearing loss. This disorder involves a gradual deterioration of the sensory receptors in the cochlea, leading to gradual loss of hearing. It is the most common form of hearing loss in older adults, affecting about 25% of people by the age of 60 or 70. Men are affected more often than women. Typically both ears are affected, and the patient has difficulty hearing high-pitched tones as well as normal conversation. Presbycusis is thought to be caused by factors such as prolonged exposure to loud noise, infection, injury, certain medications, and some diseases. Hearing loss can be treated effectively, however, with a hearing aid.

Tinnitus. Tinnitus is more commonly called a ringing in the ears. It can, however, take several forms, including a buzzing, whistling, or hissing sound. The most common causes of tinnitus are damage to the hearing receptors from noise or toxins, age-related changes in the organs of the ear, and use of aspirin. Tinnitus can affect people at any age but is more common as people get older. If tinnitus becomes chronic, the patient may find relief by listening to music or other distracting sounds or by using a device similar to a hearing aid that masks the noise with more pleasant sounds.

Surgery

Surgery is used to treat a variety of diseases and disorders. Surgery may be performed to repair wounds and broken bones or to repair or remove diseased or injured tissues,

PROCEDURE 23.4

Assisting With a Needle Biopsy

Objective: To remove tissue from a patient's body so that it can be examined in a laboratory

OSHA Guidelines

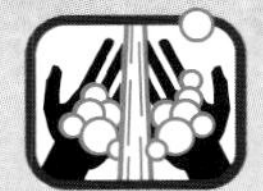
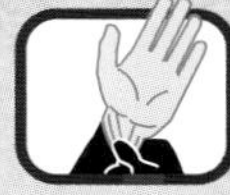
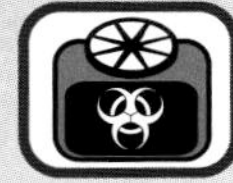

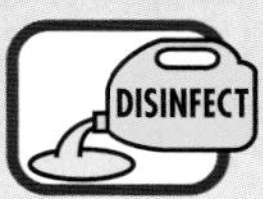

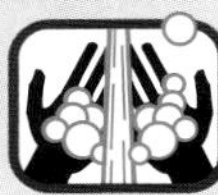

Materials: Sterile drapes, tray or Mayo stand, antiseptic solution, cotton balls, local anesthetic, disposable sterile biopsy needle or disposable sterile syringe and needle, sterile sponges, specimen bottle with fixative solution, laboratory packaging, sterile wound-dressing materials

Method

1. Identify the patient and introduce yourself; instruct the patient as needed.
2. Wash your hands and assemble the necessary materials.
3. Prepare the sterile field and instruments.
4. Put on examination gloves.
5. Cleanse the biopsy site. Prepare the patient's skin.
6. Remove the gloves, wash your hands, and put on clean examination gloves.
7. Assist the doctor as she injects anesthetic.
8. During the procedure, help drape and position the patient.
9. If you will be handing the doctor the instruments, remove the gloves, perform a surgical scrub, and put on sterile gloves.
10. Place the sample in a properly labeled specimen bottle, complete the laboratory requisition form, and package the specimen for immediate transport to the laboratory.
11. Dress the patient's wound site.
12. Properly dispose of used supplies and instruments.
13. Clean and disinfect the room according to OSHA guidelines.
14. Remove the gloves and wash your hands.

organs, and limbs. Some surgeons specialize in one field, such as ophthalmology or cardiology, and others are general surgeons.

Assisting a general or specialty surgeon requires familiarity with body systems. You should also understand presurgical procedures such as patient education, operating room preparation, and skin preparation; surgical assisting procedures such as maintaining asepsis; and postsurgical responsibilities such as decontaminating the operating room and dressing wounds.

A relatively simple surgical procedure is a tissue biopsy. There are several types of biopsies. A surgeon performs an incisional, or open, biopsy by making an incision and removing a piece of tissue. A needle biopsy is performed by removing tissue with a needle inserted into the growth or area through the skin. A surgeon performs needle aspiration by removing fluid from a lump or cyst with a needle. You may be asked to assist during these types of surgery. Procedure 23-4 describes the steps in assisting with a needle biopsy.

During a biopsy, Universal Precautions and sterile technique must be maintained. Always place the specimen in a prepared, labeled container provided by the laboratory. Transport it according to laboratory instructions, attaching the proper accompanying forms. After the biopsy you might assist with or perform the cleaning and bandaging of the site.

Urology

A urologist diagnoses and treats disorders and diseases of the urinary system in both males and females as well as the male reproductive system. Urologists also perform surgical procedures such as hernia repairs and vasectomies. A vasectomy is a sterilization procedure for men in which a section of each vas deferens is removed.

In a urologist's office, you would assist with general examinations; collect and process urine, blood, and other specimens; obtain cultures; and participate in patient education about conditions as well as about presurgical and postsurgical care. You must understand the urinary system and the diseases and disorders you are likely to encounter.

Urology Examinations

You must be thorough when you take a patient's history for a urologist. Much information about urinary problems is obtained by questioning the patient about changes in frequency or urgency of urination, difficulty or pain with

Educating the Patient

Testicular Self-Examination

Testicular cancer is rare, but when it occurs, it usually affects men between the ages of 29 and 35. The American Cancer Society recommends that all men perform a monthly testicular self-examination (TSE) from age 15 onward to increase the chances of early detection. Although testicular cancer is one of the most curable cancers, early detection is vital to its treatment.

A man who perceives an abnormality during TSE should be examined by a physician right away. TSE should be performed after a warm shower or bath, when scrotal skin is relaxed.

1. The man first observes the testes for changes in appearance, such as swelling. He then manually examines each testicle, gently rolling it between the fingers and thumbs of both hands to feel for hard lumps (see Figure 23-21).
2. After examining each testicle, the man should locate the area of the epididymis and spermatic cord. This area can be felt as a cordlike structure originating at the top back of each testicle.

Warning signs of testicular cancer include a heavy or dragging feeling in the groin, enlargement of one testicle, and a dull ache in the groin.

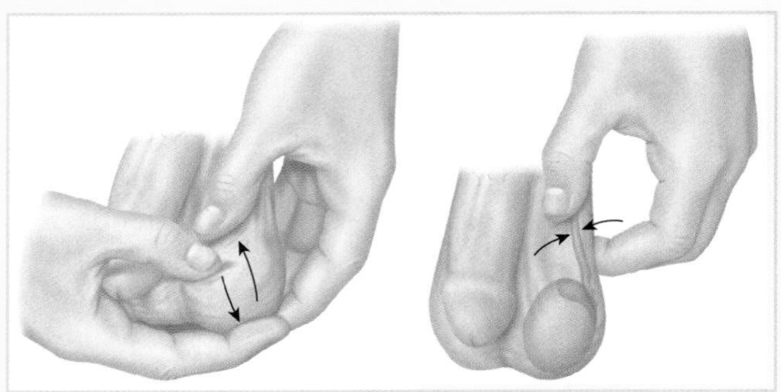

Figure 23-21. Males from age 15 onward should perform a monthly testicular self-examination.

urination (dysuria), and incontinence. The physical examination usually includes palpation of the kidneys and bladder and visual inspection of the external genitalia. Women are examined in the lithotomy position, and men are usually seated when the examination begins.

During examination of the male reproductive system, the urologist inspects and palpates the patient's penis and scrotum. The genitalia are usually examined with the patient standing and the chest and abdomen draped. The doctor usually examines the inguinal region for a hernia and, in men over 40, checks the prostate gland. This gland is examined by digital insertion into the rectum.

The doctor instructs the patient as needed in performing regular testicular self-examination (TSE). This instruction, discussed in the Educating the Patient section, may also be your responsibility.

Diagnostic Testing

Urologists sometimes use imaging techniques, such as CT scans and MRIs. Pyelography is an x-ray of the kidney area with an iodine-based contrast agent. It is used to diagnose renal (kidney-related) disorders. Urologists also use several other diagnostic techniques.

Urine and Blood Tests. Urinalysis is the most common test ordered in a urology practice. Urine can be tested for the presence of bacteria, blood, and other substances. Blood testing is also done for a variety of reasons, including monitoring for dysfunctions of the prostate gland and for certain sexually transmitted diseases (STDs). The Leydig's cell test is a blood test used to assess testosterone levels.

Semen Analysis and Smears. Semen samples may be obtained to determine fertility or to evaluate the success of a vasectomy. The patient usually collects these samples at home, but you may be required to provide a container, written instructions, and laboratory paperwork. Smears are used in diagnosing infections.

Cystometry. Cystometry is used to measure urinary bladder capacity and pressure. Using a catheter passed through the urethra, the doctor fills the bladder with carbon dioxide gas. The test results are examined to diagnose disorders of bladder function.

Cystoscopy. In cystoscopy the physician examines the walls of the bladder and urethra by visualization and inspection. A special viewing instrument, called a cystoscope, is used for this procedure. The cystoscope is inserted into the bladder through the urethra.

Testicular Biopsy. Testicular biopsy, a hospital procedure, involves obtaining a tissue sample of a mass for laboratory examination. The patient will need your emotional support because he will most likely be very anxious about the nature of the lump.

Career Opportunities

Surgical Technologist

To gain medical assistant credentials, you must fulfill the requirements of either the American Association of Medical Assistants (for a Certified Medical Assistant) or the American Medical Technologists (for a Registered Medical Assistant). After obtaining your medical assistant certification or registration, you may wish to acquire additional skills in specialty areas through course work or on-the-job training. Although this course work or training may not lead to an additional certification or degree, it will enable you to expand your role in the medical office and advance your career as the demand for health professionals increases.

Skills and Duties

The surgical technologist, sometimes called a surgical technician or operating room technician, is a vital member of the surgical team. He assists surgeons, nurses, and other surgical staff before, during, and after an operation.

Prior to an operation the technologist sets up the operating room. He sterilizes and prepares instruments and supplies and arranges them for the surgical staff. He also checks all operating room equipment to make sure the machines are fully functional.

The surgical technologist also prepares the patient for surgery. He washes the surgical site and shaves the area if necessary. He then transports the patient to the operating room and lifts her to position her on the table, requesting assistance if needed. He may apply antiseptic to the incision site and arrange sterile drapes around the site to create a sterile field. He may also help surgeons, nurses, and staff scrub up and dress in their gowns, gloves, and masks.

During the operation the surgical technologist observes vital signs, checks charts, and passes instruments and supplies to nurses and surgeons. He wears a mask and other personal protective equipment during the operation. He also may operate the lights, suction machines, or diagnostic equipment and help prepare specimens for transport to the laboratory or apply dressings to the patient's wound.

Following the operation the technologist lifts and transfers the patient to the recovery room, requesting assistance if needed. He then cleans and disinfects the operating room, restocking supplies as needed.

Workplace Settings

Surgical technologists typically work in hospital operating rooms. Some surgical technologists also work in clinics, surgery centers, or physicians' and dentists' offices where outpatient surgery is performed. A few are employed privately by surgeons who use their own surgical teams for specialized work.

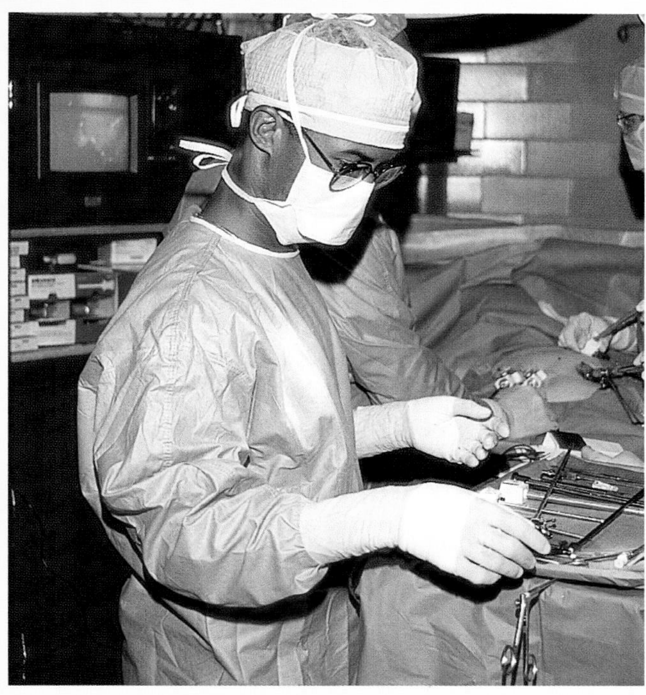

Surgical technologists usually work a standard 40-hour week. They may also be placed on call for emergencies during nights and weekends.

Education

The Committee on Allied Health Education and Accreditation of the American Medical Association recognizes 130 programs for surgical technologists. Programs are offered by colleges and universities, hospitals, vocational schools, and the military. They range from 9 months to 2 years in duration and offer the graduate a certificate, diploma, or associate degree.

After graduating from a program, surgical technologists may voluntarily take an examination to receive professional certification from the Liaison Council on Certification for the Surgical Technologist. Certification must be renewed every 6 years.

Where to Go for More Information

American Hospital Association
One North Franklin
Chicago, IL 60606
(312) 422-3000
www.aha.org

Association of Surgical Technologists
7108-C South Alton Way
Englewood, CO 80112
(303) 694-9130
www.ast.org

or to repair an injury. Other procedures may be elective, or optional. Removal of a wart, skin tag (a small outgrowth of skin, occurring frequently on the neck as people get older), or other small growth for cosmetic reasons is an elective procedure. Some of the common minor surgical procedures you may assist the doctor with include the following:

- Repair of a laceration
- Irrigation and cleaning of a puncture wound
- Wound debridement
- Removal of foreign bodies
- Removal of small growths
- Removal of a nail or part of a nail
- Drainage of an abscess
- Collection of a biopsy specimen
- Cryosurgery
- Laser surgery
- Electrocauterization

Common Surgical Procedures

Many surgical procedures are routinely performed in a doctor's office. You may perform some of these procedures on your own. For example, you may change dressings for surgical wounds, and under doctor's orders you may remove sutures (commonly called stitches) or staples after wounds have healed. Any procedure that requires an **incision** (a surgical wound made by cutting into body tissue) must be performed by a doctor.

Draining an Abscess. An **abscess** is a collection of pus (white blood cells, bacteria, and dead skin cells) that forms as a result of infection. A protective lining can form around an abscess and prevent it from healing. In such a case the physician may make an incision in the lining of the abscess. The physician may allow the abscess to drain on its own or insert a drainage tube.

Obtaining a Biopsy Specimen. A **biopsy specimen** is a small amount of tissue removed from the body for examination under a microscope. The specimen must be placed in a preservative, most commonly a 10% **formalin** solution (a dilute solution of formaldehyde), to prevent changes in the tissue. Most biopsies involve cutting the tissue. A **needle biopsy** uses a needle and syringe to aspirate (withdraw by suction) fluid or tissue cells. (Procedure 23-4 in Chapter 23 describes how to assist with a needle biopsy.) All specimens require preservation, whether obtained by cutting or by aspiration using a needle and syringe.

Caring for Wounds. A wound is any break in the skin. The break may be accidental or intentional, as from a surgical procedure. There are several types of accidental wounds. A **laceration** is a jagged, open wound in the skin that can extend down into the underlying tissue. The jagged edges may have to be cut away before the wound is closed. A **puncture wound** is a deep wound caused by a sharp object. (See Chapter 26 for further information on types and care of accidental wounds.) Both surgical and accidental wounds require special care to prevent infection. Proper wound care that promotes healing without infection is discussed in the Caution: Handle With Care section.

Cleaning a Wound. The first step in preventing a nonsurgical wound from becoming infected is careful cleansing. The wound must be thoroughly cleaned with soap and water. Then it must be irrigated with sterile saline solution or sterile water that is applied with a syringe and needle. **Debridement,** the removal of debris or dead tissue from the wound, may be necessary to expose healthy tissue.

Wound Healing. It is important to know how a wound heals so that you can care for it properly. A wound heals in three phases: lag phase, proliferation phase, and maturation phase. During the initial phase, or **lag phase,** bleeding is reduced as blood vessels in the affected area constrict. White blood cells and blood components play an important role in this phase. They seal the wound, clot the blood that has seeped into the area, and remove bacteria and debris from the wound. The wound contracts under the clot or scab that forms.

During the second phase, or **proliferation phase,** new tissue forms. Skin cells at the edges of the wound begin to move together to close off the wound. The scab that often forms over a wound actually slows down this movement of skin cells. The edges of the wound do eventually come together and form a continuous layer, closing off the wound.

The **maturation phase** (the third phase) involves the formation of scar tissue. Scar tissue is important for closing large, gaping, or jagged wounds. The continuous layer of skin cells formed during the second phase becomes thicker and pushes off the scab, leaving a scar. Scar tissue contains no nerves or blood vessels and lacks the resilience of skin.

The proliferation phase is sped up if the edges of an incision or nonsurgical wound are **approximated**—brought together so the tissue surfaces are close. This intervention protects the area from further contamination and minimizes scab and scar formation. Small wounds can be held together with butterfly closures or sterile strips. Larger wounds or those subject to strain may require suturing or stapling.

Closing a Wound. **Sutures** are surgical stitches used to close a wound. Suture materials, or **ligature,** can be either absorbable or nonabsorbable. The body breaks down absorbable sutures, so they do not require removal after the wound has healed. They are typically made of catgut (a sterile strand made of collagen fibers usually obtained from sheep or cow intestines). If a wound is particularly deep, the doctor may need to suture in layers, from inside to outside. In this case absorbable sutures are used for the inner suturing. Removable (nonabsorbable) sutures are generally used for the outside layer. Nonabsorbable ligature must be removed after wound healing is well under

CAUTION *Handle With Care*

Conditions That Interfere With Fast, Effective Wound Healing

The goals for treating both surgical and nonsurgical wounds are similar: they are to heal the wound without infection and to preserve normal skin function and appearance. Nonsurgical wounds often involve conditions that do not promote fast, effective healing. In these cases the wound requires special attention to ensure good results.

Many types of nonsurgical wounds may contain foreign material that can lead to infection. For example, a child may have a deep laceration from landing on a dirty, broken bottle when falling off a bicycle. These types of wounds always need vigorous cleaning. Some need debridement, or the removal of dead tissue or foreign material.

Wounds heal better when the edges are brought closely together, or approximated. Jagged edges in a laceration make approximation harder. It is also difficult to approximate crushed tissue, as you would see with fingers closed in a car door. Crushing disrupts a tissue's blood supply by rupturing blood vessels throughout the affected area. A physician might debride this type of wound with a scalpel to remove severely damaged tissue and achieve a clean wound edge before suturing.

After a surgical or nonsurgical wound is closed and sutured, it is essential to keep the wound clean and dry. Maintaining this condition serves a number of purposes. Most important is the prevention of infection. Infection delays the healing process and can have other serious consequences.

A sutured wound heals more quickly and smoothly when no scab forms because the migrating skin cells encounter no barrier to their movement. Proper postoperative care, including daily cleaning with soap and water or a mild antiseptic, keeps a wound scab-free. Although skin cells migrate across the space of a wound more easily in a somewhat moist environment, a wet wound offers the ideal conditions for bacteria to grow and cause infection. Covering a wound with antiseptic ointment and a clean, dry dressing keeps the wound slightly moist yet helps prevent infection.

Wound healing may be delayed in a number of instances not directly related to the surgery or injury. The presence of any of the following conditions can put a patient at risk for wound-healing problems. Wounds in such patients may require extra attention and care.

- Poor circulation: This condition results in inadequate supplies of nutrients, blood cells, and oxygen to the wound, all of which delay the healing process.
- Aging: Physiologic changes that occur with age can decrease a person's resistance to infection.
- Diabetes: Patients with diabetes experience changes in the walls of their arteries that result in poor circulation to peripheral tissues. These patients may also have a decreased resistance to infection.
- Poor nutrition: Patients who are undernourished, particularly those who are deficient in protein or vitamin C, do not have the physiologic resources for vigorous healing.
- High levels of stress: An increase in stress-related hormones can decrease resistance to infection.
- Weakened immune system: Patients who are on certain medications or who have certain chronic diseases may have weakened immune systems, putting them at increased risk of infection.
- Obesity: When someone is obese, the circulation directly under the skin is often poor, leading to slow healing.
- Smoking: Nicotine constricts the blood vessels in the skin, reducing circulation to the area of the wound and slowing healing.

way. Nonabsorbable sutures may be made of silk, nylon, or polyester. Suture materials come in thicknesses ranging from size 11-0 (smallest) to size 7 (largest). The needle is already attached to most prepackaged ligature.

Staples may be used to bring the edges of a wound together if there is considerable stress on the incision. For example, a long and deep surgical wound or a wound across the leg would have a strong tendency to gape open if not firmly secured. Surgical staples look somewhat like ordinary staples. They are inserted into the skin with a disposable staple unit.

Special Minor Surgical Procedures

Some types of minor surgical procedures require special surgical instruments. These procedures include laser surgery, cryosurgery, and electrocauterization. They all remove excess or abnormal tissue, as in the case of warts or skin lesions. These procedures usually require surgical aseptic technique because they break the integrity of the skin.

Laser Surgery. A laser emits an intense beam of light that is used to cut away tissue. Laser surgery is sometimes preferred over conventional surgery because it causes less damage to surrounding healthy tissue than does conventional surgery. Laser surgery also promotes quick healing and helps prevent infection.

When a laser is used in an office setting, close blinds and shades to keep out stray light. Remove any items that could catch fire if they came in contact with the laser beam. Cover any shiny or reflective surfaces. Make sure that everyone in the room, including the patient, wears special safety goggles to protect the eyes. Post a standard laser warning placard in the entryway to the room, per Occupational Safety and Health Administration (OSHA) regulations.

Position, drape, and prepare the patient as you would for conventional surgery. Place gauze around the surgical site, and assist the physician with administration of a local anesthetic if requested. The physician uses the laser to vaporize the unwanted tissue; vaporized tissue is cleared away by the vacuum hose portion of the unit (see Figure 24-1). You may be asked to apply pressure to control any bleeding. Clean the wound with an antiseptic, and apply a sterile dressing. Give the patient the normal instructions on wound care, including the recommendation to protect the site from exposure to the sun.

Cryosurgery. The use of extreme cold to destroy unwanted tissue is called **cryosurgery.** Cryosurgery is often used to remove skin lesions and lesions on the cervix. Before cryosurgery inform the patient that an initial sensation of cold will be followed by a burning sensation. Instruct the patient to remain as still as possible to prevent damage of nearby tissue.

The doctor may freeze the tissue by touching it with a cotton-tipped applicator dipped in liquid nitrogen or by spraying it with liquid nitrogen from a pressurized can. Sometimes a special cryosurgical instrument is used, most often during surgery on the cervix.

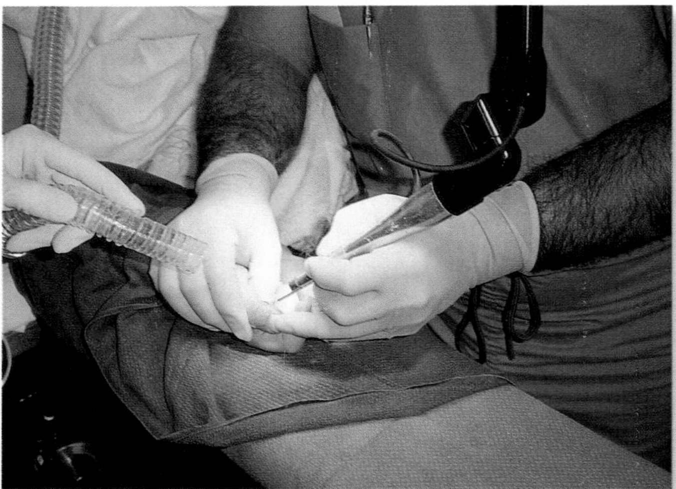

Figure 24-1. Suction eliminates vaporized tissue as a physician uses a laser to remove a wart from a patient's hand.

Make the patient aware that more than one freezing cycle may be necessary. A local anesthetic is usually not required because the cold itself reduces sensation in the area. After the procedure the area is cleaned with an antiseptic, and a sterile dressing may be applied. An ice pack may be applied to reduce swelling, and pain relievers may be given for pain.

Reassure the patient that some pain, swelling, or redness is normal after a cryosurgical procedure. Encourage the patient to use ice and pain relievers as necessary. Let the patient know that a large, painful, bloody blister may form. Left undisturbed, the blister usually ruptures in about 2 weeks. It should be left intact to promote healing and prevent infection. The patient should call the doctor if a blister becomes too painful. Be sure to provide the patient with complete wound-care instructions.

Electrocauterization. **Electrocauterization** is a technique whereby a needle, probe, or loop heated by electric current destroys the target tissue. A physician may use this technique to remove growths such as warts, to stop bleeding, and to control nosebleeds that either will not subside or continually recur.

Several types of electrocautery units are in use. Some are small, often handheld, units powered by battery or by ordinary household electric current. Other, larger units are designed for countertop placement or for mounting on a wall. Some units use disposable probes, whereas others employ reusable ones.

With certain units a grounding pad or plate is placed somewhere on the patient's body (or under it) during the procedure. This grounding completes the circuit and prevents electric shock to the patient, the physician, and staff members. Reassure the patient that grounding causes no discomfort.

A local anesthetic may be administered before the procedure. A scab or crust generally forms over the area. Healing may take 2 to 3 weeks. General wound-care instructions are appropriate for this procedure, except that a dressing may be omitted to keep the area drier.

Instruments Used in Minor Surgery

The type of minor surgical procedure determines which surgical instruments are used. Surgical instruments have specific purposes and may be classified by function.

Cutting and Dissecting Instruments

Cutting and dissecting instruments have sharp edges and are used to cut (incise) skin and tissue. Figure 24-2 illustrates some of the basic cutting and dissecting instruments

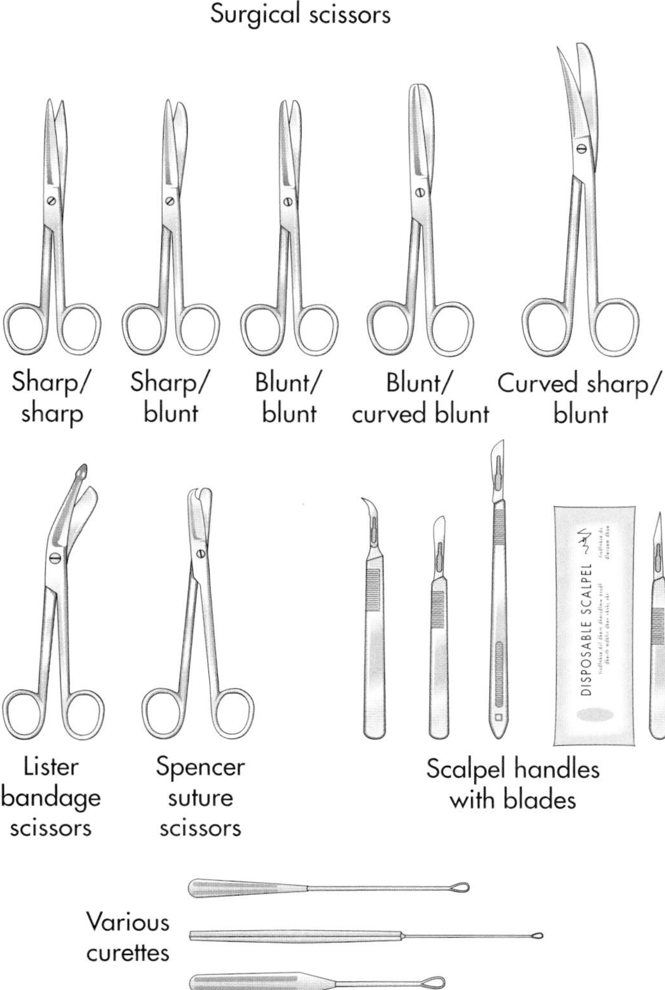

Figure 24-2. These are typical cutting and dissecting instruments used in minor surgical procedures.

you will encounter. You must be careful when cleaning, sterilizing, and storing these instruments to avoid injuring yourself and to protect the instruments' sharp edges.

Scalpels. A scalpel consists of a handle that holds a disposable blade. Scalpel handles are either reusable or disposable and vary in width and length. A scalpel's specific use determines the shape and size of its blade. General-purpose scalpels have wide blades and a straight cutting surface. A no. 15 blade is the most common one for performing minor procedures.

Scissors. Surgical scissors come in various sizes. They may be straight or curved and have either blunt or pointed tips. Tissue scissors must be sharp enough to cut without damaging or ripping surrounding tissue. Suture scissors have blunt points and a curved lower blade. The lower blade is inserted under the suture material to cut it. Bandage scissors are used to remove dressings. They have a blunt lower blade so that the skin next to the dressing is not injured. Clippers are scissorlike instruments used for cutting nails or thick materials.

Curettes. The doctor uses a curette for scraping tissue. Curettes come in a variety of shapes and sizes. They consist of a circular blade—actually a loop—attached to a rod-shaped handle. The blade is blunt on the outside and sharp on the inside. The inner part of the blade may also be serrated. Serrated blades may be used to take Pap smears (Papanicolaou smears) and to perform ear irrigations where a large amount of cerumen has accumulated.

Grasping and Clamping Instruments

Special instruments are used for grasping and clamping tissue. Grasping instruments are used to hold surgical materials or to remove foreign objects, such as splinters, from the body. Clamping instruments are used to apply pressure and close off blood vessels. They are also used to hold tissue and other materials in position. Figure 24-3 shows some common grasping and clamping instruments.

Forceps. Forceps are instruments that are most often used to grasp or hold objects. Grasping types are usually shaped like tweezers and include thumb forceps and tissue forceps. Thumb forceps, also called smooth forceps, vary in shape and size. The blades of thumb forceps are tapered to a point and have small grooves at the tip. Tissue forceps (serrated forceps) have one or more fine teeth at the tips of the blades. When closed, these forceps hold tissue firmly. Holding forceps have handles with ratchets that lock the teeth in a closed position. Dressing, or sponge, forceps have ridges to hold a sponge or gauze when it is used to absorb body fluids.

Hemostats. The most commonly used surgical instruments are hemostats. These surgical clamps vary in size and shape. Hemostats are typically used to close off blood vessels. The serrated jaws of hemostats taper to a point. Like holding forceps, hemostats have handles that lock on ratchets, holding the jaws securely closed.

Towel Clamps. Towel clamps are used to keep towels in place during a surgical procedure. This stability is important in maintaining a sterile field.

Retracting, Dilating, and Probing Instruments

Retracting instruments are used to hold back the sides of a wound or incision. Dilating and probing instruments may be used to enlarge, examine, or clear body openings, body cavities, or wounds. The shapes of these instruments vary with their functions. Some typical retracting, dilating, and probing instruments are shown in Figure 24-4.

Retractors. The use of retractors allows greater access to and a better view of a surgical site. Some retractors must be held open by hand, whereas others have ratchets or locks to keep them open.

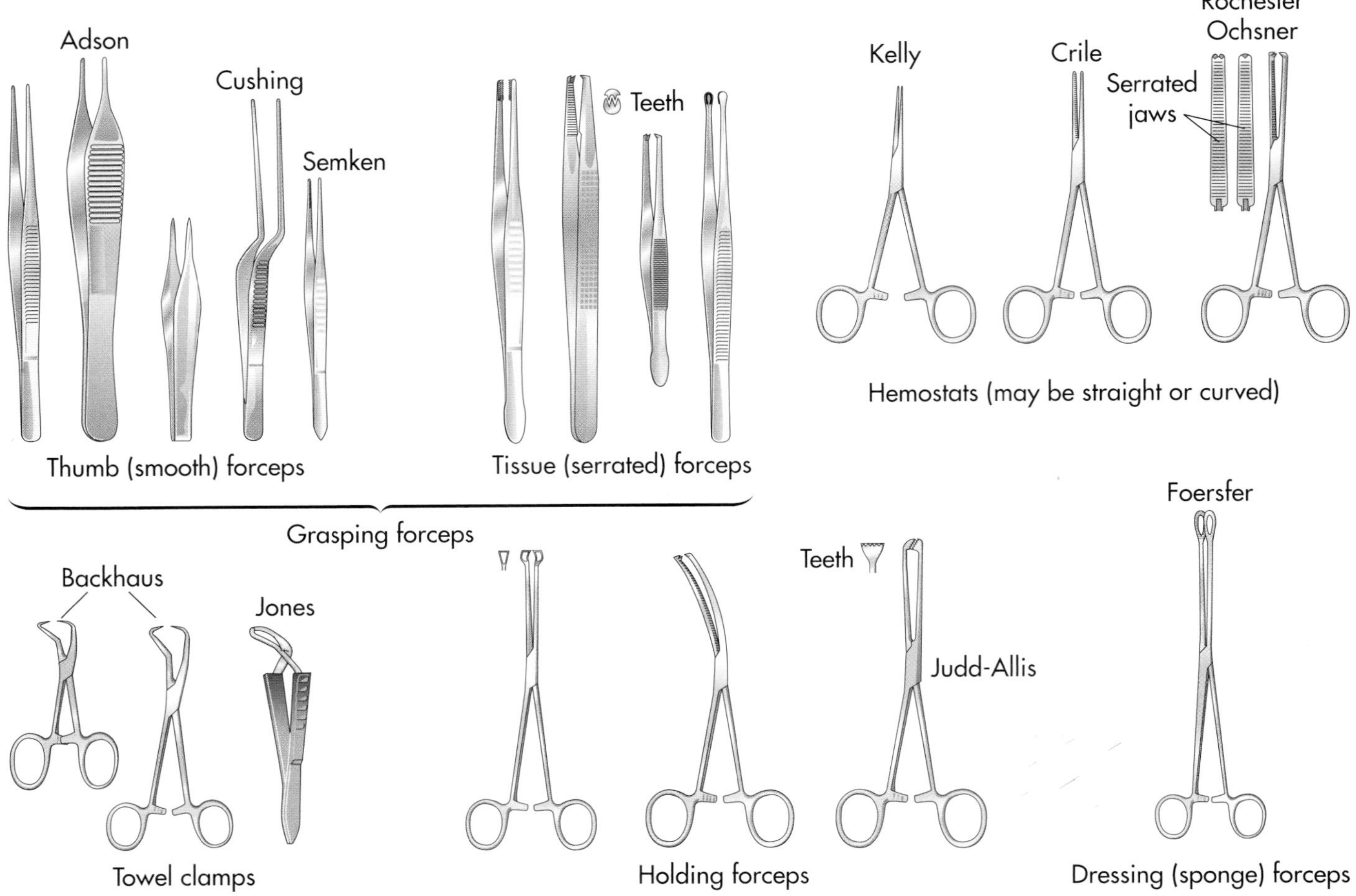

Figure 24-3. These are typical grasping and clamping instruments used in minor surgical procedures.

Dilators. Dilators are slender, pointed instruments. They are used to enlarge a body opening, such as a tear duct.

Probes. A surgical probe is a slender rod with a blunt tip shaped like a bulb. Probes are used to explore wounds or body cavities and to locate or clear blockages.

Suturing Instruments

Suturing instruments are used to introduce suture materials into and retrieve them from a wound. Some carry the suture material, whereas others manipulate the suture carriers. Examples of suturing instruments are shown in Figure 24-5.

Suture Needles. Surgical suture needles carry suture material, also called ligature, through the tissue being sutured. They are either pointed or blunt at one end. They may have an eye at the other end to hold suture materials. Ligature often comes prepackaged with the needle already connected. Prepackaged suture needles with attached ligature have no eye and produce less trauma to the tissue being sutured than do suture needles with eyes.

Suture needles may be straight, or they may be curved to allow deeper placement of sutures. Taper point needles (needles that taper into a sharp point) are used to suture tissues that are easily penetrated. They create only very small holes, thus minimizing leakage of tissue fluids. Cutting needles (needles that have at least two sharpened edges) are used on tough tissues that are not easily penetrated, such as skin.

Several measurements are used to determine the size of a surgical needle. Needle length is the distance from the tip to the end, measuring along the body of the needle. Chord length is the straight-line distance from the tip to the end of the needle. (Chord length is not the same as needle length in curved needles.) The radius of a curved needle is determined by mentally continuing the curve of the needle into a full circle and finding the distance from the center of the circle to the needle body. The diameter is the thickness of the needle. Needle size generally corresponds to the size of suture material used. Smaller needles are used for delicate procedures, such as eye surgery or repairing a facial laceration. Larger needles are used for suturing wounds of less delicate parts of the body, such as the hands or legs.

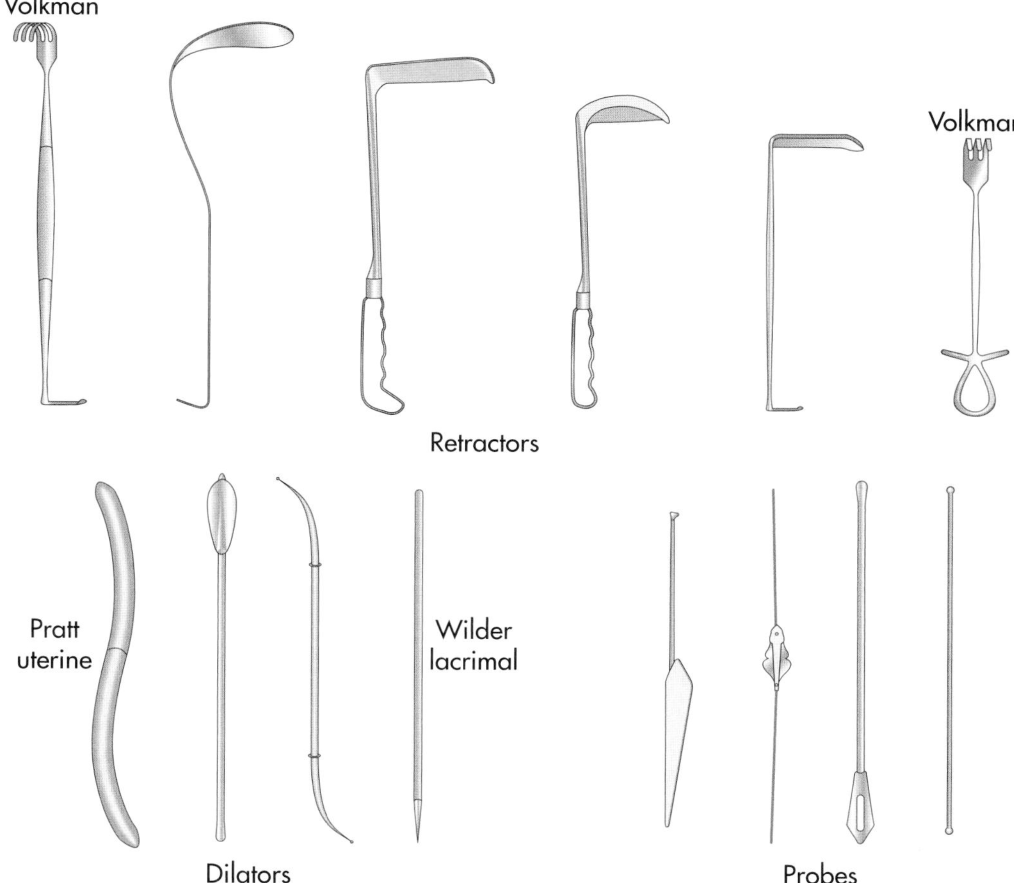

Figure 24-4. These are typical retracting, dilating, and probing instruments used in minor surgical procedures.

Needle Holders. Curved suture needles require special instruments to hold, insert, and retrieve them during suturing. Most needle holders look like hemostats with short, sturdy jaws.

Syringes and Needles

Sterile syringes and needles are used to inject anesthetic solutions, withdraw fluids, or obtain biopsy specimens. The size of the syringe and needle varies with the intended use. For example, a needle used to perform a biopsy is generally larger than needles used for most injections. (Syringes and needles used for injections are discussed and illustrated in Chapter 33.) Both syringes and needles are provided in individual sterile envelopes.

Instrument Trays and Packs

All the surgical instruments needed for a specific procedure are usually assembled beforehand. They are then sterilized together in a pack. Certain surgical supplies necessary for the procedure (such as gauze) are included in the pack because they, too, must be sterile. Surgical trays can be quickly set up with these instrument packs. Individually wrapped items may also be added as needed.

These are common types of instrument trays:

- Laceration repair tray (see Figure 24-6)
- Laceration repair with debridement tray
- Incision and drainage tray
- Foreign body or growth removal tray
- **Onychectomy** (nail removal) tray
- Vasectomy (male sterilization procedure) tray
- Suture removal tray
- Staple removal tray

Asepsis

Maintaining asepsis during surgical procedures is always a priority. It is critical to the health and safety of both the patient and the health-care professional. The two levels of aseptic technique are medical asepsis (clean technique) and surgical asepsis (sterile technique). Chapter 1 describes in detail the two types of asepsis. You will use both levels of asepsis when assisting with minor surgery.

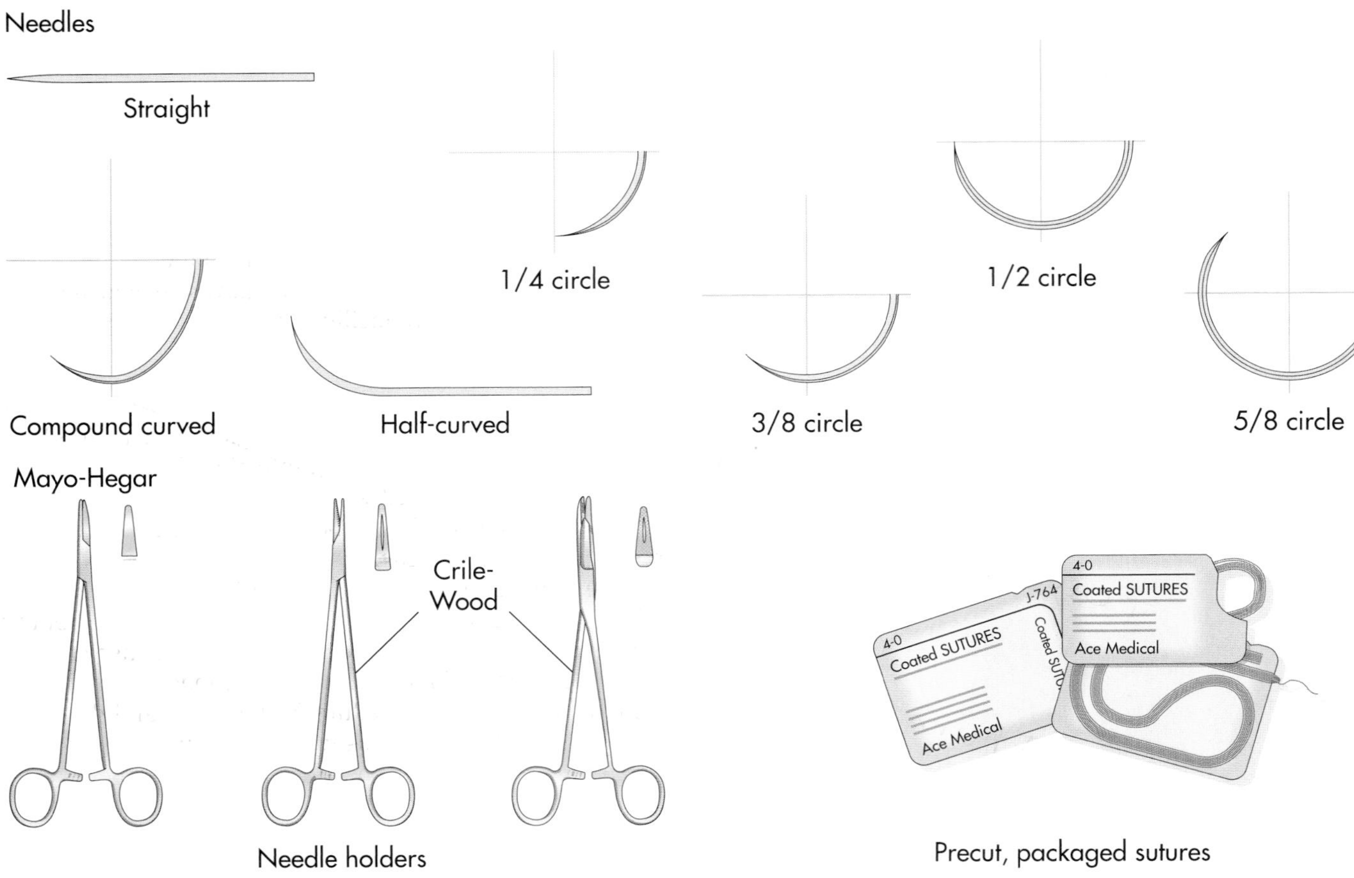

Needles

Straight

1/4 circle

1/2 circle

Compound curved

Half-curved

3/8 circle

5/8 circle

Mayo-Hegar

Crile-Wood

Needle holders

4-0 Coated SUTURES Ace Medical

Precut, packaged sutures

Figure 24-5. These are typical suturing instruments.

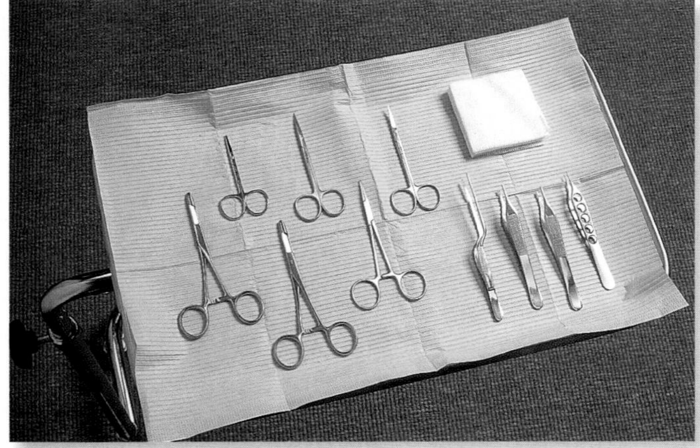

Figure 24-6. This laceration tray contains scissors, several pairs of forceps, a needle holder, suture material, and sterile gauze.

Medical Asepsis

Medical asepsis involves procedures to reduce the number of microorganisms and thus prevent the spread of disease. These procedures do not necessarily eliminate microorganisms. Hand washing is always the first line of defense against spreading disease. The use of antimicrobial agents (agents that kill microorganisms or suppress their growth) and personal protective equipment are also part of medical asepsis. Other practices include proper handling and disposal of sharps and biohazardous materials.

Personal Protective Equipment. Personal protective equipment, or PPE, includes all items used as a barrier between the wearer and potentially infectious or hazardous medical materials. PPE includes gloves, gowns, and masks and protective eyewear or face shields (Figure 24-7). OSHA regulations regarding PPE are discussed in detail in Chapter 1.

Gloves are of particular importance during surgical procedures. You should wear properly sized latex or vinyl gloves during any procedure that might expose you to potentially infectious or hazardous materials. (Gloves that are too big can catch on instruments or equipment and cause accidents.) When you wear gloves, you also protect the patient from any infectious organisms on your hands.

Both vinyl and latex gloves can prevent contamination of the hands with bacteria. Many health-care institutions prefer latex gloves. However, the incidence of latex allergy among health-care professionals has grown. Allergic reactions to latex can range from a skin rash to shock and even death. Many health-care institutions are switching to less

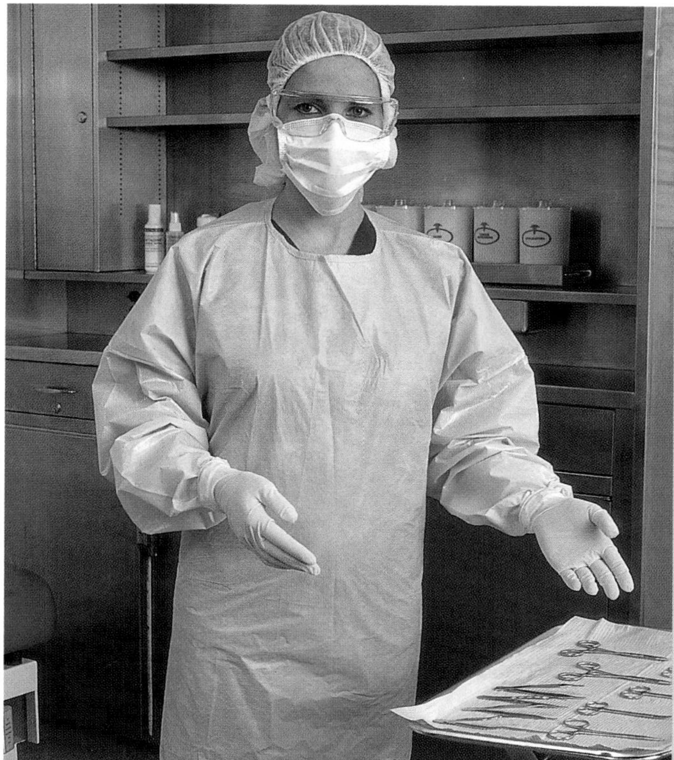

Figure 24-7. Personal protective equipment provides a barrier between infectious or hazardous medical materials and the wearer.

allergenic latex gloves, such as low-powder and powderless varieties. The powder in the gloves, which makes them easier to put on, is one of the primary sources of latex allergy. The latex protein that causes the allergy mixes with the powder. When the gloves are removed, the powder containing the latex protein becomes airborne and is inhaled.

Other steps to prevent latex allergy include changing gloves frequently, thoroughly drying hands after washing, and frequently applying lotion to the hands. If you notice symptoms of a latex allergy, you should consider consulting an allergist. You should also discuss your symptoms with your supervisor, who will recommend that you switch to hypoallergenic or vinyl gloves. If you have an allergy, the health-care facility where you are employed is required to provide nonlatex gloves for your use.

Sharps and Biohazardous Waste Handling and Disposal. Sharp medical and surgical instruments have great potential for transmitting infection through cuts and puncture wounds. Used scalpels, needles, syringes, and other sharp objects should be disposed of in a puncture-resistant sharps container.

All items other than sharps that have come in contact with tissue, blood, or body fluids must be disposed of in a leakproof plastic bag or container. The container must either be red or be labeled with the orange-red biohazard symbol. The proper procedure for handling and disposing of sharps and biohazardous waste is discussed in detail in Chapter 1.

Surgical Asepsis

In contrast to medical asepsis, the purpose of **surgical asepsis** is to eliminate all microorganisms. Surgical asepsis does not just reduce the quantity of microorganisms but completely eliminates them. View the Caution: Handle With Care section that contains rules for sterile technique.

CAUTION *Handle With Care*

Rules for Sterile Technique

A sterile field is an area used during surgical asepsis or a sterile technique that is free of microorganisms. Sterile fields are prepared for minor surgical procedures. To maintain sterility throughout the procedure, follow the surgical technique and adhere to these rules:

1. The contact of a sterile area or article with a nonsterile article renders it nonsterile.
2. If there is a doubt about the sterility of an article or area, it is considered nonsterile.
3. Unused, opened sterile supplies must be discarded or resterilized.
4. Packages are wrapped or sealed in such a way that they can be opened without contamination.
5. The edges of wrappers (1-inch margin) covering sterile supplies, the outer lips of bottles, or flasks containing sterile solutions are not considered sterile.
6. When a sterile surface or package becomes wet, it is considered contaminated.
7. Reaching over a sterile field when you are not wearing sterile clothing contaminates the area.
8. When wearing sterile gloves, keep your hands between your shoulders and your waist to maintain sterility.
9. Even in a sterile gown, your back is considered contaminated; do not turn your back on a sterile field.

PROCEDURE 24.1

Creating a Sterile Field

Objective: To create a sterile field for a minor surgical procedure

OSHA Guidelines: This procedure does not involve exposure to blood, body fluids, or tissues.

Materials: Tray or Mayo stand, sterile instrument pack, sterile transfer forceps, cleaning solution, sterile drape, additionally packaged sterile items as required

Method

1. Clean and disinfect the tray or Mayo stand.
2. Wash your hands and assemble the necessary materials.
3. Check the label on the instrument pack to make sure it is the correct pack for the procedure.
4. Check the date and sterilization indicator on the instrument pack to make sure the pack is still sterile (Figure 24-8).
5. Place the sterile pack on the tray or stand, and unfold the outermost fold away from yourself.
6. Unfold the sides of the pack outward, touching only the areas that will become the underside of the sterile field.
7. Open the final flap toward yourself, stepping back and away from the sterile field (Figure 24-9).
8. Place additional packaged sterile items on the sterile field.
   - Ensure that you have the correct item or instrument and that the package is still sterile.

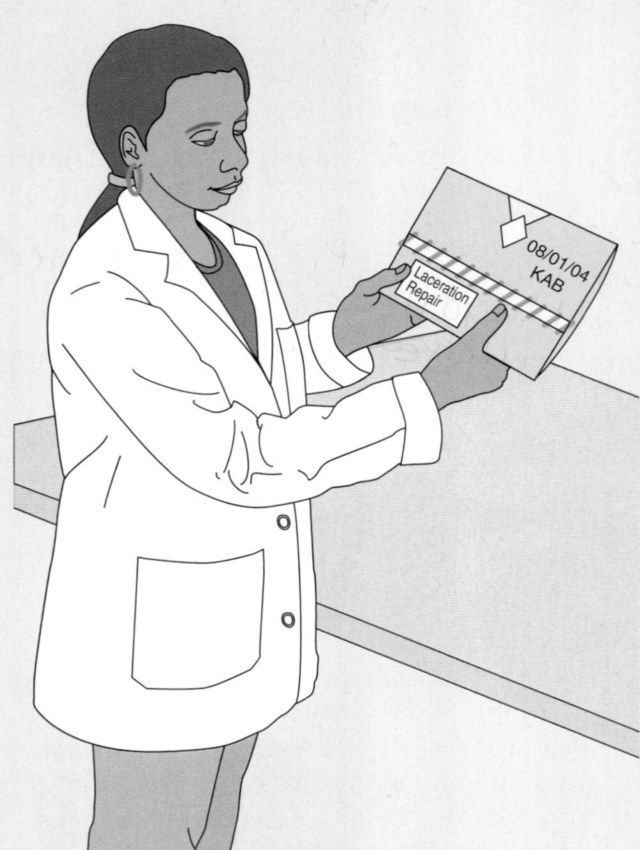

Figure 24-8. Before you open it, confirm that you have the correct instrument pack and that it has not expired.

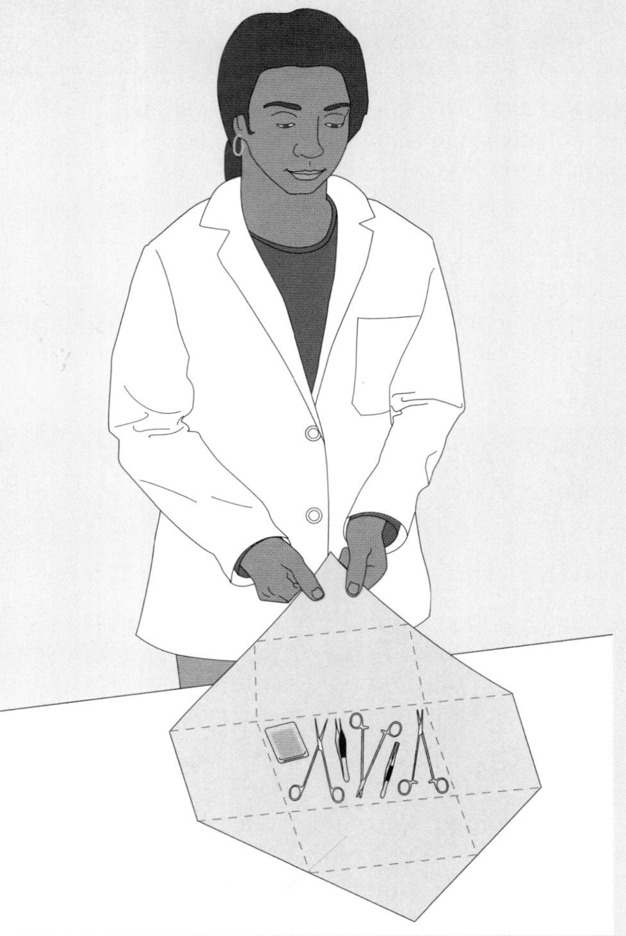

Figure 24-9. The fully open instrument pack constitutes a sterile field.

continued →

PROCEDURE 24.1

Creating a Sterile Field *(continued)*

- Stand away from the sterile field.
- Grasp the package flaps and pull apart about halfway. Bring the corners of the wrapping beneath the package, paying attention not to contaminate the inner package or item.
- Hold the package over the sterile field with the opening down; with a quick movement, pull the flap completely open and snap the sterile item onto the field.

9. Place basins and bowls near the edge of the sterile field so you can port liquids without reaching over the field (Figure 24-10).

10. Use sterile transfer forceps if necessary to add additional items to the sterile field (Figure 24-11).

11. If necessary, don sterile gloves after a sterile scrub to arrange items on the sterile field.

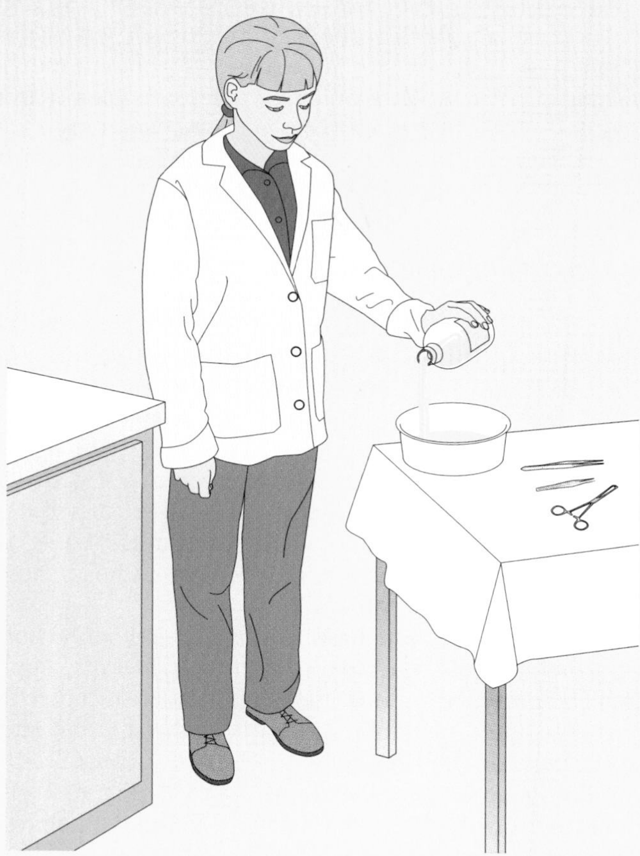

Figure 24-10. Pour a sterile solution into a sterile bowl near the edge of the sterile field without touching the rim of the bowl, splashing the solution, or reaching over the field.

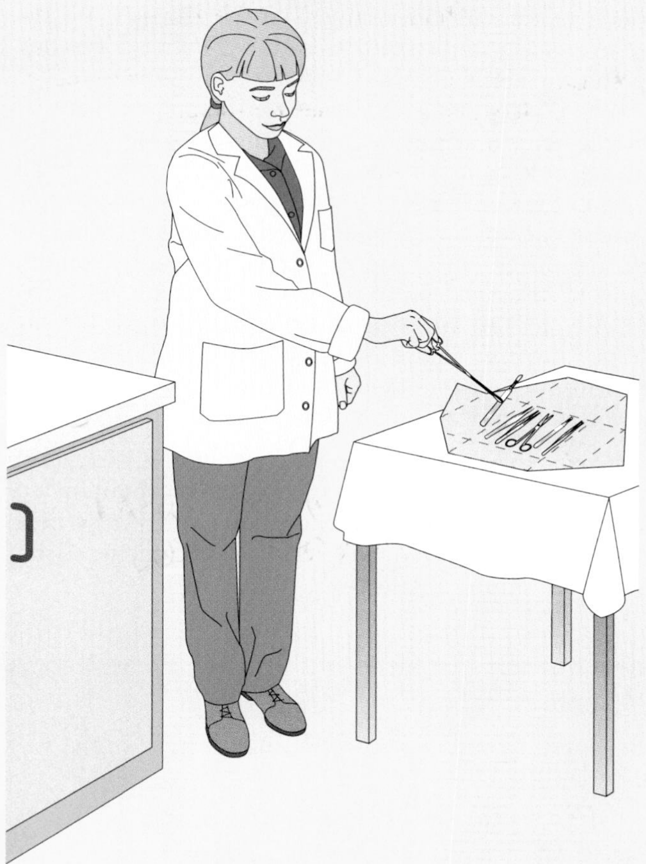

Figure 24-11. You can place sterile items on the sterile field by using transfer forceps.

Common procedures involving sterile technique that you will be expected to perform include the following:

- Creating a sterile field
- Adding sterile items to the sterile field
- Performing a surgical scrub
- Putting on sterile gloves
- Sanitizing, disinfecting, and sterilizing equipment

Creating a Sterile Field. A **sterile field** is an area free of microorganisms that will be used as a work area during a surgical procedure. Always be aware that in the following instances the sterile field is considered to become contaminated and must be redone:

- An unsterile item touches the field
- Someone reaches across the field
- The field becomes wet

The sterile field is often set up on a **Mayo stand,** a movable stainless steel instrument tray on a stand. You should adjust the stand so the tray is above waist level. Remember, items placed below waist level are considered contaminated. Before beginning, disinfect the Mayo stand with 70% isopropyl alcohol, and allow it to dry.

To create the sterile field, cover the stand with two layers of sterile material. This material can be sterile disposable drapes, separately sterilized muslin towels, or the muslin towels that the surgical instruments are wrapped in before autoclaving to produce office-sterilized sterile instrument packs. Commercially prepared sterile instrument packs, usually with disposable paper wrappings, are also used to create a sterile field. Procedure 24-1 describes how to prepare a sterile field and how to open sterile packages.

When assembling the necessary supplies, place all unsterile items that may be used during the procedure outside the sterile field. Unsterile items include items that are sterile on the inside but not on the outside, such as a sterile gauze pack or sterile liquid such as alcohol, saline, or peroxide inside an unsterile bottle. Unsterile supplies should be arranged on a counter away from the sterile field. A typical arrangement of unsterile items used in surgery is shown in Figure 24-12. If you place an unsterile item within the sterile field, the field is no longer sterile, and you must repeat the entire process.

Adding Sterile Items to the Sterile Field. The outer 1 inch of the sterile field is considered contaminated. Therefore, before you add sterile items to the sterile field, carefully plan where you will place the instruments so that they are within the sterile field.

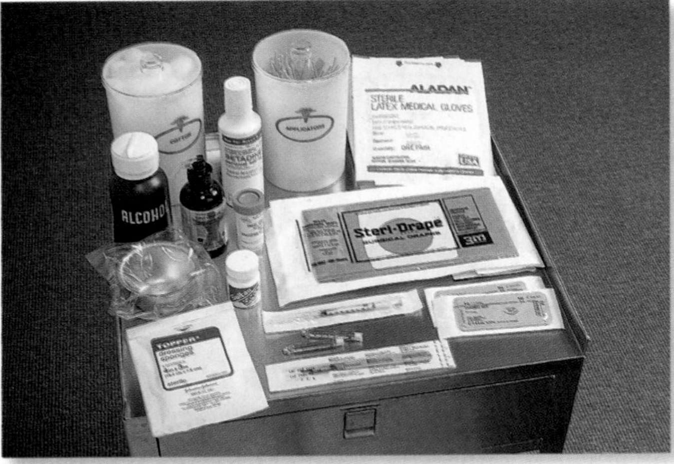

Figure 24-12. For each surgical procedure, unsterile surgical supplies must be gathered and arranged in an area separate from the sterile field.

Instruments and Supplies. If you have used sterile disposable drapes or separately sterilized muslin towels to create the sterile field, you will need to add the necessary instruments. Stand away from the sterile field, and open the sterile instrument pack in the manner described in Procedure 24-1. Place the pack on a counter or hold it open in your hand. Transfer and arrange the instruments on the sterile field with sterile transfer forceps (see Figure 24-11). Avoid reaching across the sterile field.

If you must add other items to the field, open them using the same method. Stand away from the sterile field. As you unwrap the item, gather the corners of the wrapping beneath it. You can place the contents on the sterile field by using sterile transfer forceps or by using the sterile inside of the wrapping to prevent your hands from touching the item. Place basins or bowls near the edge of the sterile field so you can pour liquids without reaching over the field.

Some instruments are sterilized individually in autoclave bags, and sterile supplies are often prepackaged. Stand away from the sterile field as you open an individual bag or package. You can pull the flaps of the packaging partway apart, then snap (remove from position by a sudden movement) the item onto the sterile field from a distance of 8 to 12 inches. Alternatively, you can use sterile forceps to grasp and place the items in the sterile field.

Pouring Sterile Solutions. Sterile solutions are often required during the surgical procedure to rinse or wash the wound. Sterile solutions can be added to the sterile field after the sterile instruments. Several sterile solutions are commonly used during minor surgical procedures. These include sterile water and physiological (normal) saline (0.9% sodium chloride).

Bottles of these sterile solutions come in a variety of sizes. You should choose the smallest size that will meet the solutions needed during the procedure. Using the smallest size possible minimizes the cost because unused solutions must be discarded.

When pouring a solution, cover the label on the bottle with the palm of your hand to keep the label dry. Pour a small amount of the liquid into a liquid waste receptacle to clean the lip of the bottle. As you pour the solution into a sterile bowl on the field, hold the bottle at an angle so that you do not reach over the sterile area (see Figure 24-10). Hold the bottle fairly close to the bowl without touching it. Pour the contents slowly to avoid splashing the drape, which would contaminate the field.

When a sterile solution bottle is opened and may be used again during the procedure, do not let any unsterile object touch the inside of its cap. To accomplish this, place the cap on a clean location in the same position it was in on the bottle (the sterile inside of the cap facing down).

Performing a Surgical Scrub and Donning Sterile Gloves. If you assist in a surgical procedure, you must perform a surgical scrub and wear sterile surgical gloves. You may wonder why a surgical scrub is necessary if you are planning to wear sterile gloves. The answer is that there is always the possibility that a glove may be punctured. If the skin is as clean as possible, the risk of contamination from a punctured glove is minimized. Nevertheless, if a glove is damaged during a sterile procedure, you must consider anything touched by that glove to be contaminated. Contaminated items must be resterilized or replaced before you continue.

A surgical scrub removes microorganisms more effectively than does routine hand washing. Routine hand washing removes bacteria present on the skin's surface, whereas the surgical scrub removes bacteria in deeper layers of the skin—where the hair follicles and oil-producing glands are. Procedure 24-2 describes the process.

Sterile gloves are required for many procedures. You don sterile gloves after you perform the surgical scrub. The process is described in Procedure 24-3.

Remember that once you are wearing sterile gloves, you may touch only the items in the sterile field. Therefore, you must remove any drape covering the sterile instrument tray before you glove. Sterile gloves provide a small margin of safety in preventing contamination. You must keep your movements controlled and precise to work within that margin to protect the sterile area.

Sanitizing, Disinfecting, and Sterilizing Equipment. Many supplies used in a doctor's office are disposable. Most surgical instruments, however, are made of steel and are reusable. Preparing surgical instruments for reuse involves cleaning them with soap and water (a process called sanitization), then disinfecting and/or sterilizing them, depending on how the equipment will be used. (These procedures are described more fully in Chapter 2.)

Wearing gloves, first clean surgical instruments with soap and water to remove dirt and debris. Then rinse and dry them. After you have sanitized the instruments, disinfect them. If you cannot wash surgical instruments immediately after use, place them directly in disinfectant.

The most common disinfecting agents are chemicals and boiling water. Remember that disinfection kills many microorganisms but does not kill bacterial spores and some viruses. For this reason instruments used in surgical procedures are always sterilized. It is also common to sterilize surgical instruments, even when they will be used in nonsurgical procedures, to reduce the possibility of infection.

Autoclaving is the most common method of sterilization. The autoclave kills microorganisms and spores by means of steam under pressure. The dry heat oven provides another method of sterilization. This technique is preferred for sterilizing sharp instruments, because the moist heat in the autoclave may damage cutting edges.

The Chemiclave is another type of sterilization equipment. It uses alcohol under pressure rather than steam. Cold sterilization methods involve lengthy periods of soaking in sterilizing chemicals. Gas sterilization with ethylene oxide is sometimes used for equipment that might be damaged by heat or moisture. The drawback with ethylene oxide gas is that it is highly toxic to humans and the environment. Because of this potential danger, gas sterilization is generally used only in hospital and manufacturing environments.

Preoperative Procedures

You must complete a number of steps before a surgical procedure. The steps include performing various preliminary duties, preparing the surgical room, and physically preparing the patient for surgery.

Preliminary Duties

You will perform several preliminary tasks before the surgery. They include providing **preoperative** (prior to surgery or "preop") instructions to the patient, completing various administrative tasks, and easing the patient's fears.

Preoperative Instructions. When a patient is scheduled for a minor surgical procedure in the doctor's office, you must explain the preoperative instructions. You should also be prepared to answer the patient's questions about the procedure and about possible risks. The patient may ask you, rather than the doctor, such questions or may need clarification of information provided by the doctor.

A patient may need to follow certain dietary and fluid restrictions before a minor surgical procedure. Not eating or drinking for a specific period of time is a common restriction. There may also be restrictions on what medications a patient may take, because of the administration of an anesthetic during the procedure. You will need to tell non-English-speaking patients to bring along a family member or other interpreter who can help them understand the forms they must sign and their instructions.

You should instruct the patient to wear either comfortable, loose-fitting clothes that will not interfere with the procedure or clothing that can be removed easily. In most cases patients also need to arrange for someone to drive them home after a procedure.

Administrative and Legal Tasks. You must ensure that all the necessary paperwork is completed before surgery. Routine administrative tasks include completing the required insurance forms and obtaining prior authorization from the patient's insurance company.

Make absolutely certain that the patient reads, understands, and signs the surgical consent form. The patient needs a clear understanding of what to expect during and after the surgery to give informed consent as required by law. Sometimes surgery is performed on a child or a patient with limited understanding of legal documents. In such cases the consent form must be signed by the patient's parent or legal guardian.

Failure to obtain the necessary paperwork prior to a surgical procedure can cause serious legal problems. The doctor and other staff members could be held legally liable if problems were to develop during or after the procedure.

PROCEDURE 24.2

Performing a Surgical Scrub

Objective: To remove dirt and microorganisms from under the fingernails and from the surface of the skin, hair follicles, and oil glands of the hands and forearms

OSHA Guidelines: This procedure does not involve exposure to blood, body fluids, or tissues.

Materials: Dispenser with surgical soap, sterile surgical scrub brush, orange stick, sterile towels

Method

1. Remove all jewelry and roll up your sleeves to above the elbow.
2. Assemble the necessary materials.
3. Turn the water on and adjust it so that it is warm.
4. Wet your hands from the fingertips to the elbows. You must keep your hands higher than your elbows to prevent water from running down your arms and contaminating the washed area.
5. Apply surgical soap, and for 2 minutes scrub your hands, fingers, areas between the fingers, wrists, and forearms with the scrub brush, using a firm circular motion (Figure 24-13).
6. Rinse from fingers to elbows, always keeping your hands higher than your elbows (Figure 24-14).
7. Use the orange stick to clean under your fingernails, and rinse your hands again.
8. Apply more surgical soap, and again use the brush to completely scrub your hands, fingers, areas between the fingers, wrists, and forearms. Scrub for at least 3 minutes, and then rinse from fingers to elbows again.
9. Thoroughly dry your hands and forearms with sterile towels, working from the hands to the elbows (Figure 24-15).
10. Turn off the faucet with the foot or knee pedal. Use a clean paper towel if a foot or knee pedal is not used.

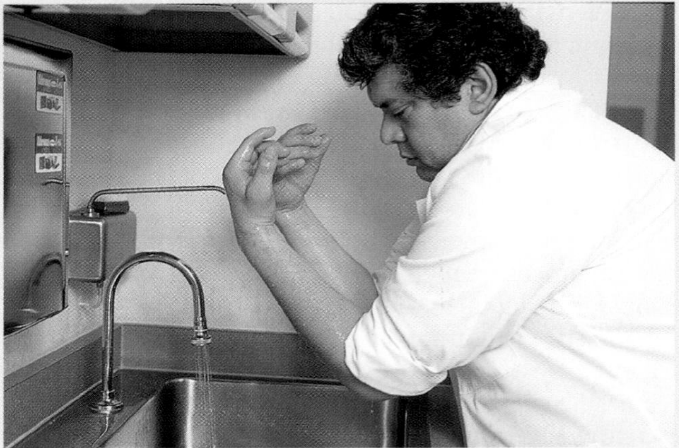

Figure 24-14. Keep your hands above your elbows while rinsing from fingertips to elbows.

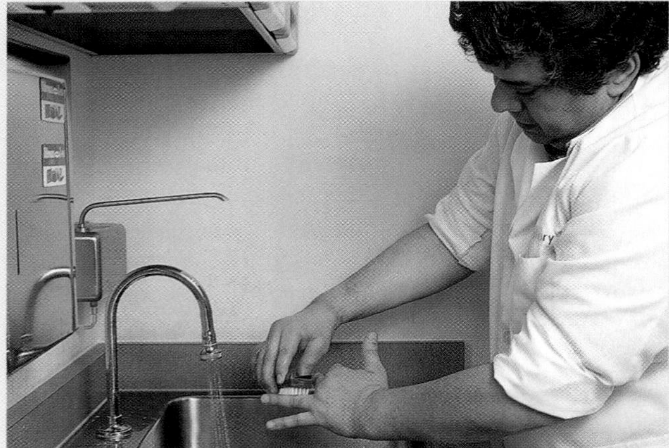

Figure 24-13. Use the scrub brush to work the surgical soap into your fingers, then your wrists, and then your forearms with a firm, circular motion.

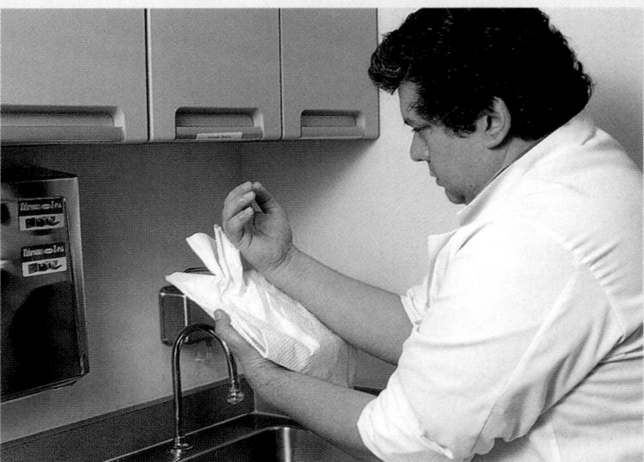

Figure 24-15. Dry your hands thoroughly before carefully drying your forearms.

PROCEDURE 24.3

Donning Sterile Gloves

Objective: To don sterile gloves without compromising the sterility of the outer surface of the gloves

OSHA Guidelines: This procedure does not involve exposure to blood, body fluids, or tissues.

Materials: Correctly sized, prepackaged, double-wrapped sterile gloves

Method

1. Obtain the correct size gloves.
2. Check the package for tears, and ensure that the expiration date has not passed.
3. Perform a surgical scrub.
4. Peel the outer wrap from gloves and place the inner wrapper on a clean surface above waist level (Figure 24-16).
5. Position gloves so the cuff end is closest to your body.
6. Touch only the flaps as you open the package.
7. Use instructions provided on inner package, if available.
8. Do not reach over the sterile inside of the inner package.
9. Follow these steps if there are no instructions:
   a. Open the package so the first flap is opened away from you.
   b. Pinch the corner and pull to one side.
   c. Put your fingertips under the side flaps and gently pull until the package is completely open.
10. Use your nondominant hand to grasp the inside cuff of the opposite glove (the folded edge). Do not touch the outside of the glove. If you are right-handed, use your left hand to put on the right glove first, and vice versa.
11. Holding the glove at arm's length and waist level, insert the dominant hand into the glove with the palm facing up. Don't let the outside of the glove touch any other surface (Figure 24-17).
12. With your sterile gloved hand, slip the gloved fingers into the cuff of the other glove.
13. Pick up the other glove, touching only the outside. Don't touch any other surfaces (Figure 24-18).
14. Pull the glove up and onto your hand. Ensure that the sterile gloved hand does not touch skin (Figure 24-19).
15. Adjust your fingers as necessary, touching only glove to glove.
16. Do not adjust the cuffs because your forearms may contaminate the gloves.
17. Keep your hands in front of you, between your shoulders and waist. If you move your hands out of this area, they are considered contaminated.

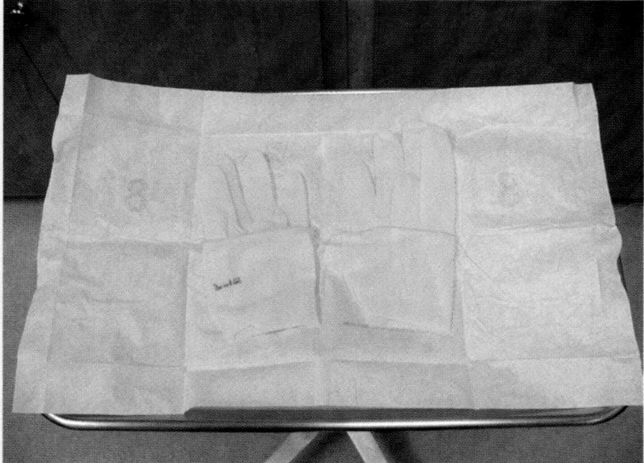

Figure 24-16. You must put these sterile gloves on without reaching across the sterile surfaces of the gloves or the sterile inner wrap of the pack.

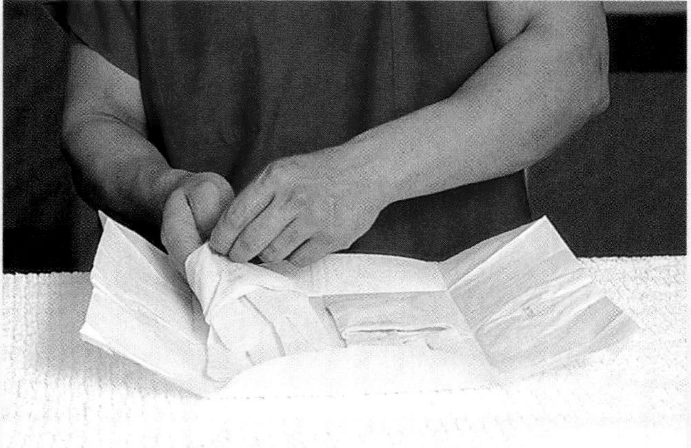

Figure 24-17. Your palm should face up as you slide your dominant hand into the first glove.

continued ⟶

PROCEDURE 24.3

Donning Sterile Gloves *(continued)*

18. If contamination or the possibility of contamination occurs, change gloves.

19. Remove gloves the same way you remove clean gloves, by touching only the inside.

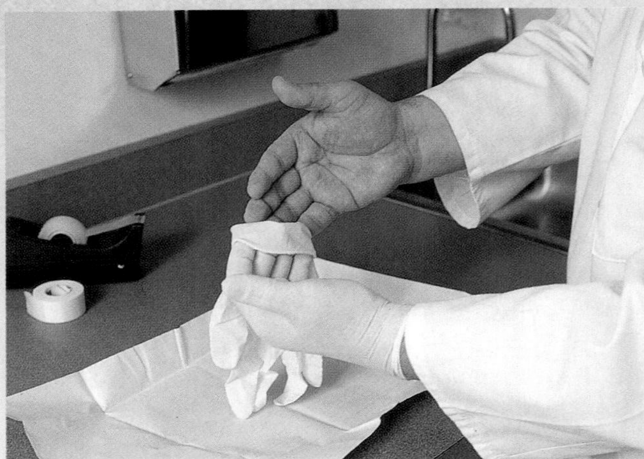

Figure 24-18. Your gloved fingers secure the remaining glove while you slip it over your nondominant hand.

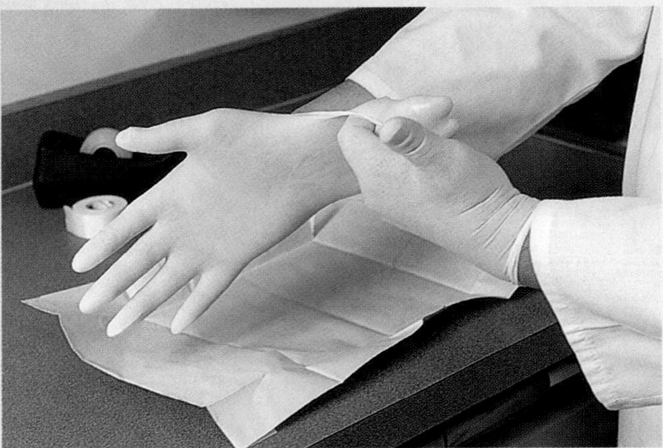

Figure 24-19. Unfold the cuff over your arm while touching only the sterile surface of the glove.

It is common practice to call the patient the day before the surgery to confirm the appointment. This call also provides a chance to ensure that the patient follows the preoperative instructions. You may be responsible for making this call.

Easing the Patient's Fears. Knowing what to expect during and after a surgical procedure will ease patients' fears. This information allows them to plan their daily activities and, if necessary, to arrange for help at home during the recovery period.

Some offices may have educational materials such as brochures, fact sheets, or videotapes about the procedure the patient will undergo. The availability of such materials varies with the practice specialty and the frequency with which the procedure is performed. You may assist in preparing or acquiring these materials if your office's policy includes such participation for medical assistants. This type of information is extremely helpful to the patient. It may increase patient compliance with the pre- and postoperative instructions.

Much of a patient's fear about a surgical procedure can be overcome if you spend sufficient time before the procedure explaining what to expect. Be prepared to answer the patient's questions honestly, calmly, and confidently. Your calm and knowledgeable manner will reassure the patient. If the answer to a question requires experience or knowledge beyond your own, pass the question on to the doctor.

Preparing the Surgical Room

Prior to surgery the doctor should inform you of specific instructions concerning patient preparation. He will also tell you what special equipment or supplies are necessary for the procedure.

Because patients are likely to feel anxious before a procedure, it is best to have everything ready in the surgical room before you escort the patient into the room. Make sure the room is clean, neat, and free of waste from previous procedures. The examining table should have been cleaned and disinfected, and surface barriers (table paper and pillow covers) should have been changed.

Check to see that there is adequate lighting. Make sure that all equipment and supplies necessary for the procedure are available. Check the date and sterilization indicator on sterilized packs and supplies. Sterile packs are typically considered unsterile if more than 1 month has passed since they were originally sterilized.

You will then wash your hands, put on examination gloves, and prepare the sterile field as outlined in Procedure 24-1. The sterile field and the instruments should be draped with a sterile towel.

Preparing the Patient

Just before the surgery, various concerns must be addressed and procedures completed in sequence. The initial tasks are followed by gowning and positioning the patient and preparing the patient's skin for surgery.

Initial Tasks. Before leading the patient into the surgical room, find out whether he has followed the presurgical instructions. Restrictions on food and fluid intake are of particular concern. It is also important to ask what medications the patient is taking and whether he has taken that day's dosage.

Measure the patient's vital signs. Ask if there are any symptoms or problems the doctor should know about before the surgery. If any unusual signs or symptoms are present, notify the doctor. The doctor will want to examine the patient before proceeding.

Check the chart for medication orders, such as pain medication or a tranquilizer to calm the patient. Medications should be administered at this time so that they will take effect before surgery.

Gowning and Positioning the Patient. Some procedures require the patient to disrobe and put on a gown to expose the surgical site. If this is the case, you should offer to assist, if appropriate, or leave the room while the patient changes. You should then help the patient onto the table and into the position required for the procedure. You may use one or more small pillows to make the patient as comfortable as possible. Then adequately drape the patient to retain body heat and preserve personal dignity.

Sterile drapes are also used to create a sterile field on a patient's body around the surgical site. Drapes come in a variety of sizes and styles. A fenestrated drape has a round or slitlike opening cut out in the center to provide access to the surgical site.

Surgical Skin Preparation. Proper preparation of the patient's skin before surgery reduces the number of microorganisms and the risk of infection. The prepared area should extend 2 inches beyond the surgical field—the area exposed in the center of the fenestrated drape. This extra margin allows for draping without contaminating the field.

Cleaning the Area. Before proceeding with the surgical skin preparation, wash your hands and put on examination gloves. Place a plastic-backed drape under the surgical site to absorb any liquids. Clean the site first with antiseptic soap and sterile water, using forceps and gauze sponges dipped in the solution. Begin at the center of the surgical site, and work outward in a firm, circular motion (Figure 24-20). Discard the gauze sponge after each complete pass. Clean in concentric circles until you cover the full preparation area. Continue the process, repeating as necessary, for at least 2 minutes or the amount of time specified in the office's procedure manual. Cleaning takes more time if a wound is dirty or contains foreign materials. When procedures are performed on a hand or foot, clean the entire hand or foot.

Shaving the Area. Depending on office policy, you may be required to shave the surgical site to remove hair. Shaving often causes many small wounds on the skin, however, and may increase the risk of infection. Because of this fact some experts feel that hair should not be removed unless it is thick enough to interfere with surgery. Alternatively, hair may be trimmed with scissors or smoothed out of the way.

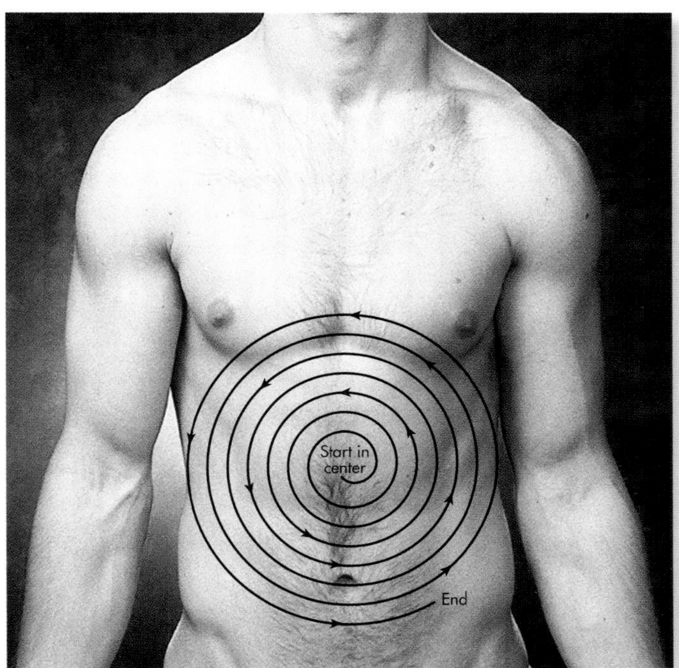

Figure 24-20. Use concentric circles to clean the surgical site and apply antiseptic solution.

When shaving is indicated, use a disposable razor and soap for lubrication. Shave in the direction in which the hair grows, and include the same area you cleaned beforehand. When you finish, rinse the area with sterile water and allow it to air-dry. You may also pat the area dry with sterile gauze, starting at the surgical site and moving outward in a circular motion.

Applying the Antiseptic. Next apply antiseptic solution to the area. Antiseptics are agents that are applied to the skin to limit the growth of microorganisms and to help prevent infection. Povidone iodine (Betadine) is most commonly used, but chlorhexidine gluconate (Hibiclens) or benzalkonium chloride (Zephiran Chloride) may also be used, particularly if the patient is allergic to iodine. Swab an area 2 inches larger than the surgical field with the antiseptic solution in a circular outward motion, starting at the surgical site. This is the same motion that is used for cleaning the surgical site. For surgery on a hand or foot, swab the entire hand or foot. Allow the antiseptic to air-dry; do not pat it dry—that would remove some of the solution's antiseptic properties.

When the area is dry, treat it as a sterile field. Instruct the patient not to touch the area. Cover the area with a sterile fenestrated drape, from front to back. Avoid reaching over the field.

At this point notify the physician that the patient is ready. Then prepare yourself to assist with the surgery.

Intraoperative Procedures

Intraoperative procedures are procedures that take place during surgery. You may be asked to perform a wide variety of unsterile and sterile tasks during surgery, such as preparing local anesthetic for the doctor, monitoring the patient, processing specimens, and handing instruments to the doctor. The doctor may also ask you to explain to the patient step by step what will be done next during the procedure.

Administering a Local Anesthetic

Before beginning the surgical procedure, the physician will administer a local anesthetic. Some local anesthetics are injected. An injected anesthetic is packaged in a sterile **vial** (a small glass bottle with a self-sealing rubber stopper). Other local anesthetics come in a cream, gel, or spray form. These anesthetics are **topical** (applied directly to the skin) and affect only the area to which they are applied.

Lidocaine (Xylocaine) is the most commonly used anesthetic. It is often used as a topical gel anesthetic. Tetracaine hydrochloride (Pontocaine), a long-acting anesthetic, is injected.

The physician administers the local anesthetic by injection or by applying it directly to the skin. The choice of administration methods depends on how invasive or painful the procedure is likely to be.

Topical Application. Anesthetic gels, creams, and sprays may be used topically in certain surgical procedures. A topical anesthetic is useful when the pain will be mild or when only the upper layers of the skin are affected. It is common to use such agents to anesthetize the area of a small laceration prior to suturing. Sometimes an anesthetic cream is applied before a local anesthetic is injected. This application reduces or eliminates the pain caused by the injection. A topical anesthetic must usually remain on the skin for 10 to 15 minutes for the area to become sufficiently anesthetized.

Injections. If a local anesthetic is to be injected, it is typically administered after the skin is prepared but before the patient is draped. In some cases, however, the anesthetic is injected prior to skin preparation to allow time for it to take effect. In either case it is important to note the time of anesthetic administration in the patient's chart.

If the doctor is already wearing sterile gloves, you may be asked to assist in administering the anesthetic. Administering anesthetic is an unsterile task because the outside of the vial is unsterile. When performing this task, follow proper procedure to protect the sterility of the doctor's gloves and the anesthetic solution.

First check the label of the anesthetic vial three times to confirm that it is the correct solution. Clean the vial's rubber stopper with 70% isopropyl alcohol, and leave the cotton or gauze on top of the stopper. Present the requested needle and syringe to the doctor by peeling half the outer wrapper away and allowing the doctor to remove them from the wrapper.

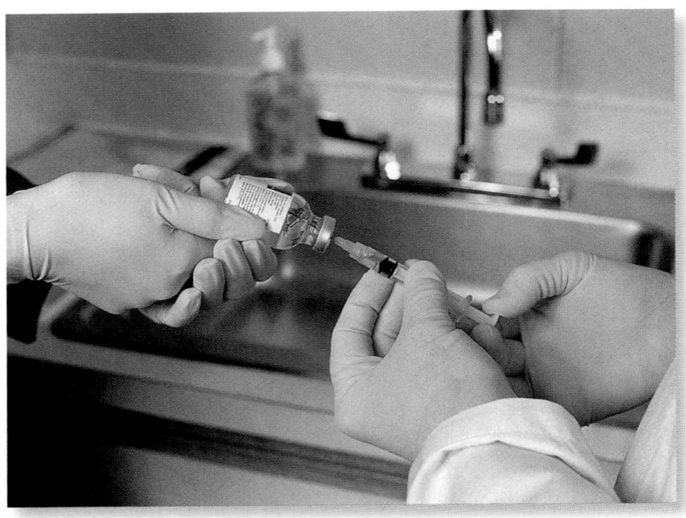

Figure 24-21. You must hold the anesthetic vial firmly to allow the physician to puncture the rubber stopper with the needle.

Remove the cotton or gauze from the rubber stopper, and hold the vial so the doctor can verify that it is the proper medication. Turn the vial upside down, and hold it securely around the base, without touching the sterile stopper. Be sure to hold the vial in front of you at shoulder height. Because significant force will be necessary to push the needle through the rubber stopper, you should brace the wrist of the hand holding the vial with your free hand. Hold the vial firmly so the doctor can withdraw the anesthetic from it (Figure 24-21).

Potential Side Effects of the Anesthetic. You should inform the patient of possible reactions to the anesthetic medication. Although rare, reactions may include dizziness, loss of consciousness, seizures, or cardiac arrest. Adverse reactions can occur if the anesthetic dose is too high or if it is absorbed too quickly. They can also occur if the patient is taking other medications that should not be mixed with the anesthetic. It is vital to document all medications (including over-the-counter ones) that the patient is taking at the time of the surgery.

Use of Epinephrine. Epinephrine is a sterile solution that is sometimes injected along with an anesthetic. Epinephrine constricts the blood vessels, making them narrower. This constriction reduces bleeding and prolongs the action of the local anesthetic. Epinephrine is used if the site of surgery is an area with many small blood vessels that are expected to bleed profusely (such as the head). Reducing bleeding makes it easier to see and to repair the wound. (Epinephrine should be used with caution, however, in patients with heart disease or respiratory disease.)

When epinephrine is combined with the anesthetic to reduce bleeding, it prolongs the anesthesia because epinephrine slows the rate at which anesthetic spreads into the tissue. This effect may or may not be desirable. Epinephrine should not be used in areas such as the fingers, toes, nose, or ears, where it could also compromise the local blood supply. There is some concern that epinephrine may increase wound infection rates.

Assisting the Physician During Surgery

Your role in surgical assisting depends on the type of surgery and the physician's preference. You may assist the physician in one of two capacities. You may serve as a **floater**, an unsterile assistant who is free to move about the room and attend to unsterile needs. Alternatively, you may serve as a **sterile scrub assistant**, who assists in handling sterile equipment during the procedure. The duties are different for the two functions. Procedure 24-4 outlines the tasks performed by both sterile and unsterile assistants.

The Floater. First the surgical room is set up and the patient is prepared. If you are assisting as a floater (sometimes called a circulator), you will perform a routine scrub and put on examination gloves. Remember that you cannot touch sterile items in the sterile field because you have not performed a surgical scrub and are not wearing sterile gloves.

Monitoring and Recording. One of the most important duties of a floater is to monitor the patient during the procedure. You must measure vital signs regularly and observe the patient for reactions to the anesthetic. Record all observations in the patient's chart. Also write down any information or notes the doctor requests. You must keep a record of time, including when the anesthetic is administered, when the procedure begins, and when the procedure is completed.

Processing Specimens. When you serve as a floater during surgery, the doctor may ask you to receive and process specimens for laboratory examination. Most tissues are placed in a 10% formalin solution to preserve them before they are sent to the laboratory. Half-fill the specimen container with the formalin solution ahead of time. Remove the lid of the specimen container without touching the rim. Hold the container out toward the doctor so she can place the tissue directly into it without contaminating the sample (Figure 24-22).

The container should be labeled with the following information:

- The patient's name and the doctor's name
- The date and time of collection
- The body site from which the specimen was obtained
- Your initials

If more than one specimen is obtained from a patient, place each specimen in a separate container. Label each container with the necessary information, along with a number to indicate the order in which the specimens are obtained (no. 1, no. 2, and so on). You will also fill out a laboratory requisition slip to send along with the specimen(s). Specimen containers should be red in color or labeled with the biohazard symbol. Specimen containers should be placed in specially designed bags for transport.

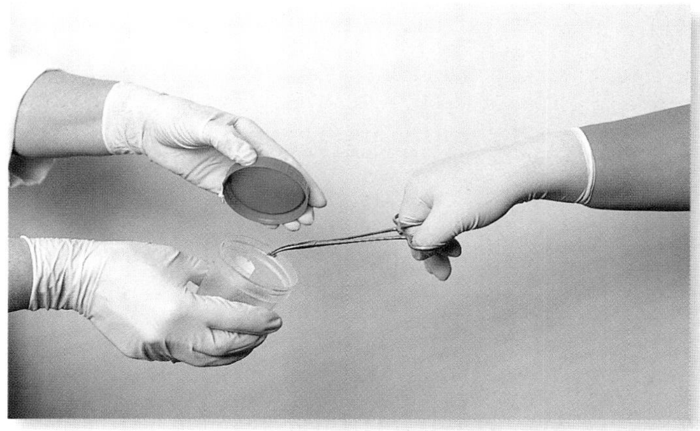

Figure 24-22. Be sure to hold the specimen container so that the doctor can place the tissue in it without touching the rim or the outside of the container with the tissue.

Other Duties. As a floater you may also be asked to perform a number of other duties, including these:

- Assisting with the injection of additional anesthetic
- Adding additional sterile items to the sterile tray
- Pouring sterile solutions
- Keeping the surgical area clean and neat during the procedure
- Repositioning the patient as necessary
- Adjusting lighting

The Sterile Scrub Assistant. When you serve as a sterile scrub assistant, you perform a surgical scrub and wear sterile gloves. You may be asked to perform a variety of tasks under sterile conditions. Remember not to touch unsterile items after putting on sterile gloves.

Handling Instruments. Your first duty as a sterile scrub assistant is, typically, to close the instruments on the sterile tray because they are normally left in the open position during sterilization. Your next duty is to rearrange the instruments on the tray. Instruments should be arranged in the order in which they will be used or according to the doctor's preference. Instruments are generally used in the following sequence:

- Cutting instruments
- Grasping instruments
- Retractors
- Probes
- Suture materials
- Needle holders and scissors

PROCEDURE 24.4

General Assisting Procedures for Minor Surgery

Objective: To provide assistance to the doctor during minor surgery while maintaining clean or sterile technique as appropriate

OSHA Guidelines

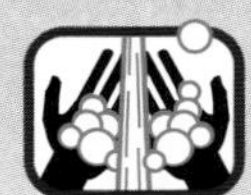
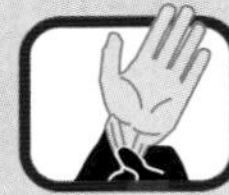

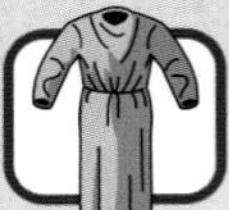
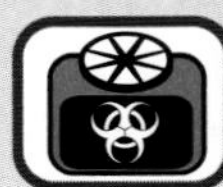
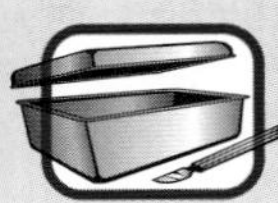

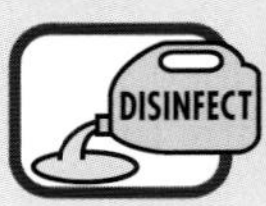

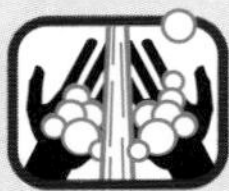

Materials: Sterile towel, tray or Mayo stand, appropriate instrument pack(s), needles and syringes, anesthetic, antiseptic, sterile water or normal saline, small sterile bowl, sterile gauze squares or cotton balls, specimen containers half-filled with preservative, suture materials, sterile dressings and tape

Method

Floater (Unsterile Assistant)

1. Perform routine hand washing and put on examination gloves.
2. Monitor the patient during the procedure; record the results in the patient's chart.
3. During the surgery assist as needed.
4. Add sterile items to the tray as necessary.
5. Pour sterile solution into a sterile bowl as needed.
6. Assist in administering additional anesthetic.
   a. Check the medication vial three times.
   b. Clean the rubber stopper with alcohol (write the date opened when using a new bottle); leave cotton or gauze on top.
   c. Present the needle and syringe to the doctor.
   d. Remove the cotton or gauze from the vial, and show the label to the doctor.
   e. Hold the vial upside down, and grasp the lower edge firmly; brace your wrist with your free hand. (This firmly supports the vial to sustain the force of the needle being inserted into the rubber stopper.)
   f. Allow the doctor to fill the syringe.
7. Receive specimens for laboratory examination.
   a. Uncap the specimen container; present it to the doctor for the introduction of the specimen.
   b. Replace the cap and label the container.
   c. Treat all specimens as infectious.
   d. Place the specimen container in a transport bag or other container.
   e. Complete the requisition form to send the specimen to the laboratory.

Sterile Scrub Assistant

1. Perform a surgical scrub and put on sterile gloves. (Remember to remove the sterile towel covering the sterile field and instruments before gloving.)
2. Close and arrange the surgical instruments on the tray.
3. Prepare for swabbing by inserting gauze squares into the sterile dressing forceps.
4. Pass the instruments as necessary.
5. Swab the wound as requested.
6. Retract the wound as requested.
7. Cut the sutures as requested.

Floater or Sterile Scrub Assistant (After Surgery)

1. Monitor the patient.
2. Put on clean examination gloves, and clean the wound with antiseptic.
3. Dress the wound.
4. Remove the gloves and wash your hands.
5. Give the patient oral postoperative instructions in addition to the release packet.
6. Discharge the patient.
7. Put on clean examination gloves.
8. Properly dispose of used materials and disposable instruments.
9. Sanitize reusable instruments and prepare them for disinfection and/or sterilization as needed.
10. Clean equipment and the examination room according to OSHA guidelines.
11. Remove the gloves and wash your hands.

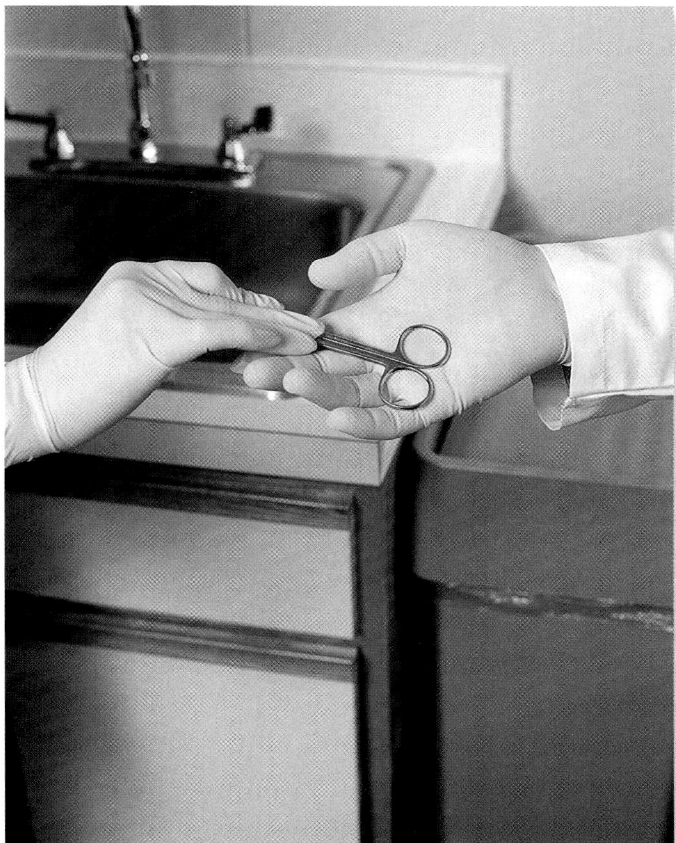

Figure 24-23. Holding the scissors by the hinge, slap the handles into the doctor's hand.

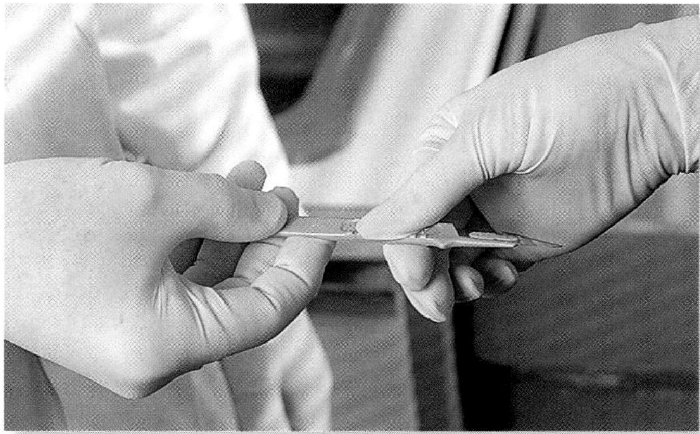

Figure 24-24. Hold a scalpel above and just behind the cutting edge as you pass the handle into the palm of the doctor's hand.

Prepare for swabbing by placing several sterile gauze squares in the dressing forceps. They will then be ready when needed. As the sterile scrub assistant, you will be asked to pass instruments to the doctor during the procedure. You must hold instruments so that the doctor can grasp them securely and will not need to reposition them in her hands. At the same time, the instruments must be handled properly to maintain their sterility.

When passing scissors and clamps, hold them by the hinge (Figure 24-23). You will have a clear view of the tip of the instrument, and the doctor will have full use of the handles. Firmly slap the instrument handles into the doctor's extended palm. The doctor's hand will close around the handles as a reflex action to the slapping. This technique reduces the risk of dropping an instrument. If the scissors or clamp is curved, the curve should follow the same curve as the doctor's hand.

When passing a scalpel, hold it above and just behind the cutting edge of the blade so the doctor can grasp the entire handle (Figure 24-24). Pass a needle holder with suture material so that the needle is pointing up, and hold the end of the suture material with your other hand to prevent the material from becoming tangled in the handles.

Other Duties. As a sterile scrub assistant, you may also be asked to swab fluids from a wound or to retract the edges of a wound to help the doctor view the area. While the doctor is closing the wound, you may be required to cut the suture material after each stitch. The doctor may not verbalize every request to you. With practice and after experience with a particular doctor, you will learn how to respond to the doctor's actions.

When cutting suture materials, leave $\frac{1}{8}$ inch of the material above the knot. This excess material prevents the suture from coming untied. It also leaves the material short enough so that it does not bother the patient.

Postoperative Procedures

You will be responsible for the patient's **postoperative** ("postop") follow-up after the surgical procedure. Your duties may include immediate care of the patient, proper cleaning of the surgical room, and follow-up care of the patient.

Immediate Patient Care

Patient care is your top priority as a medical assistant. Except for intravenous medications, you will administer postoperative medications that the physician requests for the patient. You will also ensure that the patient remains lying down on the examining table for the prescribed length of time after the procedure. During this period continue to monitor the patient's vital signs, and watch for adverse reactions. It is important to document your observations in the patient's chart.

Dressing the Wound. You may also dress the wound during the monitoring period. **Dressings** are sterile materials used to cover an incision. They serve a number of functions. They protect the wound from further injury and keep the wound clean, thus preventing infection. Dressings also reduce bleeding, absorb fluid drainage, reduce discomfort to the patient, speed healing, and reduce the possibility of scarring. Gauze dressings are the most common type of dressings and come in a variety of sizes and shapes.

Before dressing the wound, put on clean examination gloves. Clean the site with povidone iodine (Betadine), and allow it to dry. If ordered by the physician, apply antibiotic ointment over the wound. Place the sterile dressing over the site, and secure it appropriately.

Bandaging the Wound. It may be necessary to apply a bandage (a clean strip of gauze or elastic material) over the dressing to help hold it in place. Bandages may also be used to improve circulation, to provide support or reduce tension on a wound or suture and prevent it from reopening, or to prevent movement of that area of the body. Adhesive tape may also be used for these purposes. Some patients are allergic to the adhesive, but most tapes are now hypoallergenic. The patient is usually more comfortable after a bandage or adhesive tape has been applied.

Postoperative Instructions. After the procedure, provide oral postoperative instructions to the patient. You may do this during the monitoring part of the postoperative period or afterward. These instructions include guidelines for pain management and instructions for wound care. Postoperative information also includes dietary or activity restrictions, if any, and when to come in for a follow-up appointment. It is a good idea to ask patients to repeat what you say so that you know they understand the information.

Instructions are often also provided in writing and may be part of a complete postoperative information packet. You may be asked to help prepare or update packet materials, especially if you routinely assist patients as they recover from minor surgery. A postoperative information packet might include the following information:

- Proper wound-care instructions
- Suggestions for pain relief and reduction of swelling, such as medications and hot or cold packs
- Dietary restrictions
- Activity restrictions
- Timing for a follow-up appointment or an appointment card

Wound-care instructions include details on dressing changes, which will vary depending on the depth and size of the wound. Generally a patient should clean the wound daily with soap and water or dilute hydrogen peroxide (3%) and allow it to air-dry. The patient should then apply an antibiotic cream and place a dry, sterile dressing over the wound. Except when cleansing the wound, the patient should keep it dry. The dressing should be replaced if it gets wet. Although cleansing aids wound healing, a wet dressing provides bacteria and other contaminants with access to the wound.

Descriptions, and often illustrations, of normal and infected incisions are an important part of wound-care instructions. The patient should call the physician if any signs of infection are noted. The instructions should also encourage the patient to protect the incision from exposure to the sun. This guideline is advisable for as long as 3 to 6 months to prevent the incision line from becoming darker than surrounding skin.

The length of time it takes for a wound to heal varies with the site, the patient's age, and the severity of the wound. Each patient therefore needs specific instructions on how long to continue with the dressings and when to return for suture or staple removal.

Patient Release. Notify the doctor when the patient is stabilized and ready to leave. The doctor may want to further observe and instruct the patient. Be sure to offer assistance if the patient needs help getting dressed.

Then help the patient check out. Schedule the next appointment for the patient. Make sure the patient has the correct discharge packet. Confirm arrangements to transport the patient home. Finally, assist the patient to the car or other transport if this is part of office procedure.

If a patient insists on driving himself home, enter this information on the chart. Indicate the time and have the patient initial the entry. This documentation is important for legal reasons. It would clarify liability should an accident occur as a result of a reaction to the surgery or the anesthetic.

Surgical Room Cleanup

If there is time during the monitoring period, begin to clean up the surgical area. If time is not available then, perform the cleanup routine after the patient has been released.

Until the reusable instruments can be cleaned, place them in a disinfectant soak that has anticoagulant properties. A reusable sharps container is generally used for this purpose for surgical instruments. Place disposable waste in the sharps or biohazardous waste container. Clean the counters, examining table, and trays according to OSHA guidelines by disinfecting them. A 10% chlorine bleach solution, which is one part household bleach to nine parts water, is commonly used. Disinfect small pieces of nonsurgical equipment (stethoscopes, thermometers, and so on) with 70% isopropyl alcohol. Replace paper table and pillow covers at this time, along with necessary supplies.

Follow-Up Care

During a follow-up appointment the physician examines the patient's surgical wound. You may be asked to change the dressing or remove the wound closures.

Typically, suture or staple removal takes place 5 to 10 days after minor surgery. The sutures or staples are ready for removal when a clean, unbroken suture line is observed. There should be no scabs, no seepage from the wound, and no visible opening. Any of these signs may indicate unhealed areas. Suture removal is described in Procedure 24-5. Staple removal is similar, except that staple removal forceps, rather than forceps and scissors, are used to remove the staples.

PROCEDURE 24.5

Suture Removal

Objective: To remove sutures from a healing wound while maintaining sterile technique and protecting the integrity of the closed wound

OSHA Guidelines

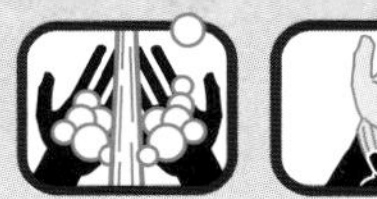
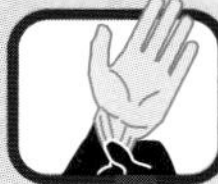
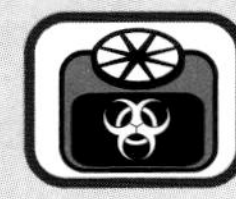
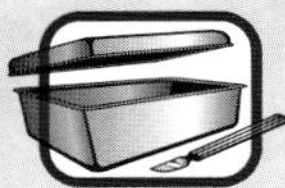

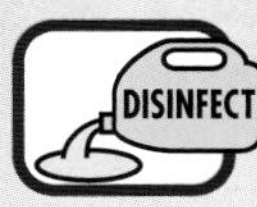

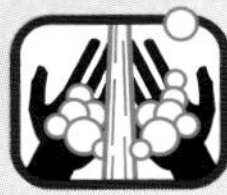

Materials: Tray or Mayo stand, suture removal pack (suture scissors and thumb forceps), sterile towel, antiseptic solution, hydrogen peroxide (3%), two small sterile bowls, sterile gauze squares, sterile strips or butterfly closures, sterile dressings and tape

Method

1. Clean and disinfect the tray or Mayo stand.
2. Wash your hands and assemble the necessary materials.
3. Check the date and sterilization indicator on the suture removal pack.
4. Unwrap the suture removal pack, and place it on the tray or stand to create a sterile field.
5. Unwrap the sterile bowls and add them to the sterile field.
6. Pour a small amount of antiseptic solution into one bowl, and pour a small amount of hydrogen peroxide into the other bowl.
7. Cover the tray with a sterile towel to protect the sterile field while you are out of the room.
8. Escort the patient to the examination room and explain the procedure.
9. Perform a routine scrub, remove the towel from the tray, and put on examination gloves.
10. Remove the old dressing.
    a. Lift the tape toward the middle of the dressing to avoid pulling on the wound.
    b. If the dressing adheres to the wound, cover the dressing with gauze squares soaked in hydrogen peroxide. Leave the wet gauze in place for several seconds to loosen the dressing.

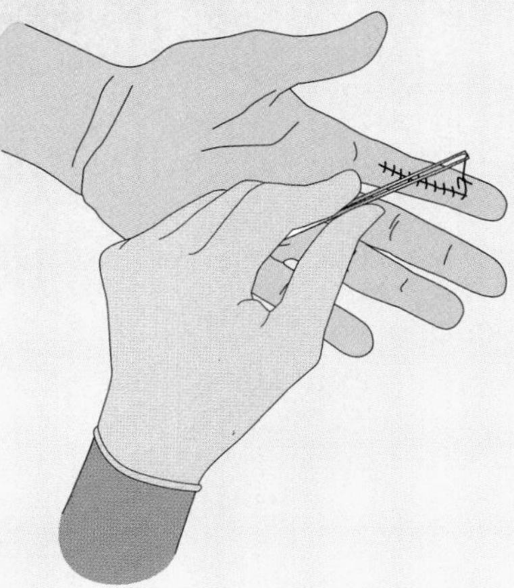

Figure 24-25. Without pulling on the wound, lift the suture knot away from the skin to make room for the suture scissors.

    c. Save the old dressing for the doctor to inspect.
11. Inspect the wound for signs of infection.
12. Clean the wound with gauze pads soaked in antiseptic, and pat it dry with clean gauze pads.
13. Remove the gloves and wash your hands.
14. Notify the doctor that the wound is ready for examination.
15. Once the doctor indicates that the wound is sufficiently healed to proceed, put on clean examination gloves.
16. Place a square of gauze next to the wound for collecting the sutures as they are removed.
17. Grasp the first suture knot with forceps.
18. Gently lift the knot away from the skin to allow room for the suture scissors (Figure 24-25).
19. Slide the suture scissors under the suture material, and cut the suture where it enters the skin (Figure 24-26).
20. Gently lift the knot up and toward the wound to remove the suture without opening the wound (Figure 24-27).
21. Place the suture on the gauze pad, and inspect to ensure that the entire suture is present.
22. Repeat the removal process until all sutures have been removed.

continued ⟶

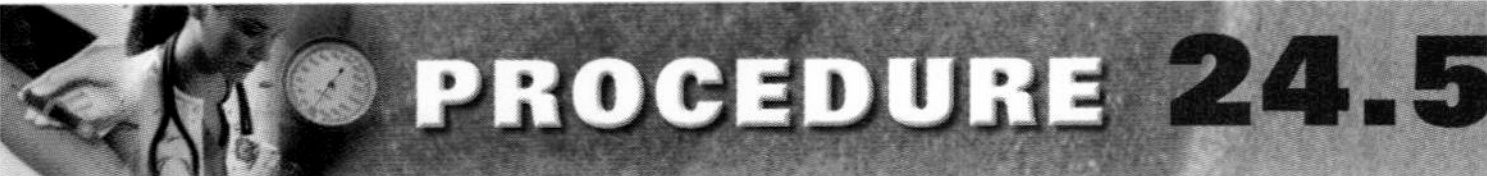

PROCEDURE 24.5

Suture Removal *(continued)*

23. Count the sutures and compare the number with the number indicated in the patient's record (Figure 24-28).
24. Clean the wound with antiseptic, and allow the wound to air-dry.
25. Dress the wound as ordered, or notify the doctor if the sterile strips or butterfly closures are to be applied.
26. Observe the patient for signs of distress, such as wincing or grimacing.
27. Properly dispose of used materials and disposable instruments.
28. Remove the gloves and wash your hands.
29. Instruct the patient on wound care.
30. In the patient's chart, record pertinent information, such as the condition of the wound and the type of closures used, if any.
31. Escort the patient to the checkout area.
32. Put on clean gloves.
33. Sanitize resuable instruments and prepare them for disinfection and/or sterilization as needed.
34. Clean the equipment and examination room according to OSHA guidelines.
35. Remove the gloves and wash your hands.

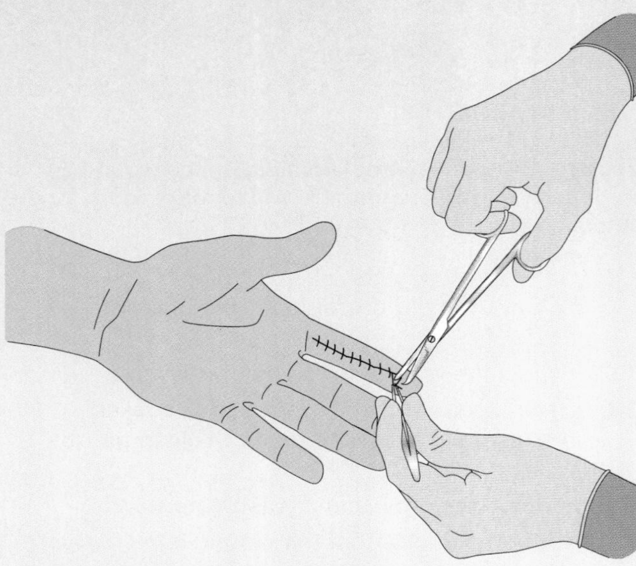

Figure 24-26. Cut the suture material as close as possible to its entry point in the skin.

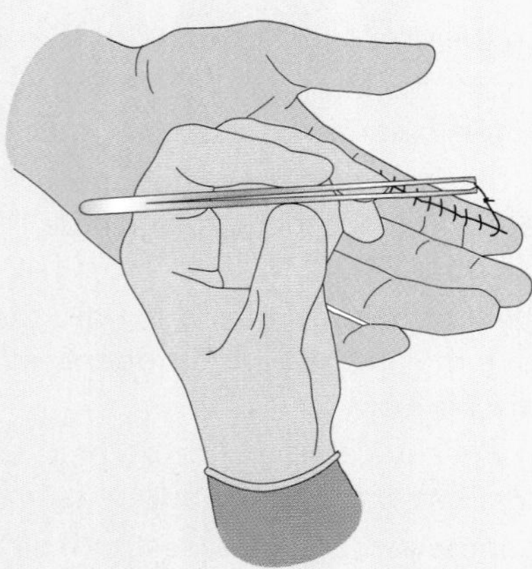

Figure 24-27. Remove the suture by lifting the knot up and toward the wound.

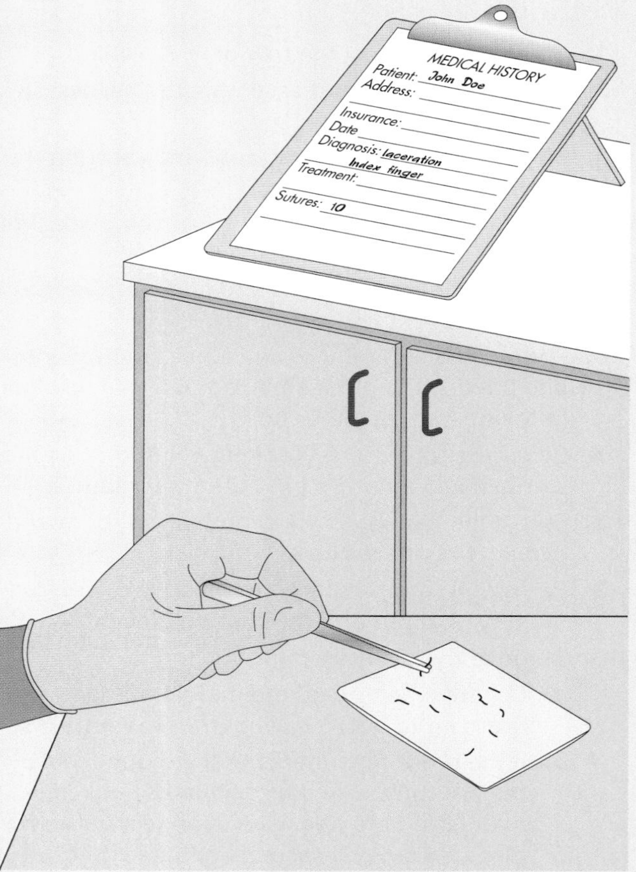

Figure 24-28. Compare the number of sutures removed with the recorded number of sutures placed.

Summary

As the doctor's assistant in minor surgical procedures, you perform many functions. Your responsibilities during the patient's preoperative and postoperative care, however, are just as important.

Before surgery you provide the patient with preoperative instructions, make sure the necessary administrative and legal forms are completed, help prepare the patient emotionally, and set up the surgical room. You then confirm that the patient has followed all preoperative instructions and physically prepare the patient for surgery.

During the procedure you follow proper medical and surgical aseptic techniques. Your actual responsibilities vary with the role you play as a floater or a sterile scrub assistant for a particular surgery. At all times you ensure the safety and comfort of the patient and are knowledgeable enough to function as the doctor's "right hand" during the procedure.

After the surgery you provide the postoperative patient with care and instruction that will help ensure prompt healing. Then you clean the surgical room and prepare it for the next procedure.

REVIEW

CHAPTER 24

CASE STUDY QUESTIONS

Now that you have completed this chapter, review the case study at the beginning of the chapter and answer the following questions:

1. How could you reduce the patient's apprehension?
2. What would you say to her before the physician arrives to perform the minor surgery?

Discussion Questions

1. Explain the stages of wound healing and the benefit of approximation.
2. List five different categories of surgical instruments by function, give an example of each, and describe how instruments in each category are used.
3. List three minor surgical procedures you may assist with in the doctor's office. Name one procedure you may perform on your own.

Critical Thinking Questions

1. What might you say to ease the fears of an anxious patient who is about to undergo a laceration repair?
2. Explain the procedure you would follow if you were functioning as a sterile scrub assistant and your glove was punctured while you were handling instruments during a surgical procedure.
3. Explain how to make sure that a patient has understood the postoperative instructions for wound care.
4. A patient arrives at the clinic with a laceration to the left thumb that occurred while she was washing dishes. She is holding a bloody paper towel on the thumb. She states, "I cannot take this towel off—the blood will gush right out of the cut. It just would not stop bleeding." What should you do?
5. A patient will need to have a minor surgical procedure done next week at your clinic. What administrative tasks must you perform before the procedure?

Application Activities

1. Using instrument flash cards or actual instruments, choose and list the types of instruments you would need during a procedure to clean and repair a laceration.
2. Working with one or two classmates, practice opening a sterile pack and creating a sterile field. Practice adding additional instruments and a sterile bowl to the sterile field. Offer suggestions to each other for improving your techniques.
3. With a partner, practice handing surgical instruments to each other. The receiver should look the other way while receiving the instrument. This approach simulates actual conditions in which the doctor may be concentrating on a procedure rather than looking at the instrument. This approach also tests the ability of the person handing the instrument to use proper technique.
4. With a partner, practice preparing a site for surgery. Obtain the necessary equipment to clean the site, apply antiseptic, and drape. Follow the procedure steps carefully, paying close attention to your cleaning technique. Be certain to use concentric circles. Practice various surgical sites, and evaluate each other's technique. Note: You may choose not to use actual soap and antiseptic for practice in order to avoid irritation.

Internet Activity

Use the Internet to learn more about surgical instruments and to create your own personal flash cards. Use picture search engines such as **www.google.com** and **www.ixquick.com** to search for pictures of various instruments used in different procedures. Once you find a picture you would like to print, right-click on it and save it in a folder for later printing.

CHAPTER 25

Assisting With Cold and Heat Therapy and Ambulation

AREAS OF COMPETENCE

2003 Role Delineation Study

ADMINISTRATIVE

Administrative Procedures

- Schedule, coordinate, and monitor appointments
- Schedule inpatient/outpatient admissions and procedures

CLINICAL

Fundamental Principles

- Screen and follow up patient test results

GENERAL

Professionalism

- Work as a member of the health-care team

Communication Skills

- Serve as liaison

Instruction

- Instruct individuals according to their needs
- Explain office policies and procedures

KEY TERMS

cryotherapy
diathermy
erythema
fluidotherapy
gait
goniometer
hydrotherapy
mobility aid
physical therapy
posture
range of motion (ROM)
therapeutic team
thermotherapy
traction

CHAPTER OUTLINE

- General Principles of Physical Therapy
- Cryotherapy and Thermotherapy
- Hydrotherapy
- Exercise Therapy
- Traction
- Mobility Aids
- Referral to a Physical Therapist

OBJECTIVES

After completing Chapter 25, you will be able to:

25.1 Explain how medical assistants might assist with some forms of physical therapy.
25.2 Describe ways to test joint mobility, muscle strength, gait, and posture.
25.3 Discuss the benefits of cold and heat therapies.
25.4 List contraindications to cold and heat therapies.

OBJECTIVES *(Continued)*

25.5 Identify various cold and heat therapies.
25.6 Demonstrate how to perform cold and heat therapies.
25.7 Describe hydrotherapy methods.
25.8 Identify several methods of exercise therapy.
25.9 Compare different methods of traction.
25.10 Demonstrate how to teach a patient to use a cane, a walker, crutches, and a wheelchair.

Introduction

Applying cold and heat therapy and assisting patients with ambulation are common responsibilities of a medical assistant. These activities are part of the field of physical therapy. For a full program of physical therapy, a physician generally refers a patient to a licensed physical therapist. However, a physician may request that you assist with some forms of physical therapy, including:

- Applying cold and heat
- Teaching basic exercises
- Demonstrating how to use a cane, walker, and crutches
- Demonstrating how to use a wheelchair
- Discussing with the patient specific therapies for use at home

CASE STUDY

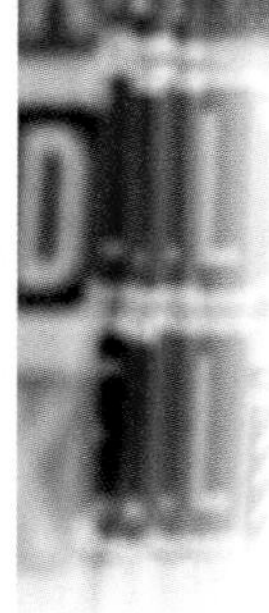

While on vacation, a 28-year-old male had a mountain biking accident that resulted in a broken leg and other injuries. He went to the local emergency room for treatment and was instructed to follow up with his primary care physician on arriving home. Three days after the accident, he presents in your office with crutches and a cast on his left leg. Using the crutches, he stumbles and almost falls as you ask him back to the examination area. You also notice a dry, crusted, bloody injury on his left forearm.

As you read this chapter, consider the following questions:

1. What type of teaching do you think this patient will need?
2. What type of therapy may be necessary for the crusted bloody injury on his forearm, and how would you perform it?

General Principles of Physical Therapy

Physical therapy is a medical specialty for the treatment of musculoskeletal, nervous, and cardiopulmonary disorders. A physical therapist uses a variety of treatments, including cold, heat, water, exercise, massage, and traction. Some physical therapy regimens combine two or more treatments. Exercising in a pool, for example, combines the use of water and exercise. In addition, the physical therapist actively promotes patient education and rehabilitation programs.

Physical therapy benefits patients in several ways. It restores and improves muscle function, builds strength, increases joint mobility, relieves pain, and increases circulation. Physical therapy is used to treat various disorders, including arthritis, stroke, lower-back pain, muscle spasms, muscle injuries or diseases, pressure sores, skin disorders, and burns.

Assisting Within a Therapeutic Team

Many people who require physical therapy are recovering from traumatic injuries or dealing with chronic illnesses. They may therefore be receiving therapeutic attention from several different specialists. Physicians, nurses, medical assistants, and other specialists who work with patients dealing with chronic illness or recovery from major injuries make up a **therapeutic team.** When you work with such patients, your responsibilities may include:

- Coordinating the patient's schedule of sessions with different specialists
- Making referrals, as directed by the physician
- Explaining a specialist's treatment approach to the patient
- Communicating the physician's findings to the specialist

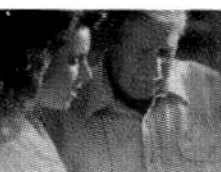

Educating the Patient

Specialized Therapies and Their Benefits

Health-care professionals recognize the contribution of specialized therapies to a patient's recovery. Because many people do not know about these specialized therapies, you may be called on to explain them to patients. You can educate patients about potential benefits of art therapy or other specialized therapies. When specialized therapies are ordered, patients will be more at ease if they know what to expect. You can help when necessary by explaining the following types of therapies and their advantages.

- In art therapy, patients learn to express themselves visually through drawing, painting, and sculpture. Art therapy aids both physical and mental healing; provides a recreational outlet; improves mobility and fine motor coordination; provides an outlet for expressing fears or other emotions that patients may be unaware of or unable or unwilling to express verbally; helps relieve anxiety; allows patients to focus on something other than their physical condition; and encourages patients to take better care of themselves. To aid in the art therapy process, encourage patients to relax and give this approach time to work. Although the benefits of art therapy may be evident immediately, they are just as likely to be perceived only after the course of therapy is well under way.
- In music therapy, patients listen to and create music to calm themselves and to alleviate anxiety. This therapy is often used with surgical patients and patients with chronic pain.
- In dance therapy, patients participate in dance to improve balance, flexibility, strength, and quality of life.
- In writing therapy, patients express themselves through a chosen form of writing such as poetry or a journal.
- In crafts therapy, patients express themselves by using a variety of media to create handiworks.
- In pet therapy, patients play with, groom, or walk a pet. Pets provide companionship and the opportunity to nurture.
- In aquatic therapy, patients swim in a therapeutic pool equipped with a ramp and a lift so that it is accessible to all. Many patients who cannot walk when on land can move their legs remarkably well in water.
- In horticultural therapy, patients work with plants and flowers to bring beauty into their daily lives and to help improve their balance, strength, memory, and socialization skills.
- In equestrian therapy, patients ride horses to help develop strength, coordination, and muscle tone and to improve balance.

- Documenting the specialist's treatments and findings for the physician
- Reinforcing the specialist's instructions for the patient
- Answering the patient's questions

To fulfill these responsibilities, you must have a working knowledge of therapy techniques. If, for example, the physician refers a patient to an art therapist, you would set up an art therapy appointment and explain in general terms what the patient can expect. The Educating the Patient section offers basic information about various specialized therapies.

Besides learning the basic information you need to know about physical therapy, you will want to keep up-to-date on emerging techniques. You may want to become proficient in some of these new techniques. By expanding your knowledge and skills, you increase your value as a member of the therapeutic team.

Assisting With Patient Assessment

Before the doctor prescribes physical therapy, she assesses the patient's physical abilities and condition. She inspects and palpates the patient's joints and muscles and tests the patient's joint mobility, muscle strength, gait, and posture. You will typically assist with these tests. In some cases the doctor may direct you to perform them.

Joint Mobility Testing. People usually assume that their joints are mobile until stiffness or injury limits them. When a patient complains of these difficulties, the doctor may ask you to assist in testing range of motion. **Range of motion (ROM)** is the degree to which a joint is able to move, measured in degrees with a protractor device called a universal **goniometer** (Figure 25-1). The measurement of joint mobility is known as goniometry, a noninvasive test that is frequently performed in doctors'

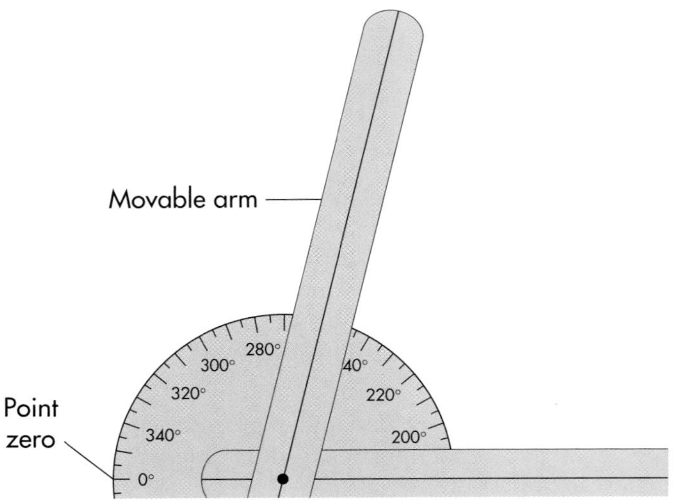

Figure 25-1. A universal goniometer is a protractor with a movable pointer that measures degrees of joint movement.

offices and that requires the patient to move each major joint in various ways. The specific movements that are evaluated are described in Table 25-1 and Figure 25-2. The doctor may ask you to assist with goniometry. After special training, you may be asked to perform goniometry. When performing goniometry, you measure the joints from the head to the feet, comparing each joint measurement with a standard measurement (in degrees of movement) for that joint.

Muscle Strength Testing. The physician tests muscle strength to determine the amount of force the patient is able to exert with a muscle or group of muscles. This test is usually done at the same time as ROM testing. It may be performed by the physician with your assistance, or once you have had special training, the physician may ask you to perform it yourself.

Like the ROM test, the muscle strength test is usually done from head to foot. The patient is asked to resist the pressure that you or the physician applies to each muscle or group of muscles (usually near a joint). Strength is rated according to a five-point scale.

TABLE 25-1 Range of Motion Movements Measured by Goniometry

Term	Description	Example
Abduction	Movement away from midline of body or movement away from axis of limb	Raising arm straight out to side
Adduction (opposite of abduction)	Movement toward midline of body or movement toward axis of limb	Lowering raised arm down to side
Circumduction	Circular movement of body part	Performing arm circles
Dorsiflexion	Upward or backward movement of body part	Flexing foot—toes pointing upward
Eversion	Outward movement of body part	Moving ankle—sole of foot turning outward
Extension	Movement that spreads apart two body parts or that opens joint	Straightening leg after being in bent-knee position
Flexion (opposite of extension)	Movement that brings together two body parts or that closes joint	Bending leg at knee
Inversion (opposite of eversion)	Inward movement of body part	Moving ankle—sole of foot turning inward
Plantar flexion (opposite of dorsiflexion)	Downward movement of body part	Flexing foot—toes pointing downward
Pronation	Twisting movement that brings palm face down	Turning wrist so palm faces down
Rotation	Movement of body part around axis	Turning head from side to side
Supination (opposite of pronation)	Rotating movement that brings palm facing upward	Turning wrist so that palm faces upward

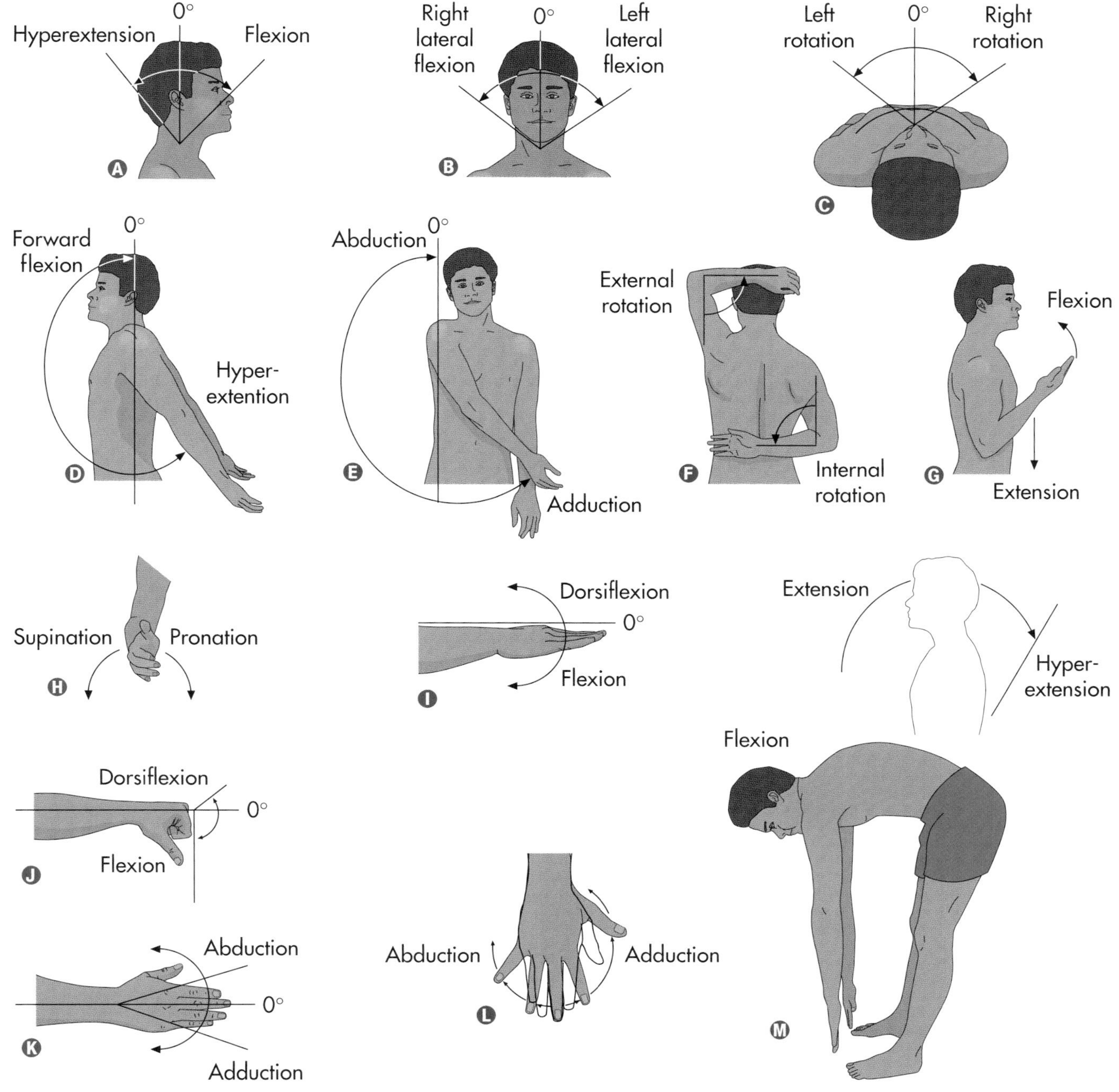

Figure 25-2. When you measure joint ROM, begin at the head and work down to the feet.

Typically, a patient can move a joint a certain distance and can easily resist the pressure you apply. The patient usually has equal strength on both sides of the body. If the patient has weakness, however, a medical problem may be indicated. The physician must be made aware of weaknesses so that he can use this information to develop a treatment plan.

Gait Testing. **Gait** is the way a person walks. A normal gait has two phases: stance and swing (Figure 25-3). A typical stance phase begins with the right heel strike (when the patient's right heel meets the floor). As the foot rocks forward and the toes meet the floor, the right foot flattens and bears the body's weight. In midstance the patient lifts the left foot. Then the right foot begins to push off by flexing the toes and lifting the heel off the floor.

The swing phase begins with the right foot poised to begin the swing as the left heel strikes the floor. Then the right foot clears the floor and swings forward. In midswing

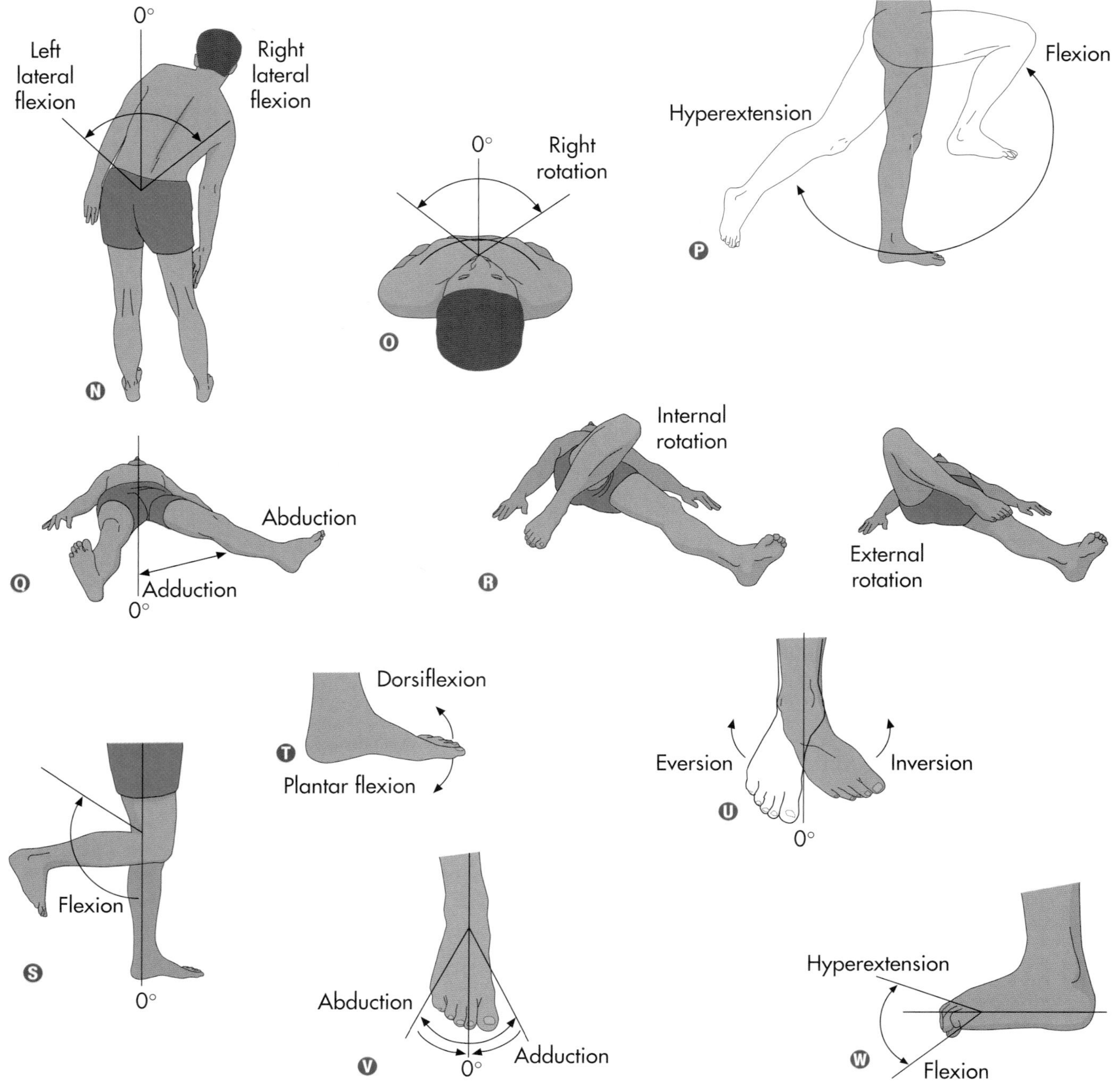

Figure 25-2. (continued)

it passes the left foot. At the end of the swing, the right foot slows, and heel strike occurs again.

Generally, a physician or physical therapist assesses a patient's gait. To do so, the physician asks the patient to walk away, turn around, and walk back. Assessment of gait includes an appraisal of the patient's length of stride, balance, coordination, direction of knees (inward or outward), and direction of feet (inward or outward).

Posture Testing. **Posture** is body position and alignment. The doctor assesses posture by looking at the patient's spinal curve from the sides, back, and front. Normally, the thoracic spine has a convex (outward) curve, and the lumbar spine has a concave (inward) curve. The doctor also notes the symmetry of alignment of the shoulders, knees, and hips.

To assess alignment and degree of straightness of the spine, the doctor asks the patient to bend at the waist and let the arms dangle freely. To assess knee position, the doctor asks the patient to stand with both feet together to determine whether the knees are at the same height, facing forward, and symmetrical.

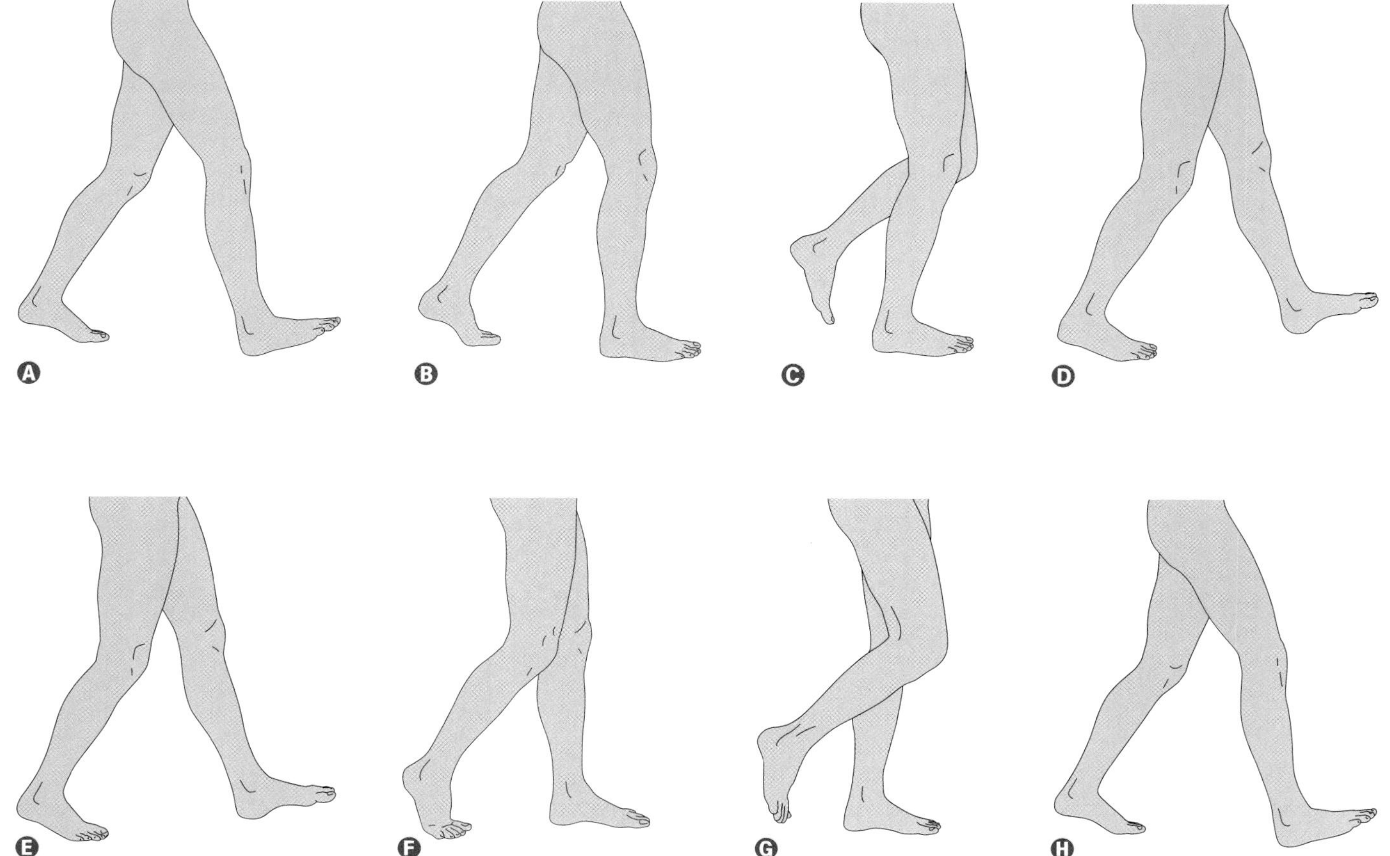

Figure 25-3. These are the two phases of gait. Illustrations (a) through (d) show the movements of the stance phase; illustrations (e) through (h) show the movements of the swing phase: (a) right heel strike, (b) flat right foot, (c) midstance, (d) push off with right foot, (e) right foot poised, (f) left heel strike, (g) midswing, (h) right heel strike.

Cryotherapy and Thermotherapy

Applying cold to a patient's body for therapeutic reasons is called **cryotherapy.** This type of therapy can be administered in a number of ways. Treatments may be dry or wet, and they may be chemical or natural. Examples of dry cold applications are ice bags and ice packs. Wet cold applications include cold compresses and ice massage.

Applying heat to a patient's body for therapeutic reasons is called **thermotherapy.** As with cryotherapy, thermotherapy can be administered in a variety of ways. Examples of devices used in dry heat treatments are electric heating pads, hot-water bottles, and heat lamps. Moist heat treatments include hot soaks and the use of hot compresses and hot packs.

Factors Affecting the Use of Cryotherapy and Thermotherapy

To choose a cold or heat therapy for a patient, the physician considers the therapy's purpose, the location and condition of the affected area, and the patient's age and general health. After choosing a therapy, the physician may direct you to apply the cold or heat treatment and to teach the patient and family how to continue the therapy at home.

Performed correctly, cold and heat therapies generally promote healing. These therapies can, however, cause side effects in some patients. Therefore, you need to exercise caution when applying the therapies. You also need to be aware of conditions that contraindicate (make inadvisable) cold or heat therapies. Table 25-2 summarizes circumstances that warrant precautions or contraindications for the therapies as well as possible side effects. When performing any cold or heat therapy, you should consider the age of the patient, treatment location, patient problems with circulation or sensation, and individual temperature tolerance.

Age. Age is an important consideration because young children and elderly patients usually are more sensitive than others to cold and heat. When administering cryotherapy or thermotherapy, stay with the patient during its application to check the patient's skin frequently for excessive paleness or redness.

Treatment Location. Thin-skinned areas that are usually covered with clothing (such as the back, chest, and

TABLE 25-2 Contraindications, Precautions, and Side Effects Related to Cold and Heat

Therapy	Precautions	Contraindications	Side Effects
Dry and moist cold applications	Poor circulation, extreme age or youth, arthritis, impaired sensation (insensitivity to cold)	Inability to tolerate weight of device, pain caused by application (more common with moist cold)	Numbness, pain, very pale or bluish skin, blood clots (rare)
Dry and moist heat applications	Impaired kidney, heart, or lung function; arteriosclerosis and atherosclerosis; impaired sensation (insensitivity to heat); extreme age or youth; pregnancy	Possibility of hemorrhage; malignancy; acute inflammation, such as appendicitis; severe circulation problems; pain caused by weight of device	Burns (especially with heat lamps), increased respiratory rate, lowered blood pressure

abdomen) are more sensitive to cold and heat therapies than other areas, such as the face and hands. Use caution around any broken skin (as with a wound), because it is susceptible to further tissue damage from cryotherapy or thermotherapy.

Circulation or Sensation Impairment. Patients with diabetes or cardiovascular disease may have impaired circulation or sensory perception. These impairments may prevent such patients from sensing that a treatment is too cold or too hot. These patients require close monitoring during cryotherapy or thermotherapy. Carefully observe their skin to determine the treatment's therapeutic effect.

Temperature Tolerance. Tolerance of temperature extremes varies greatly from person to person. Some people are unusually sensitive to cold or to heat. Listen carefully to patients for any indication of temperature intolerance during treatment. Cases of intolerance should be reported to the physician, who may decide to change the treatment.

Principles of Cryotherapy

The application of cryotherapy causes blood vessels to constrict and involuntary muscles of the skin to contract. These physiologic responses can have the following results:

- Prevention of swelling by limiting edema, or fluid accumulation in body tissue
- Control of bleeding by constricting blood vessels
- Reduction of inflammation by slowing blood and fluid movement in the affected area
- Provision of an anesthetic effect for pain by reducing inflammation
- Reduction of pus formation by inhibiting microorganism activity
- Lowering of body temperature

Administering Cryotherapy

Cryotherapy is highly effective in alleviating swelling, pain, inflammation, and bleeding caused by various types of injuries. For best results, cryotherapy should be used frequently (about 20 minutes every hour) for the first 48 hours after an injury. As cold is applied, the skin becomes cool and pale because blood vessels constrict, decreasing the blood supply to the area. The decreased blood supply also reduces tissue metabolism, oxygen use, and waste accumulation.

Dry Cold Applications. Dry cold applications include ice bags, ice collars, and chemical ice packs. An ice bag is a rubber or plastic bag with a locking lid. An ice collar is a rubber or plastic kidney-shaped bag that is specially curved to fit around the back of the neck.

A chemical ice pack is usually a flat plastic bag containing a semifluid chemical (Figure 25-4). Ice packs come in various sizes and types. Some are disposable, whereas others can be stored in a freezer and reused. The chemical prevents them from freezing solid, allowing them to be

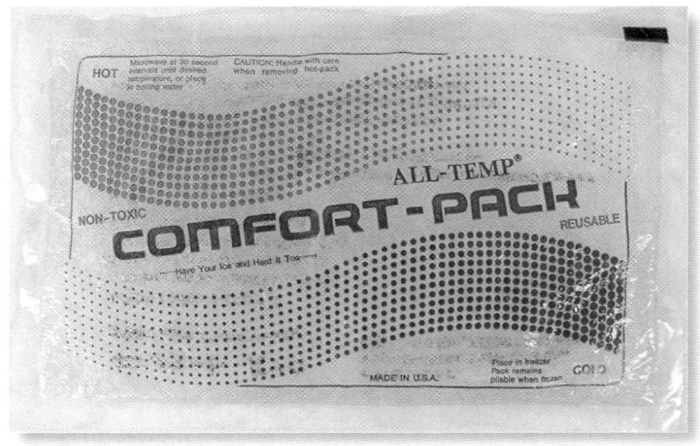

Figure 25-4. This chemical pack can be frozen, boiled, or microwaved for cold or heat therapy.

molded to the area to be treated. Chemical ice packs may require squeezing or shaking to activate the cooling action. Most packs remain cold for 30 to 60 minutes. Some ice packs come with a soft covering; others must be wrapped in a cloth before they are applied to the skin.

Wet Cold Applications. Wet cold applications include cold compresses and ice massage. A cold compress is a cloth or gauze pad moistened with ice water. It may be used to treat the pain associated with a toothache, tooth extraction, eye injury, or headache. The ice used in ice massage may be a cube wrapped in a plastic bag or water frozen in a paper cup. The combination of the cold temperature and the motion of the massage can provide therapeutic relief for the localized pain resulting from a sprain or strain. Although cold causes muscles to contract, the pain-relieving effect can help a patient relax. The procedure for administering cryotherapy is outlined in Procedure 25-1.

Principles of Thermotherapy

The application of thermotherapy causes blood vessels to dilate (expand), which increases the blood supply to the area. Increased blood supply brings about an increased tissue metabolism that carries oxygen and nutrients to the cells of the area being treated. Increased metabolism carries toxins and wastes away from the cells. During thermotherapy, the treated skin becomes warm and develops **erythema** (redness) as the capillaries in the deep layers of the skin fill with blood. These physiologic responses can have the following results:

- Relief of pain and congestion
- Reduction of muscle spasms
- Muscle relaxation
- Reduction of inflammation
- Reduction of swelling by increasing the fluid absorption from the tissues

Administering Thermotherapy

Thermotherapy is highly effective in relieving pain, congestion, muscle spasms, and inflammation and promoting muscle relaxation. However, if heat is applied for too long, it may increase skin secretions that soften the skin and lower resistance. Heat that is too extreme can burn the skin or increase edema. Always monitor patients receiving thermotherapy, particularly children and elderly patients. The three basic types of thermotherapy are dry heat, moist heat, and diathermy. The general principles for administering the following types of thermotherapy are outlined in Procedure 25-2.

Dry Heat Therapies. There are several types of dry heat therapy. They include the use of chemical hot packs, heating pads, hot-water bottles, heat lamps with infrared or ultraviolet bulbs, and fluidotherapy.

Chemical Hot Pack. A chemical hot pack is a disposable, flexible pack of chemicals that becomes hot when you activate it by kneading or slapping it. After activating the pack, cover it with a cloth, and place it on the patient's skin in the area being treated. Chemical hot packs are pliable and conform to body contours. For best results, follow the manufacturer's directions.

Heating Pad. A heating pad is a flat pad with electrical coils between layers of soft fabric. When turned on, the coils provide localized heat. The physician should specify the heating pad temperature (low, medium, or high) and the length of time the pad should be applied.

Before applying a heating pad, cover it with a pillowcase or towel, check to be sure the cord is not frayed, and plug it into an electrical outlet. Make sure the patient's skin is dry. Then turn on the pad, and set the temperature selector switch to the specified temperature. The patient should never lie on top of a heating pad.

Hot-Water Bottle. A hot-water bottle is a flat, flexible, plastic or rubber bottle with a stopper. Fill the bottle with hot water, using a thermometer to make sure the water temperature does not exceed 125°F. For children under the age of 2 years and for elderly patients, the temperature should range from 105° to 115°F. For older children, a safe temperature is 115° to 125°F. Fill the bottle halfway; then compress it to expel air. The half-filled bottle can conform to the area to be treated. A half-filled bottle is also lighter than a full one and therefore more comfortable for the patient. Cover the bottle with a cloth or pillowcase before you apply it.

After you apply the hot-water bottle, check with the patient to make sure the temperature is not too hot. Check the temperature frequently, and replace the hot water as needed. Each time you remove the bottle, check the patient's skin to make sure that it is merely warm to the touch.

Heat Lamp. A heat lamp uses an infrared or ultraviolet bulb to provide heat. When the lamp is turned on, infrared rays heat and penetrate the skin's surface to a depth of 3 to 5 millimeters. To avoid burning the skin, place an infrared heat lamp 2 to 4 feet from the area being treated. Treatment usually lasts for 20 to 30 minutes or as directed by the physician.

Although ultraviolet rays produce little heat, they can burn the skin and damage the eyes. They are used to kill bacteria and to promote vitamin D formation. Ultraviolet rays stimulate epithelial cells and cause blood vessels to overfill, increasing the skin's defenses against bacterial infections. Ultraviolet lamps are used to treat acne, psoriasis, pressure sores, and wound infections.

Before recommending the use of an ultraviolet lamp, the physician assesses the patient's sensitivity and determines the treatment duration. Treatments typically range from 30 seconds to a few minutes. The duration is usually increased in 10-second intervals. Because ultraviolet rays can burn the skin, monitor the patient closely. Do not leave the room during the treatment. Both you and the patient must wear goggles to prevent harm to the eyes.

Fluidotherapy. **Fluidotherapy** is a relatively new technique for stimulating healing, particularly in the hands

PROCEDURE 25.1

Administering Cryotherapy

Objective: To reduce pain and swelling by administering cryotherapy safely

OSHA Guidelines

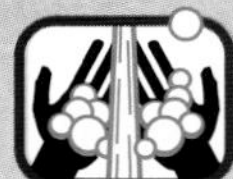 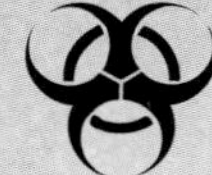 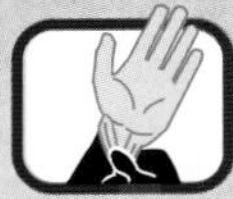

Materials: Gloves, cold application materials required for order: ice bag, ice collar, chemical cold pack, washcloth or gauze squares, or ice

Method

1. Double-check the physician's order. Be sure you know where to apply therapy, the proper temperature for the application, and how long it should remain in place.
2. Identify the patient, and explain the procedure and its purpose. Ask if the patient has any questions.
3. Have the patient undress and put on a gown, if required; provide privacy or assistance as needed.
4. Wash your hands and put on gloves. Utility gloves and a laboratory coat may be necessary depending on the temperature and type of treatment.
5. Position and drape the patient properly.
6. Remove any dressing covering the area and place in the biohazardous waste container.
7. Check the temperature on all applications before and during the treatment. As necessary, cool devices to provide therapeutic temperatures and then reapply them.
8. Prepare the therapy as ordered.
   - Ice bag or collar
     - **a.** Check the ice bag or collar for leaks.
     - **b.** Fill the ice bag or collar two-thirds full with ice chips or small ice cubes. Finish filling the ice bag or collar with water and then drain it so as to smooth the edges of the ice and help the device conform to the patient's body, which will better conduct the cold. Compress the container to expel any air or water and then close it.
     - **c.** Dry the bag or collar completely and cover it with a towel to absorb moisture and provide comfort.
   - Chemical ice pack
     - **a.** Check the pack for leaks.
     - **b.** Shake or squeeze the pack to activate the chemicals, or use a cold chemical pack taken from a refrigerator or freezer.
     - **c.** Cover the pack with a towel.
   - Cold compress
     - **a.** Place large ice cubes and a small amount of water in the basin. Large pieces do not melt as quickly as smaller ones, so they should last the length of the procedure.
     - **b.** Place the washcloth or gauze squares in the basin.
     - **c.** Moisten and wring them out.
9. Place the device on the patient's affected body part. If you are using a compress, place an ice bag on it, if desired, to keep it colder longer.
10. Ask the patient how the device feels. Explain that the cold is of great benefit, although it may be somewhat uncomfortable.
11. Leave the device in place for the length of time ordered by the physician. Periodically check the skin for color, feeling, and pain. If the area becomes excessively pale or blue, numb, or painful, remove the device and have the physician examine the area.
12. Remove the application and observe the area for reduced swelling, redness, and pain. Replace the patient's dressing if necessary.
13. Help the patient dress, if needed.
14. Remove equipment and supplies, properly discarding used disposable materials and arranging for the appropriate sanitization, disinfection, and/or sterilization of reusable equipment and materials as needed.
15. Remove the gloves and wash your hands.
16. Document the treatment and your observation in the patient's chart. If you teach the patient or the patient's family how to use the device, document your instructions.

PROCEDURE 25.2

Administering Thermotherapy

Objective: To administer thermotherapy safely

OSHA Guidelines

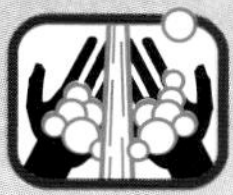
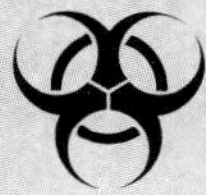
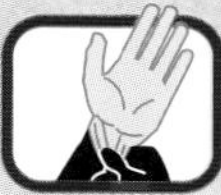

Materials: Gloves, towels, blanket, heat application materials required for order: chemical hot pack, heating pad, hot-water bottle, heat lamp, container and medication for hot soak, container and gauze for hot compress

Method

1. Double-check the physician's order. Be sure you know where to apply therapy, the proper temperature for the application, and how long it should remain in place.
2. Identify the patient, and explain the procedure and its purpose. Ask if the patient has any questions.
3. Have the patient undress and put on a gown, if required; provide privacy or assistance as needed.
4. Wash your hands and put on gloves. Utility gloves and a laboratory coat may be necessary depending on the temperature and type of treatment.
5. Position and drape the patient properly.
6. Remove any dressing covering the area and place in the biohazardous waste container.
7. Check the temperature on all applications before and during the treatment. As necessary, reheat devices or solutions to provide therapeutic temperatures and then reapply them.
8. Prepare the therapy as ordered.
   - Chemical hot pack
     - **a.** Check the pack for leaks.
     - **b.** Activate the pack. (Check manufacturer's directions.)
     - **c.** Cover the pack with a towel.
   - Heating pad
     - **a.** Turn the heating pad on, selecting the appropriate temperature.
     - **b.** Cover the pad with a towel or pillowcase.
     - **c.** Make sure the patient's skin is dry, and do not allow the patient to lie on top of the heating pad.
   - Hot-water bottle
     - **a.** Fill the bottle one-half full with hot water of the correct temperature—usually 110°F to 115°F. Use a thermometer. The physician can provide information on the ideal temperature water that should be used, which will depend on the area being treated.
     - **b.** Expel the air and close the bottle.
     - **c.** Cover the bottle with a towel or pillowcase.
   - Heat lamp
     - **a.** Place the lamp 2 feet to 4 feet away from the treatment area.
     - **b.** Follow the treatment time as ordered.
   - Hot soak
     - **a.** Select a container of the appropriate size for the area to be treated.
     - **b.** Fill the container with hot water that is no more than 110°F. Use a thermometer. Add medication to the container if ordered.
   - Hot compress
     - **a.** Soak a washcloth or gauze in hot water. Wring it out.
     - **b.** Frequently rewarm the compress to maintain the temperature.
9. Place the device on the patient's affected body part, or place the affected body part in the container. If you are using a compress, place a hot-water bottle on top, if desired, to keep it warm longer.
10. Ask the patient how the device feels. During any heat therapy, remember that dilated blood vessels cause heat loss from the skin and that this heat loss may make the patient feel chilled. Be prepared to cover the patient with sheets or blankets.
11. Leave the device in place for the length of time ordered by the physician. Periodically check the skin for redness, blistering, or irritation. If the area becomes excessively red or develops blisters, remove the patient from the heat source and have the physician examine the area.
12. Remove the application and observe the area for reduced pain, inflammation, and swelling. Replace the patient's dressing if necessary.

continued ⟶

PROCEDURE 25.2

Administering Thermotherapy *(continued)*

13. Help the patient dress, if needed.
14. Remove equipment and supplies, properly discarding used disposable materials and arranging for the appropriate sanitization, disinfection, and/or sterilization of reusable equipment and materials as needed.
15. Remove the gloves and wash your hands.
16. Document the treatment and your observation in the patient's chart. If you teach the patient or the patient's family how to use the device, document your instructions.

and feet. The patient places the affected body part in a container of glass beads that are heated and agitated with hot air. Although the therapy is dry, its effect is similar to that of a therapy using water.

Moist Heat Applications. Moist heat is often used to soften dried, crusted exudates (discharges from body tissues) for easy removal. Moist heat applications include hot soak, hot compress, hot pack, and paraffin bath.

Hot Soak. With hot-soak therapy, the patient places the affected body part—usually an arm or leg—in a container of plain or medicated water that has been heated to no more than 110°F. A hot soak should last about 15 minutes.

Hot Compress. A compress is a piece of gauze or cloth suitable for covering a small area. After soaking the compress in hot water, wring it out and apply it to the area to be treated. Keep the compress warm either by placing a hot-water bottle on top of it or by frequently rewarming the compress in hot water.

Hot Pack. A hot pack is a large canvas bag filled with heat-retaining gel that is used on a large body area. Like a hot compress, a hot pack retains heat after being placed in hot water.

Paraffin Bath. A paraffin bath is a receptacle of heated wax and mineral oil. It is used to reduce pain, muscle spasms, and stiffness in patients with arthritis and similar disorders. The patient's affected area is dipped repeatedly into the mixture until the area is covered with a thick coat of wax. The wax remains on the area for about 30 minutes and then is peeled off. Particularly useful for joints, the paraffin bath has the added benefit of leaving the skin warm, flexible, and soft. Some erythema may result.

Diathermy. **Diathermy** is a type of heat therapy in which a machine produces high-frequency waves that achieve deep heat penetration in muscle tissue. The heat helps decrease joint stiffness, dilate blood vessels, relieve muscle spasms, and reduce discomfort from sprains and strains. Three types of diathermy are ultrasound, shortwave, and microwave. Equipment for these therapies is continually being improved. Be sure to familiarize yourself with the manufacturer's instructions regarding the specific equipment in your office.

Ultrasound. Ultrasound is the most common type of diathermy. It projects high-frequency sound waves that are converted to heat in muscle tissue. This type of diathermy is used to treat sprains, strains, and other acute ailments.

Ultrasound diathermy may be administered by rubbing a gel-covered transducer over the skin in circular patterns. It may also be administered to a body part under water. Do not use ultrasound in areas where bones are near the skin's surface, because it could cause bone damage.

Shortwave. Shortwave diathermy uses radio waves that travel through the body between two condenser plates and are converted to heat in the tissues. This type of diathermy is used to treat acute, subacute, and chronic inflammation. Treatment duration typically ranges from 20 to 30 minutes. Do not use shortwave diathermy on a patient who has a pacemaker.

Microwave. Microwave diathermy uses microwaves to provide heat deep in body tissues. Contraindications include use on patients with pacemakers, use in combination with wet dressings, or use in high dosages on patients with swollen tissue. Also, never use microwave diathermy near metal implants, because the reaction between metal and microwaves could cause burns.

Hydrotherapy

Hydrotherapy is the use of water to treat physical problems. It is typically performed in the physical therapy department of a hospital, in an outpatient clinic, or at home. Common forms of hydrotherapy include the use of whirlpools and contrast baths and underwater exercises.

Whirlpools

Whirlpools are tanks in which water is agitated by jets of air under pressure. Whirlpools vary in size from small (capable of accommodating only one body part) to very

Career Opportunities

Physical Therapist Assistant

To gain medical assistant credentials, you must fulfill the requirements of either the American Association of Medical Assistants (for a Certified Medical Assistant) or the American Medical Technologists (for a Registered Medical Assistant). After obtaining your medical assistant certification or registration, you may wish to acquire additional skills in specialty areas through course work or on-the-job training. Although this course work or training may not lead to an additional certification or degree, it will enable you to expand your role in the medical office and advance your career as the demand for skilled health professionals increases.

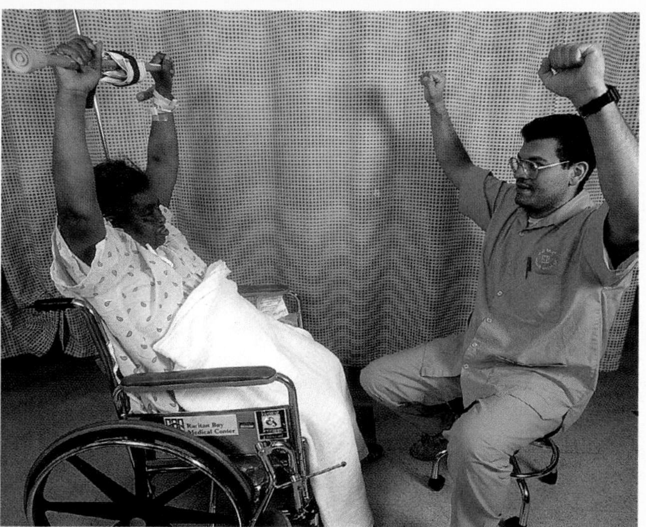

Skills and Duties

A relatively new profession, physical therapist assisting was first developed in the late 1960s because of the overwhelming interest in the potential of physical therapy in rehabilitation. The goal of physical therapy is to restore or increase physical movement and strength. A physical therapist assistant helps patients improve their physical function when it has been impaired by injury, disease, birth defects, or other causes. Physical therapist assistants often work as part of a team of therapeutic specialists, which may include physicians, physical therapists, occupational therapists, and sometimes social workers.

Working under the supervision of a physical therapist, the assistant carries out the treatments and exercises prescribed by the therapist. She may administer cold and heat therapy, massage, or ultraviolet light to decrease pain and relax muscles. In addition, she helps the patient perform physical exercises to build muscle strength and stamina and to increase mobility. When helping patients exercise, the physical therapist assistant often works in swimming pools or with gym equipment, such as stationary bicycles, weights, and parallel bars. She may take measurements, such as vital signs or range of motion, to help evaluate patients' progress.

The physical therapist assistant may also fit assistive devices for patients who have lost limbs or need mobility training. She routinely teaches them how to use and care for wheelchairs, walkers, braces, and artificial arms and legs. In all cases she records patients' progress for the physical therapist to evaluate. In addition, the physical therapist assistant may perform administrative office work, such as scheduling therapy sessions and maintaining records, and may prepare both equipment and patients for therapy.

Because the job can be physically demanding, people entering this career should be physically fit. Good communication skills are also important.

Workplace Settings

Physical therapist assistants most often work in hospitals and rehabilitation centers. They may also work in nursing homes, physicians' offices, or clinics. Most work 40-hour weeks, although some are employed part-time.

Education

A physical therapist assistant requires less education than a physical therapist. In most states she must complete an accredited 2-year associate degree program at a junior or community college. In 36 states physical therapist assistants must also become licensed by passing a written examination. License renewal differs from state to state.

Where to Go for More Information

American Physical Therapy
Association/Foundation for Physical Therapy
1111 North Fairfax Street
Alexandria, VA 22314
(703) 684-2782
www.apta.org

National Rehabilitation Association
633 South Washington Street
Alexandria, VA 22314
(703) 836-0850
www.nationalrehab.org

large (capable of accommodating a wheelchair or full-body submersion). The action of the agitated water in a whirlpool generates a hydromassage, which relaxes muscles and increases circulation. Whirlpools are also used to cleanse and debride (remove foreign matter and dead tissue from) the skin of patients with wounds, ulcers, or burns.

Contrast Baths

Contrast baths are separate baths, one filled with hot water and the other with cold water. The patient alternately moves the treated body part quickly from one bath to the other. This treatment induces relaxation, stimulates improved circulation (which speeds up healing), and results in greater mobility.

Underwater Exercises

Underwater exercises are usually performed in a warm swimming pool. They are prescribed for patients with joint injuries, burns, and arthritis. Because the water's buoyancy takes pressure off the joints, underwater exercises are particularly useful for patients with painful or limited movement. Combined with the movement of the water around the body, the exercises promote relaxation and increased circulation.

Exercise Therapy

For many patients, exercise is as important as medications or other treatments. Exercise offers both preventive and therapeutic benefits. As a patient ages, exercise helps promote flexibility, mobility, muscle tone, and strength. Exercise is a primary treatment for fractures, arthritis, and some respiratory disorders; it can minimize symptoms or help slow disease progression. For patients who have had surgery, stroke, burns, or amputation, regular exercise therapy can help prevent problems caused by inactivity.

A doctor orders exercise therapy for many reasons. Exercise improves or restores general health and is especially therapeutic when a patient is weak from illness. Explain to patients that exercise will help them to:

- Improve muscle tone and strength
- Regain range of motion (ROM) after an injury
- Prevent ROM from diminishing in chronic conditions
- Prevent or correct physical deformities
- Promote neuromuscular coordination
- Improve circulation
- Relieve stress
- Lower cholesterol levels
- Aid in the resumption of normal daily activities

Exercise therapy is commonly used for treating sports injuries. Exercise therapy for injured athletes is described in the Educating the Patient section. This type of therapy focuses primarily on regaining muscle strength and flexibility in the injured area.

Role of the Medical Assistant

As a medical assistant, you may have several roles in exercise therapy. As an information resource for the patient and family, you must understand various types of exercise programs and the patient's specific treatment plan. You may also serve as a source of support and encouragement when exercise programs are long and difficult. You may, for example, assist with ROM exercises and teach the patient and family how to perform them at home.

When teaching patients about exercises, give them illustrations of the exercises. Include with each illustration written instructions on the number of times to perform the exercise, as prescribed by the doctor.

After demonstrating each exercise, have patients perform it while you watch and give direction. Patients are more likely to perform exercises properly at home if they can perform them correctly in your presence. It is also helpful for patients' caregivers or family members to watch and perform the exercises to become familiar with them.

Types of Exercise

Before a patient begins an exercise program, the doctor evaluates the patient's heart and lung function and overall physical condition. The doctor adjusts the level of exercise accordingly and may prescribe other forms of physical therapy, such as cryotherapy, thermotherapy, or hydrotherapy. Careful preparation by the doctor and patient before beginning a program of exercise therapy helps prevent injuries. Some measures to prevent and treat common exercise therapy problems are outlined in Table 25-3. A doctor may also refer a patient to a physical therapist, who will develop an exercise program specifically for that patient. Types of exercises in therapeutic programs include active mobility, passive mobility, aided mobility, active resistance, isometric, and ROM.

Active Mobility Exercises. Active mobility exercises are self-directed exercises that the patient performs without assistance. Their purpose is to increase muscle strength and function. They often require equipment such as a stationary bicycle or a treadmill.

Passive Mobility Exercises. In passive mobility exercises the physical therapist or a machine moves a patient's body part. The patient does not actively assist in these exercises. Patients who require passive mobility exercises may have neuromuscular disability or weakness. Passive mobility exercises can help retain patients' ROM and improve their circulation.

Aided Mobility Exercises. Aided mobility exercises are self-directed exercises. The patient performs them with the aid of a device such as an exercise machine or a therapy pool.

Active Resistance Exercises. In active resistance exercises the patient works against resistance (counterpressure). Resistance is provided manually by the therapist

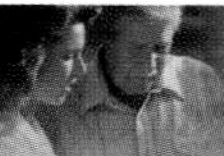

Educating the Patient

The Injured Athlete

The risk of injury is associated with most sports, but some sports carry a greater risk of serious injury than others. Many sports-related injuries affect joints—in the neck, shoulders, elbows, wrists, hands, knees, ankles, and feet.

You may be called on to educate injured athletes and to start them on the road to recovery. To do so, you need to understand the mind of the athlete. Why do many athletes get injured in the first place? Here are some reasons.

- The sport they participate in has a high injury rate.
- They return to a sport before their injuries are completely healed.
- They become impatient with a physical therapy regimen.
- They do not work at gradual muscle strengthening.

When does your job begin? After diagnosing the injury, the physician will probably refer the athlete to a sports medicine center or other physical therapy setting, where an individualized program will be set up. As a medical assistant, you will often be responsible for counseling an athlete about the physical therapy program she will be entering. Here are some basic rules that you can communicate.

- Follow the physical therapy regimen set up by the physician or physical therapist—even if it is tedious or time consuming.
- Use only the equipment specified by the therapist: free weights, weight-training equipment, stationary bike, other aerobic equipment, or swimming pool. The physical therapist recommends the designated equipment based on the type of injury. Using other equipment could cause further injury or interfere with healing.
- Do not rush the therapy in an attempt to recover more quickly.
- Work slowly to strengthen muscles and improve flexibility.
- Continue exercises at home as instructed.
- Be patient.

Explain to the athlete how the physical therapy program will be presented. Knowing what to expect from the physical therapist can improve the athlete's compliance. Here are some explanations you might offer.

- The therapist will demonstrate exercises and then watch you perform them.
- The therapist may increase the number of repetitions or the amount of resistance (weight) but probably not both at the same time.
- The therapist will provide handouts illustrating the exercises, along with instructions on how to perform them.
- The therapist may provide an activity log to help you chart your progress.

An athlete who is impatient with a physical therapy regimen and returns to a sport before an injury has completely healed has an increased risk of repeated injury. Impress on the athlete the importance of the physical therapy process. Emphasize the need for gradual strengthening and healing over a period of time. To help the athlete in the long run, focus on recovery from injury and on the need to prevent recurrent injury.

TABLE 25-3 Preventing and Treating Common Problems of Exercise Therapy

Problem	Prevention Methods	Treatment
Muscle strain	Beginning with gentle warm-up exercises	Rest and application of ice followed by heat
Muscle aches	Keeping track of number of repetitions and amount of weight (resistance), if used; increasing number of repetitions or amount of weight slowly	Rest, soaking in hot bath to relieve aches
Impatience with slowness of progress	Discussing expectations with patient; setting realistic goals with patient; stressing necessity of avoiding recurrent injury, which would prolong recovery	Creation of goal sheet, noting small successes as therapy progresses

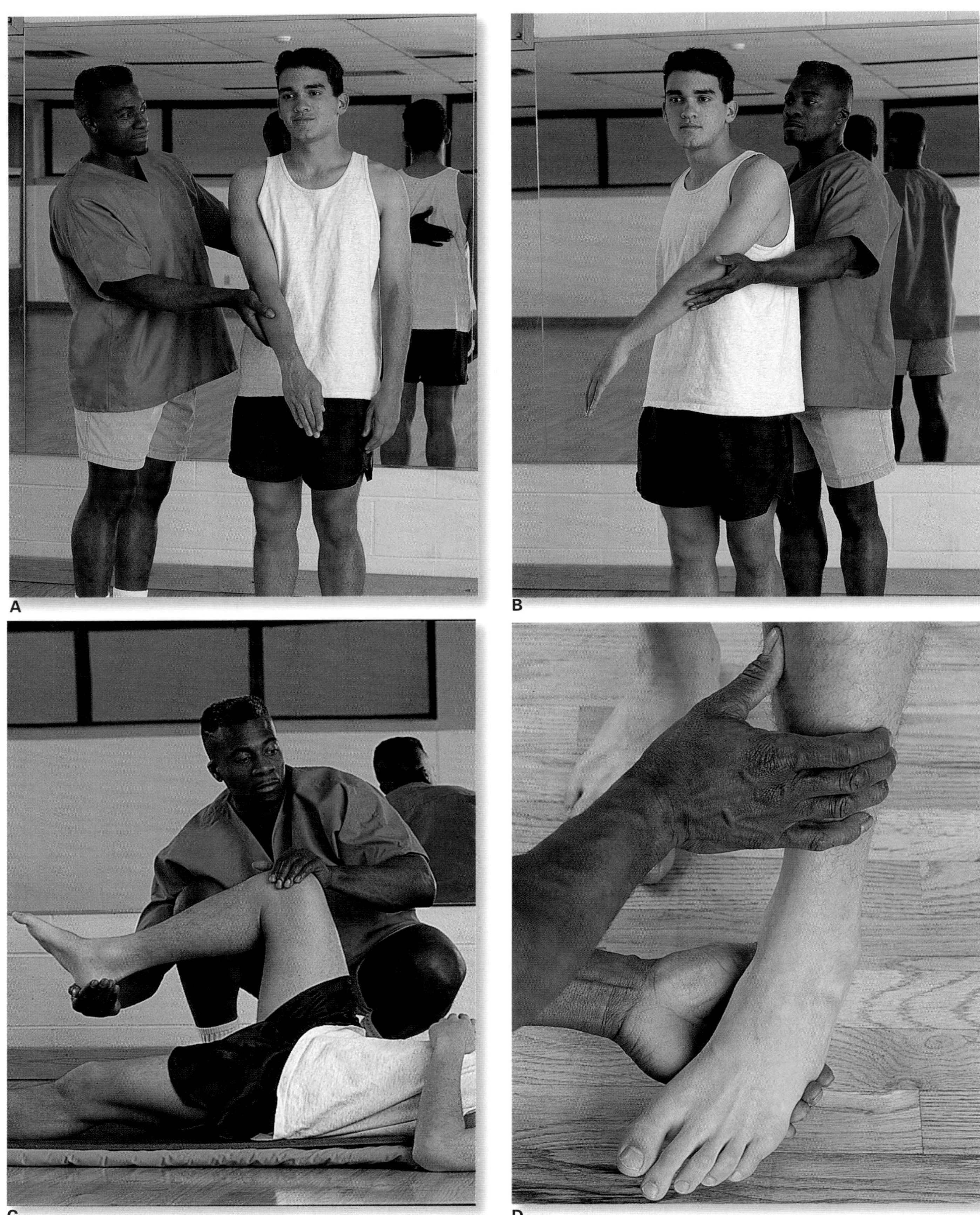

Figure 25-5. A medical assistant helps a patient perform typical ROM exercises: (a) shoulder abduction; (b) back rotation; (c) hip flexion; (d) toe abduction.

or mechanically by an exercise machine. These exercises increase the patient's muscle strength.

Isometric Exercises. During isometric exercises the patient relaxes and then contracts the muscles of a body part while in a fixed position. Isometric exercises can maintain the patient's muscle strength when a joint is temporarily or permanently immobilized.

ROM Exercises. ROM exercises move each joint through its full range of motion. These exercises should be done slowly and gently. Doing them too quickly or too soon after an injury can cause pain, fracture, or bleeding into the joint. For this reason a physical therapist assesses the patient and determines a recommended regimen of ROM exercises. You may be asked to educate the patient and caregiver or family about the regimen.

ROM exercises are typically prescribed after a joint injury. The physical therapist may recommend that the joint be moved in its full range of motion three times, twice a day. ROM exercises are also recommended for elderly people, to improve circulation and muscle function. The therapist will prescribe one of two types of ROM exercises for patients:

1. Active range-of-motion exercises: performed by the patient without assistance
2. Passive range-of-motion exercises: performed by the patient with the help of another person or a machine

Active and passive ROM exercises do not build muscle strength but do improve flexibility and mobility. Typical ROM exercises are illustrated in Figure 25-5.

Electrical Stimulation

Electrical stimulators deliver controlled amounts of low-voltage electric current to motor and sensory nerves to stimulate muscles. Electrical stimulation helps prevent atrophy in muscles that cannot move voluntarily by causing the muscles to contract involuntarily (on impulse) and relax. Frequent and regular electrical stimulation also aids in healing injured joints and in revitalizing muscles.

Electrical stimulation can help retrain a patient to use injured muscles by creating a perceivable connection between the stimulus (muscle movement) and the area of the brain that controls those muscles. If a limb does not function because of injury or disease, this therapy can give the patient hope that injured muscles are not dead. Hope often encourages a patient to work harder and to cooperate in the physical therapy regimen, which can be long and arduous. Electrical stimulation units that patients can wear are being developed for people with spinal cord injuries to help them retrain affected muscles.

Traction

Traction is the pulling or stretching of the musculoskeletal system to treat fractured bones and dislocated, arthritic, or other diseased joints. It is traditionally performed by a therapist in a specially equipped setting. A physical therapist may set up traction in the patient's home and visit regularly to ensure that the equipment is used and maintained properly. Traction may be used to:

- Create and maintain proper bone alignment
- Reduce or prevent joint stiffening and abnormal muscle shortening
- Correct deformities
- Relieve compression of vertebral joints
- Reduce or relieve muscle spasms

Although you will not be setting up or performing traction, you should know about its types and uses. This information will prepare you to answer basic questions from patients and family members.

Manual Traction

The physical therapist performs manual traction by using his hands to pull a patient's limb or head gently. Pulling stretches the muscles and separates the joints, allowing for greater motion and less stiffening. Manual traction is used with patients who have muscle spasms, stiffness, and arthritis.

Static Traction

To perform static traction (also called weight traction), the therapist places a patient's limb, pelvis, or chin in a harness. The harness is then attached to weights through a system of pulleys. This type of traction is commonly used to relieve muscle spasms.

Skin Traction

During skin traction, the therapist wraps foam rubber or other types of pads around both sides of a limb and then attaches the pads to pulleys and weights. Elastic bandages are used to secure the foam. This type of traction uses limited weight to prevent injury to the skin while decreasing painful muscle spasms. It may be set up in a patient's home or an inpatient facility.

Skeletal Traction

Skeletal traction is performed in inpatient facilities on patients whose injuries require long traction time and heavy weights. During surgery a surgeon inserts pins, wires, or tongs into bones. After surgery the pins, wires, or tongs are attached to pulleys and weights to provide continuous traction.

Mechanical Traction

Mechanical traction uses a special device that pulls and relaxes intermittently. The therapist sets the time intervals between contractions and relaxations. Mechanical traction is used to promote relaxation.

Mobility Aids

Mobility aids (also called mobility assistive devices) include canes, walkers, crutches, and wheelchairs. These devices are designed to improve patients' ability to ambulate, or move from one place to another.

The appropriate aid depends on the patient's disability, muscle coordination, strength, and age. The patient may need a device temporarily—perhaps crutches after a sprain—or permanently—such as a wheelchair in the case of permanent paralysis.

Canes

Canes come in several styles, including standard, tripod, and quad-base (Figure 25-6). All styles are lightweight, made of wood or aluminum, and have a rubber tip or tips at the bottom. They provide support and help patients maintain balance. Canes are especially useful for patients with weaknesses on one side of the body (possibly due to a stroke), joint disability, or neuromuscular defect.

A standard cane is best for a patient who needs only a small amount of support. Its curved handle is convenient, allowing the patient to hang it from a pocket or a doorknob. When the patient uses a standard cane, however, the curved handle concentrates most of the patient's weight in one small area of the hand. To avoid stressing the hand in this way, some standard canes have a T-shaped handle, which distributes pressure on the hand more evenly.

Tripod canes have three legs, and quad-base canes have four. The multiple legs create a wide base of support, making them more stable than a standard cane. Tripod and

PROCEDURE 25.3

Teaching a Patient How to Use a Cane

Objective: To teach a patient how to use a cane safely

OSHA Guidelines: This procedure does not involve exposure to blood, body fluids, or tissues.

Materials: Cane suited to the patient's needs

Method

Standing From a Sitting Position

1. Instruct the patient to slide his buttocks to the edge of the chair.
2. Tell the patient to place his right foot against the right front leg of the chair and his left foot against the left front leg of the chair. (This provides him with a wide, stable stance.)
3. Instruct the patient to lean forward and use the armrests of the chair to push upward. Caution the patient not to lean on the cane.
4. Have the patient position the cane for support on the strong side of his body.

Walking

1. Teach the patient to hold the cane on the strong side of her body with the tip(s) of the cane 4 to 6 inches from the side of her strong foot. Remind the patient to make sure the tip is flat on the ground.
2. Have the patient move the cane forward approximately 12 inches and then move her affected foot forward, parallel to the cane.
3. Next have the patient move her strong leg forward past the cane and her weak leg.
4. Observe as the patient repeats this process.

Ascending Stairs

1. Instruct the patient to always start with his strong leg when going up stairs.
2. Advise the patient to keep the cane on the strong side of his body and to use the wall or rail for support on the weak side.
3. After the patient steps on the strong leg, instruct him to bring up his weak leg and then the cane.
4. Remind the patient not to rush.

Descending Stairs

1. Instruct the patient to always start with her weak leg when going down stairs.
2. Advise the patient to keep the cane on the strong side of her body and to use the wall or rail for support on the weak side.
3. Have the patient use the strong leg and wall or rail to support her body, bending the strong leg as she lowers the weak leg and cane to the next step. She can move the cane and weak leg simultaneously, or she can move the cane first, followed by the weak leg.
4. Instruct the patient to step down with the strong leg.

Walking on Snow or Ice

Suggest that the patient try a metal ice-gripping cane or a ski pole. These can be dug into the snow or ice to prevent slipping.

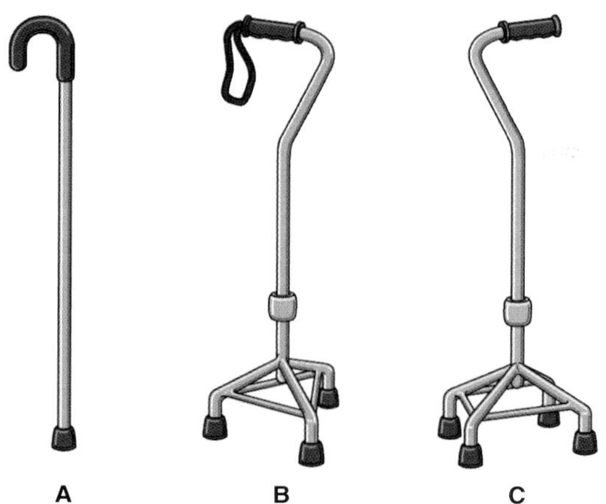

Figure 25-6. Shown here are three types of canes: (a) standard; (b) tripod; and (c) quad-base. Borrowed from McGraw-Hill *Health Care Science Technology* by Booth, 2004.

quad-base canes can stand alone, freeing up the patient's hands when she sits down. These canes are bulkier and more difficult to pick up and put down than a standard cane, however. Both styles have T-shaped handles.

After determining the most suitable cane for the patient, the physical therapist adjusts the cane's height. When the cane is the correct height, the patient's elbow is flexed at 20° to 25°, and the patient stands tall while using the cane (instead of leaning on it for support). The therapist makes sure that the handle is the right size for the patient's hand and instructs the patient on how to use the cane. If directed, you may do the teaching or reinforce it, as discussed in Procedure 25-3.

Walkers

A walker is an aluminum frame that is open on one side and has four widely placed legs with rubber tips. The legs are adjustable for various heights. Some models are designed to fold up for storage. To use a walker, the patient stands within the frame and leans on the upper bar, which has a handgrip on each side. The frame is lightweight, so it is easy for most patients to use.

Typically, a walker is used by older patients who are too weak to walk unassisted or who have balance problems. The walker is designed to give these patients a sense of stability as they ambulate. In tight spaces or in areas with throw rugs, however, a walker may be difficult to manage. A patient who is too weak to pick up the walker may use a walker on wheels. Wheeled walkers have brakes for safety. Patients should never slide a walker that does not have wheels because the movement could easily result in a fall.

A physical therapist selects a walker that suits the patient's abilities and height. A walker should reach the patient's hipbone. Although the physical therapist usually trains the patient in the use of a walker, you may be asked to do this, or you may need to reinforce the information presented in Procedure 25-4.

Crutches

Crutches allow a patient to walk without putting weight on the feet or legs by transferring that weight to the arms. Crutches are made of aluminum or wood. Aluminum crutches are lighter and usually more expensive than those made of wood. Pediatric crutches are available for children. The two basic types of crutches are axillary and Lofstrand. Procedure 25-5 provides the steps for teaching patients how to use crutches.

Axillary crutches reach from the ground to the armpit. Each crutch has a rubber tip on the bottom to prevent slipping. This type of crutch is designed for short-term use by patients with such injuries as a sprained ankle.

Lofstrand, or Canadian, crutches reach from the ground to the forearm, and each one has a rubber tip on the bottom to prevent slipping. For additional support, this type has a handgrip extension attached at a 90° angle and a metal cuff that fits securely around the patient's forearm. Lofstrand crutches are geared for long-term use by patients with such disorders as paraplegia.

Measuring the Patient for Crutches. To prevent back pain and nerve injury to the armpits and palms, crutches must be measured to fit each patient. Axillary crutches that are too long can put pressure on nerves in the armpit, causing a condition called crutch palsy (muscle weakness in the forearm, wrist, and hand). They can also force the patient's shoulders forward, causing strain on the back and making ambulation difficult. Crutches that are too short force the patient to bend forward during ambulation, causing back pain or imbalance, which can lead to falls.

Before a patient who uses crutches leaves the office, make sure the crutches fit properly and that the patient is comfortable walking with them. To confirm that the fit is correct, check for the following conditions.

- The patient is wearing the type of shoes he will wear when walking.
- The patient is standing erect with feet slightly apart.
- The crutch tips are positioned 2 to 4 inches in front of the patient's feet and 4 to 6 inches to the side of each foot.
- The axillary supports allow 2 to 3 finger-widths between supports and armpits. (Use wing nuts and bolts to adjust crutches.)
- The handgrips are positioned to create 30° flexion at the elbows. (Use wing nuts and bolts to adjust; use a goniometer to check flexion.) See Figure 25-7.

Crutch Gaits. To teach a patient how to stand and walk with crutches, you must learn the crutch gaits, or walks. First show the patient the standing, or tripod, position. To

PROCEDURE 25.4

Teaching a Patient How to Use a Walker

Objective: To teach a patient how to use a walker safely

OSHA Guidelines: This procedure does not involve exposure to blood, body fluids, or tissues.

Materials: Walker suited to the patient's needs

Method

Walking

1. Instruct the patient to step into the walker.
2. Tell the patient to place her hands on the handgrips on the sides of the walker.
3. Make sure the patient's feet are far enough apart so that she feels balanced.
4. Instruct the patient to pick up the walker and move it forward about 6 inches.
5. Have the patient move one foot forward and then the other foot.
6. Instruct the patient to pick up the walker again and to move it forward. If the patient is strong enough, explain that she may advance the walker after moving each leg rather than waiting until she has moved both legs.

Sitting

1. Teach the patient to turn his back to the chair or bed.
2. Instruct the patient to take small, careful steps and to back up until he feels the chair or bed at the back of his legs.
3. Instruct the patient to keep the walker in front of himself, let go of the walker, and place both his hands on the arms of the chair or on the bed.
4. Teach the patient to balance himself on his arms while lowering himself slowly to the chair or bed.

Ascending and Descending Stairs

1. Teach the patient not to use a walker when going up or down stairs.
2. Tell the patient to use the railing and a small quad-base cane instead of the walker.
3. Instruct the patient to ask her caregiver to place the walker at the top or bottom of the stairs as appropriate. It will then be ready for the patient to use after she has gone up or down the stairs.

do this, have the patient stand erect and look straight ahead. The patient should place the crutch tips 4 to 6 inches in front of her feet and 4 to 6 inches away from the side of each foot. See Figure 25-8.

To determine the proper gait for a patient, you will make a preteaching assessment of the patient's muscle coordination and physical condition. In general, instruct a patient to use a slow gait in crowded areas or when feeling tired. The patient can use a faster gait in open places or when feeling more energetic. Using various gaits and speeds enables the patient to exercise different muscle groups and improve overall conditioning.

Four-Point Gait. The four-point gait is a slow gait used only when a patient can bear weight on both legs. Because this gait has three points of contact with the ground at all times, it is stable and safe. It is especially useful for patients with leg muscle weakness, spasticity, or poor balance or coordination. To teach this gait, have the patient start in the tripod position. Then outline the following steps, as illustrated in Figure 25-9.

1. Move the right crutch forward.
2. Move the left foot forward to the level of the left crutch.
3. Move the left crutch forward.
4. Move the right foot forward to level of the right crutch.

Three-Point Gait. The three-point gait is used when a patient cannot bear weight on one leg but can bear full weight on the unaffected leg. This gait allows the patient's weight to be carried alternately by the crutches and by the unaffected leg. It is appropriate for amputees, patients with tissue or musculoskeletal trauma (such as a fractured or sprained leg), and those recovering from leg surgery. The patient must have good muscle coordination and arm strength, however. To teach this gait, have the patient start in the tripod position. Then give the patient the following instructions, as illustrated in Figure 25-9b.

1. Move both crutches and the affected leg forward.
2. Move the unaffected leg forward while weight is balanced on both crutches.

Two-Point Gait. The two-point gait is faster than the four-point gait and is used by patients who can bear some weight on both feet and have good muscle coordination and balance. To teach this gait, have the patient start in the

PROCEDURE 25.5

Teaching a Patient How to Use Crutches

Objective: To teach a patient how to use crutches safely

OSHA Guidelines: This procedure does not involve exposure to blood, body fluids, or tissues.

Materials: Crutches suited to the patient's needs

Method

1. Verify the physician's order for the type of crutches and gait to be used.
2. Wash your hands, identify the patient, and explain the procedure.
3. Elderly patients or patients with muscle weakness should be taught muscle strength exercises for their arms.
4. Have the patient stand erect and look straight ahead.
5. Tell the patient to place the crutch tips 2 to 4 inches in front of and 4 to 6 inches to the side of each foot.
6. When instructing a patient to use an axillary crutch, make sure the patient has a 2-inch gap between the axilla and the axillary bar and that each elbow is flexed 25° to 30°.
7. Teach the patient how to get up from a chair:
   a. Instruct the patient to hold both crutches on his affected or weaker side.
   b. Have the patient slide to the edge of the chair.
   c. Tell the patient to push down on the arm of the chair on his stronger side.
   d. Advise the patient to put the crutches under his arms and press toward his ribs.
8. Teach the patient the required gait. Which gait the patient will use depends on the muscle strength and coordination of the patient. It also depends on the type of crutches, the injury, and the patient's condition. Check the physician's orders, and see Figures 25-9 and 25-10 for examples.
9. Teach the patient how to ascend stairs:
   a. Start the patient close to the bottom step, and tell her to push down with her hands.
   b. Instruct the patient to step up on the first step with her good foot.
   c. Tell the patient to step up to the same step with her crutches and then with her other foot. Advise the patient to keep her crutches with her affected limb.
   d. Remind the patient to check her balance before she proceeds to the next step.
10. Teach the patient how to descend stairs:
    a. Have the patient start at the edge of the steps with his hips beneath him.
    b. Instruct the patient to bring his crutches and then the affected foot down first. Advise the patient to bend at the hips and knees to prevent leaning forward, which could cause him to fall.
    c. Tell the patient to bring his unaffected foot to the same step.
    d. Remind the patient to check his balance before he proceeds. In some cases, a handrail may be easier and can be used with both crutches in one hand.
11. Give the patient the following general information related to the use of crutches:
    a. Report to the physician any tingling or numbness in the arms, hands, or shoulders.
    b. Support body weight with the hands.
    c. Always stand erect to prevent muscle strain.
    d. Look straight ahead when walking.
    e. Generally, move the crutches not more than 6 inches at a time to maintain good balance.
    f. Check the crutch tips regularly for wear; replace the tips as needed.
    g. Check the crutch tips for wetness; dry the tips if they are wet.
    h. Check all wing nuts and bolts for tightness.
    i. Wear flat, well-fitting, nonskid shoes.
    j. Remove throw rugs and other unsecured articles from traffic areas.
    k. To elevate an injured leg when sitting, use a crutch to support the thigh.
    l. To support the body when fatigued, place the back against a wall, and divide weight between the back and the strong leg and foot.
    m. Report an unusual pain in the affected leg.

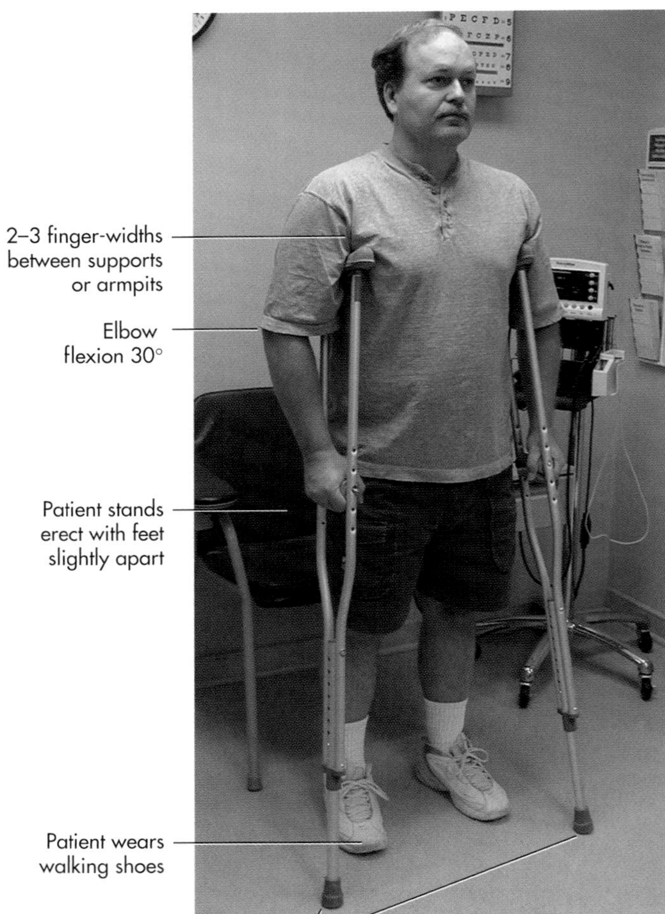

Figure 25-7. Use these guidelines when measuring a patient for crutches.

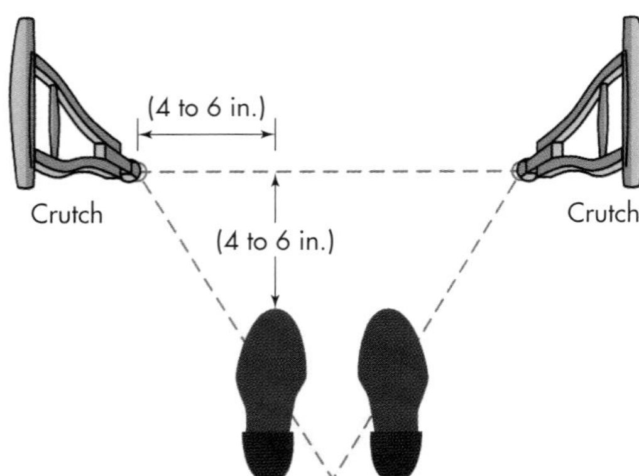

Figure 25-8. This the correct beginning position for the patient's feet and crutches when you are teaching a patient to walk with crutch. Borrowed from McGraw-Hill *Health Care Science Technology* by Booth, 2004.

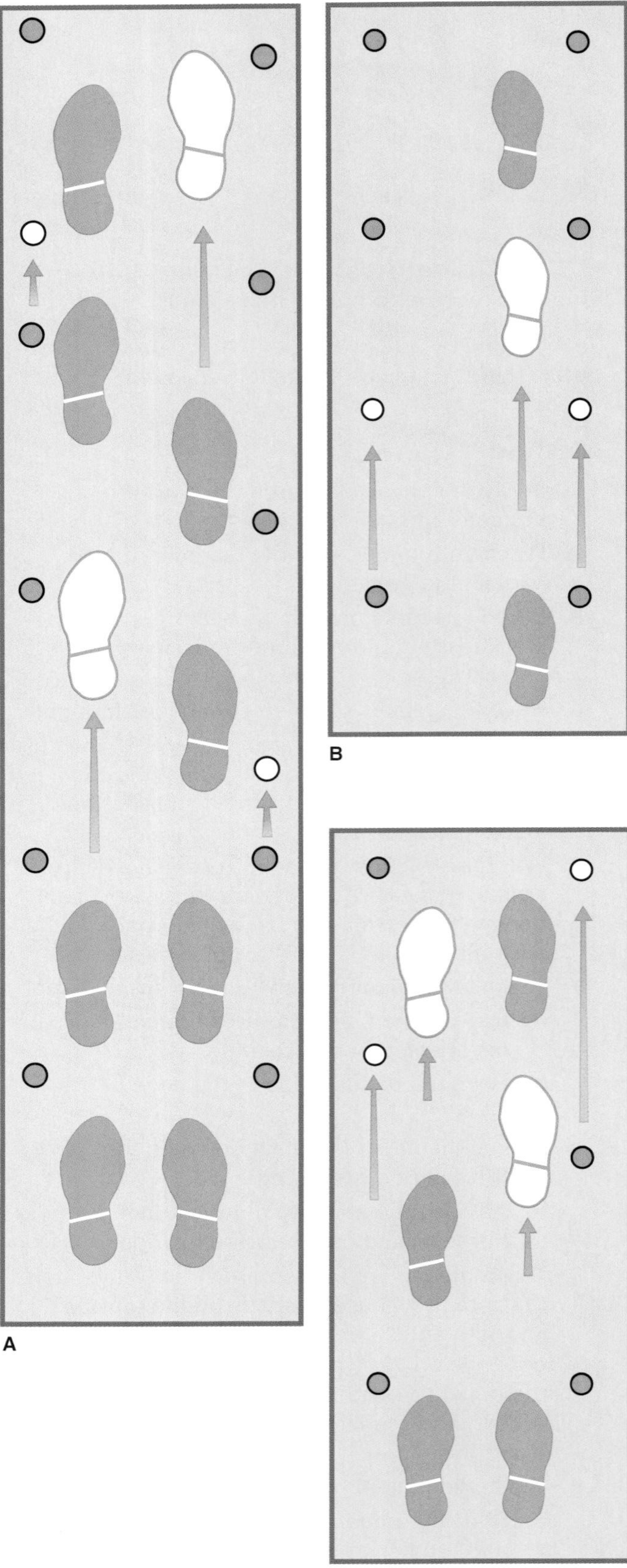

Figure 25-9. Crutch gaits include (a) four-point gait, (b) three-point gait, and (c) two-point gait.

tripod position. Then outline the following steps, as illustrated in Figure 25-9c.

1. Move the left crutch and the right foot forward at the same time.
2. Move the right crutch and the left foot forward at the same time.

Swing Gaits. Patients with severe disabilities, such as leg paralysis or deformity, may use one of two swing gaits: the swing-to gait or the swing-through gait (Figure 25-10a and b). To teach the swing-to gait, have the patient start in the tripod position. Then outline the following steps.

1. Move both crutches forward at the same time.
2. Lift the body and swing to the crutches.
3. End with the tripod position again.

To teach the swing-through gait, have the patient start in the tripod position. Then go over the following steps.

1. Move both crutches forward.
2. Move the body and swing past the crutches.

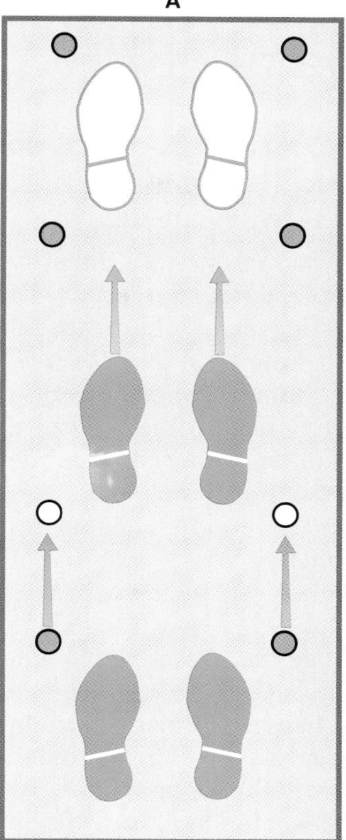

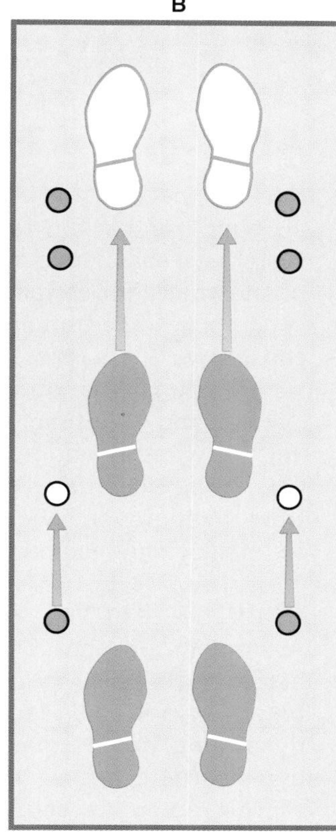

Figure 25-10. Patients with severe disabilities may walk with crutches using (a) the swing-to gait or (b) the swing-through gait.

Wheelchairs

Wheelchairs range from small, folding models to large, motorized ones. Depending on the patient's disability and the length of time the wheelchair will be needed, the physical therapist will select an appropriate wheelchair.

When patients come to the medical office in a wheelchair, the doctor may not be able to examine them adequately if they remain in their wheelchair. If this is the case, you will be responsible for transferring the patients from the wheelchair to the examining table and back to the wheelchair after the examination. To ensure their safety and yours, follow the steps in Procedure 20-3 in Chapter 20. Here are some reminders on preventing injury.

- Ask for help if the patient is weak, heavy, or unstable.
- Explain to the patient the steps of transfer you will use.
- Before starting the transfer, make sure that the wheelchair is in the locked position and that the patient is sitting at the front of the wheelchair seat.
- When you lift, use the large muscles in your thighs, which are stronger than your back muscles.
- When lifting, bend from the knees and keep your back straight.
- Count to 3 and enlist the patient's help on the count of 3.

Educating the Patient

Alternative Therapies

Some patients will choose to consult alternative practitioners for pain relief, for help with chronic problems, and for improvement of overall health. If a patient shows interest in an alternative therapy, encourage the patient to view it as a complementary therapy to the doctor's primary medical treatment. Be aware that some doctors consider alternative therapies incompatible with conventional medicine.

Acupuncture

Acupuncture originated in China more than 5000 years ago, but it was not introduced in the United States until the early 1970s. Acupuncture is a system of healing that uses special needles inserted into points on the body to alleviate pain, to increase energy and balance, and to treat diseases of the heart,

Educating the Patient

Alternative Therapies *(continued)*

muscles, nerves, and eyes. Many people believe that acupuncture can aid the digestive and reproductive systems, treat chemical addictions, and take the place of anesthesia for certain surgical procedures.

Inform patients considering acupuncture that licensing varies from state to state. Some states have no licensing, while others stipulate that only medical doctors and chiropractors may practice acupuncture. You will want to caution patients considering acupuncture to be sure that the practitioner has graduated from an approved school and, if required, has passed a state licensing examination.

Aromatherapy

Aromatherapy uses essential oils from plants and herbs, such as peppermint, eucalyptus, chamomile, rosemary, and lavender. It is used to relieve pain, to induce sleep, and to treat stress, skin conditions, digestive disorders, and a variety of other conditions.

Aromatherapy actually is not limited to aroma, because many of the oils are readily absorbed through the skin. You will want to caution patients considering aromatherapy that some practitioners recommend internal application of the oils. This practice is not sanctioned in the United States. In general, medical doctors have not incorporated aromatherapy into their treatments.

Biofeedback Training

Biofeedback training uses simple electronic devices that measure selected changes in the body, such as muscle activity, brain wave activity, and cardiovascular activity. A trained expert views a readout of the patient's responses during relaxation and during stress. The readout is a scan of electronic information on paper.

Biofeedback training teaches the patient to control breathing, heart rate, and blood pressure. The purpose of the training is to improve the patient's responses to stress or pain and to alleviate other problems, such as muscular dysfunctions, back pain, sleep disorders, hyperactivity, gastrointestinal disorders, headaches, and fatigue. Counsel the patient who is considering biofeedback to find a practitioner who is certified.

Bodywork

Bodywork includes massage, deep-tissue manipulation, movement therapies, shiatsu, acupressure, and reflexology. All forms of bodywork aim to improve the body's structure and function. Patients often seek bodywork to help soothe injured muscles and joints, reduce pain, stimulate circulation, and promote relaxation.

Chiropractic

Chiropractic is a holistic approach to health that treats disease by manipulating the spinal column. The philosophy of chiropractic is that the nervous system can help the body heal itself. Some patients seek out chiropractors for relief of musculoskeletal problems, including misalignment of the spine. Inform patients that chiropractic is becoming increasingly accepted in the medical community and that more chiropractors are on staff at hospitals and becoming involved in sports medicine than there were in the past. You will also want to tell patients, however, that some physicians do not agree with the philosophy of chiropractic for treatment of musculoskeletal conditions.

Craniosacral Therapy

In craniosacral therapy, the bones of the skull are manipulated through rhythmic motions that shift the pressure of the cerebrospinal fluid. Craniosacral therapy is used to treat headaches and ear infections as well as more serious conditions, such as stroke, spinal cord injury, and cerebral palsy.

Homeopathy

Homeopathy uses natural substances from plants, minerals, and animals to stimulate the body's physical healing. Homeopathic remedies are based on the principle that "like cures like," which means that the same substance that in large doses causes an illness, in minute doses cures it. Because these substances are often greatly diluted, many people consider homeopathy to be a safe, nontoxic form of medicine. The Food and Drug Administration recognizes homeopathic substances and regulates their production and dispensation to the public.

Naturopathy

Naturopathy treats conditions by using the body's natural mechanisms of healing. Diet, herbs, and preventive techniques are its hallmarks. Naturopathy advocates changing one's lifestyle, reducing stress, participating in regular exercise, and consuming a high-fiber diet.

Referral to a Physical Therapist

If the doctor refers the patient to a physical therapist or other specialist, you may be asked to contact the specialist directly or to give the patient a written order and information about contacting the specialist. Keep a file with information about the therapists that your office uses. In the file, note the forms and information each therapist requires. If you speak to the therapist, be sure to inform the doctor and to document the referral in the patient's chart. The therapist may be an independent practitioner or may be employed by a hospital, clinic, or home health-care agency.

In addition to physical therapy, some patients may decide to try alternative therapies, such as acupuncture, chiropractic, or biofeedback training. Although some doctors believe that alternative therapies provide some benefits, such as pain relief, many doctors do not. See the Educating the Patient section for information on a variety of alternative therapies.

Summary

Physical therapy is a medical specialty that helps patients who have musculoskeletal and neurological disorders. It produces therapeutic effects through physical and mechanical processes, patient education, and rehabilitation programs.

Before prescribing physical therapy, the physician must assess a patient's joint mobility, muscle strength, gait, and posture. Depending on the patient's needs, the physician may decide to include cryotherapy, thermotherapy, or hydrotherapy in the physical therapy program. The physician or physical therapist may also recommend exercise therapy, massage, or traction. If the patient has difficulty with ambulation, the physical therapist may indicate a mobility aid such as a cane, a walker, crutches, or a wheelchair.

As a medical assistant, you may be asked to help a patient with cryotherapy or thermotherapy, range-of-motion (ROM) exercises, hydrotherapy, and other treatments. You may also need to teach a patient how to use mobility aids. Working directly with patients to help alleviate their pain and improve their mobility will reward you with immediate and long-term satisfaction.

REVIEW

CHAPTER 25

CASE STUDY QUESTIONS

Now that you have completed this chapter, review the case study at the beginning of the chapter and answer the following questions:

1. What type of teaching do you think this patient will need?
2. What type of therapy may be necessary for the crusted bloody injury on his forearm, and how would you perform it?

Discussion Questions

1. Identify three conditions that can be treated with cryotherapy, and give two examples of dry cold applications and two examples of wet cold applications.
2. Identify three conditions that can be treated with thermotherapy. Give two examples of dry heat applications and two examples of moist heat applications.
3. Explain how to teach a patient the four-point, three-point, and two-point crutch gaits.

Critical Thinking Questions

1. Your patient's physical therapist has prescribed hydrotherapy three times a week. Although the patient can drive, he tells you that he cannot keep his appointments because his wife has Alzheimer's disease and should not be left alone. How could you help solve this problem?
2. When teaching patients how to use a walker, what changes to their home environment would you suggest to ensure their safety?
3. Describe how you can improve your skills in applying physical therapy and how you can keep informed about new therapies and techniques.
4. A 76-year-old man arrives at the clinic using a walker. As he enters the examination room, you notice that he is pushing the walker and not lifting it. What should you do?
5. The physician asks you to teach a client how to perform upper body ROM exercises. What teaching techniques would you use?

Application Activities

1. With a partner, prepare and apply one type of cryotherapy and one type of thermotherapy to each other. Check the treatments after 5, 10, and 20 minutes. Evaluate the skin, and report how it looks and feels. Evaluate your partner's technique.
2. Teach a classmate how to use a cane to walk up and down stairs. Ask the classmate to critique your instructions. Exchange roles and critique your classmate's instructions.
3. Measure crutches for three different classmates. Teach each one a different gait. Then have a classmate measure crutches for you and teach you a gait.

Internet Activity

1. Take a virtual field trip to the National Library of Medicine's reference Web site at **www.nlm.nih.gov/medlineplus/** and complete the following activities:
   a. Go the topic page titled Rehabilitation and find out more about art therapy or some other specialized therapy.
   b. Search for information about a specific injury of a part of the body such as the wrist, arm, elbow, knee, or back. Find out the common treatment and latest research regarding the type of injury you choose.

CHAPTER 26

Medical Emergencies and First Aid

AREAS OF COMPETENCE

2003 Role Delineation Study

CLINICAL

Patient Care

- Adhere to established patient screening procedures
- Obtain patient history and vital signs
- Recognize and respond to emergencies

GENERAL

Professionalism

- Prioritize and perform multiple tasks

Instruction

- Locate community resources and disseminate information

CHAPTER OUTLINE

- Understanding Medical Emergencies
- Preparing for Medical Emergencies
- Accidental Injuries
- Common Illnesses
- Less Common Illnesses
- Common Psychosocial Emergencies
- The Patient Under Stress
- Educating the Patient
- Disasters
- Bioterrorism

OBJECTIVES

After completing Chapter 26, you will be able to:

26.1 Discuss the importance of first aid during a medical emergency.
26.2 Describe the purpose of the emergency medical services (EMS) system and explain how to contact it.
26.3 List items found on a crash cart or first-aid tray.
26.4 List general guidelines to follow in emergencies.
26.5 Compare various degrees of burns and their treatments.
26.6 Demonstrate how to help a choking victim.
26.7 Demonstrate cardiopulmonary resuscitation (CPR).
26.8 Demonstrate four ways to control bleeding.

KEY TERMS

automated external defibrillator (AED)
bioterrorism
cast
chain of custody
concussion
contusion
crash cart
dehydration
dislocation
epistaxis
hematemesis
hematoma
hyperglycemia
hypoglycemia
hypovolemic shock
palpitations
recovery position
septic shock
splint
sprain
strain
stroke
tachycardia
ventricular fibrillation
xiphoid process

OBJECTIVES *(Continued)*

26.9 List the symptoms of heart attack, shock, and stroke.

26.10 Explain how to calm a patient who is under extreme stress.

26.11 Describe your role in responding to natural disasters and those caused by humans.

Introduction

Emergencies of all types can occur when you are working as a medical assistant. Patients may come to your facility with an acute illness or an injury. You may have to handle a phone call from a patient who has an urgent physical or psychological problem. Additionally, you could experience a disaster—anything from a simple office fire to a bomb threat or bioterrorism. As a medical assistant you must be prepared to determine the urgency and handle any emergency that arises. Remember to stay calm and think through each situation in order to respond appropriately and create the best outcome.

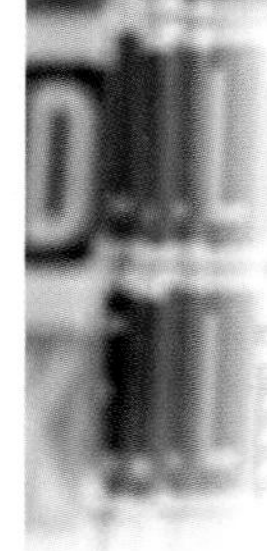

CASE STUDY

While you are working as a medical assistant in a busy office practice, the following three things occur at the same time:

1. You have a telephone call waiting for you; a woman wants to speak to you regarding her 4-year-old daughter. According to the administrative assistant, who took the call, the daughter has a fever of 103°F, and the mother wants to know how much acetaminophen or aspirin she can give her.
2. A 56-year-old male in room 2 comes out of the room to tell you that his chest is hurting and he is having difficulty breathing.
3. Three patients are waiting to be seen, and you have only the patient in room 2 ready for the physician. The other two examination rooms are empty.

As you read this chapter, consider each situation and determine the order in which you will respond. Explain your decisions.

Understanding Medical Emergencies

A medical emergency is any situation in which a person suddenly becomes ill or sustains an injury that requires immediate help by a health-care professional. Your prompt action in a medical emergency could prevent permanent disability or even death.

You may see life-threatening medical emergencies in the health-care setting. For example, a patient in the waiting room may have chest pains that could indicate a heart attack is imminent. You may see emergencies that are not life-threatening, such as a coworker sustaining a minor injury on the job. You may also encounter emergencies outside the office. For example, a family member might cut a finger while using a kitchen knife, or a patron in a restaurant might choke on a piece of food. Your quick response is vital in all of these situations.

In or out of the office, a medical emergency may require you to perform first aid. First aid is the immediate care given to someone who is injured or suddenly becomes ill, before complete medical care can be obtained. Prompt and appropriate first aid can:

- Save a life
- Reduce pain
- Prevent further injury
- Reduce the risk of permanent disability
- Increase the chance of early recovery

Because most emergencies do not occur in a medical office, your role in patient education is critical. The more you teach patients about first aid and the proper way to respond to emergencies, the better equipped they will be to handle accidental injuries and illnesses.

Preparing for Medical Emergencies

How well prepared you are for an emergency can mean the difference between life and death for a patient. You must be able to perform procedures quickly and correctly. Keeping your skills up-to-date will enable you to handle medical emergencies effectively.

Just as important is your ability to ensure that the medical office where you work is ready to handle whatever emergencies arise. This preparedness will depend on your own organizational skills and knowledge of community resources.

Preparing the Office

You must first establish with the doctor which duties are expected of you and of other office personnel in case of an emergency and determine what resources are available. One of your most important allies will be the local emergency medical services (EMS) system. An EMS system is a network of qualified emergency services personnel who use community resources and equipment to provide emergency care to victims of injury or sudden illness.

Posting Emergency Telephone Numbers. Although the telephone number for the local EMS system is 911 in many parts of the country, some areas may not have 911 service. Post the area's EMS system telephone number at every telephone and on the **crash cart** (the rolling cart of emergency supplies and equipment) or first-aid tray. Every office employee should know this number. If the community has no EMS system, post the telephone number of the local ambulance or rescue squad. You should also post the telephone numbers of the nearest fire company, police station, poison control center, women's shelter, rape hotline, and drug and alcohol center.

When you call the EMS system for medical assistance and transport, speak clearly and calmly to the dispatcher. Be prepared to provide the following information:

- Your name, telephone number, and location
- Nature of the emergency
- Number of people in need of help
- Condition of the injured or ill patient(s)
- Summary of the first aid that has been given
- Directions on how to reach the location of the emergency

Do not hang up until the dispatcher gives you permission to do so.

Common Emergency and First-Aid Supplies. The crash cart or tray contains basic drugs, supplies, and equipment for medical emergencies. Most crash carts also contain a first-aid kit with supplies for managing minor injuries and ailments. Figure 26-1 lists the usual items in a first-aid kit. The actual contents of the crash cart or tray may vary slightly from practice to practice. Become familiar with these contents and know where they are located in the office. Procedure 26-1 describes how to check and restock the essential items on a crash cart.

Contents of a First-Aid Kit

- Absorbent cotton (sterile)
- Adhesive dressings in various sizes
- Adhesive tape
- Airway or mouthpiece
- Analgesics, such as aspirin or acetaminophen
- Antiseptic solution
- Antiseptic wipes
- Calamine lotion
- Chemical hot and cold packs
- Diphenhydramine (Benadryl™)
- Disposable gloves
- Elastic bandages in various sizes
- First-aid book
- Liquid form glucose tablets
- Personal protective equipment: gloves, mask and goggles or face shield, gown, shower cap, booties, pocket mask or mouth shield
- Scissors
- Splints in various sizes
- Sterile gauze pads in various sizes
- Sterile rolls of gauze
- Sugar packets
- Triangular bandage
- Tweezers
- Waterproof flashlight with extra batteries

Figure 26-1. These supplies are often included in a first-aid kit.

Guidelines for Handling Emergencies

A medical emergency requires you to take certain steps. You are not responsible for diagnosing or providing medical care other than first aid. You are expected, however, to note the presence of serious conditions that threaten the patient's life. Then take appropriate action, but perform only those procedures that you have been trained to perform.

Patient Emergencies. Assess the situation and surroundings to determine whether it is safe for you to assist. If safe, put on the appropriate personal protective equipment (PPE), such as gloves. Next, do an initial assessment to detect and immediately correct any life-threatening problems of the airway, breathing, and circulation. Corrections of life-threatening problems are essential to survival. There are six steps in the initial assessment: (1) form a general impression of the patient, (2) determine the patient's level of responsiveness, (3) assess the airway, breathing, and circulation status of the patient, sometimes referred to as the ABCs, (4) determine the priority or urgency of the patient's condition, (5) conduct a focused exam, and (6) document a history. Procedure 26-2 provides guidelines for performing these six steps.

PROCEDURE 26.1

Stocking the Crash Cart

Objective: To ensure that the crash cart includes all appropriate drugs, supplies, and equipment needed for emergencies

OSHA Guidelines: This procedure does not involve exposure to blood, body fluids, or tissues.

Materials: Protocol for or list of crash cart items, crash cart

Method

1. Review the office protocol for or list of items that should be on the crash cart.
2. Verify each drug on the crash cart, and check the amount against the office protocol or list. Restock those that were used, and replace those that have passed their expiration date. Some typical crash cart drugs are listed here:
   - Activated charcoal
   - Atropine
   - Dextrose 50%
   - Diazepam (Valium)
   - Digoxin (Lanoxin)
   - Diphenhydramine hydrochloride (Benadryl)
   - Epinephrine, injectable
   - Furosemide (Lasix)
   - Glucagon
   - Glucose paste or tablets
   - Insulin (regular or a variety)
   - Intravenous dextrose in saline and intravenous dextrose in water
   - Isoproterenol hydrochloride (Isuprel), aerosol inhaler and injectable
   - Lactated Ringer's solution
   - Lidocaine (Xylocaine), injectable
   - Methylprednisolone tablets
   - Nitroglycerin tablets
   - Phenobarbital, injectable
   - Phenytoin (Dilantin)
   - Saline solution, isotonic (0.9%)
   - Sodium bicarbonate, injectable
   - Sterile water for injection
3. Check the supplies on the crash cart against the list. Restock items that were used, and make sure the packaging of supplies on the cart has not been opened. Some typical crash cart supplies are listed here:
   - Adhesive tape
   - Constricting band or tourniquet
   - Dressing supplies (alcohol wipes, rolls of gauze, bandage strips, bandage scissors)
   - Intravenous tubing, venipuncture devices, and butterfly needles
   - Personal protective equipment
   - Syringes and needles in various sizes
4. Check the equipment on the crash cart against the list, and examine it to make sure that it is in working order. Restock equipment that is missing or broken. Some typical crash cart equipment is listed here:
   - Airways in assorted sizes
   - Ambu-bag, a trademark for a breathing bag used to assist respiratory ventilation
   - Defibrillator (electrical device that shocks the heart to restore normal beating)
   - Endotracheal tubes in various sizes
   - Oxygen tank with oxygen mask and cannula
5. Check miscellaneous items on the crash cart against the list, and restock as needed. Some typical miscellaneous crash cart items are listed here:
   - Orange juice
   - Sugar packets

Telephone Emergencies. Sometimes a patient or a patient's family member calls the medical office with an emergency. If you are responsible for handling telephone calls, be prepared to triage the injuries by telephone. Triaging is the classification of injuries according to severity, urgency of treatment, and place for treatment.

To handle emergency calls, follow the practice's telephone triage protocols. For example, if a parent calls to say her daughter has broken her arm and the child's bone is visible, tell her to call the local EMS system for immediate care and transport to the hospital. If, however, a parent calls to say her son swallowed half a bottle of baby bath, tell her to remain calm and give her the telephone number of the poison control center. Depending on circumstances, you may offer to make the necessary telephone call yourself.

PROCEDURE 26.2

Performing an Emergency Assessment

Objective: To assess a medical emergency quickly and accurately

OSHA Guidelines

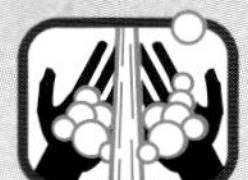 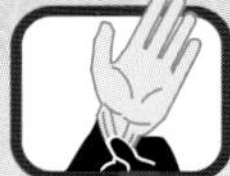 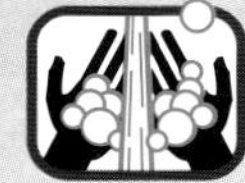

Materials: Patient's chart, pen, gloves

Method

1. Put on gloves.
2. Form a general impression of the patient, including his level of responsiveness, level of distress, facial expressions, age, ability to talk, and skin color.
3. If the patient can communicate clearly, ask what happened. If not, ask someone who observed the accident or injury.
4. Assess an unresponsive patient by tapping on his shoulder and asking, "Are you OK?" If there is no response, proceed to the next step.
5. Assess the patient's airway. If necessary, open the airway by using the head tilt–chin lift maneuver. If you suspect a neck injury, use the jaw thrust maneuver.
6. Assess the patient's breathing. If the patient is not breathing, then perform rescue breathing.
7. Assess the patient's circulation. Determine if the patient has a pulse. Is there any serious external bleeding? Perform CPR as needed (Procedure 26-8). Control any significant bleeding (Procedure 26-5).
8. If all life-threatening problems have been identified and treated, perform a focused exam. Start at the head and perform the following steps rapidly, taking about 90 seconds.
   a. Head: Check for deformities, bruises, open wounds, tenderness, depressions, and swelling. Check the ears, nose, and mouth for fluid, blood, or foreign bodies.
   b. Eyes: Open the eyes and compare the pupils. They should be the same size.
   c. Neck: Look and feel for deformities, bruises, depressions, open wounds, tenderness, and swelling. Check for a medical alert bracelet.
   d Chest: Look and feel for deformities, bruises, open wounds, tenderness, depressions, and swelling.
   e Abdomen: Look and feel for deformities, bruises, open wounds, tenderness, depressions, and swelling.
   f. Pelvis: Look and feel for deformities, bruises, open wounds, tenderness, depressions, and swelling.
   g Arms: Look and feel for deformities, bruises, open wounds, depressions, tenderness, and swelling. Compare the arms for any differences in size, color, or temperature.
   h Legs: Look and feel for deformities, bruises, open wounds, depressions, tenderness, and swelling. Compare the legs for any differences in size, color, or temperature.
   i. Back: Look and feel for deformities, bruises, open wounds, depressions, tenderness, and swelling.
9. Check vital signs and observe the patient for pallor (paleness) or cyanosis (a bluish tint). If the patient is dark-skinned, observe for pallor or cyanosis on the inside of the lips and mouth.
10. Document your findings and report them to the doctor or emergency medical technician (EMT).
11. Assist the doctor or EMT as requested.
12. Remove your gloves and wash your hands.

Adhere to the following general guidelines in any emergency situation.

- Stay calm
- Reassure the patient
- Act in a confident, organized manner

Personal Protection. Whenever you administer first aid and emergency treatment, try to reduce or eliminate the risk of exposing yourself and others to infection. Follow Standard Precautions and assume that all blood and body fluids are infected with blood-borne pathogens. To protect yourself and others, take the following basic precautions. Include PPE in your first-aid kit at work and at home. Standard PPE includes gloves, goggles and mask or face shield, gown, cap, and booties. A pocket mask or mouth shield provides personal protection when you perform rescue breathing. Plan to use specific PPE based on the condition of the patient. Table 26-1 provides examples of PPE to use in various

TABLE 26-1 Personal Protective Equipment for Emergencies

Equipment	Conditions for Use	Sample Emergencies Requiring Equipment
Gloves	Chance of contact with blood or other body secretion or excretion during emergency	Open wound, eye trauma
Goggles and mask or face shield and possibly shower cap	Chance of blood or other body secretion or excretion being splattered, coughed, or sprayed onto the mucus membranes of the eyes, mouth, or nose	Bleeding, vomiting, most emergency care for small children (because of squirming)
Gown and possibly booties	Chance of contact with excessive bleeding or secretion and excretion	Childbirth, severe nosebleed
Pocket mask or mouth shield	Needed for CPR or rescue breathing	Heart attack, respiratory arrest

emergency situations. When in doubt, wear more PPE than you may think is called for.

Wear gloves if you expect hand contact with blood, body fluids, mucous membranes, torn skin, or potentially contaminated articles or surfaces. In addition, if you have any cuts or lesions, wear PPE over the affected area.

Minimize splashing, splattering, or spraying of blood or other body fluids when performing first aid. If blood or other body fluids splash into your eyes, nose, or mouth, flush the area with water as soon as possible.

Wash your hands thoroughly with soap and water after removing the gloves. Also wash other skin surfaces that have come in contact with blood or other body fluids. Do not touch your mouth, nose, or eyes, and do not eat or drink after providing emergency care until you have washed your hands thoroughly. If you have been exposed to blood or other body fluids, be sure to tell the doctor. You may need postexposure treatment.

Documentation. Document all office emergencies in the patient's chart. Be sure to include your assessment, treatment given, and the patient's response. If the patient was transported to another facility, record the location. Include the date and time with the documentation, as well as your signature and credentials.

Accidental Injuries

No matter where you encounter an emergency, your knowledge and certifications should enable you to provide first aid for the patient until a physician or EMT arrives. To help you become familiar with how to handle various emergency situations, the following sections present accidental injuries, common illnesses, and less common illnesses.

Accidental injuries that may call for emergency medical intervention include the following:

- Bites and stings
- Burns
- Choking
- Ear trauma
- Eye trauma
- Falls
- Fractures, dislocations, sprains, and strains
- Head injuries
- Hemorrhaging
- Multiple injuries
- Poisoning
- Weather-related injuries
- Wounds

Bites and Stings

Dog and cat bites and bee, wasp, and hornet stings are fairly common. Less common are snakebites and spider bites, which you are more likely to encounter in certain parts of the country, such as Florida or the Southwest, than in other areas.

Animal Bites. An animal bite may bruise the skin, tear it, or leave a puncture wound. A wound that tears the skin should be seen by a doctor and may need to be reported to the police, animal control officer, and local health department. If the animal can be found, it should be checked for rabies. Then, depending on the animal's rabies vaccination status, the animal may need to be quarantined. If the animal is a probable carrier of rabies and cannot be found, the doctor may administer antirabies serum to the patient as a precaution.

Dogs, cats, skunks, squirrels, raccoons, bats, and foxes are more likely to carry rabies than are other animals. Hamsters, gerbils, guinea pigs, and mice are rarely infected by the rabies virus.

Human bites can raise concerns about transmitting the human immunodeficiency virus (HIV) or hepatitis B virus. HIV can be transmitted only if the bite breaks the skin and if the biter has bleeding gums. Hepatitis B virus may be transmitted by a human bite that punctures the skin. In this case a series of three injections is required to immunize against hepatitis B.

Immediate care for bites calls for washing the area thoroughly with antiseptic soap and water. (If the bite caused a puncture wound, try to make it bleed to flush out bacteria. Then wash the area with soap and water.) Apply an antibiotic ointment and a dry, sterile dressing. The doctor will administer tetanus toxoid if the patient has not received it in the last 7 to 10 years.

Insect Stings. Insect stings are merely a nuisance to most patients. The site of the sting can become red, swollen, itchy, and painful. If the patient was stung by a honeybee, you must first remove the stinger, because it still has the ability to release venom. Remove the stinger by scraping the skin with a credit card or other flat, hard, sharp object. Be careful not to release more venom. Avoid using your fingers or tweezers, because squeezing the stinger may force more venom into the wound. (If you cannot remove the stinger, call the physician.) Wash the skin with soap and water. Apply ice to the site after the stinger is removed to reduce the pain and swelling. Later apply a paste of baking soda or a dressing soaked in aloe vera juice or vinegar to reduce discomfort and itching.

A sting can be deadly to a patient who is allergic to the insect venom, because anaphylaxis can develop. The symptoms of and treatment for anaphylaxis are described later in this chapter.

Snakebites. Poisonous snakes in the United States include rattlesnakes, water moccasins (or cottonmouths), copperheads, and coral snakes. Because snakes are cold-blooded, they often lie on rocks to warm themselves. Most bites occur when a person steps onto, sits down on, or reaches over or between rocks where a snake is sunning itself.

The bites of most poisonous snakes produce similar symptoms: one or two puncture marks, pain, and swelling at the site; rapid pulse; nausea; vomiting; and perhaps unconsciousness and seizures. If possible, get a description of the snake so the EMS team or the hospital can procure the proper antivenin (a substance that counteracts the snake poison) ahead of time. Snakebites are dangerous, but with proper intervention, they rarely lead to death.

If a patient has been bitten by a snake that may be poisonous, call a doctor or the EMS system. If the patient must walk, have him walk slowly to prevent dispersion of the poison through the circulation. To care for a poisonous snakebite while you await help, wash the area gently with soap and water. Then apply a clean or sterile dressing. If possible, immobilize the injured part, and position it below heart level. Do not apply ice or a tourniquet, and do not cut or suction the wound.

Spider Bites. Only two types of spiders in the United States are a serious threat to health: the black widow spider, which has a red hourglass mark on its abdomen, and the brown recluse spider, which has a violin-shaped mark on its back. The black widow bite causes swelling and pain at the site as well as nausea, vomiting, rigid abdomen, fever, rash, and difficulty breathing or swallowing. The brown recluse bite causes severe swelling and tenderness and, eventually, ulceration along the nerve closest to the location of the bite.

You are not expected to classify spiders and their bites accurately. Therefore, any patient bitten by a spider must be seen by a physician. To care for a patient with a spider bite, wash the area thoroughly with soap and water. Apply an ice pack to the area to reduce swelling and pain. If possible, keep the area below heart level to prevent the poison from spreading. Healing of the bite can sometimes take several months.

Burns

Burns involve tissue injury that occurs from heat, chemicals, electricity, or radiation. Be sure that you teach patients about emergency treatment for burns as well as any follow-up care prescribed by the physician.

Types of Burns

Thermal Burns. Thermal burns may be caused by contact with hot liquids, steam, flames, radiation, and excessive heat from fires or hot objects. Call the EMS team immediately for victims of such burns. To stop the burning process, use water to cool a burning substance, or use a wet cloth or blanket to put out the fire.

Chemical Burns. Chemical burns are more likely to affect workers at chemical or industrial facilities than individuals in the home. To treat this type of burn, flood the area with large amounts of water and then cover it with a dry dressing. Call the EMS team to transport the patient to the hospital.

Electrical Burns. Electrical burns are injuries from exposure to electrical currents, including lightning. These burns occur at the site where the electricity enters the body and where the current exits the body and enters the ground. Along the current's pathway, extensive tissue damage can occur from heat followed by chemical changes to nerve, muscle, and heart tissue. Call the EMS team immediately for these types of injuries.

Classifications of Burns. The severity of a burn is determined by the depth and extent of the burn area, the source of the burn, the age of the patient, body regions burned, and other patient illnesses and injuries. When classifying burns, use the categories *minor, moderate,* and *major.* These categories take into account all the factors that determine severity. For example, a burn might be considered minor although it damages all skin layers if it affects only a small area of one leg on an otherwise healthy person. A major burn includes any burn in children younger than age 2, electrical burns, burns complicated by fractures or serious trauma, and burns on the hands, face, feet, or perineum.

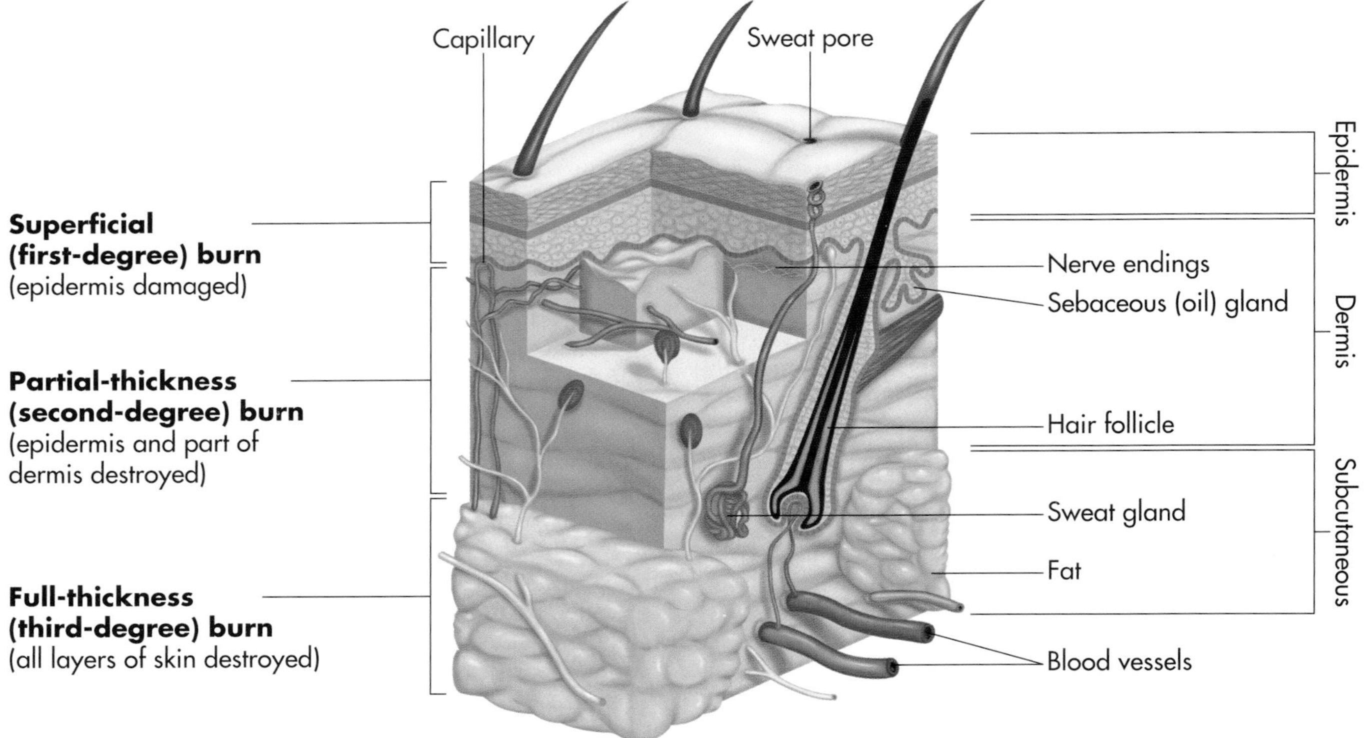

Figure 26-2. The depth of skin damage is one factor used to determine the severity of burns.

Burns classified according to the depth of skin damage are called superficial, partial thickness, and full thickness (Figure 26-2). In a superficial burn, formally called a first-degree burn, the epidermis is damaged and the skin is reddened. Blisters result from a second-degree burn, in which part of the dermis is destroyed. A third-degree burn damages all the skin layers.

Superficial (First-Degree) Burns. A superficial burn causes pain and makes the surrounding skin turn red. It is equivalent to a sunburn. Treat first-degree burns by applying cold-water dressings or by immersing the affected area in cold water. Gently pat the area dry, and apply a dry, sterile dressing. Do not use greasy ointments, butter, or other substances because they prevent oxygen from reaching the wound and will have to be scrubbed off before any treatment can be administered. Scrubbing would be very painful.

Partial-Thickness (Second-Degree) Burns. Partial thickness burns extend deeper into the skin than first-degree burns. They cause blistering along with pain and redness. Immerse second-degree burns in cold water until the pain subsides. Then gently pat the area dry, taking care not to break blisters, and apply a dry, sterile dressing. Do not apply antiseptic ointment unless the doctor orders it. If the arms or legs are affected, elevate them to reduce swelling.

Full-Thickness (Third-Degree) Burns. Full thickness burns, such as those received in a fire, involve all layers of skin and demand immediate emergency medical assistance. While you wait for the EMS team, do not remove charred or adhered clothing from the patient. Cover the burns and adhered clothing with thick, sterile dressings. If the hands, arms, or legs are burned, elevate them above the heart. Keep the patient warm and provide reassurance. Check to see whether the patient is suffering from smoke inhalation. Signs of smoke inhalation include difficulty breathing (often accompanied by coughing), smoky-smelling breath, or black residue in the patient's mouth and nose. If any of these signs are present, gently move the patient into a sitting position and monitor her breathing. Third-degree burns are usually not painful at first because of nerve damage.

Estimating the Extent of the Burn. Various methods are used to estimate the extent of the burn area (Figure 26-3). To calculate the amount of skin surface burned on an adult, use the rule of nines. This rule assigns each of the following areas 9% of the body surface: the head and neck, each upper limb, the chest, the abdomen, the upper back, the lower back and buttocks, the front of each lower limb, and the back of each lower limb. These areas make up 99% of the body's surface. The genital region is the remaining 1%. The figures to use when making calculations in children and infants are shown in Figure 26-3.

Choking

Choking occurs when food or a foreign object blocks a person's trachea, or windpipe. The main symptom of a choking emergency is the inability to speak. A choking person who cannot talk may give the universal sign of choking—a hand up to the throat and a fearful look. If you see someone giving the universal sign, be prepared to act promptly.

PROCEDURE 26.3

Foreign Body Airway Obstruction in a Responsive Adult or Child *(continued)*

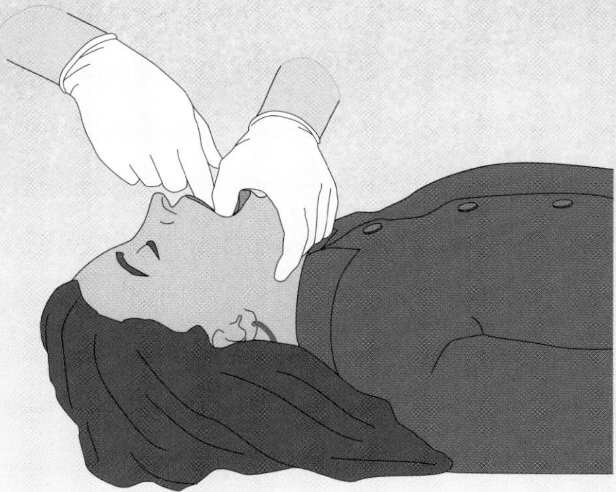

Figure 26-6. Use a finger sweep to remove a foreign object from the mouth. Do not perform a blind finger sweep on children or infants.

9. Kneel by the patient's thighs and place the heel of one hand just above the navel. Place the other hand on top and push into the abdomen, inward and upward. Once again, if the patient is obese or pregnant, position your hands over the breastbone. Perform 15 compressions for an adult and 5 for a child.
10. Return to the head and repeat steps 6 through 9 until the foreign body is removed or until trained personnel arrive to relieve you.
11. If the foreign body is removed, open the airway and check for breathing. If the patient is not breathing, perform two rescue breaths.
12. Check for signs of circulation and start CPR if necessary (Procedure 26-8).

PROCEDURE 26.4

Foreign Body Airway Obstruction in a Responsive Infant

Objective: To correctly relieve a foreign body from the airway of an infant

OSHA Guidelines: This procedure does not involve exposure to blood, body fluids, or tissues.

Materials: Choking infant

Caution: Never perform this procedure on an infant who is not choking.

Method

1. Assess the infant for signs of severe or complete airway obstruction, which include:
   a. Sudden onset of difficulty in breathing.
   b. Inability to speak, make sounds, or cry.
   c. A high-pitched, noisy, wheezing sound, or no sounds while inhaling.
   d. Weak, ineffective coughs.
   e. Blue lips or skin.
2. Hold the infant with his head down, supporting the body with your forearm. His legs should straddle your forearm and you should support his jaw and head with your hand and fingers. This is best done in a sitting or kneeling position (Figure 26-7).
3. Give up to five back blows with the heel of your free hand, as shown in Figure 26-7. Strike the infant's back forcefully between the shoulder blades. At any point, if the object is expelled, discontinue the back blows.
4. If the obstruction is not cleared, turn the infant over as a unit, supporting the head with your hands and the body between your forearms (Figure 26-8).
5. Keep the head lower than the chest and perform five chest thrusts. Place two fingers over the breastbone (sternum), above the xiphoid. Compress the chest upward toward the head. Stop the compressions if the object is expelled.

continued →

PROCEDURE 26.4

Foreign Body Airway Obstruction in a Responsive Infant *(continued)*

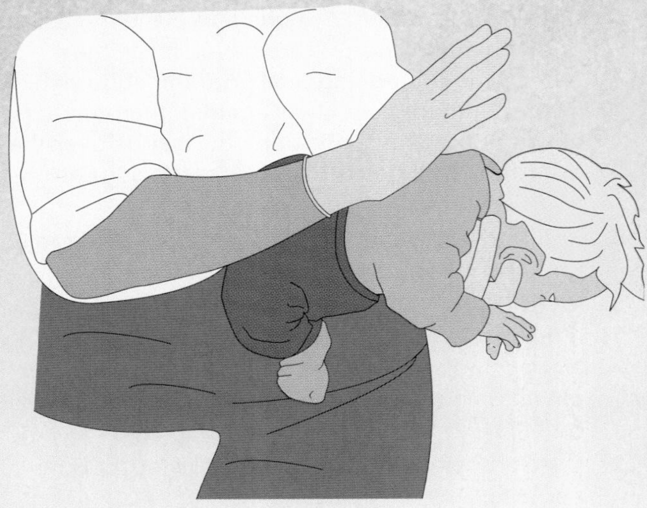

Figure 26.7. Use back blows for a choking infant. *Source: Glencoe Health Care Science Technology,* Booth 2004, p.113, Figure 4-21.

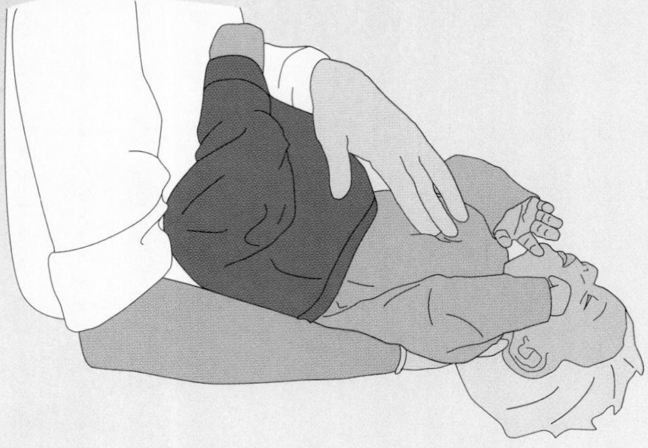

Figure 26.8. Keep the infant head and neck supported.

6. Alternate back blows and chest thrusts until the object is expelled or until the infant becomes unconscious. If the infant becomes unconscious, call EMS or have someone do it for you.
7. Open the infant's mouth by grasping both the tongue and the lower jaw between the thumb and fingers, and pull up the lower jawbone. If you see the object, remove it using your smallest finger. Do not use blind finger sweeps on an infant.
8. Open the airway and attempt to provide rescue breaths. If the chest does not rise, reposition the airway (both head and chin) and try to provide another rescue breath.
9. If the rescue breaths are unsuccessful, give five back blows and five chest thrusts.
10. Repeat steps 7 through 9 until rescue breaths are effective, and then continue CPR as necessary.

to the hospital, and document the fall and injury in the patient's chart.

If the fall results in only a bump, apply ice and observe for bruises and swelling. Give the patient time to collect himself. Be sure to notify the doctor, who should examine the patient. Then document the fall, the injury, and the treatment in the patient's chart.

Falls are not limited to the physician's office, of course. Follow these procedures wherever you encounter someone who has fallen.

Fractures, Dislocations, Sprains, and Strains

A fracture is a break in a bone. Fractures are categorized in several ways (Figure 26-9). Complete fractures go across the entire bone; incomplete fractures go through only part of the bone. Comminuted fractures are those in which the bone has broken into several fragments. In a greenstick fracture, the bone is bent, but only one side is fractured. Greenstick fractures occur most often in children because their bones are still soft and pliable. A fracture is closed if it does not cause a break in the skin. In open fractures, the bone breaks through the skin.

A **dislocation** is the displacement of a bone end from the joint. Both fractures and dislocations usually result from accidents or sports injuries. They can cause pain, tenderness, loss of function, deformity, swelling, and discoloration. The injury is usually diagnosed by x-ray.

Treatment of fractures and dislocations depends on factors such as the nature of the injury and the patient's age and physical condition. The basic emergency steps are:

- Immobilization to reduce pain and continuing damage to soft tissue
- Reduction, or moving the bone back into the proper position, for some fractures

Complete fracture

Incomplete fracture

Closed fracture

Open fracture

Greenstick fracture

Comminuted fracture

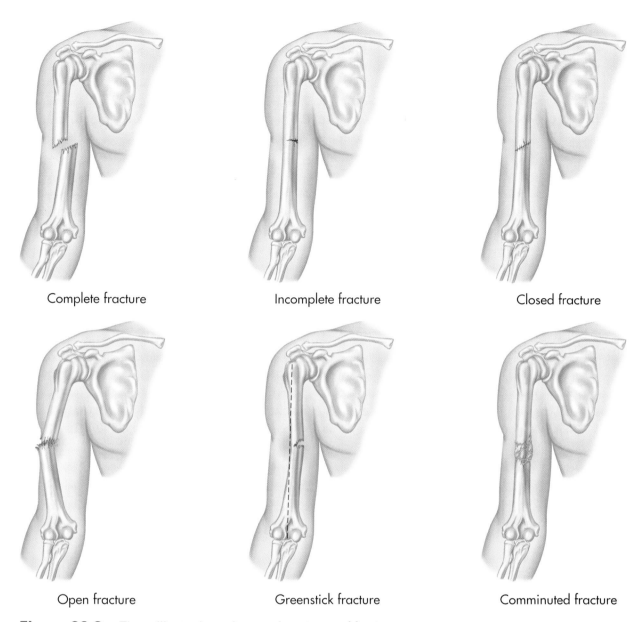

Figure 26-9. These illustrations show various types of fractures.

Immobilization is sometimes provided by the application of a splint or cast. The purpose of both splints and casts is to keep an injured body part in place and protect it as it heals. A **splint** is an appliance used for conditions that do not require rigid immobilization or, as a temporary measure, for those in which swelling is anticipated. A **cast** is a rigid, external dressing, usually made of plaster or fiberglass, that is molded to the contours of the body part to which it is applied. You may assist the physician with the application of a cast (Figure 26-10). You may also educate the patient about these basic elements of cast care.

- Report any of the following to the physician immediately: pain, swelling, discoloration of exposed portions, lack of pulsation and warmth, or the inability to move exposed parts
- Keep the casted extremity elevated for the first day

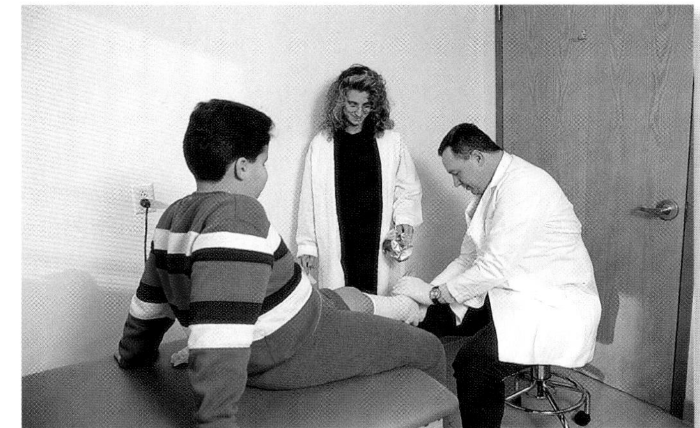

Figure 26-10. Patients should be instructed to keep the cast dry and to notify the physician if they have pain or unusual sensations.

- Avoid indenting the cast until it is completely dry
- Check the movement and sensation of the visible extremities frequently
- Restrict strenuous activities for the first few days
- Avoid allowing the affected limb to hang down for any length of time
- Do not put anything inside the cast
- Keep the cast dry
- Follow the physician's orders regarding restrictions of activities

Sprains and strains often result from sports injuries and accidents. A **sprain** is an injury characterized by partial tearing of a ligament that supports a joint, such as the ankle. A sprain may also involve injuries to tendons, muscles, and local blood vessels and contusions of the surrounding soft tissue. A **strain** is a muscle injury that results from overexertion. For example, back strain may occur when a person carries a heavy load.

Symptoms of a sprain include swelling, tenderness, pain during movement, and local discoloration. If you suspect a sprain, splint the joint, apply ice, and call the EMS system if needed. Inform the patient that an x-ray may be required to confirm that there is no fracture. A strain causes pain on motion. In most cases it should be examined by a physician, who may prescribe rest, application of heat, and a muscle relaxant.

Head Injuries

Head injuries include concussions, contusions, fractures, intracranial bleeding, and scalp hematomas and lacerations. Some head injuries can be life-threatening and require immediate medical attention.

Concussion. A **concussion** is a jarring injury to the brain. It is the most common type of head injury. Someone who has a concussion may lose consciousness. Temporary loss of vision, pallor (paleness), listlessness, memory loss, or vomiting can also occur. Symptoms may disappear rapidly or last up to 24 hours. A concussion may produce slow intracranial bleeding. Teach the patient and the patient's family basic precautions after this type of injury. See the Educating the Patient section for more information on concussions.

Severe Head Injuries. Contusions, fractures, and intracranial bleeding cause symptoms similar to, but more profound than, symptoms of concussions. Symptoms to look for are leakage of clear or bloody fluid from the ears or nose, seizures, and respiratory arrest. A patient with a severe head injury requires immediate hospitalization. Your priority is to maintain the patient's airway and to begin rescue breathing or CPR if needed.

Scalp Hematomas and Lacerations. A **hematoma** is a swelling caused by blood under the skin. A scalp hematoma causes a bump on the head. This swelling can

Educating the Patient

Concussion

Because a concussion can cause intracranial bleeding, handle gently a patient who is being treated for this type of injury. If bleeding is slow, it might take up to 24 hours to produce symptoms. Because intracranial bleeding may require brain surgery, use the following patient education guidelines to help ensure patient safety after a concussion.

- Inform the patient that the first 24 hours after the injury are the most critical.
- Tell the patient to refrain from strenuous activity, to rest, and to return to regular activity gradually.
- Instruct the patient to avoid using pain medicines other than acetaminophen, unless the drugs are approved by the physician.
- Advise the patient to eat lightly, especially if nausea and vomiting occur.
- Tell a family member to check on the patient every few hours. The family member should make sure the patient knows his own name, his location, and the name of the family member.
- Instruct the family member to call for medical assistance immediately if the patient exhibits any of these warning signs:
  - Any symptom that is getting worse, such as headaches, sleepiness, or nausea, including nausea that doesn't go away
  - Changes in behavior, such as irritability or confusion
  - Dilated pupils (pupils that are bigger than normal) or pupils of different sizes
  - Trouble walking or speaking
  - Drainage of bloody or clear fluids from ears or nose
  - Vomiting
  - Seizures
  - Weakness or numbness in the arms or legs
  - A less serious head injury in a patient taking blood thinners or who has a bleeding disorder such as hemophilia

PROCEDURE 26.5

Controlling Bleeding

Objective: To control bleeding and minimize blood loss

OSHA Guidelines

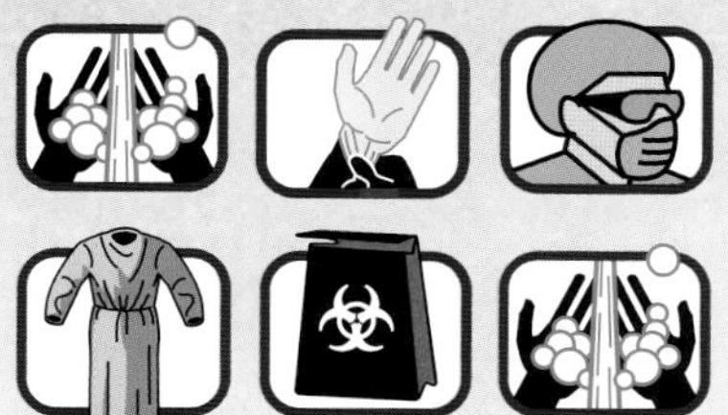

Materials: Clean or sterile dressings

Method

1. If you have time, wash your hands and put on examination gloves, face protection, and a gown to protect yourself from splatters, splashes, and sprays.
2. Using a clean or sterile dressing, apply direct pressure over the wound.
3. If blood soaks through the dressing, do not remove it. Apply an additional dressing over the original one.
4. Elevate the body part that is bleeding.
5. If direct pressure and elevation do not stop the bleeding, apply pressure over the nearest pressure point between the bleeding and the heart (Figure 26-11). For example, if the wound is on the lower arm, apply pressure on the brachial artery. For a lower-leg wound, apply pressure on the femoral artery in the groin.
6. When the doctor or EMT arrives, assist as requested.
7. After the patient has been transferred to a hospital, properly dispose of contaminated materials.
8. Remove the gloves and wash your hands.

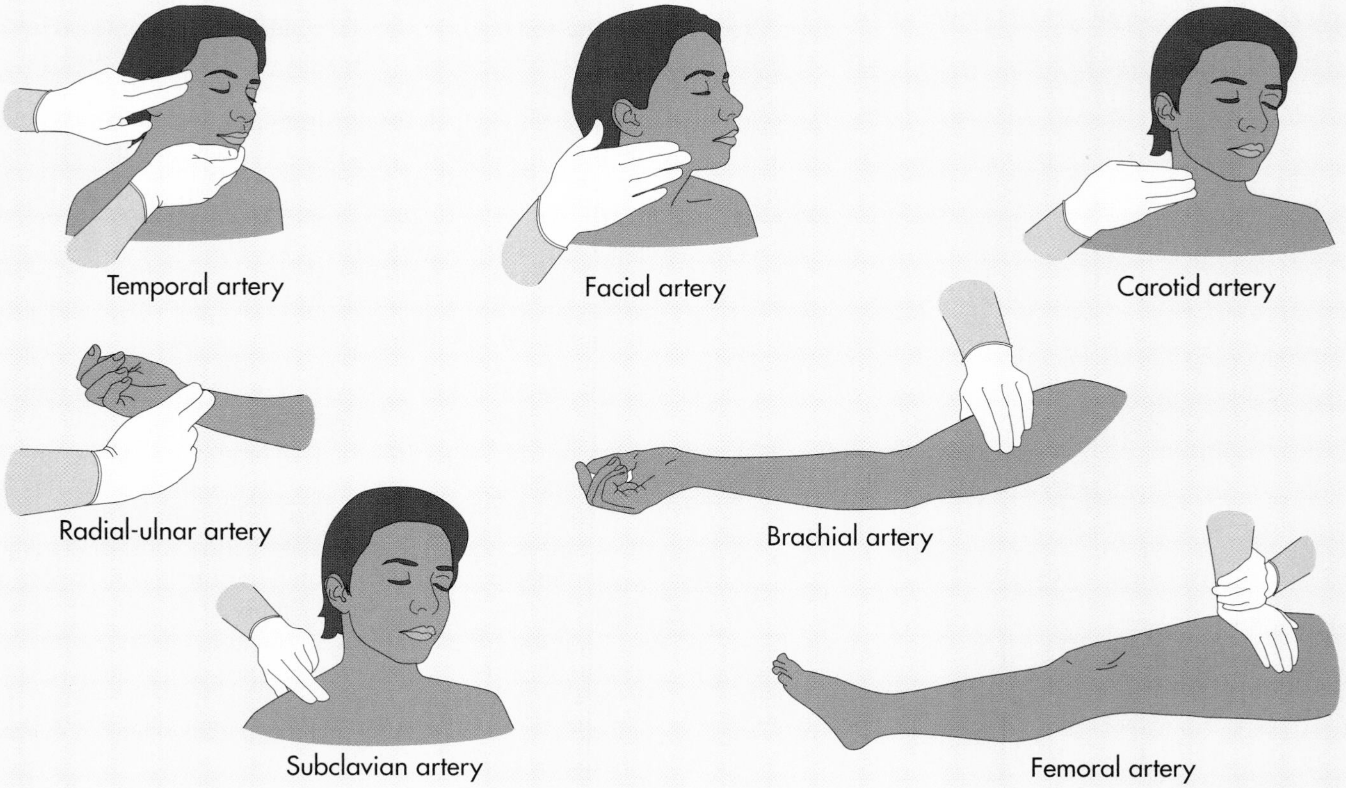

Figure 26-11. Apply pressure on these pressure points to stop bleeding.

be reduced by applying ice immediately after the injury. Because blood vessels in the scalp are close to the skin, scalp lacerations often bleed profusely and look worse than they really are. Apply direct pressure to stop bleeding from a scalp laceration, wash the area with soap and water, and apply a dry, sterile dressing over the area.

Hemorrhaging

Hemorrhaging (heavy or uncontrollable bleeding) is generally the result of an injury. It may also be caused by an illness. The first-aid treatment remains the same in both cases. Bleeding can be internal or external. When administering first aid to a patient who may have internal bleeding, cover the patient with a blanket for warmth, keep the patient quiet and calm, and get medical help immediately.

Control external bleeding to prevent rapid blood loss and shock. Use direct pressure, apply additional dressings as needed, elevate the bleeding body part, and put pressure over a pressure point, as described in Procedure 26-5 and as illustrated in Figure 26-11. Then transport the patient to an emergency care facility.

As a last resort, if medical help is more than an hour away, you may need to use a tourniquet (Figure 26-12) to save a person's life. You apply a tourniquet over the main pressure point just above the wound and tighten the tourniquet until the bleeding stops. Many people do not recommend applying a tourniquet in any situation because it may be difficult to judge when a person's life is at stake. Keep in mind that application of a tourniquet to a person's limb almost surely leads to loss of the limb.

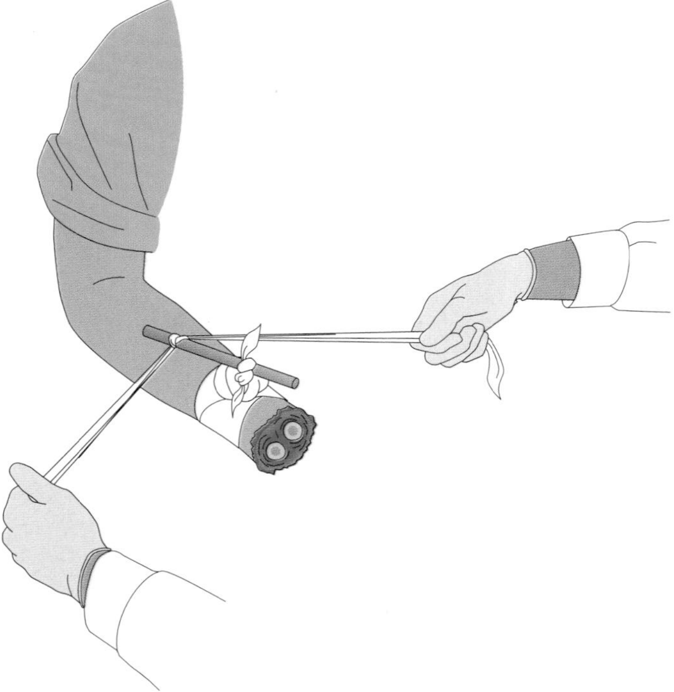

Figure 26-12. Apply a tourniquet only as a last resort, that is, if bleeding cannot be stopped and the patient is likely to die as a result.

Multiple Injuries

Sometimes a patient sustains more than one type of injury—for example, an arm fracture, head injury, lacerations, and internal bleeding. Multiple injuries often result from a car accident or a fall. If you need to assist a patient with multiple injuries, assess the ABCs and perform CPR if needed. Then call (or have someone else call) the EMS system or the physician. Once you have ensured an open airway, breathing, and circulation, perform first aid for the most life-threatening injuries first.

Poisoning

A poison is a substance that produces harmful effects if it enters the body. Poisoning is serious and it can result in death or permanent injury if immediate medical care is not provided.

In addition to being able to handle a poisoning emergency, you need to educate patients in how to do the same. You should teach them about the symptoms of and treatment for the different types of poisoning. Provide them with pamphlets that describe the procedures to follow and stickers with the telephone number of the regional poison control center.

The majority of accidental poisonings happen to children under the age of 5. Young children are not necessarily put off by strong smells or burning sensations when they swallow something. Common causes of poisoning in children are household cleaning products, household plants, and medications. Poisons can also be caused by improperly prepared or contaminated food. These types of poisons are ingested, or swallowed.

Poisoning that results from coming in contact with plants, such as poison ivy, poison sumac, and poison oak, is common and generally fairly minor. This type of poisoning is referred to as absorbed poisoning. It can be serious, however, if the poisoning occurs over a large surface of the body.

Poisons can also be inhaled. This situation occurs when a person inhales a poisonous gas such as carbon monoxide or the fumes from burning poisonous plants.

Ingested Poisons. Poison that is swallowed remains in the stomach only a short time. Most of it is absorbed while in the small intestine. Symptoms of poisoning include abdominal pain and cramping; nausea; vomiting; diarrhea; odor, stains, or burns around or in the mouth; drowsiness; and unconsciousness. You should also suspect poisoning if packages containing poisonous substances are near a person who has one or more of these symptoms.

It is extremely important to call a poison control center (if available), hospital emergency room, doctor, or the EMS system for instructions if you think a patient has swallowed a poison. When you call, you will need to know the following:

- The patient's age
- The name of the poison

- The amount of poison swallowed
- When the poison was swallowed
- Whether or not the person has vomited
- How much time it will take to get the patient to a medical facility

Poisons vary in their toxicity. Some cause damage right away, whereas others cause damage several hours later. If the patient is alert and not having convulsions, follow these steps.

1. Call the regional poison control center.
2. Induce vomiting with ipecac syrup if directed by the poison control center.
3. Seek immediate medical attention.

Do not induce vomiting unless directed by a medical authority. The patient may have ingested a strong acid, alkali, or petroleum product, such as chlorine bleach or gasoline. These products may cause further damage to the throat and esophagus during vomiting. If you do not know what the patient ingested, never induce vomiting.

Turn the patient on her left side. This position delays stomach emptying by several hours and prevents aspiration if the patient vomits. Take both poison container and vomited material to the hospital for inspection.

Food poisoning, another type of ingested poisoning, can occur when bacteria produce toxins in food. Botulism, for example, results from eating improperly canned or preserved foods that have been contaminated with the bacterium *Clostridium botulinum*. Symptoms appear within 12 to 36 hours after eating contaminated food. Initial symptoms include dry mouth, sore throat, weakness, vomiting, and diarrhea.

Food poisoning is often difficult to detect because the signs and symptoms vary greatly. A patient with food poisoning usually has abdominal pain, nausea, vomiting, gas, frequent bowel sounds, and diarrhea. Chills, joint pain, and excessive sweating may also occur. If you suspect that a patient has food poisoning, call the poison control center, and arrange for immediate transport to the hospital.

Absorbed Poisons. Most people have had the red, itchy rash that results from contact with poison ivy, poison sumac, or poison oak. In some people, however, the rash may be accompanied by a generalized swelling, burning eyes, headache, fever, and abnormal pulse or respirations.

To treat a patient who has come in contact with an absorbed poison, call the regional poison control center. Have the patient immediately remove all contaminated clothing. Then wash the affected skin thoroughly with soap and water, drench it with alcohol, and rinse well. To help relieve symptoms, apply wet compresses soaked with calamine lotion. Also suggest baths in colloidal oatmeal or applications of a paste made from 3 teaspoons baking soda and 1 teaspoon water to soothe the itching. If the rash is severe, the doctor may prescribe a corticosteroid ointment. Tell the patient to seek medical assistance if a fever or swelling develops.

Inhaled Poisons. A patient may inhale poisons by breathing air contaminated by chemicals in the workplace or by a malfunctioning stove or furnace in the home. The patient may not realize she has been exposed to a poisonous gas until symptoms arise. Even then, a patient may merely suspect the flu, because some symptoms of inhalation poisoning mimic those of influenza. Common symptoms include headache, tinnitus (ringing in the ears), angina (chest pain), shortness of breath, muscle weakness, nausea, vomiting, confusion, and dizziness, followed by blurred or double vision, difficulty breathing, unconsciousness, and cardiac arrest. Also, a patient who has facial burns may have sustained an inhalation injury.

To treat poisoning by inhalation, first get the patient into fresh air. Have someone call the EMS system or the regional poison control center. Loosen tight-fitting clothing and wrap the patient in a blanket to prevent shock. Check the patient's ABCs and begin CPR if needed. Expect the EMS team to treat the patient with 100% oxygen.

Carbon monoxide is a major cause of inhalation poisoning in the home. It is a colorless and odorless natural gas produced by incomplete combustion of organic fuels, such as coal, wood, or gasoline. Carbon monoxide is especially dangerous in closed spaces because, when inhaled, it replaces oxygen in the blood. If you suspect carbon monoxide poisoning, look for clues in the environment such as a malfunctioning furnace or a car engine left running in a closed space such as a garage.

Mild carbon monoxide poisoning can cause headache and flulike symptoms without fever. Moderate poisoning may cause tinnitus, drowsiness, severe seizures, coma, and cardiopulmonary problems. Because the gas is odorless, people are often unaware they are being poisoned. They may fall asleep, lapse into unconsciousness, and die.

Weather-Related Injuries

Exposure to extreme cold, extreme heat, and the sun's damaging rays can cause weather-related injuries. These injuries may require emergency medical attention.

Frostbite. When body tissues are exposed to below-freezing temperatures, frostbite can occur. Frostbite causes ice crystals to form between tissue cells, and these crystals enlarge as they extract water from the cells. Frostbite also causes obstruction to the blood supply in the form of blood clots. This aspect of frostbite prevents blood from flowing to the tissues and causes additional, severe damage to cells.

Symptoms of frostbite include white, waxy, or grayish yellow skin. The affected body part feels cold, tingling, and painful. The skin surface may feel crusty and the underlying tissue soft in comparison. If the frostbite is deep, the body part may feel cold and hard and not be sensitive to pain. Blisters may appear after rewarming.

Treat frostbite by wrapping warm clothing or blankets around the affected body part or placing it in contact with another body part that is warm. Do not rub or massage the affected area, or you may cause further damage to the frozen tissue. Call for medical assistance. If you are in a remote area, use the wet rapid rewarming method. This method involves placing the affected part in warm (100° to 104°F) water. Hot water should be added at regular intervals to keep the temperature of the bath stable. As an alternative method, you can heat the affected area with warm compresses. Because warming may cause pain, administer aspirin or acetaminophen. Continue rewarming for 20 to 40 minutes. After the affected area becomes soft, place dry, sterile gauze between skin surfaces, such as between the toes or the fingers or between the ear and the side of the head. Do not massage the skin or break blisters.

Heatstroke. Heatstroke results from prolonged exposure to high temperatures and humidity. This condition may lead to excessive loss of fluids (dehydration) and insufficient blood in the circulatory system (hypovolemic shock). High body temperature can damage tissues and organs throughout the body. If untreated, the patient will die. People most susceptible to heatstroke are children, the elderly, athletes, and patients who are obese, are diabetic, or have circulatory problems or other chronic illnesses.

Symptoms of heatstroke include hot, dry skin; high body temperature; altered mental state; rapid pulse; rapid breathing; dizziness; and weakness. If you suspect that a patient has heatstroke, check the patient's ABCs, and call the EMS system. Move the patient to a cool place, and remove outer clothing unless it is made of light cotton or other light fabric. Also, cool the patient with any means available, such as gentle spraying with a hose, movement to an air-conditioned place, vigorous fanning, or application of a wet sheet. If the humidity is above 75%, place ice packs on the patient's groin and armpits. Stop cooling when the patient's mental state improves. Keep the patient's head and shoulders slightly elevated.

Sunburn. Do not dismiss a sunburn as trivial. It is a burn that can cause redness, tenderness, pain, swelling, blisters, and peeling skin. It can lead to skin damage or cancer later in life.

Soak sunburned skin in cool water to help reduce the heat. Apply cold compresses, and later calamine lotion, to bring relief from the burning sensation. Have the patient elevate the legs and arms to prevent swelling. The patient should also drink plenty of water and take a pain reliever.

Educate the patient about the importance of using sunscreen and reapplying it every 2 to 3 hours when outdoors. Advise the patient to stay out of direct sunlight between 10:00 A.M. and 2:00 P.M., because the sun's rays are strongest during that period.

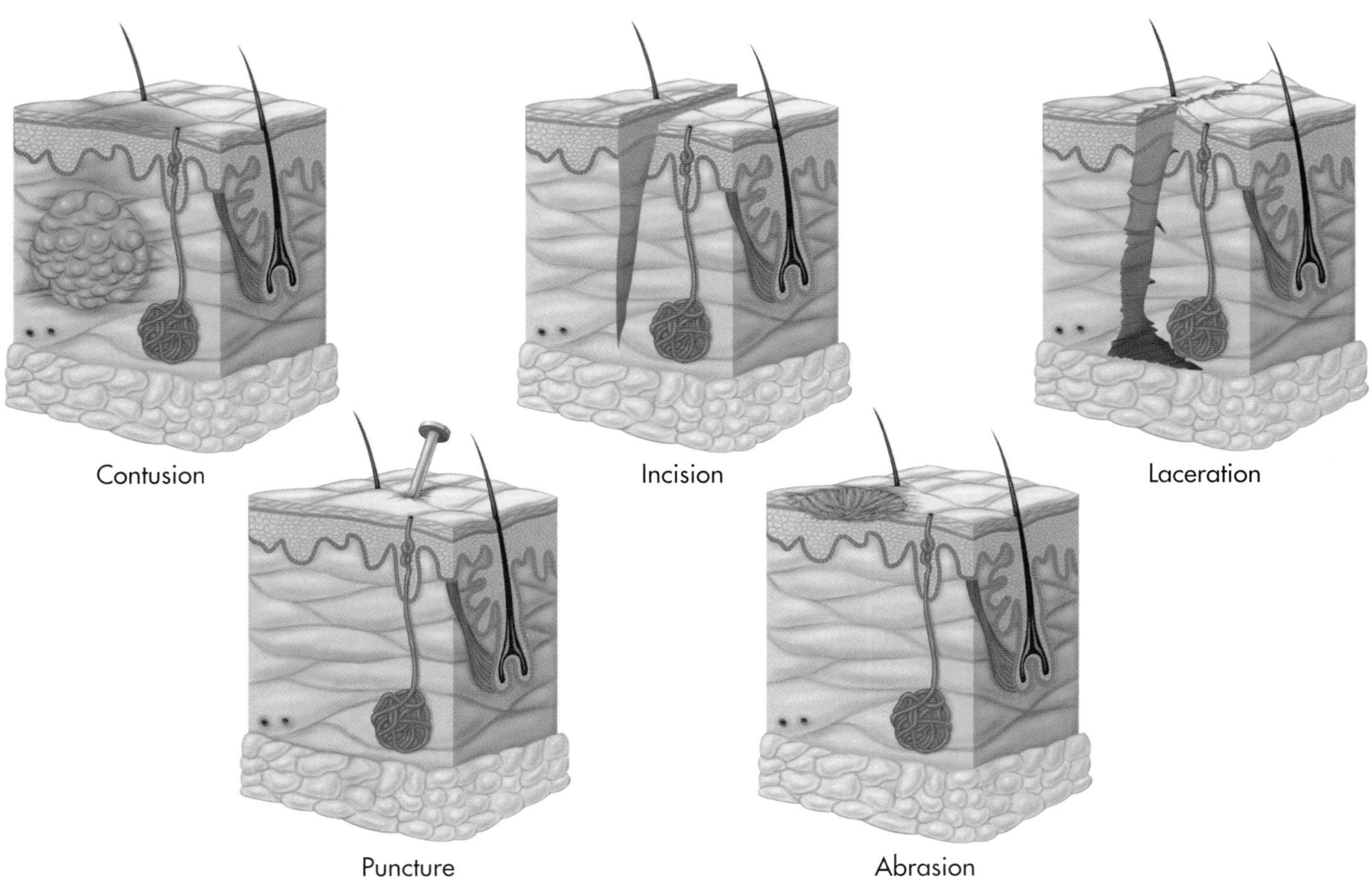

Figure 26-13. Different types of wounds produce different degrees of tissue damage.

Wounds

A wound is an injury in which the skin or tissues under the skin are damaged. Wounds can be either open or closed. Figure 26-13 shows the various types of wounds.

Open Wounds. An open wound is a break in the skin or mucous membrane. Types of open wounds include incisions, lacerations, abrasions, and punctures.

Incisions and Lacerations. An incision is a clean and smooth cut, such as that from a kitchen knife. A laceration has jagged edges, as may result when a child steps on a piece of broken glass in the sand at the beach. Care of minor incisions and lacerations involves controlling bleeding by covering the wound with a clean or sterile dressing and applying direct pressure. After the bleeding stops, clean and dress the wound. Procedure 26-6 explains how to clean minor wounds. Teach the patient the importance of keeping the wound clean and checking for signs of infection, such as heat, redness, pain, and swelling.

If the wound is deep and involves muscle, tendons, the face, the genitals, the mouth, or the tongue, control the bleeding with direct pressure to the wound (with a sterile dressing or clean cloth held against its surface), elevation,

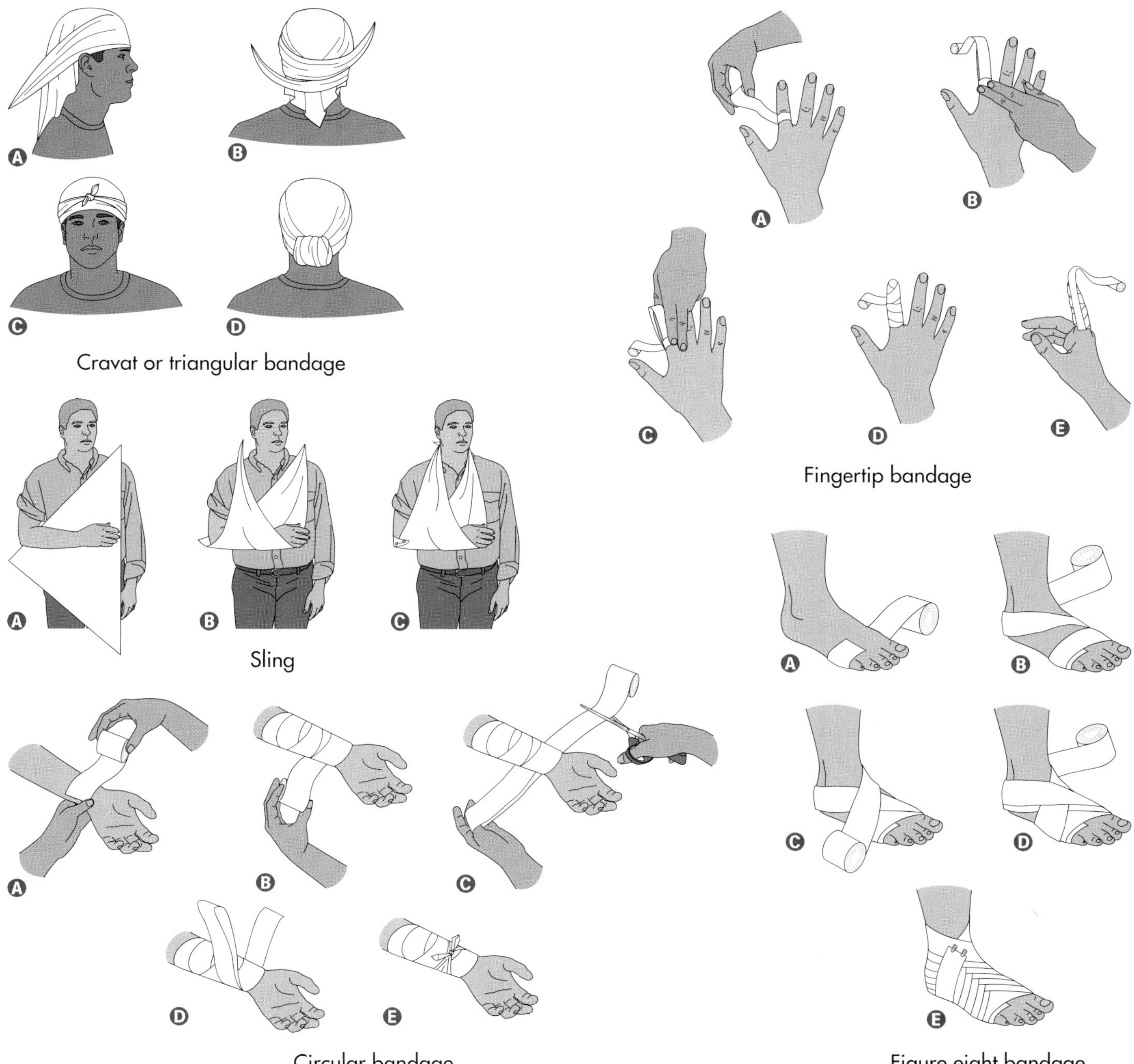

Figure 26-14. Apply a bandage, as needed, to a wound.

PROCEDURE 26.6

Cleaning Minor Wounds

Objective: To clean and dress minor wounds

OSHA Guidelines

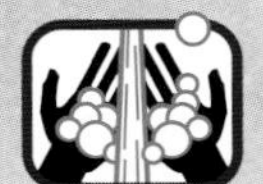
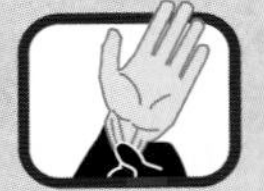

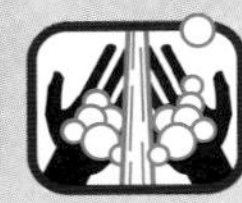

Materials: Sterile gauze squares, basin, antiseptic soap, warm water, sterile dressing

Method

1. Wash your hands and put on examination gloves.
2. Dip several gauze squares in a basin of warm, soapy water.
3. Wash the wound from the center outward to avoid bringing contaminants from the surrounding skin into the wound. Use a new gauze square for each cleansing motion.
4. As you wash, remove debris that could cause infection.
5. Rinse the area thoroughly, preferably by placing the wound under warm, running water.
6. Pat the wound dry with sterile gauze squares.
7. Cover the wound with a dry, sterile dressing. Bandage the dressing in place.
8. Properly dispose of contaminated materials.
9. Remove the gloves and wash your hands.
10. Instruct the patient on wound care.
11. Record the procedure in the patient's chart.

and use of pressure points. Contact the doctor and, if necessary, the EMS system.

Abrasions. An abrasion is a scraping of the skin, as when someone slides across gravel during a softball game. Abrasions require washing with soap and water. Be sure to remove all the dirt and debris to prevent tattooing (dark discoloration under the skin). Minor abrasions do not need a dressing or bandage, but large ones do. Various types of bandaging are shown in Figure 26-14. As with any wound, teach the patient to watch for signs of infection.

Punctures. A puncture wound is a small hole created by a piercing object, such as a bullet, knife, nail, or animal tooth. Puncture wounds are a potential breeding ground for tetanus bacteria, because the bacteria can live and thrive in the absence of oxygen. Allow the wound to bleed freely for a few minutes to help wash out bacteria. Then clean the wound with soap and water, and apply a dry, sterile dressing. If the patient has not had a tetanus toxoid immunization in the past 7 to 10 years, inform the physician so that one can be ordered.

Closed Wounds. A closed wound is an injury that occurs inside the body without breaking the skin. Closed wounds, which are usually called **contusions** (bruises), are caused by a blunt object striking the tissue. This action produces broken blood vessels and internal, localized bleeding (hematoma) below the area that has been struck. Treat such a wound with cold compresses to reduce swelling. The affected area will turn from black and blue to green to yellow as blood pigments oxidize. Inform the patient that these color changes are part of the normal healing process.

Common Illnesses

A variety of common illnesses frequently call for emergency medical intervention. As a patient educator, you can help ensure that patients recognize the symptoms of these illnesses and know when to call for medical assistance. Teaching patients the importance of following physician's orders for follow-up care is also your responsibility. Common illnesses include the following:

- Abdominal pain
- Asthma
- Dehydration
- Diarrhea
- Fainting
- Fever
- Hyperventilation
- Nosebleed
- Tachycardia
- Vomiting

Abdominal Pain

Acute abdominal pain that occurs suddenly and is accompanied by fever may indicate an emergency that requires surgery. The pain may involve spasmodic contractions. It may feel knifelike or ache dully, and it may be localized or may radiate. The location of the pain gives clues to its cause. Acute pain in the right upper quadrant, for example, may signal a gallbladder attack. Pain in the right lower quadrant may indicate appendicitis.

Other causes include internal hemorrhage, intestinal perforation or obstruction, peptic ulcer, and hernia. In women, pelvic pain can indicate a gynecologic problem. Obviously, trauma to the area, such as wounds or blows, can produce acute abdominal pain.

While waiting for patient transport, have the patient lie on his back with his knees flexed (unless there is a wound or swelling in the abdomen). This position lets the abdominal muscles relax. Keep the patient quiet and warm, and act calm and concerned. Do not give anything by mouth, and keep an emesis basin handy in case the patient vomits. Do not apply heat to the abdomen because heat may exacerbate inflammation. Monitor the patient's pulse and consciousness, and check for signs of shock.

Asthma

Asthma is a common disorder caused by spasmodic narrowing of the bronchi. It is often an inherited tendency—that is, several members of one family may suffer from it. A patient who is having an acute attack wheezes, coughs, and is short of breath. She may become frightened and feel as if she cannot get enough air. If you spot an asthma attack, check the patient's ABCs, and notify the doctor at once. You may assist the patient in using a respiratory inhaler if she carries one with her. If directed, administer a mininebulizer treatment with a bronchodilator (drug that opens the bronchi), such as albuterol (Proventil) or epinephrine.

Dehydration

Dehydration results from a lack of adequate water in the body. The body's fluid intake is not sufficient to meet its fluid needs. Severe dehydration can result from vomiting, excessive heat and sweating, diarrhea, or lack of food or fluid intake. The following are symptoms of dehydration:

- Extreme thirst
- Tiredness
- Light-headedness
- Abdominal or muscle cramping
- Confusion (especially in elderly people)

Perform the following steps to administer first aid to a dehydrated person.

1. Move the victim into the shade or to a cool area.
2. To replace lost fluids, give the victim water, tea, fruit juice, a commercial electrolyte replacement fluid, or clear broth.
3. If symptoms persist or are accompanied by nausea, diarrhea, or convulsions, call for the EMS system or a physician.

Diarrhea (Acute)

Acute diarrhea can be caused by an intestinal infection, food poisoning, a bowel disorder, or the side effects of medication. Severe diarrhea causes dehydration and dangerous electrolyte imbalances that can lead to shock. Symptoms of shock include rapid pulse, low blood pressure, and pale, clammy skin.

Help the patient lie on his back and elevate his legs. Report the patient's condition to the doctor. As directed, prepare to assist in administering intravenous fluids to correct dehydration and restore electrolytes and to draw blood for testing.

Fainting (Syncope)

Fainting, or syncope, is a partial or complete loss of consciousness. It usually follows a decrease in the amount of blood flow to the brain. Before fainting, patients may feel weak, dizzy, cold, or nauseated. They may perspire or look pale and anxious.

If you are with a patient who feels as if she is going to faint, tell her to lower her head between her legs and to breathe deeply. Stay with her until the feeling passes. If the patient is having difficulty breathing or faints, lay her flat on her back with her feet slightly elevated. Loosen tight clothing and apply a cold cloth to her face. Observe the patient carefully, monitoring her breathing and level of consciousness. Observe for weakness in her arms and legs. Let her rest for at least 10 minutes after she regains full consciousness. Notify the physician that the patient fainted.

If your efforts do not revive a patient who has fainted, call the physician and the EMS system. The patient may be slipping into a coma.

Fever

Fever is a common clinical sign that often indicates infection. Mild or moderate fever can accompany a cold or an upset stomach. It can usually be managed with aspirin or acetaminophen. A fever of 106°F or higher (hyperthermia) is dangerous, however, because irreversible brain damage can occur if the fever is not lowered immediately.

If a patient's temperature is dangerously high, you must proceed at once to check the other vital signs and the level of consciousness. Notify the doctor and be prepared to start rapid cooling measures. Place ice packs on the groin and axilla, or give the patient a tepid sponge bath. If the patient is a child, be prepared to manage seizures (discussed later in this chapter).

Hyperventilation

Some patients who are under a great deal of stress lack the skills to deal with the stress effectively. They may seem anxious, frazzled, and more emotional than average patients. Patients under stress may begin to hyperventilate, or breathe too rapidly and too deeply. This breathing disturbs the normal balance of oxygen and carbon dioxide in the blood, and the carbon dioxide concentration falls below normal levels. Patients who are hyperventilating may also feel light-headed and as if they cannot get enough air. In addition, they may have chest pain and feel apprehensive.

Move a hyperventilating patient to a quiet area. Have the patient sit quietly and visualize a calm and serene environment, such as a beach or the mountains. With a calm and soothing voice, coach the patient to take slow, normal breaths.

Nosebleed

Nosebleed, or **epistaxis,** can occur for a variety of reasons. They include blowing the nose too hard, local irritation or dryness, frequent sneezing, fragile or superficial blood vessels, high blood pressure, a blow to the nose, and a foreign body in the nose. Nosebleeds are common in children, especially at night.

Treat a nosebleed by having the patient sit up with the head tilted forward to prevent blood from running down the back of the throat. Next, have the patient gently pinch the nostrils shut at the bottom for at least 5 minutes. If that does not stop the bleeding, apply an ice pack or cold compress to the nose and face, and continue to pinch the nostrils. If the bleeding cannot be controlled, arrange for transport to the office or to a hospital for cauterization or nasal packing.

Tachycardia

Tachycardia is a rapid heart rate, generally in excess of 100 beats per minute. A patient with tachycardia may report having **palpitations,** unusually rapid, strong, or irregular pulsations of the heart. He may feel as if his heart is pounding. Help the patient lie down, take his vital signs, and if instructed, obtain an electrocardiogram (ECG). (Electrocardiography is discussed in Chapter 34.) If tachycardia is accompanied by low blood pressure and lightheadedness, notify the physician immediately. These symptoms indicate that the patient could faint or go into shock. Remain with the patient and keep him calm. If directed, obtain another ECG.

Vomiting

Vomiting is a symptom common to many disorders, ranging from food poisoning to various infections. When severe, it can lead to dehydration and dangerous changes in electrolyte levels, especially in patients who are very young, very old, or diabetic or who also have diarrhea. Because these problems can be severe, notify the doctor and provide appropriate care. Procedure 26-7 describes how to provide emergency care for a patient who is vomiting.

PROCEDURE 26.7

Caring for a Patient Who Is Vomiting

Objective: To increase comfort and minimize complications, such as aspiration, for a patient who is vomiting

OSHA Guidelines

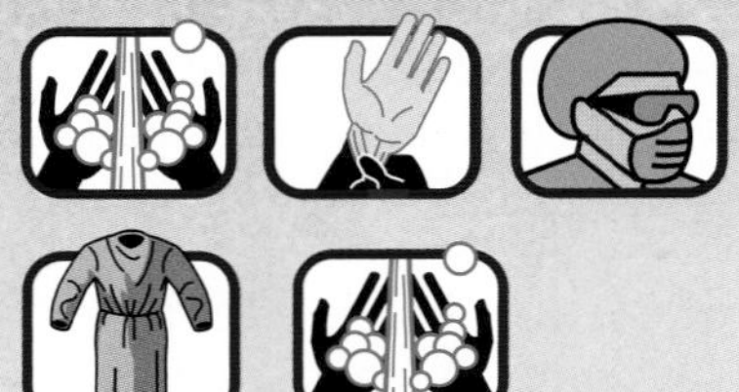

Materials: Emesis basin, cool compress, cup of cool water, paper tissues or a towel, and (if ordered) intravenous fluids and electrolytes and an antinausea drug

Method

1. Wash your hands and put on examination gloves and other PPE.
2. Ask the patient when and how the vomiting started and how frequently it occurs. Find out whether she is nauseated or in pain.
3. Give the patient an emesis basin to collect vomit. Observe and document its amount, color, odor, and consistency. Particularly note blood, bile, undigested food, or feces in the vomit.
4. Place a cool compress on the patient's forehead to make her more comfortable. Offer water and paper tissues or a towel to clean her mouth.
5. Monitor for signs of dehydration, such as confusion, irritability, and flushed, dry skin. Also monitor for signs of electrolyte imbalances, such as leg cramps or an irregular pulse.
6. If requested, assist by laying out supplies and equipment for the physician to use in administering intravenous fluids and electrolytes. Administer an antinausea drug if prescribed.
7. Prepare the patient for diagnostic tests if instructed.
8. Remove the gloves and wash your hands.

Less Common Illnesses

Even though some illnesses are less common than those previously discussed, you should still be familiar enough with them so that you can handle them effectively if a physician or EMT is not immediately available. Educate patients about symptoms they may encounter that require emergency medical intervention as well as about the importance of follow-up care when they are recovering from such illnesses. Less common illnesses that may require emergency medical intervention include the following:

- Anaphylaxis
- Bacterial meningitis
- Diabetic emergencies
- Gallbladder attack
- Heart attack
- Hematemesis
- Obstetric emergencies
- Respiratory arrest
- Seizures
- Shock
- Stroke
- Toxic shock syndrome
- Viral encephalitis

Anaphylaxis

Anaphylaxis, or anaphylactic shock, is a severe, often life-threatening allergic reaction. The reaction can be immediate or delayed up to 2 hours. It happens to people who have become sensitized to certain substances. For example, it can result from eating a type of food, being stung by an insect, or taking a particular type of medication, such as penicillin.

The first sign of anaphylaxis usually comes from the patient's skin. It becomes itchy, turns red, feels hot, and develops hives. The face may also become puffy. The throat may swell so that the patient has trouble breathing and swallowing and feels as if he has a "lump in the throat." Other symptoms include pallor, perspiration, and a weak, rapid, irregular pulse. If you detect these symptoms or if the patient becomes restless, has a headache, or says that his throat feels as if it is closing up, take the following steps immediately.

Check the patient's ABCs and then notify the doctor. As directed, administer epinephrine, oral antihistamines, and oxygen, and help the patient sit up. After the patient receives epinephrine, monitor his vital signs every 2 to 3 minutes. Note skin color and monitor the airway. If he does not recover quickly, arrange for immediate transport to the hospital.

When severely allergic patients stabilize, the doctor prescribes an epinephrine autoinjector for patients to carry with them. You are responsible for teaching patients how to use this device. See the Educating the Patient section in Chapter 33 for directions.

Because of the possibility of anaphylaxis, a patient who has just received any type of injection should routinely be kept in the office for 20 to 30 minutes of observation. This procedure reduces the possibility that an allergic reaction to the medication will occur while the patient is unattended.

A less severe allergic reaction to drugs or certain foods may cause sneezing, itching, slight swelling of the skin, rash, or hives. This type of reaction can usually be controlled with diphenhydramine hydrochloride (Benadryl) or another antihistamine. The patient should be monitored closely, however, to make sure the condition does not progress to anaphylaxis.

Bacterial Meningitis

Bacterial meningitis is almost always a complication of another bacterial infection, such as otitis media (middle ear infection) or pneumonia. Therefore, first find out whether the patient currently has or recently has had a bacterial infection. The signs of bacterial meningitis are fever, chills, headache, neck stiffness, and vomiting. If the patient has these signs and then develops a fever of 102°F, becomes less alert, has altered respirations, or experiences seizures, the infection has progressed to a dangerous state.

If these signs are present, assess the patient's ABCs and notify the physician of the change in the patient's condition. Expect to arrange for transport to the hospital, where the patient will be treated with intravenous antibiotics.

Diabetic Emergencies

Diabetes is a fairly common disorder of carbohydrate metabolism (see Chapter 23). The body needs insulin, a hormone secreted by the pancreas, to use blood sugar to fuel body cells. Insulin secretion is impaired in patients with diabetes.

You can teach patients who have diabetes or who are at risk for diabetes how to recognize early signs of **hypoglycemia** (low blood sugar) and **hyperglycemia** (high blood sugar) before these conditions become medical emergencies. Symptoms of hypoglycemia include dizziness; headache; hunger; weakness; full, rapid pulse; and pallor. Symptoms of hyperglycemia include dry mouth, intense thirst, muscle weakness, and blurred vision. You should also be familiar with the signs and symptoms of the two most common diabetic emergencies you will encounter: insulin shock and diabetic coma.

Insulin Shock. Insulin shock is basically very severe hypoglycemia, in which a patient has too little sugar in the blood. Insulin shock occurs when insulin levels are so high that they move too much sugar from the blood into cells. Symptoms include rapid pulse; shallow respiration; hunger; profuse sweating; pale, cool, clammy skin; double vision; tremors; restlessness; confusion; and possibly fainting. Insulin shock can usually be corrected with administration of some form of sugar (candy, juice, or regular soda for a conscious patient or a sprinkle of table sugar

Career Opportunities

CPR Instructor

To gain medical assistant credentials, you must fulfill the requirements of either the American Association of Medical Assistants (for a Certified Medical Assistant) or the American Medical Technologists (for a Registered Medical Assistant). After obtaining your medical assistant certification or registration, you may wish to acquire additional skills in specialty areas through course work or on-the-job training. Although this course work or training may not lead to an additional certification or degree, it will enable you to expand your role in the medical office and advance your career as the demand for skilled health professionals increases.

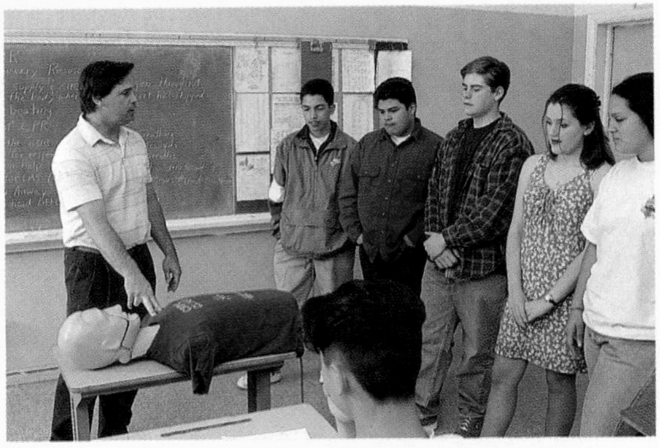

Skills and Duties

A CPR (cardiopulmonary resuscitation) instructor provides people with the knowledge and skills necessary to help save a person's life in an emergency. He teaches his students how to:

- Call for help.
- Help sustain life.
- Reduce pain.
- Minimize the consequences of injury or sudden illness until professional medical help arrives.

To teach a CPR class, an instructor must plan and coordinate the course in conjunction with a local American Red Cross unit or American Heart Association affiliate. He demonstrates the appropriate skills to his students and observes their technique. He then provides constructive feedback as they learn skills and make decisions regarding the appropriate action to take in an emergency.

The instructor is responsible for identifying participants who are having difficulty with the skills. He must develop effective strategies to help these students meet the course objectives. At the end of the course, the CPR instructor submits completed course records to the local American Red Cross chapter or American Heart Association affiliate.

Workplace Settings

CPR instructors teach classes in a variety of settings, including schools and universities, community rooms, camps, religious institutions, and medical clinics. Some employers, such as operators of swimming pools, camps, and day-care facilities, may require CPR instruction as a condition of employment.

Education

Red Cross To be certified as a CPR instructor by the Red Cross, you must be at least 17 years old. In addition, you must complete two Red Cross courses. The first, the instructor candidate training course, provides instruction in teaching methods, evaluation, and reporting. After completing this course, you will be awarded an instructor candidate training certificate, which qualifies you to take the first aid and CPR instructor course. You must then pass a written test with a grade of 80% or better to gain certification. CPR instructors must teach one class every 2 years for recertification from the Red Cross.

American Heart Association The American Heart Association also provides training for CPR instructors. You must first pass the basic life support course for health-care providers, which teaches CPR skills. You then must take the instructor course, which covers teaching methods. After passing the instructor course, you must coteach a CPR class with an experienced instructor, who will monitor your performance. You will then become an approved instructor. CPR instructors affiliated with the American Heart Association are required to teach a minimum of two classes a year. The association has no minimum age to become an instructor.

National Safety Council The National Safety Council is another option that offers training to become a CPR instructor. Typically, you must first complete a CPR and AED provider training course and then take an instructor course. With successful completion of the instructor course you will be monitored by an experienced instructor before you are issued instructor status. The path to become a CPR instructor however is flexible depending on your background. Instructors must teach two CPR classes a year to maintain their instructor status.

CPR instructors may be paid or work as volunteers. There is no specific salary range for the job.

Where to Go for More Information

American Heart Association
National Center
7272 Greenville Avenue
Dallas, TX 75231-4596
(800) 242-8721, or call your local center

American Red Cross
17th and D Streets, NW
Washington, DC 20006
(202) 728-6400, or call your local chapter

National Safety Council
1121 Spring Lake Dr.
Itasca, IL 60143
www.nsc.org or call your local chapter

on the tongue for an unconscious patient). If the cause of a diabetic emergency is unknown, give sugar. Patients will improve quickly if the cause is insulin shock and will not be harmed if the cause is diabetic coma, provided they are then transported to the hospital.

Diabetic Coma. Diabetic coma is the end result of severe hyperglycemia, in which a patient has too much sugar in the blood. It occurs when insulin levels are insufficient to move blood sugar into body cells. Its symptoms include rapid, deep gulping breaths; flushed, warm, dry skin; thirst; acetone breath (a sweet or fruity odor from the mouth); and disorientation or confusion. If you suspect diabetic coma, notify the doctor at once, and expect to arrange transport to the hospital.

Gallbladder Attack (Acute)

A classic acute gallbladder attack occurs after a person eats a high-fat meal rich in cholesterol. The patient may wake up in the night with acute abdominal pain (gallbladder colic) in the right upper quadrant. The pain is caused by inflammation of the gallbladder, usually related to gallstones obstructing the cystic duct, through which bile is secreted by the gallbladder. The pain may radiate to the back between the shoulder blades or be localized in the epigastric region (the upper central region of the abdomen) and the front chest area. The attack may be accompanied by nausea and vomiting. The pain is usually so severe that the patient seeks medical attention; many patients think they are having a heart attack.

Gallbladder attacks caused by gallstones are more common among women who are over age 40 and obese, and the frequency of attacks increases with age (especially after age 65). Diagnosis is usually made with the help of ultrasonography. The patient may require surgery to remove the gallstones.

Heart Attack

A heart attack, or **myocardial infarction (MI)**, occurs when the blood flow to the heart is reduced as a result of blockage in the coronary arteries or their branches. Chest pain is the cardinal symptom of a heart attack. The patient may describe the pain as crushing, burning, heavy, aching, or like that of indigestion. The pain may radiate down the left arm or into the jaw, throat, or both shoulders. It may be accompanied by shortness of breath, sweating, nausea, and vomiting. The patient may be pale and have a feeling of doom. If you cannot easily detect pallor (paleness) because the patient has dark skin, check the patient's inner lip for paleness. Elderly patients may experience atypical symptoms of a heart attack, such as jaw pain, because responses to pain diminish during the aging process. The pain of a heart attack is not relieved by nitroglycerin.

If you think a patient is having a heart attack, notify the physician and EMS system immediately. Do not let the patient walk. Loosen tight clothing and have the patient sit up to aid breathing. The physician may order you to administer oxygen at 4 to 6 liters per minute; make sure that no one in the area is smoking. Stay with the patient, observe the ABCs, and begin CPR if required (Procedure 26-8). If directed, obtain an ECG. Take apical and radial pulses, as instructed by the physician. Be prepared to obtain medication from the crash cart or use a defibrillator if required.

Ventricular fibrillation (VF) is an abnormal heart rhythm. It is the most common cause of cardiac arrest. During VF the heart's rhythm becomes chaotic and the heart does not pump blood. The treatment for VF is defibrillation using a medical device called a defibrillator. This device works by delivering an electrical shock to the heart, which interrupts the chaotic rhythm. Defibrillators are effective only if used within minutes of the patient's collapse. An **automated external defibrillator (AED)** is a computerized defibrillator programmed to recognize VF and other lethal heart rhythms (Figure 26-15). These devices are found in many public places, including airports, but may also be used at the clinic where you are employed.

To use an AED, attach the adhesive electrode pads to the client's chest in a specific arrangement as determined by the manufacturer. Look at the illustration on the electrode's packing or machine. Activate the AED, and it will analyze the rhythm of the heart and determine if a shock is required. Pressing the "Shock" button will deliver an electrical charge to the patient's heart by way of the AED's electrode wires, which are attached to the chest.

In order to use an AED, you must be properly trained. Training is included as part of the CPR courses of the American Red Cross and the American Heart Association. Obtaining CPR and first aid certification will be an asset to you as a medical assistant.

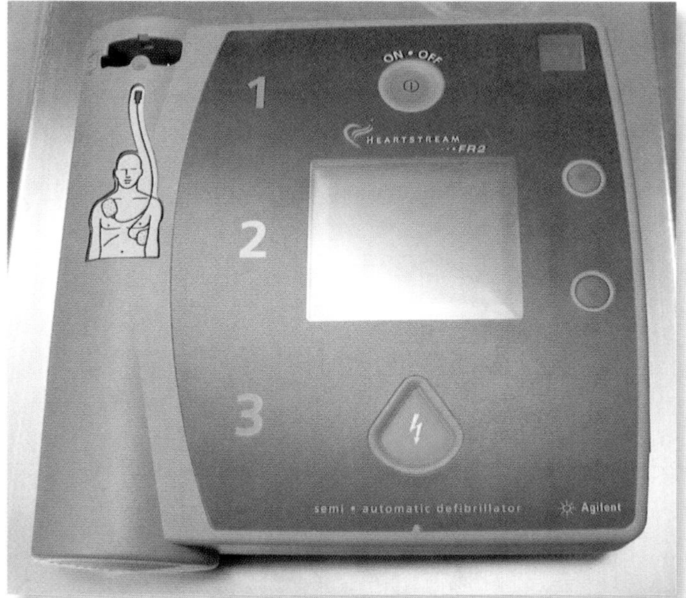

Figure 26-15. An automated external defibrillator delivers an electric current to the heart to stop a chaotic rhythm such as ventricular defibrillation.

PROCEDURE 26.8

Performing Cardiopulmonary Resuscitation (CPR)

Objective: To provide ventilation and blood circulation for a patient who shows none

OSHA Guidelines

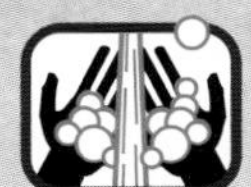 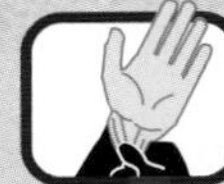 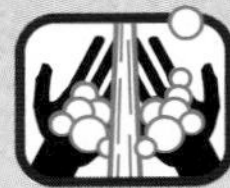

Materials: Mouth shield, or if not in the office, a piece of plastic with a hole for the mouth

Method

1. Check responsiveness:
   - Tap shoulder.
   - Ask "Are you OK?"
2. If patient is unresponsive, call 911 or the local emergency number or have someone place the call for you.
3. Open the patient's airway:
   - Tilt the patient's head back, using the head tilt–chin lift maneuver (Figure 26-16). Use the jaw thrust if the patient has a suspected neck or back injury (Figure 26-17). Look in mouth and remove any obvious obstructions.
4. Check for breathing:
   - Place your ear next to the patient's mouth, turn your head, and watch the chest.
   - Look for the chest to rise and fall, listen for sounds coming out of the mouth or nose, and feel for air movement.

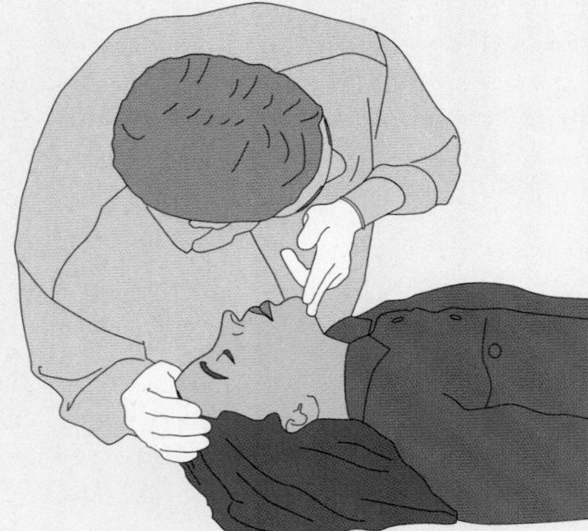

Figure 26-16. Use the head tilt–chin lift maneuver to open an airway.

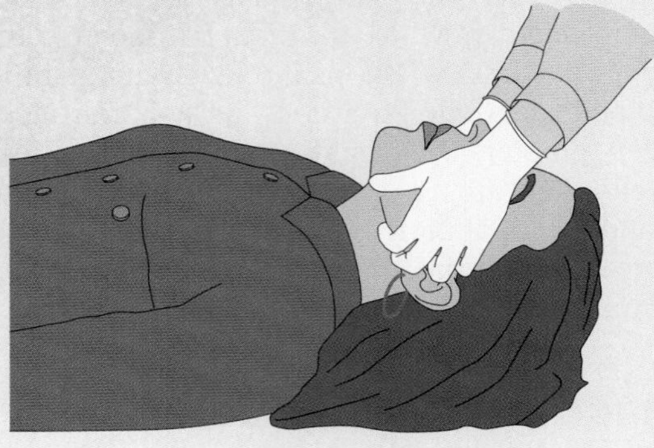

Figure 26-17. Use the jaw thrust maneuver for a patient with a neck injury.

   - If the patient is breathing, place him in the **recovery position:**
     - Kneel beside the patient and place the arm closest to you straight out from the body. Position the far arm with the back of the hand against the patient's near cheek.
     - Grab and bend the patient's far knee.
     - Protecting the patient's head with one hand, gently roll him toward you by pulling the opposite knee over and to the ground.
     - Position the top leg to balance the patient onto his side.
     - Tilt his head up slightly so that the airway is open. Make sure that his hand is under his cheek. Place a blanket or coat over the person, and stay close until help arrives.
   - If the patient is not breathing or has inadequate breathing, give two slow rescue breaths, which should be given at two seconds per breath using one of three methods:
     1. Mouth-to-mouth or mouth-to-nose rescue breathing (Figures 26-18 and 26-19):
        - Place your mouth around the patient's mouth and pinch the nose, or close the patient's mouth and place your mouth around the patient's nose.
        - Deliver two slow breaths. Use a face shield.
     2. Mouth-to-mask device (Figure 26-20).
     3. Bag-valve-mask ventilation (Figure 26-21).
   - Ensure the adequate rise and fall of the patient's chest. If his chest does not rise, reposition the airway and try again. If on the

continued ⟶

PROCEDURE 26.8

Performing Cardiopulmonary Resuscitation (CPR) *(continued)*

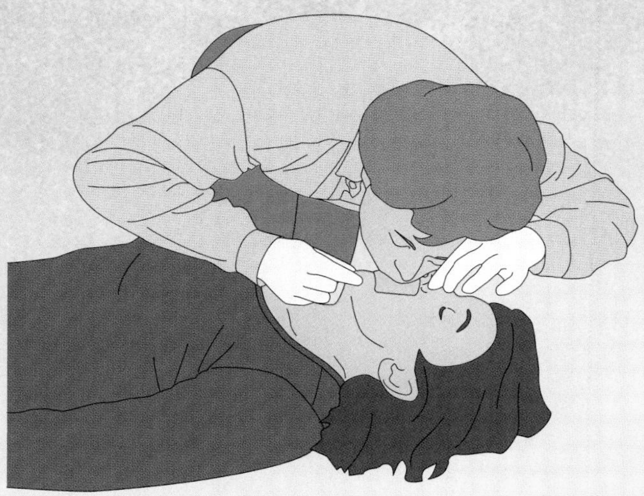

Figure 26-18. Perform mouth-to-mouth rescue breathing.

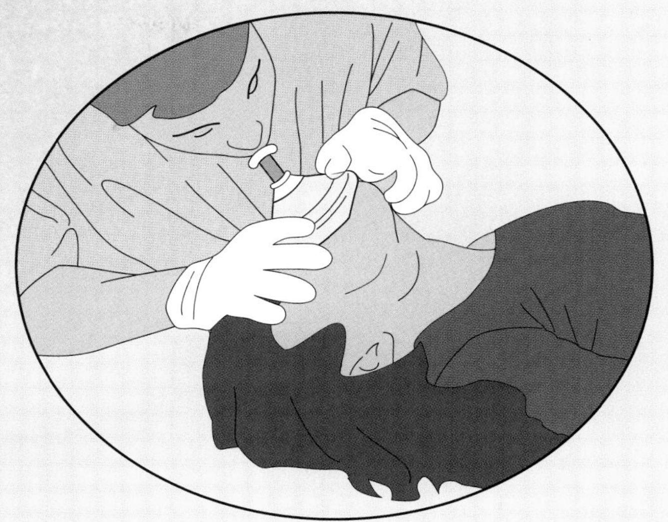

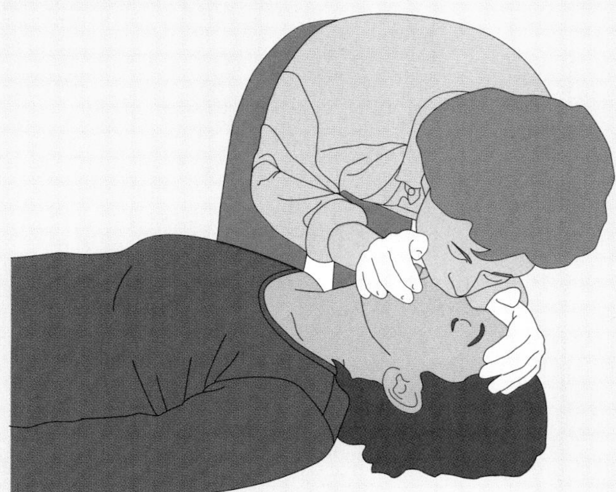

Figure 26-19. Use mouth-to-nose breathing if mouth-to-mouth breathing is not possible.

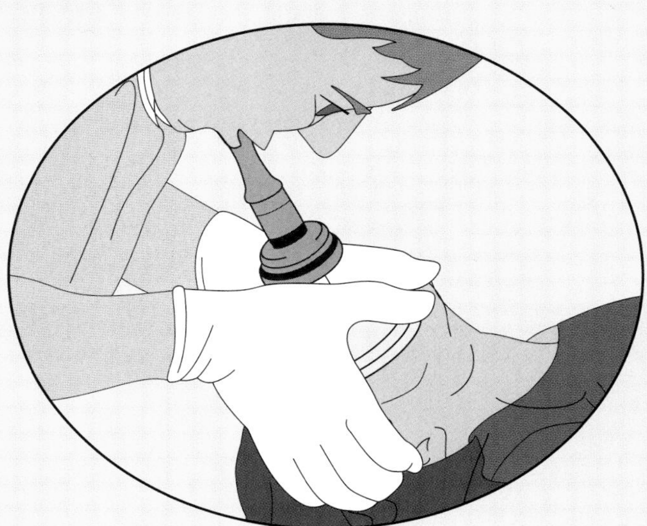

Figure 26-20. The side or the head technique can be used when performing mouth-to-mask ventilations. *Source: Glencoe Health Care Science Technology,* Booth 2004, p. 98.

second attempt the chest does not rise, your patient may have an airway obstruction. See Procedure 26-3.

5. Check for signs of circulation.
   - Check for adequate breathing, coughing, movement, and normal skin color.
   - Check for a carotid pulse:
     - Locate the patient's windpipe or trachea with your index and middle fingers.
     - Slide your fingers into the groove between the windpipe and the side of neck.
     - Feel for a pulse for a complete 5 to 10 seconds.
   - If the patient is not breathing but other signs of circulation are present, give rescue breaths at a rate of one every 5 seconds.
   - If you cannot determine whether the patient has a pulse or signs of circulation, start CPR

continued ⟶

PROCEDURE 26.8

Performing Cardiopulmonary Resuscitation (CPR) *(continued)*

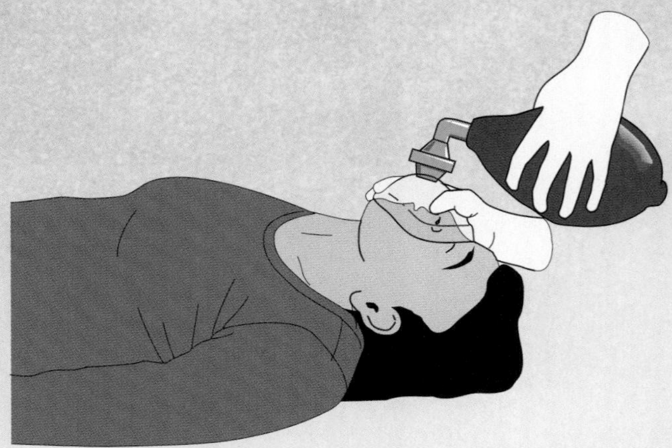

Figure 26-21. When using the bag-valve-mask ventilation, circle the top edges of the mask with your thumb and index finger and use your other three fingers to lift the jaw and open the airway.

Source: Glencoe Health Care Science Technology, Booth 2004, p.101, Figure 4-8.

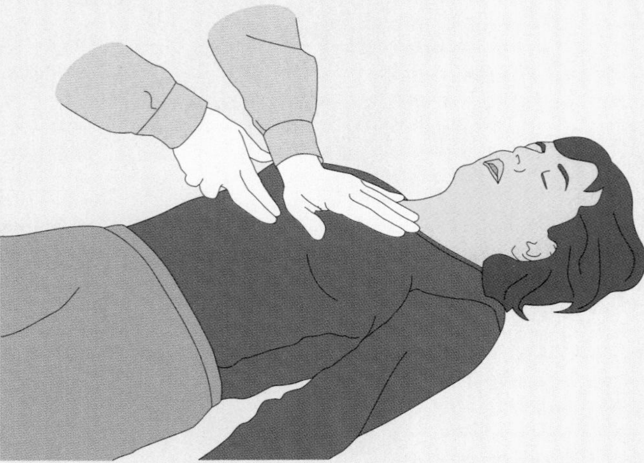

Figure 26-22. Place your hands above the xiphoid process.

and prepare to use an AED if an AED is available and you are trained to use it.

6. Perform CPR.

- Place two fingers on the lower end of the patient's rib cage, on the side closest to you.
- Slide your fingers up the patient's rib cage to the notch where the ribs meet the lower sternum.
- Place the heel of one hand just above your two fingers on the lower half of the sternum, and then place your other hand on top of the first.

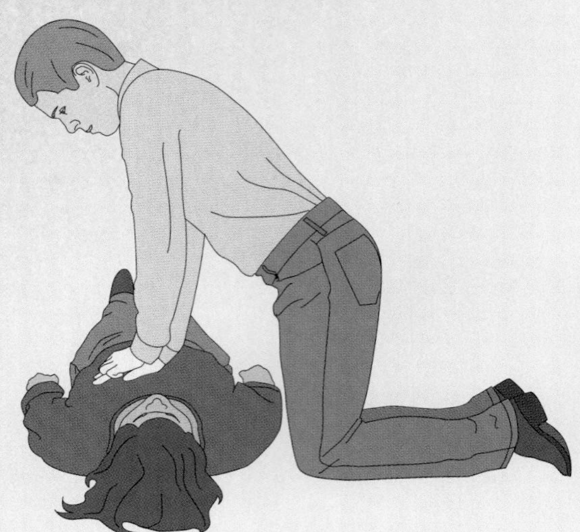

Figure 26-23. Align your shoulders directly over the victim's sternum, with your elbows locked.

The proper location for chest compression is between the nipples (Figure 26-22).

- Lean forward so your shoulders are over the patient, keeping your arms straight (Figure 26-23).
- Keep the heel of your hand on the patient's chest but make sure your fingers are kept off the chest.
- Give 15 chest compressions at a rate of 100 compressions per minute, followed by 2 slow rescue breaths for an adult.
- Push down on the sternum1½ to 2 inches with each compression.
- Allow the chest to return to its normal state between compressions.
- Continue cycles of 15:2 (15 chest compressions and 2 rescue breaths) for a total of four cycles or approximately one minute.

7. Recheck circulation.

- After four cycles of 15:2, which is about one minute, recheck the patient for signs of circulation.
- If the patient is not breathing and has no signs of circulation, resume CPR cycles beginning with chest compressions.
- If signs of circulation are present but patient is not breathing, give 1 rescue breath every 5 seconds.
- Recheck for signs of circulation every few minutes.

Hematemesis

Hematemesis is the vomiting of blood. A patient who vomits bright red blood may have a gastrointestinal disorder, such as a bleeding ulcer. A patient who vomits blood that looks like coffee grounds may have slow bleeding into the stomach.

Quickly check the vital signs of a patient with hematemesis. If pulse and breathing are rapid and blood pressure is low, the patient may be going into shock. Notify the doctor immediately, and get the crash cart to help the doctor start an intravenous line to replace lost fluid. Then call the EMS system.

Obstetric Emergencies

If you work in an obstetric practice, you may see emergencies that are unique to this specialty. Although the physician handles most obstetric emergencies, you can assist by asking the patient specific questions about her problem so that the physician can decide what treatment is necessary.

Set up written protocols to handle these situations. For example, if the patient calls from home and reports gushing vaginal bleeding, your protocol may be to call the EMS system for her and tell her to lie down with her feet elevated. If the patient has a miscarriage, have her bring the expelled tissue with her to the office or hospital.

If you work in an obstetrician's office, you must also know how to assist a physician with an emergency childbirth. If there is no physician present when the emergency occurs, however, whether it is inside or outside the office, summon help and begin the procedure on your own. Never try to delay delivery when a birth is imminent. Procedure 26-9 describes how to assist with an emergency childbirth.

Respiratory Arrest

Respiratory arrest, or lack of breathing, is usually preceded by symptoms of respiratory distress. Symptoms include difficulty breathing, rapid breathing, palpitations, racing pulse, high or low blood pressure, sweating, pale or bluish skin, and decreasing level of consciousness. If a patient shows these symptoms, notify the doctor right away. If the patient develops respiratory arrest, have someone call the doctor and the EMS system while you perform CPR as described in Procedure 26-8.

Seizures

A **seizure,** or convulsion, is a series of violent and involuntary contractions of the muscles. Seizures are usually related to brain malfunctions that can result from diseased or injured brain tissues. A seizure may be caused by high fever, epilepsy (a brain disorder that causes seizures with varying severity), meningitis, diabetic states, and many other medical problems.

Follow this emergency care for seizure patients.

1. Remove objects that may cause injury.
2. Place the patient on the floor or the ground. If possible, position him on his side with his head turned to the side to help keep the airway open and unobstructed by the tongue. This position is especially important if the patient vomits, to prevent aspiration of vomitus into the lungs.
3. Loosen restrictive clothing, and never place anything in the patient's mouth.
4. Protect the patient from injury, but do not try to hold him still during convulsions.
5. After convulsions end, keep the patient at rest, positioned for drainage from the mouth.
6. Make sure the patient is breathing. If he is not, begin rescue breathing.
7. Take vital signs and monitor respirations closely.
8. Move the patient to an examination room, or have him taken to a medical facility.

Shock

Generally speaking, shock is a life-threatening state associated with failure of the cardiovascular system. It can bring to a stop all normal metabolic functions. This condition prevents the vital organs from receiving blood.

Early symptoms of shock include restlessness; irritability; fear; rapid pulse; pale, cool skin; and increased respiratory rate. Treat a patient in shock by elevating the feet 8 to 12 inches. If you suspect a head injury, however, keep the patient flat or elevate the head and shoulders slightly. Monitor the patient's ABCs and take steps to control bleeding. If the patient is chilly, wrap the patient in a blanket. Call the EMS system.

Several types of shock are possible. Anaphylactic shock, or anaphylaxis, is usually associated with an allergic reaction, as previously discussed. Hypovolemic shock and septic shock are two other types of shock.

Hypovolemic Shock. **Hypovolemic shock** results from insufficient blood volume in the circulatory system. It occurs after an injury that causes major fluid loss. Hemorrhage or burns can cause this type of fluid loss. Patients with hypovolemic shock must be transported to an emergency facility immediately.

Septic Shock. **Septic shock** results from massive, widespread infection that affects the ability of the blood vessels to circulate blood. Common causes are urinary tract infection (especially in older adults), postpartum infection, and a variety of infections in patients with immunosuppression (as caused by chemotherapy or acquired immunodeficiency syndrome [AIDS]).

Stroke (Brain Attack)

A **stroke,** or cerebrovascular accident (CVA), occurs when the blood supply to the brain is impaired. This impairment

PROCEDURE 26.9

Assisting With Emergency Childbirth

Objective: To assist in performing an emergency childbirth

OSHA Guidelines

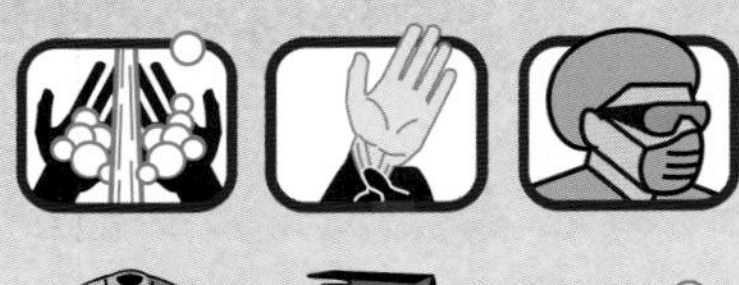

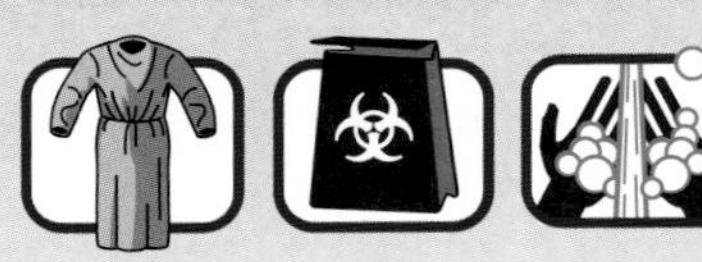

Materials: Clean cloths, sterile or clean sheets or towels, two sterile clamps or two pieces of string boiled in water for at least 10 minutes, sterile scissors, plastic bag, soft blankets or towels

Method

1. Ask the woman her name and age, how far apart her contractions are (about two per minute signals that the birth is near), if her water has broken, and if she feels straining or pressure as if the baby is coming.
2. Help remove the woman's lower clothing.
3. Explain that you are about to do a visual inspection to see if the baby's head is in position. Ask the woman to lie on her back with her thighs spread, her knees flexed, and her feet flat. Examine her to see if there is crowning (a bulging at the vaginal opening from the baby's head) (see Figure 26-24).
4. If the head is crowning, childbirth is imminent. Place clean cloths under the woman's buttocks, and use sterile sheets or towels (if they are available) to cover her legs and stomach.
5. Wash your hands thoroughly and put on examination gloves. If other PPE is available, put it on now.
6. At this point the physician would begin to take steps to deliver the baby, and you would position yourself at the woman's head to provide emotional support and help in case she vomited. If no physician is available, position yourself at the woman's side so that you have a constant view of the vaginal opening.
7. Talk to the woman and encourage her to relax between contractions while allowing the delivery to proceed naturally.
8. Position your gloved hands at the woman's vaginal opening when the baby's head starts to appear. Do not touch her skin.
9. Place one hand below the baby's head as it is delivered. Spread your fingers evenly around the baby's head to support it so that it does not touch the mother's anal area. Use your other hand to help cradle the baby's head (see Figure 26-25). Never pull on the baby.
10. If the umbilical cord is wrapped around the baby's neck, gently loosen the cord and slide it over the baby's head.

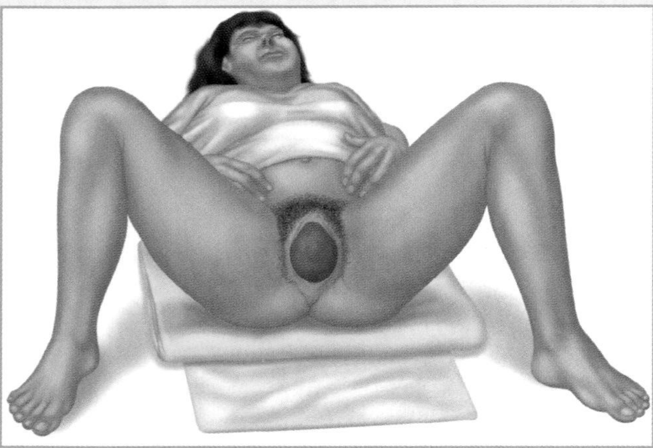

Figure 26-24. Crowning occurs when part of the baby's head becomes visible with each contraction.

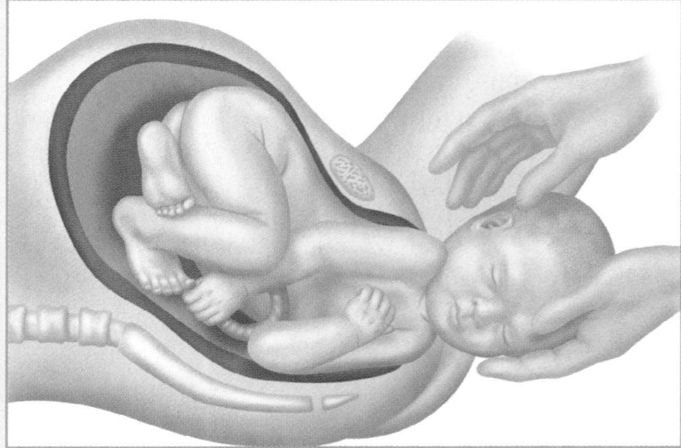

Figure 26-25. Support the baby's head with one hand while using the other hand to cradle the baby's head.

continued ⟶

PROCEDURE 26.9

Assisting With Emergency Childbirth *(continued)*

11. If the amniotic sac has not broken by the time the baby's head is delivered, use your finger to puncture the membrane. Then pull the membranes away from the baby's mouth and nose.
12. Wipe blood or mucus from the baby's mouth with a clean cloth.
13. Continue to support the baby's head as the shoulders emerge. The upper shoulder will deliver first, followed quickly by the lower shoulder.
14. After the feet are delivered, lay the baby on his side with the head slightly lower than the body. Keep the baby at the same level as the mother until you cut the umbilical cord.
15. If the baby is not breathing, lower the head, raise the lower part of the body, and tap the soles of the feet. If the baby is still not breathing, begin rescue breathing through the mouth and nose as directed in this chapter.
16. To cut the cord, wait several minutes, until pulsations stop. Use the clamps or pieces of string to tie the cord in two places.
17. Use sterilized scissors to cut the cord in between the placement of the two clamps or pieces of string.
18. Within 10 minutes of the baby's birth, the placenta will begin to expel. Save it in a plastic bag for further examination.
19. Keep the mother and baby warm by wrapping them in towels or blankets. Do not touch the baby any more than necessary.
20. Massage the mother's abdomen just below the navel every few minutes to control internal bleeding.
21. Arrange for transport of the mother and baby to the hospital.

may cause temporary or permanent damage, depending on how long the brain cells are deprived of oxygen.

A minor stroke can cause headache, confusion, dizziness, tinnitus, minor speech difficulties, personality changes, weakness of the limbs, and memory loss. A major stroke typically produces loss of consciousness, paralysis on one side of the body, difficulty swallowing, loss of bladder and bowel control, slurred or garbled speech, and unequal pupil size.

If a patient has a stroke in the office, notify the physician at once, and call the EMS system. Maintain the patient's airway by turning the head toward the affected side to allow secretions to drain out rather than be aspirated. Loosen tight clothing. If directed by the physician, monitor vital signs and administer oxygen.

Toxic Shock Syndrome

Toxic shock syndrome (TSS) is an acute infection caused by the bacterium *Staphylococcus aureas.* The toxin produced by the bacterium can enter the body through a break in the skin or through the uterus. Although the infection is most common in menstruating women who are using tampons at the time of onset, the link between tampon use and TSS is unclear.

TSS symptoms include high fever, intense muscle aches, vomiting, diarrhea, headache, bouts of violent shivering, vaginal discharge, red eyes, and a decreased level of consciousness. A sign specific to TSS is a deep red rash on the palms of the hands and the soles of the feet. This skin then sloughs off. A menstruating patient with these symptoms should be instructed to remove the tampon immediately and replace it with a sanitary napkin.

TSS is treated in the medical office with intravenous antibiotics and fluids. The patient will require hospitalization, however.

Viral Encephalitis

Viral encephalitis is a severe inflammation of the brain caused directly by a virus or secondary to a complication resulting from a viral infection. Viral encephalitis may result from an epidemic, or it may arise sporadically. This condition requires accurate identification and prompt treatment. Symptoms develop suddenly, beginning with fever, headache, and vomiting. They quickly progress to stiff neck and back, decreased level of consciousness (from drowsiness to coma), and paralysis and seizures.

The level of consciousness must be monitored frequently in a patient with viral encephalitis. Prepare the patient for treatment with antiviral drugs, and arrange for transport to a hospital for a spinal tap and other diagnostic tests.

TABLE 26-2 Resources for Patient Assistance

Resource	Contact Information
Al-Anon and Alateen	www.al-anon.alateen.org/ 888-4AL-ANON (425-2666) WSO@al-anon.org
Alcoholics Anonymous	www.alcoholics-anonymous.org/ 212-870-3400 PO Box 459, Grand Central Station New York, NY 10163
Child Abuse Hotline	www.childhelpusa.org/ 800-422-4453 or 480-922-8212 Fax: 480-922-7061 15757 N. 78th Street Scottsdale, AZ 85260
Mothers Against Drunk Driving (MADD)	www.madd.org/ 800-GET-MADD (438-6233) MADD National Office 511 E. John Carpenter Frwy, Suite 700 Irving, TX 75062
Narcotics Anonymous	www.na.org/ 818-773-9999 Fax: 818-700-0700 World Service Office in Los Angeles PO Box 9999 Van Nuys, CA 91409
National Center on Child Abuse and Neglect	www.ojjdp.ncjrs.org/pubs/fedresources/ag-05.html 202-205-8586 Fax: 202-260-9351 PO Box 1182 Washington, DC 20013-1182
National Institute for Alcohol Abuse and Alcoholism (NIAAA)	www.niaaa.nih.gov/ 6000 Executive Boulevard, Willco Building Bethesda, MD 20892-7003
National Coalition Against Domestic Violence	www.ncadv.org/ 800-799-SAFE (7233)
National Committee to Prevent Child Abuse	www.childabuse.org/ Childhelp USA National Child Abuse Hotline: 1-800-4-A-CHILD (422-4453)
National Council on Child Abuse and Family Violence	www.nccafv.org/ 202-429-6695 FAX: 831-655-3930 1025 Connecticut Ave. NW, Suite 1012 Washington, DC 20036 info@NCCAFV.org
National Domestic Violence Hotline	www.ndvh.org/ 800-787-3224

continued ⟶

TABLE 26-2 Resources for Patient Assistance (*continued*)

Resource	Contact Information
National Families in Action Drug Information Center	www.nationalfamilies.org/ 404-248-9676 Fax: 404-248-1312 2957 Clairmont Road NE, Suite 150 Atlanta, GA 30329
National Institutes on Drug Abuse	www.nida.nih.gov/ 301-443-1124 6001 Executive Boulevard, Room 5213 Bethesda, MD 20892-9561 Information@lists.nida.nih.gov
National Organization for Victim Assistance	www.try-nova.org/ 800-TRY-NOVA (879-6692) 1730 Park Road NW Washington, DC 20010
Students Against Destructive Decisions	www.saddonline.com/ 877-SADD-INC (723-3462) Fax: 508-481-5759 PO Box 800 Marlborough, MA 01752

Common Psychosocial Emergencies

You will probably encounter psychosocial emergencies in the medical office at some point. These may result from drug or alcohol abuse, spousal abuse, child abuse, or elder abuse. Handle these situations as you were directed in Chapters 18 and 22. If you encounter patients who have overdosed on drugs, exhibit violent behavior, mention suicide, or have been raped, follow the specific clinical responsibilities described in this section.

You may also be responsible for referring patients with psychosocial emergencies to resources in the community. Some of these resources are listed in Table 26-2.

A patient who is overdosing on drugs can suffer serious medical problems and can even die. If a patient who has taken an overdose is brought to the medical office, call the EMS system immediately, and arrange for transport to the hospital.

Patients on drugs may become violent during withdrawal from the substance or while under the influence. If, at any time, a patient becomes aggressive or threatening, follow office protocol for handling violent behavior. The protocol should state when to call the police, how to document the incident, and when to notify the insurance carrier.

During a psychosocial emergency, a patient may tell you he is so depressed that he has thought about killing himself. Allow the patient to talk freely. Listen carefully without interrupting. Whenever a patient mentions suicide or talks about life in ways that make you suspect suicidal tendencies, discuss your suspicions with the physician. Take comments on suicide seriously, no matter how casual they may seem.

Victims of rape may be of any age and either gender, but more than 90% are women. If a patient says she has been raped, provide privacy. Limit the number of people who ask her questions. She may feel traumatized, embarrassed, and fearful. Do not make her go through the office routine at this time.

If the physician asks you to speak to the patient, explain to her that you are legally required to contact the police so that they can file a report. The patient can decide later whether she wishes to press charges.

Contact the local rape hotline, and request that a rape counselor come to the office to stay with the patient during the examination and police report procedures. The physician should be familiar with state laws for collecting specimens and the protocol for caring for a rape victim.

The procedure of ensuring that a specimen is obtained from the victim and is correctly identified, that the specimen is under the uninterrupted control of authorized personnel, and that the specimen has not been altered or replaced is called establishing **chain of custody.** This procedure is required for medicolegal issues such as evidence of rape as well as for drug tests for illicit drug use. If the chain between the victim and the specimen cannot be proved to have remained unbroken, the specimen must be considered invalid.

CHAIN OF CUSTODY FORM

MADISON CLINICAL LABORATORY

195 North Parkway
Madison, WA 90869
(608) 555-3030

SPECIMEN I.D. NO:

STEP 1—TO BE COMPLETED BY COLLECTOR OR EMPLOYER REPRESENTATIVE.

Employer Name, Address, and I.D. No.: ______ OR Medical Review Officer Name and Address: ______

Donor Social Security No. or Employee I.D. No.: ______

Donor I.D. verified: ❒ Photo I.D. ❒ Employer Representative ______ Signature

Reason for test: (check one) ❒ Preemployment ❒ Random ❒ Postaccident ❒ Periodic ❒ Reasonable suspicion/cause ❒ Return to duty ❒ Other (specify)

Test(s) to be performed: ______ Total tests ordered: ☐

Type of specimen obtained: ❒ Urine ❒ Blood ❒ Semen ❒ Other (specify)

Submit only one specimen with each requisition.

STEP 2—TO BE COMPLETED BY COLLECTOR.

For urine specimens, read temperature within 4 minutes of collection.
Check here if specimen temperature is within range. ❒ Yes, 90°–100°F/32°–38°C
Or record actual temperature here: ______

STEP 3—TO BE COMPLETED BY COLLECTOR.

Collection site: ______ Address ______
City ______ State ______ Zip ______ Phone ______
Collection date: ______ Time: ______ ❒ a.m. ❒ p.m.

I certify that the specimen identified on this form is the specimen presented to me by the donor identified in step 1 above, and that it was collected, labeled, and sealed in the donor's presence.

Collector's name: ______ Signature of collector ______

STEP 4—TO BE INITIATED BY DONOR AND COMPLETED AS NECESSARY THEREAFTER.

Purpose of change	Released by Signature	Received by Signature	Date
A. Provide specimen for testing			
B. Shipment to Laboratory			
C.			

Comments:

STEP 5—TO BE COMPLETED BY THE LABORATORY:

Specimen package seal(s) intact when received in lab? ❒ Yes ❒ No. If no, explain.
Laboratory receiver's initials ______

Copy 1 - Original - Must accompany specimen to laboratory.

Figure 26-26. The chain of custody form provides documentation that specific specimen collection safeguards have been followed.

The first link in the chain of custody is collecting the specimen. Semen specimens are commonly collected for typing in a rape examination. Other samples collected from the victim's body and clothing may include hair and skin that can help identify the offender.

Proper specimen identification is important. Without it, the chain of custody is broken at the beginning. If you are responsible for collecting the specimen, you must be sure the specimen is collected from the correct patient and that no one tampers with it. The chain of custody form (see Figure 26-26) must be completed correctly, and the patient may be required to sign or initial the form as well.

Multiple copies of the form are used as a safeguard system. One copy, usually the original, accompanies the specimen in a sealed envelope. Another copy is attached to the outside of the envelope so that each person who handles the specimen can initial the form. A third copy is usually retained in the patient's file.

These general procedures help maintain an intact chain of custody. Always refer to your office's procedures to make sure you are meeting all relevant requirements.

The Patient Under Stress

In emergency situations patients and family members are under a great deal of stress. You must realize that people react differently to emergency situations. You can learn how to detect signs of extreme stress by being alert for patients whose behavior varies from that previously observed or who cannot focus or follow directions.

Your role during many emergency situations may be to keep victims and their families and friends calm. You can promote calmness by listening carefully and giving your full attention. Your first priority, at all times, is the victim's well-being. If he is very distraught, for example, hold his hand while the doctor examines him. If one of his relatives is crying and causing him to become emotional, suggest that the relative do something to help—for example, fill out paperwork in another room.

You may face special challenges when communicating with victims during emergencies. Victims may not speak your language, or they may have a visual or hearing impairment. In such instances, follow these guidelines.

- Use gestures throughout the process for non-English-speaking victims. Continue to speak, however, because they may be able to understand some English.
- Tell patients who have visual impairments what you are going to do before you do it, and maintain voice and touch contact while caring for them.
- Ask patients who have hearing impairments whether they can read lips. If they can, speak slowly to them and never turn away while you are speaking. If they cannot read lips, communicate by writing and using gestures. At all times try to remain face-to-face and keep direct physical contact.

Educating the Patient

During minor medical emergencies, after major emergencies have been resolved, and during routine office visits, you can educate patients about ways to prevent and handle various medical emergencies. For example, you might tell them how to contact the local American Red Cross office, post notices of upcoming classes that the Red Cross offers, and encourage patients and family members to learn basic first aid. You might also develop a first-aid kit checklist and make it available to patients and families.

Make sure that all family members, including children, are familiar with the local EMS system and know how to contact it in an emergency. Suggest that families keep emergency numbers by the telephone. In addition, teach parents how to childproof their home for children of various ages. Remember that childproofing differs for different children—for example, for children who can crawl as opposed to children who can walk.

Provide brief, easy-to-read handouts to reinforce the information you present to patients. Prepare handouts in multiple languages if you provide care for non-English-speaking patients. Find and use patient education resources for the types of patients seen by the practice. For example, if you work in an obstetric office, obtain educational materials for pregnant and postpartum patients from companies that provide pregnancy-related products. Ask company representatives what materials are available. Many companies provide free videos and booklets.

Disasters

Your skills in dealing with emergencies, including first-aid and CPR training, will be an enormous help to your community in the event of a disaster. To be fully effective, you must also be familiar with standard protocols for responding to disasters. Table 26-3 shows ways that you can help in certain types of disasters. You may even want to participate in fire or other disaster drills to familiarize yourself with emergency procedures.

Disasters can occur in any community. Two of the most common types of disasters are floods and hurricanes. One of the biggest floods in the United States occurred in the Midwest in the summer of 1993. Even before national disaster relief personnel could respond, local medical personnel were called to the scene to triage injured and displaced residents. In this type of disaster, many people suffer from emotional shock (which often results in physical problems), injuries, and illnesses. These people require skilled medical assistance.

Bioterrorism

Bioterrorism is the intentional release of a biologic agent with the intent to harm individuals. The CDC defines a biologic agent as a weapon when it is easy to disseminate,

TABLE 26-3 Assisting in Disasters

Type of Disaster	Action to Take
Weather disaster, such as flood or hurricane	Report to the community command post. Have your credentials with you. Receive an identifying tag or vest and assignment. Accept only an assignment that is appropriate for your abilities. Expect to be part of a team. Document what medical care each victim receives on each person's disaster tag.
Office fire	Activate the alarm system. Use a fire extinguisher if the fire is confined to a small container, such as a trash can. Turn off oxygen. Shut windows and doors. Seal doors with wet cloths to prevent smoke from entering. If evacuation is necessary, proceed quietly and calmly. Direct ambulatory patients and family members to the appropriate exit route. Assist patients who need help leaving the building.

has a high potential for mortality, can cause a public panic or social disruption, and requires public health preparedness. There are numerous biologic agents identified as weapons, including anthrax, tularemia, smallpox, plague, and botulism. The CDC maintains an Internet site with current information about identified biologic agents at www.bt.cdc.gov.

Physicians' offices will be on the front lines should a biologic agent be intentionally released. It will be up to physicians and their staff to sound the alarm to public

PROCEDURE 26.10

Performing Triage in a Disaster

Objective: To prioritize disaster victims

OSHA Guidelines

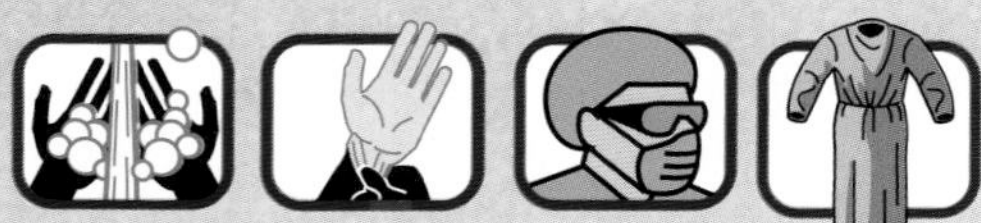

Materials: Disaster tag and pen

Method

1. Wash your hands and put on examination gloves and other PPE if available.
2. Quickly assess each victim.
3. Sort victims by type of injury and need for care, classifying them as emergent, urgent, nonurgent, or dead.
4. Label the emergent patients no. 1, and send them to appropriate treatment stations immediately. Emergent patients, such as those who are in shock or who are hemorrhaging, need immediate care.
5. Label the urgent patients no. 2, and send them to basic first-aid stations. Urgent patients need care within the next several hours. Such patients may have lacerations that can be dressed quickly to stop the bleeding but can wait for suturing.
6. Label nonurgent patients no. 3, and send them to volunteers who will be empathic and provide refreshments. Nonurgent patients are those for whom timing of treatment is not critical, such as patients who have no physical injuries but who are emotionally upset.
7. Label patients who are dead no. 4. Ensure that the bodies are moved to an area where they will be safe until they can be identified and proper action can be taken.

officials that something may be amiss. Physicians and medical assistants should be vigilant about cases that present themselves as well as common trends in syndromes. Be on the lookout for unusual patterns in affected patients. Indications of a bioterrorist attack might include many patients having been in the same place at the same time or an unusual distribution for common illnesses, such as an increase in chickenpox-like illness in adults that might be smallpox.

If you suspect that bioterrorism is responsible for an illness, report your suspicians to the physician. It is the responsibility of your facility to immediately contact the local public health department. The information about the patient should be recorded, and appropriate tests should be performed. The laboratory should be notified of the potential for bioterrorism. Additionally, consultations with specialists and discussions of all findings are necessary when bioterrorism is suspected. The following is a list of clues of a bioterroristic attack as defined by the American College of Physicians—American Society of Internal Medicine.

- Unusual temporal or geographic clustering of illness
- Unusual age distribution of common disease, such as an illness that appears to be chickenpox in adults but is really smallpox
- A large epidemic with greater caseloads than expected, especially in a discrete population
- More severe disease than expected
- Unusual route of exposure
- A disease that is outside its normal transmission season or is impossible to transmit naturally in the absence of its normal vector
- Multiple simultaneous epidemics of different diseases
- A disease outbreak with health consequences to humans and animals
- Unusual strains or variants of organisms or antimicrobial resistance patterns

In any disaster, you may be asked to perform triage. When you perform triage, you give each injured victim a tag that classifies the person as emergent (needing immediate care), urgent (needing care within several hours), nonurgent (needing care when time is not critical), or dead. The triage process is outlined in Procedure 26-10.

Summary

A medical emergency can occur anywhere—in a doctor's office, at home, in a restaurant, or on the street. The more you learn about handling each type of medical emergency, the more valuable your contributions to the situation become. You can make a substantial, positive difference in the health and lives of people who face medical emergencies to which you respond.

Always notify the doctor or the local EMS system when you encounter a medical emergency. Do not, at any time, perform procedures you have not been trained to do. Use common sense, assess the situation and the patient's condition, and provide first aid until a doctor or EMT arrives.

Patients having a medical emergency are often under extreme stress. Remember to stay calm and communicate clearly. Communicating with non-English-speaking patients and those with visual or hearing impairments requires special skills. You can develop these skills through educational and training programs you seek out or during routine office visits with these patients.

You may not be present when medical emergencies occur, so patients need to know how to respond to emergency circumstances. Take every opportunity to educate patients about preventing and responding to medical emergencies. Remember to draw on community resources when you provide information or support to patients and their families. There will always be opportunities to expand your knowledge, skills, and network for dealing with medical emergencies in your medical assisting work.

REVIEW

CHAPTER 26

CASE STUDY QUESTIONS

Now that you have completed this chapter, review the case study at the beginning of the chapter. Consider each situation and determine the order in which you will respond. Explain your decisions.

Discussion Questions

1. What should you do to prepare the medical office for emergencies?
2. How would you assist a person who was bleeding from accidental injuries if you had no personal protective equipment with you?
3. Why should you be certified in first aid and CPR?
4. A patient falls to the floor holding his chest in one of the examination rooms. What should you do?
5. A screaming young child is carried into your clinic with blood all over his left leg. The blood is dripping on the floor as the child is brought into the examination room. What should you do?

Critical Thinking Questions

1. A 27-year-old male patient with diabetes comes to the office for treatment of an upper respiratory infection. While in the waiting room, he begins to sweat profusely and becomes restless and confused. What should you do and why?
2. One of the office secretaries confesses to you that she has become addicted to painkillers. She asks for your help, but she does not want you to tell anyone about her problem because she is afraid of losing her job. What should you do?
3. A 39-year-old female patient has visited your office many times. Today, however, you notice that she is disheveled and anxious. After you greet her, she describes general, nonspecific complaints in a sad, tired tone of voice. What should you do?
4. An infant has been burned on his entire chest and the left arm. What percentage of his body is burned? An adult has the same burns. What percentage of her body has been burned?

Application Activities

1. Demonstrate first aid for choking, using mock abdominal thrusts on a classmate. Switch roles and have the classmate demonstrate the variations needed for a pregnant or obese patient. Critique each other's technique.
2. Demonstrate on a classmate how to stop bleeding from a large laceration on the lower arm. Switch roles and critique each other's technique.
3. As a class, divide into one large group and one small group. Students in the large group should role-play victims of a natural disaster such as an earthquake. Students in the small group should role-play medical assistants helping at the scene of the disaster. The victims should describe and role-play their conditions. On the basis of the descriptions and apparent conditions, the medical assistants should perform triage on the group of victims.
4. With a partner, practice applying bandages to each other. Use Figure 26-14 as a reference. After each bandage is applied, check it for correctness, and check the skin color and circulation of each area bandaged.

Internet Activity

Research the Internet for the latest information about one possible bioterroristic threat. Create a brochure or report regarding the agent you research. You can start your research at the CDC Web site at **www.bt.cdc.gov.**

SECTION 5

PHYSICIAN'S OFFICE LABORATORY PROCEDURES

CHAPTER 27

Laboratory Equipment and Safety

KEY TERMS

artifact
biohazard symbol
centrifuge
Certificate of Waiver tests
Clinical Laboratory Improvement Amendments of 1988 (CLIA '88)
compound microscope
control sample
electron microscope
hazard label
objectives
ocular
oil-immersion objective
optical microscope
photometer
physician's office laboratory (POL)
proficiency testing program
qualitative test response
quality assurance program
quality control program
quantitative test result
reagent
reference laboratory
standard
10× lens

AREAS OF COMPETENCE

2003 Role Delineation Study

CLINICAL

Fundamental Principles

- Apply principles of aseptic technique and infection control
- Comply with quality assurance practices
- Screen and follow up patient test results

Diagnostic Orders

- Collect and process specimens

GENERAL

Legal Concepts

- Prepare and maintain medical records
- Implement and maintain federal and state health-care legislation and regulations
- Comply with established risk management and safety procedures
- Recognize professional credentialing criteria

CHAPTER OUTLINE

- The Role of Laboratory Testing in Patient Care
- The Medical Assistant's Role
- Use of Laboratory Equipment
- Safety in the Laboratory
- Quality Assurance Programs
- Communicating With the Patient
- Record Keeping

OBJECTIVES

After completing Chapter 27, you will be able to:

27.1 Describe the purpose of the physician's office laboratory.
27.2 List the medical assistant's duties in the physician's office laboratory.
27.3 Identify important pieces of laboratory equipment.
27.4 Operate a microscope.
27.5 Identify the regulatory controls governing procedures completed in the physician's office laboratory.
27.6 Identify measures to prevent accidents.

OBJECTIVES *(Continued)*

27.7 Describe correct waste disposal procedures.

27.8 Describe the need for quality assurance and quality control programs.

27.9 Maintain accurate documentation, including all logs related to quality control.

27.10 List common reference materials to consult for information on procedures performed in the physician's office laboratory.

27.11 Communicate with patients regarding test preparation and follow-up.

27.12 Identify the medical assistant's record-keeping responsibilities.

Introduction

Laboratory testing of patients' specimens is an integral component of patient care. Medical assistants often find a role in the clinical laboratory setting, either in the physician's office or a hospital setting. This chapter will introduce you to various types of common laboratory equipment and their use. You will learn about safety in the laboratory mandated by OSHA regulations and steps to aid in preventing accidents. A discussion of the Clinical Laboratory Improvement Amendments of 1988 and this law's impact on the laboratory setting is included in this chapter for your understanding of quality assurance, quality control procedures, and required record keeping.

CASE STUDY

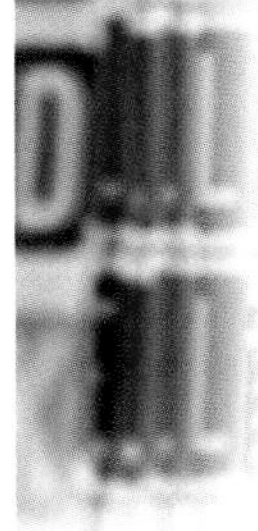

You have been employed as a medical assistant in a physician's office for approximately a year, and part of your duties include the performance of waived laboratory tests in the POL. The POL is supervised by a pathologist and is also staffed by a full-time medical laboratory technologist. When you arrive at the office one morning, you are informed by the office manager that the laboratory technologist has called in sick and that you will have to take over the performance of the Level I testing in addition to the waived testing. You have never been trained for the Level I testing, you do not know how to operate the instruments for this testing, nor are you familiar with the proper quality control procedure.

As you read this chapter, consider the following questions:

1. What is a POL?
2. What enactment regulates laboratories, personnel, and the testing they perform?
3. What is the difference between waived testing and Level I testing?
4. Does quality control have an impact on laboratories? If so, how?
5. Should you perform the testing as requested? Why or why not?

The Role of Laboratory Testing in Patient Care

Laboratory analysis of blood, urine, or other body fluids and substances provides three kinds of information about a patient. First, regular monitoring through laboratory tests, such as those that are part of an annual examination, can help a physician identify possible diseases or other problems. Second, specific tests can help confirm or contradict a physician's initial diagnosis. Third, laboratory testing can help a physician determine and monitor the proper dosage of a patient's medication.

Kinds of Laboratories

Some physicians prefer to have all laboratory tests performed by a **reference laboratory,** a laboratory owned and operated by an organization outside the practice. Other physicians choose to have some tests completed by the reference laboratory and some completed in the office in the **physician's office laboratory (POL).**

There are advantages and disadvantages to each method of managing laboratory analyses. Reference laboratories often have technological resources beyond those available in the POL. Using a reference laboratory frees a physician's staff from testing duties and allows more time for patient care. Furthermore, some managed care companies have contracts with laboratory companies that require their subscribers to use a specific reference laboratory. On the other hand, processing tests in the POL produces quicker turnaround and eliminates the need for the patient to travel to other test locations.

The Purpose of the Physician's Office Laboratory

Office policy determines which tests, if any, will be performed at your location and which tests will be performed by a reference laboratory. A POL, such as the one shown in Figure 27-1, is responsible for accurate and timely processing of routine tests, usually involving blood or urine, and for reporting test results to the physician. (A reference laboratory offers a complete range of tests in all specialties and subspecialties: cytology, toxicology, immunology, blood banking, urinalysis, histology, serology, chemistry, microbiology, and hematology.)

A POL usually processes chemical analyses, hematologic tests, microbiologic tests, and urinalyses. Chemical analyses are performed on blood and its components, urine, and other body fluids. Hematologic tests usually use samples of whole blood to identify problems with the count, size, or shape of blood cells that could indicate disease. Microbiologic tests examine blood, urine, sputum, reproductive fluids, and fluids from wounds to identify the presence of pathogenic organisms such as bacteria, viruses, fungi, protozoans, and parasites. Semen may be examined microscopically to determine sperm levels, appearance, and motility. Urinalysis includes chemical analysis of the urine sample, analysis of its physical characteristics, and microscopic examination of the sample to detect disease states.

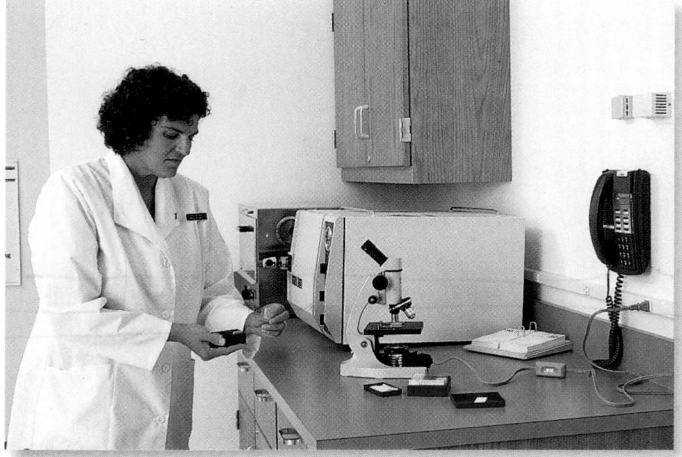

Figure 27-1. A physician's office laboratory (POL) may be simple or elaborate, depending on what tests the office performs.

The Medical Assistant's Role

As a medical assistant, you may be responsible for processing tests done in the POL, including preparing the patient for the test, collecting the sample, completing the test, reporting the results to the physician, and communicating information about the test from the physician to the patient. Your role in the POL requires you to integrate a great deal of information to serve both the physician and the patient effectively. You will need to master the following subjects:

- Use of laboratory equipment
- Regulations governing laboratory practices and procedures
- Precautions for accident prevention
- Waste disposal requirements
- Housekeeping and maintenance routines
- Quality assurance and control procedures
- Technical aspects of specimen collection and test processing, including expected results
- Communication with patients
- Reporting of test results to the physician
- Record keeping of test specimens, procedures, and results
- Inventory and ordering of equipment and supplies
- Use of reference materials in the POL
- Screening and follow-up of test results

Use of Laboratory Equipment

Learning to use a specific piece of equipment may take the form of on-the-job training, or you may attend training programs conducted by manufacturers' representatives at your location or at their training centers. You must be familiar with the operation of common laboratory equipment. You may routinely use the following equipment:

- Autoclave
- Centrifuge
- Microscope
- Electronic equipment
- Equipment used for measurement

Autoclave

A steam autoclave is used to sterilize, or eradicate all organisms on, the surfaces of instruments and equipment before they are used on a patient or in testing procedures. Use of the autoclave is discussed in Chapter 2.

Centrifuge

A **centrifuge** is a device for spinning a specimen at high speed until it separates into its component parts. The centrifuge in a POL is generally used to separate whole blood samples into blood components or to prepare urine samples for examination. Use of a centrifuge is described in greater detail in Chapter 30.

Microscope

The instrument used most often in a POL is the microscope. Common uses of the microscope are the examination of blood smears and identification of microorganisms in body fluid samples.

The usual microscope in a POL is an **optical microscope** (Figure 27-2). An optical microscope uses light, concentrated through a condenser and focused through the object being examined, to project an image. Most optical microscopes in POLs are **compound microscopes,** which use two lenses to magnify the image created by the condensed light.

You may see images that have been produced by an electron microscope in a research or reference laboratory. Instead of using a beam of light, the **electron microscope** uses a beam of electrons. Whereas the best optical microscopes can magnify an image several thousand times, an electron microscope can magnify an image several million times. Use of this highly specialized piece of equipment requires extensive training. An electron microscope is not usually found in the POL because it is expensive and unnecessarily sophisticated for routine specimen examination.

You must be able to operate an optical microscope correctly. First you need to become familiar with the component parts.

Oculars. The **oculars** are the eyepieces through which you view the image. A microscope is either monocular, with a single eyepiece, or binocular, with two eyepieces. You can adjust the oculars on a binocular microscope to compensate for differences in visual acuity between your right and left eyes. You can also adjust the distance between oculars to match the distance between your eyes. The ocular contains a magnifying lens that usually magnifies an image ten times. Such a lens is called a **10× lens.**

Objectives. The ocular or oculars lead to the nosepiece, which contains the **objectives.** An objective contains another magnifying lens. Generally, microscopes used in the POL have a three-piece objective system. The three objectives are mounted on a swivel base, the nosepiece. An objective is moved into position directly under the ocular when needed.

Two of the objectives are dry objectives, which means there is air space between the specimen under examination and the objective. Condensed light passes through the specimen and the air space above the specimen as it travels toward the objective lens. These dry objectives are low- and high-power lenses, usually 10× and 40× respectively. When the low-power objective lens is combined with the ocular lenses, the total magnification factor is 100× (10× times 10×). The high-power lens and ocular lenses yield a magnification factor of 400×.

The third objective is an **oil-immersion objective.** It is designed to be lowered into a drop of immersion oil placed directly above the prepared specimen under examination. This design eliminates the air space between the microscope slide and the objective, where some of the light scatters beyond the objective. Placing the end of the objective in oil reduces the loss of light. A much sharper, brighter

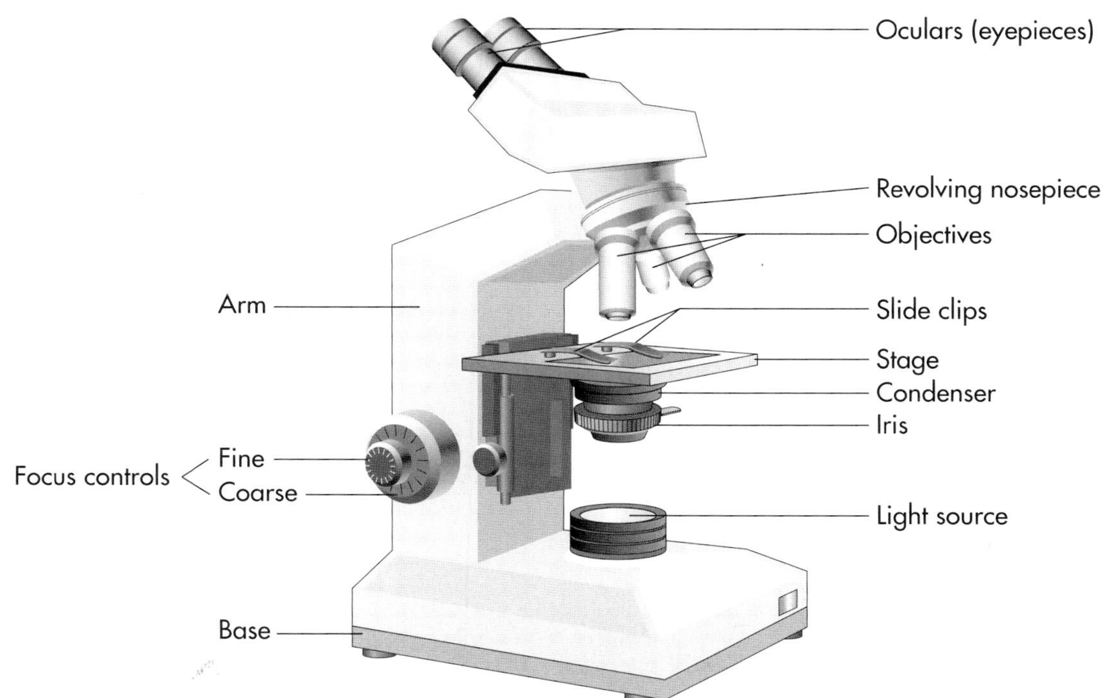

Figure 27-2. The microscope is the most heavily used piece of equipment in a POL.

Medical Laboratory Assistant

To gain medical assistant credentials, you must fulfill the requirements of either the American Association of Medical Assistants (for a Certified Medical Assistant) or the American Medical Technologists (for a Registered Medical Assistant). After obtaining your medical assistant certification or registration, you may wish to acquire additional skills in specialty areas through course work or on-the-job training. Although this course work or training may not lead to an additional certification or degree, it will enable you to expand your role in the medical office and advance your career as the demand for skilled health professionals increases.

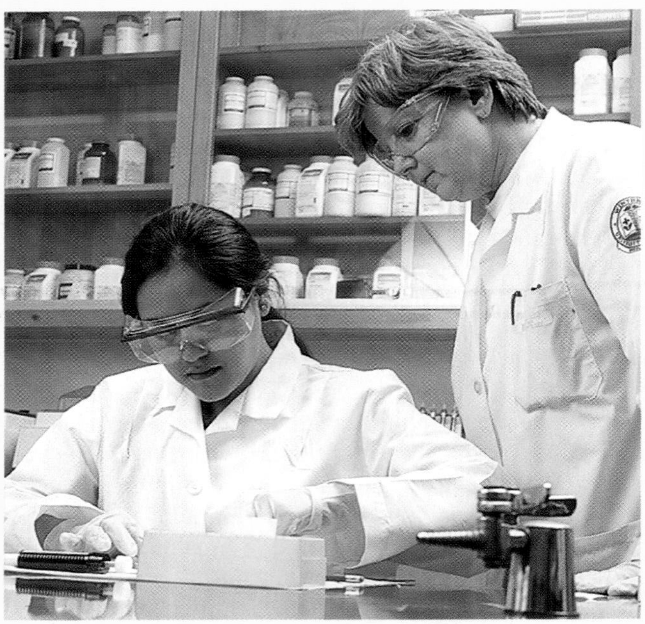

Skills and Duties

A medical laboratory assistant conducts laboratory tests on specimens of body fluids and tissue. Samples may be tested to diagnose disease, to develop new treatments to combat disease, or to evaluate the success of existing treatments. A medical laboratory assistant works under the supervision of a medical laboratory technician or physician.

The assistant uses sophisticated laboratory equipment to collect, process, and analyze samples of body fluids and tissue. The assistant may prepare slides of the samples for viewing under the microscope or may separate components within the samples for further testing. As part of the testing process, the assistant labels all samples and fills out reports of the analyses for the physician. Sterilization of instruments and checking functionality of equipment may be part of the medical assistant's duties.

The range of tests performed by a particular medical laboratory assistant will vary, depending on the type of laboratory. For example, an assistant who works in a small rural laboratory may perform a wide variety of tests, whereas an assistant working in a large reference laboratory may only perform tests of a single type. Some procedures require specialized knowledge and training. A medical laboratory assistant's education and experience will determine the complexity of the tests that may be performed.

Workplace Settings

Medical laboratory assistants usually work in a hospital, clinic, or research center. An increasing number are also finding work at medical laboratories that run tests for hospitals and physicians. Medical laboratory assistants usually work a standard 40-hour week, although hospital laboratories sometimes require some evening and weekend shifts.

Education

A medical laboratory assistant must have a high school diploma or the equivalent. Some assistants acquire their additional training on the job, but most are trained in a certified program. The Commission on Accreditation of Allied Health Education Programs certifies more than 100 training programs, which range in length from 1 to 2 years, at vocational schools and community colleges. In some cases students may be able to combine courses in medical assisting with a liberal arts program to gain an associate's degree in medical laboratory technology.

Certification as a medical laboratory assistant is not required, but it is helpful in getting a job and advancing to other positions. In addition, some states require that medical laboratory assistants, along with all other laboratory staff, be licensed.

Where to Go for More Information

American Medical Technologists
710 Higgins Road
Park Ridge, IL 60068
(847) 823-5169

American Society of Clinical Pathologists
2100 West Harrison Street
Chicago, IL 60612
(312) 738-1336

National Accrediting Agency for Clinical Laboratory Services
8410 West Bryn Mawr Avenue, Suite 670
Chicago, IL 60631
(312) 714-8880

image results, allowing for greater magnification. An oil-immersion objective has a magnification factor of 100×. Combined with the ocular lenses, the total magnification factor is 1000×. The oil-immersion objective is used for specimens that need extreme magnification, such as blood smears and bacteriological slides.

Arm and Focus Controls. The ocular(s) and objectives, collectively referred to as the body tube, are attached to the base of the microscope by the arm. When moving a microscope, use one hand to grasp the arm and the other hand to support the base. (Never carry a microscope with one hand or by just the arm.) If the microscope has an electrical cord, make sure it is loosely coiled and secured with a wire tie or an elastic band.

The microscope arm is also the location of the focus controls. There are two focus controls: coarse and fine. These controls move the body tube up and down to bring into focus the object being examined.

Stage and Substage. The objectives and oculars are focused on a specimen placed on the stage of the microscope. The stage is the platform on which rests the specimen slide, held in place by metal clips. Under the stage is the substage containing the condenser, which concentrates the light being directed through the sample, and the iris. The iris is a diaphragm that opens and closes like the shutter of a camera to increase or decrease the amount of light illuminating the specimen. The stage is controlled by the stage mechanisms, which control left-right and forward-backward movements of the stage, allowing you to examine different areas of the specimen without reseating the slide.

Light Source. Under the stage and substage assemblies is the light source. Most POL microscopes use a built-in electric light source, and most of these are equipped with controls that allow you to adjust the light intensity. In place of a built-in light source, older microscopes use a mirror, which gathers and focuses light from a microscope lamp onto the specimen.

Specimen Slides and Coverslip. Although the specimen slide is not technically part of the microscope assembly, it is necessary for using the microscope. All specimens must be placed on slides. Many specimens also require a coverslip, or cover glass. The slide and coverslip support and position the specimen. They also prevent contamination of the microscope by the specimen. Specimens that are to be stained or immersed in oil, such as blood smears, do not require coverslips.

Using an Optical Microscope. To use an optical microscope, you must be able to focus it using each of the three objectives. Procedure 27-1 describes how to operate an optical microscope correctly.

You will also be responsible for the proper care and maintenance of the optical microscope in your office. Related concerns and techniques are described in the Caution: Handle With Care section.

Electronic Equipment

Electronic equipment is used in the POL because it is more accurate, safer, and more efficient than manual methods; generally requires little maintenance; and does not require extensive training prior to its use. A wide variety of tasks,

CAUTION *Handle With Care*

Care and Maintenance of the Microscope

The microscope is the workhorse of the POL. For it to provide trouble-free service, however, it must be well cared for. Dust, oil, and other contaminants cause major problems with microscopes. Careless cleaning and haphazard storage will also eventually cause problems. These problems may include mechanical difficulties with the microscope or contamination of the specimen being examined. Foreign objects visible through a microscope, but unrelated to the specimen, are called **artifacts** and may be misinterpreted when the specimen is examined.

Clean the microscope after each use. Inspect the body tube, arm, and stage to make sure they are free from dust and other contaminants. Clean the ocular and objective lenses with lens paper, not tissue or other products. Tissue fibers are a common artifact. The eyepiece is an area in which skin oil, dust, and eye makeup may collect, posing a risk of disease transmission and making images difficult to see. Use lens-cleaning products according to the manufacturer's guidelines. Excess amounts of these products may dissolve the cement holding the lenses in place, rendering the microscope useless.

When not in use, the microscope should be stored under its plastic cover. If there is a power cord, wrap it loosely around the base, and secure it with a twist tie or elastic band. Lower the low-power objective close to the stage and center the stage.

If the microscope must be moved, hold it by the arm, and support it under the base. Carry the cord so that it does not dangle and pose a tripping hazard. Place the microscope on a sturdy table or bench, away from the edge.

PROCEDURE 27.1

Using a Microscope

Objective: To correctly focus the microscope using each of the three objectives for examination of a prepared specimen slide

OSHA Guidelines

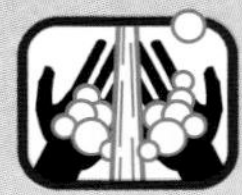 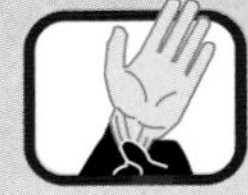 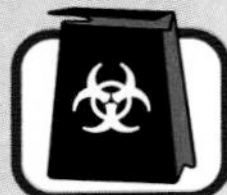
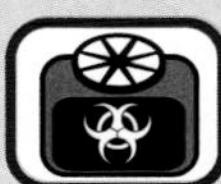 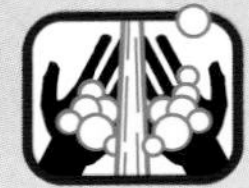

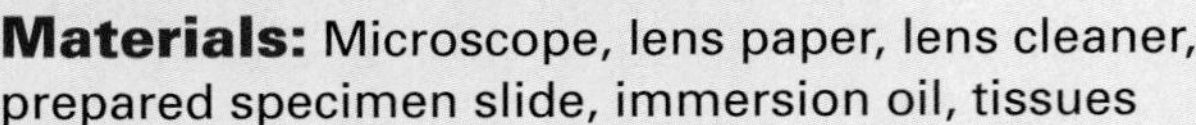

Materials: Microscope, lens paper, lens cleaner, prepared specimen slide, immersion oil, tissues

Method

1. Wash your hands and put on examination gloves.
2. Remove the protective cover from the microscope. Examine the microscope to make sure that it is clean and that all parts are intact.
3. Plug in the microscope and make sure the light is working. If you need to replace the bulb, refer to the manufacturer's guidelines. (Be sure to note bulb replacements in the maintenance log for the microscope.) Turn the light off before cleaning the lenses.
4. Clean the lenses and oculars with lens paper. Avoid touching the lenses with anything except lens paper. Pay careful attention to the oculars. They are easily dirtied by dust and eye makeup. If a lens is particularly dirty, use a small amount of lens cleaner. Oil-immersion lenses are prone to oil buildup if not cleaned properly. Too much lens cleaner, however, can loosen the cement that holds the lens in place.
5. Place the specimen slide on the stage. Slide the edges of the slide under the slide clips to secure the slide to the stage (Figure 27-3).
6. Adjust the distance between the oculars to a position of comfort. You have correctly adjusted the oculars when the field you see through the eyepieces is a merged field, not separate left and right fields.
7. Adjust the objectives so that the low-power (10×) objective points directly at the specimen slide, as shown in Figure 27-4. Before swiveling the objective assembly, be sure you have sufficient space for the objective. Raise the body tube by using the coarse adjustment control,

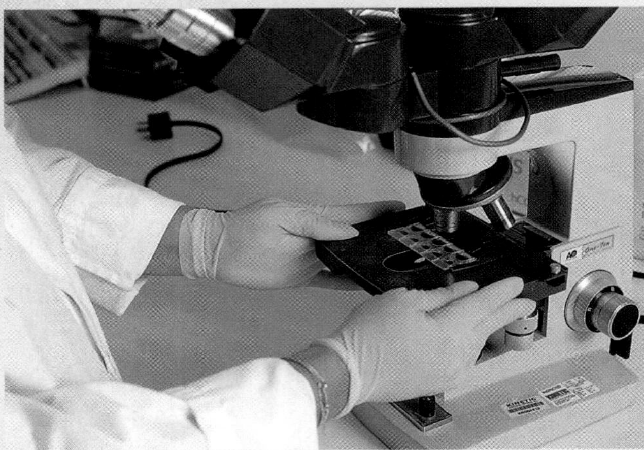

Figure 27-3. Carefully secure the specimen slide on the stage of the microscope.

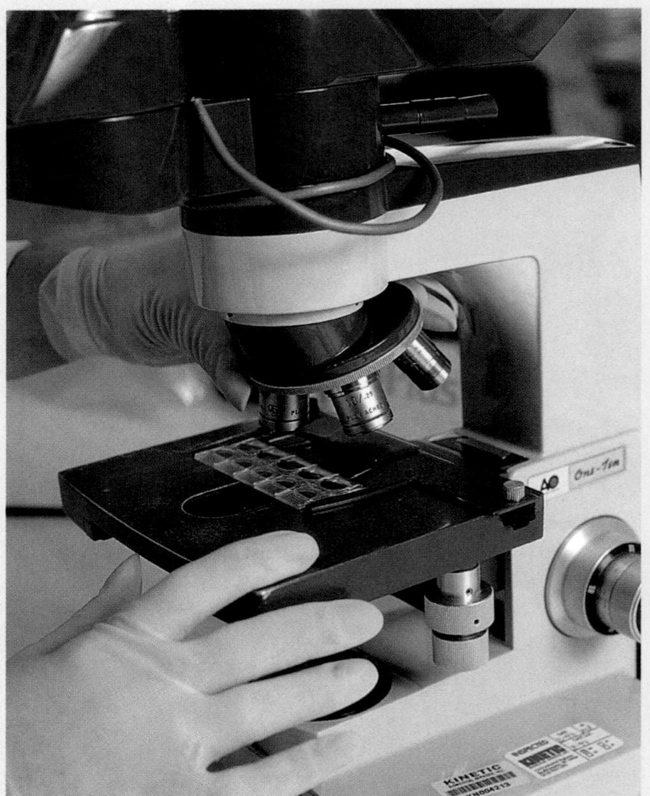

Figure 27-4. Move the low-power objective into position above the specimen slide.

continued ⟶

PROCEDURE 27.1

Using a Microscope *(continued)*

and lower the stage as needed. If the objective assembly is too close to the stage, you may hit the specimen slide and crack it. The specimen is then contaminated and cannot be used. The objective may also be damaged.

8. Turn on the light and, using the iris controls, adjust the amount of light illuminating the specimen so that the light fills the field but does not wash out the image. (At this point you are not examining the specimen image for focus but adjusting the overall light level.)
9. Observe the microscope from one side, and slowly lower the body tube to move the objective closer to the stage and specimen slide. This adjustment is shown in Figure 27-5. If you used the stage controls to lower the stage away from the objectives, you may also need to adjust those controls. Again, take care not to strike the stage with the objective. The objective should almost meet the specimen slide but not touch it.
10. Look through the oculars and use the coarse focus control to slowly adjust the image. If necessary, adjust the amount of light coming through the iris.
11. Continue using the fine focus control to adjust the image. When the image is correctly adjusted, the specimen will be clearly visible, and the field illumination will be bright enough to show details but not so bright that it is uncomfortable to view.
12. Switch to the high-power (40×) objective. Most microscopes can be switched from the low-power objective to the high-power objective without your having to use the coarse focus adjustments again. Use the fine focus controls to view the specimen clearly.
13. Rotate the objective assembly so that no objective points directly at the stage and specimen slide. You will now have enough room to apply a small drop of immersion oil to the slide. (Only dry slides, without coverslips, are used with the oil-immersion objective.)
14. Apply a small drop of immersion oil to the specimen slide, as shown in Figure 27-6.
15. Swing the oil-immersion (100×) objective over the stage and specimen slide. Gently lower the objective so that it is surrounded by the immersion oil.

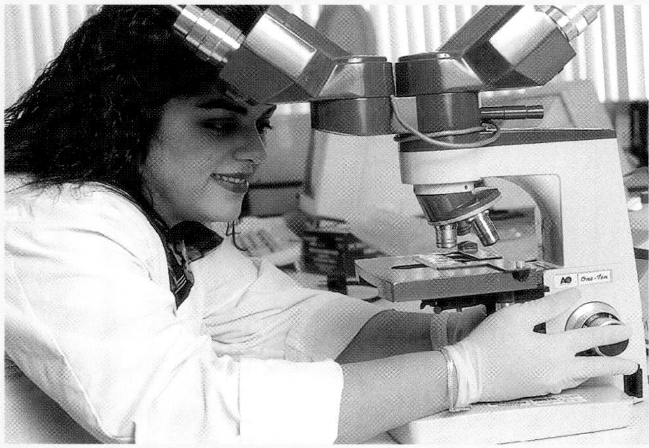

Figure 27-5. When lowering the objective toward the stage and specimen slide, observe the microscope from the side to be sure you do not hit the stage with the objective and crack the slide.

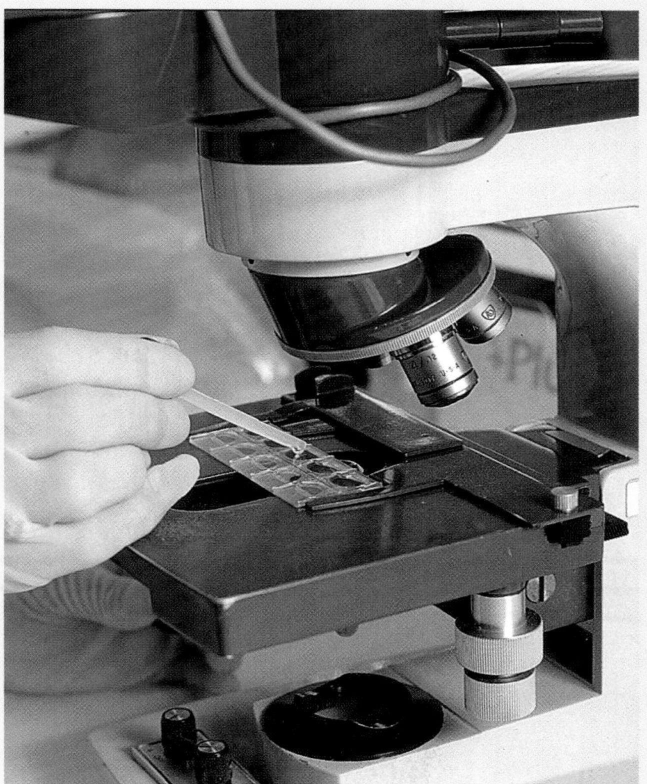

Figure 27-6. Place a small drop of immersion oil directly on the dry specimen.

continued ⟶

PROCEDURE 27.1

Using a Microscope *(continued)*

16. Examine the image and adjust the amount of light and focus as needed. To eliminate air bubbles in the immersion oil, gently move the stage left and right.
17. After you have examined the specimen as required by the testing procedure, lower the stage and raise the objectives.
18. Remove the slide. Dispose of it or store it as required by the testing procedure. If you must dispose of the slide, be sure to use the appropriate biohazardous waste container. If you must store the slide, remove the immersion oil with a tissue.
19. Clean the microscope stage, ocular lenses, and objectives (Figure 27-7). Be careful to remove all traces of immersion oil from the stage and oil-immersion objective.
20. Turn off the light. Unplug the microscope if that is your laboratory's standard operating procedure.
21. Rotate the objective assembly so that the low-power objective points toward the stage. Lower the objective so that it comes close to but does not rest on the stage.
22. Cover the microscope with its protective cover. Check the work area to be sure you have cleaned everything correctly and disposed of all waste material.
23. Remove the gloves and wash your hands.

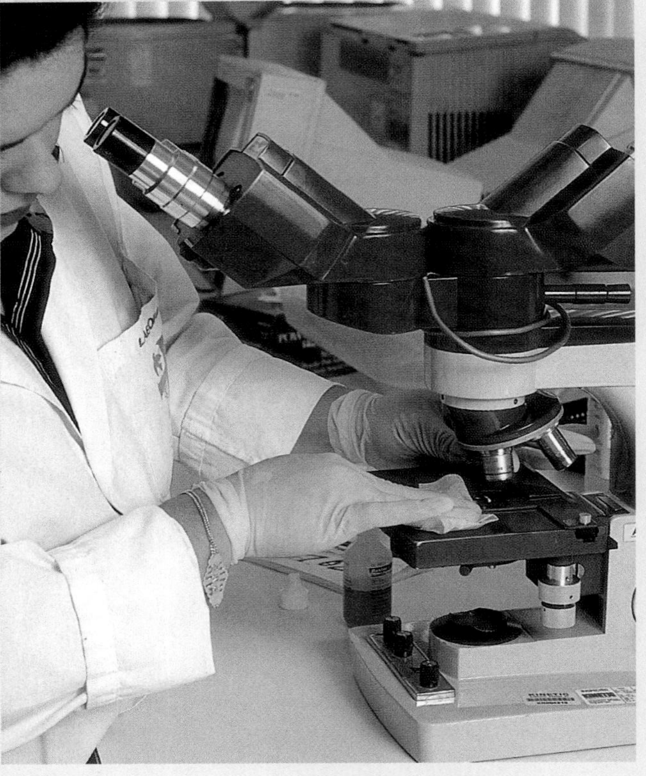

Figure 27-7. You need to remove all traces of immersion oil when you clean the microscope stage, ocular lenses, and objectives.

such as record keeping and retrieval, cell counting, and complex chemical analyses, are performed with electronic equipment. Manufacturers' instructions for operation and maintenance must be followed to ensure safety, efficiency, and reliable results.

A **photometer,** which measures light intensity, is a basic electronic component of many pieces of analytic laboratory equipment. A handheld glucometer (Figure 27-8), for example, contains a photometer that measures reflected light. A glucometer is used by patients with diabetes and by clinical personnel to monitor blood glucose levels.

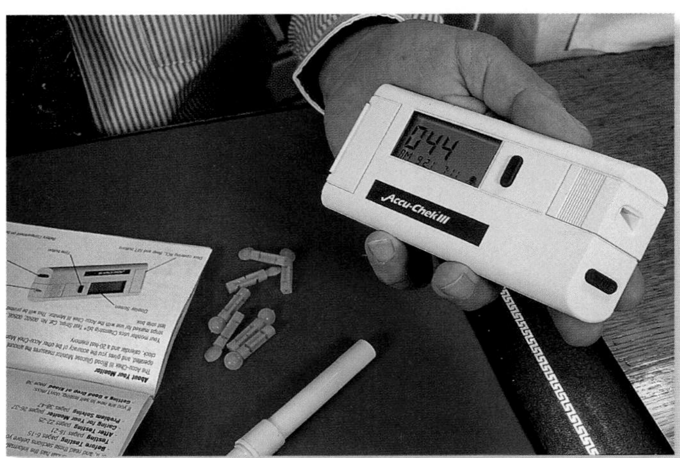

Figure 27-8. A handheld glucometer translates the amount of reflected light into the level of glucose in a blood sample.

Equipment Used for Measurement

Precise measurement is critical in the POL because it produces accurate test results. Much of the measurement required in the POL is built into the electronic equipment or premeasured kits you will use. You still must perform various measurements, however, when blood, semen, urine, and other body fluids are analyzed using manual tests. Some reagents also require measuring.

Metric system units are commonly used in the POL. For information on metric system weight, height, and temperature measurements, see Chapter 19. To learn how to convert between measurement systems, see Chapter 33.

A variety of equipment is used to provide accurate measurements. You must take these measurements carefully for them to be of value in the final test results. Other types of measuring equipment include:

- Pipettes, either mechanical or manual, which are used to measure small amounts of liquids
- Volumetric or graduated flasks or beakers, which are used to measure the relatively large amounts of liquids necessary for reagents
- A hemocytometer, which is a slide calibrated to the exact measurements needed to count blood cells and sperm under a microscope
- Thermometers, generally in degrees centigrade, which are used to provide legal documentation that refrigerators, bacterial incubators, and other appliances maintain the precise temperature range required for accurate laboratory work

Safety in the Laboratory

Safety is a primary concern in any laboratory environment. It is especially important in a physician's office laboratory because patients as well as laboratory workers may be at risk. For your own protection, as well as that of patients and coworkers, you must always be aware of and observe guidelines for laboratory safety.

Occupational Safety and Health Administration

The Occupational Safety and Health Administration (OSHA) was created within the Department of Labor as a result of legislation passed in 1970 (the Occupational Safety and Health Acts) to protect the safety of employees in the workplace. OSHA's duties include the creation and enforcement of both general safety standards and standards for specific industries and operations. In general, if a specific standard exists, its guidelines must be followed, but if no specific standard has been developed, the "general duty clause" takes effect. This clause requires an employer to maintain a workplace free from hazards that are recognized as likely to cause death or serious injury. OSHA also acts to enforce guidelines developed by the Centers for Disease Control and Prevention (CDC), in particular the guidelines for Universal Precautions. Copies of these guidelines can be obtained from many sources, including local OSHA offices; the CDC in Atlanta, Georgia; many industrial organizations throughout the country; and the Internet.

Important regulations or guidelines with which you should be familiar as you work as a medical assistant include the following:

- Universal Precautions
- Hazard Communication Standard
- OSHA Bloodborne Pathogens Standard
- Hazardous Waste Operations and Emergency Response Final Rule
- Needlestick Safety and Prevention Act

Universal Precautions. As discussed in Chapter 1 and elsewhere, the general concept behind Universal Precautions is to assume that all blood, blood products, human tissue, and certain body fluids (including semen, vaginal secretions, saliva from dental procedures, cerebrospinal fluid, synovial fluid, pleural fluid, peritoneal fluid, pericardial fluid, and amniotic fluid) are contaminated with blood-borne pathogens. (Breast milk is not on the official list of transmission agents covered by Universal Precautions, but it is treated as such because it is believed that HIV has been transmitted from mother to child through breast milk.)

It has become common practice in the medical office to use Universal Precautions when handling all body fluids, excretions, and secretions. If you have any doubt about whether you need to take precautions, take them. Even though some substances do not present a risk of transmitting blood-borne pathogens, they may present a high risk of transmitting bacteria, viruses, or parasites. Follow these guidelines.

- Wear gloves when handling all body fluids, secretions, and excretions.
- Change gloves every time you move from patient to patient as you collect specimens for testing.
- Wash your hands immediately after removing used gloves.
- Wear other protective gear such as eye protection and face masks during procedures in which there is a risk that droplets or spray may come in contact with your eyes, nose, or mouth.
- Take special care to avoid injury from sharp or pointed instruments or equipment. Although gloves protect you from surface exposure to potentially infected substances, they offer little protection against exposure from needlesticks or cuts. Never use needles or other sharp instruments unnecessarily.
- Use only recommended instruments and equipment. A once common laboratory technique that has been discontinued is the use of a mouth pipette (a type of calibrated glass or plastic straw) to transfer specimens. Under no circumstances should you use a mouth pipette to transfer blood from one collection device to another.
- Take care to prevent spills and splashes when transporting specimens to the laboratory and when moving specimens in the laboratory.
- If a work surface becomes contaminated because of spilling or splashing, disinfect the area completely,

using an approved solution such as 10% bleach, before beginning any other procedure.

- Dispose of waste products carefully and correctly.
- Be sure to remove protective gear before leaving the laboratory.

Hazard Communication Standard. The Hazard Communication Standard requires that employees receive training regarding workplace hazards, including how to interpret documentation about hazardous substances that pose an exposure threat. Hazardous materials must be correctly labeled, and employees must have access to information about the materials. The information must include the measures that employees can take to protect themselves against harm from these substances.

Biohazard Labels. All containers used to store waste products, blood, blood products, or other specimens that may be contaminated with blood-borne pathogens are considered biohazardous. They must be clearly marked with the **biohazard symbol,** as shown in Figure 27-9. The biohazard symbol label must be bright orange-red and clearly lettered so that no one can mistake the meaning of the warning. Labels should be securely attached to containers.

In addition to individual biohazard labels that identify particular containers, warning signs must be posted in the laboratory itself. These signs, such as the one shown in Figure 27-10, identify the presence of biohazardous material and list important safeguards to follow.

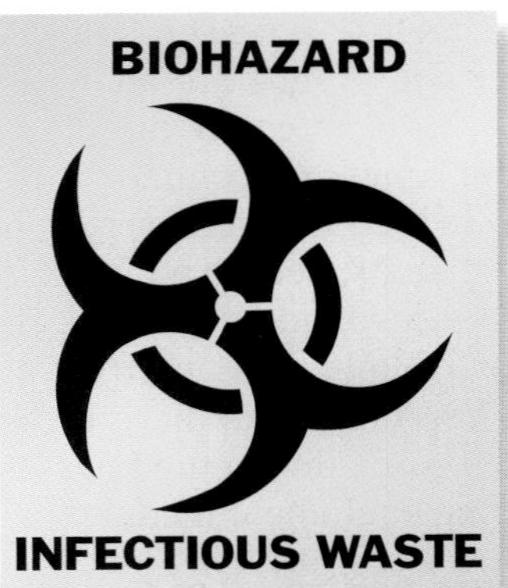

Figure 27-9. The biohazard symbol identifies material that has been exposed to potentially contaminated substances such as blood, blood products, or other body fluids.

Material Safety Data Sheets. **Material Safety Data Sheets (MSDSs)** contain information about hazardous chemicals or other substances. A sample MSDS is shown in Figure 27-11. Each MSDS must contain the following

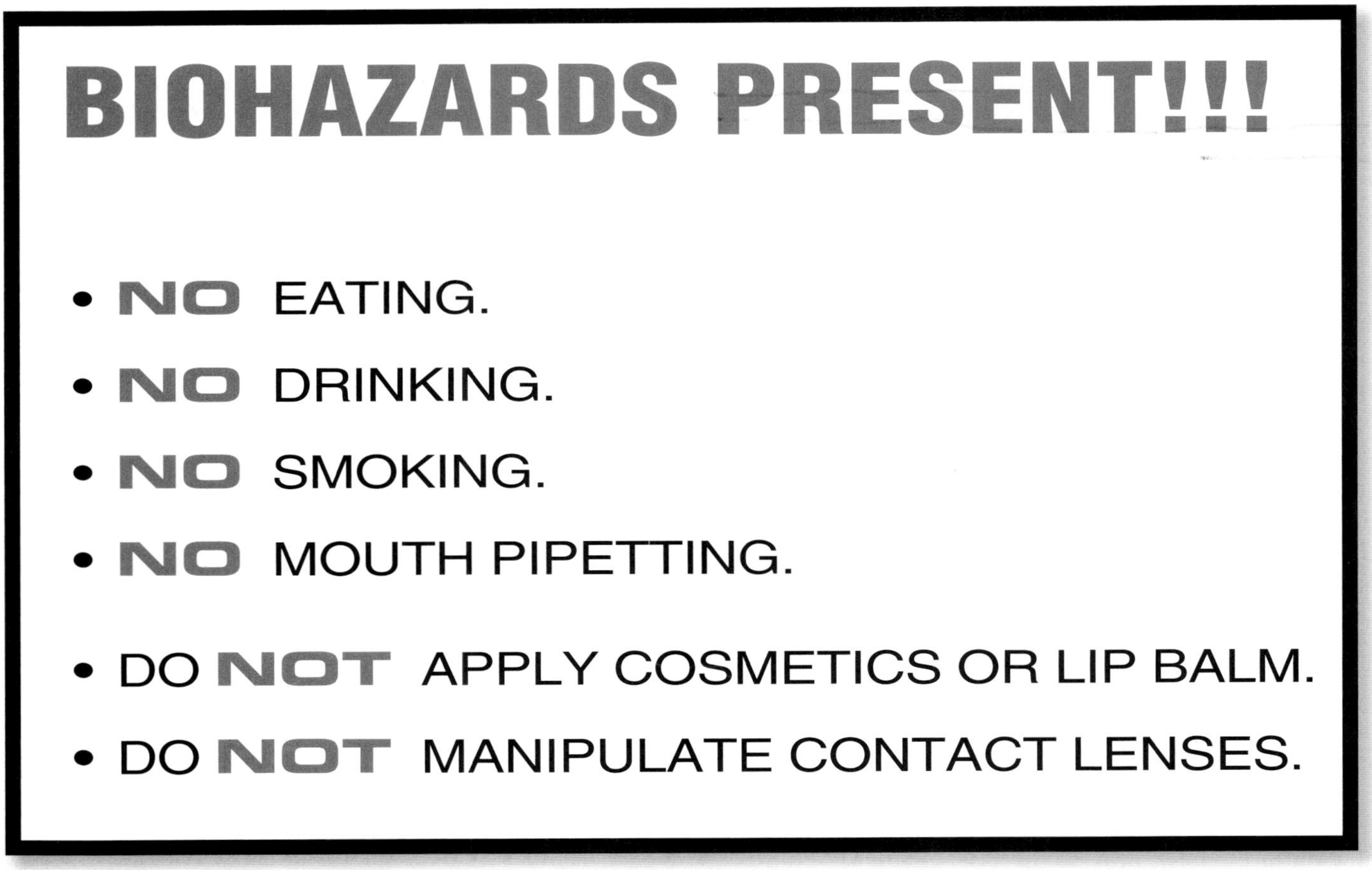

BIOHAZARDS PRESENT!!!

- **NO** EATING.
- **NO** DRINKING.
- **NO** SMOKING.
- **NO** MOUTH PIPETTING.
- DO **NOT** APPLY COSMETICS OR LIP BALM.
- DO **NOT** MANIPULATE CONTACT LENSES.

Figure 27-10. The biohazard warning sign alerts personnel to the presence of potentially contaminated substances and advises them about safety guidelines.

MATERIAL SAFETY DATA SHEET

WAVICIDE-01

Date Issued:

SECTION 1 — IDENTIFICATION

Manufacturers Name and Address: Wave Energy Systems, Inc.
25 Mansard Court
Wayne, NJ 07470

Phone: 1-800-252-1125
Fax: (201) 633-1023

Product Name: WAVICIDE-01 (2.5% aqueous glutaraldehyde solution)

Product Code: 0104 (case of 4 gallons) or 0112 (case of 12 quarts)

Product Type/General Information: Chemical Sterilant/Disinfectant

EPA Registration Number: 15136-1

Chemical Name: (active ingredient) 2.5% glutaraldehyde

Hazardous Chemicals: *Glutaraldehyde*
Routes of entry: *Inhalation* ✓ *Skin/Eye* ✓ *Ingestion* ✓

PRECAUTIONARY LABELING
(HMIS Rating System)

Health	3
Flammability:	0
Reactivity:	0
Physical Hazard:	None

The New Jersey Poison Control Center has been provided information for use in medical emergencies involving this product. Call 1-800-962-1253.

SECTION 2 — HAZARDOUS INGREDIENTS/IDENTITY INFORMATION

WAVICIDE-01 contains the following hazardous ingredients at concentrations greater than 1.0%:

CHEMICAL COMPONENTS	CAS%	% w/v	OSHA PEL	ACGIH TLV
Glutaraldehyde (active ingredient)	111-30-8	2.5	0.2 ppm[1]	0.2 ppm

WAVICIDE-01 contains no hazardous ingredients listed as carcinogens or potential carcinogens by the National Toxicology Program (NTP), International Agency on Cancer (IARC) or OSHA, and present at a concentration greater than 0.1%:

[1] The OSHA Permissible Exposure Level (PEL) for glutaraldehyde was invalidated in 1992 by court order. However, the PEL may remain valid in some OSHA approved state plans, and also can be enforced by federal OSHA under its General Duty Clause.

SECTION 3 — PHYSICAL/CHEMICAL CHARACTERISTICS

Boiling Point:	100°C/212°F	**Evaporation Rate:**	0.81 (Butyl Acetate = 1)
Specific Gravity:	1.005 - 1.013	**Solubility (H_2O):**	Complete
Vapor Pressure:	16.9 mm Hg	**Appearance & Color:**	A clear, slightly yellow liquid with typical aldehyde odor and added lemon scent.
Melting point:	N/A	**pH:**	Approximately 6.30
Vapor Density:	1.1 (air = 1)	**Molecular Weight:**	100.11 (glutaraldehyde)
Freezing Point:	0°C/32°F (same as water)	**Odor Threshold:**	0.04 ppm, detectable (ACGIH)

SECTION 4 — FIRE AND EXPLOSION HAZARD DATA

Flash Point (Test Method): None (Tag Closed Cup ASTM D 56)

Special Fire Fighting Procedures: Self-Contained Breathing Apparatus (SCBA) and protective clothing should be worn when fighting chemical fires.

Unusual Fire and Explosion Hazards: None known

Extinguishing Media: Carbon dioxide, foam, dry chemical.

SECTION 5 — REACTIVITY DATA

Stability: Unstable______ Stable __✓__ **Hazardous Polymerization:** May Occur______ Will Not Occur __✓__

Hazardous Decomposition Products: Thermal decomposition may produce carbon dioxide and or carbon monoxide.

Conditions and Materials to Avoid: Alkaline (pH > 10) and acidic (pH < 3) materials catalyze an aldol-type condensation (exothermic but not expected to be violent). Avoid High temperatures above 40°C/104°F and or evaporation of H_2O.

Figure 27-11. This two-page Material Safety Data Sheet (MSDS), as required by OSHA, contains important information about each hazardous substance used in the POL. (Courtesy of Wave Energy Systems, Inc., Wayne, NJ.) (continued)

Date Issued:

SECTION 6 HEALTH HAZARD DATA

Routes of Entry: *Inhalation:* ✓ *Skin:* ✓ *Ingestion:* ✓ *Eyes:* ✓

Signs and Symptoms Associated With Overexposure (one-time or repeated):

Ingestion: May cause irritation and possibly chemical burns of the mouth, throat, stomach and esophagus. May produce discomfort in the mouth, throat, chest and abdomen, nausea, vomiting, diarrhea, dizziness, faintness, drowsiness, thirst and weakness.

Eyes: Solution contact may cause damage, including severe corneal injury, which could permanently impair vision if prompt first-aid and medical treatment are not obtained. Vapors may cause stinging sensation in the eye with excess tear production, blinking, and redness of the conjuntiva.

Skin: Direct solution contact may cause skin irritation or aggravation of an existing dermatitis. May also cause skin to turn a harmless yellow or brown color.

Inhalation: Vapor is irritating to the respiratory tract. May cause stinging sensations in the nose and throat, chest discomfort and tightening, difficulty with breathing and headache. May also aggravate pre-existing asthma and pulmonary disease.

Emergency and First Aid Procedure:

Ingestion: DO NOT INDUCE VOMITING. Drink large quantities of water and call a physician immediately
NOTE TO PHYSICIAN: Probable mucosal damage from oral exposure may contraindicate the use of gastric lavage.

Eyes: Immediately flush eyes with water and continue washing for at least 15 minutes. Obtain medical attention immediately, and follow up with an ophthalmologist.

Skin: Immediately remove contaminated clothing and flush skin with soap and water for a minimum of 15 minutes. If irritation persists, seek medical attention. Wash or discard contaminated clothing.

Inhalation: Remove to fresh air. Give artificial respiration if not breathing. If breathing is difficult, oxygen may be given by qualified personnel. If irritation persists, seek medical help.

Medical Conditions Generally Aggravated by Overexposure: See above.

SECTION 7 PRECAUTIONS FOR SAFE HANDLING AND USE

Steps to be Taken if Material is Released or Spilled: Wear suitable protective equipment, including nitrile gloves, chemically resistant gown or apron, and protective eyewear (safety glasses or shield). A full face respirator , or half-face respirator with gas proof goggles, both worn with organic vapor cartridges, is recommended for small spills. A respirator is essential for large spills, or if you experience discomfort watery eyes, nasal or respiratory irritation) due to inadequate ventilation. For **small spills of 1 gallon or less**, gather up a bucket, household ammonia, and a sponge or mop. Don protective equipment and mix approximately 1 cup of ammonia with 1 cup of water in the bucket. Mop or sponge the ammonia mixture into the spill until thoroughly combined (about 2 minutes). Wipe or mop up resulting mixture and discard down the drain with a copious amount of water. Rinse bucket, mop or sponge with water, and give spill area a final wipe or mop with fresh water. Re-rinse all equipment, and allow spill area to dry. For **large spills of more than 1 gallon**, remove people from immediate spill area, and isolate until cleaned up. Don protective equipment including a respirator with organic vapor cartridges. Contain spill with absorbent material, ie. towels. Add approximately 228 grams of sodium bisulfite powder per gallon of WAVICIDE-01 spilled (aqueous sodium hydroxide and ammonium will also neutralize glutaraldehyde). With a sponge, mix neutralizing chemical into spill, and allow 5 minutes for deactivation to occur. Discard resulting mixture according to your facility's waste disposal guidelines. Mop spill area with fresh water. Rinse out all equipment (bucket, mop, towels) with large amounts of water. If paper towels were used, dispose of in a tightly closed trash bag. Let spill area dry, and if possible increase ventilation. Once glutaraldehyde odor is below allowable levels (TLV), the area may be released from isolation.

Waste Disposal Method: Dispose of WAVICIDE-01 after 30 days of re-use, or the MEC Indicator shows the solution is below it's minimum effective concentration (1.7% w/v), which ever is sooner. This may be accomplished by pouring solution down drain in accordance with state and local regulations. Flush with a large quantity of water. Do not reuse empty containers. Rinse thoroughly with water and dispose of in trash.

Precautions to be Taken in Handling and Storing: WAVICIDE-01 should be stored in it's original sealed container at controlled room temperature (15°C/50°F to 30°C/85°F).

Precautionary Labeling: Avoid contact with eyes, prolonged and repeated contact with skin, and contamination with food.

SECTION 8 TRANSPORTATION DATA & ADDITIONAL INFORMATION

Proper Shipping Name: 2.5% Glutaraldehyde Solution	**DOT (ground):** Not regulated	**IATA (air):** Not Regulated	**IMO (ocean):** Not Regulated
Hazard Class: None	**Labels:** None needed **Packaging:** None	**ID#:** None	**Special Instructions:** None	**Reportable Quantity:** None

SECTION 9 CONTROL MEASURES

Eye Protection: Safety glasses, goggles or face shield recommended when working with WAVICIDE-01. An eye wash, and full face respirator with organic vapor cartridges or half face respirator with gas proof goggles and organic vapor cartridges should be available for emergency situations.

Ventilation: WAVICIDE-01 should be used in closed containers with tight fitting lids. The working area should be large enough with ventilation necessary to keep the level of atmospheric glutaraldehyde below the Threshold Limit Value (TLV). If the solution vapors are irritating to eyes and nose, the TLV is probably being exceeded, and additional ventilation may be necessary. A fume hood or self contained fume absorber may be appropriate for this purpose. Any ventilation should pull fumes away from worker and towards the floor.

Skin Protection: Nitrile gloves and a chemical resistant gown or apron should be worn when working with WAVICIDE-01. Rubber boots may be needed to contain large spills.

Respiratory Protection: None required if glutaraldehyde vapor levels are below the TLV. A full face respirator with organic vapor cartridges or SCBA should be available for emergencies.

SECTION 10 SPECIAL REQUIREMENTS

None

Figure 27-11. Material Safety Data Sheet (continued)

information about the product it describes:

- Substance name, as it appears on the container label
- Chemical name(s) of each ingredient
- Common name(s) of each ingredient
- Chemical characteristics of the product (boiling point, specific gravity, melting point, appearance, odor)
- Physical hazards posed by the product (fire, vapor pressure)
- Health hazards posed by the product (carcinogenicity [ability to cause cancer], routes and methods of entry, signs and symptoms of exposure)
- Guidelines for safe handling of the substance
- Emergency and first-aid procedures to be followed in the event of exposure

Hazard Labels. In addition to the MSDS, each hazardous substance must be identified with a hazard label. A **hazard label** is a shortened version of the MSDS that is permanently affixed to the substance container. A sample hazard label is shown in Figure 27-12.

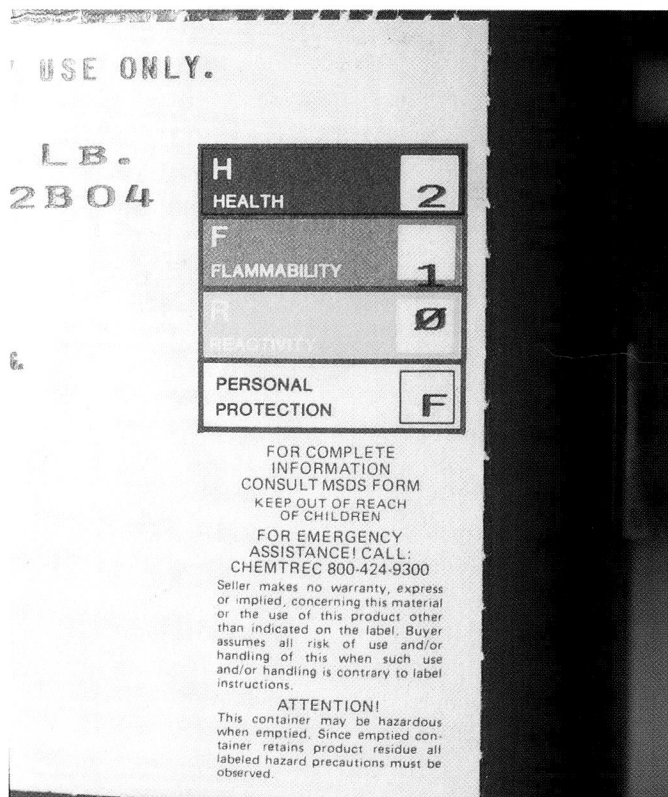

Figure 27-12. A hazard label is a condensed version of the MSDS and displays important information about a substance. It must be permanently affixed to the substance container.

OSHA Bloodborne Pathogens Standard. The OSHA Bloodborne Pathogens Standard identifies methods for reducing the risk of transmission of blood-borne pathogens, specifically the hepatitis B virus (HBV) and the human immunodeficiency virus (HIV). HIV is the virus that causes acquired immunodeficiency syndrome (AIDS). The standard identifies laboratory procedures that must be followed to prevent occupational exposure. It also describes the procedure that must be followed in the event of exposure to one of these viruses. To be in compliance with this standard, an employer must meet the following requirements.

- A written OSHA Exposure Control Plan must be created and updated annually or whenever procedures that require exposure to potentially contaminated material are added or changed. The plan must be available to all employees and to authorized OSHA authorities.
- Training must be provided to all employees describing the documentation mandated by the standard. This documentation includes the symptoms, methods of transmission, and epidemiology of infectious diseases caused by blood-borne pathogens. Employees must also be instructed in the use of personal protective equipment, Universal Precautions, and engineering controls designed to prevent exposure. Procedures to follow in the event of exposure or emergency situations must also be part of the training.
- The employer must make hepatitis B vaccine available at no charge to all employees who are at risk for occupational exposure. Employees must either receive the vaccination or decline it in writing. The employer must maintain documentation of vaccinations and refusals. Employees who initially decline the vaccine are free to reverse their decision at any point during their employment.

Hazardous Waste Operations and Emergency Response Final Rule. OSHA regulations also extend to the disposal of waste products generated during laboratory procedures. Hazardous waste products include the following:

- Blood
- Blood products
- Body fluids
- Body tissues
- Cultures
- Vaccines, killed or attenuated (live but weakened)
- Sharps
- Gloves
- Specula
- Inoculating loops
- Paper products contaminated with body fluids

Hazardous waste must be disposed of in properly constructed and labeled containers. Containers for sharps must be puncture-proof, leak-resistant, and rigid

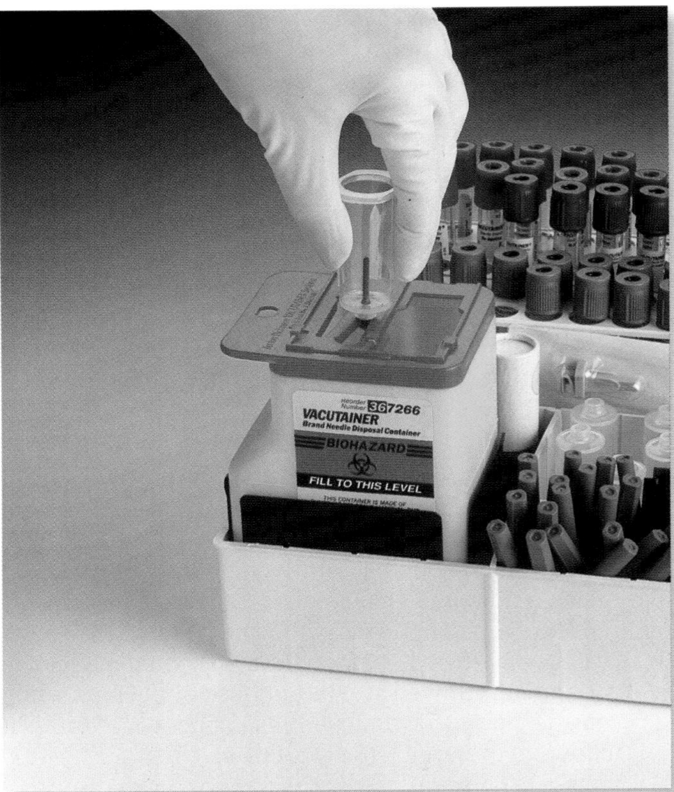

Figure 27-13. A sharps disposal container is a receptacle for used needles, lancets, specimen slides, and other disposable pointed or edged instruments, supplies, and equipment.

(Figure 27-13). Needles should be dropped into the sharps container without bending, breaking, or recapping them and with as little extra handling as possible. Other waste must be placed in plastic bags clearly labeled to identify the infectious contents. All biohazardous waste containers should be placed as close as possible to the area in which the waste is generated. This last procedure is followed to reduce the risk of spillage on the way to the disposal container.

Needlestick Safety and Prevention Act. In response to the Needlestick Safety and Prevention Act, which was signed into law in November 2000, OSHA revised the Bloodborne Pathogens Standard. The additional provisions to the standard are:

- Health-care employers must evaluate new safety-engineered control devices on an annual basis and implement the use of devices that reasonably reduce the risk of needlestick injuries
- Health-care facilities must maintain a detailed log of sharps injuries that are incurred from contaminated sharps
- Health-care employers must solicit input from employees involved in direct patient care to identify, evaluate, and implement engineering and work practice controls

Accident Prevention Guidelines

Work in the POL exposes you to hazards of four main types: physical, fire and electrical, chemical, and biologic. The following safeguards reduce the risk in one or more of these hazard categories. For example, by handling chemical containers carefully and correctly, you protect yourself from harmful chemical exposure as well as from physical injury from broken glass or other materials.

Physical Safety. There are many ways to ensure physical safety in the laboratory. You must understand and apply all the appropriate safeguards. Because accidents can happen, however, post emergency numbers in multiple locations throughout the laboratory. Once each quarter, make sure the numbers are accurate and up-to-date.

Some safeguards come under the heading of common sense. Their application requires no special knowledge.

- Walk, do not run, in the laboratory. Be careful when carrying objects through the laboratory, especially when approaching blind corners.
- Close all cabinet and closet doors and all desk and worktable drawers.
- Never use damaged equipment or supplies, such as cracked or chipped glassware.
- Do not overextend your reach when attempting to grasp supplies. Use only approved equipment, such as stepladders or stools, to reach high shelves. Do not climb onto chairs, desks, or tables to reach anything.
- When lifting an object, squat close to the object. Keep your back straight but not rigid. Lift the item by pushing up with your legs, not by pulling with your back. Hold the load firmly with both hands, close to your body. If necessary, put on a back-support belt before attempting to move heavy loads.

Being aware of the laboratory environment will help you protect your health and well-being. For example:

- Adjust your seat to the correct position to prevent back strain.
- If you are using a computer, take frequent breaks to reduce eyestrain and hand cramping.
- Do not eat or drink in the laboratory, and do not store food there. Never use laboratory supplies, such as beakers or flasks, for eating or drinking.
- Do not put anything in your mouth while working in the laboratory. (Some people have a habit of chewing on the end of their pencils, for example.)
- Do not apply makeup or lip balm or insert contact lenses in the laboratory.
- Familiarize yourself with the location of the first-aid kit. If you are responsible for the kit in your area, check it weekly to make sure that it is adequately stocked with supplies and that expiration dates on medications have not passed.
- Familiarize yourself with the location and operation of the emergency eyewash and shower stations.

Wear appropriate protective gear and clothing in the laboratory. Use heat-resistant mitts or gloves to prevent burns. Wear sturdy, low-heeled, closed-toe shoes with rubber soles to prevent injury if you drop or spill something and to avoid slipping. Do not wear dangling jewelry or loose clothing that could get caught in laboratory equipment. Keep hair pulled back or covered for the same reason.

When you work with laboratory equipment, always follow manufacturers' guidelines. For example, wait for centrifuges to stop spinning before you open them.

Many laboratory materials and supplies require special handling and precautions.

- Store caustic chemicals and other hazardous substances below eye level to reduce the risk of upsetting the container and spilling the substance into your eyes.
- Do not attempt to grasp bottles, jars, or other containers if your hands or the containers are wet.
- Close containers immediately after use.
- Clean up spills immediately. If the floor is wet, either dry it or use appropriate warning devices to alert others to the hazard.
- Clean up broken glass with a broom. Do not handle the debris. If the material is biohazardous, use tongs or forceps to pick up the glass. Package the pieces in a sturdy container with a label identifying the contents.

Fire and Electrical Safety. The equipment and materials used in the POL make it especially vulnerable to fire and electrical hazards. It is critical for you to know how to respond to a fire or electrical accident.

- Familiarize yourself with the location of all fire extinguishers and fire blankets in the laboratory. Review the floor plan, noting the location of fire exits.
- Make sure you know how to operate the fire extinguishers.
- Participate in all office fire drills.
- Familiarize yourself with the location of circuit breakers and emergency power shutoffs.

It is, of course, never acceptable to smoke in the laboratory. Keep your area clear of clutter such as boxes or empty storage containers. Such materials can feed, or even start, a fire. The following safeguards reduce electrical hazards.

- Avoid using extension cords. If they must be used, be sure the circuit is not overloaded. Tape extension cords to the floor to avoid tripping.
- Repair or replace equipment that has a broken or frayed cord.
- Dry your hands before working with electrical devices.
- Do not position electrical devices near sinks, faucets, or other sources of water. Be sure electrical cords do not run through water.

Work in the laboratory may sometimes require that you use a flame. Special precautions are essential in such circumstances.

- If you must use an open flame, extinguish it immediately after use.
- When using an open flame, be careful to keep your hair, clothing, and jewelry away from the flame source.
- If you must use a chemical in a procedure that requires an open flame, double-check the MSDS to identify the level of risk of fire for that chemical. If necessary, bring a fire extinguisher to the area in which you will be working.
- Never lean over an open flame.
- Never leave an open flame unattended.
- Turn off gas valves immediately after use. If you must use an open flame in the vicinity of a gas valve, always double-check to be sure the gas is off. Make sure there is adequate ventilation.

Chemical Safety. Familiarize yourself with the MSDS and hazard label of every chemical you will use during a procedure. If the MSDS indicates the need for special equipment or conditions to use a chemical safely, be sure you meet the requirements before beginning to work with the substance. General precautions as you prepare include the following.

- Wear protective gear to prevent harm to your skin or damage to your clothing. (Be sure to remove the protective gear before leaving the laboratory.)
- Always carry chemical containers with both hands as you gather supplies.
- Make sure you work in an area that is properly ventilated.

When you are ready to begin work, adhere to these guidelines.

- If you must smell the chemicals you are using, do not hold them directly under your nose. Instead, hold them a few inches away, and fan air across them and toward your nose.
- Work inside a fume hood if the chemical vapor is hazardous.
- Wear a personal ventilation device when working with certain chemicals, as specified by the MSDS.
- Never combine chemicals in ways not specifically required in test procedures.
- Mouth pipetting is prohibited at all times.
- If you are combining acids with other substances, always add the acid to the other substance. Adding substances to acid increases the risk of splashing.
- If you encounter a spill of an unknown chemical substance, do not pour any other chemicals on it. Clean it up following strict hazardous waste control procedures. Never touch an unknown substance with your bare hands.

Biologic Safety. You will work with test specimens that may be contaminated with blood-borne or other pathogens. Treat every specimen as if it were contaminated.

- Follow Universal Precautions.
- If you have any cuts, lesions, or sores, do not expose yourself to potentially contaminated material. Consult your supervisor if you have any doubt about whether you can safely perform test procedures.
- Wash your hands before and after every procedure and whenever you come in contact with a potentially contaminated substance.
- Wear gloves at all times. Use other protective gear as appropriate to prevent exposing your eyes, nose, and mouth to potentially contaminated material.
- Mouth pipetting is prohibited at all times. Use specially made rubber suction bulbs to draw specimens mechanically.
- Work in a biologic safety cabinet (similar to a fume hood) when completing procedures that are likely to generate droplet sprays or splashes of potentially contaminated material.
- When transferring a blood specimen from a collection tube to another container, cover the tube stopper with an absorbent pad or a commercial stopper remover to prevent spray or splatter from the tube. Do not rock the stopper back and forth, because this could cause the tube to break. Always remove the stopper by opening it away from your face so that the vapor pressure flows away from you. Place the stopper on a sterile gauze pad while you work with the collection tube. Do not allow the stopper to come in contact with other work surfaces. Keep the collection tube stoppered unless you are actively using it.
- Establish clean and dirty areas in the laboratory. Place all used instruments and equipment in the dirty area for sanitization, disinfection, and sterilization.
- Disinfect your work area at least once a day with a 10% bleach solution or a germ-killing solution approved by the Environmental Protection Agency (EPA). If a spill occurs, immediately disinfect the work area.
- Dispose of waste products immediately.
- Dispose of needles in the appropriate sharps container. Do not bend, break, or recap a used needle, and never reuse a disposable needle.
- If an instrument or piece of equipment must be serviced, be sure it has been decontaminated first.
- If you use a bleach solution for disinfection, change it daily.

Accident Reporting. Despite all precautions, accidents still occur in the laboratory. Armed with an understanding of the materials with which you are working and basic first-aid procedures, you should be able to deal with most emergencies. Your office should also have written procedures to follow in the event of an accident. Familiarize yourself with the procedures beforehand so that you will know what to do if an accident occurs.

Your first responsibility is to ensure your safety and that of your colleagues and patients. If someone is injured as a result of an accident, administer first aid if required, and take steps to ensure that appropriate health-care personnel take charge of the injured person.

If exposure to spilled chemicals or other substances does not pose a threat, clean up the spill. Take precautions to prevent any of the spilled substances from coming in contact with your skin or clothes. Use appropriate cleaning products for spilled chemicals. Do not touch broken pieces of glass with your hands. Use tongs or a broom and dustpan to pick up the pieces.

Disinfect the surfaces on which the substance spilled. Soaking surfaces with a 10% bleach solution, made fresh each day, is usually sufficient to remove any contamination from blood, blood products, or body fluids.

Report the accident to your supervisor or other personnel as required by your office's policies. If the accident involves exposure to blood or blood products, OSHA regulations require that several steps be followed:

1. Immediate cleaning of the area, including disinfection of contaminated surfaces and sterilization of contaminated instruments and equipment
2. Notification of a designated emergency contact, as identified in your office's safety manual
3. Documentation of the incident on a form similar to that shown in Figure 27-14, including the names of all parties involved, the names of witnesses, a description of the incident, and a record of medical treatments given to those involved
4. Medical evaluation and follow-up examination of the employees involved
5. Written evaluation of the medical condition of the involved individuals as well as testing for infection, provided that such testing does not violate confidentiality regulations

Housekeeping

There is a high risk of serious contamination in the laboratory. Laboratory housekeeping duties are designed to reduce the risk of disease transmission. Great care must be taken to ensure that these duties are done correctly and regularly. Guidelines to ensure good operating procedures and to reduce the risk of infection are as follows:

- Refer to your office's written policies and procedures to ensure that you are performing housekeeping duties correctly and according to schedule.
- Immediately clean up spills or splashes of potentially contaminated material. Depending on the material,

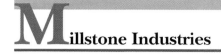

Millstone Industries

Central State Division
Incident Report

Name of Injured Employee ______

Department ______ Job Title ______

Supervisor ______

Date of Accident ______ Time ______

Nature of Injury ______

Was injured acting in a regular line of duty? ______

Was first aid given? ______ By whom? ______

Was designated emergency contact notified? ______

Did injured receive medical treatment? ______

Was injured tested for infection? ______ If no, why not? ______

Did injured go to ER? ______ Other? ______

Did injured leave work? ______ Date ______ Hour ______ A.M. P.M.

Did injured return to work? ______ Date ______ Hour ______ A.M. P.M.

Other Parties Involved ______

Names of Witnesses ______

Describe where and how accident occurred. ______

What, in your opinion, caused the accident? ______

Has anything been done to prevent a similar accident? ______

Has the hazard causing the injury been reported by telephone or in writing? ______

______ Date ______ Employee's Signature

______ Date ______ Supervisor's Signature

IF TREATMENT IS NEEDED, TAKE THE ORIGINAL AND DUPLICATE OF THIS FORM TO THE EMERGENCY ROOM.

This part for Employee Health Office use only

Was incident investigated? ______

Has injured had follow-up medical care? ______

Comments ______

Original copy to Employee Health Office *Duplicate copy to supervisor*

Figure 27-14. In the event of an accident or exposure incident in the POL, OSHA regulations require completion of an incident report form.

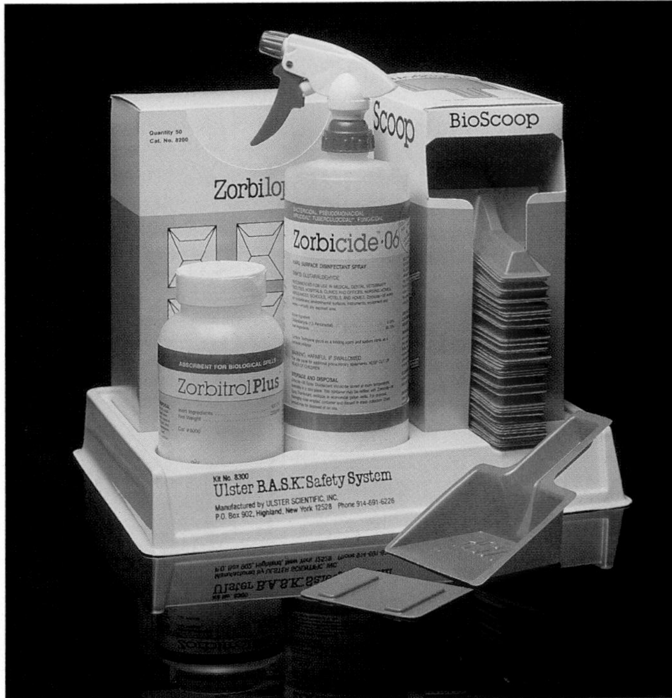

Figure 27-15. Certain substances require cleanup with specially formulated products such as these.

you may need to use special hazardous waste control products, such as those shown in Figure 27-15. Be sure to dry the area if appropriate, or clearly indicate that the area is still wet.

- Clean laboratory equipment immediately after use. Contaminants often become hard to remove if they are left on for a long time.
- Dispose of waste products carefully and correctly. Use extreme caution when handling and disposing of sharps. Procedure 27-2 describes how to dispose of biohazardous waste properly.

Quality Assurance Programs

The operation of a POL can have a significant impact on the health of the patients who depend on the medical practice for care. Accurate testing of specimens from patients is a primary concern. A **quality assurance program** is designed to monitor the quality of the patient care that a medical laboratory provides.

Clinical Laboratory Improvement Amendments

In response to public concern over the accuracy of laboratory tests, Congress enacted the **Clinical Laboratory Improvement Amendments of 1988 (CLIA '88).** This law placed all laboratory facilities that conduct tests for diagnosing, preventing, or treating human disease or for assessing human health under federal regulations administered by the Health Care Financing Administration (HCFA) and the CDC. State governments have the ability to implement their own standards, which must be at least as stringent as federal standards. If your state has its own standards, your office will operate under those standards. The state health department provides information about which standards to follow in a given locale.

CLIA '88 has had a major impact on office laboratories. Because of the complexity of the regulations and the expense required to meet them, many doctors have closed their laboratories or sharply reduced the number of tests they perform. Several attempts have been made to change the federal legislation, including an effort to exempt POLs from the regulations. As the health-care debate continues, you may see changes in laboratory operations as a result of changes in CLIA '88 regulations.

As updated and implemented in 1992, CLIA '88 standards apply to four areas of laboratory operation: standards, fees, enforcement, and accreditation programs. Most of the regulations relate to laboratory standards. The specific standards that must be met depend on the test. Tests have been divided into three categories, based on complexity. They are Certificate of Waiver tests; Level I tests, of moderate complexity; and Level II tests, of high complexity.

Certificate of Waiver Tests. The **Certificate of Waiver tests,** as listed in Figure 27-16, are laboratory tests defined as follows.

- The tests pose an insignificant risk to the patient if they are performed or interpreted incorrectly

Certificate of Waiver Tests

Urine tests

- Urinalysis by dipstick (reagent strip) or tablet reagent (nonautomated) for bilirubin, glucose, hemoglobin, ketone, leukocytes, nitrite, pH, protein, specific gravity, and urobilinogen
- Ovulation (visual color comparison tests)
- Pregnancy (visual color comparison tests)

Blood tests

- Erythrocyte sedimentation rate (ESR), nonautomated
- Hemoglobin by copper sulfate, nonautomated
- Spun microhematocrit
- Blood glucose (using devices approved by the FDA for home use)
- Fecal occult blood
- Hemoglobin by single analyte instruments automated

Figure 27-16. A POL that performs only these tests is exempt from CLIA '88 standards once the POL has been granted a Certificate of Waiver.

PROCEDURE 27.2

Disposing of Biohazardous Waste

Objective: To correctly dispose of contaminated waste products, including sharps and contaminated cleaning and paper products

OSHA Guidelines

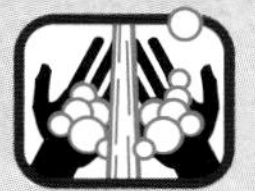
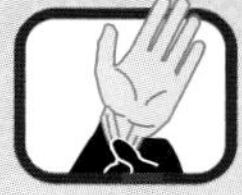
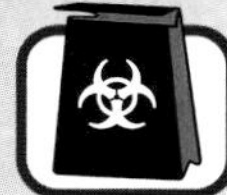
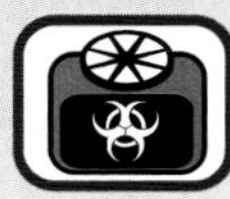
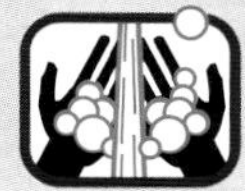

Materials: Biohazardous waste containers, gloves, waste materials

Method

To dispose of sharps or other materials that pose a danger of cutting, slicing, or puncturing the skin:

1. While wearing gloves, hold the article by the unpointed or blunt end.
2. Drop the object directly into an approved container. (If you are using an evacuation system, unscrew the needle and allow it to drop into the receptacle.) The container should be puncture-proof, with rigid sides and a tight-fitting lid.
3. If you are disposing of a needle, do not bend, break, or attempt to recap the needle before disposal. If the needle is equipped with a safety shield, slide the shield over the needle, and drop the entire assembly into the sharps container.
4. When the container is two-thirds full, replace it with an empty container. Depending on your office's procedures, the container and its contents may be sterilized before further disposal, or they may be collected by an authorized waste management agency.
5. Remove the gloves and wash your hands.

To dispose of contaminated paper waste:

1. While wearing gloves deposit the materials in a properly marked biohazardous waste container. A standard biohazardous waste container has an inner plastic liner, either red or orange and marked with the biohazard symbol, and a puncture-proof outer shell, also marked with the biohazard symbol.
2. If the container is full, secure the inner liner and place it in the appropriate area for biohazardous waste. (Biohazardous waste must be held in an area separate from regular waste and trash.)
3. Remove the gloves and wash your hands.

- The procedures involved are simple and accurate to such a degree that the risk of obtaining incorrect results is minimal
- The tests have been approved by the Food and Drug Administration (FDA) for use by patients at home

If laboratory management decides to perform these tests only, the office may apply for a Certificate of Waiver. When the certificate is granted, the laboratory is exempt from meeting various CLIA '88 standards that apply to the other two test categories. Such laboratories, however, are subject to the following: (1) random inspections to ensure that laboratories operating under a Certificate of Waiver are performing only those tests that qualify for the waiver and (2) investigation of the laboratory if there is any reason to believe the laboratory is not operating safely or if there have been complaints against the laboratory.

Level I Tests. Level I tests are moderately complex and make up approximately 75% of all tests performed in the laboratory. Among these tests are blood cell counts and cholesterol screening. Test procedures falling into the Level I category include studies involving bacteriology, mycobacteriology, mycology, parasitology, virology, immunology, chemistry, hematology, and immunohematology.

A laboratory that performs Level I tests must be run by a pathologist who has an MD or PhD degree. Technicians performing the tests must have training beyond the high school level as defined by CLIA '88 regulations. All personnel must participate in a quality assurance program for laboratory procedures, and the laboratory is subject to periodic unannounced inspections and proficiency testing.

Level II Tests. Level II tests are considered high-complexity procedures. They include more complicated tests in the specialties and subspecialties included in Level I; any test in clinical cytogenics, histopathology, histocompatibility, and cytology; and any test not yet categorized by the CMS. Manufacturers' guidelines for testing products are often the best source for discovering the CMS determination for a test. The CMS publishes a directory of all Level I and Level II tests.

Like a laboratory that conducts Level I tests, a laboratory that conducts Level II tests is subject to inspection, proficiency testing, and participation in a quality assurance program, and it must be headed by a medical doctor or a scientist who has a PhD degree. Testing procedures can be performed only by qualified laboratory personnel, whose training exceeds that provided by high schools and is defined by CLIA '88 regulations.

Components of Quality Assurance

Every quality assurance program must include the following components, in a measurable and structured system, to satisfy CLIA '88 requirements:

- Quality control
- Instrument and equipment maintenance
- Proficiency testing
- Training and continuing education
- Standard operating procedures documentation

Quality Control and Maintenance

A **quality control program** is one component of a quality assurance program. The focus of the quality control program is to ensure accuracy in test results through careful monitoring of test procedures. To be in compliance with quality control standards, a laboratory must follow certain procedures.

Calibration. Testing equipment must be calibrated regularly, in accordance with manufacturers' guidelines. Calibration ensures that the equipment is operating correctly. Each calibration must be recorded in a quality control log, such as the one shown in Figure 27-17. Calibration routines are performed on a set of standards. A **standard** is a specimen, like the patient specimens you would normally process with the equipment except that the value for each standard is already known. The calibration procedure requires that the test equipment yield the correct results for the standards supplied. Calibration routines are run on the standards alone, never with patient samples. They are used exclusively to ensure that the equipment is performing according to manufacturers' specifications.

Control Samples. **Control samples** are similar to standards in that they are specimens like those taken from a patient and have known values. Unlike standards, however, control samples are used every time before a patient sample is processed. Using a control sample serves as a check on the accuracy of the test. If the control tests do not fall within the manufacturer's prescribed ranges, patient samples are not analyzed, which prevents erroneous results.

The control samples for certain laboratory procedures show normal (negative) and abnormal (positive) results. Generally, positive and negative control samples are used with tests that yield a **qualitative test response** (the substance being tested for is either present or absent).

Other control samples are formulated to show when results fall within a normal range. These samples are used for tests that yield **quantitative test results** (the concentration of a test substance in a specimen). At least two control samples containing different concentrations of the test substance should be run for quantitative tests.

Reagent Control. Control samples or standards are also run every time you open a new supply of testing products, such as staining materials, culture media, and reagents. **Reagents** are chemicals or chemically treated substances used in test procedures. A reagent is formulated to react in specific ways when exposed under specific conditions. One example of a reagent is the chemically coated strip used in blood glucose monitoring. A visual change on the reagent strip (also called a dipstick) occurs in the presence of glucose in a blood sample. To ensure

Quality Control Daily Log

Name of Unit	Glucose Control Solution	Strip Lot No./ Exp. Date	Low Control Value 35–65 mg/dL	High Control Value 175–235 mg/dL	Analyzed By	Date	Remedial Action Taken If Control Values Abnormal	Retest After Remedial Action Taken
XYZ Glucometer	Check-strip control solution	Lot 851 10/15/99	39 mg/dL	230 mg/dL	MSM	1/17/99		
Mitchell Drugs Glucometer	Check-strip control solution	Lot 851 10/15/99	50 mg/dL	267 mg/dL	MSM	1/17/99	Machine cleaned	220 mg/dL high value
XYZ Glucometer	Check-strip control solution	Lot 851 10/15/99	Unable to read	Unable to read	LMC	1/18/99	Battery changed	38 mg/dL low 198 mg/dL high
Mitchell Drugs Glucometer	Check-strip control solution	Lot 851 10/15/99	45 mg/dL	226 mg/dL	LMC	1/18/99		

Figure 27-17. The quality control log shows the completion of every quality control check conducted on a piece of equipment.

Urine Reagent Strip Control Log										Control Solution	Exp. Date ______		Lot # ______	
Reagent Strip / Lot # & Exp. Date	Test	Specific Gravity	pH	Protein	Glucose	Ketone	Bilirubin	Blood	Nitrite	Urobilinogen	Control Test Date	Remedial Action Taken If Reading Is Abnormal	Retest Date	Technician Initials
	Reagent Strip Expected Range													
	Test Results													
	Reagent Strip Expected Range													
	Test Results													

Figure 27-18. The reagent control log shows the quality testing performed on every batch or lot of reagent products.

the quality of reagents, you should keep a reagent control log. If a defective reagent test is identified, it can be tracked to its source. A sample reagent control log is shown in Figure 27-18.

Maintenance. Testing instruments and equipment must be properly maintained, and all maintenance procedures must be documented. Follow manufacturers' guidelines for performing instrument and equipment maintenance. A maintenance log provides a complete record of all work performed on an instrument or a piece of equipment (Figure 27-19).

Documentation. A quality control program depends first on careful adherence to procedures designed to identify problems with equipment calibration, errors in testing procedures, and defective testing supplies. The second component of a quality control program is the careful documentation of all procedures. Besides maintaining the quality control log, the reagent control log, and the equipment maintenance log, you will also complete the following records as part of a quality control program:

- Reference laboratory log, which lists specimens sent to another laboratory for testing
- Daily workload log, which shows all procedures completed during the workday

Proficiency Testing

All laboratories that perform Level I and Level II tests as identified by CLIA '88 must participate in a proficiency testing program. **Proficiency testing programs** measure the accuracy of test results and adherence to standard operating procedures. Generally, proficiency tests include two parts: (1) a control sample from the proficiency testing

Acme Medical Supplies
Equipment Maintenance Record

Practice Russo and Russo Medical Associates
Name of Equipment Acme Microscope Model ABC-123
Location Lab **Purchase Date** 12/1/04

Date	Cleaning	Maintenance/Repair	Technician Initials
6/5	Microscope	Cleaned	CJC
6/11	Microscope high objective	Cleaned	DWM
6/14	Microscope	Changed bulb	CJC
6/16	Microscope eyepiece	Lens cover replaced	CJC
6/17	Microscope high objective	Cleaned	CJC

Figure 27-19. A maintenance log must be kept for every piece of laboratory equipment. All work done on the equipment must be recorded in the log.

organization engaged by your laboratory and (2) forms that must be completed to record the steps in the testing procedure. The control sample is processed normally, under the same conditions as any patient sample. The results, the forms, and sometimes the control samples are returned to the proficiency testing organization, which then informs your office of whether it has passed or failed the test. A passing mark means that your laboratory can continue to perform that particular test. A failing mark can mean that your laboratory must discontinue that test and possibly other tests as well.

Training, Continuing Education, and Documentation

One of your employer's responsibilities is to provide opportunities for employee training and continuing education. Another is to provide written reference materials and documentation for all procedures conducted in the POL. Your responsibility is to consult reference materials and take part in available training to keep your skills sharpened and up to date.

It may seem unnecessary to refer to written instructions for procedures that you do many times a day. Changes can be made in a procedure for many reasons, however, and you must be aware of these changes. Here are some reference materials with which you should be familiar:

- Material Safety Data Sheets
- Standard operating procedures
- Safety manuals
- Equipment manufacturers' user or reference guides
- Clinical Laboratory Technical Procedure Manuals
- Regulatory documentation (OSHA standards, CLIA '88 requirements)
- Maintenance and housekeeping schedules

Filling Out a Laboratory Requisition Form

As a medical assistant, it is your responsibility to ensure that the laboratory requisition form is properly completed. Missing information can lead to improper testing or lost results. The completed form should be included with the specimen collected or sent with the patient to the laboratory. Be sure to include the following information on all requisitions:

- Patient's full name, sex, date of birth, and address
- Patient's insurance information
- Physician's name, address, and phone number
- Source of the specimen
- Date and time of the specimen collection
- Test(s) requested
- Preliminary diagnosis
- Any current treatment that might affect the results

See Figure 27-20 for a sample laboratory requisitions form.

Communicating With the Patient

In your job as a medical assistant, you will be involved with patients before they submit samples for laboratory testing, during the specimen collection procedure, and after the physician has interpreted the test results. It is your responsibility to ensure that patients understand what is expected of them every step of the way.

Before the Test

Certain tests require patients to prepare by fasting or restricting fluid intake. It is your duty to explain test preparations. Use simple, nontechnical language and check with patients to be sure they understand the information. In some cases providing a written instruction sheet may be helpful.

Explaining the reason for the preparation can help ensure compliance or unearth potential problems. For example, if you explain to a patient that he is to refrain from drinking anything for a particular period, he might ask whether that includes the water he uses to take a certain medication. You can then make sure the patient receives the answers he will need for carrying out the physician's orders in light of his own circumstances.

If you are the person who collects specimens, you need to determine whether patients have correctly completed the required test preparations. Test results are invalid in some cases if patients fail to follow test preparation guidelines. When preparations have not been completed correctly, discuss the situation with the physician or other appropriate staff member as required by your office to determine whether the specimen should still be collected. If the specimen is not collected, document the reason the test was not carried out as requested. Review the guidelines for specimen collection with the patient, and schedule another appointment if appropriate.

During Specimen Collection

The instructions you deliver to patients during specimen collection vary with the nature of the specimen. Always deliver instructions clearly and in language patients can understand. Do not assume that patients do not need to hear the instructions, even if they have had the test before. Explain what you must do and what patients must do before moving to each new step in the process.

Patients are understandably nervous during many collection procedures. In addition to communicating technical information, you should provide any helpful advice

LAB USE ONLY	Laboratory Name & Address	Requesting Physician Information
Acct #		Address
DATE		
		Phone Number
TIME		

Patient Information Patient Name (Last)	(First)		(MI)	Date of Birth / /
Address	City, State		Zip	Phone Number
Patient I.D. Number	Responsible Party (Last)	(First)	(Phone)	□ Male □ Female
Social Security Number	Physician			Specimen Collection Date Time

Bill: Check One □ Our account □ Medicare □ Insurance Co./Patient		
Complete the Following Information for Billing a Patient and/or a Third Party Agency		
Policy Holder Name	Policy Holder Address: Policy Holder Phone Number:	Relation □ Self □ Spouse □ Child □ Other __________________
Insurance Co. Name	Address Insurance Co.	City , State, Zip
Employer		
Policy / Group #		
	PATIENT or GUARDIAN SIGNATURE:	DATE:

CHECK DESIRED TESTS **PLEASE PROVIDE ICD=9-CM#**

√	ORGAN DISEASE PANELS, BLOOD	ICD-9	√	TEST, BLOOD	ICD-9	√	TEST, BLOOD	ICD-9	√	TEST, URINE	ICD-9
	ACUTE HEP. A,B,C			ESR			WBC with diff			U/A Routine	
	BASIC METABOLIC			EBV			PT				
	THYROID			FBS			PTT				
	ELECTROLYTES			Grp A β-Hem strep			Bleeding time				
	HEPATIC FUNCTION			Hgb			PCO_2				
	LIPID PROFILE			Hct			PO_2				
	RENAL FUNCTION			HgbA1c			CO_2				
	TEST, BLOOD			HIV antibodies			HCO_3			**MICROBIOLOGY**	
	ACE			Insulin			Ca^{++}			AFB culture	
	ADH			Iron			Cl^-			C & S	
	ALT			Ketone bodies						Chlamydia screen	
	AFP			LD						Endocervical culture	
	Amylase			pH						GC screen	
	Acetone			Phenylalanine						Gram stain	
	AST			K^+ and Na^+			**TEST, URINE**			O & P	
	Bilirubin			Proteins, Albumin			Cys			Strep A culture	
	BUN			Proteins, Fibrinogen			CrCl			Throat culture	
	CEA			PSA			Glucose			Urine culture	
	Calcium, total			RBC			HCG			Viral culture	
	Carbon dioxide, total			Sickle cells			UBG			Wound culture	
	Cholesterol, total			TSH			UFC				
	Cholesterol, HDLs			T3			UK				
	Cholesterol, LDLs			T4			UNA				
	CK			Uric Acid			Uosm				
	CMV			WBC			UUN				

Figure 27-20. The laboratory requisition form must be accurately completed.

that may make the test easier. Also provide reassurance as appropriate. For example, if a patient asks whether the blood-drawing procedure is painful, explain that a sharp stick or stinging sensation may be experienced when the needle is inserted but that no pain should be felt after that. Let the patient be your guide in determining how much information to provide. Some people want to know every detail, whereas others prefer to know as little as possible.

One important aspect of communicating with patients about testing procedures is your nonverbal communication skills. Even if you deliver accurate technical information and answer every question patients have, there can still be a breakdown in communication if your nonverbal signals do not support your verbal message. Follow these guidelines to ensure that your nonverbal actions are helping, not hindering, the communication process.

- Strike a balance between a strict, businesslike attitude and overly familiar friendliness. Your actions must impress on the patient that you are well informed about the procedure involved and that you care about the patient's understanding of it.
- Treat the patient with respect. Address the patient by name, using the appropriate courtesy title unless you have been invited to use the patient's first name or the patient is a child. Provide privacy during specimen collection. Privacy needs may be met by using a separate room or contained area for drawing blood, for example; a private bathroom is best for collecting urine specimens.
- Recognize that the patient may be under stress because of the test procedure or the pending results. Some patients may be familiar with the test procedures, but others may not know what to expect. You may need to repeat instructions or explain what you are doing more than one time. Remain calm and patient—never be abrupt or condescending.
- Direct your attention to the patient, particularly during a procedure that might be uncomfortable, such as drawing blood. Unless an emergency develops, pay attention to nothing else at that time.

After Specimen Collection

If the patient must follow particular guidelines after you collect the specimen, explain them. Commonly, posttest instructions deal with care of venipuncture sites, signs and symptoms of infection, additional or continuing dietary restrictions, and the schedule for further testing if it is necessary.

When the Test Results Return

When you receive the tests results, do not communicate them to the patient but to the doctor. Only the doctor is qualified to interpret test results for the patient. Your role in reporting results comes after the doctor examines the test information and prepares a report. Sometimes the doctor discusses the results with the patient. At other times you will be asked to convey the test results to the patient along with instructions from the doctor. Answer only those patient questions that are within the range of your knowledge and experience. If the patient needs more information than you can provide, refer the patient to the doctor.

Record Keeping

The importance of accurate and complete record keeping can be summed up in one statement: If it is not written down, it was not done. This motto applies to all your duties as a medical assistant. Besides recording information about quality control and equipment maintenance, you may be called on to handle inventory control, record test results in patient records, and keep track of every specimen that passes through your hands. You may need to use standard abbreviations for measures when recording test results. Figure 27-21 provides a list of common abbreviations used in the laboratory.

Inventory Control

You will be responsible for taking inventory of equipment and supplies to ensure that the POL never runs out of them. To do so, you will keep a list of items that are used routinely and reordered systematically. Establish a regular

Abbreviations for Common Laboratory Measures

cm = centimeter
cm^3 = cubic centimeter
dL = deciliter
fl oz = fluid ounce
g = gram
L = liter
lb = pound
m = meter
mg = milligram
mL = milliliter
mm = millimeter
mm Hg = millimeters of mercury
oz = ounce
pt = pint
QNS = quantity not sufficient
qt = quart
U = unit
wt = weight

Figure 27-21. You may encounter these common abbreviations when recording patients' test results.

schedule for counting items in the POL, perhaps every week or so. Then estimate when you will probably need to reorder an item—and put the date on your calendar.

Patient Records

When recording test results, it is your responsibility to identify unusual findings. Many offices require that out-of-range test results be circled or underlined in red. Follow the procedure established by your office. Test results are not communicated to the patient until the physician has had the opportunity to review the information. The physician usually initials or otherwise marks the records after examining them.

Specimen Identification

All specimens must be clearly identified with the patient's name, the patient's identification code if your office uses one, the date and time the specimen was collected, the initials of the person who collected the specimen, the physician's name, and other information as required by the test procedure or your office. If you encounter an unidentified or incorrectly identified specimen, you must make an effort to track it to its source. The specimen will probably be discarded or destroyed, however, because there is no guarantee that it was identified correctly. Even if you do manage to identify it, it may have been compromised in some way.

Summary

The physician's office laboratory offers many opportunities for interesting and satisfying work in your role as a medical assistant. Those opportunities carry with them the responsibility to maintain and improve your technical skills; to stay abreast of technological, legislative, and regulatory developments; to take every precaution to prevent the transmission of disease and the occurrence of accidents or emergency situations; and to seek ways to improve the quality of patient care.

Keeping a level head and applying common sense will go a long way toward making your work in the laboratory efficient and accurate. Take time to do a procedure correctly the first time. Avoid shortcuts—they lead to mistakes and lost time.

The quantity of information you will need to learn, integrate, and convey to the patient through your actions and educational efforts may be daunting at first. As you gain understanding and confidence in your skills, however, much of it will become routine.

REVIEW

CHAPTER 27

CASE STUDY QUESTIONS

Now that you have completed this chapter, review the case study at the beginning of the chapter and answer the following questions:

1. What is a POL?
2. What enactment regulates laboratories, personnel, and the testing they perform?
3. What is the difference between waived testing and Level I testing?
4. Does quality control have an impact on laboratories? If so, how?
5. Should you perform the testing as requested? Why or why not?

Discussion Questions

1. Identify five common physical hazards in the laboratory and the steps you can take to eliminate them.
2. What responsibilities does an employer have under the OSHA Bloodborne Pathogens Standard?
3. A common instrument used in laboratories is a microscope. Identify the component parts of a microscope.
4. What information must be included on MSOSs for chemicals?
5. When laboratory results return for a patient, how should the report be routed?

Critical Thinking Questions

1. While you are holding a vial of blood, it slips out of your hand and breaks. What should you do?
2. How could a physician's office laboratory be more advantageous than a reference laboratory? What advantages does a reference laboratory afford?
3. What types of accident prevention guidelines fall under a commonsense heading?
4. What nonverbal communication techniques can you use when you are instructing patients during the specimen collection process?

Application Activities

1. Examine a prepared slide under a microscope. With a partner, practice bringing the slide specimen into focus with each objective. Partners should check each other's work.
2. Obtain a Material Safety Data Sheet, and review the information on it. Explain to another student what hazards the substance poses, what measures can be taken to avoid injury from the substance, and what steps should be taken in the event of an accident.
3. With another student acting as your patient, explain the preparations necessary for a common blood test. Prepare a set of written instructions, but before giving them to the "patient," ask him to repeat the oral instructions you gave. Compare the patient's version to your written instructions to see how clearly you conveyed the preparation information.

Internet Activity

Use the Internet to access the Web site for the American Society of Clinical Pathologists and American Medical Technologists. Provide a description of the educational requirements that you need in order to take their examinations and become a medical laboratory assistant.

CHAPTER 28

Introduction to Microbiology

AREAS OF COMPETENCE

2003 Role Delineation Study

CLINICAL

Fundamental Principles

- Apply principles of aseptic technique and infection control
- Comply with quality assurance practices

Diagnostic Orders

- Collect and process specimens
- Perform diagnostic tests

Patient Care

- Obtain patient history and vital signs

GENERAL

Legal Concepts

- Document accurately

CHAPTER OUTLINE

- Microbiology and the Role of the Medical Assistant
- How Microorganisms Cause Disease
- Classification and Naming of Microorganisms
- Viruses
- Bacteria
- Protozoans
- Fungi
- Multicellular Parasites
- How Infections Are Diagnosed
- Specimen Collection
- Transporting Specimens to an Outside Laboratory
- Direct Examination of Specimens
- Preparation and Examination of Stained Specimens
- Culturing Specimens in the Medical Office
- Determining Antimicrobial Sensitivity
- Quality Control in the Medical Office

OBJECTIVES

After completing Chapter 28, you will be able to:

28.1 Define microbiology.
28.2 Describe how microorganisms cause disease.
28.3 Describe how microorganisms are classified and named.
28.4 Explain how viruses, bacteria, protozoans, fungi, and parasites differ and give examples of each.

KEY TERMS

acid-fast stain
aerobe
agar
anaerobe
antimicrobial
bacillus
coccus
colony
culture
culture and sensitivity (C and S)
culture medium
etiologic agent
facultative
fungus
gram-negative
gram-positive
Gram's stain
KOH mount
microbiology
mold
mordant
O and P specimen
parasite
protozoan
qualitative analysis
quality control (QC)
quantitative analysis
smear
spirillum
stain
vibrio
virus
wet mount
yeast

OBJECTIVES *(Continued)*

28.5 Describe the process involved in diagnosing an infection.

28.6 List general guidelines for obtaining specimens.

28.7 Describe how throat culture, urine, sputum, wound, and stool specimens are obtained.

28.8 Explain how to transport specimens to outside laboratories.

28.9 Describe two techniques used in the direct examination of culture specimens.

28.10 Explain how to prepare and examine stained specimens.

28.11 Describe how to culture specimens in the medical office.

28.12 Explain how cultures are interpreted.

28.13 Describe how to perform an antimicrobial sensitivity determination.

28.14 Explain how to implement quality control measures in the microbiology laboratory.

Introduction

Humans are surrounded by tiny living organisms invisible to the naked eye. For the most part, these microorganisms cause no problems; however, when they are pathogenic in nature or are displaced from their natural environment, they can cause infections and disease. This chapter addresses the different life forms of microorganisms and how they may be identified; it also teaches you the proper collection technique for common types of specimens. You will learn about the processes involved in identifying microorganisms, the types of culture media used for these processes, how antimicrobial testing is done, and how quality control fits into ensuring reliable patient results.

CASE STUDY

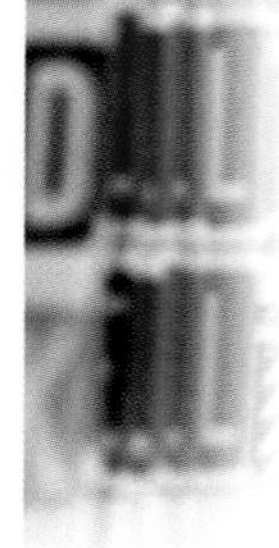

You awoke this morning with a scratchy sore throat and slight fever. You decide to go to work at the doctor's office because you don't really feel that bad, but as the morning progresses, so do your symptoms. You ask the doctor for permission to have a throat culture obtained, and with approval, you ask another medical assistant to collect the specimen. While the specimen is being collected, you can't help but notice that the swab touches your lips and tongue, but not the back of your throat. The rapid strep test is negative, so the doctor does not prescribe any medication for you. The next morning when you arise, you feel much worse and have a temperature of 102.8°. When you return to the office, the doctor briefly examines you and decides to repeat the test; this one is properly collected and the results come back as positive for strep throat. You are then prescribed antibiotics and sent home to rest.

As you read this chapter, consider the following questions:

1. What is the proper technique for collecting a throat specimen?
2. Why do you think the first test result came back as negative?
3. What organism is responsible for causing strep throat?
4. What complications may have developed if you had not had another throat culture obtained and been prescribed antibiotics?

Microbiology and the Role of the Medical Assistant

Microbiology is the study of microorganisms—simple forms of life that are microscopic (visible only through a microscope) and are commonly made up of a single cell. Microorganisms are found everywhere. Some microorganisms are normally found on the skin and within the human body; they are called normal flora. They do not typically cause disease. Instead, they perform a number of important functions. For example, microorganisms in the intestines produce vitamins and help digest food. They also help protect the body from infection.

Many microorganisms cause infections. These microorganisms are referred to as pathogenic, or disease-causing. Infections can be mild, as in the case of the common cold. Infections can, however, sometimes lead to serious conditions. The proper diagnosis and treatment of infections are essential to restoring good health.

You may assist the physician in performing a number of microbiologic procedures that aid in diagnosing and treating infectious diseases. The types of microbiologic procedures you may be required to perform in the medical office include obtaining specimens or assisting the physician in doing so, preparing specimens for direct examination by the physician, and preparing specimens for transportation to a microbiology laboratory for identification.

Some physicians' offices have their own laboratories and are equipped to perform certain microbiology procedures. If you work in such an office, you may be required to perform additional microbiologic procedures.

How Microorganisms Cause Disease

Anton van Leeuwenhoek first observed single-celled organisms through a microscope more than 300 years ago. It was not until much later, however, that microorganisms were identified as the cause of disease, through the works of scientists such as Louis Pasteur and Robert Koch.

Microorganisms can cause disease in a variety of ways. They may use up nutrients or other materials needed by the cells and tissues they invade. Microorganisms may damage body cells directly by reproducing themselves within cells, or the presence of microorgan-isms may make body cells the targets of the body's own defenses. Some microorganisms produce toxins, or poisons, that damage cells and tissues. Infecting microorganisms, or toxins they produce, may remain localized or may travel throughout the body, damaging or killing cells and tissues. The resulting symptoms include local swelling, pain, warmth, and redness along with generalized symptoms of fever, tiredness, aches, and weakness. Infection by certain organisms may also cause skin reactions, gastrointestinal upset, or other symptoms.

Pathogenic organisms can be transmitted from one person to another in one of two ways:

1. Through direct person-to-person contact, such as touching
2. Through indirect contact, as with vectors, contaminated objects, droplets expelled in the air, or contaminated food or drink

The microorganisms that make up normal flora, in addition to intact skin and mucous membranes, act as a barrier against infection by certain pathogens. Even these protective microorganisms, however, can cause infection if they invade other areas of the body.

Classification and Naming of Microorganisms

There are many different types of microorganisms, several of which can cause disease. Scientists classify microorganisms on the basis of their structure. Common classifications of microorganisms include the following:

- Subcellular, which consist of hereditary material, either deoxyribonucleic acid (DNA) or ribonucleic acid (RNA), surrounded by a protein coat
- Prokaryotic, which have a simple cell structure with no nucleus and no organelles in the cytoplasm
- Eukaryotic, which have a complex cell structure containing a nucleus and specialized organelles in the cytoplasm

Table 28-1 lists the characteristics that distinguish these classifications as well as the types of microorganisms found in the classifications. Types of microorganisms include the following:

- Viruses
- Bacteria
- Protozoans
- Fungi
- Multicellular parasites

These types may be further divided into special groups that share certain characteristics. For example, within the bacteria are the special groups mycobacteria and rickettsiae, within each of which the members share distinct characteristics.

Specific microorganisms are named in a standard way, using two words. The first word refers to the genus (a category of biologic classification between the family and the species) to which the microorganism belongs. The second word refers to the particular species of the organism. Each species represents a distinct kind of microorganism. For

TABLE 28-1 Classifications of Microorganisms

Classification	Characteristics	Examples
Subcellular	Noncellular Nucleic acid surrounded by protein coat	Viruses
Prokaryotic cells	Simple structure Single chromosome No organelles	Bacteria
Eukaryotic cells	Highly structured Nucleus and cytoplasm Organelles	Protozoans, fungi, parasites

example, within the bacteria is the *Staphylococcus* genus. Then within that genus are various species such as *Staphylococcus aureus* and *Staphylococcus epidermidis.* Although the two bacteria belong to the same genus, they differ greatly in their ability to cause disease. The first letter of the genus is always capitalized, and the species name is always written in all lowercase letters.

Viruses

Viruses are among the smallest known infectious agents. They cannot be seen with a regular microscope. Viruses are a simpler life form than the cell, consisting only of nucleic acid surrounded by a protein coat, as shown in Figure 28-1. Because of this fact, viruses can live and grow only within the living cells of other organisms.

Many viruses cause disease in people. Viruses are the cause of many of the common illnesses and conditions seen frequently in the medical office, including the common cold, influenza, chickenpox, croup, hepatitis, mononucleosis, and warts. Other illnesses caused by viruses are acquired immunodeficiency syndrome (AIDS), mumps, rubella, measles, encephalitis, and herpes. Vaccines are available to protect people from many of these viruses.

Bacteria

Bacteria are single-celled prokaryotic organisms that reproduce very quickly and are one of the major causes of disease. Under the right conditions—the right temperature, the right nutrients, and moisture—bacterial cells can double in number in 15 to 30 minutes. This rapid reproduction is one reason why untreated infections can be dangerous.

Classification and Identification

There are many different kinds of bacteria and many ways to identify them. Bacteria can be classified according to their shape, their ability to retain certain dyes, their ability to grow with or without air, and certain biochemical reactions. Table 28-2 lists some of the major groups of bacteria, with distinguishing characteristics and a few examples.

Shape. The most common way to classify bacteria is according to their shape. A **coccus** (plural, cocci) is spherical, round, or ovoid; a **bacillus** (plural, bacilli) is rod-shaped;

A

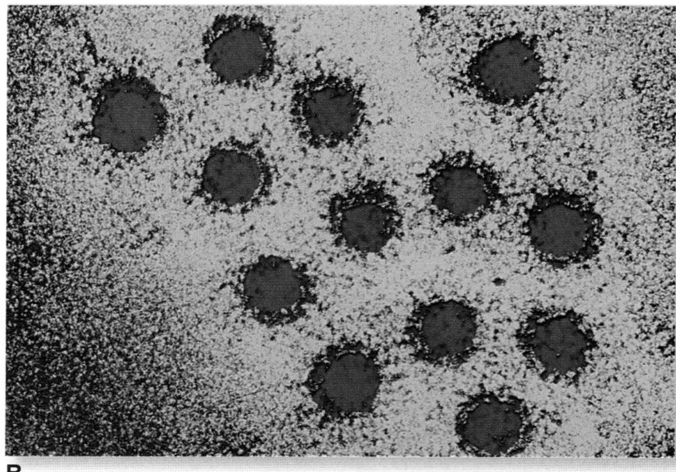

B

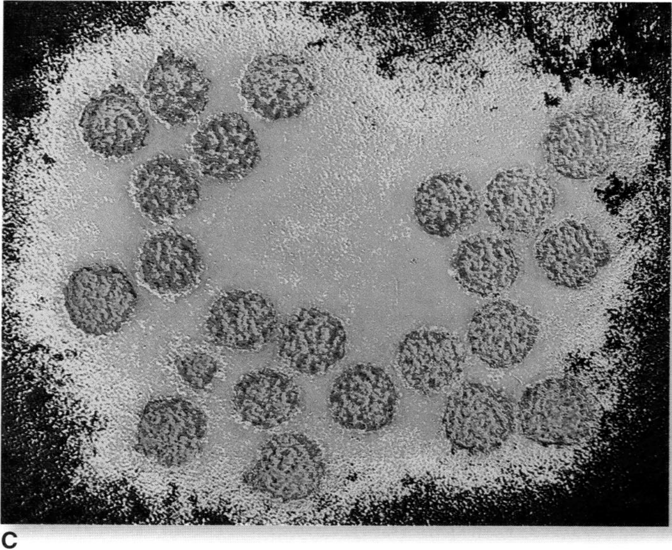

C

Figure 28-1. Three types of viral diseases often seen in medical offices are (a) influenza, (b) hepatitis, and (c) warts.

TABLE 28-2 Some Major Groups of Bacteria

Shape	Characteristic	Genus	Species
Gram-Positive Bacteria			
Spherical, round, or ovoid	Grow in clusters Grow in chains	*Staphylococcus* *Streptococcus*	*aureus epidermidis* *pyogenes pneumoniae*
Straight rod	Are aerobic Are anaerobic	*Bacillus* *Clostridium*	*subtilis* *botulinum tetani*
Gram-Negative Bacteria			
Spherical, round, or ovoid	Are aerobic	*Neisseria*	*meningitidis gonorrhoeae*
Straight rod	Are aerobic	*Pseudomonas* *Haemophilus*	*aeruginosa* *influenzae*
	Are facultative	*Escherichia* *Salmonella* *Shigella*	*coli* *typhi* *dysenteriae*
Comma	Are facultative	*Vibrio*	*cholerae*
Spiral	Move by undulating	*Treponema*	*pallidum*
Other Groups			
Straight, curved, or branched rod	Are acid-fast	*Mycobacterium*	*tuberculosis*
Variable	Have no rigid cell wall Are intracellular parasites	*Mycoplasma* *Rickettsia*	*pneumoniae* *rickettsii*
Spherical, round, or ovoid	Are intracellular parasites	*Chlamydia*	*trachomatis*

a **spirillum** (plural, spirilla) is spiral-shaped; and a **vibrio** (plural, vibrios) is comma-shaped. Figure 28-2 illustrates the four shapes.

- Cocci can be further divided into three types. Staphylococci are grapelike clusters of cocci commonly found on the skin. One species of this microorganism causes a variety of infections, including boils, acne, abscesses, food poisoning, and a type of pneumonia. Diplococci are pairs of cocci. The causative agents for gonorrhea and some forms of meningitis are diplococci. Streptococci are cocci that grow in chains. These microorganisms are responsible for infections such as strep throat, certain types of pneumonia, and rheumatic fever.
- Bacilli, or rod-shaped bacteria, are responsible for a wide variety of infections, including gastroenteritis, tuberculosis, pneumonia, whooping cough, urinary tract infections, botulism, and tetanus.
- Spirilla, or spiral-shaped bacteria, are responsible for infections such as syphilis and Lyme disease.
- Vibrios, or comma-shaped bacteria, are responsible for diseases such as cholera and some cases of food poisoning.

Ability to Retain Certain Dyes. In addition to their shape, bacteria are commonly classified by how they react to certain stains. A **stain** is a solution of a dye or group of dyes that imparts a color to microorganisms. The most common staining procedure in use today is the **Gram's stain,** a method of staining that differentiates bacteria according to the chemical composition of their cell walls. This procedure is often performed in the medical office. Another important stain is the **acid-fast stain,** a staining procedure for identifying bacteria with a waxy cell wall. The bacteria that cause tuberculosis can be stained with this procedure.

Ability to Grow in the Presence or Absence of Air. Bacteria that grow best in the presence of oxygen are referred to as **aerobes.** Those that grow best in the absence of oxygen are referred to as **anaerobes.** Organisms that can grow in either environment are referred to as being **facultative.** Although most common bacteria are aerobes, many of the bacteria that make up the normal flora of the body are anaerobes. Not surprisingly, anaerobes are often responsible for infections within the body.

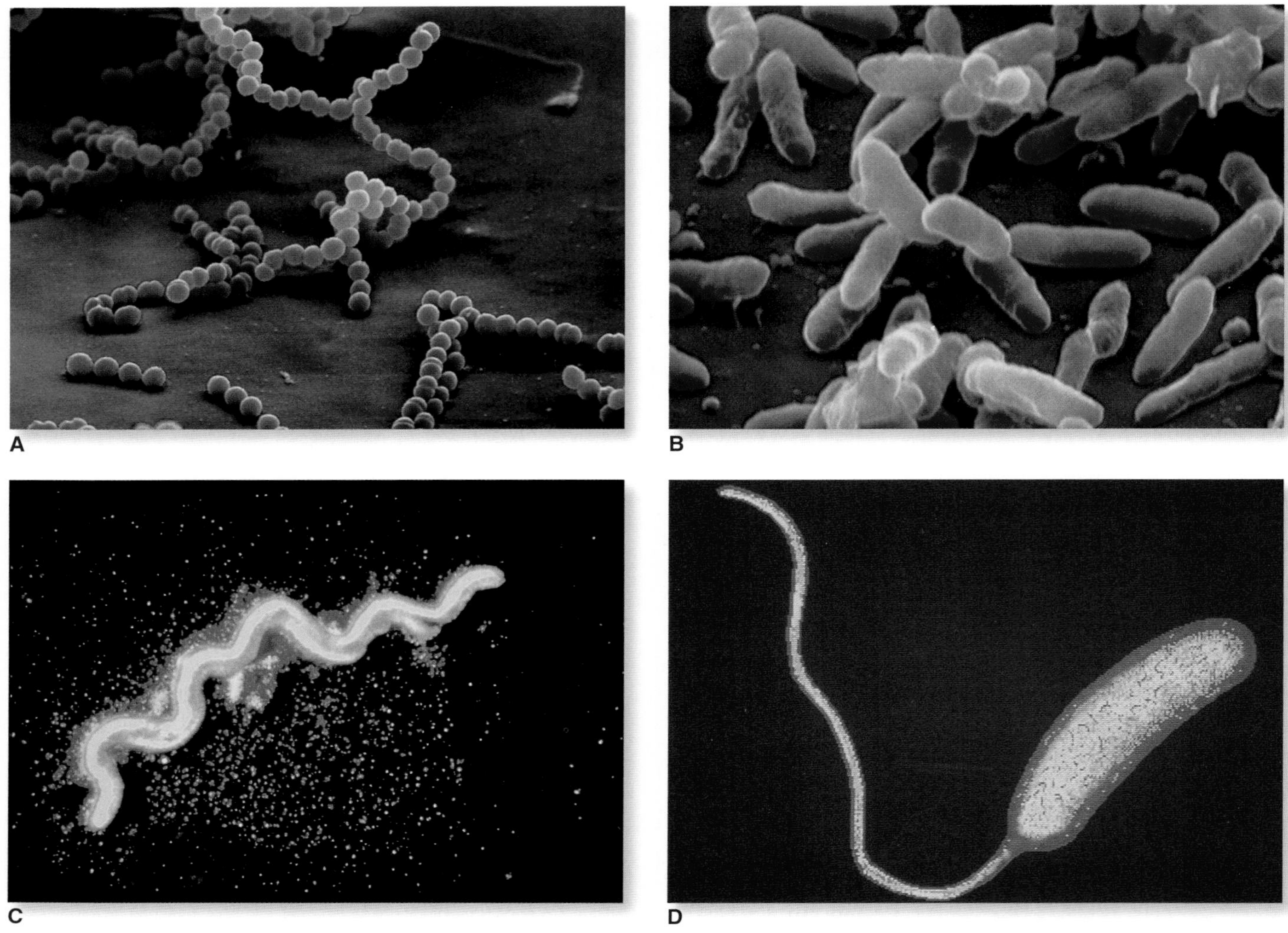

Figure 28-2. The four bacterial classifications by shape are (a) coccus, (b) bacillus, (c) spirillum, and (d) vibrio.

Biochemical Reactions. Many closely related bacteria can be differentiated from one another only by certain biochemical reactions that occur within the bacterial cell. One way to identify a particular bacterial strain is to look at what type of sugars the bacteria can use as food.

Special Groups of Bacteria

Several groups of bacteria have certain characteristics that set them apart from most other bacteria. These include the mycobacteria, rickettsiae, chlamydiae, and mycoplasmas.

Mycobacteria. Mycobacteria are rod-shaped bacilli with a distinct cell wall that differs from that of most bacteria. Certain types of mycobacteria cause disease in humans. For example, *Mycobacterium tuberculosis* causes the respiratory disease tuberculosis, and *Mycobacterium leprae* causes leprosy.

Rickettsiae. Rickettsiae are very small bacteria that can live and grow only within other living cells. Rickettsiae are commonly found in insects such as ticks and mites but may be transmitted to humans through bites. Rickettsiae are responsible for diseases such as Rocky Mountain spotted fever and typhus.

Chlamydiae. Chlamydiae are organisms that differ from other bacteria in the structure of their cell walls. Like rickettsiae, they can live and grow only within other living cells. In humans, chlamydiae can cause venereal disease, eye disease, certain types of pneumonia, and certain types of heart disease.

Mycoplasmas. Mycoplasmas are small bacteria that completely lack the rigid cell wall of other bacteria. These bacteria cause a variety of human diseases, including venereal disease and a form of pneumonia.

Protozoans

Protozoans are single-celled eukaryotic organisms that are generally much larger than bacteria. Protozoans are found in soil and water, and most do not cause disease in people. Certain protozoans are pathogenic, however, and cause diseases such as malaria (see Figure 28-3), amebic dysentery (a type of diarrhea), and trichomoniasis vaginitis (a type of venereal disease). Protozoal diseases are a leading cause of death in developing countries because the lack of proper sanitation in some areas promotes their spread. These diseases are also common in patients with depressed immune systems.

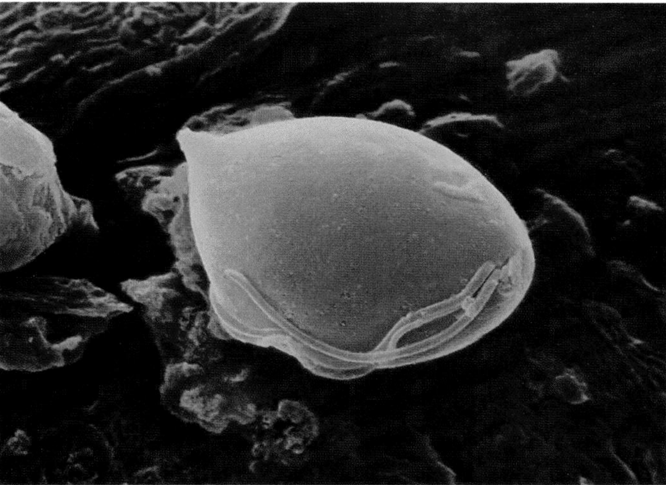

Figure 28-3. The protozoan *Trichomonus vaginalis* causes a venereal disease in humans.

Fungi

A **fungus** (plural, fungi) is a eukaryotic organism that has a rigid cell wall at some stage in the life cycle. Fungi that grow mainly as single-celled organisms that reproduce by budding are referred to as **yeasts,** whereas fungi that grow into large, fuzzy, multicelled organisms that produce spores are called **molds.** Figure 28-4 shows the differences between these two types of fungi.

Most fungi do not cause disease in humans. Of those that do, the majority produce superficial infections such as athlete's foot (tinea pedis), ringworm, thrush, and vaginal yeast infections. Fungi can produce serious, life-threatening illness, however, when they infect the body's internal tissues. This kind of infection can occur when patients have a depressed immune system, as in patients who are undergoing treatment for cancer and patients with AIDS.

Multicellular Parasites

A **parasite** is an organism that lives on or in another organism and uses that other organism for its own nourishment, or for some other advantage, to the detriment of the host organism. Viruses, rickettsiae, chlamydiae, and some protozoans are parasitic. Multicellular organisms can also be parasitic, and some of these organisms are microscopic during all or part of their lives. An infection caused by a parasite is called an infestation. Multicellular parasites that cause human disease include certain worms and insects, as illustrated in Figure 28-5.

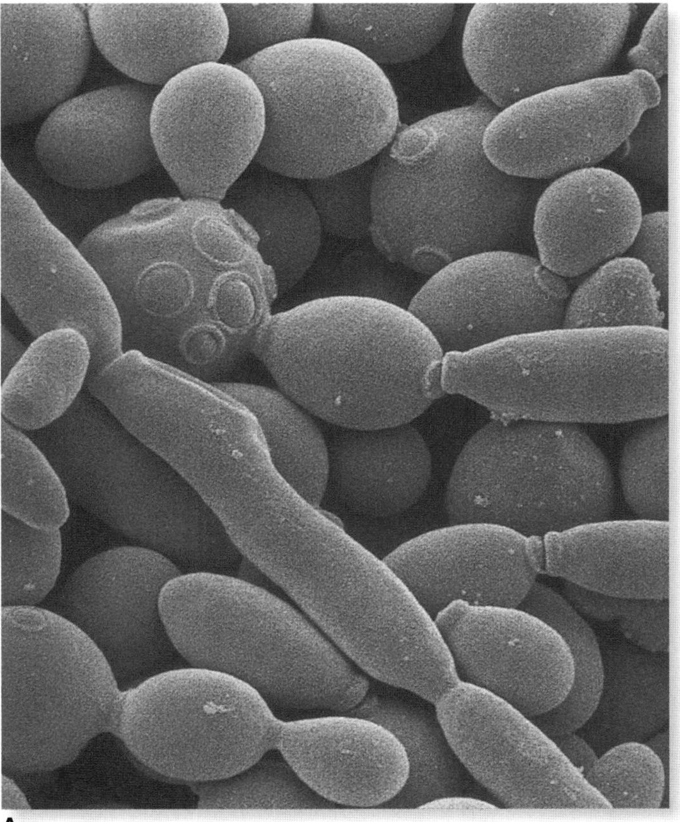

A

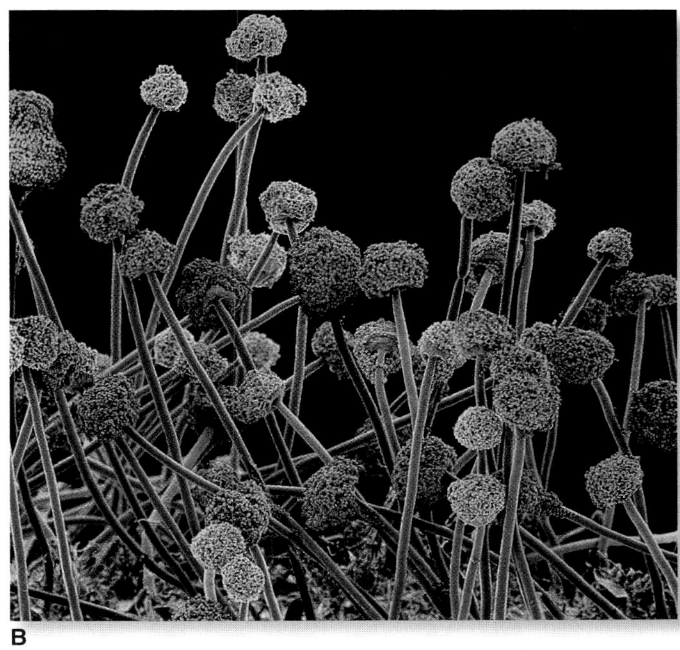

B

Figure 28-4. Because fungi lack the ability to make their own food, they depend on other life forms. (a) Single-celled fungi are called yeasts. (b) Multicelled fungi are called molds.

Parasitic Worms

People can be infected with a parasitic worm by ingesting its eggs or an immature form of the worm or by having the parasite penetrate the skin. As with the protozoans, infestation by these parasites is more common in developing nations that have poor sanitation.

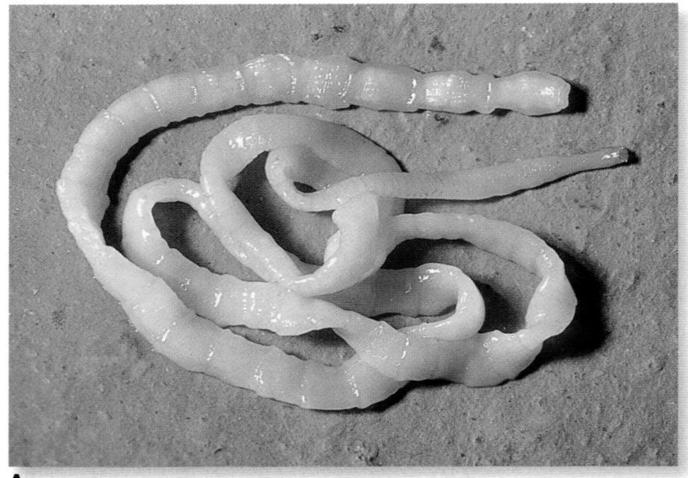

A

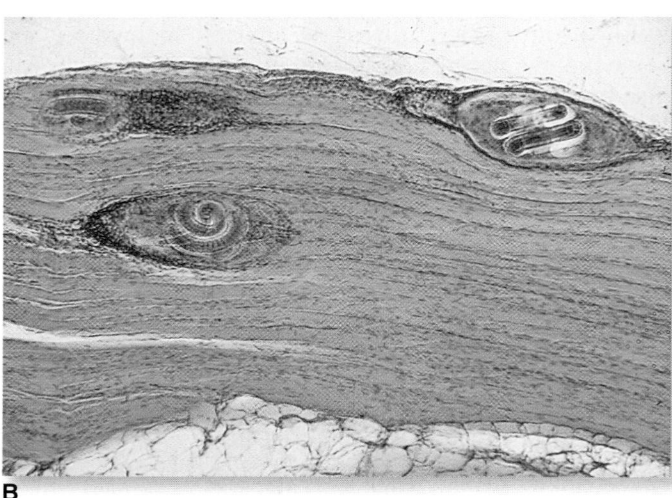

B

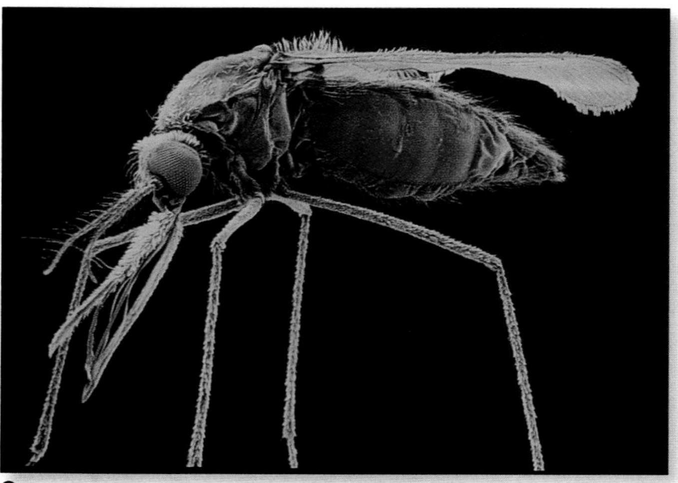

C

Worms that infect people include roundworms, flatworms, and tapeworms. Roundworms can occur in the intestines, as in the case of pinworms, a common infection in children. Other roundworms, such as *Trichinella,* are found in muscle tissue. *Trichinella spiralis,* which causes the infection trichinosis, enters the human body in infected meat eaten raw or insufficiently cooked. People may also get flatworms and tapeworms by eating undercooked meats. A trained medical professional must inspect a patient's stool for the presence of the parasite or its eggs to diagnose an intestinal infection with a parasitic worm.

Parasitic Insects

Insects that can bite or burrow under the skin include mosquitoes, ticks, lice, and mites. These insects spread many viral, bacterial (including rickettsial), and protozoal dis-

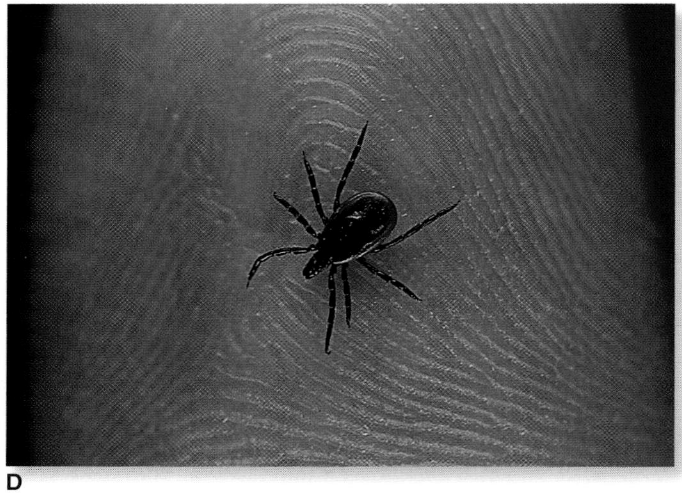

D

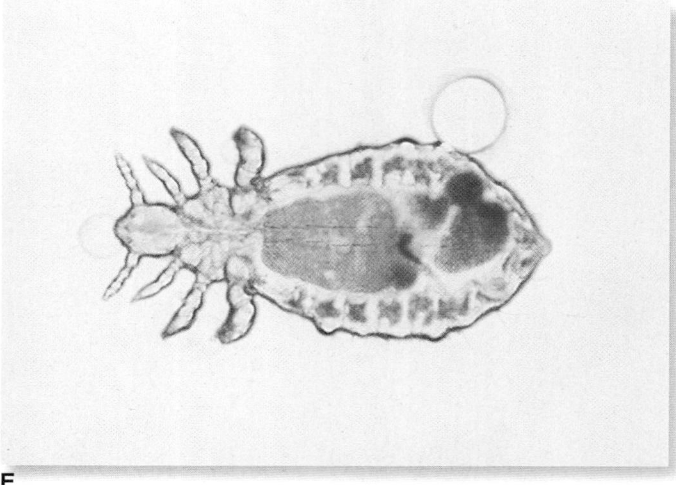

E

Figure 28-5. Parasitic worms, such as (a) tapeworms and (b) *Trichinella,* cause disease in humans when they are ingested. Parasitic insects, such as (c) mosquitoes, (d) deer ticks, and (e) mites, cause disease by biting or burrowing into the skin.

eases. The causative organisms can live in the insects' bodies and enter people's bodies when they are bitten by the insects. Such diseases include Lyme disease, malaria, Rocky Mountain spotted fever, and encephalitis. Infestations such as scabies that are caused by some lice and mites are considered parasitic diseases.

How Infections Are Diagnosed

To assist with the diagnosis and treatment of an infection, you must work closely with other members of the medical team. The basic steps in diagnosis and treatment are summarized in Figure 28-6.

Step 1. Examine the Patient

When a patient comes into the office with signs or symptoms that suggest an infection, begin by taking the patient's vital signs and noting the patient's complaints. On the basis of these findings and examination of the patient, the doctor can make a presumptive, or tentative, clinical diagnosis.

In many cases signs and symptoms of a particular infection are so characteristic of the disease that the doctor need not perform additional tests to reach a diagnosis. An example might be a case of chickenpox or mumps. At other times, however, the doctor needs to gather additional information to confirm a diagnosis and determine the cause.

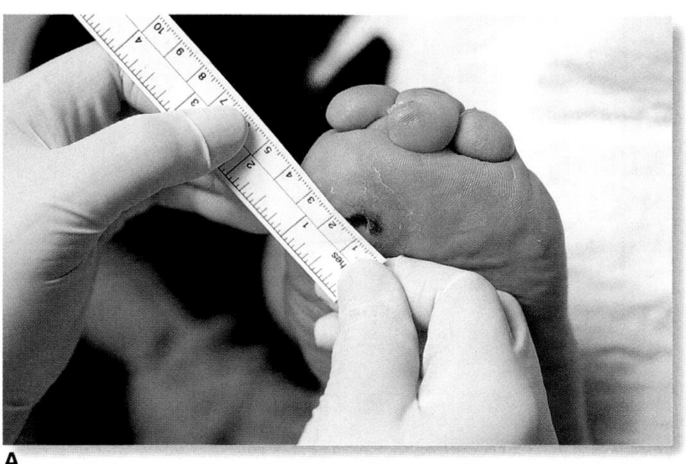

A

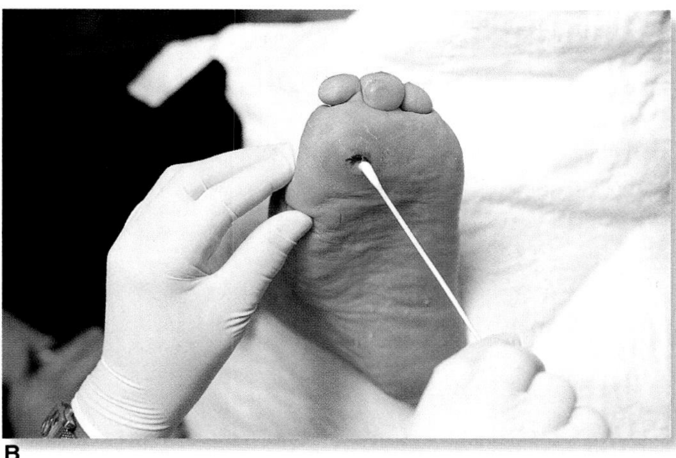

B

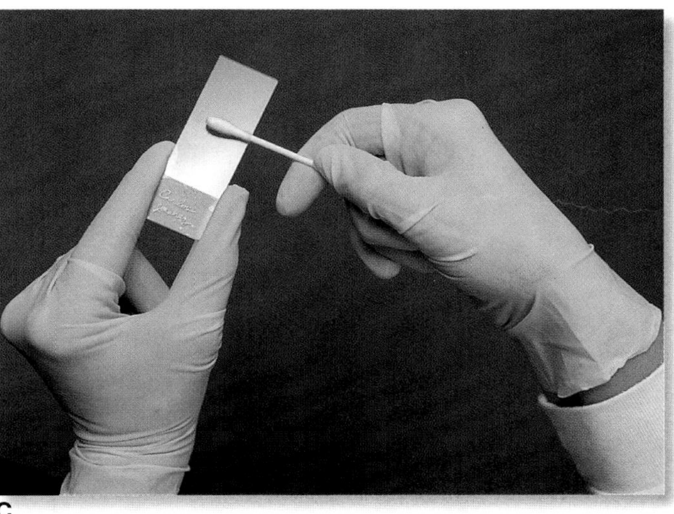

C

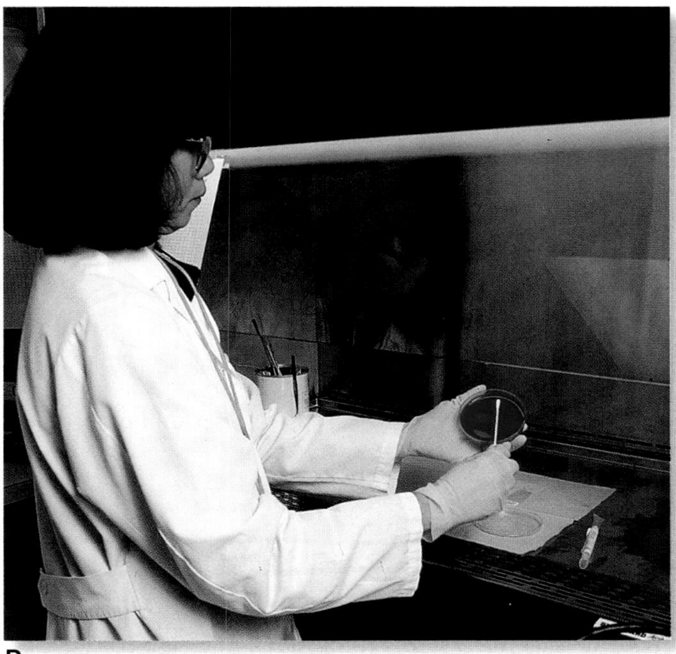

D

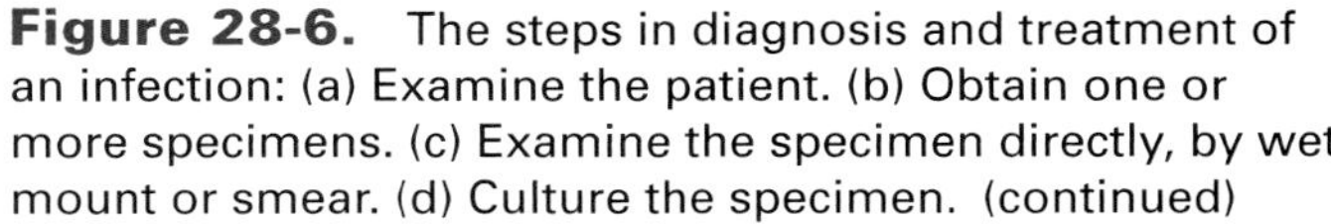

Figure 28-6. The steps in diagnosis and treatment of an infection: (a) Examine the patient. (b) Obtain one or more specimens. (c) Examine the specimen directly, by wet mount or smear. (d) Culture the specimen. (continued)

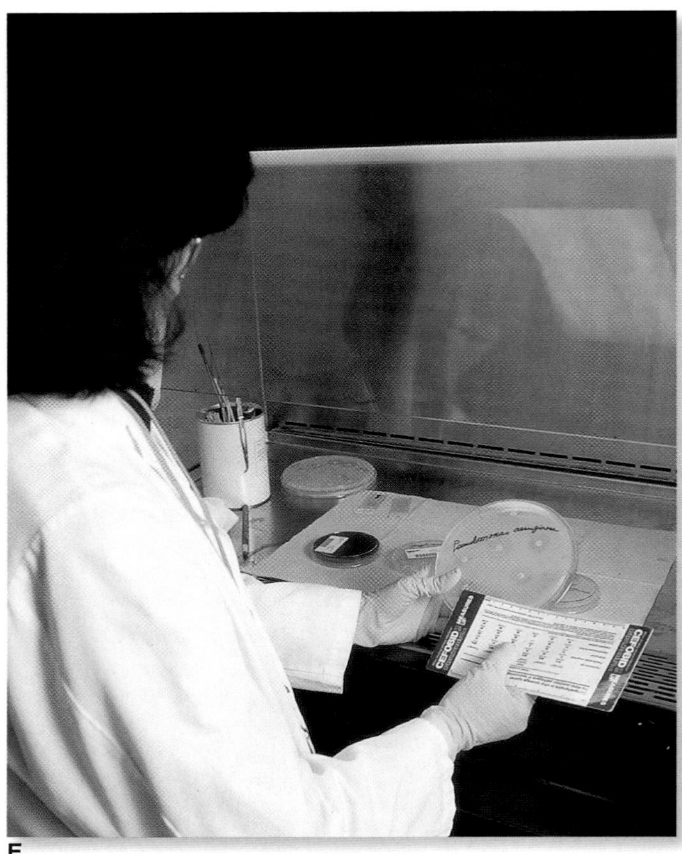

E

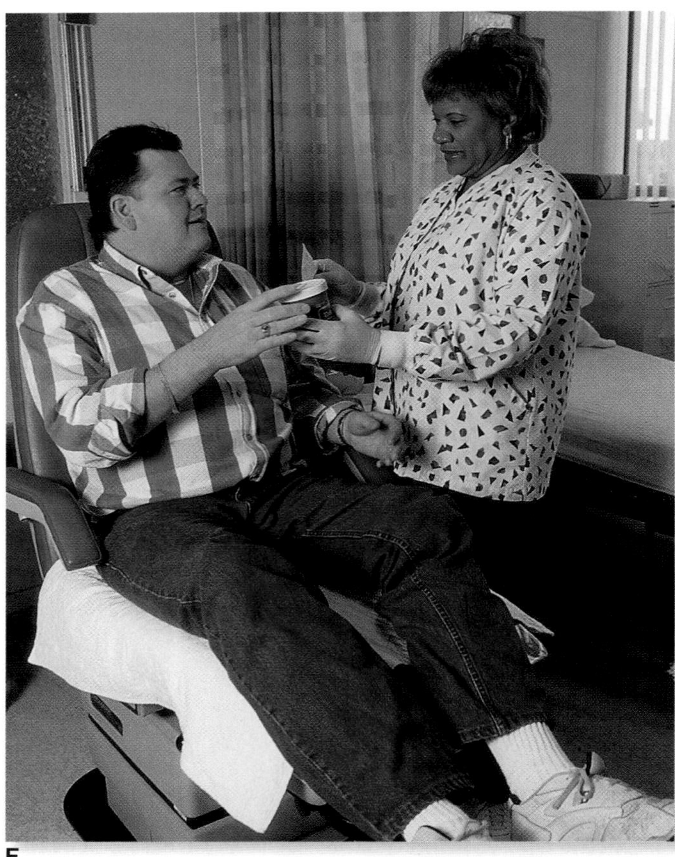

F

Figure 28-6. (continued)
(e) Determine the culture's antibiotic sensitivity. (f) Treat the patient as ordered by the physician.

Step 2. Obtain One or More Specimens

To determine the cause of an infection, you may need to obtain material from one or more areas of the patient's body. Label each specimen properly and include with it the physician's presumptive diagnosis. If the sample is to be transported to an outside laboratory, ensure that it is transported in such a way that any pathogenic organisms remain alive (and safely contained) during transit.

Step 3. Examine the Specimen Directly

You must sometimes obtain more than one specimen from each site. The doctor or specially trained laboratory or microbiology personnel will then directly examine one specimen under the microscope. The specimen may be viewed in one of two ways:

1. As a **wet mount,** a preparation of a specimen in a liquid that allows the organisms to remain alive and mobile while they are being identified
2. As a **smear,** in which a specimen is spread thinly and unevenly across a slide

If you make a smear, allow it to dry, and stain or treat it as ordered before it is examined microscopically. In some cases direct examination allows the doctor to make a presumptive diagnosis of the offending microorganism.

Step 4. Culture the Specimen

If the physician still needs a more definitive identification of the microorganism, you may perform a **culture,** in which a sample of the specimen is placed in or on a substance that allows microorganisms to grow. A **culture medium** is a substance that contains all the nutrients a particular type of microorganism needs. Most media come in the form of a semisolid gel. The particular medium is chosen according to the site from which the specimen was obtained and the suspected cause of infection. After you inoculate (place a sample of the specimen in or on) the medium, place it in an incubator (a chamber that can be set to a specific temperature and humidity) to allow the microorganism to grow.

The culture is examined visually and microscopically after a specified time, and a preliminary identification is made. The physician sets up additional tests to confirm the identification of the microorganism that has been isolated from the specimen. See Table 28-3 for information on specific microbial diseases and the body systems they

TABLE 28-3 Microbial Diseases

System	Disease	Causative Organism	Route of Transmission	Signs and Symptoms
Integumentary System	Anthrax	*Bacillus anthracis*	Inhalation or ingestion of spores; consumption of contaminated food	Fever, chills, night sweats, cough, shortness of breath, fatigue, muscle aches, sore throat
	Skin infections	*Staphylococcus aureus*	Direct contact of individuals colonized or infected with this bacteria; hand hygiene is the single most important step in controlling spread of these bacteria	Minor: pimples, boils Major: septicemia, surgical wound infection, necrotizing fasciitis
	Chickenpox	*Varicella-zoster virus*	Droplets spread through coughing and sneezing	Skin rash of blister-like lesions, usually on the face, scalp, or trunk
Respiratory System	Pneumonia	*Haemophilus influenzae* *Streptococcus pneumoniae* *Mycoplasma pneumoniae*	Direct contact with respiratory droplets	Fever, decreased breath sounds, shortness of breath, increased heart rate (tachycardia), increased respiratory rate (tachypnea)
	Legionellosis • Legionnaire's disease (severe form) • Pontiac fever (mild form)	*Legionella pneumophila*	Breathing water mists contaminated with *Legionella* bacteria (spa, air conditioner, shower)	Fever, chills, and a cough; muscle aches, headache, tiredness, loss of appetite, and occasionally diarrhea
	Tuberculosis	*Mycobacterium tuberculosis*	Respiratory droplet spread	Bad cough that lasts longer than 2 weeks, pain in the chest, coughing up blood or sputum (phlegm from deep inside the lungs), weakness, fatigue, weight loss, no appetite, chills, fever, and night sweats
	Pertussis	*Bordetella pertussis*	Contact with respiratory droplets	Typically manifested in children with paroxysmal spasms of severe coughing, whooping, and post-tussive vomiting
	Diphtheria	*Corynebacterium diphtheriae*	Person-to-person spread through respiratory tract secretions	Sore throat; low-grade fever; adherent membrane of the tonsils, pharynx, or nose; neck swelling

continued →

TABLE 28-3 Microbial Diseases *(continued)*

System	Disease	Causative Organism	Route of Transmission	Signs and Symptoms
Respiratory System	Influenza	Influenza A and B virus	Respiratory droplet spread	Fever (usually high), headache, extreme tiredness, dry cough, sore throat, runny nose, and muscle aches; gastrointestinal symptoms include nausea, vomiting, and diarrhea
	Common cold	Rhinoviruses	Respiratory droplet spread	Runny nose; sneezing; sore throat; mild, hacking cough
	Severe acute respiratory syndrome (SARS)	SARS-associated coronavirus (SARS-CoV)	Close person-to-person contact	High fever (temperature greater than 100.4°F [38.0°C]), headache, overall feeling of discomfort, body aches, dry cough, pneumonia
Gastrointestinal System	Salmonellosis	*Salmonella enteritidis*	Consumption of contaminated food (raw eggs, chicken, or beef)	Fever, abdominal cramps, and diarrhea beginning 12 to 72 hours after consuming a contaminated food or beverage
	Typhoid fever	*Salmonella typhi*	Fecal oral	Sustained high fever (103° F–104°F), weakness, stomach pains, headache, loss of appetite
	E.coli diarrhea	*Escherichia coli* O157:H7	Eating contaminated foods (ground beef, raw milk)	Severe bloody diarrhea and abdominal cramps
	Cholera	*Vibrio cholerae*	Drinking contaminated water or eating contaminated food	Severe disease characterized by profuse watery diarrhea, vomiting, leg cramps, dehydration, and shock
	Botulism	*Clostridium botulinum*	Consuming improperly canned food contaminated with botulinum	Double vision, blurred vision, drooping eyelids, slurred speech, difficulty swallowing, dry mouth, and muscle weakness
	Mumps	Mumps virus (paramyxovirus)	Airborne and direct contact with infected respiratory droplets	Fever, headache, muscle ache, and swelling of the lymph nodes close to the jaw

continued ⟶

TABLE 28-3 Microbial Diseases *(continued)*

System	Disease	Causative Organism	Route of Transmission	Signs and Symptoms
Gastrointestinal System	Hepatitis A Hepatitis B Hepatitis C	Hepatitis A virus Hepatitis B virus Hepatitis C virus	Hepatitus A: fecal oral Hepatitus B: blood and body fluids Hepatitus C: blood and body fluids	Symptoms are similar for each: Jaundice, fatigue, abdominal pain, loss of appetite, nausea, diarrhea, fever, joint pain, dark urine
Genitourinary System	Chlamydia	*Chlamydia trachomatis*	Sexual contact	Usually silent; can have mild symptoms of abnormal vaginal discharge or a burning sensation when urinating
	Gonorrhea	*Neisseria gonorrhea*	Sexual contact	Mucopurulent endocervical or urethral exudate
	Syphilis	*Treponema pallidum*	Sexual contact; can be passed to the fetus from an infected woman	Single sore, usually firm, round, small, and painless, that appears at the spot where syphilis entered the body
	Genital herpes	Herpes simplex viruses type 1 (HSV-1) and type 2 (HSV-2)	HSV-1: oral and genital contact HSV-2: sexual contact	Genital sores, flu-like symptoms including fever and swollen glands
Nervous System	Meningitis	*Neisseria meningitides* *Streptococcus pneumoniae* *Haemophilus influenzae*	Direct contact with respiratory secretions from a carrier	High fever, headache, stiff neck, nausea, vomiting, photophobia, confusion, and sleepiness
	Toxoplasmosis	*Toxoplasma gondii*	Accidental ingestion of cat feces, ingestion of contaminated raw or undercooked meat or contaminated water	Swollen lymph glands or muscle aches and pains that last for a month or more
	Poliomyelitis	Polioviruses 1, 2, and 3	Person-to-person, fecal or oral	Ranges from asymptomatic to symptomatic, including acute flaccid paralysis, quadriplegia, respiratory failure, and rarely, death
	Rabies	Rabies virus	Bite of a rabid animal	Fever, headache, confusion, sleepiness, or agitation

continued ⟶

TABLE 28-3 Microbial Diseases *(continued)*

System	Disease	Causative Organism	Route of Transmission	Signs and Symptoms
Blood and Immune System	Plague	*Yersinia pestis*	Flea-borne from infected rodents to humans; respiratory droplets from cats and humans with pneumonic plague	Bubonic plague: enlarged, tender lymph nodes, fever, chills, and prostration Septicemic plague: fever, chills, prostration, abdominal pain, shock, and bleeding into skin and other organs Pneumonic plague: fever, chills, cough, and difficulty breathing; rapid shock
	Rocky Mountain spotted fever	*Rickettsia rickettsii*	Tick-borne ixodid ticks infected with *R. rickettsii*	Fever, nausea, vomiting, severe headache, muscle pain, lack of appetite, rash, abdominal pain, joint pain, and diarrhea
	Lyme disease	*Borrelia burgdorferi*	Tick-borne deer ticks infected with *Borrelia burgdorferi*	Fever, headache, fatigue, and myalgia
	Mononucleosis	Epstein-Barr virus	Contact with saliva of infected person	Fever, sore throat, and swollen lymph glands
	HIV/AIDS	Human immunodeficiency virus	Blood and body fluids	The following *may be* warning signs of infection with HIV: rapid weight loss; dry cough; recurring fever or profuse night sweats; profound and unexplained fatigue; swollen lymph glands in the armpits, groin, or neck; diarrhea that lasts for more than a week; white spots or unusual blemishes on the tongue, in the mouth, or in the throat; pneumonia; red, brown, pink, or purplish blotches on or under the skin or inside the mouth, nose, or eyelids; memory loss, depression, and other neurological disorders
	Malaria	*Plasmodium: P. falciparum, P. vivax, P. ovale,* or *P. malariae*	Mosquito-borne from Anopheles mosquito infected with *P. malariae*	Fever and influenza-like symptoms, including chills, headache, myalgias, and malaise

Source: Centers for Disease Control, Health Topics A to Z. Atlanta, Georgia, 2003. http://www.cdc.gov/health/default.htm

affect. Most microbiology laboratories and some physicians' office laboratories are equipped to grow routine bacterial cultures and some fungal cultures. Physicians' office laboratories, in particular, may have to send out other types of cultures, such as virus cultures, to a specialized laboratory for identification.

Step 5. Determine the Culture's Antibiotic Sensitivity

In many cases of bacterial infection, a **culture and sensitivity (C and S)** is performed. This procedure involves culturing a specimen and then testing the isolated bacterium's susceptibility (sensitivity) to certain antibiotics. The results help the doctor determine which antibiotics might be most effective in treating the infection.

Step 6. Treat the Patient as Ordered by the Physician

On the basis of identification of the microorganism and antibiotic sensitivity, if determined, the physician can prescribe an **antimicrobial.** This agent, which kills microorganisms or suppresses their growth, should help clear up the patient's infection.

Specimen Collection

Perhaps the most important step in isolating and identifying a microorganism as the cause of an infection is collecting the specimen. If you do not collect the specimen properly, the organism may not grow in culture so that it can be identified. The result may be an untreated infection. Furthermore, if the specimen becomes contaminated during collection and the contaminant is mistakenly identified as the cause of the infection, the patient may receive incorrect or even harmful therapy.

In addition to vaginal specimens (discussed in detail in Chapter 22), the most common types of culture specimens involve the following:

- Throat
- Urine
- Sputum
- Wound
- Stool

Specimen-Collection Devices

To help ensure optimal recovery of microorganisms, you must use the appropriate collection device or specimen container. This container is usually provided by the laboratory where the specimen is going to be analyzed. Special collection devices are available for the collection of sputum, urine, and stool specimens, as shown in Figure 28-7. These containers are designed with large openings to allow collection of the specimen with minimal chance of contamination. They also have tight-fitting caps to prevent leakage and contamination.

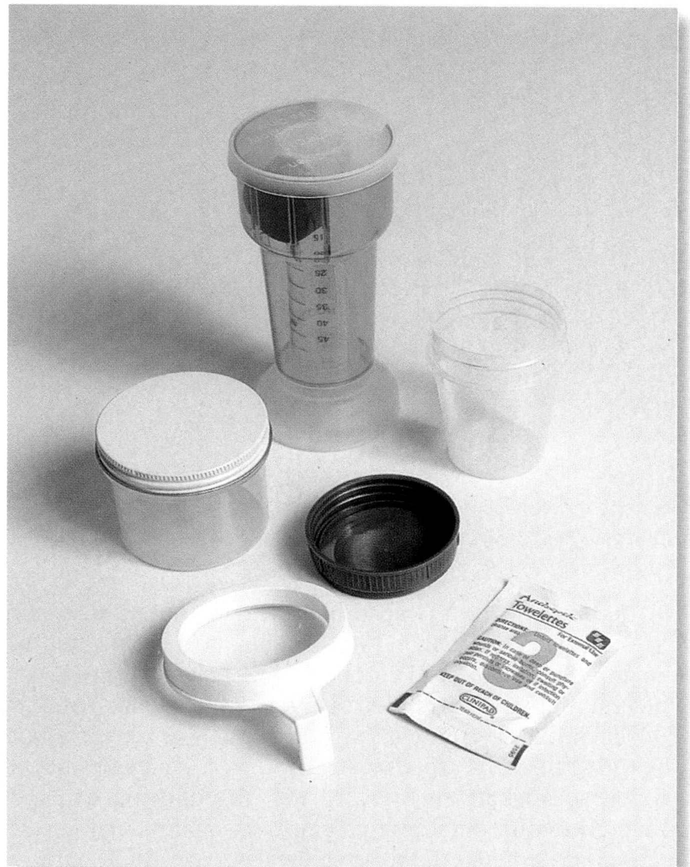

Figure 28-7. You may use specially designed collection containers to collect sputum, urine, and stool specimens.

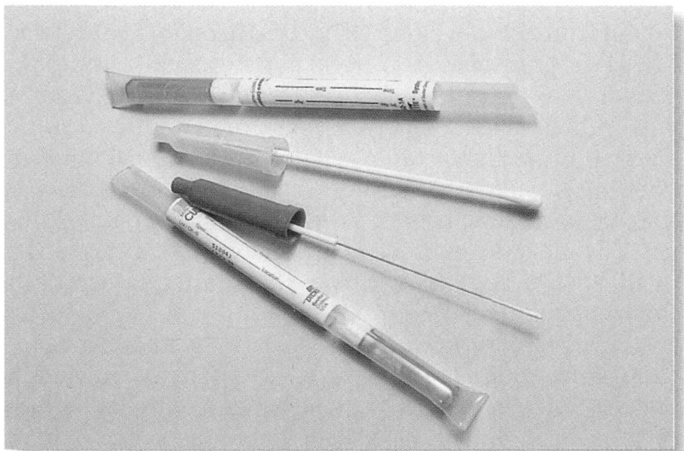

Figure 28-8. Sterile swabs vary in size and in material.

Sterile Swabs. The most common device for obtaining cultures is the sterile swab. They vary in the absorbent material at the tip and in the composition of the shaft (Figure 28-8).

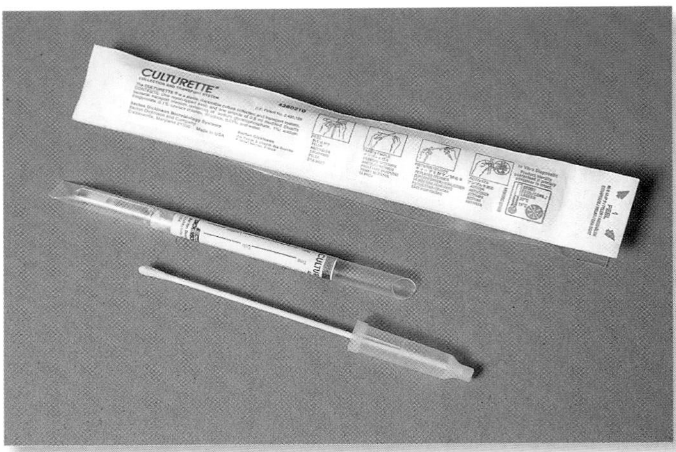

Figure 28-9. The CULTURETTE is used to obtain and transport microbiologic specimens to outside laboratories. (Courtesy of Becton Dickinson Microbiology Systems)

Although cotton is absorbent, it is no longer used for culture swabs because natural chemicals in cotton inhibit the growth of certain microorganisms. Polyester, rayon, or calcium alginate fibers are preferred. Most swabs used to collect routine specimens have a wooden or plastic shaft for rigidity. There are also swabs with a small tip and a flexible wire shaft made especially for culturing hard-to-reach areas and obtaining pediatric specimens. Some collection containers contain two swabs—one for a culture and one for a smear.

Collection and Transport Systems. Sterile, self-contained systems for obtaining and transporting specimens are commercially available from many suppliers. The CULTURETTE Collection and Transport System, manufactured by Becton Dickinson Microbiology Systems of Sparks, Maryland, is a well-known example. The unit, shown in Figure 28-9, contains a polyester swab and a small, thin-walled vial of transport medium in a plastic sleeve. If a specimen will not be tested within 30 minutes after it is obtained, the swab is replaced in the sleeve, and the vial is crushed between the thumb and the index finger. The moisture and nutrients provided by the transport medium help keep the bacteria alive during transport to the laboratory.

Several collection systems are also available for culturing anaerobic organisms. These systems provide a means of generating an oxygen-free environment so that the anaerobic organisms remain viable (alive and able to reproduce) during transport.

Specimen-Collection Guidelines

To collect specimens properly, you should follow a number of general guidelines.

- Obtain the specimen with great care to avoid causing the patient harm, discomfort, or undue embarrassment. If patients are to collect specimens on their own, give them clear, detailed instructions along with the proper container.
- Collect the material from a site where the organism is most likely to be found and where contamination is least likely to occur. For example, the best location to obtain a specimen for diagnosing strep throat is at the back of the throat in the area of the tonsils. A properly collected sputum specimen should contain mucus that is coughed up from the respiratory tract, but it should not contain saliva, which is a contaminant.
- Obtain the specimen at a time that allows optimal chance of recovery of the microorganism. Knowledge of the infectious disease process allows the doctor to determine the best time to collect a specimen. For example, certain viruses are more readily isolated during the early, symptomatic stage of an illness.
- Use appropriate collection devices, specimen containers, transport systems, and culture media to ensure optimal recovery of microorganisms. The purpose of such equipment and materials is to preserve the viability of any microorganisms so that they will grow in culture. Special collection devices are available for certain body areas or suspected pathogens.
- Obtain a sufficient quantity of the specimen for performing the requested procedures. If, for example, both a culture and a direct examination of a swabbed specimen will be done, you must collect two specimens. Each procedure requires its own sample.
- Obtain the specimen before antimicrobial therapy begins. If the patient is already taking an antibiotic, note this fact on the laboratory request form, or ask the doctor whether you should obtain the specimen.

After correctly collecting the specimen, you must label the container and include the appropriate requisition form. The label should contain the following information:

- Patient's name and identification number (if appropriate)
- Source (collection site) of the specimen
- Date and time of collection
- Doctor's name
- Your initials (if you obtained the specimen)

The requisition form should include the following information:

- Patient's name, address, and identification number
- Patient's age and gender
- Patient's insurance billing information
- Type and source of the microbiologic specimen (for example, discharge from wound, big toe)
- Date and time of microbiologic specimen collection
- Test requested
- Medications the patient is currently receiving
- Doctor's presumptive diagnosis
- Doctor's name, address, and phone number
- Special instructions or orders

Throat Culture Specimens

A microbiologic procedure frequently performed in a medical office is obtaining a throat culture. The doctor may request a culture on patients with signs or symptoms of an upper respiratory, throat, or sinus infection. Identification of the microorganism responsible for the infection allows the doctor to treat the patient as effectively as possible.

In most cases the doctor wants to determine whether the patient has strep throat, an infection caused by the bacterium *Streptococcus pyogenes.* It is particularly important to diagnose and treat this infection because, left untreated, strep throat can lead to complications such as rheumatic fever. Rheumatic fever is an inflammation of the heart tissue that occurs more frequently in school-age children than in any other population.

When you obtain a throat culture specimen, you must avoid touching any structures inside the mouth, because this will contaminate the specimen. The correct technique for obtaining a throat culture specimen is outlined in Procedure 28-1.

Many doctors order rapid strep tests done if strep is suspected. Antigen-antibody test kits for strep are available in a variety of brands. They provide immediate indications of the presence of the strep antigen on a throat swab, sparing the patient the expense and waiting period associated with having a culture done.

If your office does not culture microbiologic specimens, you need to use a sterile collection system to obtain the specimen. If your office has the equipment to perform its own cultures, use a sterile swab and inoculate a culture plate directly with the swab. Specimens to be evaluated in the office should be cultured immediately after collection.

Urine Specimens

To minimize contaminants in urine specimens, it is important to obtain a clean-catch midstream specimen. You must process urine specimens within an hour of collection or refrigerate them to prevent continued bacterial growth. (Collection of urine specimens for culturing is discussed in detail in Chapter 29.)

Sputum Specimens

To obtain sputum specimens, have the patient expectorate (cough up) mucus from the lungs into a wide-mouthed specimen container. Beforehand, instruct the patient to avoid contaminating the specimen with saliva. If sputum specimens are not cultured right away, they should be refrigerated.

Observe Universal Precautions whenever you handle sputum samples. Wear a face shield or mask and goggles when collecting such a specimen, especially if the patient is coughing. Even when tuberculosis is not suspected, the potential for transmission of this type of bacteria always exists.

Wound Specimens

You usually obtain specimens from infected wounds and lesions by swabbing. The procedure is similar to that of a throat culture. Be sure you obtain representative material from a deep area and a surface area of the wound without contaminating the swab by touching areas outside the site.

Stool Specimens

If the physician suspects that the patient has certain diseases, such as cancer or colitis or bacterial, protozoal, or parasitic infections, you may need to obtain stool specimens. The collection technique varies with the suspected microorganism. Although both you and the patient may be embarrassed to discuss instructions for collecting stool specimens, do not let this interfere with proper specimen collection.

Patients must collect stool specimens properly so they are not contaminated with urine or water from the toilet, both of which can lead to inaccurate results. Patients can collect stool specimens on a clean paper plate, in a clean waxed-paper carton, or in a container or on collection tissue that you provide. Another way to collect a stool specimen is to place plastic wrap loosely over the toilet seat with enough material to form a collection pocket in the middle. Patients then use a tongue depressor to place a portion of the sample in a specimen container with a tight-fitting lid.

Suspected Bacterial Infection. Bacterial infections caused by species of the *Shigella* or *Salmonella* genus can cause loose, bloody, or mucus-tinged stools. A doctor who suspects that a patient has one of these types of infections may request that a stool specimen be obtained for culture.

Successful recovery of these pathogenic bacteria from a stool specimen depends on timely inoculation of special culture media. The doctor may request obtaining a sample in the office whenever possible to avoid delay in processing the specimen. Several types of culture media promote the growth of intestinal pathogens while suppressing the growth of other microorganisms.

Suspected Protozoal or Parasitic Infection. In cases of a suspected protozoal or parasitic infection, the physician may request what is known as an **O and P specimen,** short for an ova and parasites specimen. This type of stool sample is examined for the presence of certain forms of protozoans or parasites, including their eggs (ova).

When a physician requests an O and P test, obtain both a fresh and a preserved stool specimen. A fresh specimen is examined both macroscopically and microscopically for the presence of microorganisms. A preserved specimen is also necessary because certain forms of these organisms are destroyed within a short time after leaving the body and may not be detected in the fresh specimen. You must always obtain a preserved specimen when stool samples are sent to an outside laboratory.

Special stool collection kits are available. They contain a specimen container for a fresh sample along with vials

PROCEDURE 28.1

Obtaining a Throat Culture Specimen

Objective: To isolate a pathogenic microorganism from the throat or to rule out strep throat

OSHA Guidelines

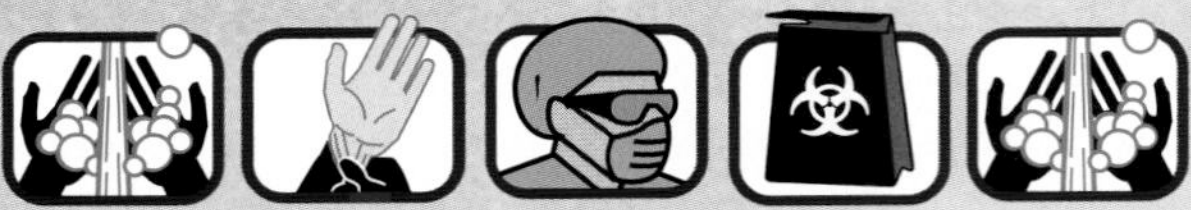

Materials: Tongue depressor, sterile collection system or sterile swab plus blood agar culture plate

Method

1. Identify the patient, introduce yourself, and explain the procedure.
2. Assemble the necessary supplies; label the culture plate if used.
3. Wash your hands and put on examination gloves and goggles and a mask or a face shield. (The patient may cough while you swab the throat.)
4. Have the patient assume a sitting position. (Having a small child lie down rather than sit may make the process easier. If the child refuses to open the mouth, gently squeeze the nostrils shut. The child will eventually open the mouth to breathe. Enlist the help of the parent to restrain the child's hands if necessary.)
5. Open the collection system or sterile swab package by peeling the wrapper halfway down; remove the swab with your dominant hand.
6. Ask the patient to tilt back her head and open her mouth as wide as possible.
7. With your other hand, depress the patient's tongue with the tongue depressor.
8. Ask the patient to say "Ah."
9. Insert the swab and quickly swab the back of the throat in the area of the tonsils (Figure 28-10), twirling the swab over representative areas on both sides of the throat. (Avoid touching the uvula, the soft tissue hanging from the roof of the mouth, because touching it will make the patient gag and will contaminate the specimen.)
10. Remove the swab and then the tongue depressor from the patient's mouth.
11. Discard the tongue depressor in a biohazardous waste container.

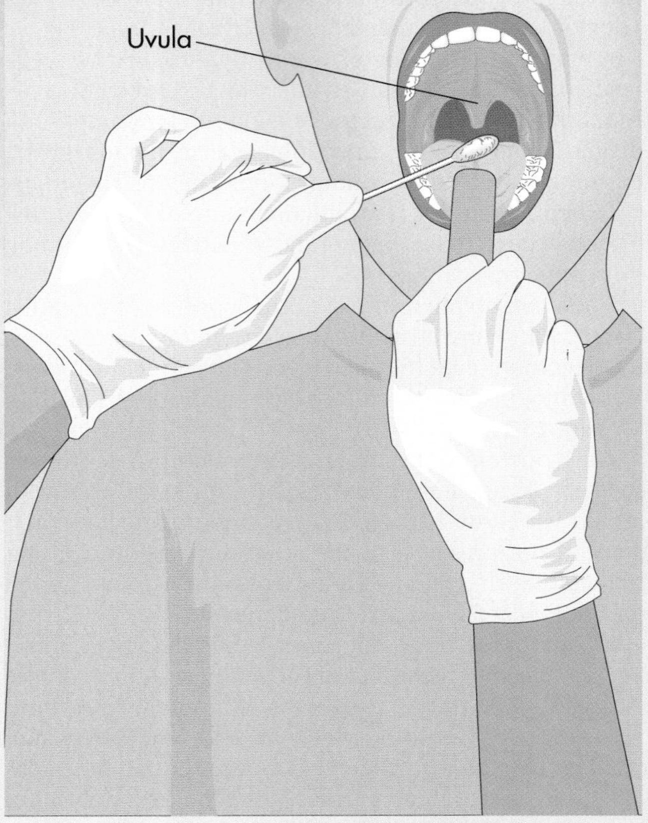

Figure 28-10. When obtaining a throat culture specimen, swab the back of the throat in the area of the tonsils on each side, taking care to avoid touching the uvula.

To transport the specimen to a reference laboratory:

12. Immediately insert the swab back into the plastic sleeve, being careful not to touch the outside of the sleeve with the swab.
13. Crush the vial of transport medium to moisten the tip of the swab (Figure 28-11).

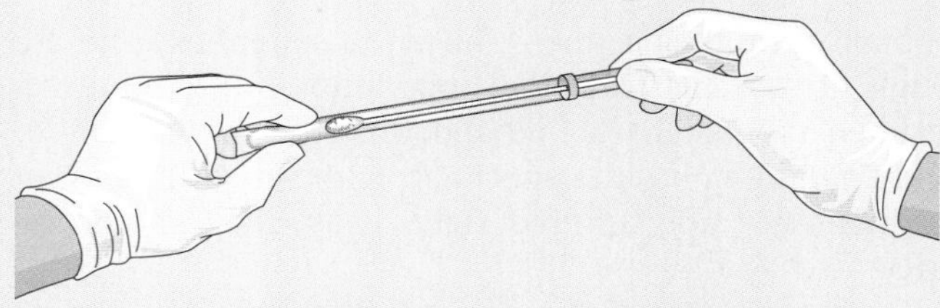

Figure 28-11. The transport medium released from the crushed capsule keeps microorganisms alive while in transit to the laboratory for culturing.

continued ⟶

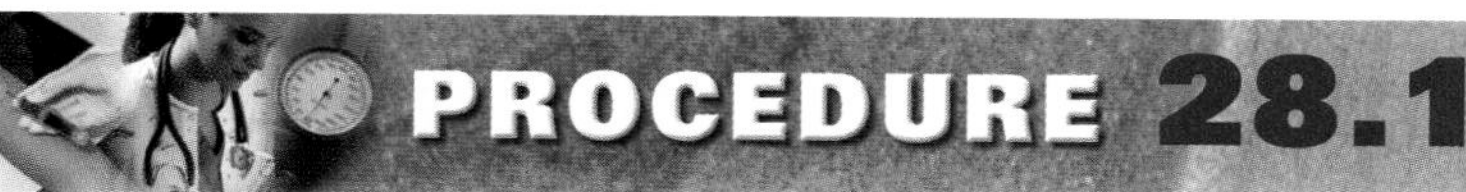

Obtaining a Throat Culture Specimen *(continued)*

14. Label the collection system and arrange for transport to the laboratory.

To prepare the specimen for evaluation in the physician's office laboratory:

12. Immediately inoculate the culture plate with the swab, using a back-and-forth motion.

13. Discard the swab in a biohazardous waste container.

14. Place the culture plate in the incubator.

When finished with all specimens:

15. Remove the gloves and wash your hands.

16. Document the procedure in the patient's chart.

of two types of preservatives, formalin (a dilute solution of formaldehyde) and polyvinyl alcohol (PVA). Instruct the patient to place the stool sample in the specimen container and to mix portions of the specimen in each of the preservative vials. The laboratory will examine all specimens for the presence of microorganisms.

When a physician suspects that a patient has a protozoal or parasitic infection, he will request that a series of at least three stool specimens be examined. Three specimens are required because different diagnostic forms of the microorganism may be present in the stool at different times. The presence of the microorganism could be missed with only one sample. Because certain medications can interfere with detection of these microorganisms, the patient may be asked to refrain from using medications such as antidiarrheal compounds, antacids,

PROCEDURE 28.2

Preparing Microbiologic Specimens for Transport to an Outside Laboratory

Objective: To properly prepare a microbiologic specimen for transport to an outside laboratory

OSHA Guidelines

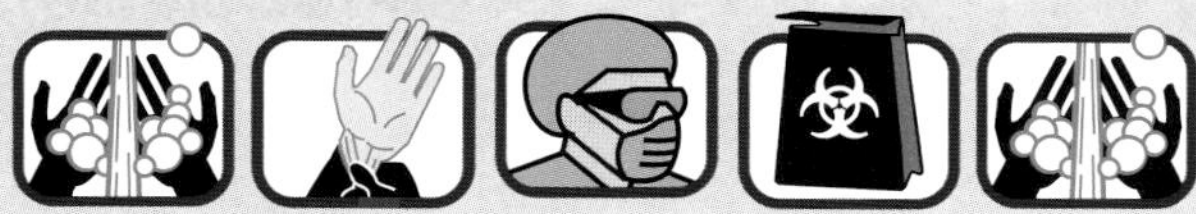

Materials: Specimen-collection device, requisition form, secondary container or zipper-type plastic bag

Method

1. Wash your hands and put on examination gloves (and goggles and a mask or a face shield if you are collecting a microbiologic throat culture specimen).
2. Obtain the microbiologic culture specimen.
   a. Use the collection system specified by the outside laboratory for the test requested.
   b. Label the microbiologic specimen-collection device at the time of collection.
   c. Collect the microbiologic specimen according to the guidelines provided by the laboratory and office procedure.
3. Remove the gloves and wash your hands.
4. Complete the test requisition form.
5. Place the microbiologic specimen container in a secondary container or zipper-type plastic bag.
6. Attach the test requisition form to the outside of the secondary container or bag, per laboratory policy.
7. Log the microbiologic specimen in the list of outgoing specimens.
8. Store the microbiologic specimen according to guidelines provided by the laboratory for that type of specimen (for example, refrigerated, frozen, or 37°C).
9. Call the laboratory for pickup of the microbiologic specimen, or hold it until the next scheduled pickup.
10. At the time of pickup ensure that the carrier takes all microbiologic specimens that are logged and scheduled to be picked up.
11. If you are ever unsure about collection or transportation details, call the laboratory.

and mineral oil laxatives for at least a week before samples are obtained.

Transporting Specimens to an Outside Laboratory

Many physicians' offices do not perform microbiologic testing. They choose to send their culture specimens to an outside laboratory. In addition, many specialized microbiologic procedures cannot be performed routinely in the office laboratory and must be sent out. One example of a specialized procedure is a virus culture. Culturing and identifying viruses require special techniques and equipment that are almost never found in a physician's office laboratory. Culturing a specimen for bacteria such as chlamydia is also a procedure that requires special techniques.

Your Main Objectives

When you collect and transport a microbiologic specimen to an outside laboratory, you have three main objectives:

1. To be sure you follow the proper collection procedures and use the proper collection device. Most laboratories have specific directions for sample collection and packaging that you must follow. A laboratory may even provide specific containers in which to collect and transport samples. If you collect or package any specimens improperly, the laboratory may not accept them for testing.
2. To maintain the samples in a state as close to their original as possible. You must take specific steps to prevent them from deteriorating.
3. To protect anyone who handles a specimen container from exposure to potentially infectious material. To do so, ensure that the specimen container has a tight-fitting lid. As extra protection against leakage, place the specimen container in a secondary container or zipper-type plastic bag. The laboratory usually provides such a bag.

Methods of Transportation

Specimens that are to be tested by an outside laboratory may be transported there in one of three ways:

1. During regularly scheduled daily pickups by the laboratory
2. During an as-needed pickup by the laboratory
3. Through the mail

Pickup by the laboratory is the most reliable and timely method of transporting microbiologic specimens. Although each laboratory has its own procedure, the general steps for preparing specimens for transport to a laboratory are outlined in Procedure 28-2.

Sending Specimens by Mail

There may be times when you must send a specimen through the mail to a special reference laboratory for a test that is not normally done by a local laboratory. The U.S. Postal Service accepts a package containing microbiologic specimens as long as the total volume of specimen material is less than 50 milliliters and it is packaged under strict regulations specified by the U.S. Public Health Service.

When sending specimens through the mail, pack them securely with adequate cushioning material to prevent

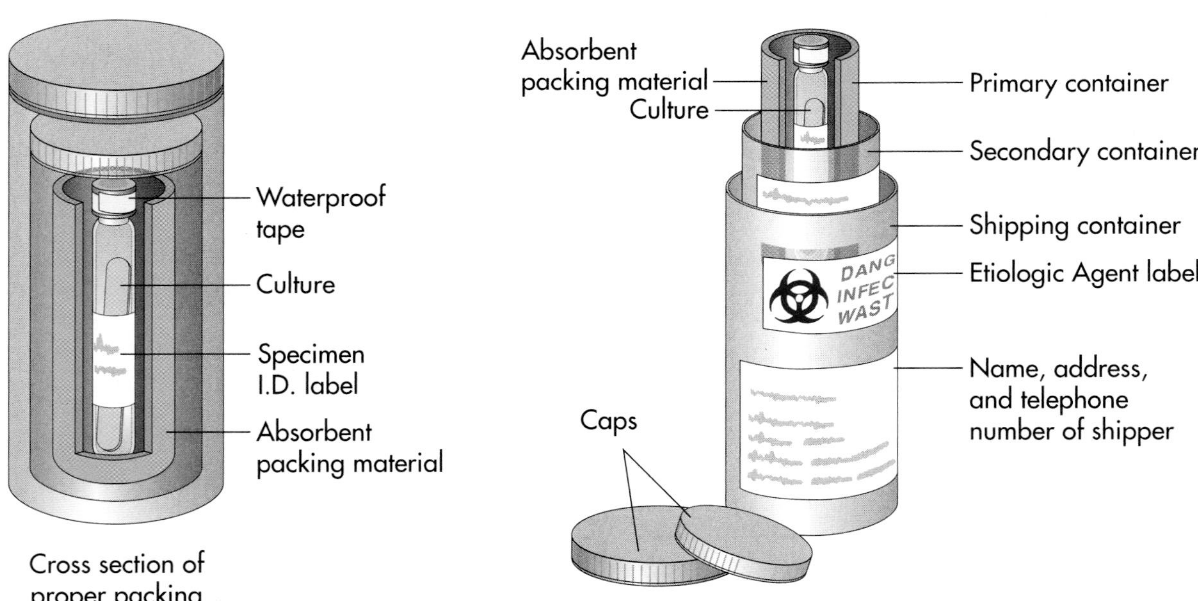

Figure 28-12. When packaging and labeling a specimen for mail delivery, you must follow the procedures set by the CDC, based on U.S. Public Health Service regulations.

breakage and leakage. Leakage can not only contaminate the specimen but also put mail handlers at risk of contamination with infectious materials. The proper technique for packaging and labeling microbiologic specimens is outlined by the CDC and shown in Figure 28-12.

Securely close the primary culture container, and surround it with enough absorbent packing material to absorb the entire fluid contents if the container were to leak. Place these items together in a secondary container, commonly a metal container with a screw-top or snap-on lid. Then place the secondary container in an outer shipping carton made of cardboard or Styrofoam.

In addition to the address label, microbiologic specimens sent through the mail must have an Etiologic Agent label affixed to the package, as shown in Figure 28-12. This label uses the biohazard symbol to alert the mail carrier as to the nature of the contents. The term **etiologic agent** refers to a living microorganism or its toxin that may cause human disease.

Direct Examination of Specimens

At times, the physician may directly examine the specimen under a microscope to detect the presence of microorganisms or to identify them. The physician may perform this procedure in the office to get the information needed to initiate treatment immediately.

Two types of procedures that allow direct examination of microbiologic specimens are preparing wet mounts and preparing potassium hydroxide (KOH) mounts. You may be required to perform these procedures as part of your duties.

PROCEDURE 28.3

Preparing a Microbiologic Specimen Smear

Objective: To prepare a smear of a microbiologic specimen for staining

OSHA Guidelines

Materials: Glass slide with frosted end, pencil, specimen swab, Bunsen burner, forceps

Method

1. Wash your hands and put on examination gloves.
2. Assemble all the necessary items.
3. Use a pencil to label the frosted end of the slide with the patient's name.
4. Roll the specimen swab evenly over the smooth part of the slide, making sure that all areas of the swab touch the slide (Figure 28-13).

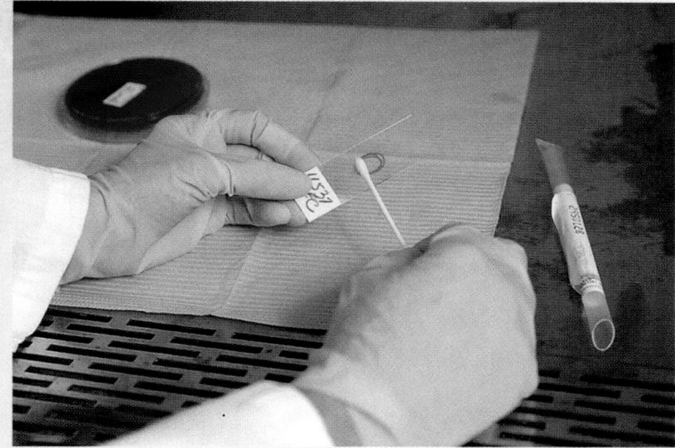

Figure 28-13. Rolling the swab ensures that representative microorganisms collected on it are deposited on the slide.

5. Discard the swab in a biohazardous waste container. (Retain the microbiologic specimen for culture as necessary or according to office policy.)
6. Allow the smear to air-dry. Do not wave the slide to dry it, because this may spread pathogens or contaminate the slide.
7. Heat-fix the slide by holding the frosted end with forceps and passing the clear part of the slide, with the smear side up, through the flame of a Bunsen burner three or four times. (Your office may use an alternate procedure for fixing the slide, such as flooding the smear with alcohol, allowing it to sit for a few minutes, and either pouring off the remaining liquid or allowing the smear to air-dry. Pap smear slides must be fixed with a chemical spray within 10 seconds. Chlamydia slides come with their own fixative.)
8. Allow the slide to cool before the smear is stained.
9. Return the materials to their proper location.
10. Remove the gloves and wash your hands.

Wet Mounts

A wet mount permits quick identification of many microorganisms. Wet mounts are easy to prepare.

1. Wearing examination gloves, mix a small amount of the specimen with a drop of normal saline (0.9% sodium chloride [NaCl] solution) on a glass slide.
2. Apply a coverslip over the mixture.
3. Provide the doctor with the slide for direct examination under the microscope.

If you obtain a specimen from a body site that is normally sterile, detection of microorganisms on a wet mount immediately tells the doctor whether there is infection. Wet mounts are also useful in determining whether a microorganism is motile, or able to move, which helps in identifying the microorganisms.

Potassium Hydroxide (KOH) Mounts

A **KOH mount** is a type of mount used when a physician suspects that a patient has a fungal infection of the skin, nails, or hair. It is difficult to visualize a fungus directly in these types of specimens because the body produces a tough, hard protein called keratin that often masks any fungus present. The chemical potassium hydroxide (KOH) is added to the specimen to dissolve the keratin and allow visualization of any fungus.

PROCEDURE 28.4

Performing a Gram's Stain

Objective: To make bacteria present in a specimen smear visible for microscopic identification

OSHA Guidelines

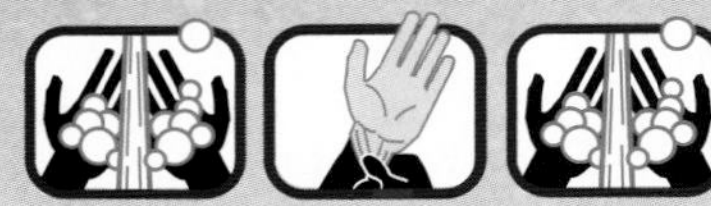

Materials: Heat-fixed smear, slide staining rack and tray, crystal violet dye, iodine solution, alcohol or acetone-alcohol decolorizer, safranin dye, wash bottle filled with water, forceps, blotting paper or paper towels (optional)

Method

1. Assemble all the necessary supplies.
2. Wash your hands and put on examination gloves.
3. Place the heat-fixed smear on a level staining rack and tray, with the smear side up.
4. Completely cover the specimen area of the slide with the crystal violet stain (Figure 28-14a). (Many commercially available Gram's stain solutions have flip-up bottle caps that allow you to dispense stain by the drop. If the stain bottle you are using does not have an attached dropper cap, use an eyedropper.)
5. Allow the stain to sit for 1 minute; wash the slide thoroughly with water from the wash bottle (Figure 28-14b).
6. Use the forceps to hold the slide at the frosted end, tilting the slide to remove excess water.
7. Place the slide flat on the rack again, and completely cover the specimen area with iodine solution (Figure 28-14c).
8. Allow the iodine to remain for 1 minute; wash the slide thoroughly with water (Figure 28-14d).
9. Use the forceps to hold and tilt the slide to remove excess water.
10. While still tilting the slide, apply the alcohol or decolorizer drop by drop until no more purple color washes off (Figure 28-14e). (This step usually takes no more than 10 seconds.)
11. Wash the slide thoroughly with water (Figure 28-14f); use the forceps to hold and tip the slide to remove excess water.
12. Completely cover the specimen with safranin dye (Figure 28-14g).
13. Allow the safranin to remain for 1 minute; wash the slide thoroughly with water (Figure 28-14h).
14. Use the forceps to hold the stained smear by the frosted end, and carefully wipe the back of the slide to remove excess stain.
15. Place the smear in a vertical position and allow it to air-dry. (The smear may be blotted lightly between blotting paper or paper towels to hasten drying [Figure 28-14i]. Take care not to rub the slide, or the specimen may be damaged.)
16. Sanitize and disinfect the work area.
17. Remove the gloves and wash your hands.

continued ⟶

PROCEDURE 28.4

Performing a Gram's Stain *(continued)*

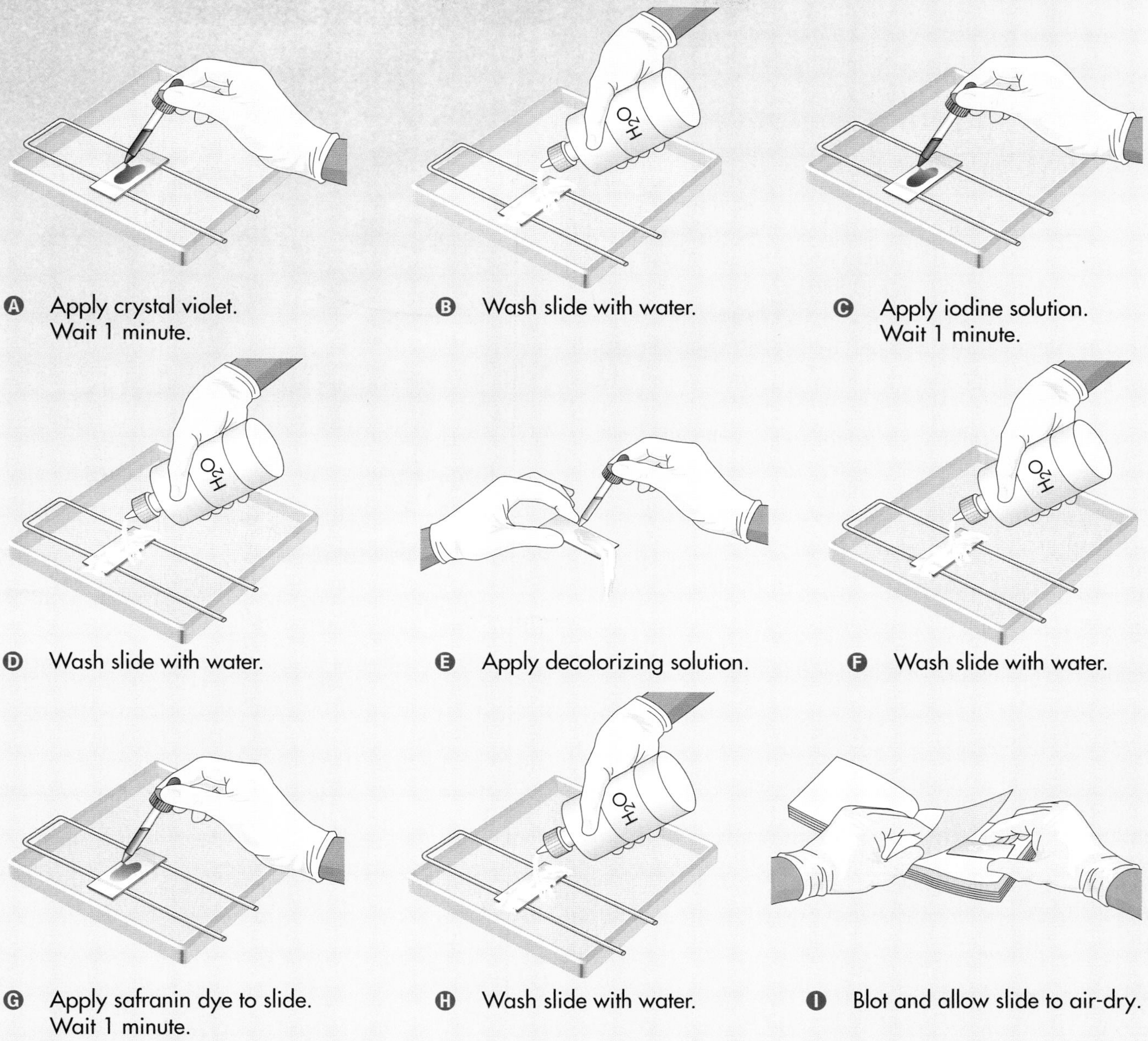

A Apply crystal violet. Wait 1 minute.

B Wash slide with water.

C Apply iodine solution. Wait 1 minute.

D Wash slide with water.

E Apply decolorizing solution.

F Wash slide with water.

G Apply safranin dye to slide. Wait 1 minute.

H Wash slide with water.

I Blot and allow slide to air-dry.

Figure 28-14. The procedure for performing a Gram's stain on a microbiologic specimen involves covering the specimen with a series of stains, water washes, and alcohol in a specific order, for precise periods of time.

To prepare a KOH mount, follow these steps.

1. Wearing examination gloves, suspend the specimen of skin, hair, or nails in a drop of 10% KOH on a glass slide.
2. Apply a coverslip.
3. Allow the specimen to sit at room temperature for 30 minutes to dissolve the keratin. To speed up this process, gently heat (do not boil) the slide in the flame of a Bunsen burner.
4. Provide the physician with the slide to examine for microscopic evidence of fungal structures.

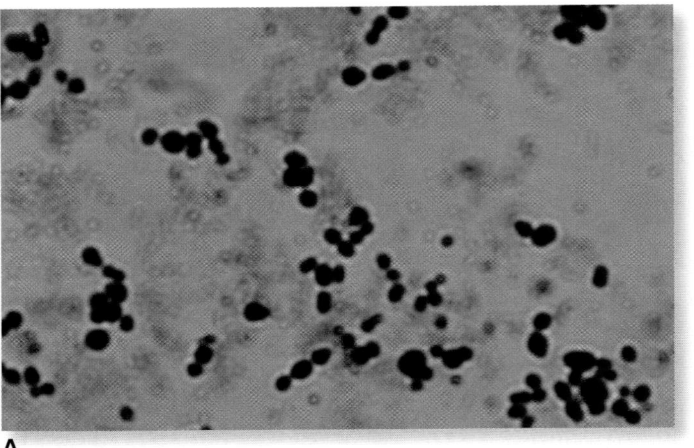

A

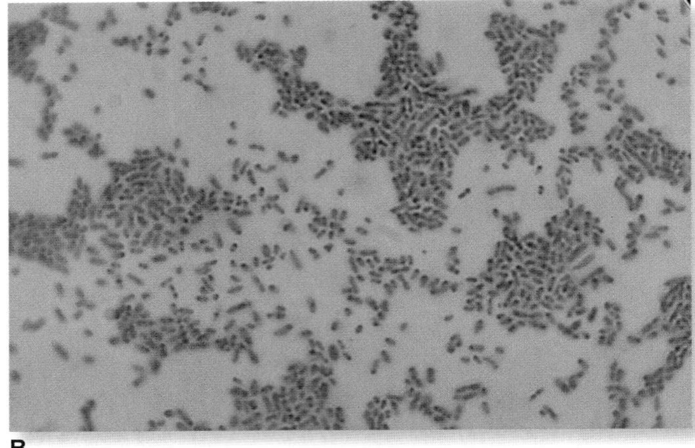

B

Figure 28-15. (a) Gram-positive organisms appear blue or violet after staining. (b) Gram-negative organisms appear red.

Preparation and Examination of Stained Specimens

Although wet mounts are a useful tool for detecting microorganisms, microorganisms and their structures can be seen more clearly when you stain them with a dye or group of dyes. As with wet mounts and KOH mounts, the doctor can make a quick, tentative diagnosis with stained specimens. A stained specimen also enables the doctor to differentiate between types of infections, such as bacterial and yeast infections, or between bacterial infections of one type and another. Stains also help doctors identify microorganisms that have grown on culture plates.

Preparation of Smears

The first step in staining a microbiologic specimen is to prepare a smear. To do so, simply apply a small amount of the specimen to a glass slide. Allow the sample to dry, and briefly heat the slide to "fix" the sample to the slide so that it does not wash off during the staining process. The steps in preparing a specimen smear are described in detail in Procedure 28-3.

Gram's Stain

The stain that is most frequently used for microscopic examination of bacteriologic specimens is the Gram's stain. A Gram's stain is a simple procedure that you can easily perform in the medical office. The steps for performing a Gram's stain are outlined in Procedure 28-4.

A Gram's stain involves performing a series of staining and washing steps on the heat-fixed smear. First, apply a purple stain called crystal violet (also known as gentian violet) to the smear. After washing the slide in water, apply iodine. The iodine acts as a **mordant,** a substance that can intensify or deepen the response of a specimen to a stain. Iodine helps bind the dye to the bacterial cell wall. After washing the slide again in water, apply a decolorizing solution (alcohol or acetone-alcohol). Certain bacterial species retain the purple dye even after the decolorizer is added. These bacteria appear blue or violet and are referred to as being **gram-positive.**

Other bacteria lose their purple color when the decolorizer is added. To allow the physician to visualize these bacteria, apply a red counterstain (safranin) to the smear. Bacteria that lose the purple color and pick up the red color of the safranin are referred to as being **gram-negative.** Figure 28-15 illustrates gram-positive and gram-negative bacteria.

On the bases of a bacterium's staining characteristics and the shape and arrangement of cells, the physician can make a presumptive identification of an organism. For example, clusters of cocci that appear gram-positive typically suggest an infection with staphylococci.

Besides bacteria, other types of microorganisms, such as protozoans and parasites, can often be visualized with the Gram's stain. Since the Gram's stain is typically not the best type of stain for these microorganisms, however, the physician may order another type of stain.

Culturing Specimens in the Medical Office

If your medical office is equipped with a laboratory and if you have the necessary on-the-job training or additional courses, you may be required to culture certain specimens. It is, however, becoming more common for doctors' offices to send specimens to outside laboratories because of Clinical Laboratory Improvement Amendments of 1988 (CLIA '88) guidelines and the additional requirements concerning personnel and administrative work.

Culturing involves placing a sample of the specimen on or in a specialized culture medium. This medium contains nutrients that enable microorganisms such as bacteria and fungi to grow. The medium is placed in an incubator set at 37°C (body temperature), the optimal temperature for growth. As the microorganism multiplies, a **colony**—a distinct group of the organisms—can be seen on the surface of the culture medium. The microorganism is identified according to the colony appearance, its staining characteristics, and certain biochemical reactions.

Culture Media

Culture media come in liquid, semisolid, and solid forms. In the medical office you will most likely work with a semisolid. The medium contains **agar,** a gelatin-like substance derived from seaweed that gives the medium its consistency. This form of medium comes commercially prepared in culture plates—round, covered glass or plastic dishes also called petri dishes.

When using petri dishes, handle them only on the outside, so that they do not become contaminated. You can avoid introducing contaminants by storing the petri dishes with the agar side up. Use the palm of your hand to pick up the agar-containing part of the dish when you are ready to inoculate it with a specimen.

Types of Media. Many different types of semisolid media are commercially available. The type of medium used for culturing depends on the type of suspected organism and the site from which the specimen is obtained. Some types allow the growth of only certain kinds of bacteria while inhibiting the growth of others. These types are referred to as selective media. Selective media are commonly used for specimens that normally contain bacteria, such as stool or vaginal samples.

Other types of media support the growth of most organisms and are referred to as nonselective media. The most common type of culture medium used in the laboratory is blood agar, a nonselective medium. Blood agar gets its red color from sheep's blood. Comparing the growth of a specimen on selective and nonselective media often provides important information about the microorganisms present.

You will typically use a blood agar plate when you culture a throat swab specimen. The organism that causes strep throat (*Streptococcus pyogenes*) can be identified when it grows on blood agar because it destroys the blood cells in the agar, leaving a clear zone surrounding each colony. This process of red blood cell destruction is referred to as hemolysis.

Special Culture Units. Small physicians' office laboratories often use commercial culture units with specific culturing purposes. Units for performing rapid urine culture, such as Uricult (manufactured by Orion Diagnostica, Somerset, New Jersey), are typical. Uricult consists of a small vial that has a double-sided paddle attached to a screw-on top (Figure 28-16). Each side of the paddle contains a different type of medium on its surface. To culture a urine specimen, simply dip the media paddle into the clean-catch midstream urine specimen or catheterized

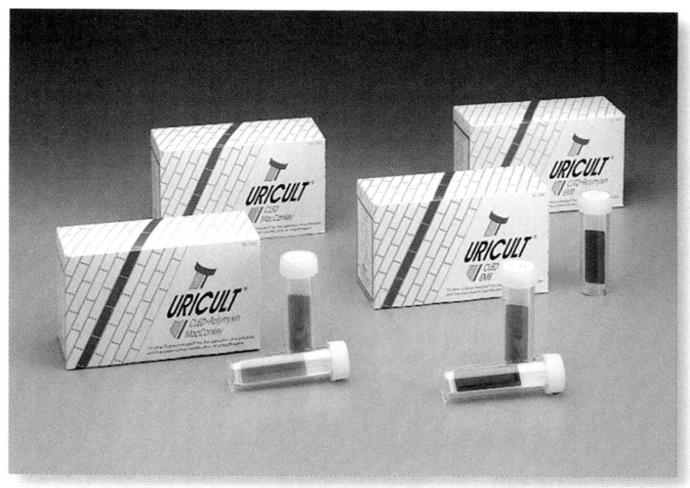

Figure 28-16. One common urine culture device consists of a lid and attached double-sided paddle that screws into a vial.

specimen, coating both sides of the paddle. Then remove the paddle from the specimen, screw it into the vial, and place it upright in the incubator for 18 to 24 hours. If bacteria are present, they will grow on the surfaces of the media. Other units for culturing urine, throat specimens, vaginal specimens, and blood are also simple to use. These units usually enable you to obtain an estimate of the number of bacteria in the sample in addition to identifying the bacteria.

Inoculating a Culture Plate

Inoculating a culture plate involves transferring some or all of the specimen onto the plate. Before inoculating a plate, label it on the bottom (agar side) rather than the lid, because the lid can be lost or switched. Label the plate with the patient's name, doctor's name, source of the sample, date and time of inoculation, and your initials. You can apply a label or write the information with a grease pencil or permanent marker.

In the case of a specimen swab, inoculate the plate by streaking the swab across the plate. Bacterial colonies can be identified by their appearance. This determination of the type of pathogen is referred to as a **qualitative analysis** of the specimen.

To perform a qualitative analysis of a specimen such as urine, introduce only a small portion of the specimen onto the plate. A calibrated inoculating loop is used for this purpose. A loop is a small circle of wire or plastic attached to a long handle. When this loop is dipped into the specimen, a small amount of liquid can be transferred to the plate.

In addition, you may need to perform a separate determination of the number of bacteria present in specimens such as urine. This determination is referred to as a **quantitative analysis.** A quantitative analysis is important

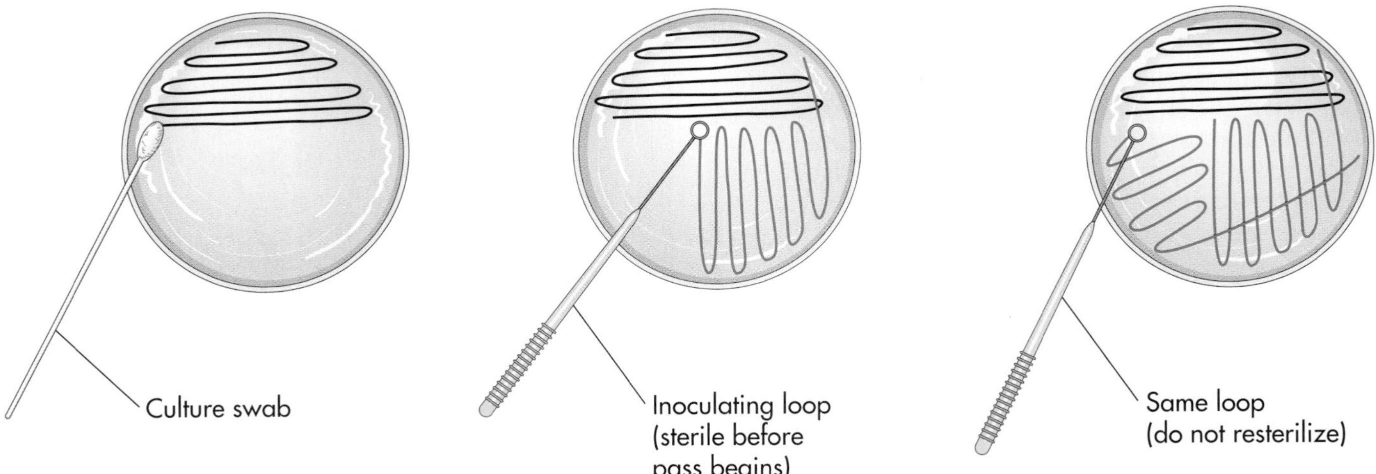

Figure 28-17. When inoculating a plate for qualitative analysis, roll and streak the culture swab or inoculating loop of specimen material across one-third of the surface of the culture plate. Begin the next pass with a sterile loop.

with a specimen such as urine because a few bacteria may contaminate a urine sample during collection. A true infection is confirmed by the presence of a certain number of bacteria; any number beneath this level is typically considered contamination.

Inoculating for Qualitative Analysis. To inoculate an agar plate for qualitative analysis, perform the first pass with a culture swab (as with a throat culture) or an inoculating loop (as with a urine culture). If you use a culture swab, roll and streak it back and forth across an area covering roughly one-third of the culture plate to deposit the microorganisms. When using an inoculating loop, spread the material by streaking the loop across one-third of the plate in the same back-and-forth pattern. Figure 28-17 shows the correct pattern for inoculating a plate.

Because there may be a great many microorganisms in the specimen, you need to streak the inoculated (first-pass) area with a sterile loop to separate out individual colonies that can be identified on the remaining areas of the culture plate. Unless you use a sterile disposable loop, first sterilize the loop by heating it in a bacterial loop incinerator until it glows red. Allow the loop to cool, and pass it once across the inoculated area of the plate to pick up a small number of microorganisms. Then streak it in a back-and-forth pattern over the second one-third of the plate. Next pass it once across the second inoculated area of the plate, and streak it back and forth over the last one-third of the plate. Each successive pass serves to reduce the concentration of the microorganisms. This procedure allows isolated colonies, or colony-forming units, to be observed in the area of the last pass of the loop, as Figure 28-18 shows.

For throat cultures, the physician may simply want you to screen the sample to see whether streptococcal organisms are present. You may not need to use a loop to spread the microorganisms; the swab will be sufficient, as described in Procedure 28-1, when preparing the specimen for screening.

Inoculating for Quantitative Analysis. To perform a quantitative analysis of a urine specimen, use a calibrated loop to withdraw a portion of urine from the sample. The circle on a calibrated loop is a precise size that picks up an exact volume of liquid when it is dipped into the specimen. For example, calibrated loops may allow you to pick up either 0.01 or 0.001 milliliter of liquid.

When you perform a quantitative analysis, be sure the urine specimen is well mixed before taking the sample. Mixing is required because the microorganisms may settle to the bottom of the specimen cup. Sterilize, cool, and dip the calibrated loop into the sample. Transfer the entire volume to the surface of an agar plate by making a single streak down the center of the plate. Next spread the specimen evenly across the plate at a right angle to the initial streak, using the same loop (without sterilizing it). Turn the plate and spread the material again, at a right angle to the

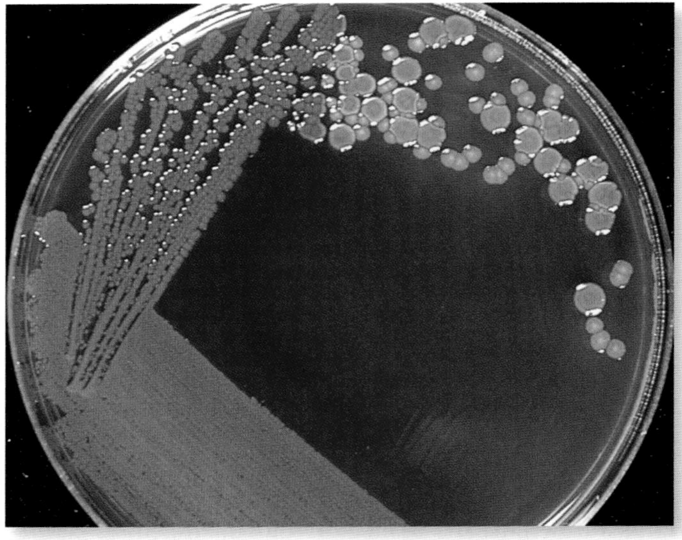

Figure 28-18. You can see individual colony-forming units in the last third of an inoculated culture plate.

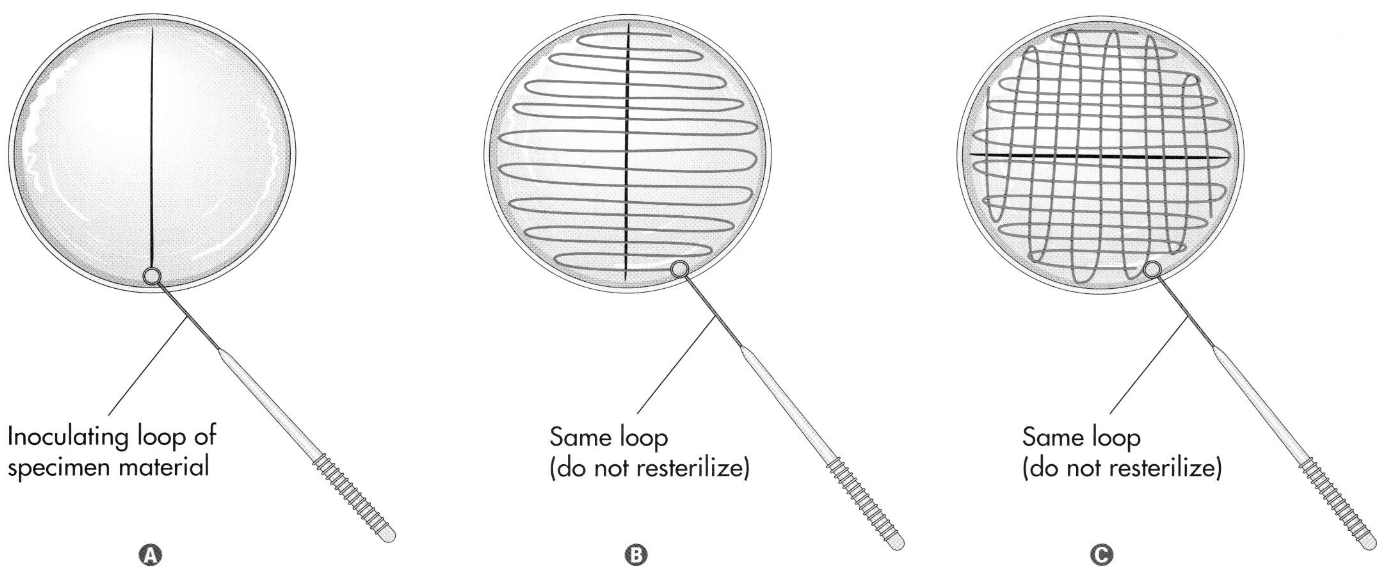

Figure 28-19. When inoculating a plate for quantitative analysis, (a) streak the loop down the center of the plate. Next (b) streak the loop at right angles to the first inoculation. Then (c) turn the plate 90°, and streak the entire surface once more.

last streak, over the entire surface. Figure 28-19 illustrates this technique.

After the microorganisms are allowed to grow for 24 hours, estimate the number of microorganisms by counting the number of colonies that appear on the surface of the plate. For example, if you use a 0.001 milliliter loop to streak the plate and 50 colonies grow, multiply the 50 colonies by 1000 to obtain the number of colonies per milliliter. In this case you would estimate that there are 50,000 colony-forming units per milliliter of urine. You must be especially careful that your counts and calculations are correct so that the doctor has accurate information on which to base a diagnosis.

Incubating Culture Plates

After inoculating a plate, place it in an incubator set at 35° to 37°C (human body temperature) to allow the bacteria to grow. Plates are always incubated with the agar side up, so that any moisture that collects in the plate will fall on the inside of the lid and not on the growing surface of the agar. How long plates are allowed to grow varies with the type of culture. Most bacteria grow sufficiently within 24 hours, but some require 48 hours. Fungi typically take longer to grow than bacteria and may grow at a slightly lower temperature (35° to 36°C).

Interpreting Cultures

After incubation, cultures are assessed for growth and are interpreted. Pathogens may be identified at this time. This process requires considerable skill and practice because pathogens must often be differentiated from normal flora. This step may be performed by the physician, a microbiologist, or a technician who has been properly trained to do so through on-the-job training or additional course work. The Tips for the Office section discusses the types of qualifications and training you need to interpret cultures.

The process of interpreting a culture typically involves several determinations. The characteristics of the colonies growing on the agar are noted, along with their relative numbers. In addition, any changes in the media surrounding the colonies are noted, because these changes may reflect certain characteristics of the microorganism.

The physician decides at this point whether additional procedures are required. In the case of a throat culture, the presence of colonies of a characteristic shape, size, and color, surrounded by areas of hemolysis, suggests strep throat, as shown in Figure 28-20. A Gram's stain and

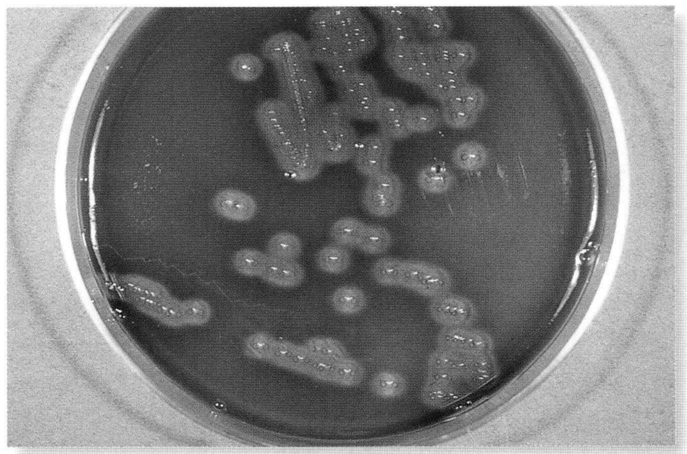

Figure 28-20. A positive strep throat culture contains distinctive colonies surrounded by areas of hemolysis.

Tips for the Office

Obtaining Additional Training in Microbiology

Identifying microorganisms in culture specimens requires considerable skill and practice. In a microbiology laboratory, these tests may be performed by medical technologists (MTs), medical laboratory technicians (MLTs), or other health professionals, including medical assistants who have received special training.

These classifications differ in the amount of education and training required. Medical technologists, also called clinical laboratory scientists, must earn a bachelor's degree and undergo 1 year of clinical training. Medical laboratory technicians must have completed a 2-year program at an accredited college (or the equivalent amount of course work), be a graduate of an accredited professional school or armed forces school, or hold certification in another related field while completing specific on-the-job training. Certification for both MTs and MLTs requires successful completion of a national certifying examination. In addition to certification, some states require MTs and MLTs to obtain a state license to work in a laboratory.

As part of their training, MTs and MLTs routinely receive instruction in microbiology. They also learn the clinical laboratory skills involved in identifying microorganisms. As part of your current medical assistant curriculum, you are learning the basic principles of microbiology and some of the techniques of specimen collection and processing. To be able to perform microbiologic tests, such as sensitivity tests, and interpret cultures of specimens, however, you would need additional training.

You can learn these types of skills and advance your career by taking part in the continuing education programs your office has to offer. Local colleges or schools of allied health may also offer clinical microbiology courses. Such a course will enable you to become proficient in performing microbiologic identification. All laboratories, including those in the doctor's office, require employees to participate in a proficiency testing program, according to guidelines set forth by the Clinical Laboratory Improvement Amendments of 1988 (CLIA '88).

Developing clinical skills in the area of microbiology can be challenging and satisfying. These skills will contribute to your office's efficiency and ability to provide high-quality patient care. Additional training in microbiology will also enhance your career by making you more valuable to any medical practice or facility.

determination of bacterial shape may be all that is necessary for a confirmed diagnosis. Many cultures, however, require additional biochemical and, in some cases, serologic tests for definitive identification of the pathogen.

Determining Antimicrobial Sensitivity

After a particular bacterial (or sometimes fungal) pathogen is identified, the organism's sensitivity (also called susceptibility) to several different antimicrobial agents must be determined. This information enables the doctor to choose an agent for treating the infection that is likely to be effective in curing it. If your office does not perform antimicrobial sensitivity tests but, instead, receives reports on them from reference laboratories, the results are reported as sensitive (no growth), intermediate (little growth), or resistant (overgrown).

Performing an antimicrobial sensitivity test involves taking a sample of the isolated pathogen, suspending it in a small amount of liquid medium, and streaking it evenly on the surface of a culture plate. Small disks of filter paper containing various antimicrobial agents are placed on top of the inoculated agar plate. Although this step can be done manually using sterile forceps, a special dispenser that is often used places all the disks down at once (Figure 28-21).

The plate is then incubated at 37°C, and the results are evaluated the following day. If a particular antimicrobial

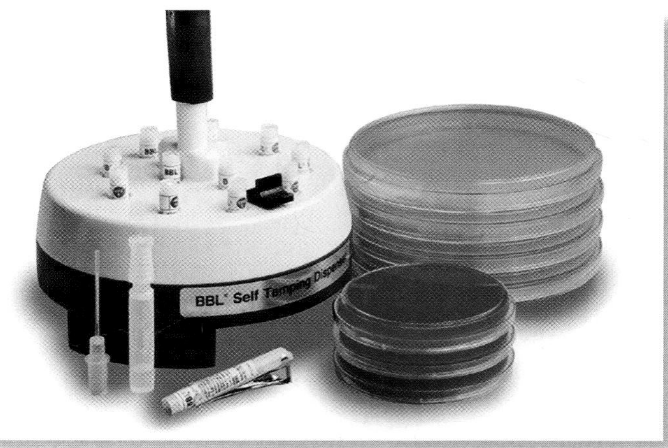

Figure 28-21. Antimicrobial disk dispensers simplify placement of antimicrobial disks, help ensure that each disk contains a single antimicrobial agent, and reduce the probability of contaminating the culture.

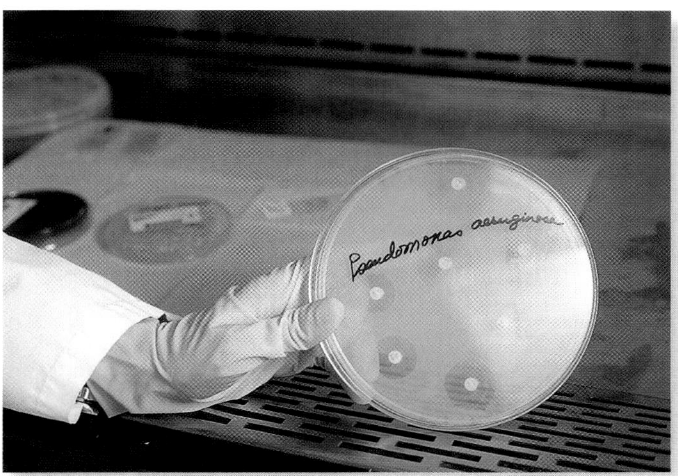

Figure 28-22. The effectiveness of different antimicrobial agents against an organism is apparent when an antimicrobial sensitivity test is performed.

agent is effective against the microorganism, there will be a clear zone around the disk, indicating that the growth was inhibited in the area of the agent, as seen in Figure 28-22. If there is growth right up to the disk, it means that the agent is not effective against the organism. Each zone is measured in millimeters and compared to a standard chart to determine the degree of effectiveness of the antimicrobial agent. The doctor uses these results to choose an effective antimicrobial agent to treat the patient.

Many bacterial identification systems are now available as automated systems. These systems are used at most larger institutions and reference laboratories. They require special instrumentation that has the capability to identify the organism. This instrumentation also determines the antibiotic susceptibility, a procedure known as MIC (minimum inhibitory concentration). This susceptibility testing is performed in special welled plates that test the organism against an antibiotic dilution to determine the minimum antibiotic concentration that is required to inhibit bacterial growth.

Quality Control in the Medical Office

Medical offices are required to have a **quality control (QC)** system in place, which is an ongoing system to evaluate the quality of medical care being provided. Although quality is sometimes difficult to define, most people would agree that high-quality care involves achieving the best possible medical outcome for each patient while attending to both the patient's and the family's needs. Quality control in the medical office provides an objective means of defining, monitoring, and correcting potential problems that affect the quality of care.

Part of quality control in the medical office includes risk management, which is the development of strategies for helping to minimize the chances of accidents or the risk of infection. These strategies include following general safety rules and regulations and Universal Precautions. Keep in mind that, in practice, medical offices use Universal Precautions when obtaining and handling all types of specimens, not only those capable of transmitting bloodborne pathogens.

Quality control involves an ongoing assessment of the reliability and quality of the work performed. As with all laboratory procedures, quality control in the microbiology laboratory of a medical office is particularly important in achieving quality assurance.

Quality Control in the Microbiology Laboratory

Quality control is necessary in several areas in a microbiology laboratory. All media, staining solutions, and reagents (chemicals and chemically treated substances used in test procedures) should be evaluated frequently for effectiveness. Media must also be evaluated for sterility. Equipment such as refrigerators, freezers, and incubators should be properly maintained, cleaned, and checked for accuracy of temperature. The essential components of a quality control program as established by the College of American Pathologists are outlined in the Tips for the Office section.

The Impact of CLIA '88

In addition to an internal quality control program, all laboratories must incorporate the appropriate policies and procedures to comply with CLIA '88. (See Chapter 27 for a full discussion of CLIA '88.) A substantial part of these requirements involves proper documentation of laboratory policies and procedures, materials, and personnel qualifications and training. If a laboratory has a good quality control program in place, it is likely that the required guidelines are already being followed.

In addition, any laboratory that performs certain procedures must enroll and participate in an approved proficiency testing program. A proficiency testing program monitors the quality of a laboratory's test results. The procedures in a microbiology laboratory that require proficiency testing include those classified as moderately complex or highly complex. An example of a moderately complex procedure is performing a culture and sensitivity test.

Proficiency testing involves culturing, identifying, and determining the sensitivity of blind specimen samples, that is, samples that are unknown to laboratory personnel. The results are then checked for accuracy. If you perform these types of procedures in the medical office, you may be asked to participate in the proficiency testing program.

Tips for the Office

Guidelines for a Quality Control Program in a Microbiology Laboratory

To maintain the highest possible standards of patient care and safety, all facets of a medical laboratory must be checked and monitored. The essential components of a quality control program in a microbiology laboratory include the following:

- Developing an up-to-date procedures manual. This manual is one of the most important documents in the laboratory. The procedures manual directs day-to-day activities and ensures that proper procedures are followed. It should include all general policies, regulations, and procedures, including those involving quality control and the transport of specimens to outside laboratories. The manual should be placed in a binder and kept in a location where all employees can refer to it. At least once a year, the laboratory director or supervisor should update and revise the manual.
- Monitoring laboratory equipment. A quality control program should include a preventive maintenance program for all laboratory equipment to ensure proper functioning. All equipment should be checked and cleaned at regular intervals. Temperatures of refrigerators, freezers, heating blocks, water baths, and incubators should be checked daily with an accurate standardized thermometer. Autoclaves should be tested each week with a spore strip to check sterility, and pH meters must be tested for accuracy using pH-calibrating solutions. A tachometer should be used to check the revolutions per minute of serology rotators and centrifuges. (All centrifuges must have lids.) Safety hoods should be checked two to four times per year to make certain that they permit adequate air flow. The results of all quality control tests should be documented each time a test is performed.
- Monitoring media, supplies, and reagents. Media should be periodically checked for sterility and the ability to grow certain strains of stock organisms. Stains and reagents should also be checked with control organisms to ensure accurate results. Each culture tube, plate of medium, and reagent should be labeled as to its content and its preparation and expiration dates.
- Ensuring qualified personnel. Only qualified personnel should be hired, and employees should be offered an effective continuing education program. All personnel should be given the opportunity to learn new skills. This procedure benefits the laboratory and can also help advance employees' careers. Proficiency testing of blind samples may be used as teaching exercises and should be made available to all interested personnel.
- Ensuring adequate space. One issue of quality control and safety in the laboratory that is often overlooked is the allocation of sufficient work space for personnel. A minimum of 100 square feet of work space for each full-time equivalent employee is recommended. Safety and high-quality performance are enhanced when there is sufficient space to perform each task.

Summary

A variety of microorganisms can cause infection. They are a major cause of disease in humans. As a medical assistant, you play an important role in the diagnosis and treatment of infection.

Collecting a microbiologic specimen is the most important step in diagnosing an infection. To ensure accurate results, you must use the correct collection device and technique. Then you must process the specimen or transport it to the laboratory in a timely manner to enable recovery of microorganisms.

The process of identification often begins when the doctor examines the fresh or stained specimen. Most specimens are cultured and incubated, and the resultant growth is evaluated. The antibiotic sensitivity of an isolated pathogen can then be determined to aid the doctor in making treatment decisions.

Quality control in the microbiology laboratory is an important factor in ensuring high-quality medical care. The focus and attention you bring to this part of your work will pay handsome dividends in terms of patient care, laboratory safety, and personal satisfaction. Developing your clinical skills will be an asset to the office and will allow you to advance in your career.

REVIEW

CHAPTER 28

CASE STUDY QUESTIONS

Now that you have completed this chapter, review the case study at the beginning of the chapter and answer the following questions:

1. What is the proper technique for collecting a throat specimen?
2. Why do you think the first test result came back as negative?
3. What organism is responsible for causing strep throat?
4. What complications may have developed if you had not had another throat culture obtained and been prescribed antibiotics?

Discussion Questions

1. What are the different classifications of microorganisms, and how do the classifications differ?
2. List the common sites from which cultures may be obtained.
3. What information should be included on a laboratory requisition form when sending a specimen to an outside laboratory?

Critical Thinking Questions

1. Gram's stain is a procedure performed to stain bacteria for microscopic examination. What are the reagents used to perform this test? Identify the staining characteristics of gram-positive and gram-negative organisms.
2. What are the basic steps for diagnosing and treating infections?
3. Why are cotton-tipped swabs no longer used as sterile specimen collection devices?

Application Activities

1. With your instructor's approval, practice performing a throat culture on a partner.
2. Use one of your throat culture specimens to inoculate a blood agar plate. Incubate the culture and observe the appearance of normal throat flora.
3. Fill out a laboratory request form for a microbiology test being sent to a reference laboratory.

CHAPTER 29

Collecting, Processing, and Testing Urine Specimens

KEY TERMS

anuria
bilirubinuria
cast
catheterization
clean-catch midstream urine specimen
crystal
drainage catheter
enzyme immunoassay (EIA)
first morning urine specimen
glycosuria
hematuria
hemoglobinuria
myoglobinuria
nocturia
oliguria
phenylketonuria (PKU)
proteinuria
random urine specimen
refractometer
splinting catheter
supernatant
timed urine specimen
24-hour urine specimen
urinalysis
urinary catheter
urinary pH
urine specific gravity
urobilinogen

AREAS OF COMPETENCE

2003 Role Delineation Study

CLINICAL

Fundamental Principles

- Apply principles of aseptic technique and infection control

Diagnostic Orders

- Collect and process specimens
- Perform diagnostic tests

GENERAL

Communication Skills

- Adapt communications to individual's ability to understand

CHAPTER OUTLINE

- The Role of the Medical Assistant
- Anatomy and Physiology of the Urinary System
- Obtaining Specimens
- Urinalysis

OBJECTIVES

After completing Chapter 29, you will be able to:

29.1 Describe the characteristics of urine, including its formation, physical composition, and chemical properties.
29.2 Explain how to instruct patients in specimen collection.
29.3 Identify guidelines to follow when collecting urine specimens.
29.4 Describe proper procedures for collecting various urine specimens.
29.5 Explain the process of urinary catheterization.
29.6 List special considerations that may require you to alter guidelines when collecting urine specimens.
29.7 Explain how to maintain the chain of custody when processing urine specimens.
29.8 Explain how to preserve and store urine specimens.
29.9 Describe the process of urinalysis and its purpose.

OBJECTIVES *(Continued)*

29.10 Identify the physical characteristics present in normal urine specimens.

29.11 Identify the chemicals that may be found in urine specimens.

29.12 Identify the elements categorized and counted as a result of microscopic examination of urine specimens.

Introduction

The routine analysis of a urine specimen is a simple, noninvasive diagnostic test that provides a health-care provider with a window to a patient's health. Many significant conditions may be noted with the assessment of the physical, chemical, and microscopic examinations of a patient's specimen. This chapter reviews the function of the urinary system and the formation of urine. You will learn about various types of urine specimens and how to properly instruct or assist patients with the collection of these specimens. Additionally, you will learn how to correctly process a specimen, including a random specimen and a chain of custody drug screen. You will learn to identify normal and abnormal constituents of urine samples and what may cause these abnormal elements to be present in a specimen.

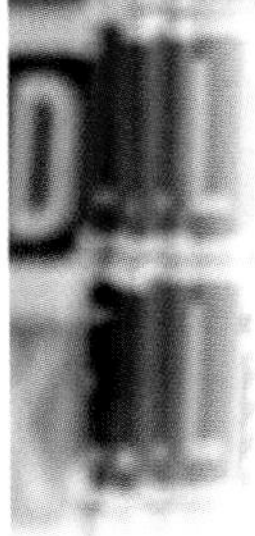

CASE STUDY

As a medical assistant, you are performing reagent chemical strip analyses on patient specimens when you discover a specimen that is more than two hours old and has been sitting at room temperature during this time. When you remove the lid from the container, the odor very evident to you is ammonia-like and foul. The chemical strip indicates positive protein, positive nitrite, and positive bacteria. The microscopic analysis reveals 4+ bacteria but no evidence of white blood cells.

As you read this chapter, consider the following questions:

1. What is the maximum length of time that a urine specimen should be left at room temperature? If analysis cannot be performed within that maximum length of time, how should the specimen be handled?
2. An ammonia-like or foul odor associated with a specimen ordinarily indicates what condition or disease?
3. Does the chemical analysis confirm your suspicion associated with the odor?
4. Given the circumstances, can you trust the results on this specimen?

The Role of the Medical Assistant

You will help collect, process, and test urine specimens. To perform your duties, you need to know about the anatomy and physiology of the kidneys, how urine is formed, and what its normal contents are. This information will help you collect various specimen types, process them, and perform urinalysis on them. Dealing with a variety of patient groups who require special care, including elderly patients and pediatric patients, will also be an important part of your job as a medical assistant.

Although you will not generally be dealing with bloodborne pathogens when obtaining and processing urine specimens, you will deal with potentially infectious body waste. For this reason you must take precautions to protect yourself, the patient, and others in the environment from transmitting disease-causing microorganisms. Most medical offices use Universal Precautions when dealing with urine. (See Chapters 1, 2, and 3 for detailed information on these precautions.) During all procedures you must be sure to wear adequate personal protective equipment (PPE), handle and dispose of specimens properly, dispose of used supplies and equipment properly, and sanitize, disinfect, and/or sterilize all reusable equipment.

Anatomy and Physiology of the Urinary System

The urinary system comprises two kidneys, two ureters, a bladder, and a urethra. The kidneys are located behind the peritoneum on either side of the lumbar spine. They remove excess water from the body and waste products from the

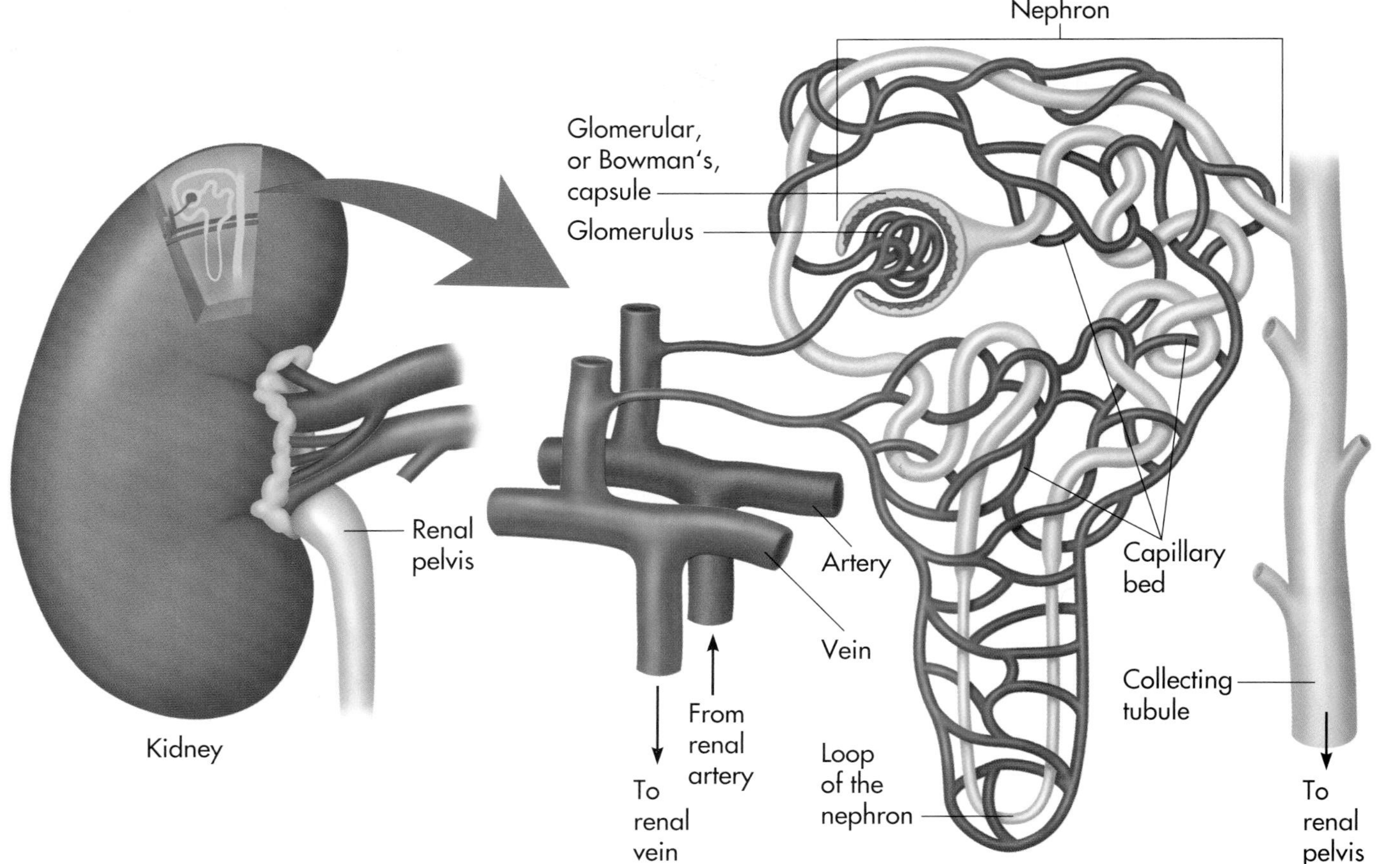

Figure 29-1. Urine is formed in the nephron, a long tubular structure, during a complex filtering process.

blood in the form of urine. The urine then drains through the ureters and into the urinary bladder. The urinary bladder stores urine until it leaves the body through the urethra. The ureters, bladder, and urethra make up the urinary tract.

Formation of Urine in the Kidney

Urine formation is essentially a filtering process that occurs in the nephrons. Nephrons are the structural and functional units of the kidney (Figure 29-1). Each kidney contains about a million nephrons, each of which is capable of forming urine.

Glomerular filtration occurs as blood moves through a tight ball of capillaries called the glomerulus. The glomerular capsule (Bowman's capsule) surrounds the glomerulus. Filtered fluid collects in this capsule, which is the functional beginning of the nephron. A capillary bed surrounds the winding tubule that makes up the rest of the nephron structure. Reabsorption of water, nutrients, and some electrolytes returns these substances to the blood as the filtered fluid passes through the long tubule. Other electrolytes and some additional substances are secreted from the blood into the tubule. Urine is the fluid that flows out of the nephron into the collecting tubule, passes through the funnel-shaped renal pelvis, leaves the kidney, and is carried down the ureter to the bladder.

The specific function of the nephron is to remove certain end products of metabolism from the blood plasma. Because the nephron allows for reabsorption of water and some electrolytes back into the blood, the nephron also plays a vital role in maintaining normal fluid balance in the body.

Physical Composition and Chemical Properties

Urine is made up of 95% water and 5% waste products and other dissolved chemicals. Components other than water include urea, uric acid, ammonia, calcium, creatinine, sodium, chloride, potassium, sulfates, phosphates, bicarbonates, hydrogen ions, urochrome, urobilinogen, a few red blood cells, and a few white blood cells. If a patient is taking any drugs that are excreted renally, the drugs may also show up in the urine. Urine in males may contain a few sperm cells. Table 29-1 provides a list of abbreviations commonly used in urine analysis and testing.

Obtaining Specimens

It is essential to collect, store, and preserve urine specimens in ways that do not alter their physical, chemical, or microscopic properties. You must follow guidelines each

TABLE 29-1 Abbreviations Common to Urine Analysis and Testing

ADH	antidiuretic hormone	RBCs	red blood cells
BIL; bili; BR	bilirubin	SPG; sp gr; sp.gr.	specific gravity
BJP	Bence Jones proteins	U/A	urinalysis
Ca	calcium	UBG	urobilinogen
CC	clean catch (urine)	U/C	urine culture
CCMS	clean catch, midstream (urine)	UC	urinary catheter
CL VOID	clean voided specimen (urine)	UC&S	urine culture and sensitivity
CrCl	creatinine clearance	UcaV	urinary calcium volume
CSU	catheter specimen (urine)	UCRE	urine creatinine
Cys	cysteine	UFC	urinary free cortisol
CYS	cystoscopy	UK	urine potassium
EMU	early morning urine(s)	Una	urinary sodium
HCG; hcg; hCG	human chorionic gonadotropin	Uosm	urine osmolarity
IVP	intravenous pyelogram	UTI	urinary tract infection
K	potassium	UUN	urinary urea nitrogen
pH	hydrogen ion concentration	UV	urinary volume
PKD	polycystic kidney disease	Vol	volume
PKU	phenylketonuria	WBCs	white blood cells

time you obtain specimens and instruct patients in the proper guidelines to follow.

General Collection Guidelines

When you collect urine specimens from patients, follow these guidelines.

- Make sure you are following the procedure that is specified for the urine test that will be performed.
- Use the type of specimen container indicated by the laboratory. If a patient must bring in a specimen, be sure that the container is provided by the physician's office or that the container is appropriate for the testing protocol.
- Label the specimen container before giving it to the patient or on receipt of a container that the patient provides. Include the patient's name, the physician's name, the date and time of collection, and the initials of the person collecting the sample. Label the side of the specimen container, not the lid, because lids may be lost or switched.
- If the patient is having an invasive test, such as catheterization, always explain the procedure to the patient completely, using simple, clear language.
- If you are assisting in the collection process, wash your hands before and after the procedure, and wear gloves during the procedure.
- Complete all necessary paperwork, recording the collection in the patient's chart and making sure you use the correct request slip for the test that has been ordered.

In many instances, patients need to collect a urine specimen at home. It is your responsibility to give patients instructions for obtaining the specific type of specimen. In addition, provide them with the following general instructions.

- Urinate into the container indicated by the laboratory. In most instances urinate into a widemouthed, throw-away, spouted specimen container as instructed. Do not add anything to the container except the urine.
- If the collection container contains liquid or powdered preservative, do not pour it out.
- If any of the preservative spills on you, wash the area immediately and contact the physician's office.
- Always refrigerate the labeled collection container or keep it in a cooler or pail filled with ice.
- Be sure to keep the lid on the container.

Specimen Types

Many different tests are performed on urine. You may need to obtain different types of specimens for different tests. Specimens vary in two ways: in the method used to collect them and in the time frame in which they are collected.

Whenever you collect a specimen, you must follow the steps in the procedure exactly—or have the patient follow them exactly. Quality assurance is essential in the physician's office laboratory. As discussed in Chapter 27, control samples must be used every time you test patient specimens. These are the types of urine specimens:

- Random
- First morning
- Clean-catch midstream
- Timed
- 24-hour

Random Urine Specimen. The **random urine specimen** is the most common type of sample. It is a single urine specimen taken at any time of the day. A random urine specimen is collected in a clean, dry container. If the doctor is requesting that a culture be done on the specimen, provide the patient with a sterile container.

If the collection of a random urine specimen is to be done at the doctor's office, supply the patient with a urine specimen container. Show the patient to the bathroom, and ask the patient to void a few ounces of urine into the specimen cup and to leave the cup on the sink. Retrieve the specimen when the patient leaves the bathroom and attach a properly completed label and requisition slip. Transport the specimen to the laboratory immediately. Urine specimens should be processed within 1 hour of collection. If this is not possible, refrigerate the specimens. Before processing refrigerated specimens, however, allow them to come to room temperature. If specimens will be shipped to an outside laboratory, chemical preservatives are added.

If patients are to collect a random urine specimen at home, have them use the container indicated by the laboratory. Either provide patients with a urine specimen container or instruct them to use a clean, widemouthed glass jar with a tight-fitting lid. Explain that a household dishwasher provides hot enough water to disinfect a jar adequately. Tell patients to refrigerate specimens until they bring them to the doctor's office and to keep them cool during transport.

First Morning Urine Specimen. The **first morning urine specimen** is collected after a night's sleep. This type of specimen contains greater concentrations of substances that collect over time than do specimens taken during the day. A urine specimen container or clean, dry jar is used to collect the urine as per the laboratory's request.

Clean-Catch Midstream Urine Specimen. The **clean-catch midstream urine specimen,** sometimes referred to as midvoid, may be collected and submitted for culturing to identify the number and the types of pathogens present. The presence of clinical symptoms or unexplained bacteria in a urinalysis specimen is an indication for urine culture. This method is not like other urine tests in which urine is simply voided into a specimen container. Instead, the clean-catch midstream method requires special cleansing of the external genitalia to avoid contamination by organisms residing near the urethral meatus (the external opening of the urethra). Voiding a small amount of urine into the toilet prior to collecting the midstream specimen flushes the normal flora out of the distal urethra to prevent possible contamination of the specimen. The only other way to obtain a specimen without this type of contamination is through catheterization, a procedure not routinely recommended because of the risk of infection. Procedure 29-1 describes how to collect a clean-catch midstream urine specimen and how to instruct patients to perform this technique.

Timed Urine Specimen. A physician may order a **timed urine specimen** to measure a patient's urinary output or to analyze substances (see also the discussion of the 24-hour urine specimen). First determine whether the required time period means that the patient must collect the specimen at home. If so, provide the patient with the proper collection container; written instructions on the process, including preservation of the specimen; and the following oral instructions.

- Discard the first specimen
- Then collect *all* urine for the specified time (2 to 24 hours)
- Be sure the urine does not mix with stool or toilet paper
- Keep the sample refrigerated until returning it to the physician's office or laboratory

24-Hour Urine Specimen. A **24-hour urine specimen** is collected over a 24-hour period and is used to complete a quantitative and qualitative analysis of one or more substances, such as sodium, chloride, and calcium. You need to instruct the patient in the proper collection process. If an outside laboratory will be testing the specimen, you will receive protocols for collection, preservation, and transport. See the Educating the Patient section for specific information on the 24-hour collection process.

Catheterization

A **urinary catheter** is a sterile plastic tube inserted to provide urinary drainage. Such a catheter may be inserted into the kidney, the ureter, or the bladder. **Catheterization** is the procedure during which the catheter is inserted. Catheterization is performed for various reasons, including to:

- Relieve urinary retention
- Obtain a sterile urine specimen from a patient
- Measure the amount of residual urine in the bladder to determine how much urine remains after normal voiding (Patient voids and is then catheterized; more than 50 milliliters is considered abnormal.)
- Obtain a urine specimen if the patient cannot void naturally
- Instill chemotherapy as a treatment for bladder cancer
- Empty the bladder before and during surgery and before some diagnostic examinations

PROCEDURE 29.1

Collecting a Clean-Catch Midstream Urine Specimen

Objective: To collect a urine specimen that is free from contamination

OSHA Guidelines

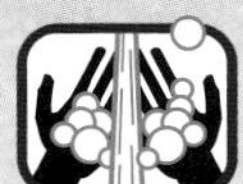 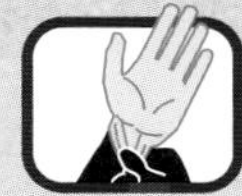 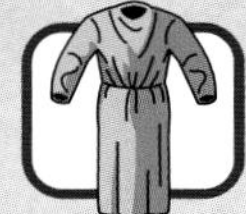 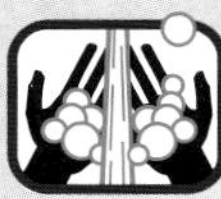

Materials: Dry, sterile urine container with lid; label; written instructions (if the patient is to perform procedure independently); antiseptic towelettes

Method

1. Confirm the patient's identity and be sure all forms are correctly completed.
2. Label the sterile urine specimen container with the patient's name, the physician's name, the date and time of collection, and the initials of the person collecting the specimen.

When the patient will be completing the procedure independently:

3. Explain the procedure in detail. Provide the patient with written instructions and the labeled sterile specimen container.
4. Confirm that the patient understands the instructions, especially not to touch the inside of the specimen container and to refrigerate the specimen until bringing it to the physician's office.

When you are assisting a patient:

3. Explain the procedure and how you will be assisting in the collection.
4. Wash your hands and put on examination gloves.

When you are assisting in the collection for female patients:

5. Remove the lid from the specimen container, and place the lid upside down on a flat surface.
6. Use three antiseptic towelettes to clean the perineal area by spreading the labia and wiping from front to back. Wipe with the first towelette on one side and discard it. Wipe with the second towelette on the other side and discard it. Wipe with the third towelette down the middle and discard it. To remove soap residue that could cause a higher pH and affect chemical test results, rinse the area once from front to back with water.
7. Keeping the patient's labia spread to avoid contamination, tell her to urinate into the toilet. After she has expressed a small amount of urine, instruct her to stop the flow.
8. Position the specimen container close to but not touching the patient.
9. Tell the patient to start urinating again. Collect the necessary amount of urine in the container. (If the patient cannot stop her urine flow, move the container into the urine flow and collect the specimen anyway.)
10. Allow the patient to finish urinating. Place the lid back on the collection container.
11. Remove the gloves and wash your hands.
12. Complete the test request slip, and record the collection in the patient's chart.

When you are assisting in the collection for male patients:

5. Remove the lid from the specimen container, and place the lid upside down on a flat surface.
6. If the patient is circumcised, use an antiseptic towelette to clean the head of the penis. Wipe with a second towelette directly across the urethral opening. If the patient is uncircumcised, retract the foreskin before cleaning the penis. To remove soap residue that could cause a higher pH and affect chemical test results, rinse the area once from front to back with water.
7. Keeping an uncircumcised patient's foreskin retracted, tell the patient to urinate into the toilet. After he has expressed a small amount of urine, instruct him to stop the flow.
8. Position the specimen container close to but not touching the patient.
9. Tell the patient to start urinating again. Collect the necessary amount of urine in the container. (If the patient cannot stop his urine flow, move the container into the urine flow and collect the specimen anyway.)
10. Allow the patient to finish urinating. Place the lid back on the collection container.
11. Remove the gloves and wash your hands.
12. Complete the test request slip, and record the collection in the patient's chart.

Educating the Patient

How to Collect a 24-Hour Urine Specimen

When a patient needs to collect a 24-hour urine specimen, you must explain the procedure thoroughly and provide explicit written instructions. Be sure the patient understands that she must collect all her urine over the 24-hour period.

Provide the patient with a labeled sterile urine container with a lid. Tell her that at the start of the observation period (usually early in the morning), she should void and discard that specimen. Then every time she voids for the next 24 hours, she must collect the entire amount in the sterile container.

Tell the patient that the urine will be tested for substances that are released sporadically into the urine. Thus, it is extremely important to avoid using a bedpan, urinal, or toilet tissue, which could retain the substances for which the test is being done. Instead, the patient should urinate directly into a small collection container and then pour the urine into the large urine specimen container. Explain that the small container must be sanitized between uses with soap and warm water.

Explain that the large specimen container may have a preservative in it to prevent contamination and other alterations in the specimen. Instruct the patient to keep the specimen covered and in the refrigerator when not in use during the collection period. Emphasize the need to deliver the specimen to the doctor's office or laboratory as soon as possible after the 24-hour period is over, keeping the specimen cool during transport.

There are two primary types of urinary catheters:

- **Drainage catheters,** which are used to withdraw fluids and include an indwelling urethral (Foley) catheter placed in the bladder, a retention catheter in the renal pelvis, a ureteral catheter, a catheter for drainage through a wound that leads to the bladder (cystostomy tube), and a straight catheter to collect specimens or instill medications
- **Splinting catheters,** which are inserted after plastic repair of the ureter and must remain in place for at least a week after surgery

Catheterization is not routinely recommended because it can introduce infection. Some states do not permit medical assistants to perform catheterization, and in most health-care institutions, only a physician or nurse can insert or withdraw a catheter. Check the protocol in your state. If you cannot perform the procedure, you may be asked to assemble the necessary supplies and to assist the physician during it.

Catheterization performed in a physician's office is usually done for diagnostic purposes. Specially prepared catheterization kits are available that contain all necessary instruments and supplies. These kits include a sterile instrument pack that is used to create a sterile field for the procedure.

If a patient is incontinent, the physician may use a bladder-drainage catheter to help drain the bladder and keep the patient dry. Another type of drainage catheter, the ureteral, is inserted into the ureter to help drain urine.

The indwelling urethral (Foley) catheter is designed to stay in place within the bladder (Figure 29-2). It consists of two tubes, one inside the other. The inside tube is connected to a balloon, which is filled with water or air to keep the catheter from slipping out of the bladder. Urine travels through the bladder and drains from the outside tube into a soft plastic container. The physician may order a leg bag to attach to the patient's thigh. To prevent backflow into the patient's bladder, the container must always be lower than the bladder.

Special Considerations

When you obtain a urine specimen from a patient or take a history of a patient who may have a urinary problem, you need to consider the patient's sex, condition, and age. Some patients may require special care during collection procedures.

Special Considerations in Male and Female Patients. Depending on the test, you may need to alter guidelines for collecting urine specimens from a male or female patient. For example, Procedure 29-1 describes how to assist in collecting a clean-catch urine specimen from a female patient and from a male patient. In addition, when you take a medical history on a male or female patient, you will need to ask particular questions as part of your assessment. For example, if a female patient leaks urine when laughing or coughing, she may have bladder dysfunction, which would affect collecting a 24-hour urine specimen.

Special Considerations in Pregnant Patients. Pregnant women normally have increased urinary frequency. They may also be prone to urinary tract infections. At each prenatal visit pregnant women must have their urine checked for abnormal levels of glucose (a screening test for diabetes) and abnormal levels of protein (a screening test for preeclampsia or renal problems).

Ask a pregnant patient whether she has any pain during urination or in the kidney area. A positive response may indicate a urinary tract infection or kidney stones.

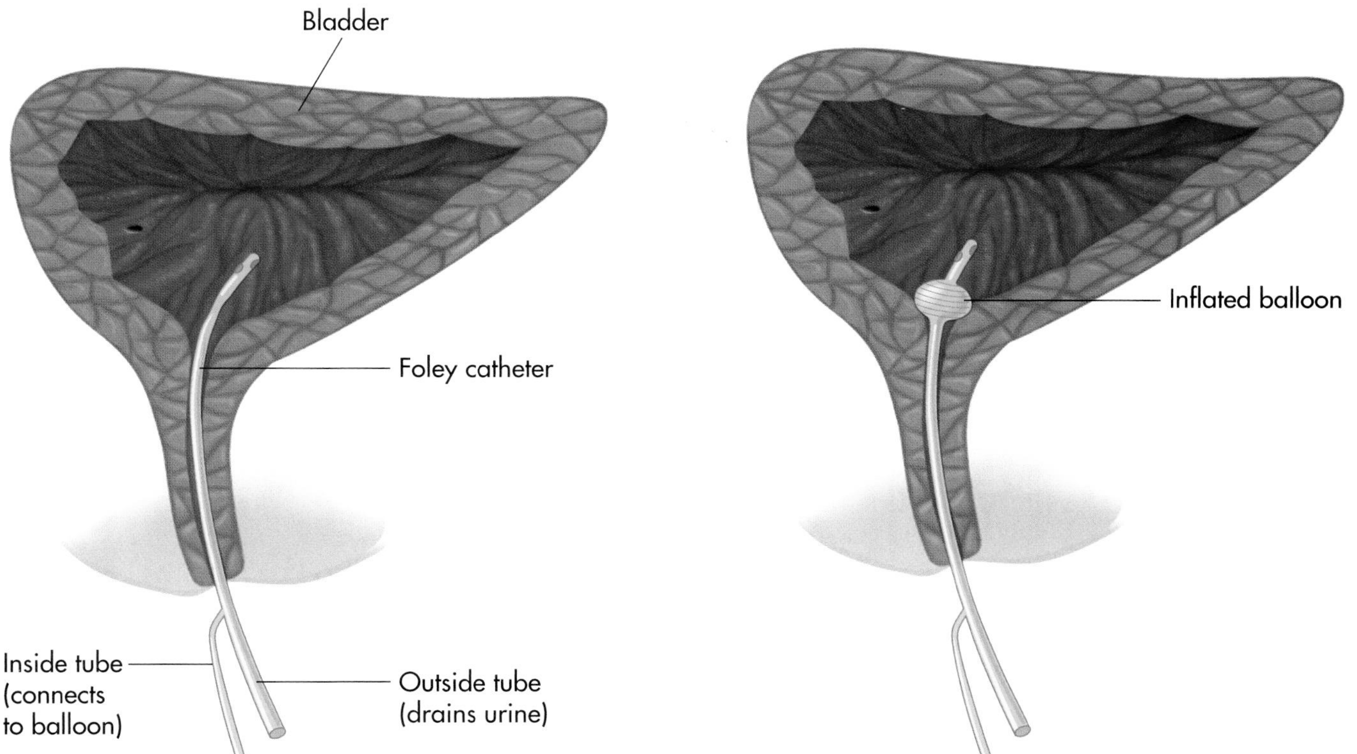

Figure 29-2. A Foley catheter stays in place within the bladder and has a collection container that is emptied periodically.

Also ask about urine leakage and whether she has previously been pregnant. Leakage may occur in a woman who has had multiple births, because the pressure of the fetus on the bladder or delivery of the baby may have weakened the patient's bladder control. Additionally, ask whether any of the babies were delivered by forceps, which can injure urinary and genital structures.

Special Considerations in Elderly Patients. When you collect urine specimens from elderly patients, you must consider several points.

- Bladder muscles weaken with age, often leading to incomplete bladder emptying and chronic urine retention, which can cause urinary tract infection, **nocturia** (excessive nighttime urination), and incontinence. Incontinence can interfere with collecting a 24-hour urine specimen.
- Weakening of the supports of the uterus may cause it to prolapse (work its way down the vaginal canal). The uterus pulls with it the vaginal walls, bladder, and rectum. This weakening, which is often the result of several childbirths, may not occur until a woman is postmenopausal. Symptoms include pressure, incontinence, and urinary retention. Normal activities, such as walking up the stairs, can aggravate the problem. This condition can interfere with collecting a 24-hour specimen.
- Find out whether the patient ever loses bladder control. If so, ask whether it occurs suddenly or whether a feeling of intense pressure precedes it. These symptoms can be a sign of weakening of the bladder muscles, which can interfere with collecting a 24-hour specimen.
- Keep in mind that some elderly patients need assistance in providing a urine specimen. For example, you may have to accompany the patient to the bathroom and hold the specimen container. (Wash your hands before and after doing so, and wear gloves while providing this help.)
- If necessary, offer repeated explanations or reminders about the procedure or the specimens that need to be provided.

Special Considerations in Pediatric Patients. When you collect a urine specimen from a pediatric patient, involve the child (if age-appropriate) and the parents or guardians. Explain the procedure thoroughly and ask specific questions, including the following.

- If the child is in diapers, ask whether there is a problem of persistent diaper rash. (Rash may indicate a change in urine composition because of renal dysfunction.)
- Is the child excessively thirsty? (In this case the patient may not be taking in enough fluids for the amount of urine being excreted. Excessive thirst, combined with increased urinary frequency and volume, is symptomatic of diabetes.)
- Has the child experienced any difficulty urinating or a urine stream change? (These signs may suggest an obstruction in the urinary tract.)

- Does the child cry when urinating? (If so, the child may have pain or burning on urination, which can indicate a urinary tract infection.)
- If the child is in diapers, ask how many diapers are wet each day. Has the number changed recently? (Responses to these questions can rule out or confirm a urine volume change. For example, a child with a fever and increased perspiration might experience decreased urine volume.)
- Has the child experienced deterioration in bladder control, such as bed-wetting (enuresis)? (The child may be under stress or may have a small bladder capacity or a urinary tract infection.)
- If the child is having problems with toilet training and is more than 4 years old, ask whether the child learned to sit, stand, and talk at the age-appropriate times. (If so, the child may have a urinary system dysfunction.)

When you collect a urine specimen from a child who is toilet-trained, follow the same procedures as for an adult. If the child is an infant or not toilet-trained, however, follow the steps outlined in Procedure 29-2.

PROCEDURE 29.2

Collecting a Urine Specimen From a Pediatric Patient

Objective: To collect a urine specimen from an infant or a child who is not toilet-trained

OSHA Guidelines

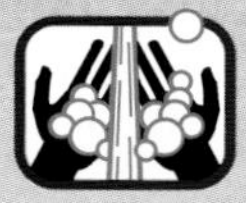 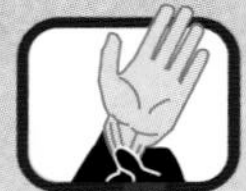 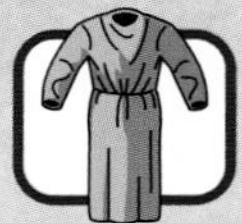 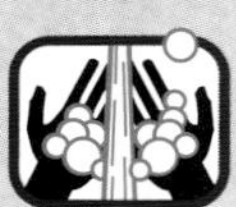

Materials: Urine specimen bottle or container, label, sterile cotton balls, soapy water, sterile water, plastic disposable urine collection bag

Method

1. Confirm the patient's identity and be sure all forms are correctly completed.
2. Label the urine specimen container with the patient's name, the physician's name, the date and time of collection, and your initials.
3. Explain the procedure to the child (if age-appropriate) and to the parents or guardians.
4. Wash your hands and put on examination gloves.
5. Have the parents pull the child's pants down and take off the diaper.
6. Position the child with the genitalia exposed.
7. Clean the genitalia. For a male patient, wipe the tip of the penis with a soapy cotton ball, and then rinse it with a cotton ball saturated with sterile water. Allow to air-dry. For a female patient, use soapy cotton balls to clean the labia majora from front to back, using one cotton ball for each wipe. Again, use cotton balls saturated in sterile water to rinse the area, and allow it to air-dry.
8. Remove the paper backing from the plastic urine collection bag, and apply the sticky, adhesive surface over the penis and scrotum (in a male patient) or vulva (in a female patient), as shown in Figure 29-3. Seal tightly to avoid leaks. Do not include the child's rectum within the collection bag or cover it with the adhesive surface.
9. Diaper the child.
10. Remove the gloves and wash your hands.
11. Check the collection bag every half-hour for urine. You must open the diaper to check; do not just feel the diaper.
12. If the child has voided, wash your hands and put on examination gloves.
13. Remove the diaper, take off the urine collection bag very carefully so that you do not irritate the child's skin, wash off the adhesive residue, rinse, and pat dry.
14. Diaper the child.
15. Place the specimen in the specimen container and cover it.
16. Remove the gloves and wash your hands.
17. Complete the test request slip, and record the collection in the patient's chart.

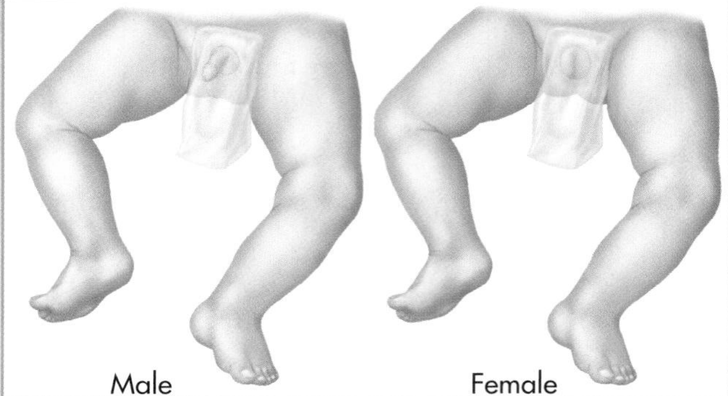

Figure 29-3. When you apply a pediatric urine bag, make sure there are no leaks.

Establishing Chain of Custody

Occasionally you may need to obtain urine specimens for drug and alcohol analysis. When you do so, you must establish a proper chain of custody.

The general approach to establishing a chain of custody is described in Chapter 26. Because of the medicolegal issues involved, it is important to follow the procedure exactly. If you alter the procedure at any point, you have broken the chain. Also, because supplying a specimen for drug or alcohol testing could be self-incriminating, it is important to thoroughly explain the procedure to donors and have them sign a consent form (Figure 29-4). The consent form may be a part of the chain of custody form (CCF), or it may be a separate form. The consent form states the purpose of the test and gives you permission to collect the specimen, prepare it for transport to the laboratory for analysis, and release the results to the agency requesting the test. Distribute copies of the CCF to the medical review officer, laboratory, patient, collector, and employer or other requesting party.

Inform the patient that medication (both prescription and nonprescription), drugs, and alcohol will show up in the test results. Encourage the patient to list on the consent form or CCF all substances consumed in the last 30 days, including what was taken and how much.

The chain of custody form, described in Chapter 26 (Figure 26-26), indicates the source of the urine sample. This form verifies that the patient whose name is on the CCF and consent forms is the same person who provided the sealed specimen sent to the laboratory. Follow Procedure 29-3 when collecting a urine sample for drug or alcohol testing.

Preservation and Storage

Proper preservation and storage of specimens are essential. Changes that affect the chemical and microscopic properties of urine occur in urine kept at room temperature for more than 1 hour. Such changes invalidate certain test results. If you leave a specimen unpreserved by any means for more than 1 hour, changes occur in the urine that affect the results of all urine testing—physical, chemical, and microscopic.

Refrigeration is the most common method for storing and preserving urine. It prevents bacterial growth in a specimen for at least 24 hours. Refrigeration can cause other changes in the urine, however, that may affect the physical characteristics of sediment and specific gravity. Bringing the specimen back to room temperature before testing will correct these problems. You can use chemical preservatives to preserve specimens, especially 24-hour specimens or those that must be sent a long distance to a laboratory.

Crossroads Medical Center
Newfield, New Jersey 07655-3213
201-555-4000

Drug Screen Consent Form

A urine drug test is required by______________________________ as part of your pre-employment screening. Please provide us with a list of all medications that you are presently taking.

____
____
____
____
____

I understand that my prospective or continued employment is contingent on a successful screening.

Date: __________ Signature:__________________________

Witness: ____

Figure 29-4. A consent form is a legal requirement when urine is collected for drug testing.

PROCEDURE 29.3

Establishing Chain of Custody for a Urine Specimen

Objective: To collect a urine specimen for drug testing, maintaining a chain of custody

OSHA Guidelines

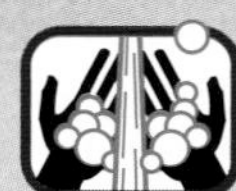
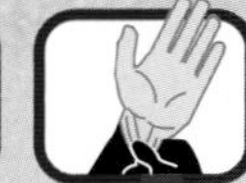
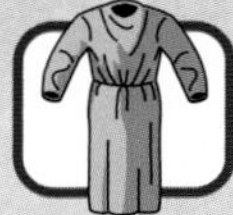
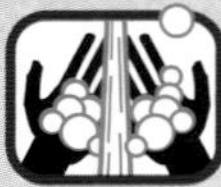

Materials: Dry, sterile urine container with lid; chain of custody form (CCF); two additional specimen containers

Method

1. Positively identify the patient. (Complete the top part of CCF with the name and address of the drug testing laboratory, the name and address of requesting company, and the Social Security number of the patient. Make a note on the form if the patient refuses to give her Social Security number). Ensure that the number on the printed label matches the number at the top of the form.
2. Ensure that the patient removes any outer clothing and empties her pockets, displaying all items.
3. Instruct the patient to wash and dry her hands.
4. Instruct the patient that no water is to be running while the specimen is being collected.
5. Instruct the patient to provide the specimen as soon as it is collected so that you may record the temperature of the specimen.
6. Remain by the door of the restroom.
7. Measure and record the temperature of the urine specimen within 4 minutes of collection. Make a note if its temperature is out of acceptable range.
8. Examine the specimen for signs of adulteration (unusual color or odor).
9. *In the presence of the patient,* check the "single specimen" or "split specimen" box. The patient should witness you transferring the specimen into the transport specimen bottle(s), capping the bottle(s), and affixing the label on the bottle(s).
10. The patient should initial the specimen bottle label(s) *after* it is placed on the bottle(s).
11. Complete any additional information requested on the form, including the authorization for drug screening. This information will include:
    - Patient's daytime telephone number
    - Patient's evening telephone number
    - Test requested
    - Patient's name
    - Patient's signature
    - Date
12. Sign the CCF; print your full name, note the date and time of the collection, and the name of the courier service.
13. Give the patient a copy of the CCF.
14. Place the specimen in a leakproof bag with the appropriate copy of the form.
15. Release the specimen to the courier service.
16. Distribute additional copies as required.

Urinalysis

Urinalysis is the evaluation of urine by various types of testing methods to obtain information about body health and disease. Urinalysis consists of three types of testing:

- Physical
- Chemical
- Microscopic

There are normal values for all tests done on urine. The normal value for a specific substance may be negative or none, or it may be a range in concentration. Urine test results within normal ranges indicate health and normality. Table 29-2 identifies normal values for a variety of urine tests. Because a urine test is a screening test, all abnormal values must be followed up with a confirmatory test.

Urinalysis is done as part of a general physical examination to screen for certain substances or to diagnose various medical conditions (Table 29-3). For example, daily urine output provides a picture of renal function. With adequate fluid intake, the average adult daily urine output is 1250 milliliters per 24 hours. When total intake and output measurements are not approximately equal, urinary tract dysfunction may be the cause.

The urinary system works with other body systems to help the body function normally. Therefore, a disorder in another body system can affect urinary function. For example, the kidneys interact with the nervous system to help regulate blood pressure and control urination. Thus, a nervous system disorder can affect the circulatory and urinary systems. The cardiovascular system delivers blood to the kidneys for filtration, and the kidneys regulate fluid balance, which helps maintain circulation of blood and

TABLE 29-2 Standard Urine Values	
Acetoacetate	None
Acetone	None
Albumin, qualitative	Negative
Albumin, quantitative	10–140 mg/L (24 hours)
Ammonia	140–1500 mg/24 hours
Bacteria (culture)	<10,000 colonies/mL
Bilirubin	Negative
Blood, occult	Negative
Calcium, quantitative	100–300 mg/24 hours
Casts	Rare/high-power field
Catecholamines, total	<100 μg/24 hours
Chloride	110–120 mEq/24 hours
Chorionic gonadotropin	Negative
Color	Pale yellow to dark amber
Creatine, nonpregnant women/men	<100 mg/24 hours (or <6% of creatinine)
Creatine, pregnant women	≤12% of creatinine
Creatinine, men	1.0–1.9 g/24 hours
Creatinine, women	0.8–1.7 g/24 hours
Crystals	Negative
Cystine and cysteine	<38.1 mg/24 hours
Estrogens, men	4–25 μg/g creatinine/24 hours
Estrogens, women	
Follicular	7–65 μg/g creatinine/24 hours
Midcycle	32–104 μg/g creatinine/24 hours
Luteal	8–135 μg/g creatinine/24 hours
Glucose, qualitative	Negative
Glucose, quantitative	50–500 mg/24 hours
Ketones	Negative
Lead	0.021–0.038 mg/L
Odor	Distinctly aromatic
pH	4.5–8.0
Phenylpyruvic acid	Negative
Phosphorus	0.4–1.3 g/24 hours
Potassium	40–80 mEq/24 hours
Protein (Bence Jones protein/free light chains)	Negative
Red blood cells	0–3/high-power field
Sodium	80–180 mEq/24 hours
Specific gravity, single specimen	1.005–1.030
Specific gravity, 24-hour specimen	1.015–1.025
Turbidity	Clear
Urea nitrogen	12–20 g/24 hours
Uric acid	0.25–0.75 g/24 hours
Urobilinogen, quantitative	1.0–4.0 mg/24 hours
Urobilinogen, semiquantitative	≤1 E. U./2 hours
Volume, adult females	600–1600 mL/24 hours
Volume, adult males	800–1800 mL/24 hours
Volume, children	3–4 times adult rate/kg
White blood cells	0–8/high-power field

myocardial function. A cardiovascular system disorder can allow blood to be delivered to the kidneys at a pressure inadequate for filtration, which would affect urinary system function.

Physical Examination and Testing of Urine Specimens

The first step in urinalysis is the visual examination of physical characteristics. Prior to starting the physical examination, it is essential to check the specimen for proper labeling. As part of quality assurance, examine it to make sure there is no visible contamination and that no more than 1 hour has passed since collection (or since the sample was refrigerated and brought back to room temperature). These physical characteristics are examined:

- Color and turbidity
- Volume
- Odor
- Specific gravity

TABLE 29-3 Common Urine Tests According to Clinical Condition

Clinical Condition or Suspected Disease	Types of Urine Testing
Acidosis	Reagent strip* for pH Specific gravity
Alkalosis (metabolic, respiratory)	Reagent strip* for pH Specific gravity
Diabetes mellitus	Odor (fruity) Microscopic examination for fatty, waxy casts Reagent strip* for ketonuria, glycosuria Specific gravity
Drug abuse	Gas chromatography; mass spectrometry**
Genitourinary infections (prostatitis, urethritis, vaginitis)	Cultures for bacteria, yeasts, parasites Microscopic examination for bacteria, RBCs
Human immunodeficiency virus (HIV)	Culture for virus (antibiotic added to kill bacteria) Other tests as indicated by specific symptoms
Hypercalcemia	Microscopic examination for calcium oxalate crystals Specific gravity
Hypertension	Microscopic examination for casts (hyaline, RBC) Specific gravity
Infectious diseases (bacterial) or other inflammatory diseases	Color and odor Cultures for bacteria, yeasts, viruses Microscopic examination for bacteria, WBCs, RBC casts (in severe cases) Reagent strip* for bacteria Turbidity
Metabolic disorders (except diabetes mellitus)	Color Microscopic examination for cystine crystals Reagent strip* for ketonuria, fructosuria, galactosuria, pentosuria, pH
Nephron disorders (nephrotic syndrome, glomerulonephritis, nephrosis, nephrolithiasis, pyelonephritis)	Color Microscopic examination for casts (epithelial, fatty, waxy, RBC), RBCs Reagent strip* for proteinuria Specific gravity Turbidity
Phenylketonuria	Color Reagent strip* for pH
Poisoning (arsenic, cadmium, lead, mercury)	Color Mass spectrometry**
Polycystic kidney disease	Proteinuria Urinary volume
Pregnancy	Reagent strip* for human chorionic gonadotropin (HCG)

continued ⟶

TABLE 29-3 Common Urine Tests According to Clinical Condition *(continued)*

Clinical Condition or Suspected Disease	Types of Urine Testing
Renal infections (acute glomerulonephritis, nephrotic syndrome, pyelonephritis, pyogenic infection)	Color Microscopic examination for epithelial cells (especially with tubular degeneration), numerous casts (granular, hyaline, WBC), RBCs, WBCs Radioimmunoassay (RIA)** Reagent strip* for bacteria, albumin Specific gravity Turbidity Urinary volume
Renal disease, renal failure, severe renal damage, acute renal failure, renal tubular degeneration	Microscopic examination for epithelial cells (especially with tubular degeneration), numerous casts (hyaline, fatty, waxy, RBC) Reagent strip* for proteinuria (albumin), pH Specific gravity Turbidity Urinary volume
Sickle cell anemia	RBC casts
Starvation, dietary imbalance, extreme change in diet, dehydration	Color Odor (fruity) Reagent strip* for ketonuria Specific gravity
Urinary tract infection or mild inflammation (cystitis, pyelonephritis)	Color and odor Cultures for bacteria, yeasts, viruses Microscopic examination for bacteria, WBC casts, RBCs, WBCs Reagent strip* for bacteria, albumin, pH Specific gravity Turbidity
Urinary obstruction (tumor, trauma, inflammation)	Color Microscopic examination for RBCs Specific gravity Urinary volume

*Federal listings of waived tests refer to these as dipstick tests.

**Drug screening and some other common urine tests must be performed by a forensic laboratory or other laboratory capable of performing gas chromatography, mass spectrometry, and radioimmunoassay.

Color and Turbidity. Normal urine ranges from pale yellow (straw-colored) to dark amber. The color, which comes from a yellow pigment called urochrome, depends on food or fluid intake, medications (including vitamin supplements), and waste products present in the urine. In general, a pale color indicates dilute urine, and a dark color indicates concentrated urine.

You will assess urine for turbidity, or cloudiness, by noting whether the urine is clear, slightly cloudy, cloudy, or very cloudy. Typically, urine is clear, although cloudy urine does not always indicate an abnormal condition.

The color of urine and any turbidity that is present can reveal medical conditions that require treatment. Table 29-4 provides more information on variations in urine color and turbidity and the possible causes or sources of these variations. Both pathologic (resulting from disease) and nonpathologic causes are noted.

Volume. Normal urine volume, or output, varies according to the patient's age. Normal adult urine volume is 600 to 1800 milliliters per 24 hours (average of 1250 millileters per 24 hours). Infants and children have smaller

TABLE 29-4 Urine Color and Turbidity: Possible Causes		
Color and Turbidity	**Pathologic Causes**	**Other Causes**
Colorless or pale straw color (dilute)	Diabetes, anxiety, chronic renal disease	Diuretic therapy, excessive fluid intake (water, beer, coffee)
Cloudy	Infection, inflammation, glomerular nephritis	Vegetarian diet
Milky white	Fats, pus	Amorphous phosphates, spermatozoa
Dark yellow, dark amber (concentrated)	Acute febrile disease, vomiting or diarrhea (fluid loss or dehydration)	Low fluid intake, excessive sweating
Yellow-brown	Excessive RBC destruction, bile duct obstruction, diminished liver-cell function, bilirubin	
Orange-yellow, orange-red, orange-brown	Excessive RBC destruction, diminished liver-cell function, bile, hepatitis, urobilinuria, obstructive jaundice, hematuria	Drugs (such as pyridium, rifampin), dyes
Salmon pink		Amorphous urates
Cloudy red	RBCs, excessive destruction of skeletal or cardiac muscle	
Bright yellow or red	RBCs (hemorrhage, myoglobin, hemoglobin), excessive destruction of skeletal or cardiac muscle, porphyria	Beets, drugs (such as phenazopyridine hydrochloride), dyes (such as food coloring and contrast media)
Dark red, red-brown	Porphyria, RBCs (menstrual contamination, hemorrhage, hemoglobin), blood from previous hemorrhage	
Green, blue-green	Biliverdin, *Pseudomonas* organisms, oxidation of bilirubin	Vitamin B, methylene blue, asparagus (for green)
Green-brown	Bile duct obstruction	
Brownish black	Methemoglobin, melanin	Drugs (levodopa)
Dark brown or black	Acute glomerulonephritis	Drugs (nitrofurantoin, chlorpromazine, iron preparations)

total urine volumes, although they produce more urine per unit of body weight. Urine volume is typically measured on a timed specimen (such as a 24-hour urine specimen) rather than a random specimen.

Oliguria, insufficient production (or volume) of urine, occurs in such conditions as dehydration, decreased fluid intake, shock, and renal disease. The absence of urine production is called **anuria.** Renal or urethral obstruction and renal failure can cause anuria.

Odor. Although the odor of urine is not typically recorded or considered a significant indicator of disease, it can provide clues about the body's condition. The odor of normal, freshly voided urine is distinct but not unpleasant and is sometimes characterized as aromatic. After urine has been standing for a while, bacteria in the specimen decompose the urea, which causes an odor similar to ammonia.

Diseases, the presence of bacteria, and particular foods (such as asparagus and garlic) can cause changes in urine odor. For example, in the presence of urinary tract infections, urine is foul-smelling, and in patients with uncontrolled diabetes, the smell is characterized as fruity (because of the presence of ketones). Phenylketonuria, a congenital metabolic disease, produces a strange, "mousy" odor in an infant's wet diaper.

Specific Gravity. **Urine specific gravity** is a measure of the concentration or amount of substances dissolved in urine. Because the kidneys remove metabolic wastes and other substances from the blood, the specific gravity of the urine they produce is an indicator of kidney function. The physician's office laboratory uses any of three methods to determine specific gravity:

1. Urinometer
2. Refractometer
3. Reagent strip (dipstick)

Specific gravity is a relative measure that is always compared to a standard. The standard for liquids is distilled water, which contains no dissolved substances.

$$\text{Specific gravity} = \frac{\text{weight of sample}}{\text{weight of distilled water}}$$

The specific gravity of distilled water is 1.000. You use special equipment to test for specific gravity (Figure 29-5).

The normal range of urine specific gravity is 1.005 to 1.030. Specific gravity fluctuates throughout the day in response to fluid intake. A first morning urine specimen normally has a higher specific gravity than a specimen provided later in the day. An increase in urine specific gravity indicates that the kidneys cannot properly dilute the urine. The urine then becomes more concentrated, causing it to darken. Increased specific gravity may indicate such conditions as a urinary tract infection, dehydration (for example, from fever, vomiting, or diarrhea), adrenal insufficiency, hepatic disease, or congestive heart failure. A decrease in the specific gravity of urine causes a lighter than normal urine color, may indicate that the kidneys cannot properly concentrate the urine, and may suggest such conditions as overhydration (excess fluid in the body), diabetes insipidus, chronic renal disease, or systemic lupus erythematosus.

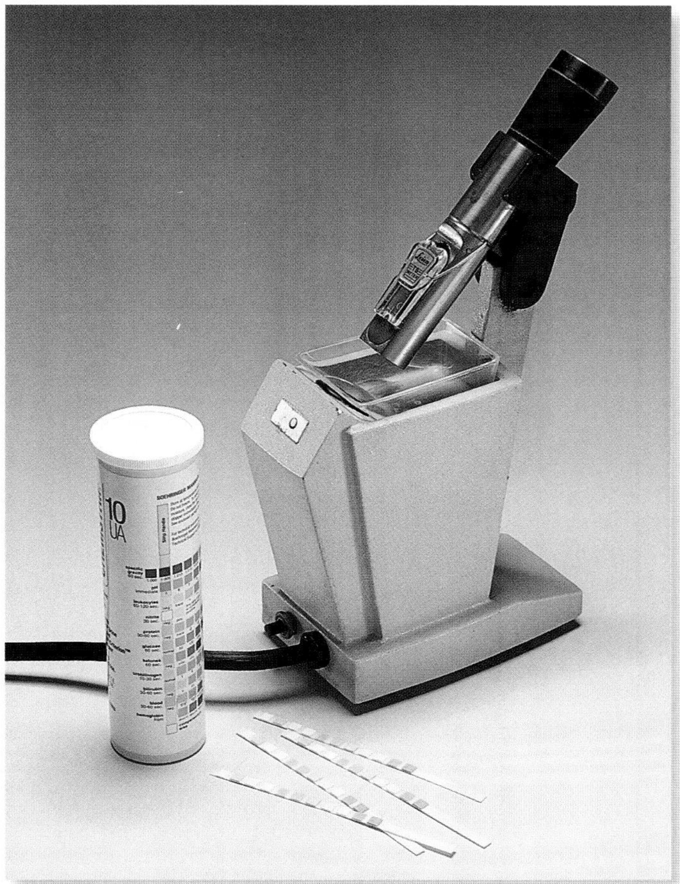

Figure 29-5. Specific gravity is commonly determined using a refractometer or reagent strips.

Refractometer Measurement. A **refractometer** is an optical instrument that measures the refraction, or bending, of light as it passes through a liquid. The degree of refraction, or refractive index, is proportional to the amount of dissolved material in the liquid. You must calibrate a refractometer each day with distilled water by setting the instrument at 1.000 with the set screw. Two standard solutions (solutions of known specific gravity) are also used to ensure accuracy. Advantages of using a refractometer to measure urine specific gravity are that the process takes little time and requires little urine. Only a drop of urine is used for this determination. Procedure 29-4 describes how to measure specific gravity with a refractometer.

Reagent Strip Measurement. You may use special reagent strips, or dipsticks, to test for specific gravity. Test pads along these plastic strips contain chemicals that react with substances in the urine and change color in precise ways. The reagent strip container includes a color chart for interpreting color changes on the test pads. When you evaluate urine specific gravity in this way, keep in mind that this type of test depends on precisely timed intervals identified by the manufacturer. Follow all directions exactly. The general steps for using reagent strips are as follows.

1. Wash your hands and put on examination gloves.
2. Identify the specimen.
3. After checking the expiration date on the reagent strip container (never use expired strips), remove a reagent strip from the container, holding the strip in your hand or placing it on a clean paper towel. Immediately replace the cap on the container.
4. Swirl the specimen to mix it thoroughly.
5. Note the time and simultaneously dip the strip into the urine and quickly remove it.
6. Draw the reagent strip across the specimen container's lip to remove excess urine.
7. Hold the strip horizontally and, after waiting for the specified time interval, compare the strip to the color chart on the container.
8. Read the value that corresponds to the matching color (for specific gravity in this case), and record the value on the laboratory report form.
9. Remove the gloves and wash your hands.
10. Place the laboratory report form in the patient's chart.

Chemical Testing of Urine Specimens

As a medical assistant, you may be asked to perform chemical tests on urine. Prior to performing chemical tests,

PROCEDURE 29.4

Measuring Specific Gravity With a Refractometer

Objective: To measure the specific gravity of a urine specimen with a refractometer

OSHA Guidelines

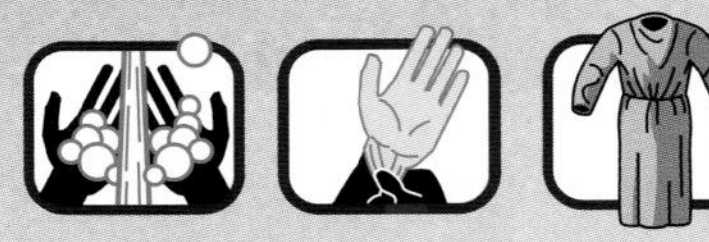

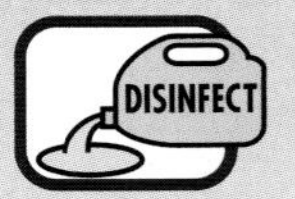

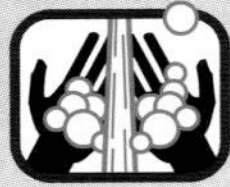

Materials: Urine specimen, refractometer, dropper, laboratory report form

Method

1. Wash your hands and put on examination gloves.
2. Check the specimen for proper labeling, and examine it to make sure that there is no visible contamination and that no more than 1 hour has passed since collection (or since the specimen has been removed from the refrigerator and brought back to room temperature).
3. Swirl the specimen to mix it thoroughly.
4. Confirm that the refractometer has been calibrated that day. If not, you must calibrate it with distilled water. You must also use two standard solutions as controls to check the accuracy of the refractometer. Follow steps 6 through 11, using each of the three samples in place of the specimen. Clean the refractometer and the dropper after each use, and record the calibration values in the quality control log.
5. Open the hinged lid of the refractometer.
6. Draw up a small amount of the specimen into the dropper.
7. Place one drop of the specimen under the cover.
8. Close the lid.

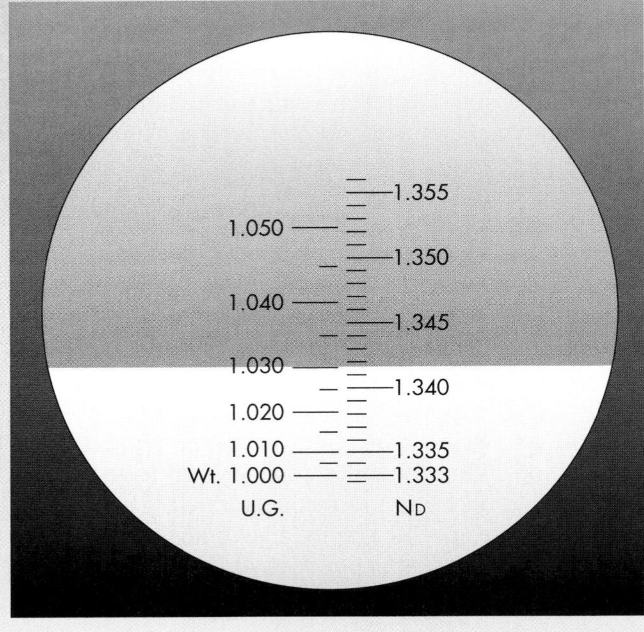

Figure 29-6. A refractometer uses light refraction to measure specific gravity.

9. Turn on the light, and look into the eyepiece of the refractometer. As the light passes through the specimen, the refractometer measures the refraction of the light and displays the refractive index on a scale on the right with corresponding specific gravity values on the left (see Figure 29-6).
10. Read the specific gravity value at the line where light and dark meet.
11. Record the value on the laboratory report form.
12. Sanitize and disinfect the refractometer and the dropper. Put them away when they are dry.
13. Clean and disinfect the work area.
14. Remove the gloves and wash your hands.
15. Record the value in the patient's chart.

always check for proper identification on the urine specimen to be tested. Chemical testing is usually done with reagent strips. It can also be performed with certain automated machines that use photometry.

The doctor orders chemical testing of urine to determine the status of body processes such as carbohydrate metabolism, liver or kidney function, or acid-base balance. Other reasons for chemical testing include determining the presence of drugs, toxic environmental substances, or infections.

Testing With Reagent Strips. As already described in the discussion of specific gravity, reagents (on plastic strips) are chemicals that react with a particular substance in urine and change color in precise ways. These changes indicate the presence of that substance and

TABLE 29-5 Some Common Chemical Analyses by Reagent Strip

Substance Test Indicates	Manufacturer of Test Strip	Name of Test Strip
Albumin (a protein)	Bayer	Albustix
		Multistix
	Boehringer Mannheim	Chemstrip
Bacteria (screen)	Bayer	Multistix
	Boehringer Mannheim	Chemstrip
Bilirubin	Bayer	Bili-Labstix
		Multistix
	Boehringer Mannheim	Chemstrip
Blood		
Red blood cells (as hemoglobin)	Bayer	Multistix
		Labstix
		Hema-Combistix
		Hemastix
	Boehringer Mannheim	Chemstrip
White blood cells (as leukocytes)	Bayer	Leucostix
		Multistix
	Boehringer Mannheim	Chemstrip
Glucose	Bayer	Clinistix
	Lilly	TesTape
Ketone bodies		
Acetoacetate	Bayer	Ketostix
		Labstix
		Multistix
	Boehringer Mannheim	Chemstrip
Acetone	Boehringer Mannheim	Chemstrip
pH	Bayer	Hema-Combistix
		Combistix
		Multistix
		Bili-Labstix
		Labstix
	Boehringer Mannheim	Chemstrip

the amount or concentration of the substance in the urine specimen. For example, when a reagent strip is used to test for ketones, the reacted color on the strip will correspond either to a specific concentration of ketone bodies, such as acetoacetic acid, or to no ketones present.

Reagent strips are used to test urine for a number of substances. In addition to ketones, these substances include nitrite, pH, blood, bilirubin, glucose, protein, and leukocytes. The tests and the usual reagent strips used in the tests are listed in Table 29-5.

There are numerous trade names for urine reagent strips, or dipsticks (for example, Multistix and Chemstrip). Not all reagents are reactive for the same chemicals. You must choose the appropriate strip according to the chemical test requested. All reagent strips are used once and discarded.

Follow the exact directions that come with the reagent strips to ensure accurate results. For quality assurance, take these basic precautions: Keep strips in tightly closed containers in a cool, dry area. Never remove them from the container until immediately before testing. Examine strips for discoloration before use; discard discolored strips. Check the expiration date on the bottle; do not use strips that have expired. Use strips within 6 months of opening the container. Every time you open a new supply of reagents, run control samples to check for proper operation.

Although the process is essentially the same for all reagent strip tests, there are variations in time intervals before reading results. Some reagent strips are designed to test for several substances at once. The basic procedure for using reagent strips for chemical tests can be found in Procedure 29-5.

PROCEDURE 29.5

Performing a Reagent Strip Test

Objective: To perform chemical testing on urine specimens (This test is used to screen for the presence of leukocytes, nitrite, urobilinogen, protein, pH, blood, specific gravity, ketones, bilirubin, and glucose.)

OSHA Guidelines

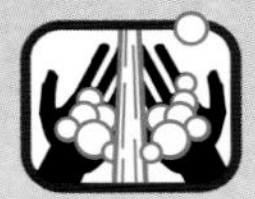
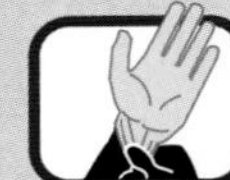
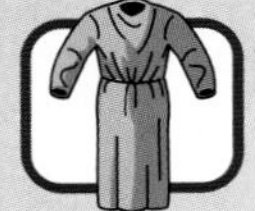
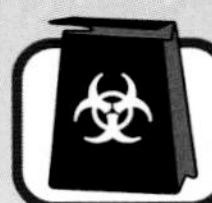
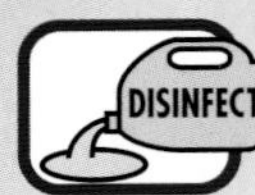

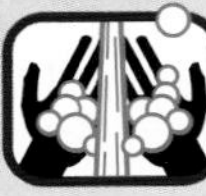

Materials: Urine specimen, laboratory report form, reagent strips, paper towel, timer

Method

1. Wash your hands and put on personal protective equipment.
2. Check the specimen for proper labeling and examine it to make sure that there is no visible contamination. Perform the test as soon as possible after collection. Refrigerate the specimen if testing will take place more than 1 hour later. Bring the refrigerated specimen back to room temperature prior to testing.
3. Check the expiration date on the reagent strip container and check the strip for damaged or discolored pads.
4. Swirl the specimen to mix it thoroughly.
5. Dip a urine strip into the specimen, making sure each pad is completely covered. Briefly tap the strip sideways on a paper towel. *Do not blot* the test pads.
6. Read each test pad against the chart on the bottle at the designated time. Note: It is important to read each pad at the appropriate time. Most reagent strip results are invalid after 2 minutes.
7. Record the values on the laboratory report form.
8. Discard the used disposable supplies.
9. Clean and disinfect the work area.
10. Remove your gloves and wash your hands.
11. Record the result in the patient's chart.

Ketone Bodies. Ketone bodies (or ketones) are intermediary products of fat and protein metabolism in the body. They include acetone, acetoacetic acid, and beta-hydroxybutyric acid. Only the first two substances can be determined by a reagent strip test. Normally, there are no ketones in urine. The presence of ketones in the urine may indicate that a patient is following a low-carbohydrate diet, or it may indicate that the patient has a condition such as starvation, excessive vomiting, or diabetes mellitus. Because ketones evaporate at room temperature, be sure to test urine immediately or cover the specimen tightly and refrigerate it until testing can be done.

pH. **Urinary pH** is a measure of the degree of acidity or alkalinity of the urine. Determination of pH can provide information about a patient's metabolic status, diet, medications being taken, and several conditions. The normal pH of freshly voided urine ranges from 5.0 to 8.0. The average urine pH is 6.0, which is slightly acidic. A pH of 7.0 is neutral, a lower pH is acidic, and a higher one is alkaline. Patients with alkaline urine may have such conditions as urinary tract infection or metabolic or respiratory alkalosis. Those with acidic urine may have such conditions as phenylketonuria or acidosis. Reagent strip, or dipstick, tests on both urine and blood are used to measure pH in the body. (See Chapter 30 for information on blood tests for pH.)

Blood. A patient who has blood in the urine may be menstruating, have a urinary tract infection, or have trauma or bleeding in the kidneys. To test for blood in urine, use a reagent strip that reacts with hemoglobin. There are two indicators on the strip. One is for nonhemolyzed blood, the other for hemolyzed blood.

Colors on the strip range from orange through green to dark blue and may indicate **hematuria** (the presence of blood in the urine) caused by cystitis; kidney stones; menstruation; or ureteral, bladder, or urethral irritation. The presence of free hemoglobin in the urine is known as **hemoglobinuria,** a rare condition caused by transfusion reactions, malaria, drug reactions, snakebites, or severe burns. Injured or damaged muscle tissue—such as occurs in crushing injuries, myocardial infarction, muscular dystrophy, or injuries during contact sports—can cause **myoglobinuria** (the presence of myoglobin in the urine). Reagent strip testing does not distinguish between these two conditions.

Bilirubin and Urobilinogen. When hemoglobin breaks down, it converts into conjugated bilirubin in the liver and then to urobilinogen in the intestines. Presence of the bile pigment **bilirubin** in the urine **(bilirubinuria)** is one of the first signs of liver disease or conditions that involve the liver. When bilirubin is present, urine turns yellow-brown to greenish orange. You usually use a reagent strip to test for bilirubin.

Although **urobilinogen** is present in the urine in small amounts, elevated levels of this colorless compound formed in the intestines may indicate increased red blood cell destruction or liver disease. Lack of urobilinogen in the urine may suggest total bile duct obstruction, as a result of which urobilinogen is not formed in the intestines or reabsorbed in the circulation. To test for urobilinogen, you use reagent strips.

Testing for either bilirubin or urobilinogen must be performed on a fresh urine specimen. Bilirubin decomposes rapidly in bright light to form biliverdin, which is not detected by the reagent strip test for bilirubin. Urobilinogen breaks down to urobilin on standing.

Glucose. Glucose is present in patients with normal urine, but only in small quantities not detectable by the reagent strip test for glucose. **Glycosuria** (the presence of significant glucose in the urine) is common in patients with diabetes. Blood is more commonly tested for glucose than urine is, because reagent strip tests may show false-negative results when used for testing urine.

Protein. Although a small amount of protein is excreted in the urine every day, an excess of protein in the urine **(proteinuria)** usually indicates renal disease. Proteinuria is also common in pregnant patients or after heavy exercise.

Nitrite. The presence of nitrite in the urine suggests a bacterial infection of the urinary tract. The test is not definitive, however, because some bacteria cannot convert nitrate to nitrite. Also, if an insufficient number of bacteria are present in the urine or if the urine has not incubated long enough in the bladder for a reaction to take place, a negative nitrite test can occur. The best urine specimen to test for nitrites is the first morning specimen.

When testing for urinary nitrite, you must test the urine immediately or refrigerate the specimen. Bacteria can multiply in a specimen that is allowed to sit at room temperature, thus causing a false-positive test result. Bacteria can also further metabolize the nitrite already produced, thus causing a false-negative result.

Leukocytes. Leukocytes appear in the urine in urinary tract or renal infections. Use strip tests for leukocyte esterase, a chemical seen when leukocytes are present, to test for leukocytes.

Phenylketones. The presence of phenylketones in a patient's urine indicates **phenylketonuria (PKU),** a genetically inherited disorder in which the body cannot properly metabolize the nutrient phenylalanine. This disorder causes phenylketones to accumulate in the bloodstream, resulting in mental retardation. PKU can be treated successfully by limiting dietary intake of phenylalanine, which makes up 5% of all natural protein, from early infancy. Although urine can be tested for the presence of phenylketones, blood testing is routine for newborns before discharge, at least 24 hours after birth.

Other Types of Chemical Testing. There are other types of chemical tests that may be performed on urine specimens. They generally involve testing for electrolytes and osmolality. Because these tests are performed in an outside laboratory rather than in a physician's office laboratory, you do not need to know the steps in each procedure.

Pregnancy Tests. Pregnancy testing is based on detecting the hormone secreted by the placenta. The name of the hormone is human chorionic gonadotropin, or HCG. The levels of HCG vary throughout pregnancy: they usually peak at about eight weeks; they drop to lower levels in the second trimester; and then detectable levels recur in the last trimester. Many commercial pregnancy tests are manufactured for use in the clinical setting and at home. These tests are sensitive, easy to perform and interpret, and give quick results. Most tests are now designed as an **enzyme immunoassay (EIA)** test, which always involves an antigen, an antibody specific for the antigen, and a second antibody conjugated to an enzyme. Newer technologies have been developed that are called membrane EIAs; in these tests, most of the reagents are incorporated into an absorbent membrane in a plastic case. Using either urine or serum, a sample is added through a chamber window where it migrates through the membrane and combines with the reagents to produce a reaction. Although the technology used in the design of these tests is quite complex, the actual test itself is easy to set up and interpret (Procedure 29-6). The tests are all designed with a control feature incorporated into the reagent pack for quality assurance of the test results.

Urine Tests for the Presence of STDs. In response to increasing numbers of sexually transmitted diseases, the CDC recommends that all sexually active females between the ages of 15 and 25 be screened annually for chlamydia. To accomplish this, several tests called nucleic acid amplification tests (NAATs) have recently been developed. These tests utilize urine samples to detect the presence of nucleic acid. Patients infected with either *Chlamydia trachomatis* or *Neisseria gonorrhoeae* will have nucleic acid in their urine. By amplifying nucleic acids specific to chlamydia and gonorrhea, the test can detect the presence of very small numbers of bacteria.

These tests have several advantages:

- Sample collection is noninvasive and easily collected.
- The tests are highly specific.
- The tests are highly sensitive. As little as one copy of bacterial nucleic acids can be detected in a urine specimen.
- Organisms do not have to be living to be detected.
- The tests are good screening tools for asymptomatic patients.

The tests also have some disadvantages:

- The tests are expensive.
- No living organisms remain for use in a follow-up culture. Therefore, positive tests must be confirmed by culture from an endocervical or urethral swab.

PROCEDURE 29.6

Pregnancy Testing Using the EIA Method

Objective: To perform the enzyme immunoassay in order to detect HCG in the urine (or serum) and to interpret results as positive or negative

OSHA Guidelines

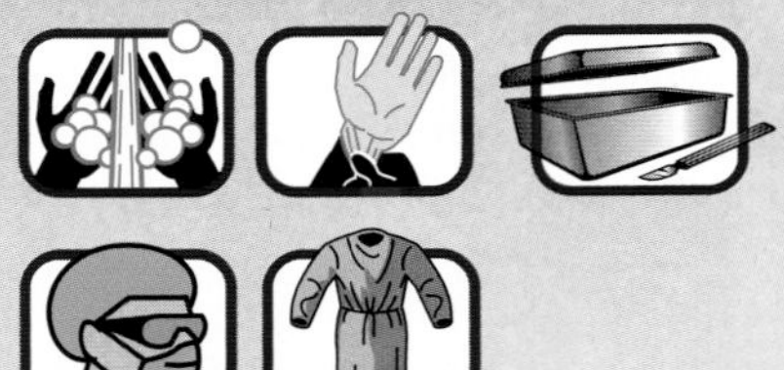

Materials: Gloves, urine specimen, timing device, surface disinfectant, pregnancy control solutions, pregnancy test kits

Method

1. Wash your hands and put on examination gloves.
2. Gather the necessary supplies and equipment.
3. If materials have been refrigerated, allow all materials to reach room temperature prior to conducting the testing.
4. Label the test chamber with the patient's name or identification number; label one test chamber for a negative and positive control.
5. Apply the urine (or serum) to the test chamber per the manufacturer's instructions.
6. At the appropriate time, read and interpret the results.
7. Document the patient's results in the chart; document the quality control results in the appropriate log book.
8. Dispose of used reagents in a biohazard container.
9. Clean the work area with a disinfectant solution.
10. Wash your hands.

Microscopic Examination of Urine Specimens

A microscopic examination of a urine sediment may be performed to view elements not visible without a microscope. You will use a centrifuge to obtain sediment for analysis. A centrifuge spins test tubes containing fluid at speeds that cause heavier substances in the fluid to settle to the bottom of the tubes.

During microscopic examination, elements that are categorized and counted include the cells, casts, crystals, yeast, bacteria, and parasites that form sediment (precipitate) after urine is centrifuged. You may use the KOVA System, manufactured by Hycor Biomedical, Irvine, California, to prepare urine sediment for microscopic examination. When you use the KOVA System, the sediment is evenly distributed to four calibrated chambers before the microscopic elements are counted. Procedure 29-7 describes how to process a urine specimen for microscopic examination of sediment.

Cells. High-power magnification is used to classify and count cells. Three types of cells are found in urine (Figure 29-7):

- Epithelial cells
- White blood cells
- Red blood cells

Epithelial Cells. Epithelial cells are classified as renal, transitional, or squamous. Renal epithelial cells can be round to oval and have a large, oval, and sometimes eccentric nucleus. Although a few of these cells appear normally in urine, several may indicate tubular damage in the kidneys.

Transitional epithelial cells line the urinary tract from the renal pelvis (the beginning of the ureter) to the upper portion of the urethra. They can be round to oval and may have a tail and, occasionally, two nuclei. Like the renal epithelial cell, a few appear normally in urine, but several may indicate tubular damage.

Squamous epithelial cells line the lower portion of the genitourinary tract. They are large, flat, irregular cells with a small, round, centrally located nucleus. They often occur in sheets or clumps and can be easily recognized under low-power magnification.

White Blood Cells. White blood cells are larger than red blood cells, have a granular appearance, and usually contain a multilobed nucleus. They are typically found in large numbers in the urine (greater than the normal zero to eight per high-power field) if inflammation is present or if the specimen was contaminated during collection.

Red Blood Cells. Red blood cells can be pale, round, nongranular, and flat or biconcave. They have no nucleus and enter the urinary tract during inflammation or injury. From zero to three red blood cells per high-power field in urine

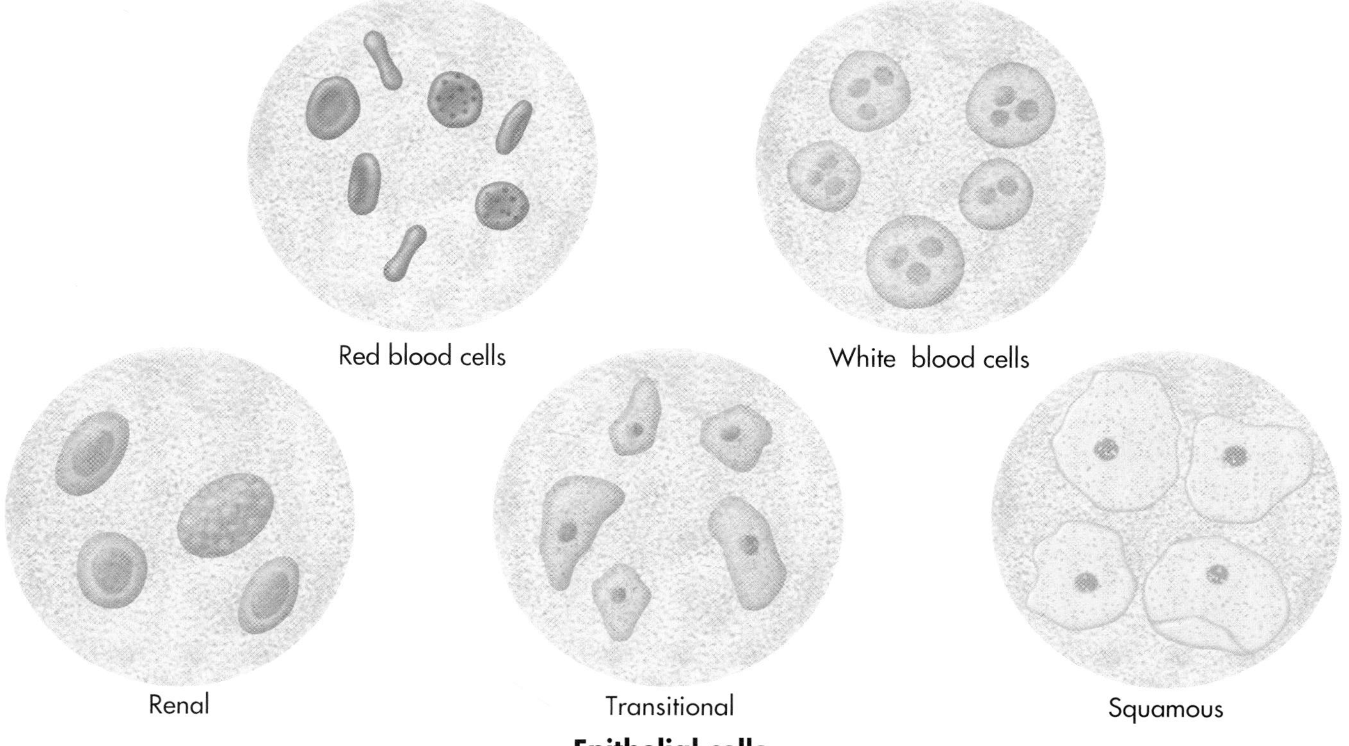

Figure 29-7. The number and types of cells found in urine constitute important diagnostic information about a patient's condition.

PROCEDURE 29.7

Processing a Urine Specimen for Microscopic Examination of Sediment

Objective: To prepare a slide for microscopic examination of urine sediment

OSHA Guidelines

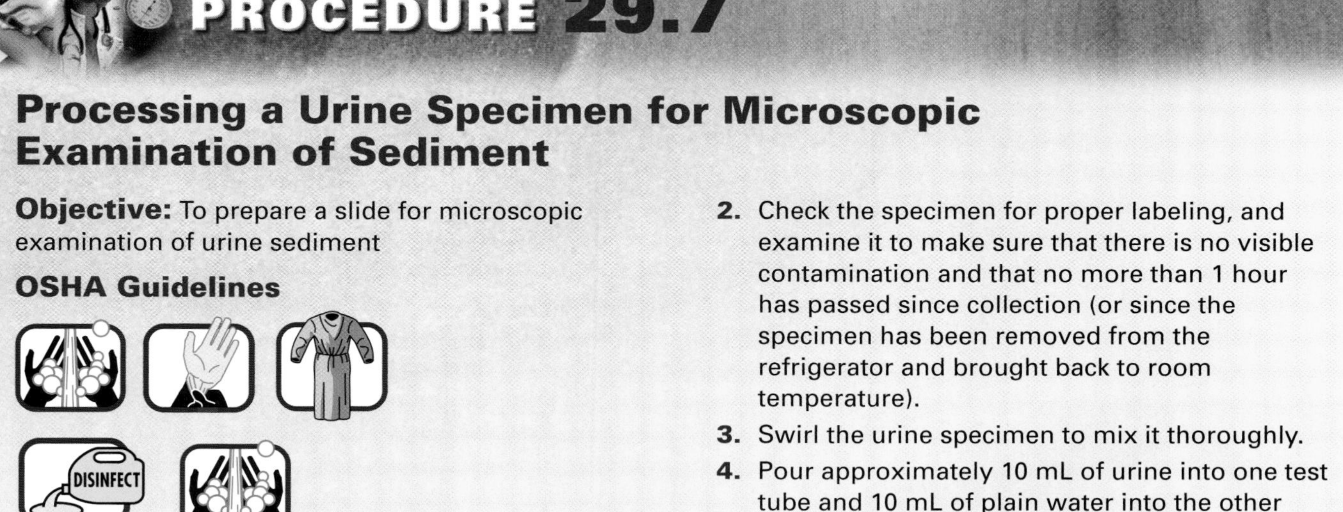

Materials: Fresh urine specimen, two glass or plastic test tubes, water, centrifuge, tapered pipette, glass slide with coverslip, microscope with light source, laboratory report form

Method

1. Wash your hands and put on examination gloves.
2. Check the specimen for proper labeling, and examine it to make sure that there is no visible contamination and that no more than 1 hour has passed since collection (or since the specimen has been removed from the refrigerator and brought back to room temperature).
3. Swirl the urine specimen to mix it thoroughly.
4. Pour approximately 10 mL of urine into one test tube and 10 mL of plain water into the other (Figure 29-8).
5. Balance the centrifuge by placing the test tubes on either side (Figure 29-9).
6. Make sure the lid is secure, and set the centrifuge timer (Figure 29-10) for 3 to 5 minutes.
7. Set the speed as prescribed by your office's protocol (usually 1500 to 2000 revolutions per minute) and start the centrifuge.

continued ⟶

PROCEDURE 29.7

Processing a Urine Specimen for Microscopic Examination of Sediment *(continued)*

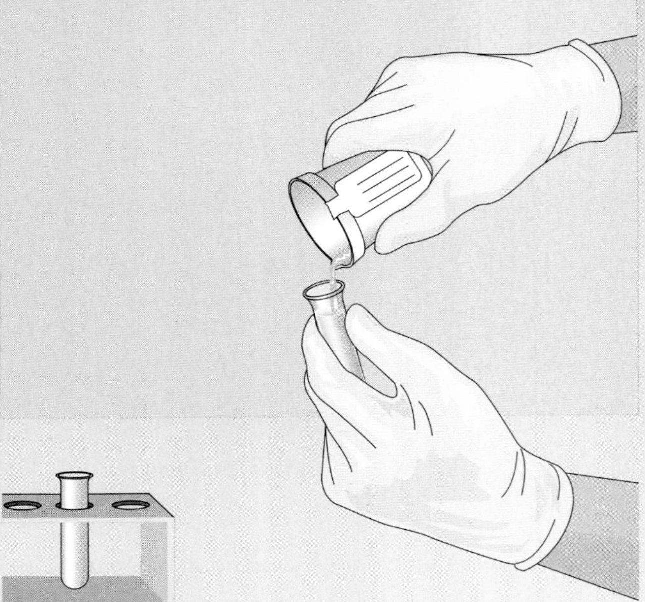

Figure 29-8. Fill one test tube with approximately 10 mL of urine and the other with 10 mL of water.

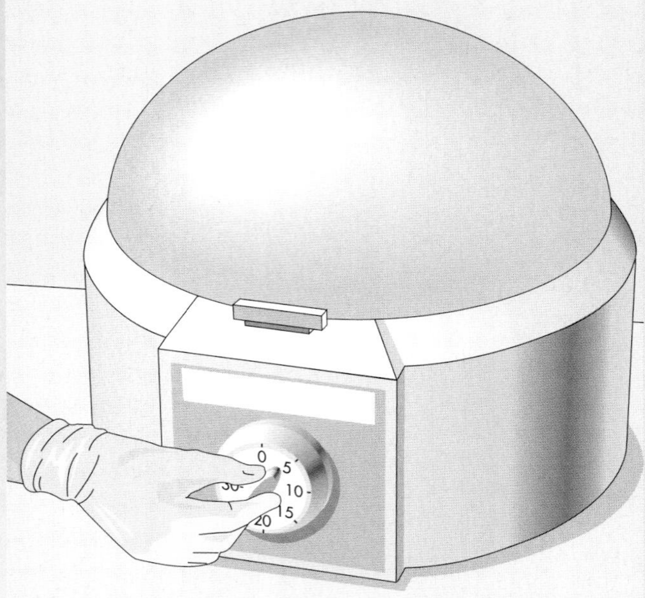

Figure 29-10. Set the centrifuge timer for 3 to 5 minutes.

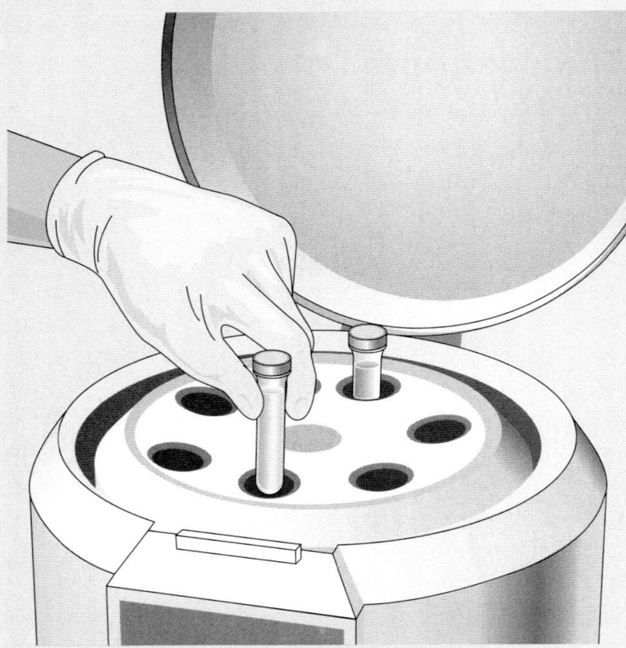

Figure 29-9. The centrifuge must be balanced by placing one test tube on each side.

8. After the centrifuge stops, lift out the tube containing the urine, and carefully pour most of the liquid portion—called the **supernatant**—down the drain in the sink (Figure 29-11).
9. A few drops of urine should remain in the bottom of the test tube with any sediment. Mix the urine and sediment together by gently tapping the bottom of the tube on the palm of your hand.
10. Use the tapered pipette to obtain a drop or two of urine sediment. Place the drops in the center of a clean glass slide.
11. Place the coverslip over the specimen, allow it to settle, and place it on the stage of the microscope.
12. Correctly focus the microscope as directed in Procedure 27-1.

Note: Most medical assistants are trained to perform this procedure only up to this point. After this, the physician usually examines the specimen. You may, however, be asked to clean the items after the

continued ⟶

PROCEDURE 29.7

Processing a Urine Specimen for Microscopic Examination of Sediment *(continued)*

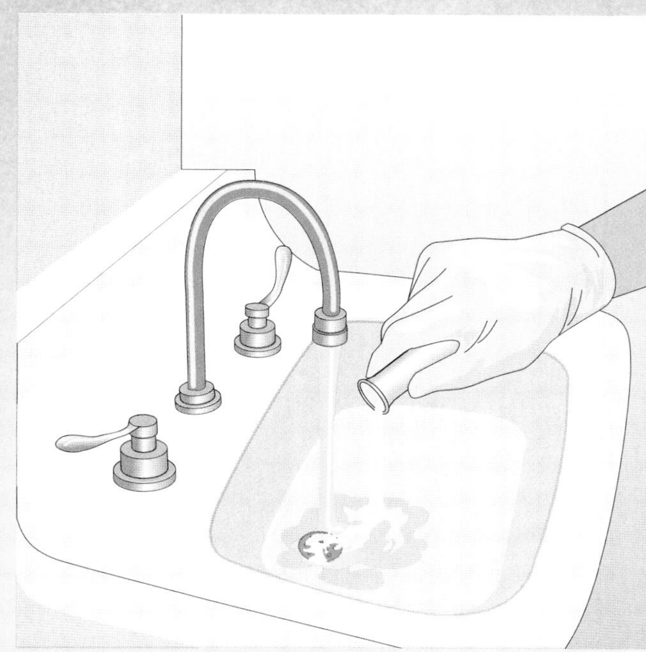

Figure 29-11. Make sure you do not lose any sediment when you pour off the urine.

examination is completed. The remaining steps are provided for your information.

13. Use a dim light and view the slide under the low-power objective.

14. Switch to the high-power objective. View any casts, cells, and crystals. Adjust the slide position so that you can view it from at least ten different fields. Turn off the light after the examination is completed.

15. Record the observations on the laboratory report form.

16. Properly dispose of used disposable materials.

17. Sanitize and disinfect nondisposable items; put them away when they are dry.

18. Clean and disinfect the work area.

19. Remove the gloves and wash your hands.

20. Record the observations in the patient's chart.

is normal. Numerous red blood cells may indicate a variety of problems, however, including urinary infection, obstruction, inflammation, trauma, or tumor.

Casts. **Casts,** which are cylinder-shaped elements with flat or rounded ends, form when protein from the breakdown of cells accumulates and precipitates in the kidney tubules and is washed into the urine. The protein then assumes the size and shape of the tubules. Casts differ in composition and size (Figure 29-12). Classified according to their appearance and composition, casts can indicate renal pathologic conditions or can be caused by strenuous exercise. Types of casts include the following:

- Hyaline casts, which are pale, transparent, and shaped like cylinders, with rounded ends and parallel sides. Composed of protein, they form because of diminished urine flow through individual nephrons. They are present in patients with kidney disease or in people who have exercised strenuously.
- Granular casts, which resemble hyaline casts and can also result from kidney disease or strenuous exercise. The granules are believed to come from degeneration of cellular inclusions.
- Red blood cell casts, which always indicate an abnormality and are hyaline casts with embedded red cells. Because of the red blood cells, these casts sometimes appear brown.
- White blood cell casts, which are hyaline casts with leukocytes. These casts typically have a multilobed nucleus and may indicate pyelonephritis, which is an inflammation of the kidney and renal pelvis.
- Epithelial cell casts, which contain embedded renal tubular epithelial cells and indicate excessive kidney damage. Causes include shock, renal ischemia, heavy-metal poisoning, certain allergic reactions, and nephrotoxic drugs. These casts are often confused with white blood cell casts.
- Waxy casts, which are rare, yellow, glassy, brittle, smooth, and homogeneous structures with cracks or fissures and squared or broken ends. These casts occur with severe renal disease.

Crystals. **Crystals,** naturally produced solids of definite form, are commonly seen in urine specimens, especially those permitted to cool. They usually do not indicate a significant disorder, except when found in large numbers

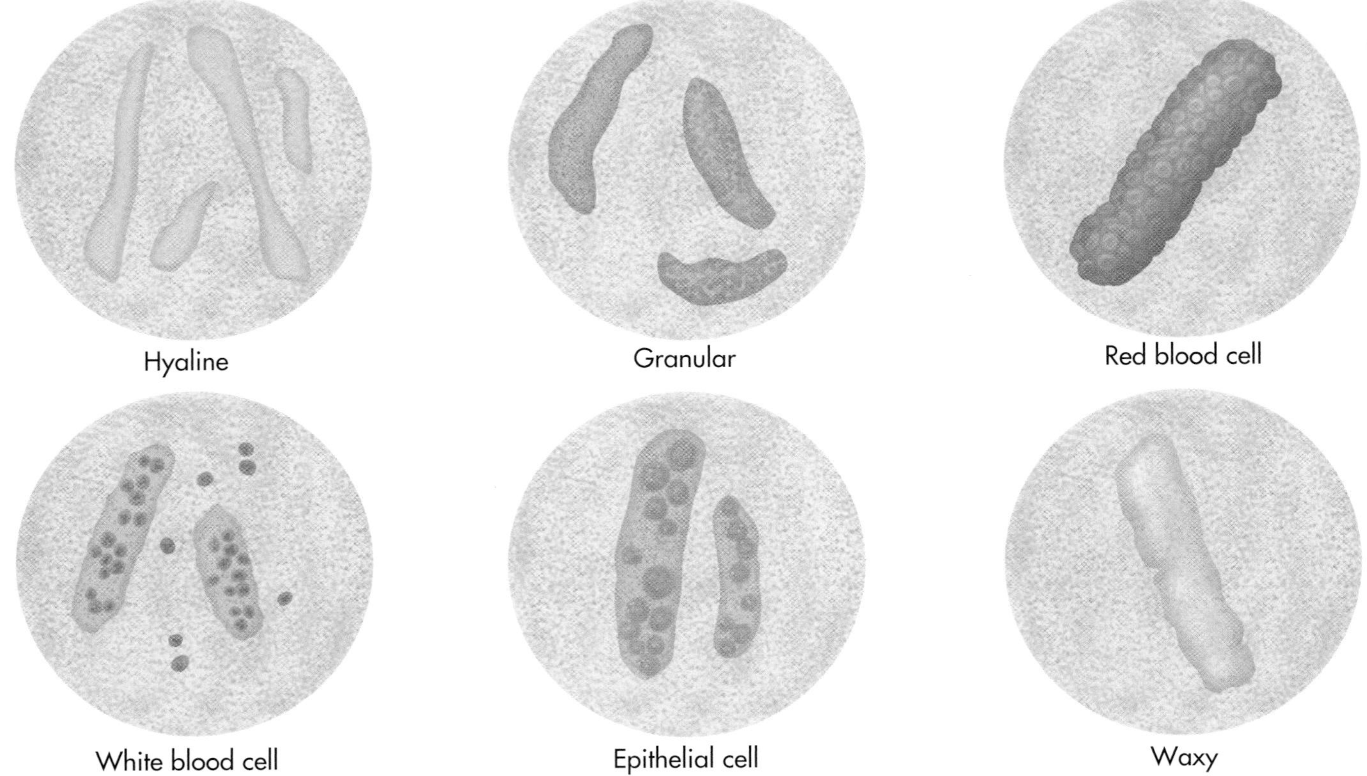

Figure 29-12. Casts, which are shaped like cylinders with flat or rounded ends, are formed when protein accumulates in the kidney tubules and is washed into the urine.

in patients with kidney stones and in a few pathologic conditions (such as hypercalcemia and some inborn errors of metabolism). Figure 29-13 shows common crystals found in urine specimens. Because different substances tend to crystallize in urine that is acidic and in urine that is alkaline, or basic, it is important to determine the pH of a patient's urine before you try to identify any crystals that are present.

Yeast Cells. Yeast cells, which are usually oval and may show budding, may be confused with red blood cells. Yeast cells in urine sediment are associated with genitourinary tract infection, external genitalia contamination, vaginitis, urethritis, and prostatitis. These cells are also commonly seen in the urine of patients with diabetes.

Bacteria. Although a few bacteria are normally found in urine, urinary tract infection may be indicated if the urine has bacteria along with a putrid odor and numerous white blood cells. Bacteria under high-power magnification appear rod- or cocci-shaped.

Parasites. The presence of parasites in sediment may signal genitourinary tract infection or external genitalia contamination. The most common urinary parasite, *Trichomonas vaginalis* (a pear-shaped protozoan with four flagella), is typically found in vaginal disorders but may also appear in males. When a urine specimen is cooled, *Trichomonas* organisms die.

Summary

The volume and physical, chemical, and microscopic characteristics of urine provide a great deal of information about a patient's health. Although invasive collection methods are sometimes necessary, routine urine specimens can be obtained by noninvasive, painless means. Urinalysis is the most common diagnostic test performed in doctors' offices.

You will have a substantial role in collecting, processing, and testing urine specimens. You will need to understand the urinary tract system and the basic characteristics of urine, including how it is formed, its physical composition, its chemical properties, and its microscopic characteristics.

Assisting patients and instructing them in the procedures required to collect different types of specimens are important aspects of your job. You must understand the purposes and procedures for collecting random specimens, first morning specimens, clean-catch midstream specimens, timed specimens, and 24-hour specimens. Throughout all collecting and processing procedures, you must practice quality assurance and employ precautions to avoid spreading disease-causing microorganisms.

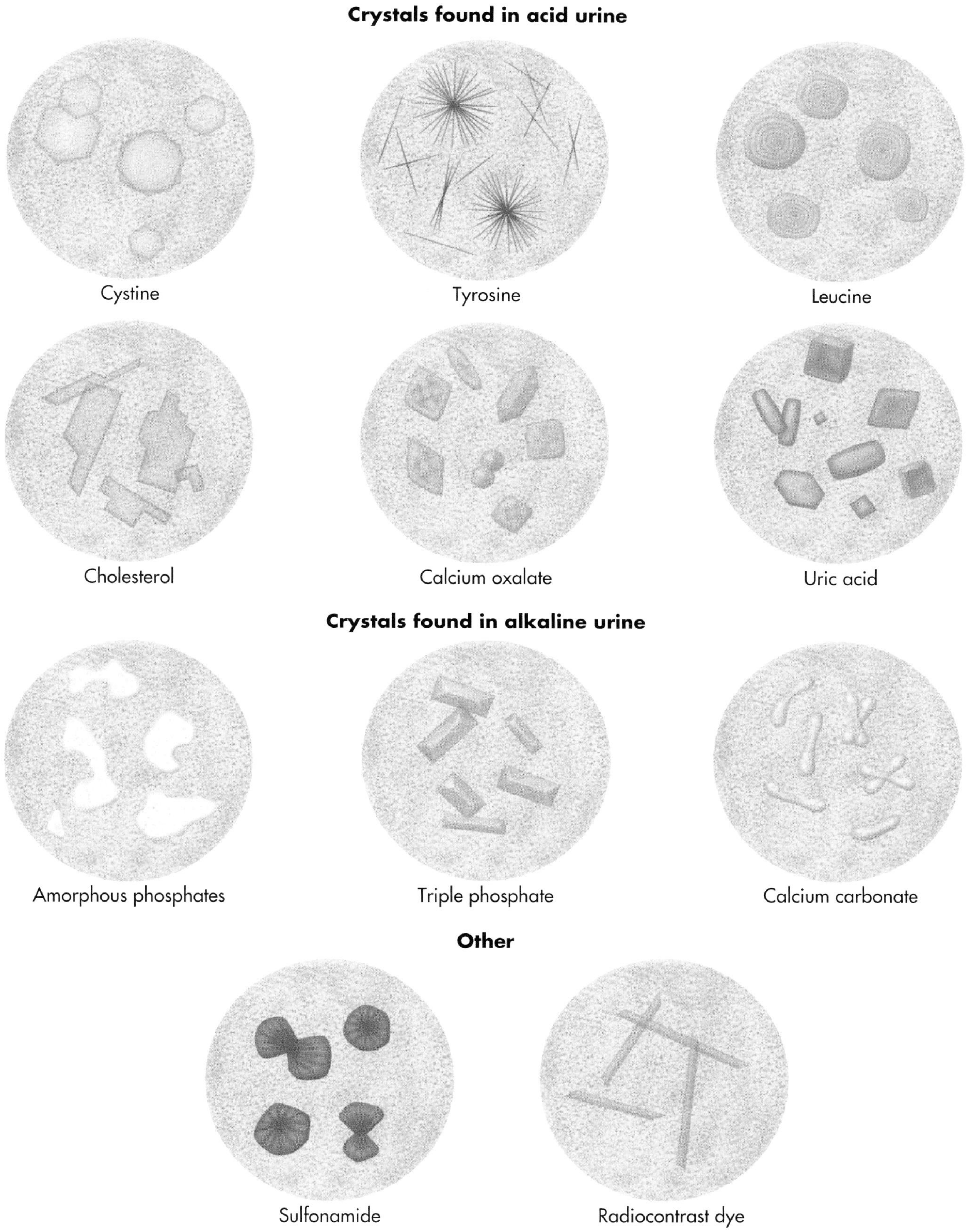

Crystals found in acid urine

Cystine

Tyrosine

Leucine

Cholesterol

Calcium oxalate

Uric acid

Crystals found in alkaline urine

Amorphous phosphates

Triple phosphate

Calcium carbonate

Other

Sulfonamide

Radiocontrast dye

Figure 29-13. You should be able to identify common crystals in urine and what they mean.

When obtaining and processing specimens, you need to follow general guidelines as well as take into account special considerations for specific groups of patients. You are responsible for ensuring that specimens are preserved and stored so that they are not contaminated or otherwise altered.

You may perform some tests on urine and prepare urine specimens for evaluation by the doctor. In either case you must be able to distinguish between normal and abnormal findings concerning the physical, chemical, and microscopic characteristics of urine.

Urinalysis provides important information to the doctor. You play a significant role in seeing that the specimen has been properly collected, processed, and tested, so that the information obtained from the analysis is useful and accurate.

REVIEW

CHAPTER 29

CASE STUDY QUESTIONS

Now that you have completed this chapter, review the case study at the beginning of the chapter and answer the following questions:

1. What is the maximum length of time that a urine specimen should be left at room temperature? If analysis cannot be performed within that maximum length of time, how should the specimen be handled?
2. An ammonia-like or foul odor associated with a specimen ordinarily indicates what condition or disease?
3. Does the chemical analysis confirm your suspicion associated with the odor?
4. Given the circumstances, can you trust the results on this specimen?

Discussion Questions

1. In the collection of a clean-catch midstream urine specimen, what purposes are served by the external cleansing of the genitalia and the voiding the first part of the specimen?
2. List the physical characteristics of a urine sample that should be observed during routine urinalysis. What would you look for in each characteristic?
3. What safeguards must be used when collecting a chain of custody specimen?

Critical Thinking Questions

1. While performing a routine examination of a urine specimen, you find that it is colorless and that the odor is fruity. What pathologic condition could cause this reaction, and which reagent strip tests could you perform to confirm the cause?
2. A 26-year-old woman provides a random urine specimen that is reddish-colored, is turbid in appearance, and shows large blood on the reagent strip. What question(s) might you ask this patient that could provide significant information about these test results?
3. What types of casts may be seen in the microscopic examination of urine specimens, and what is their significance?

Application Activities

1. Using a doll, demonstrate the correct method for applying a urine collection bag to a female infant.
2. Demonstrate the correct method for preparing a slide for microscopic examination of sediment.
3. Working with another student acting in the role of patient, explain the recommended procedure for collecting a 24-hour urine specimen. Ask appropriate questions to ensure that the "patient" understands the procedure. Then switch roles so that each student has the opportunity to play each role.

CHAPTER 30

Collecting, Processing, and Testing Blood Specimens

KEY TERMS

agranular leukocyte
B lymphocyte
buffy coat
capillary puncture
erythrocyte sedimentation rate (ESR)
formed elements
granular leukocyte
hematology
hemolysis
lancet
micropipette
morphology
packed red blood cells
phlebotomy
plasma
pyrogen
serum
T lymphocyte
venipuncture
whole blood

AREAS OF COMPETENCE

2003 Role Delineation Study

CLINICAL

Fundamental Principles

- Apply principles of aseptic technique and infection control

Diagnostic Orders

- Collect and process specimens
- Perform diagnostic tests

GENERAL

Communication Skills

- Adapt communications to individual's ability to understand

CHAPTER OUTLINE

- The Role of the Medical Assistant
- The Functions and Composition of Blood
- Collecting Blood Specimens
- Responding to Patient Needs
- Performing Common Blood Tests

OBJECTIVES

After completing Chapter 30, you will be able to:

30.1 Discuss the composition and function of blood.
30.2 Describe the process for collecting a blood specimen.
30.3 Explain the importance of confirming patients' identities and correctly identifying blood samples.
30.4 Describe how to perform venipuncture and capillary puncture procedures.
30.5 Identify the equipment and supplies required for blood-drawing procedures.
30.6 Discuss the correct procedures for disposing of waste generated during blood-drawing procedures.
30.7 Discuss common fears and concerns of patients and how to ease these fears.
30.8 Develop techniques for helping patients with special needs, including children, the elderly, patients at risk for uncontrolled bleeding, and difficult patients.
30.9 Identify common blood tests and explain their purposes.
30.10 Perform certain blood tests.

Introduction

In many health-care settings, the medical assistant is responsible for collecting blood specimens from patients and even performs some testing in the waived category. In order to properly collect the specimens, you will need to review the circulatory system and the function of blood. You will be introduced in this chapter to venipuncture and capillary collection procedures, and you will learn the appropriate supplies and equipment needed to perform these procedures. You will also learn techniques for dealing with different types of patients and how to efficiently and effectively obtain blood samples. Additionally, you will receive instruction on the performance and screening of common blood tests.

CASE STUDY

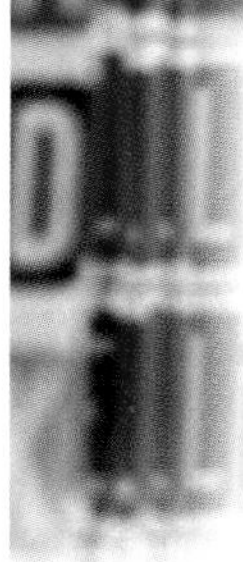

A young man comes into the office to have a PT drawn. As you examine the antecubital fossa in his arm, you don't feel confident with the vein but you attempt the phlebotomy anyway, using an evacuated system. However, the vein collapses and you are unsuccessful in your attempt. As you turn away to gather your supplies to try the collection again, he informs you that he is bleeding rather heavily from the venipuncture site and requires your attention.

As you read this chapter, consider the following questions:

1. What and where is the antecubital fossa?
2. What is the principle of the evacuated collection system?
3. How should you attempt to collect the blood on the second try?
4. What type of a blood test is a PT?
5. What could have caused the extensive bleeding this patient experienced after the venipuncture?

The Role of the Medical Assistant

The examination of blood can provide extensive information about a patient's condition. You may be asked to collect and process blood specimens for examination in your work as a medical assistant. A basic understanding of the anatomy and physiology of the circulatory system, as discussed in Chapter 10, will help you properly perform these tasks. You will also need a working knowledge of the functions of blood and the kinds of cells that make up blood tissue.

You will use several techniques to obtain blood specimens. **Phlebotomy** is the insertion of a needle or cannula (small tube) into a vein for the purpose of withdrawing blood. Phlebotomists receive special training in phlebotomy; drawing blood is the main, if not exclusive, task in their work. Smaller blood samples may be obtained by using a small, disposable instrument to pierce surface capillaries. You must be able to perform such procedures accurately so that the sample is appropriate for the ordered tests. You must also be skilled in putting the patient at ease during this procedure. Your reassuring manner, ability to handle technical problems, and careful preparation for answering many kinds of questions will be important to your success in this area.

You must understand how to process blood specimens and conduct various blood tests, particularly if you work in a laboratory. Finally, to make sure the test results are handled efficiently and accurately, you must be able to complete the necessary paperwork. All these skills are essential, regardless of whether you collect blood specimens in a physician's office laboratory (POL), hospital, or laboratory drawing station.

The Functions and Composition of Blood

The circulatory system transports blood throughout the body. The heart of the average adult pumps 8 to 12 pints of blood through more than 70,000 miles of veins, arteries, and capillaries each day. Blood is a complex and dynamic tissue that is essential to life and health.

Hematology is the study of blood, and hematologists study its functions and composition. Blood has many functions, all of which are important to the overall health of the body. Blood does all of the following:

- Distributes oxygen, nutrients, and hormones to body cells
- Eliminates waste products from body cells
- Attacks infecting organisms or pathogens
- Maintains acid-base balance
- Regulates body temperature

Blood is composed of four parts: **plasma** (the liquid in which other components are suspended), red blood cells, white blood cells, and platelets (thrombocytes). The

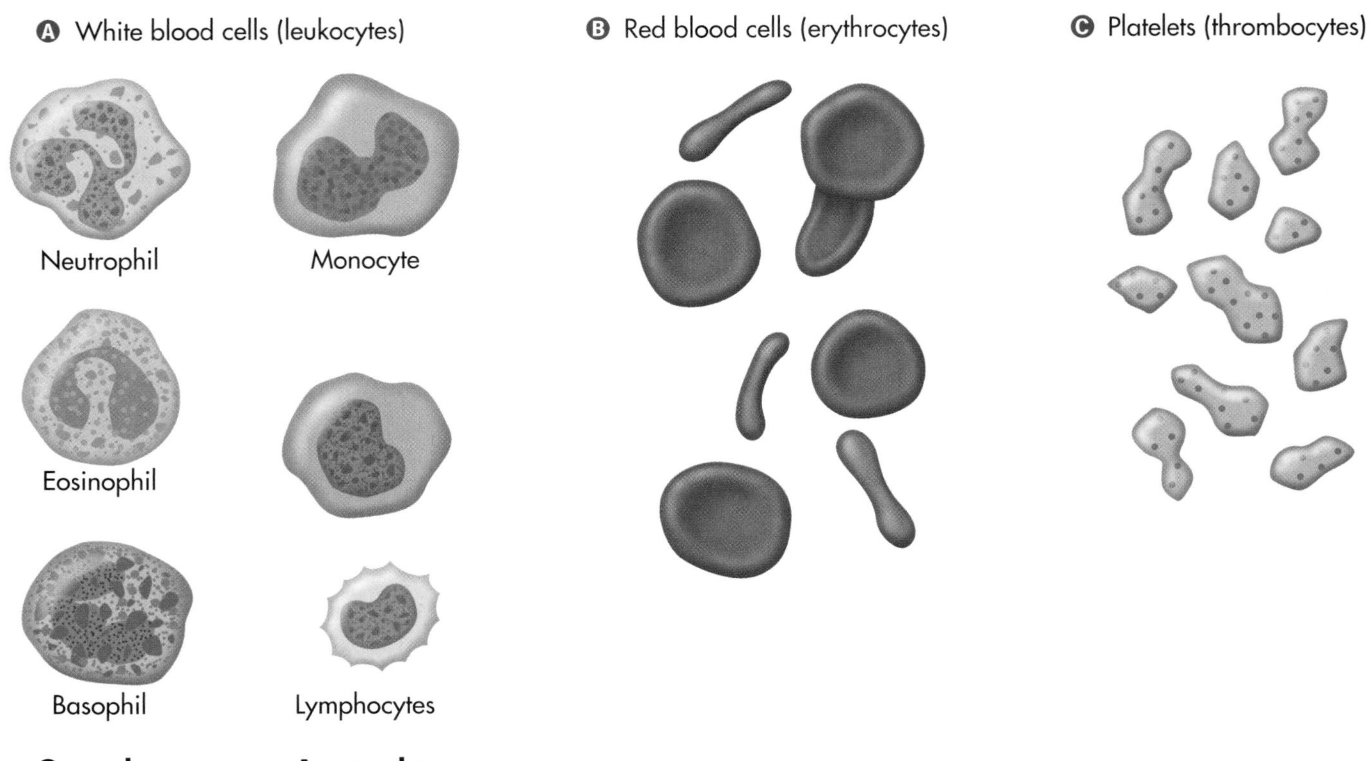

Figure 30-1. The formed elements of the blood are (a) white blood cells, (b) red blood cells, and (c) platelets.

plasma, or fluid part of blood, forms 55% of blood volume. The red blood cells, white blood cells, and platelets comprise the other 45% of blood volume, which is known as the **formed elements** (Figure 30-1). **Whole blood** is the total volume of plasma and formed elements.

Red Blood Cells

Red blood cells (RBCs), or **erythrocytes,** play a vital role in internal respiration (the exchange of gases between blood and body cells). Blood transports oxygen to body cells in two forms. About 98% of the oxygen is bound to **hemoglobin,** the main component of erythrocytes. The other 2% to 3% of the oxygen is dissolved in plasma. In addition, erythrocytes transport carbon dioxide from body cells to the lungs, although most carbon dioxide is carried in plasma. Healthy RBCs are disk-shaped and have concave sides (biconcave). Hemoglobin, a protein that contains iron, gives RBCs their rusty red color. A mature erythrocyte contains no nucleus.

White Blood Cells

White blood cells (WBCs), or **leukocytes,** protect the body against infection. (The function of WBCs as part of the body's defense against disease is discussed in Chapter 1.) Leukocytes are divided into two primary groups: **granular leukocytes** (also known as polymorphonuclear leukocytes) and **agranular leukocytes** (also known as mononuclear leukocytes). The division is based on the type of nucleus and cytoplasm in the cell. Each type of leukocyte performs a specific defense function, and the shape of each is suited to its role.

Granular Leukocytes. Granular, or polymorphonuclear, leukocytes have segmented nuclei and granulated cytoplasm. The three types of granular leukocytes are **basophils, eosinophils,** and **neutrophils.** Basophils produce the chemical histamine, which aids the body in controlling allergic reactions and other exaggerated immunologic responses. Eosinophils capture invading bacteria and antigen-antibody complexes through **phagocytosis,** or the engulfing of the invader. The number of eosinophils increases during allergic reactions and in response to parasitic infections. Neutrophils aid in phagocytosis by attacking bacterial invaders. They are also responsible for the release of **pyrogens,** which cause fever.

Agranular Leukocytes. Agranular leukocytes have solid nuclei and clear cytoplasm. The two types of agranular leukocytes are lymphocytes and monocytes. Lymphocytes are divided into two groups: B lymphocytes and T lymphocytes. **B lymphocytes** produce antibodies to combat specific pathogens. **T lymphocytes** regulate immunologic response. T lymphocytes are further classified as helper T cells and suppressor T cells. T cells are the cells attacked by human immunodeficiency virus (HIV), the virus that causes acquired immunodeficiency syndrome (AIDS). **Monocytes** are large white blood cells with oval or

Career Opportunities

Phlebotomist

To gain medical assistant credentials, you must fulfill the requirements of either the American Association of Medical Assistants (for a Certified Medical Assistant) or the American Medical Technologists (for a Registered Medical Assistant). After obtaining your medical assistant certification or registration, you may wish to acquire additional skills in specialty areas through course work or on-the-job training. Although this course work or training may not lead to an additional certification or degree, it will enable you to expand your role in the medical office and advance your career as the demand for skilled health professionals increases.

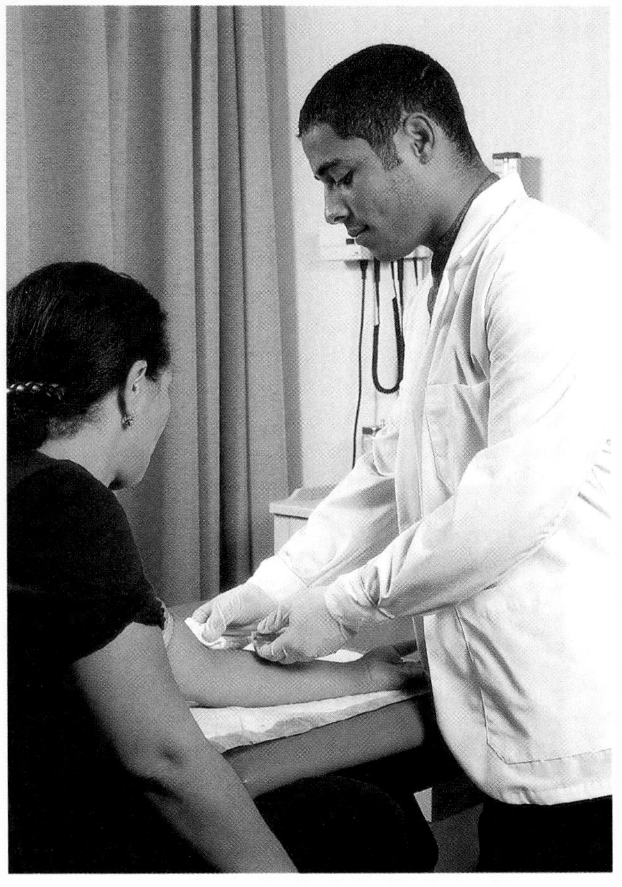

Skills and Duties

Traditionally, a phlebotomist's job has been to draw blood from patients for analysis. Today, however, phlebotomists perform many additional duties. Many phlebotomists now perform simple tests on blood samples at the patient's hospital bedside or in close proximity to the patient. This "point of care" testing speeds physician diagnoses, often reducing the length of a patient's stay in the hospital.

Other phlebotomists are trained to perform patient care functions, which differ from hospital to hospital. For example, they may run electrocardiogram equipment, change beds, deliver trays, or transport patients. While phlebotomists in the past worked primarily in the hospital laboratory, today's phlebotomists work closely with the nursing department and have more direct contact with patients.

Blood collection remains the mainstay of a phlebotomist's job. As part of this process, a phlebotomist performs administrative duties such as documenting the collected blood samples and labeling specimens. A phlebotomist may also administer a health-related questionnaire to the patient if one is required by the physician or an insurance company.

Workplace Settings

Most phlebotomists work in a hospital setting. Others are employed in laboratories, physicians' offices, and health departments. Some phlebotomists work with homebound individuals in nursing homes or private residences.

The job market for phlebotomists is good, provided that they are cross-trained in other specialties. Most institutions prefer phlebotomists who have additional training in areas such as performing blood tests.

Education

Most states require phlebotomists to be certified. The American Society of Phlebotomy Technicians (ASPT) is one of the bodies that provides certification.

To take the ASPT's national phlebotomy examination, you must either have 6 months of full-time work experience (or 1 year of part-time work experience), or graduate from an accredited phlebotomy training program. A high school diploma or general equivalency diploma (GED) is needed to enroll in such a program. To receive full certification, candidates must have at least 100 successful, documented vein punctures and 25 successful, documented skin punctures.

Where to Go for More Information

American Society of Clinical Pathologists
2100 West Harrison
Chicago, IL 60612
(312) 738-1336

American Society of Phlebotomy Technicians
P.O. Box 1831
Hickory, NC 28603
(704) 322-1334

National Phlebotomy Association
5615 Landover Road
Hyattsville, MD 20784
(301) 386-4200

horseshoe-shaped nuclei. They also defend the body by phagocytosis, recognizing and destroying foreign organisms and particles. Monocytes have a unique ability to pass through capillary walls into the body's tissues, where they perform phagocytosis.

Platelets

Platelets, or **thrombocytes,** are fragments of cytoplasm (the part of the cell that surrounds the nucleus) of megakarocytes that are smaller than either RBCs or WBCs. Platelets are irregular in shape and have no nucleus. These cell fragments are crucial to clot formation.

Plasma and Serum

Plasma is a clear, yellow liquid in which the formed elements of blood are suspended. Plasma is nearly 90% water; it also contains about 9% protein and 1% other substances in suspension (Figure 30-2). These other substances include carbohydrates, fats, gases, mineral salts, protective substances, and waste products.

Serum is the clear, yellow liquid that remains after a blood clot forms. It differs from plasma in that it does not contain fibrinogen, a protein involved in clotting. The fibrinogen converts into fibrin (a sticky protein) and traps formed elements of the blood in a clot. The process of clotting is called **coagulation.**

Blood Types or Groups

An individual's RBCs may carry one or both of two major antigens on their surface. These antigens are known as A and B. The presence or absence of these antigens determines the blood type or group to which that person's blood belongs. Blood that contains neither A nor B antigen is designated O.

In addition to antigens, an individual's blood may contain certain antibodies. Blood that carries only the A antigen contains anti-B antibodies, and blood that carries only the B antigen contains anti-A antibodies. Blood that carries neither antigen contains both anti-A and anti-B antibodies, whereas blood that carries both antigens contains neither anti-A nor anti-B antibodies.

Blood is carefully matched before a blood transfusion. If a patient is given incompatible blood, the antibodies in the patient's blood will combine with the antigens in the transfused blood. This reaction leads to clumping of the

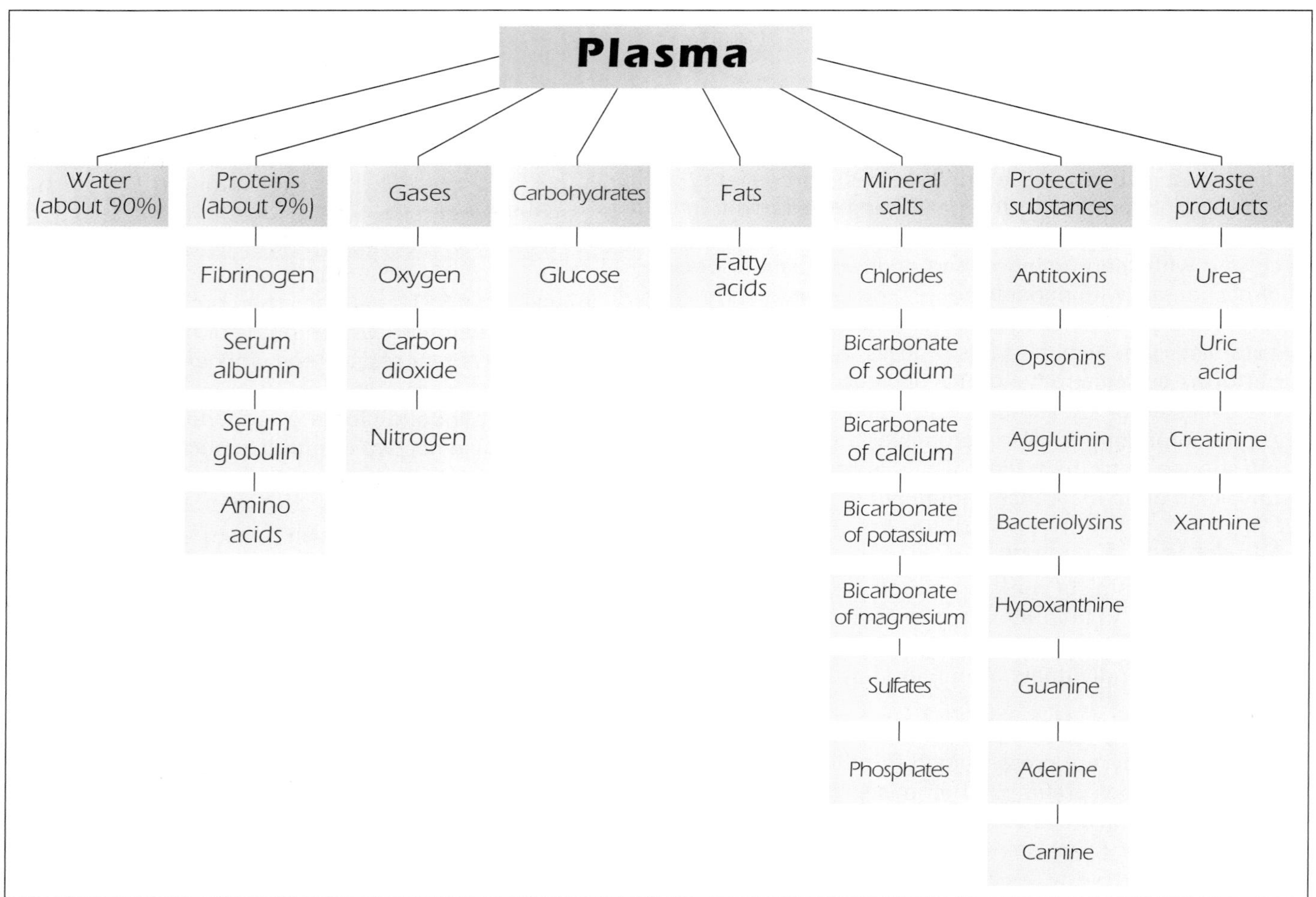

Figure 30-2. A wide variety of substances account for about 10% of plasma by volume. The remainder is water.

RBCs and possible **hemolysis** (the rupturing of red blood cells, which releases hemoglobin). The released hemoglobin can block the renal tubules and cause kidney failure and death.

Technologists can determine blood type by mixing a blood specimen with serum containing different antibodies and noting the clumping reactions that occur. The most common system for identifying blood types is the ABO system. The ABO system designates the two major antigens A and B and consists of four groups:

- A: only the A antigen (and anti-B antibodies) present
- B: only the B antigen (and anti-A antibodies) present
- AB: both A and B antigens (and neither antibodies) present
- O: neither A nor B antigen (but both antibodies) present

In addition to the ABO classification, another important blood identifier is the Rh factor. The Rh factor, so named because it was discovered through research on the rhesus monkey, is another antigen found on the surface of the RBC. Approximately 85% of people have the Rh factor in their blood, and their blood type is considered to be Rh positive (Rh+). The other 15% are Rh negative (Rh−). Like the antigens that identify the main group to which a sample belongs, the Rh antigen is also capable of generating a similar, potentially fatal, antigen-antibody reaction.

In these two classification systems, blood is identified by type and Rh factor. The following list identifies eight combinations and the approximate percentage of the population with each type, according to the American Red Cross:

- Type A+: 34%
- Type A−: 6%
- Type B+: 8%
- Type B−: 2%
- Type AB+: 3%
- Type AB−: 1%
- Type O+: 39%
- Type O−: 7%

Type O negative (O−) is considered the universal donor blood because it lacks the A, B, and Rh antigens. Type AB positive (AB+) is considered the universal recipient blood because it will not react with donated blood from any blood group. Note that recipient and donor must be compatible with regard to A and B antigens as well as the Rh factor for transfusion to be safe.

Collecting Blood Specimens

There is a standard process for drawing blood specimens. Following these steps will enable you to perform the procedure smoothly, accurately, and safely and ensure that documentation is completed properly.

Reading and Interpreting the Test Order

The first steps in preparing to draw blood for testing are to review the written testing request and to assemble the equipment and supplies. The patient should arrive with a laboratory request form if you are working in a physician's office laboratory or a laboratory drawing station. You will probably receive a test order from your supervisor if you are working in a hospital.

Reviewing the Test Order. It is essential to first review the patient's blood-collection order to determine what tests will be run. Many tests require expedited or special handling to ensure accurate results.

Your office will have specific collection procedures for each type of test. If you have any questions about these procedures, ask your supervisor. If you will be sending the blood specimen to a reference laboratory for testing, make sure you know its requirements. The cost of reprocessing a test far surpasses the extra time needed to be sure of the process requirements.

When reviewing the test order, you will need to know the meaning of certain abbreviations. Many abbreviations used in laboratory work and their meanings are presented in Figure 30-3. If you are ever in doubt or if the resources in your office or laboratory do not provide the answers you need, ask the doctor or your supervisor.

Assembling the Equipment and Supplies. Specific blood-drawing equipment and collection devices vary with the type of test. Make sure you have the appropriate equipment to collect all necessary samples if more than one test is ordered. All specimen-collection tubes, slides, and other containers should be labeled immediately after collection with the patient's name, the date and time of collection, the initials of the person collecting the specimen, and other information as required by the test procedure or your office. Some offices use an identification code for each patient.

Alcohol and cotton balls or alcohol wipes, sterile gauze, and adhesive bandages are standard supplies for procedures during which blood is drawn from a vein or capillaries. Alcohol causes inaccurate results for certain tests, however, so for these tests, povidone iodine or benzalkonium chloride is used. You will need a tourniquet (a flat, broad length of vinyl or rubber or a piece of fabric with a Velcro closure) for **venipuncture,** the puncture of a vein—performed with a needle for the purpose of drawing blood.

Preparing Patients

After you review the test order and assemble the necessary equipment and supplies, take a moment to relax, gather your thoughts, and consider your purpose. This may strike you as odd advice, but your calm and positive demeanor helps establish the best possible relationship with a patient who may be uneasy about having blood drawn. The moment you use to relax and focus may save you time and

Common Abbreviations Used in Blood Tests

Ab	antibody
ABO	classification system for four blood groups
AcAc	acetoacetate
ACE	angiotensin-converting enzyme
ACT	activated coagulation time
ACTH	adrenocorticotropic hormone
ADH	antidiuretic hormone
AFB	acid-fast bacillus
AFP	alpha-fetoprotein
Ag	antigen
AG	anion gap
A/G R	albumin-globulin ratio
AHF	antihemolytic factor
Alb	albumin
Alc	alcohol
ALG	antilymphocyte globulin
ALP; alk phos	alkaline phosphatase
ALT	alanine aminotransferase
ANA	antinuclear antibody
APAP	acetaminophen
APTT	activated partial thromboplastin time
ASA	acetylsalicylic acid (aspirin)
AST	aspartate aminotransferase
AT-III	antithrombin III
B	blood (whole blood)
Baso	basophil
BCA	breast cancer antigen
BJP	Bence Jones protein
BT	bleeding time
BUN	blood urea nitrogen
Ca; Ca^{++}	calcium
CA	cancer antigen
CBC	complete blood (cell) count
CEA	carcinoembryonic antigen
CHE	cholinesterase
CK	creatine kinase
CMV	cytomegalovirus
CN-	cyanide anion
CO	carbon monoxide
CO_2	carbon dioxide
COHb	carboxyhemoglobin
Cr	creatinine
CrCl	creatinine clearance
CT	calcitonin
DAF	decay accelerating factor
DHEA	dehydroepiandrosterone, unconjugated
Diff	differential (blood cell count)
EBNA	Epstein-Barr virus nuclear antigen
EBV	Epstein-Barr virus
EDTA	ethylenediaminetetraacetic acid
Eos	eosinophil
EP	electrophoresis
Eq	equivalent
ERP	estrogen receptor protein
ESR	erythrocyte sedimentation rate
FBS	fasting blood sugar
FFA	free fatty acids
FSH	follicle-stimulating hormone (follitropin)
FT_4	free thyroxine
FT_4I	free thyroxine index
GFR	glomerular filtration rate
GH	growth hormone
GHRH	growth hormone–releasing hormone
GnRH	gonadotropin-releasing hormone
GTT	glucose tolerance test
HA	hemagglutination
HAI	hemagglutination inhibition test
HAV	hepatitis A virus
Hb; Hgb	hemoglobin
HbCO	carboxyhemoglobin
HBV	hepatitis B virus
HCG; hCG	human chorionic gonadotropin
Hct	hematocrit
HCV	hepatitis C virus
HDL	high-density lipoprotein
HDV	hepatitis delta virus
HGH; hGH	human growth hormone
HIV	human immunodeficiency virus
HLA	human leukocyte antigen
HPV	human papilloma virus
HSV	herpes simplex virus
HTLV	human T-cell lymphotrophic virus
Ig	immunoglobulin
IgE	immunoglobulin E
INH	inhibitor

continued ⟶

Figure 30-3. These abbreviations are routinely used in blood tests.

Source: Adapted from Norbert W. Tietz, ed., *Clinical Guide to Laboratory Tests,* 3d ed. (Philadelphia: W. B. Saunders, 1995).

Common Abbreviations Used in Blood Tests (continued)

IV	intravenous	PV	plasma volume
L	liver	PZP	pregnancy zone protein
LD; LDH	lactate dehydrogenase	RAIU	thyroid uptake of radioactive iodine
LDL	low-density lipoprotein	RBC	red blood cell; red blood (cell) count
LH	luteinizing hormone	RBP	retinol-binding protein
LMWH	low-molecular-weight heparin	RCM	red cell mass
Lytes	electrolytes	RCV	red cell volume
MCV	mean cell volume	RDW	red cell distribution of width
MetHb	methemoglobin	Retic	reticulocyte
MLC	mixed lymphocyte culture	RF	rheumatoid factor; relative fluorescence unit
MONO	monocyte	Rh	rhesus factor
MPV	mean platelet volume	RIA	radioimmunoassay
MSAFP	maternal serum alpha-fetoprotein	rT_3	reverse triiodothyronine
NE	norepinephrine	S	serum
NPN	nonprotein nitrogen	Segs	segmented polymorphonuclear leukocyte
OGTT	oral glucose tolerance test	SPE	serum protein electrophoresis
P	plasma	T_3	triiodothyronine
PAP	prostatic acid phosphatase	T_4	thyroxine
PB	protein binding	TBG	thyroxine-binding globulin
PBG	porphobilinogen	TBV	total blood volume
PCT	prothrombin consumption time	TG	triglyceride
PCV	packed cell volume (hematocrit)	TRH	thyrotropin-releasing hormone
P_i	inorganic phosphate	TSH	thyroid-stimulating hormone
PKU	phenylketonuria	VDRL	Venereal Disease Research Laboratory (test for syphilis)
PLT	platelet	VLDL	very-low-density lipoprotein
PMN	polymorphonuclear (leukocyte; neutrophil)	WB	Western blot
PRL	prolactin	WBC	white blood cell; white blood (cell) count
PSA	prostate-specific antigen		
PT	prothrombin time		
PTH	parathyroid hormone		
PTT	partial thromboplastin time		

Figure 30-3. (continued)

save patients unnecessary discomfort by contributing to a quick, efficient procedure.

Greeting and Identifying Patients. Greet patients pleasantly, introduce yourself, and explain that you will be drawing some blood. It is essential to identify patients correctly before you begin the procedure. Ask patients to state their full name, and be sure you hear both the first and last names correctly. Verify that the name the patient gives is the name on the order. (In some facilities, the phlebotomist may ask for a Social Security number or a patient ID or chart number to further identify the patient.)

Confirming Pretest Preparation. The presence and level of certain substances in blood are affected by food and fluid intake or by other activities in daily life. Some tests require that the patient follow certain pretest restrictions. The purpose behind these restrictions is either to minimize the influence of the restricted food on the blood or to stress the body to see how it responds, as indicated by the blood.

One test that requires patients to follow pretest instructions closely is the glucose tolerance test, which measures a patient's ability to metabolize carbohydrates. This test is used to detect hypoglycemia and diabetes mellitus. You instruct the patient to eat a diet high in carbohydrates for the 3 days before the test and to fast for the 8 to 12 hours before the appointment. After initial blood and urine samples are taken, the patient ingests a measured dose of glucose solution. Blood and urine samples are then taken at prescribed intervals as ordered by the physician.

The glucose levels in the samples are often graphed for the physician's review.

Before you draw blood for any test, determine whether the patient has complied with pretest instructions. If the patient has not followed pretest instructions, explain that the test cannot be performed. Make a note on the order, and report the information to the physician or your supervisor.

Explaining the Procedure and Safety Precautions. Explain to the patient the procedure you will use to obtain the blood specimen for testing. Be clear and brief when you describe what you will do; too much detail leaves some patients queasy. You must follow Universal Precautions during all phlebotomy procedures, as described in the Caution: Handle With Care section. These precautions may be second nature to you, but they may raise concerns in the patient. Explain the need for each of the preventive measures you are taking in language the patient can understand. Assure the patient that these measures protect against exposure to infection.

Establishing a Chain of Custody. You will need to follow specific guidelines to establish a chain of custody for blood samples drawn for drug and alcohol analysis. (Chapter 26 explains general chain of custody procedures.) Because donating a specimen for drug and alcohol testing is potentially self-incriminating, the patient must sign a consent form for the testing. (This form is discussed in Chapter 29.) Although the clerical procedures for blood tests for drug and alcohol analysis are similar to those for urine tests, blood tests differ because you can confirm by direct observation that a blood specimen has been taken from the patient in question.

Handling an Exposure Incident. When you adhere to Universal Precautions, the risk of exposure to blood-borne pathogens is very small. Accidents can occur, however. If you suffer a needlestick or other injury that results in exposure to blood or blood products from another person, you must report the incident to the appropriate staff members immediately. Wash the injured area carefully and apply a sterile bandage. Record the time and date of the incident, the names of the people involved, and the nature of the exposure. Depending on the situation, you may receive medications. You and the other person involved will be asked to undergo blood testing and be

CAUTION ***Handle With Care***

Phlebotomy and Personal Protective Equipment

The Centers for Disease Control and Prevention (CDC) has classified all phlebotomy procedures as a risk for exposure to contaminated blood or blood products. You must use appropriate protective equipment during all phlebotomy procedures. Remember, it is up to you to protect yourself and the patient.

Gloves

Gloves are the first line of defense during a phlebotomy procedure. They protect against spills and splashing of contaminated blood. Wash your hands and put on clean examination gloves that fit snugly before you work with each patient. Remove the gloves, dispose of them in a biohazardous waste container, and wash your hands after working with each patient.

Garments

Garments such as laboratory coats and aprons can protect your clothing from spills and splashes and provide a measure of protection from contaminated materials. Some garments are designed to resist penetration by blood or blood products. You may find it necessary to wear such garments when drawing blood or performing blood tests.

Masks and Protective Eyewear

Mucous membranes are especially vulnerable to invasion by infectious agents. Use masks and protective eyewear to help safeguard mucous membranes in your mouth, nose, and eyes from infection.

Masks help protect your mouth and nose from splashes or sprays of blood or blood products. You cannot predict when exposure to blood may occur. Accidental puncture of an artery during a phlebotomy procedure could result in a spray of blood. Blood may also spray or splash accidentally during some testing protocols. Most medical assistants do not routinely wear masks for phlebotomy procedures, however, once they have achieved proficiency in performing them.

Goggles can protect your eyes from splashing and spraying during blood drawing or testing. Health-care workers in dental offices often wear goggles because patient treatments can easily expose workers to contaminated blood or bloody saliva.

Clear plastic face shields combine the protection of masks and goggles. They are often used during major surgical procedures. You may use a face shield if you do extensive testing on blood specimens. Face shields are not usually worn when drawing blood.

Personal protective equipment works two ways: it protects you from a patient's contaminated blood, and it also protects the patient from infectious agents you may be carrying. By using PPE correctly, you will make your workplace a safer place for you and the patients.

PROCEDURE 30.1

Quality Control Procedures for Blood Specimen Collection

Objective: To follow proper quality control procedures when taking a blood specimen

Materials: Necessary sterile equipment, specimen-collection container, paperwork related to the type of blood test the specimen is being drawn for, requisition form, marker, proper packing materials for transport

Method

1. Review the request form for the test ordered, verify the procedure, prepare the necessary equipment and paperwork, and prepare the work area.
2. Identify the patient and explain the procedure. Confirm the patient's identification. Ask the patient to spell her name. Make sure the patient understands the procedure that is to be performed, even if she has had it done before.
3. Confirm that the patient has followed any pretest preparation requirements such as fasting, taking any necessary medication, or stopping a medication. For example, if a fasting specimen is being taken, the patient should not have eaten anything after midnight of the day before. Some doctors' offices will let the patient drink water or black coffee, however. It often depends on the type of specimen being taken.
4. Collect the specimen properly. Collect it at the right time intervals if that applies. Use sterile equipment and proper technique.
5. Use the correct specimen-collection containers and the right preservatives, if required. For example, blood collected into a test tube with additives should be mixed immediately, or it will clot.
6. Immediately label the specimens. The label should include the patient's name, the date and time of collection, the test's name, and the name of the person collecting the specimen. Do not label the containers before collecting the specimen.
7. Follow correct procedures for disposing of hazardous specimen waste and decontaminating the work area. Used needles, for instance, should immediately be placed in a biohazard sharps container.
8. Thank the patient. Keep the patient in the office if any follow-up observation is necessary.
9. If the specimen is to be transported to an outside laboratory, prepare it for transport in the proper container for that type of specimen, according to OSHA regulations. Place the container in a clear plastic bag with a zip closure and dual pockets with the international biohazard label imprinted in red or orange. The requisition form should be placed in the outside pocket of the bag. This ensures protection from contamination if the specimen leaks. Have a courier pick up the specimen and place it in an appropriate carrier (such as an insulated cooler) with the biohazard label. Place specimens to be sent by mail in appropriate plastic containers, and then place the containers inside a heavy-duty plastic container with a screw-down, nonleaking lid. Then place this container in either a heavy-duty cardboard box or nylon bag. The words *Human Specimen* or *Body Fluids* should be imprinted on the box or bag. Seal with a strong tape strip.

involved in follow-up studies. The Occupational Safety and Health Administration (OSHA) requires every employer to have an established procedure for handling exposure incidents.

Drawing Blood

Some, but not all, states permit medical assistants to obtain blood samples. Your office will clarify which duties, if any, you may perform related to phlebotomy procedures. If your duties include collecting blood samples, you will obtain them either through venipuncture or capillary puncture. You must understand when these techniques are used and know how to perform them. Procedure 30-1 details quality control procedures for collecting blood specimens.

Venipuncture. Venipuncture requires puncturing a vein with a needle and collecting blood into either a tube or a syringe. The most common sites for venipuncture are the median cubital and cephalic veins of the forearm, although other sites may be used if the primary site is unacceptable. Figure 30-4 shows the veins in the antecubital fossa (the small depression inside the bend of the elbow) and the forearm that are used for venipuncture.

Various instruments are used to perform venipuncture. Practice using the devices so that your technique is smooth, steady, and competent.

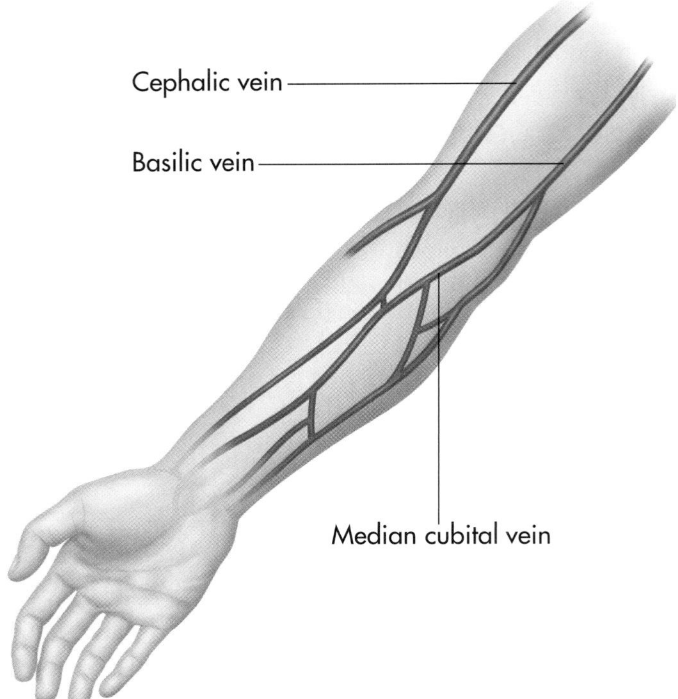

Figure 30-4. Veins commonly used for venipuncture include the cephalic vein, the basilic vein, and the median cubital vein.

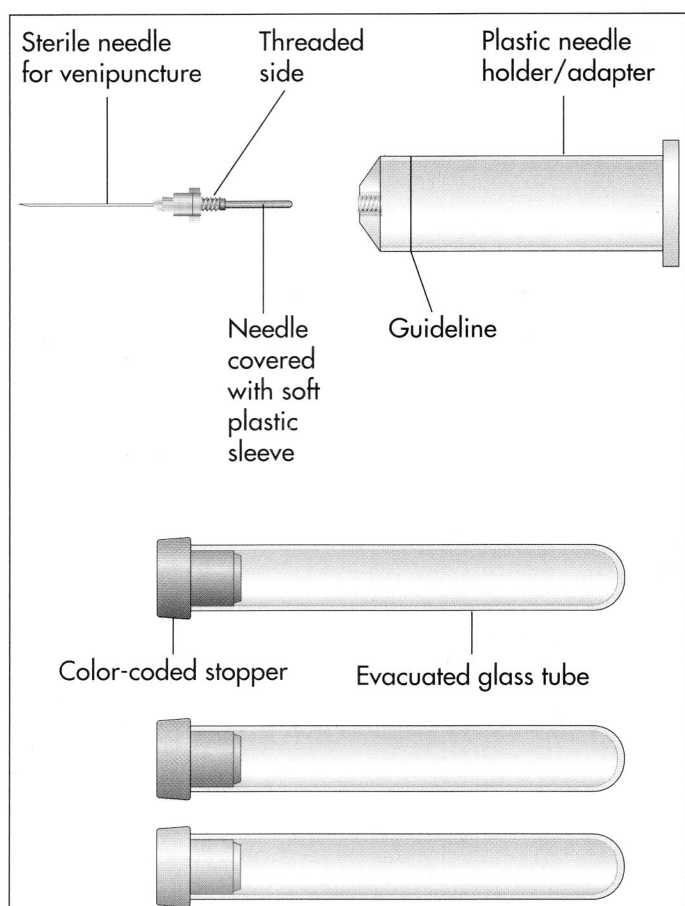

Figure 30-5. The VACUTAINER system uses interchangeable collection tubes that allow you to draw several blood specimens from the same venipuncture site.

Evacuation Systems. Evacuation systems, the most common of which is the VACUTAINER system (manufactured by Becton Dickinson VACUTAINER Systems, Franklin Lakes, New Jersey), use a special double-pointed needle, a plastic needle holder/adapter, and collection tubes (Figure 30-5). The collection tubes are sealed to create a slight vacuum. You insert the covered inner point of the needle into one end of the holder/adapter and the first collection tube into the other end. Remove the plastic cap from the outer needle of the assembled system. Hold the needle at a 15° angle to the patient's arm, and puncture the patient's vein with the needle. Then press the collection tube fully onto the covered needle tip, piercing the stopper and allowing the vacuum to help draw blood into the collection tube. Procedure 30-2 explains how to use an evacuation system to draw a blood sample.

An evacuation system has several advantages over other methods of blood collection. It is easy to collect several samples from one venipuncture site using the interchangeable vacuum collection tubes. Tubes are calibrated by evacuation to collect the exact amount of blood required. Some collection tubes are prepared with additives needed to correctly process the blood sample for testing, such as anticoagulants. Finally, because there is no need to transfer blood from a collection syringe to a sample tube, the potential for exposure to contaminated blood is reduced.

Needle and Syringe Systems. An evacuation system is not the best choice for drawing blood in every case. For example, if the patient has small or fragile veins, the vacuum created when the collection tube is pressed over the needle point can cause the veins to collapse. You may collect blood using a sterile needle and syringe assembly when an evacuation system is not suitable, such as when the patient is difficult to stick. You can use a smaller needle and control the vacuum in the syringe by pulling the plunger back slowly. Other aspects of the procedure are essentially the same, except that the blood sample is collected in the syringe and must immediately be transferred to a collection tube.

Butterfly Systems. You may also use a butterfly system, or winged infusion set, when you work with patients who have small or fragile veins. Flexible wings attached to the needle simplify needle insertion. A length of flexible tubing (either 5 or 12 inches, approximately) connects the needle to the collection device. The inserted needle remains completely undisturbed while the collection device is manipulated. Because it is motionless, the needle causes less trauma to the vein and surrounding tissue than do other systems for venipuncture. A butterfly system generally uses a smaller needle (23 gauge) than other venipuncture

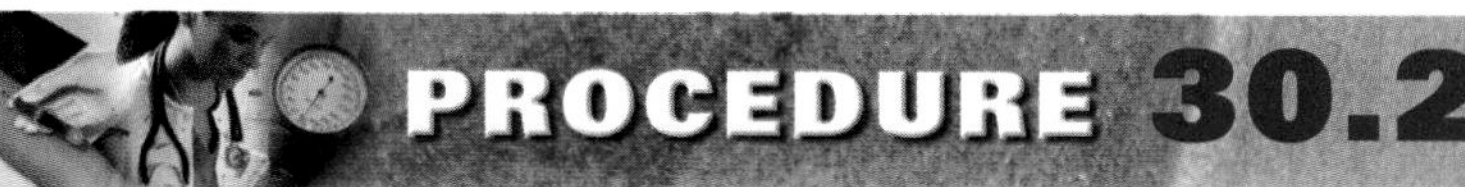

Performing Venipuncture Using an Evacuation System

Objective: To collect a venous blood sample using an evacuation system

OSHA Guidelines

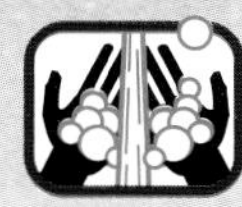
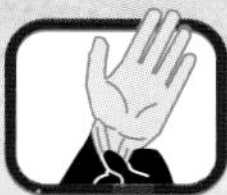
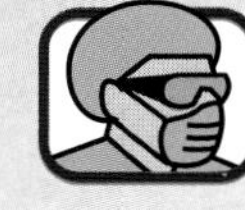
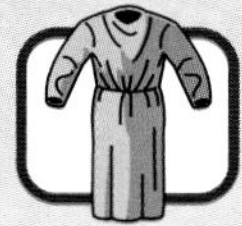
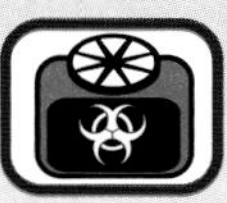

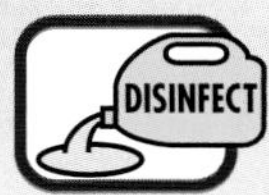

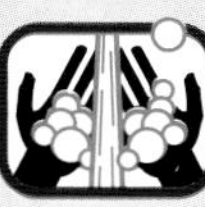

Materials: VACUTAINER components (needle, needle holder/adapter, collection tubes), antiseptic and cotton balls or antiseptic wipes, tourniquet, sterile gauze squares, sterile adhesive bandages

Method

1. Review the laboratory request form, and make sure you have the necessary supplies.
2. Greet the patient, confirm the patient's identity, and introduce yourself.
3. Explain the purpose of the procedure, and confirm that the patient has followed the physician's special instructions.
4. Make sure the patient is sitting in a venipuncture chair or is lying down.
5. Wash your hands. Put on examination gloves.
6. Prepare the needle holder/adapter assembly by inserting the threaded side of the needle into the adapter and twisting the adapter in a clockwise direction. Push the first collection tube into the other end of the needle holder/adapter until the outer edge of the collection tube stopper meets the guideline.
7. Ask the patient whether one arm is better than the other for the venipuncture. The chosen arm should be positioned slightly downward (Figure 30-6).
8. Apply the tourniquet to the patient's upper arm midway between the elbow and the shoulder. Wrap the tourniquet around the patient's arm and cross the ends. Holding one end of the tourniquet against the patient's arm, stretch the other end to apply pressure against the patient's skin. Pull a loop of the stretched end under the end held tightly against the patient's skin, as shown in Figure 30-7. The tourniquet should be tight enough to cause the veins to stand out but should not stop the flow of blood. You should still be able to feel the patient's radial pulse. Ask the patient to make a fist and release it several times to make the veins in the forearm stand out more prominently.
9. Palpate the proposed site, and use your index finger to locate the vein, as shown in Figure 30-8. The vein will feel like a small tube with some

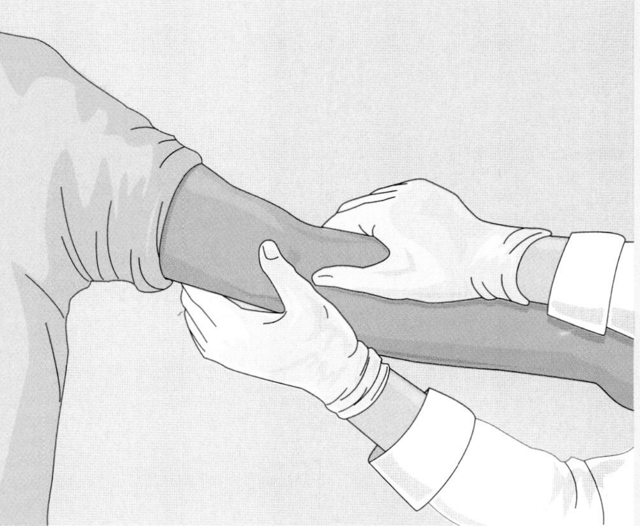

Figure 30-6. The patient's arm should be positioned slightly downward for a venipuncture.

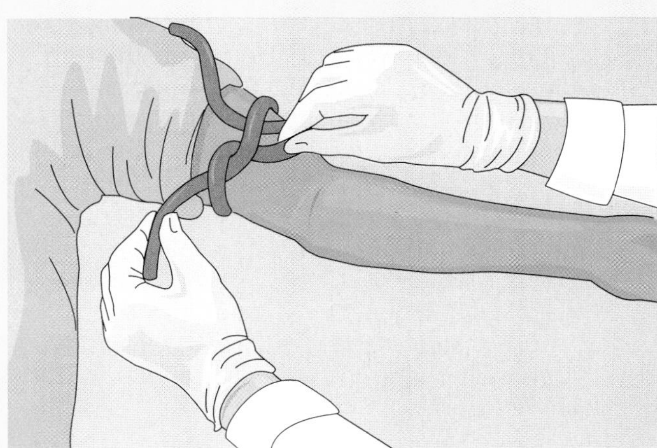

Figure 30-7. Applying a tourniquet makes it easier to find a patient's vein when you are drawing blood.

continued ⟶

PROCEDURE 30.2

Performing Venipuncture Using an Evacuation System *(continued)*

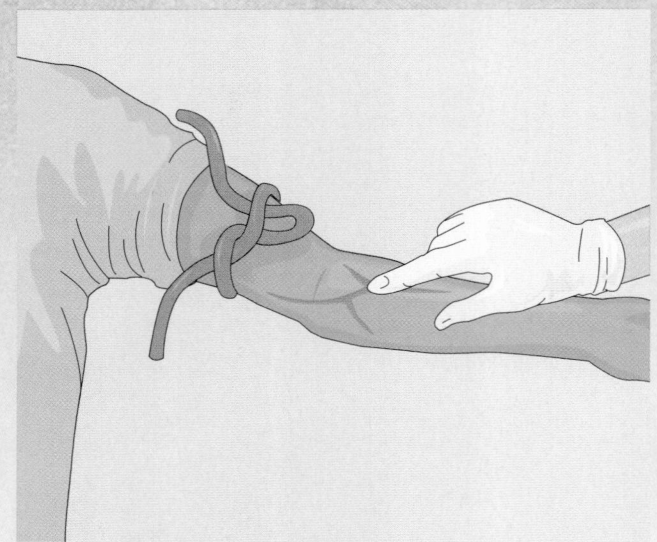

Figure 30-8. Use your index finger to locate the vein.

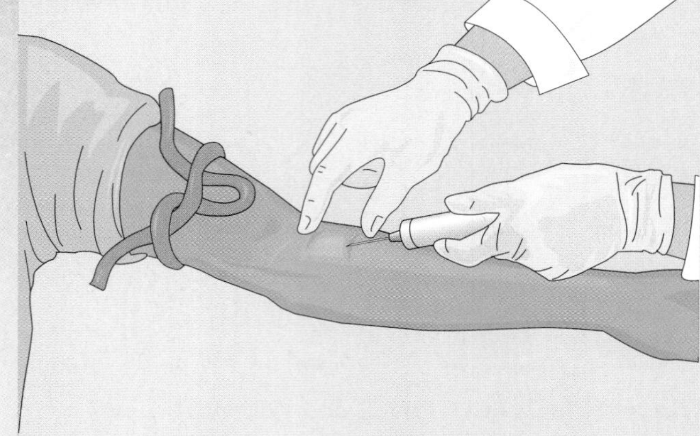

Figure 30-9. When performing venipuncture, hold the needle at a 15° angle.

elasticity. If you feel a pulsing beat, you have located an artery. If you cannot locate the vein within 1 minute, release the tourniquet and allow blood to flow freely for 1 to 2 minutes. Then reapply the tourniquet and try again to locate the vein.

10. After locating the vein, clean the area with a cotton ball moistened with antiseptic or an antiseptic wipe. Use a circular motion to clean the area, starting at the center and working outward. Allow the site to air-dry, or use the same circular motion to wipe the area dry with a sterile gauze square.
11. Remove the plastic cap from the outer point of the needle cover, and ask the patient to tighten the fist. Hold the patient's skin taut above and below the insertion site. With a steady and quick motion, insert the needle—held at a 15° angle, bevel side up, and aligned parallel to the vein—into the vein (Figure 30-9). You will feel a slight resistance as the needle tip penetrates the vein wall. Penetrate to a depth of ¼ to ½ inch. Grasp the holder/adapter between your index and great (middle) fingers. Using your thumb, seat the collection tube firmly into place over the needle point, puncturing the rubber stopper. Blood will begin to flow into the collection tube.
12. Fill each tube until the blood stops running to ensure the correct proportion of blood to additives. Switch tubes as needed by pulling one tube out of the adapter and inserting the next in a smooth and steady motion. (The soft plastic cover on the inner point of the needle retracts as each tube is inserted and recovers the needle point as each tube is removed.)
13. Once blood is flowing steadily, ask the patient to release the fist, and untie the tourniquet by pulling the end of the tucked-in loop. The tourniquet should, in general, be left on no longer than 1 minute. (Longer periods may cause hemoconcentration, an increase in the blood-cell-to-plasma ratio, and invalidate test results.) You must remove the tourniquet before you withdraw the needle from the vein. (Removing the tourniquet releases pressure on the vein.)
14. As you withdraw the needle in a smooth and steady motion, place a sterile gauze square over the insertion site (Figure 30-10). Dispose of the needle immediately. Instruct the patient to hold the gauze pad in place with slight pressure. The patient should keep the arm straight and slightly elevated for several minutes.
15. If the collection tubes contain additives, you will need to invert them slowly several times to mix the chemical agent and the blood sample.
16. Label specimens and complete the paperwork.

continued ⟶

PROCEDURE 30.2

Performing Venipuncture Using an Evacuation System *(continued)*

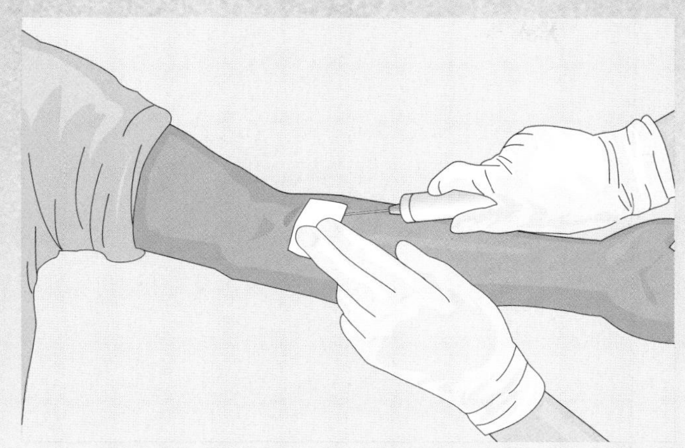

Figure 30-10. Place a sterile gauze square over the insertion site as you withdraw the needle.

17. Check the patient's condition and the puncture site for bleeding. Replace the sterile gauze square with a sterile adhesive bandage.
18. Properly dispose of used supplies and disposable instruments, and disinfect the work area.
19. Remove the gloves and wash your hands.
20. Instruct the patient about care of the puncture site.
21. Document the procedure in the patient's chart.

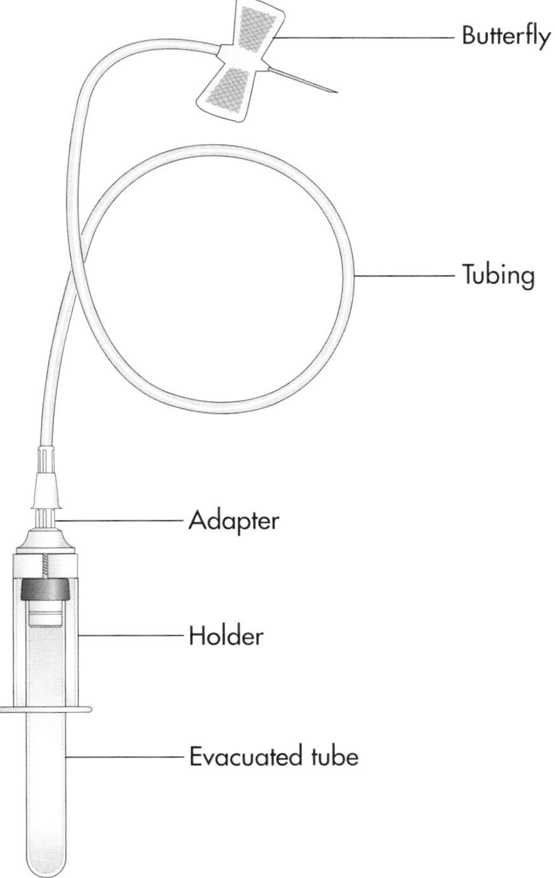

Figure 30-11. Once inserted, the needle of a butterfly system remains undisturbed during specimen collection.

techniques do. A butterfly system can be used with an evacuated collection tube or a syringe (Figure 30-11).

Collection Tubes. No matter which method is used to collect blood, the samples must immediately be mixed with the appropriate additives in the correct collection tubes before they are transported to the laboratory for testing. The stoppers of the tubes are different colors, each color identifying the type of additives (if any) they contain (Figure 30-12).

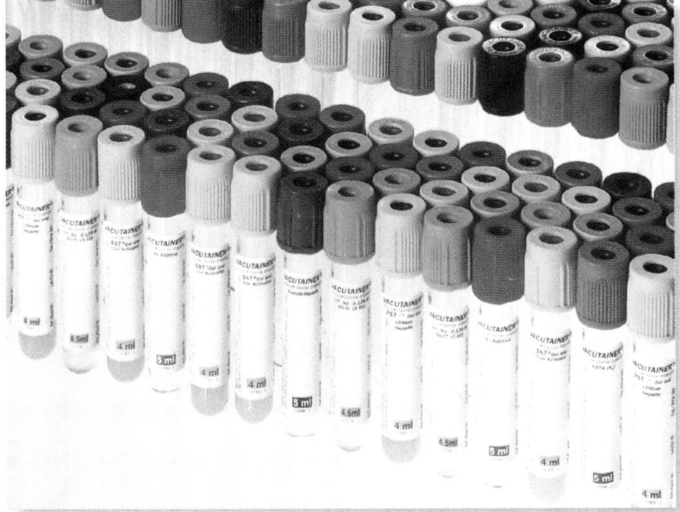

Figure 30-12. Special color-coded stoppers on collection tubes indicate which additives are present and, therefore, which types of laboratory tests may be performed on each blood specimen.

TABLE 30-1 Blood-Collection Tubes

Stopper Color	Additive	Test Types
Yellow	Sodium polyanetholesulfonate	Blood cultures
Red	None	Blood chemistries, AIDS antibody, viral studies, serologic tests, blood grouping and typing
Red/black (tiger stripes)	Silicone serum separator	Tests requiring blood serum
Blue	Sodium citrate (anticoagulant)	Coagulation studies
Green	Sodium heparin (anticoagulant)	Electrolyte studies, arterial blood gases
Lavender	Ethylenediaminetetraacetic acid (EDTA) (anticoagulant)	Hematology studies
Gray	Potassium oxalate or sodium fluoride (anticoagulant)	Blood glucose

These additives must be compatible with the laboratory process that the sample will undergo. Each laboratory may choose which tubes to use for a particular test.

Additives include anticoagulants and other materials that help preserve or process a sample for particular types of testing. When you collect a blood sample, double-check that you are using the appropriate collection tubes for the tests ordered. You must also fill the tubes in a specific order to preserve the integrity of the blood sample. Each laboratory requires a specific order of draw for collection tubes. The National Committee for Clinical Laboratory Standards also publishes its recommended order of draw. Table 30-1, identifies collection tube stopper colors, additives present in the tubes, and types of tests, in a typical order of draw.

Engineered Safety Devices. In response to the Needlestick Safety and Prevention Act, a number of engineered safety devices have been developed. These devices are intended to reduce the possibility of needlestick injuries (Figure 30-13). According to the National Institute for Occupational Safety and Health (NIOSH), the desired characteristics of engineered safety devices include the following:

- The performance of the device is reliable
- The device is easy to use, safe, and effective
- The device should be needleless when possible
- The device should either not have to be activated by the user or may be activated using only one hand
- Once the safety feature is activated, it cannot be deactivated

Procedure 30-1 details quality control procedures for collecting blood specimens.

In certain circumstances, some of these characteristics are not feasible. Drawing blood from an artery or a vein is not possible without the use of a needle. Several types of safety devices for collecting blood specimens have been developed. These include:

- Retracting needles
- Hinged or sliding shields that cover phlebotomy and winged-steel (butterfly) needles

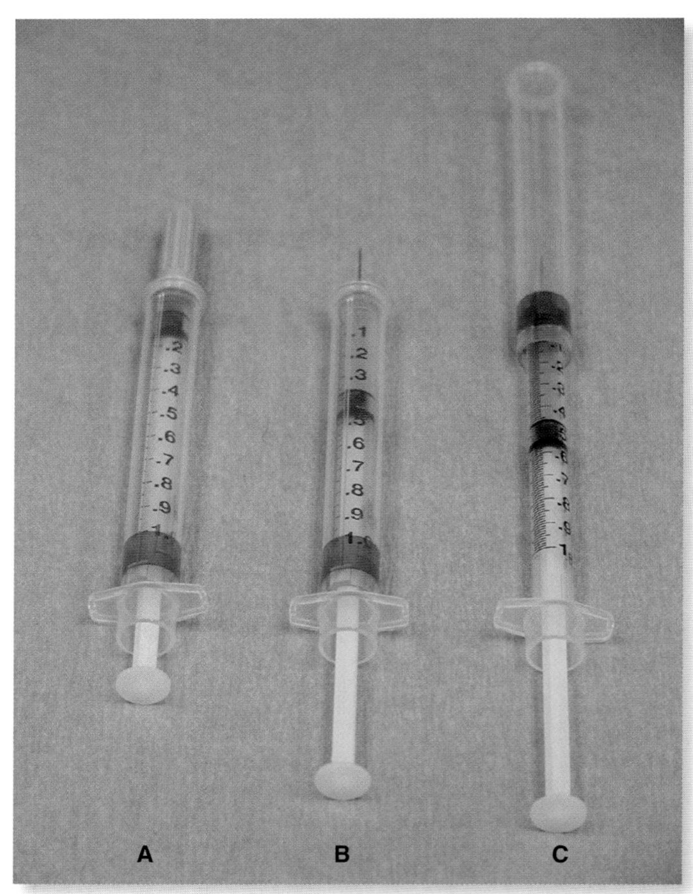

Figure 30-13. Tuberculin syringe with safety shield: (a) syringe before use, (b) syringe during injection, and (c) safety shield engaged after injection.
Photo courtesy of Total Care Programming.

- Self-blunting phlebotomy and winged-steel needles
- Retractable lancets

Studies show that these devices, when used properly, have reduced needlestick injuries. NIOSH reports a 76% reduction of injuries with self-blunting needles, a 66% reduction with hinged needle shields, and a 23% reduction with sliding shields.

In addition to advocating the use of appropriate engineered safety devices, NIOSH also recommends that healthcare workers follow these precautions:

- Recap needles only when absolutely necessary
- Ensure the safe handling and disposal of sharps prior to beginning a procedure
- Dispose of used sharps promptly using approved sharps containers
- Report all needlestick injuries
- Inform their employer of workplace hazards
- Attend yearly blood-borne pathogen training
- Follow recommended infection control practices

Capillary Puncture. **Capillary puncture** requires a superficial puncture of the skin with a sharp point. Compared with venipuncture, capillary puncture releases a smaller amount of blood. The blood may be collected in small, calibrated glass tubes. It may also be collected on glass microscope slides or applied to reagent strips (or dipsticks), which are specially treated paper or plastic strips used in specific diagnostic tests.

Capillary puncture in adults and children is usually performed on the great (middle) finger or the ring finger. (Use the patient's nondominant hand for this procedure if possible.) The puncture should be made slightly off center on the pad of the fingertip. Capillary puncture in infants is usually performed on one of the outer edges of the underside of the heel. An alternate site for both children and adults is the lower part of the earlobe, unless the patient's ear is pierced.

Lancets. Lancets are used in the capillary puncture technique. This technique is employed when the amount of blood required for a specific procedure is not very large or when technical difficulties prevent use of the venipuncture technique. A **lancet** is a small, disposable instrument with a sharp point used to puncture the skin and make a shallow incision (between 2.0 and 3.0 mm deep for an adult and no deeper than 2.4 mm for an infant). The blood welling up from the incision is then collected.

Automatic Puncturing Devices. Automatic puncturing devices are loaded with a lancet. Because the depth to which they puncture the skin is mechanically controlled, they are more accurate than the traditional lancet method. These spring-loaded devices have disposable platforms that rest on the finger. Different platforms are used, depending on the desired depth of the puncture. Both the lancet and the platform should be discarded after use. Some companies also manufacture completely disposable devices, which come individually wrapped and are used only once.

Micropipettes. A pipette is a calibrated glass tube for measuring fluids. A **micropipette** is a small pipette that holds a small, precise volume of fluid. You will use micropipettes to collect capillary blood for some tests. Capillary tubes, with a single calibration mark, are also used to collect capillary blood for certain tests. Procedure 30-3 explains how to perform a capillary puncture and collect a sample of capillary blood.

PROCEDURE 30.3

Performing Capillary Puncture

Objective: To collect a capillary blood sample using the finger puncture method

OSHA Guidelines

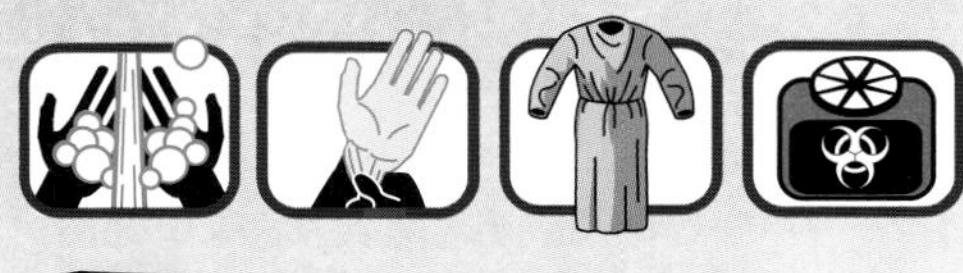

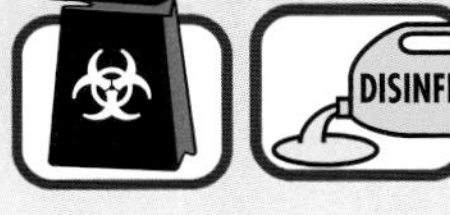

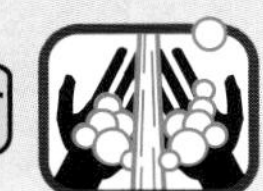

Materials: Capillary puncture device (lancet or automatic puncture device such as Autolet or Glucolet), antiseptic and cotton balls or antiseptic wipes, sterile gauze squares, sterile adhesive bandages, reagent strips, micropipettes, smear slides

Method

1. Review the laboratory request form, and make sure you have the necessary supplies.
2. Greet the patient, confirm the patient's identity, and introduce yourself.
3. Explain the purpose of the procedure, and confirm that the patient has followed the doctor's special instructions.
4. Make sure the patient is sitting in the venipuncture chair or is lying down.
5. Wash your hands. Put on examination gloves.

continued ⟶

PROCEDURE 30.3

Performing Capillary Puncture *(continued)*

6. Examine the patient's hands to determine which finger to use for the procedure. Avoid fingers that are swollen, bruised, scarred, or calloused. Generally, the ring and great (middle) fingers are the best choices. If you notice that the patient's hands are cold, you may want to warm them between your own, have the patient put them in a warm basin of water or under warm running water, or wrap them in a warm cloth. Warming the patient's hands improves circulation.
7. Prepare the patient's finger with a gentle "milking" or rubbing motion toward the fingertip. Keep the patient's hand below heart level so that gravity helps the blood flow.
8. Clean the area with a cotton ball moistened with antiseptic or an antiseptic wipe. Allow the site to air-dry, or wipe the area dry with a sterile gauze square.
9. Hold the patient's finger between your thumb and forefinger. Hold the lancet or automatic puncture device at a right angle to the patient's fingerprint, as shown in Figure 30-14. Puncture the skin on the pad of the fingertip with a quick, sharp motion. The depth to which you puncture the skin is generally determined by the length of the lancet point. Most automatic puncturing devices are designed to penetrate to the correct depth.

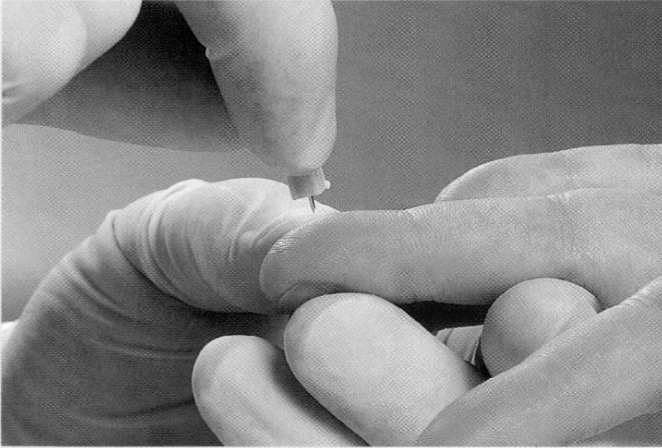

Figure 30-14. Hold the lancet or automatic puncture device at a right angle to the patient's fingerprint.

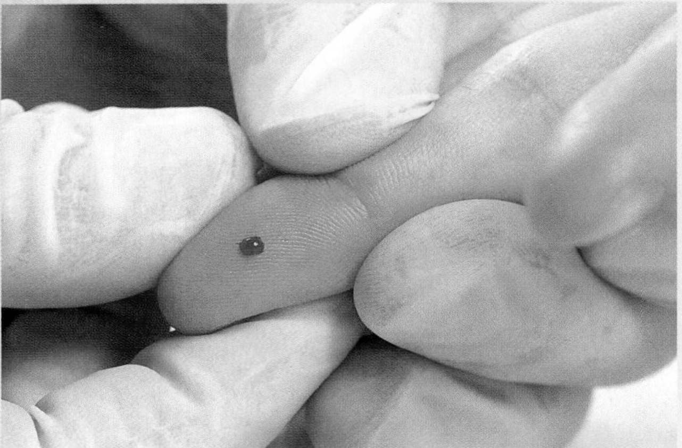

Figure 30-15. Apply steady pressure to the patient's finger, but do not milk it.

10. Allow a drop of blood to form at the end of the patient's finger. If the blood droplet is slow in forming, apply steady pressure (Figure 30-15). Avoid milking the patient's finger, because it dilutes the blood sample with tissue fluid and causes hemolysis.
11. Wipe away the first droplet of blood. (This droplet is usually contaminated with tissue fluids released when the skin is punctured.) Then fill the collection devices, as described.

    Micropipettes: Hold the tip of the tube just to the edge of the blood droplet. The tube will fill through capillary action. If you are preparing microhematocrit tubes, you need to seal one end of each tube with clay sealant. (See Procedure 30-5 for this process.)

    Reagent strips: With some reagent strips (dipsticks), you must touch the strip to the blood drop but not smear it; with other strips, you must smear it. Follow the manufacturer's guidelines.

    Smear slides: Gently touch the blood droplet to the smear slide and process the slide as described in Procedure 30-4.
12. After you have collected the required samples, dispose of the lancet immediately. Then wipe the patient's finger with a sterile gauze square (Figure 30-16). Instruct the patient to apply pressure to stop the bleeding.

continued ⟶

PROCEDURE 30.3

Performing Capillary Puncture *(continued)*

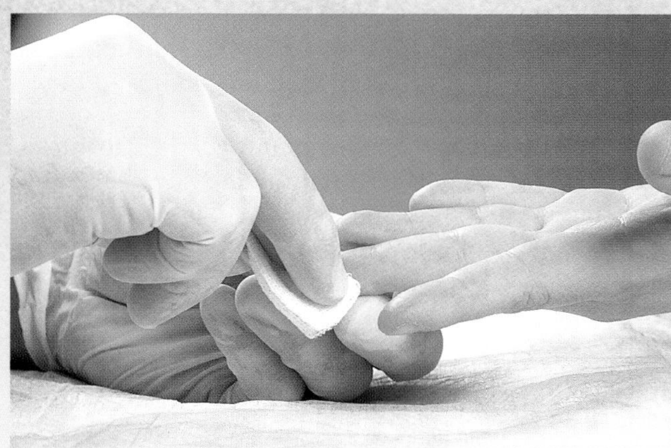

Figure 30-16. Use a sterile gauze square to wipe remaining blood from the patient's finger.

13. Label specimens and complete the paperwork. Some tests, such as glucose monitoring, must be completed immediately.
14. Check the puncture site for bleeding. If necessary, replace the sterile gauze square with a sterile adhesive bandage.
15. Properly dispose of used supplies and disposable instruments, and disinfect the work area.
16. Remove the gloves and wash your hands.
17. Instruct the patient about care of the puncture site.
18. Document the procedure in the patient's chart. (If the test has been completed, include the results.)

MICROTAINER Tubes. MICROTAINER tubes (manufactured by Becton Dickinson VACUTAINER Systems) are small plastic tubes that have a widemouthed collector, similar to a funnel, which allows blood to flow quickly and freely into the tube. Like collection tubes in an evacuation system, MICROTAINER tubes have different colored tops indicating which, if any, additives they contain.

Reagent Products. Several common tests do not require processing of fluid blood samples. For these tests, you may apply droplets of freshly collected blood to chemically treated paper or plastic reagent strips (dipsticks) or add freshly collected blood droplets to small containers holding chemicals that react in the presence of specific substances or microorganisms. Some of the blood tests performed in this way are those for determining blood glucose levels, sickle cell anemia, infectious mononucleosis, and rheumatoid arthritis.

Smear Slides. You may need to apply a drop of freshly collected blood to a prepared microscope slide for some tests. More commonly, a smear slide is prepared in the laboratory from a blood sample containing an anticoagulant, for examination under a microscope.

Responding to Patient Needs

Many patients are anxious when they have a blood test, and some patients have special needs or present special problems that make drawing blood challenging. Anxiety about blood tests may stem from a variety of concerns. Special needs may be related to a patient's age group or a medical condition. Some problems involve difficulty obtaining a blood sample or the patient's physiological or emotional response to a procedure. Being aware of possible sources of patient anxiety and understanding a wide range of special concerns can help you respond to patient needs with sensitivity and competence.

Patient Fears and Concerns

Some patients express their fears or concerns directly. Other patients ask questions that highlight their fears. Providing more information or a complete understanding is reassuring to many patients. For others, the information serves only to confuse, overwhelm, or create more fear. You must decide how much information to give each patient and be prepared to answer questions.

Patients sometimes ask questions that are not appropriate for you to answer. A patient may ask you about his prognosis, medical condition, blood type, or other medical information. It is not appropriate for you to discuss these topics with the patient. Tell the patient that only the physician can answer such questions. There are some commonly expressed fears and concerns to which you should respond, however.

Pain. The question that medical assistants performing phlebotomy probably hear most often is, Will this hurt? Never lie to a patient who asks this question. Inform the patient that he will feel a stick just as the lancet or point of the needle is inserted but that this pain goes away almost immediately. Tell a patient who seems particularly nervous to take a deep breath and let it out slowly. Also suggest that the patient focus on something else in the room or close his eyes and relax during the procedure.

A patient may express concern and report a previous unpleasant experience with blood testing. Listen to the patient's concerns. Describe what you will do to reduce discomfort and what the patient can do to be more at ease. Let the patient know that you will help him sit comfortably or lie down while the blood sample is being obtained. Tell the patient to let you know if he begins to feel lightheaded. You might also ask the patient whether one arm is better to use than the other. Many patients have had blood drawn before and can tell you which sites were successful. Consulting the patient helps the patient feel more in control and provides you with important information.

Bruises or Scars. Some patients may express fear of getting a bruise or scar from a blood test. Explain that some bruising is possible but that it will fade within a few days. Most bruising is caused by a hematoma, which occurs when blood leaks out of the vein and collects under the skin. Hematomas can be prevented by releasing the tourniquet before withdrawing the needle and applying proper pressure over the puncture site after the needle has been withdrawn. Bruising is common with fair-skinned patients. Scars, on the other hand, are unlikely.

Serious Diagnosis. Patient fears are not always rational. One fear that patients express is that the more tubes of blood you require, the more serious their condition must be. Patients may also fear that a blood test is being done to help the doctor diagnose an extremely serious disease.

You can help relieve a patient's fears by explaining that a blood test is one of the best ways to obtain an overall picture of health (emphasize health, not disease). Note that blood tests show what is normal about the blood as well as any abnormalities. You might also explain that several samples are being taken because the blood used in blood tests is processed in different ways; the blood collected for one test cannot be used in another.

Blood testing may also be done to determine how well and at what levels medications are acting in the blood. Explain that the doctor may want to see how much medication is in the blood to better manage the prescribed dosage. When a patient needs repeated tests for drug levels, explain that the tests show how the body is using the medication.

Contracting a Disease From the Procedure. Probably the greatest fear of patients undergoing blood tests is contracting HIV, AIDS, or hepatitis B virus (HBV). Although many people are now well informed about how AIDS and other serious diseases are contracted, it is understandable for a patient to worry about blood-borne pathogens. Do not dismiss the patient's concerns, and do not downplay the importance of following Universal Precautions.

Explain the precautions you will take to prevent the spread of infection. Allow the patient to see you wash your hands and put on new gloves before you begin to take the blood sample. Stress that the needle is sterile. Explain that you have not touched the needle and that it will be discarded when you finish. Let the patient see you put the needle in the sharps container.

Use this opportunity to educate the patient about the transmission of AIDS. Emphasize that AIDS, and other infections transmitted by blood, can be transmitted only when there is direct contact with contaminated blood or other body fluids. Explain that your gloves protect both you and the patient by providing a barrier to infection transmission from one person to another. Explain that your other protective equipment, such as goggles or a mask, also helps prevent the spread of infection.

Special Considerations

As you collect blood specimens, you will encounter a variety of patients, some of whom have special needs. You will find yourself in many different situations, some of them problematic. Some special needs and problematic situations are fairly common, and you must be prepared to deal with them.

Children. It is a challenge to explain blood-drawing procedures to children. Many children become visibly upset by the situation. If possible, it is best to talk with the parents or caregivers before working with the child. The adults can provide the best insight into how their child handles stressful situations.

Your primary concern when working with infants is to complete tests correctly. Because an infant's veins are often too small for adequate blood collection, the best site for drawing blood is usually the heel.

When working with children, address them directly. Speak clearly in a calm, soothing voice, and explain the procedure briefly in terms they can understand. If they ask whether the process will hurt, be honest. Very young children should be held by their parent or guardian or a coworker during a venipuncture or capillary puncture to prevent them from moving. If a child is extremely distressed, it may be best to go on to another patient while the child calms down.

After you have begun the procedure, give the child status reports such as, "We're almost finished!" and "You've been very brave." This information helps calm nervous parents or caregivers as well.

When the procedure is complete, offer a compliment on some aspect of the child's behavior. Gather your supplies and samples as quickly as possible to avoid alarming the child with the sight of blood-collection tubes. If parents or caregivers have questions, encourage them to discuss the tests with the child's physician.

Elderly Patients. The challenges presented by elderly patients may test your technical skills as well as your interpersonal skills. Physically, some older adults are frail and may not withstand blood-drawing procedures as easily as younger patients. Changes in skin condition often make elderly patients more prone to bruising and other injuries. Decreased circulation may make it difficult to collect enough blood for an adequate sampling. Elderly patients with impaired hearing may have trouble understanding instructions and answering questions. Patients with dementia may also be unable to understand what you are saying.

When you communicate with an elderly patient, speak in clear, low-pitched tones. High-pitched voices are more difficult for people with hearing impairments to understand. When asking questions, give the patient time to answer, and confirm the response to prevent misunderstandings. Avoid both overly simple yes or no questions that the patient might answer without thinking and overly complex questions that might confuse the patient. Take your time with the procedure, and explain it in language the patient can understand.

Patients at Risk for Uncontrolled Bleeding. Patients who have hemophilia or are taking blood-thinning medications are at risk for uncontrolled bleeding at the collection site. (Hemophilia is a disorder in which the blood does not coagulate at a wound or puncture site.) Be especially careful and alert as you follow the standard procedures for collecting a blood specimen. In addition, hold several gauze squares over the puncture site for at least 5 minutes to make sure bleeding has stopped completely. If uncontrolled bleeding does occur, call the physician immediately.

Difficult Patients. You may encounter a particular challenge in working with a patient either because of technical problems or because of personality issues. Being prepared for these situations is the best method for coping with them.

The Difficult Venipuncture. There will be times when you simply cannot get a good blood sample. If your first attempt at drawing blood fails, try again at another site. Give the patient (and yourself) a short break, and make an attempt on the other arm, for instance. Sometimes the veins in one arm are easier to work with than the veins in the other arm. If you cannot get a good sample on the second try, stop. Ask for assistance from your supervisor or the doctor.

Fainting Patients. It is impossible to predict which patients will have a reaction to a blood-drawing procedure. Generally, however, an ill patient is more likely to experience a reaction than a well patient. The best way to deal with this potential problem is to position every patient so that, if fainting does occur, no injury will result.

Have patients sit in a special venipuncture chair (Figure 30-17). These chairs are designed to help prevent patients from sliding to the floor in the event of fainting. If your office is not equipped with a venipuncture chair, have patients lie down on an examination table. A patient who has a history of fainting or feels ill should lie down with feet elevated or knees drawn up while you complete the procedure.

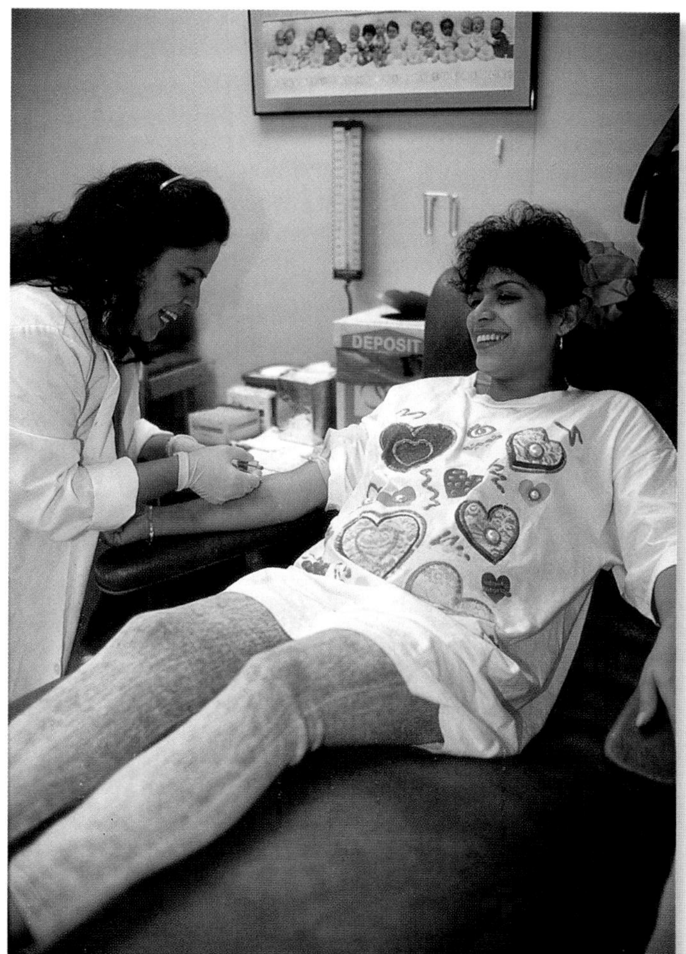

Figure 30-17. Venipuncture chairs are designed to make blood drawing easier and to prevent patients from falling if they should faint.

If a patient does faint and the needle is still in the vein, release the tourniquet and withdraw the needle quickly and steadily. Apply pressure to the site. Most people revive promptly, and no other action is required. Do not leave the patient alone. Notify the doctor that the patient fainted, and ask the doctor whether you should continue with the procedure.

If there is a more severe reaction, notify the appropriate staff member and remain with the patient. If the patient is in a chair and begins to slide out, raise the safety arm and gently lower the patient to the floor. Protect the patient's head at all times, and make sure the patient is breathing. The doctor should examine the patient before the patient is moved. Follow the doctor's instructions.

When the patient begins to recover, assist the person into a sitting position and then to a chair or couch. The patient should rest until feeling strong enough to walk—usually about 15 minutes. When the patient feels steady, take the patient to another area of the office, such as the patient reception area. At this point another staff member usually becomes responsible for the patient's care and determines when it is safe for the patient to leave.

Angry or Violent Patients. Some patients are extremely resistant to having blood drawn. Although their objections may seem illogical, remember that people often do not think as clearly in moments of high emotion as they normally do.

Encourage a patient who is mildly upset and wants to argue about the need for the blood test to let you take the sample and then discuss the situation with the doctor. If you convince the patient to submit to the test, complete the procedure quickly and accurately. Avoid arguing with the patient.

Do not force the issue with a patient who becomes violent or refuses outright to submit to the procedure. A patient does have the right to refuse testing or treatment. Under no circumstances should you attempt to physically force a patient to give a blood sample. Never endanger yourself, other patients, or your colleagues by refusing to back down from an angry or violent patient. Report the problem to the appropriate staff, make a note on the order, and follow other established procedures.

Performing Common Blood Tests

Many blood tests are routinely ordered as part of a complete general examination to determine a patient's overall health. The results of individual tests can provide information that aids in the diagnosis of specific conditions, diseases, and disorders, as noted in Table 30-2.

The number of blood tests routinely performed in POLs has declined since the implementation of Clinical Laboratory Improvement Amendments of 1988 (CLIA '88) regulations. Many POLs now perform only waivered tests. Each POL is different, however, and regulations do change. Check with your employer about what tests your office performs regularly. You should be familiar with a wide range of tests and the steps involved with each even if you do not anticipate performing them.

You may encounter several chemical substances while performing your responsibilities in the laboratory. Chemicals you might encounter in laboratory work include the following:

- Anticoagulants, which cause the blood to remain in a liquid, uncoagulated state
- Serum separators, which form a gel-like barrier between serum and the clot in a coagulated blood sample
- Stains, which color particular cells, making microscopic studies easier to complete

Anticoagulants or serum separators are always present in blood-collection tubes and do not need to be added to the sample.

You must be absolutely clear about which chemicals are used for which tests and the precise amounts involved. It is also important to understand the purpose of blood tests so you can educate patients. You must, in addition, know the range of normal test values so you can be aware of potential problems and note them for the doctor's attention. Table 30-3 shows the normal ranges for a variety of blood tests.

Hematologic Tests

Hematologic tests are commonly performed in routine blood testing. These tests can be performed on venous or capillary whole blood samples. Hematologic tests include blood cell counts, morphologic studies, coagulation tests, and the nonautomated erythrocyte sedimentation rate test.

Blood Counts. Whole blood, as described earlier, contains the formed elements (red blood cells, white blood cells, platelets) and the fluid portion (plasma). The total number of blood cells and the percentage of the whole sample that each type represents can tell the physician a great deal about a patient's condition. A physician can order an individual test or a complete blood (cell) count (CBC), which includes the following tests:

- Red blood (cell) count (RBC), which is the total number of red blood cells in a sample
- White blood (cell) count (WBC), which is the total number of white blood cells in a sample
- Differential white blood cell count, which is the number of each type of white blood cell (basophils, eosinophils, neutrophils, lymphocytes, and monocytes) in the first 100 leukocytes of a sample
- Platelet count (automated), which is the number of platelets in a sample, or a platelet estimate, which indicates whether the amount of platelets is adequate
- Hematocrit determination, which identifies how much of the volume of a sample is made up of red blood cells after the sample has been spun in a centrifuge; expressed as a percentage
- Hemoglobin determination, which measures the amount of hemoglobin in the sample

Most POLs use automated equipment for performing blood counts, but you need to know how to perform blood counts manually. This competency provides a backup for the automated instrumentation and puts you in a better position to recognize unusual findings among automated results. All manual counts are estimates. The types of blood cell counts differ in sample preparation and in the equipment and methods used.

Differential Cell Counts. You will prepare a blood smear slide and stain the smear for a differential cell count. Procedure 30-4 details preparation of a blood smear slide. When you carry out this process correctly, there will be a region of the slide where blood cells are dense but lie in a single plane (not stacked or bunched together). This is the region where the cells are counted.

A polychromatic (multicolored) stain such as Wright's stain simplifies a differential cell count. The blue and red-orange dyes (methylene blue and eosin, respectively) stain

TABLE 30-2 Common Blood Tests and the Conditions They Help Identify

Substance Identified or Quantified	Part of Blood Tested	Indication, Disease, or Disorder
Acetone	Serum or plasma	Diabetic or fasting metabolic ketoacidosis
Alanine aminotransferase (ALT)	Serum	Liver disorders
Alpha-fetoprotein (AFP)	Fetal serum	Fetal liver and gastrointestinal tract status, hepatitis
Amylase	Serum	Drug toxicity, parotid or pancreas disorders
Angiotensin-converting enzyme (ACE)	Serum	Lung cancer, sarcoidosis, acute or chronic bronchitis
Antidiuretic hormone (ADH)	Plasma	Syndrome of inappropriate ADH, Guillain-Barré syndrome, brain tumor
Aspartate aminotransferase (AST)	Serum	Liver disease (including viral hepatitis), infectious mononucleosis, damaged heart or skeletal muscle
Bilirubin	Serum	Liver disease, fructose intolerance, hypothyroidism
Blood urea nitrogen (BUN)	Serum or plasma	Kidney disorders
Cancer antigens (numbers 125, 15-3, 549, 72-4), tumor-associated glycoprotein (TAG)	Serum	Specific cancers identified, depending on antigen tested
Calcium, total (fasting)	Serum	Hyperparathyroidism, malignant disease with bone involvement
Carbon dioxide, total	Venous serum or plasma	Acidosis or alkalosis (acid-base balance)
Cholesterol, total	Serum or plasma	Hyperlipoproteinemia, coronary artery disease, atherosclerosis
Creatine kinase (CK)	Serum	Muscular dystrophies, Reye's syndrome, heart disease, shock, some neoplasms
Erythrocyte count (RBC)	Whole blood	Anemia
Erythrocyte sedimentation rate (ESR)	Whole blood	Infectious diseases, malignant neoplasms, sickle cell anemia
Glucose (fasting)	Whole blood	Pancreatic function, ability of intravenous insulin to offset diet in diabetes mellitus
Glucose (fasting—tolerance test)	Serum	Diabetes mellitus, hypoglycemia
Lactate dehydrogenase (LD)	Serum	Anemia, viral hepatitis, shock, hypoxia, hyperthermia
Leukocyte count (WBC)	Whole blood	Leukemia, infection, leukocytosis
Phenylalanine	Plasma	Hyperphenylalaninemia, obesity, phenylketonuria
Potassium (K^+) and sodium (Na^+)	Serum	Fluid-electrolyte balance
Prostatic acid phosphatase (PAP)	Serum	Prostatic cancer
Sickle cells	Whole blood	Sickle cell anemia
Thyroid-stimulating hormone (TSH), triiodothyronine (T_3), thyroxine (T_4)	Serum	Thyroid function
Uric acid	Serum	Gout, leukemia

TABLE 30-3 Normal Ranges for Blood Tests

Blood Test	Blood Component Tested	Normal Range
Blood counts		
Red blood cells (erythrocytes)		
Men	Whole blood	$4.3–5.7 \times 10^6$ cells/μL
Women	Whole blood	$3.8–5.1 \times 10^6$ cells/μL
White blood cells (leukocytes)	Whole blood	$4.5–11.0 \times 10^3$ cells/μL
Platelets	Whole blood	$150–400 \times 10^3$ cells/μL
Differential		
Neutrophils	Whole blood	60%–70%
Eosinophils	Whole blood	1%–4%
Basophils	Whole blood	0%–0.5%
Lymphocytes	Whole blood	20%–30%
Monocytes	Whole blood	2%–6%
Hematocrit (Hct)	Whole blood	
Men		39%–49%
Women		35%–45%
Hemoglobin (Hb, Hgb)	Whole blood	
Men		13.2–17.3 g/dL
Women		11.7–16.0 g/dL
Erythrocyte sedimentation rate (ESR)		
Wintrobe	Whole blood	
Men		0–5 mm/hour
Women		0–15 mm/hour
Westergren	Whole blood	
Men		0–15 mm/hour
Women		0–20 mm/hour
Coagulation tests		
Prothrombin time (PT)	Plasma	11–15 seconds
Bleeding time	Whole blood	2–7 minutes
Blood gases (collected anaerobically)		
Partial pressure of carbon dioxide ($PaCO_2$)	Arterial blood	
Men		35–48 mm Hg
Women		32–45 mm Hg
Partial pressure of oxygen (PaO_2)	Arterial blood	83–108 mm Hg
Total carbon dioxide (CO_2)	Venous serum or plasma	23–29 mEq/L
Electrolytes		
Bicarbonate (HCO_3^-)	Arterial plasma	21–28 mEq/L
	Venous plasma	27–29 mEq/L
Calcium (Ca^{++})	Serum	8.6–10.0 mg/dL
Chloride (Cl^-)	Serum, plasma	98–108 mEq/L
Potassium (K^+)	Serum	3.5–5.1 mEq/L
Sodium (Na^+)	Serum	136–145 mEq/L

continued →

TABLE 30-3 Normal Ranges for Blood Tests *(continued)*		
Blood Test	**Blood Component Tested**	**Normal Range**
Chemical and serologic tests		
Alpha-fetoprotein (AFP)	Serum	
Fetal, first trimester		20–400 mg/dL
Adult		<15 ng/mL
Alanine aminotransferase (ALT)	Serum	
Men		10–40 U/L
Women		7–35 U/L
Aspartate aminotransferase (AST, formerly SGOT)	Serum	
Men		11–26 U/L
Women		10–20 U/L
Bilirubin, total direct	Serum	0.3–1.2 mg/dL
Blood urea nitrogen (BUN)	Serum, plasma	6–20 mg/dL
Carcinoembryonic antigen (CEA)	Serum	<5.0 ng/mL
Cholesterol, total	Serum, plasma	
Men		158–277 mg/dL
Women		162–285 mg/dL
High-density lipoproteins (HDLs)	Serum, plasma	
Men		28–63 mg/dL
Women		37–92 mg/dL
Low-density lipoproteins (LDLs)	Serum, plasma	
Men		89–197 mg/dL
Women		88–201 mg/dL
Creatine kinase (CK)	Serum, plasma	
Men		38–174 U/L
Women		26–140 U/L
Creatinine	Serum, plasma	
Men		0.9–1.3 mg/dL
Women		0.6–1.2 mg/dL
Cytomegalovirus (CMV)	Serum	None
Epstein-Barr virus (EBV)	Whole blood	None
Glucose (fasting blood sugar, FBS)	Serum	74–120 mg/dL
Group A beta-hemolytic streptococci	Serum	None
Human immunodeficiency virus (HIV) antibodies	Serum, plasma	None
Insulin	Serum	<17 μU/mL
Iron, total	Serum	
Men		65–175 μg/dL
Women		50–170 μg/dL
Ketone bodies (as acetoacetate)	Serum, plasma	None

continued ⟶

Blood Test	Blood Component Tested	Normal Range
Chemical and serologic tests (continued)		
Lactate dehydrogenase (LD)	Serum, plasma	140–280 U/L
pH	Arterial blood Venous blood	7.35–7.45 7.32–7.43
Proteins Total Albumin Fibrinogen	Serum	 6.2–8.0 g/dL 3.4–4.8 g/dL 200–400 mg/dL
Uric acid Men Women	Serum	 4.4–7.6 mg/dL 2.3–6.6 mg/dL

TABLE 30-3 Normal Ranges for Blood Tests *(continued)*

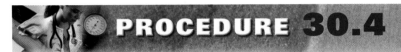

PROCEDURE 30.4

Preparing a Blood Smear Slide

Objective: To prepare a blood specimen to be used in a morphologic or other study

OSHA Guidelines

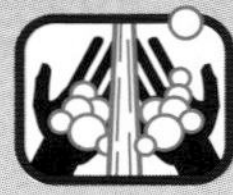
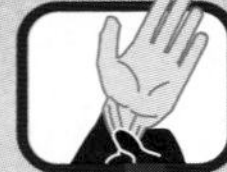

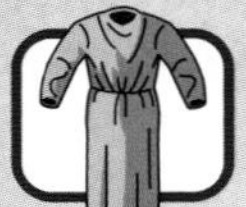
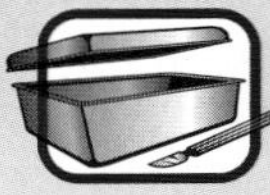

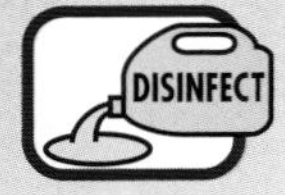

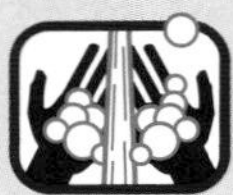

Materials: Blood specimen (either from a capillary puncture or a specimen tube containing anticoagulated blood), capillary tubes, sterile gauze squares, slide with frosted end, wooden applicator sticks

Method

1. Wash your hands and put on examination gloves.
2. If you will be using blood from a capillary puncture, follow the steps in Procedure 30-3 to express a drop of blood from the patient's finger. If you will be using a venous sample, check the specimen for proper labeling, uncap the specimen tube, and use wooden applicator sticks to remove any coagulated blood from the inside rim of the tube.
3. Touch the tip of the capillary tube to the blood specimen. The tube will take up the correct amount through capillary action.
4. Pull the capillary tube away from the sample, holding it carefully to prevent spillage. Wipe the outside of the capillary tube with a sterile gauze square to remove excess blood.
5. With the slide on the work surface, hold the capillary tube in one hand and the frosted end of the slide against the work surface with the other.
6. Apply a drop of blood to the slide, about ¾ inch from the frosted end, as shown in Figure 30-18. Place the capillary tube in a safe location to prevent spillage.
7. Pick up the spreader slide with your dominant hand. Hold the slide at approximately a 30° to 35° angle. Place the edge of the spreader

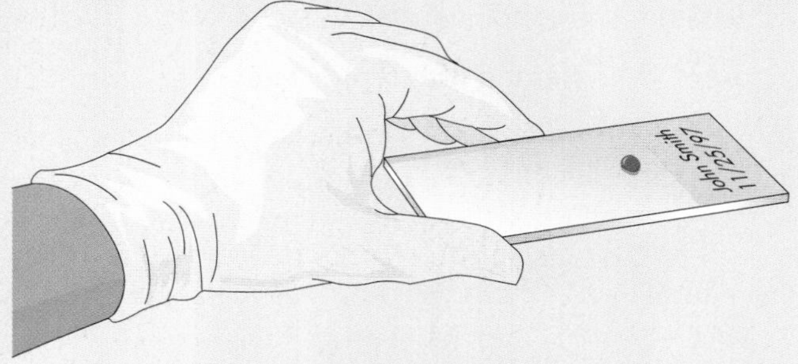

Figure 30-18. Apply a drop of blood to the slide about ¾ inch from the frosted end.

continued ⟶

PROCEDURE 30.4

Preparing a Blood Smear Slide *(continued)*

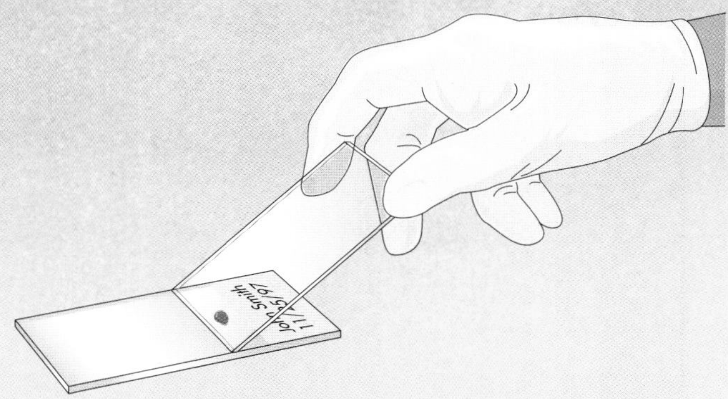

Figure 30-19. Hold the spreader slide at a 30° to 35° angle. Pull the spreader slide toward the frosted end until it touches the drop of blood.

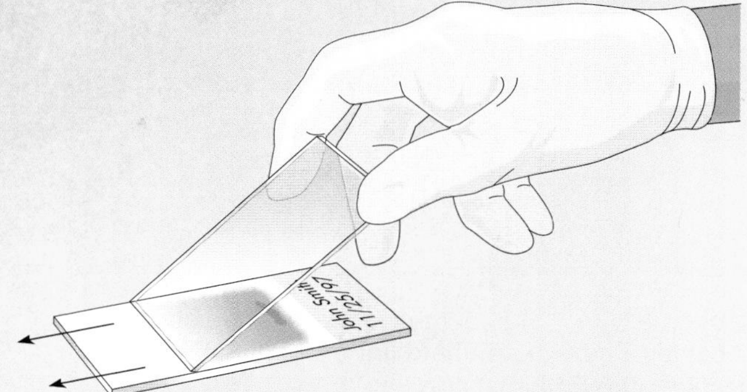

Figure 30-20. When the drop covers most of the spreader slide edge, push the spreader slide back toward the unfrosted end of the smear slide.

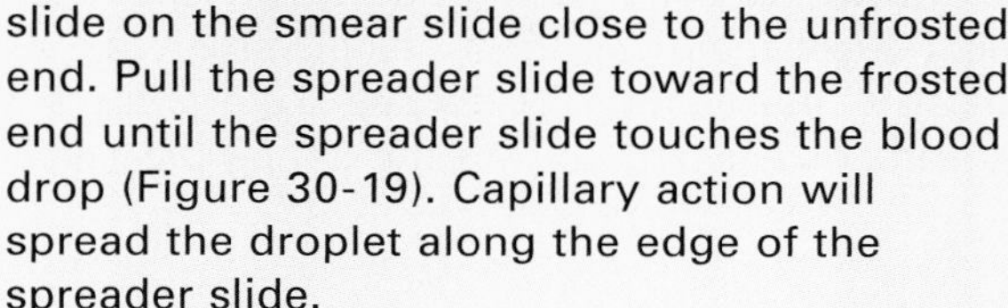

slide on the smear slide close to the unfrosted end. Pull the spreader slide toward the frosted end until the spreader slide touches the blood drop (Figure 30-19). Capillary action will spread the droplet along the edge of the spreader slide.

8. As soon as the drop spreads out to cover most of the spreader slide edge, push the spreader slide back toward the unfrosted end of the smear slide, pulling the sample across the slide behind it, as shown in Figure 30-20. Maintain the 30° to 35° angle.
9. As you near the unfrosted end of the smear slide, gently lift the spreader slide away from it, still maintaining the angle, as shown in Figure 30-21. The resulting smear should be approximately 1½ inches long, preferably with a margin of empty slide on all sides. The smear should be thicker on the frosted end of the slide.

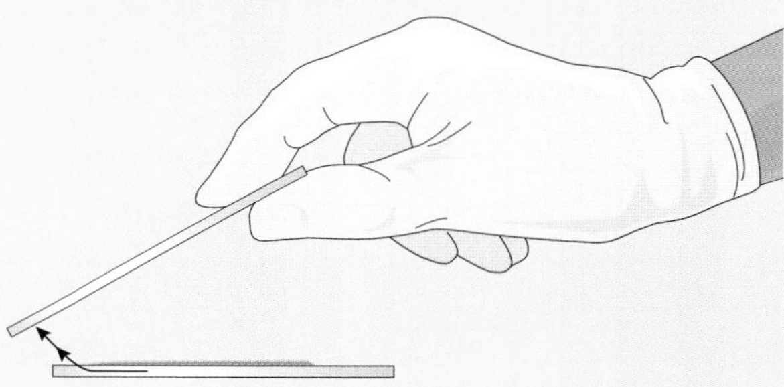

Figure 30-21. Lift the spreader slide away from the smear slide, maintaining a 30° to 35° angle. The smear should be thicker on the frosted end of the slide.

10. Properly label the slide, allow it to dry, and follow the manufacturer's directions for staining it for the required tests.
11. Properly dispose of used supplies, and disinfect the work area.
12. Remove the gloves and wash your hands.

cell structures in ways that identify each of the five types of white blood cells. When stained, neutrophils have a dark purple nucleus and pale pink cytoplasm containing fine pink or lavender granules. Basophils have a purple nucleus and light purple cytoplasm that contains large, blue-black granules. Eosinophils can be identified by the purple nucleus and the bright orange granules in pink cytoplasm. Lymphocytes appear as a large, dark purple nucleus surrounded by a small amount of blue cytoplasm. The fifth type of leukocytes, monocytes, are the largest and have gray-blue cytoplasm.

Figure 30-22 shows the zigzag pattern for counting leukocytes visible in the field when using the microscope's oil-immersion objective. A total of 100 leukocytes are counted and recorded on a differential counter. Each cell type is expressed as a percentage of the 100 leukocytes counted. The platelet count is averaged in 10 to 15 fields.

Hematocrit. You measure a patient's hematocrit percentage by collecting a small sample of the patient's blood in a microhematocrit tube, sealing the tube, and spinning

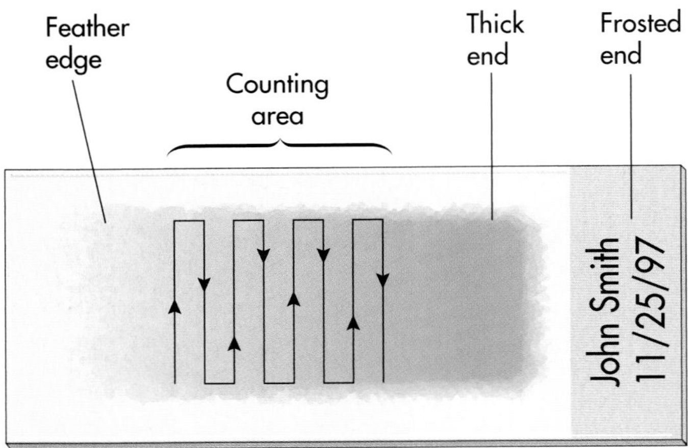

Figure 30-22. Follow this pattern when counting leukocytes visible in the field under the oil-immersion objective of the microscope.

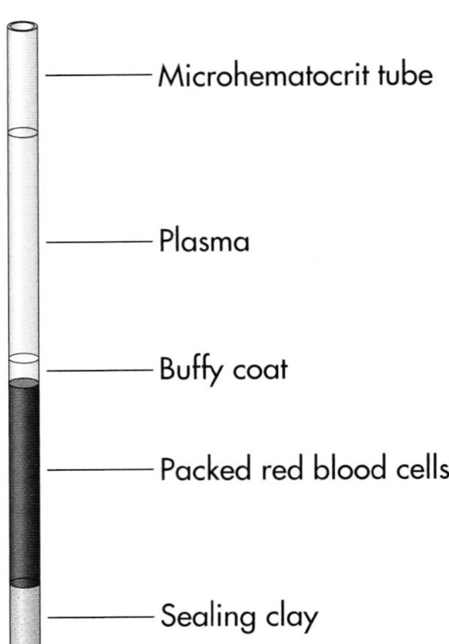

Figure 30-23. Blood in a centrifuged microhematocrit tube separates into packed red blood cells, the buffy coat, and plasma.

it in a centrifuge. This process is described in Procedure 30-5. During this process heavier red blood cells move to one end of the tube, whereas lighter plasma moves to the other end. Between the RBCs, also called the **packed red blood cells,** and the plasma is the buffy coat (Figure 30-23). The **buffy coat** contains the white blood cells and platelets.

Always run two samples of the patient's blood specimen. After removing each sample from the centrifuge, compare the column of packed RBCs with a standard hematocrit gauge. Read on the gauge the percentage of

PROCEDURE 30.5

Measuring Hematocrit Percentage After Centrifuge

Objective: To identify the percentage of a blood specimen represented by red blood cells after the sample has been spun in a centrifuge

OSHA Guidelines

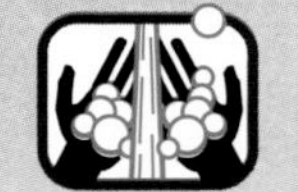 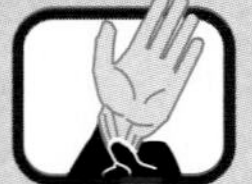  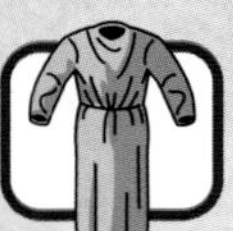

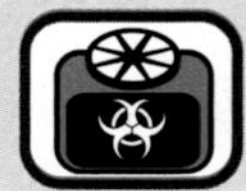 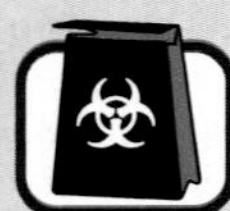 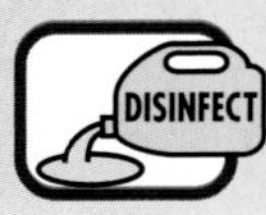

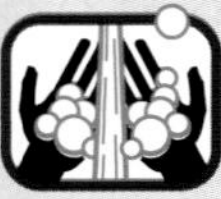

Materials: Blood specimen (either from a capillary puncture or a specimen tube containing anticoagulated blood), microhematocrit tube, sealant tray containing sealing clay, centrifuge, hematocrit gauge, wooden applicator sticks, gauze squares

Method

1. Wash your hands and put on examination gloves.
2. If you will be using blood from a capillary puncture, follow the steps in Procedure 30-3 to express a drop of blood from the patient's finger. If you will be using a venous blood sample, check the specimen for proper labeling, uncap the specimen tube, and use wooden applicator sticks to remove any coagulated blood from the inside rim of the tube.
3. Touch the tip of one of the microhematocrit tubes to the blood sample, as shown in Figure 30-24. The tube will take up the correct amount through capillary action.
4. Pull the microhematocrit tube away from the sample, holding it carefully to prevent spillage. Wipe the outside of the

continued →

PROCEDURE 30.5

Measuring Hematocrit Percentage After Centrifuge *(continued)*

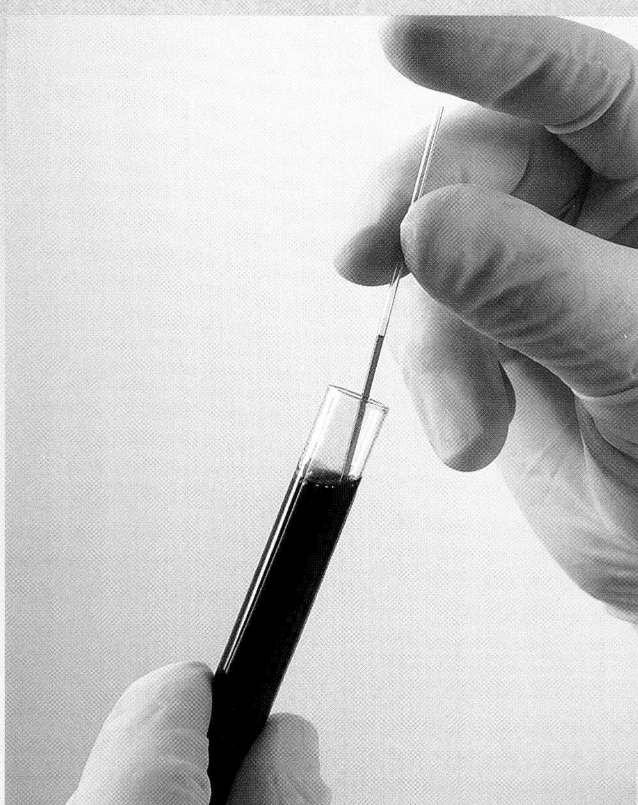

Figure 30-24. Touch the tip of one of the microhematocrit tubes to the blood specimen.

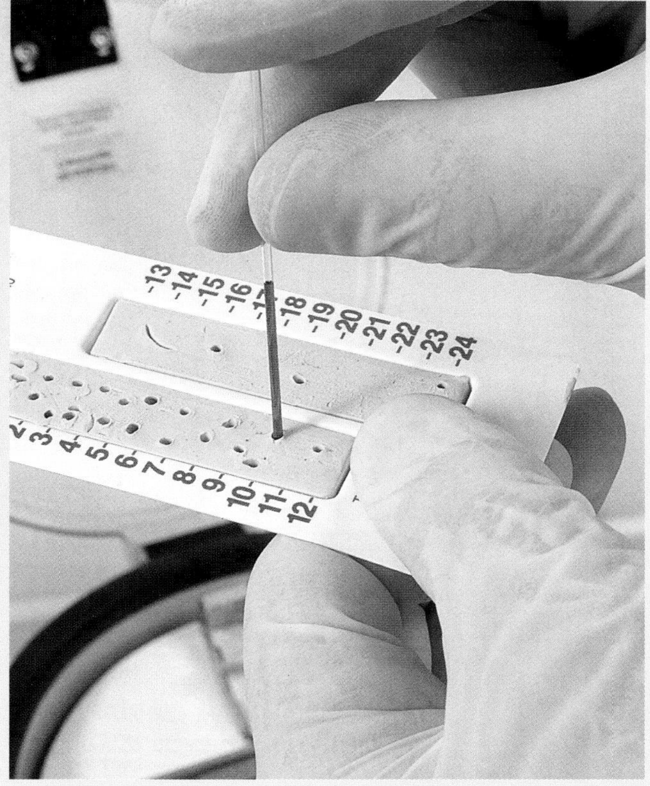

Figure 30-25. Press the end of the tube into the clay in the sealant tray.

microhematocrit tube with a gauze square to remove excess blood.

5. Hold the microhematocrit tube in one hand with a gloved finger over one end to prevent leakage, and press the other end of the tube gently into the clay in the sealant tray (Figure 30-25). The clay plug must completely seal the end of the tube.
6. Repeat the process to fill another microhematocrit tube. Tubes must be processed in pairs to maintain a balance in the centrifuge.
7. Place the tubes in the centrifuge, with the sealed ends pointing outward (Figure 30-26). If you are processing more than one sample, record the position identification number in the patient's chart to track the sample.
8. Seal the centrifuge chamber.

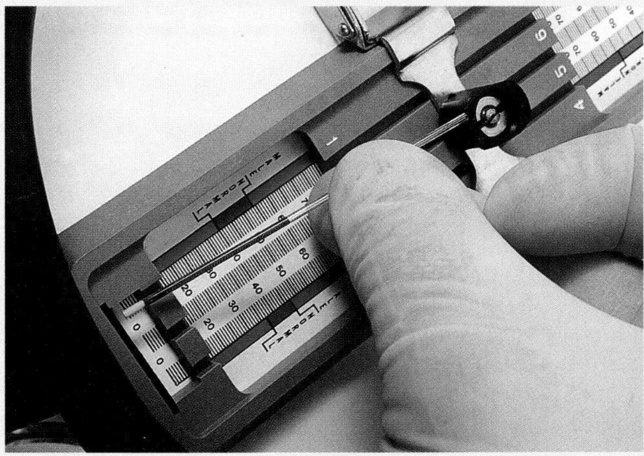

Figure 30-26. Be sure to place the tubes in the centrifuge so that the sealed ends are pointing outward.

continued ⟶

PROCEDURE 30.5

Measuring Hematocrit Percentage After Centrifuge *(continued)*

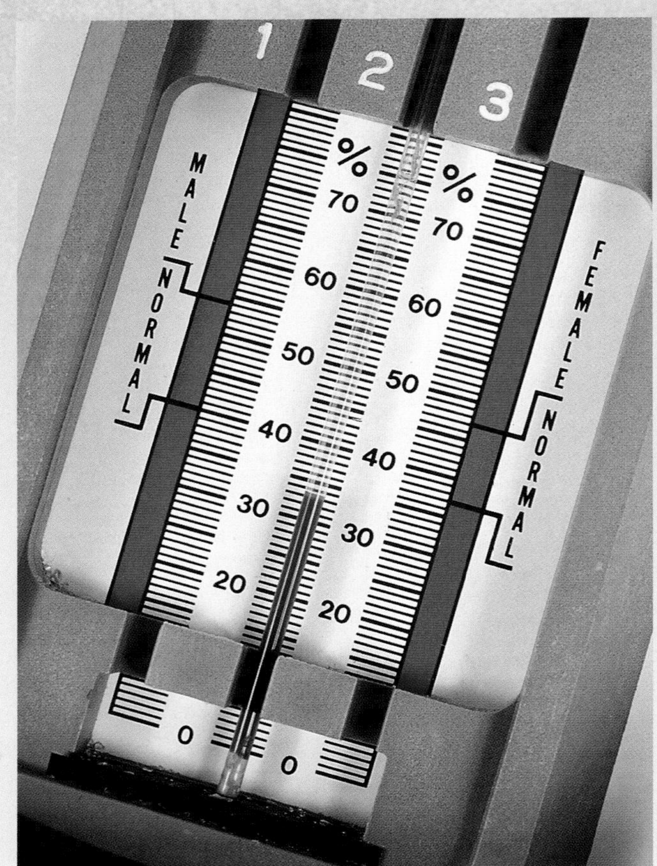

Figure 30-27. Compare the column of packed red blood cells in the microhematocrit tube with the hematocrit gauge to determine the hematocrit percentage.

9. Run the centrifuge for the required time, usually between 3 and 5 minutes. Allow the centrifuge to come to a complete stop before unsealing it.
10. Determine the hematocrit percentage by comparing the column of packed red blood cells in the microhematocrit tubes with the hematocrit gauge, as shown in Figure 30-27. Position each tube so that the boundary between sealing clay and red blood cells is at zero on the gauge. Some centrifuges are equipped with gauges, but others require separate handheld gauges.
11. Record the percentage value on the gauge that corresponds to the top of the column of red blood cells for each tube. Compare the two results. They should not vary by more than 3%. If you record a greater variance, at least one of the tubes was filled incorrectly, and you must repeat the test.
12. Calculate the average result by adding the two tube figures and dividing that number by 2.
13. Properly dispose of used supplies, and clean and disinfect the equipment and the area.
14. Remove the gloves and wash your hands.
15. Record the test result in the patient's chart. Be sure to identify abnormal results.

total blood volume represented by the RBCs. Average the readings of the two patient samples. (The samples should be within 3% of each other.)

Hemoglobin. Hemoglobin resides within the red blood cells. You will determine the concentration of hemoglobin in the blood by lysing (rupturing) the red blood cells (hemolysis) and evaluating the color of the sample. This procedure may be done with a hemoglobinometer—a handheld device that makes color evaluation less subjective than older methods of visual matching with color samples. Blood specimens mixed with a reagent, such as Drabkin's reagent, undergo a color reaction that can be quantified by reading color intensity in a photoelectric colorimeter.

Morphologic Studies. **Morphology** is the study of the shape or form of objects. A morphologic study of a blood sample can provide important information about a patient's condition. During a morphologic study on blood, a blood smear is examined, and the appearance and shape of cells in the sample are recorded. Special note is made of abnormal cell size, shape, or content and abnormal organization of cells. A morphologic study is often performed just after the differential count and platelet estimate on the same blood smear slide. Morphologic studies require special training and are not routinely done by medical assistants.

Coagulation Tests. A physician may order coagulation tests to identify potential bleeding problems before surgical procedures. A regular schedule of coagulation tests may be ordered to monitor therapeutic drug levels when a patient is receiving medications such as heparin or warfarin (Coumadin). Coagulation studies include the prothrombin time (PT) and partial thromboplastin time (PTT) tests. These tests are usually performed using automated

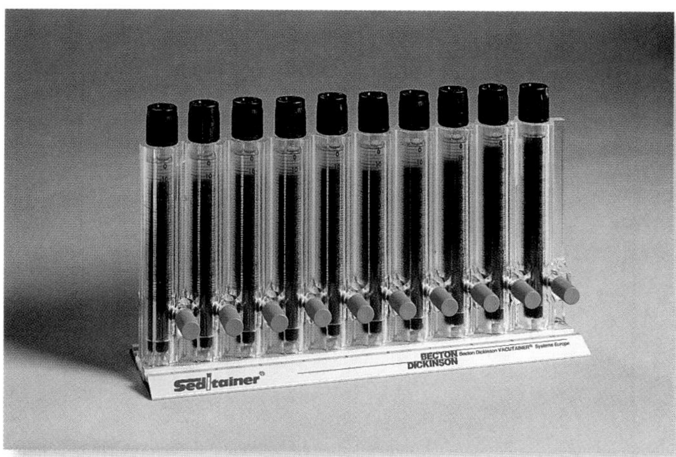

Figure 30-28. The sedimentation rack holds blood specimens steady and level for the ESR test.

devices such as the Coaguchek Plus, manufactured by Boehringer Mannheim Diagnostics, Indianapolis, Indiana. These systems monitor the changing pattern of light transmission through the sample as coagulation occurs. Medical assistants sometimes perform such coagulation studies.

Erythrocyte Sedimentation Rate. The nonautomated **erythrocyte sedimentation rate (ESR)** test measures the rate at which red blood cells, the heaviest blood component, settle to the bottom of a blood sample. You will transfer freshly collected, anticoagulated blood to a calibrated tube and place the tube in a sedimentation rack to run this test (Figure 30-28). You examine the tube an hour later to determine how far the red blood cells have fallen. Test results are recorded as millimeters per hour (mm/hr). Several standard testing systems are used, including the Westergren and Wintrobe systems. You must adhere closely to each manufacturer's instructions when using these systems, because ESR test results are sensitive to factors such as the temperature and freshness of the samples, precise position of the sample tube, and vibrations affecting the tube or the rack.

Chemical Tests

Blood chemistry analysis examines several dozen chemicals found in human blood. Tables 30-2 and 30-3 include many chemical tests on blood. Highly detailed studies are rarely performed in the POL because they require expensive, sophisticated equipment and techniques. Complex testing is also subject to strict CLIA '88 regulations that increase the administrative work and the need for more highly trained personnel. These types of tests, therefore, are commonly performed at an independent test laboratory. Automated equipment for analyzing blood chemistry, however, is becoming more available, less expensive, and simpler to operate than it was in the past. This trend makes it more likely that you may use automated equipment to perform some types of blood chemistry tests. Keeping abreast of new developments will help prepare you for possible changes in your laboratory duties.

Blood Glucose Monitoring. Some tests of blood chemistry are routinely performed in the POL. Blood glucose monitoring, for example, is often performed by a medical assistant or by a patient. Glucose monitoring systems require the use of sterile lancets to perform a capillary puncture. You will collect the blood on reagent strips that change color in accordance with glucose levels present in the blood. The level is determined either by comparing the color on the strip with color standards provided with the reagent strips or by feeding the strip into a handheld reading device. You will teach patients to perform this kind of test at home. Be sure to stress the importance of following the manufacturer's guidelines for correct operation of a testing device.

You will also teach patients and their families how to manage diabetes. This will include performing the blood glucose test, managing diet and exercise, self-monitoring for complications associated with diabetes, and additional resources for further education. See the Educating the Patient section.

Hemoglobin A1c. Another test used to monitor the health of patients with diabetes is the hemoglobin A1c test. This test measures the amount of glycosylated hemoglobin in the blood. When blood glucose levels are elevated, the glucose molecules bind with hemoglobin to form hemoglobin A1c (HgBA1c). Once HgBA1c is formed, it remains for the life of the red blood cell (90 to 120 days). This makes it a useful tool for monitoring the overall stability of the patient's blood glucose.

It is important for a patient to maintain a normal blood glucose level. Large fluctuations in blood sugar are problematic in patients with diabetes. These fluctuations can cause complications such as eye disease, stroke, renal failure, and cardiovascular disease. The HgBA1c test gives the physician a good overall picture of the patient's compliance to and the effectiveness of diabetes treatment.

There are several options for performing this test. The test may be sent to an outside reference laboratory with results available in 1 to 7 days. Some physicians' offices have the equipment necessary to perform this test in the office laboratory. These results are usually available in less than 10 minutes. Several home tests have recently become available. The patient can monitor his own HgBA1c levels, thus keeping a close watch on the efficiency of his diabetes treatment. FDA-approved home tests include:

- Bio-rad Micromat II Hemoglobin A1c Prescription Home Use Test
- Metrika A1c Now for Home Use
- Cholestech GDX A1c Test
- Provalis Diagnostics Glycosal II HBA1c
- Flex Site Diagnostics A1c at Home

Educating the Patient

Managing Diabetes

Diabetes affects an estimated 6 percent of the population, with more than 1 million newly diagnosed cases each year. In order to reduce the complications associated with diabetes, it is important for patients to maintain stable blood sugar. Proper patient education and medical care will help patients achieve this goal. As a medical assistant, you can assist patients and their families by providing them with information about diabetes that includes:

1. The risks and consequences associated with uncontrolled blood sugar. Patients whose blood sugar is unstable are at greater risk of developing the following conditions:
   - Loss of vision
   - Kidney failure
   - Heart disease
   - Nerve damage
   - Stroke
2. The patient's type of diabetes. Patients need to know the type of diabetes they have so that they can understand the type of treatment prescribed. The types of diabetes are:
   - Type I diabetes—An autoimmune disorder characterized by the body's inability to make enough insulin. Insulin is required for glucose utilization. Patients with Type I diabetes will need to take insulin daily.
   - Type II diabetes—The most common type of diabetes. Insulin is still being produced at normal levels but can no longer be utilized by the cells of the body. This causes a buildup of unused glucose in the blood. This type of diabetes is often controlled with careful diet management and increased exercise. There are also a number of oral medications used in the treatment of Type II diabetes.
   - Gestational diabetes—Develops only during pregnancy. This type of diabetes is generally managed through proper diet and exercise. Careful monitoring is important to reduce the risk of fetal complications. Women who have had gestational diabetes have an increased risk of developing Type II diabetes.
3. Maintaining proper diet and exercise. This should include:
   - Making proper food choices
   - Keeping a food diary
   - Reading food labels
   - Choosing proper food exchanges
   - Creating and implementing a routine exercise program
4. Routine self-monitoring of blood sugar and Hemoglobin A1c levels. Information should include:
   - The types of blood glucose monitors available. Figure 30-29 illustrates one type of blood glucose monitor, a glucometer.
   - Instructions on obtaining monitoring supplies
   - The number of times and the specific intervals at which blood sugar should be checked, based on individual needs and the physician's recommendations
   - Instructions on performing blood glucose testing
   - Guidelines on how to maintain a chart of blood glucose levels, including the time of day, associated meals and activities, and actual blood sugar values
   - Hemoglobin A1c monitoring. The patient should understand what Hemoglobin A1c

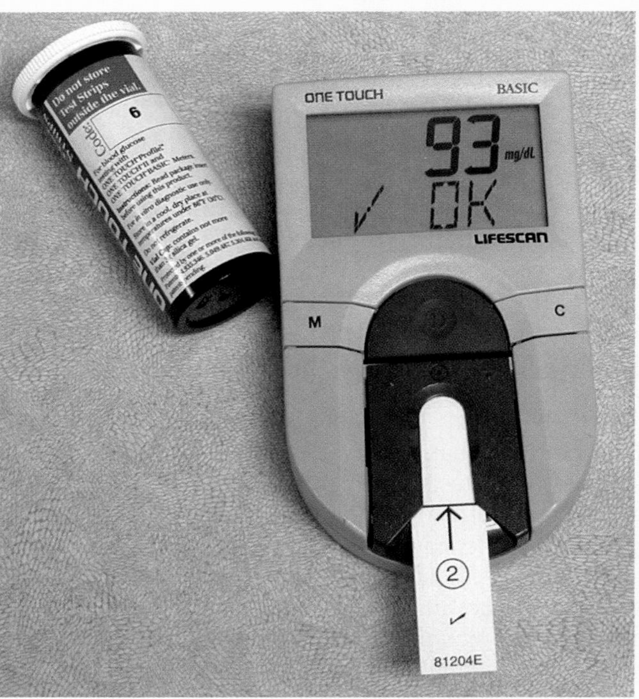

Figure 30-29. A hand-held glucometer is an important tool in helping patients manage diabetes.

continued ⟶

Educating the Patient

Managing Diabetes *(continued)*

is and why it is important to monitor these values.

- Normal (target) values for blood glucose and Hemoglobin A1c:
  - Blood glucose levels should remain between 90 and 130 mg/dl before meals and remain less than 180 mg/dl for 1 to 2 hours after a meal. Target ranges may be different for each patient. Consult with the physician about individual blood glucose levels.
  - Hemoglobin A1c is a test that shows the average amount of glucose in the blood over a three-month period. Ideally, this value should be less than 7%.

5. Symptoms of uncontrolled blood sugar. Patients need to be aware of the symptoms of both high and low blood sugar, both of which require immediate attention. Patients should test their blood sugar if any of the following occur:
   - Nausea, vomiting, or abdominal pain
   - Feeling tired all the time
   - Excessive thirst or dry mouth
   - Flushed skin
   - Confusion or difficulty thinking
6. Self-screening for complications of diabetes. Patients should be aware of the complications associated with diabetes and how to recognize them. Patients should be instructed to do the following:
   - Perform a daily foot inspection for sores
   - Recognize changes in vision
   - Recognize the symptoms of kidney failure, which include nausea, vomiting, yellow skin, and swelling of the hands and feet
   - Recognizing early signs of nerve damage, which include numbness and tingling of the arms, hands, feet, or legs; dizziness; double vision; and drooping of the eyelid or lip
7. Additional sources of information. Patients should be encouraged to continue their education about diabetes. Providing patients with additional sources of information encourages them to take an active role in controlling their diabetes. Additional sources of information include:
   - American Association of Diabetes Educators
     1-800-338-DMED
     www.aadenet.org
   - American Diabetes Association
     1-800-DIABETES
     www.diabetes.org
   - American Dietetic Association
     1-800-877-1600
     1-800-366-1655 (consumer nutrition hotline in English and Spanish)
     www.eatright.org
   - Centers for Disease Control and Prevention Division of Diabetes Translation
     1-877-232-3422
     www.cdc.gov/diabetes
   - Juvenile Diabetes Foundation International
     1-800-JDF-CURE
     www.jdfcure.org
   - National Institute of Diabetes and Digestive and Kidney Diseases
     National Diabetes Information Clearinghouse
     301-654-3327
     www.niddk.hih.gov

Testing of HgBA1c should always be done in conjunction with routine blood glucose monitoring. Daily monitoring of blood glucose helps the patient with insulin therapy and diet maintenance. HgBA1c monitoring is important in assessing the patient's overall glucose levels. The advantages of this testing include:

- No pretesting preparation. The test may be done without regard to meals.
- Better overall assessment of long-term blood glucose control. Blood glucose testing gives information about glucose levels at one point in time. HgBA1c gives information over a period of 2 to 3 months.

Patients should have their HgBA1c levels checked two to four times per year. The target range for HgBA1c levels is less than 7%. Patients whose HgBA1c levels exceed 8% are at a greater risk for the complications associated with diabetes.

Serologic Tests

Serologic tests detect the presence of specific substances in a blood sample. The terms *serologic test* and *immunoassay* refer to the introduction of an antigen or antibody into the specimen and the detection of a specific reaction to the antigen or antibody. Serologic testing methods can be used to detect disease antibodies, drugs, hormones, and vitamins in the blood and to determine blood types. They are also used to test urine and other body fluids.

Immunoassays. Although medical assistants usually do not perform immunoassays, you should be familiar with several immunoassay methods that have common applications. These methods include:

- Western blot, in which antigens are blotted onto special filter paper for examination. Western blot tests are generally used to confirm HIV infection diagnosis.
- Radioimmunoassay (RIA), in which radioisotopes are used to "tag" antibodies. RIA tests are extremely sensitive and generally performed in a reference laboratory.
- Enzyme-linked immunosorbent assay (ELISA), in which enzyme-labeled antigens and substances that can absorb antigens generate reactions to specific antibodies. These reactions are identified through visual or photoelectric color detection. HIV infection is diagnosed using an ELISA test.
- Immunofluorescent antibody (IFA) test, in which dye, visible when the sample is examined under a fluorescent microscope, colors specific antibodies.

Rapid Screening Tests. Several serologic tests have been developed for quick processing. Some, such as early pregnancy tests performed on urine, are available for home use. When you use tests of this type or explain their use to a patient, keep in mind that the manufacturer's guidelines must be carefully followed to ensure accurate results.

Summary

Successful phlebotomy procedures require not only superior technical skills but also excellent interpersonal communication skills. When you are confident in your ability to perform venipuncture and capillary puncture techniques and in your understanding of common blood tests, you impart confidence to the patient. You should know what pretest instructions the patient should follow and what the patient can expect during the test.

As a medical assistant, you may be called on to complete certain testing procedures or to explain the purpose of tests to the patient. Therefore, it is important to understand the basics of blood composition and the common blood tests a patient might undergo. You can make the difference between a successfully drawn, accurately evaluated blood specimen and one that must be drawn again from a confused, unhappy patient.

REVIEW

CHAPTER 30

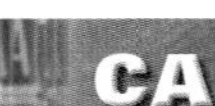

CASE STUDY QUESTIONS

Now that you have completed this chapter, review the case study at the beginning of the chapter and answer the following questions:

1. What and where is the antecubital fossa?
2. What is the principle of the evacuated collection system?
3. How should you attempt to collect the blood on the second try?
4. What type of a blood test is a PT?
5. What could have caused the extensive bleeding this patient experienced after the venipuncture?

Discussion Questions

1. Describe the various functions of blood.
2. Identify the different methods of obtaining blood from a patient.
3. A complete blood count (CBC) consists of what components?
4. Identify the major components of whole blood.

Critical Thinking Questions

1. How would you adequately prepare a patient for drawing a blood test?
2. Identify the different blood collection tubes by their stopper color, additive, and the testing usually performed with those tubes.
3. What fears or concerns may you commonly encounter when you deal with patients who are having blood drawn?

Application Activities

1. With a partner, practice each step of the capillary puncture process on each other until you can smoothly execute each step. Critique each other's work.
2. Practice creating a smoothly drawn smear slide. Have a classmate critique your work.
3. With a classmate, role-play a situation in which a medical assistant must calm a child who is fearful about having a blood test. Then switch roles and offer suggestions for improving each other's communication skills.

SECTION 6

NUTRITION, PHARMACOLOGY, AND DIAGNOSTIC EQUIPMENT

CHAPTER 31

Nutrition and Special Diets

AREAS OF COMPETENCE

2003 Role Delineation Study

GENERAL

Instruction

- Explain office policies and procedures
- Teach methods of health promotion and disease prevention
- Locate community resources and disseminate information

CHAPTER OUTLINE

- The Role of Diet in Health
- Daily Energy Requirements
- Nutrients
- Dietary Guidelines
- Assessing Nutritional Levels
- Modifying Diets
- Eating Disorders
- Patient Education

OBJECTIVES

After completing Chapter 31, you will be able to:

31.1 Explain why a medical assistant needs to understand the role of diet in health.

31.2 Describe how the body uses food.

31.3 Explain the role of calories in the diet.

31.4 Identify the seven basic food components and explain the major functions of each.

31.5 List the Dietary Guidelines for Americans.

31.6 Explain how the Food Guide Pyramid can be used to plan a nutritious, well-balanced diet.

31.7 Describe the test used to assess body fat.

31.8 Identify types of patients who require special diets and the modifications required for each group.

31.9 Identify specific modified diets that may be ordered to treat or prevent certain conditions.

31.10 Describe the warning signs, symptoms, and treatment for eating disorders.

31.11 Describe techniques the medical assistant can use to effectively educate different types of patients about nutritional requirements.

31.12 Explain the medical assistant's role in educating patients about nutrition and describe the proper documentation of patient education.

KEY TERMS

amino acid
anabolism
anorexia nervosa
antioxidant
behavior modification
bulimia
calorie
catabolism
cholesterol
complete protein
complex carbohydrate
fiber
food exchange
incomplete protein
mineral
parenteral nutrition
saturated fat
skinfold test
unsaturated fat
vitamin

Introduction

Nutrition is the process of how the body takes in and utilizes food and other sources of nutrients. It is a five-part process that includes intake, digestion, absorption, metabolism, and elimination. This chapter gives you an understanding of how a well-planned diet can lead to optimal health and well-being for your patients. You will also gain the knowledge needed to recognize the signs of illness related to diet.

CASE STUDY

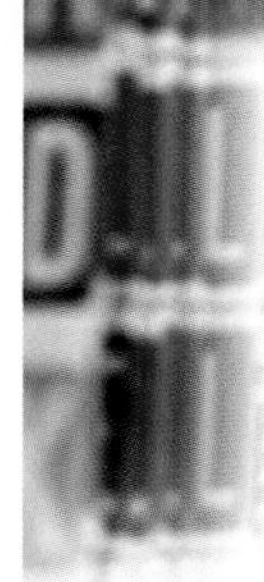

A 17-year-old female cheerleader is brought to her family doctor by her parents. As the medical assistant, you take her history and physical, noting that she has no medical problems. The patient mentions that she has a lack of interest in food because she is being "careful not to eat too many calories" so she can keep her weight down and have a chance to be head cheerleader next year. She tells you she plans to try out for a cheerleading scholarship next fall and is preparing for the competition.

You note her vital signs:

Blood pressure: 100/60
Height: 5′1″
Weight: 78 lbs.
Pulse rate: 40

She appears dehydrated and exhibits signs of muscle weakness.

As you read this chapter, consider the following questions:

1. What is the patient's probable diagnosis?
2. Do you think that the patient's attention to calorie intake is simply, as she says, preparation for the cheerleading competition?
3. Why is this patient experiencing muscle weakness?

The Role of Diet in Health

You need to know what effect food has on health so that you can help patients meet their dietary requirements. Food is the body's source of nutrients, or substances the body needs to function properly. As you study nutrition, you learn how the body uses nutrients as well as how and why people eat. People need specific types of foods to stay healthy or to regain their health after illness or surgery. People with specific conditions may also need to follow special diets.

You will work closely with the rest of the medical team to ensure that patients understand the role of diet in health and that they adhere to any diet prescribed by their physician or dietitian. A registered dietitian (RD) is a professional who uses the science of nutrition to design ways for people to obtain their optimal nourishment. Dietetics plays an important role in the health field. Dietitians work with physicians and the rest of the medical team to plan diets that are both therapeutic and realistic for patients.

Daily Energy Requirements

The human body requires the nutrients in food for three major purposes:

1. To provide energy
2. To build, repair, and maintain body tissues
3. To regulate body processes

A person's daily energy requirements depend on many factors. To understand the relationship of food to good health, you need to understand how the body uses food.

Metabolism

Food must be broken down before the body can use it. This process is an integral part of metabolism. Metabolism is the sum of all the cellular processes that build, maintain, and supply energy to living tissue. During metabolism body tissue is built up and broken down, and heat and energy are produced.

Metabolism takes place in two phases. In **anabolism,** substances such as nutrients are changed into more complex substances and used to build body tissues. In **catabolism,** complex substances, including nutrients and body tissues, are broken down into simpler substances and converted into energy. The body uses this energy to maintain and repair itself. Of the energy people get from the food they eat, about 25% is directly used for bodily functions, and the rest becomes heat.

Each person's body requires a minimal amount of nutrients to carry on a basic level of metabolism to live. Each

TABLE 31-1 Calories Burned per Hour in Selected Activities		
Activity	**120-lb Person**	**190-lb Person**
Bicycling	360	570
Football (touch)	288	456
Calisthenics	324	516
Handball	456	720
Hiking	300	480
Running (10 mph)	720	1140
Skiing		
(downhill)	426	672
(cross-country)	564	888
Soccer	456	720
Swimming	228	366
Tennis	330	522
Volleyball	258	408
Walking (2 mph)	156	252

Adapted from Marvin R. Levy et al., *Life & Health: Targeting Wellness* (New York: McGraw-Hill, 1992).

person's daily nutritional requirements vary with age, weight, percentage of body fat, activity level, state of health, and other variables. The body's metabolic rate, or speed of metabolism, can also be affected by many factors, such as pregnancy, malnutrition, and disease.

Calories

The amount of energy a food produces in the body is measured in kilocalories. A kilocalorie, commonly called a **calorie,** is the amount of energy needed to raise the temperature of 1 kilogram of water by 1°C. Foods differ in the number of calories they contain. The more calories in a food, the more available energy it has. Calories are also used to measure the energy the body uses during all activities and metabolic processes.

As mentioned, people's daily nutritional needs differ, depending on variables of age, weight, percentage of body fat, activity level, and state of health. If people eat an excess of calories—more than the body can use—the excess is stored as fat in the body. Conversely, lowering caloric intake causes the body to burn off stored fat for energy.

Depending on the food's weight (in grams) or volume, each food has a value in calories. Therefore, you can count the number of calories a person consumes by monitoring food intake and adding up the calories in each food serving. You can use a food calorie counter, such as those often found in cookbooks and in nutrition books, to look up caloric values. A calorie counter tells you, for instance, that 1 cup of cooked carrots contains 50 calories or that 1 cup of cooked corn kernels contains 130 calories. Calories are also listed on the labels of food packages.

You can estimate the number of calories a person burns during certain activities by consulting a chart similar to Table 31-1. You can see how many more calories a 190-pound person burns than a 120-pound person does during the same activity.

Nutrients

The body needs a variety of nutrients for energy, growth, repair, and basic processes. Seven basic food components provide these nutrients and work together to help keep the body healthy:

1. Proteins
2. Carbohydrates
3. Fiber
4. Lipids
5. Vitamins
6. Minerals
7. Water

As the body digests foods that contain these components, it breaks them down so that it can use them. Of the seven components, only proteins, carbohydrates, and fats contain calories and provide the body with energy. The rest perform a variety of other essential functions.

Proteins

Protein is the most essential nutrient for building and repairing cells and tissue. Therefore, it is especially important for people to get enough protein during illness and healing. Other major functions of protein are to:

- Help maintain the body's water balance
- Assist with antibody production and disease resistance
- Help maintain body heat

The body makes protein out of **amino acids,** which are natural organic compounds found in plant and animal foods. Besides being used to build and maintain tissue, protein can be broken down to produce energy, especially if other energy sources are low. Each gram of protein contains 4 calories. Excess protein is broken down by the body and contributes to fat stores.

The optimal level of protein in a healthy person's diet is 10% to 20% of total caloric intake. More protein may be required during illnesses and recovery from injury. A deficiency in protein leads to weight loss and fatigue, malnutrition, extremely dry skin, lowered resistance to infection, and interference with normal growth processes.

Complete Proteins. There are 20 amino acids that are absolutely necessary to the body. The body can make 11 of them itself, but the remaining 9—called the essential amino acids—must be obtained through diet. Proteins that contain all 9 essential amino acids are called **complete proteins.** Complete proteins are found in animal food sources such as meat, fish, poultry, eggs (both the yolk and the white), and milk.

Adults who eat meat products are advised to eat lean meats to avoid ingesting too much fat, which can be harmful. For instance, poultry, especially if it is eaten without the skin and prepared by a low-fat cooking method such as grilling, is a good lean-meat choice. Low-fat or skim milk can be substituted for whole milk (except for children under the age of 2, who need more fat in their diet than do older children and adults).

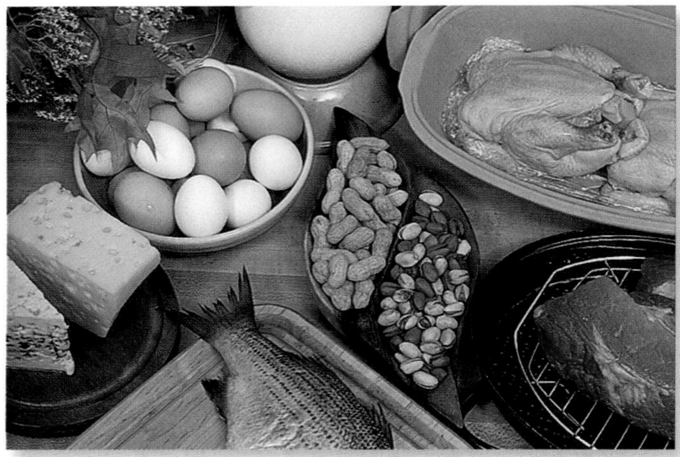

Figure 31-1. Foods such as meat, fish, poultry, eggs, and milk are complete proteins because they contain all the essential amino acids. Plant sources usually provide incomplete protein.

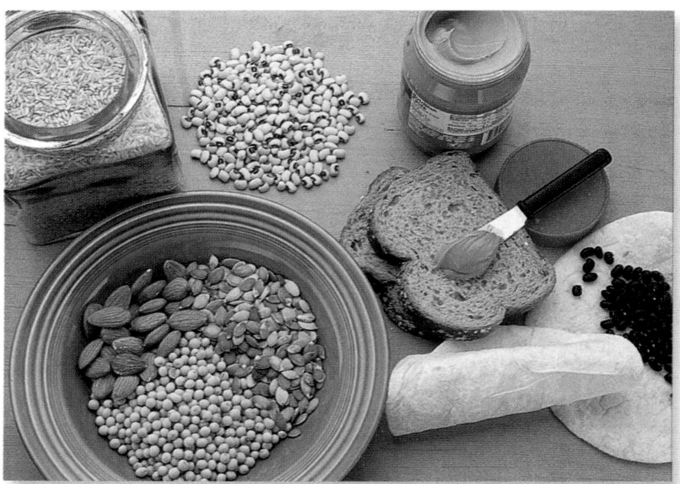

Figure 31-2. These foods, which contain incomplete protein, can be combined to make complete proteins.

Incomplete Proteins. Individual plant sources of food do not provide complete proteins. They provide **incomplete proteins**—proteins that lack one or more of the essential amino acids. Various plant sources such as nuts, dry beans, grains, and vegetables can be combined, however, to provide all nine essential amino acids. Figure 31-1 shows examples of foods containing incomplete proteins and complete proteins.

Planning for adequate protein intake and learning to combine protein foods to obtain all the essential amino acids are especially important for vegetarians (people who do not eat meat). Types of vegetarians include lacto-ovo-vegetarians, who eat no animal products except eggs and dairy products, and vegans, who eat no animal or dairy products at all. Although vegetarians may have to eat a larger quantity of foods than nonvegetarians to meet their daily nutritional needs, their diet offers advantages that include greater fiber intake and less fat. Figure 31-2 shows types of incomplete protein foods, such as rice and beans, that can be used in combination to provide complete proteins.

Carbohydrates

Carbohydrates in food provide about two-thirds of a person's daily energy needs. Carbohydrates also provide heat, help metabolize fat, and help reserve protein for uses other than supplying energy. Each gram of carbohydrate contains 4 calories. The daily requirement for carbohydrates is 50% to 60% of total caloric intake. Carbohydrate deficiency leads to weight loss, protein loss, and fatigue.

There are two basic types of carbohydrates:

1. Simple sugars, found in fruits, some vegetables, milk, and table sugar

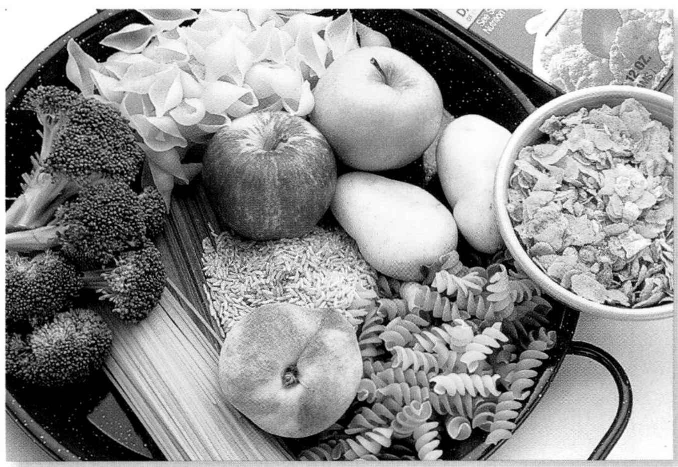

Figure 31-3. Healthful sources of carbohydrates are plentiful.

2. Complex carbohydrates, found in grain foods, such as breads, pastas, cereals, and rice; in some fruits and vegetables, such as potatoes, corn, broccoli, apples, and pears; and in legumes, such as peas, peanuts, and beans

Simple sugars are small molecules that consist of 1 or 2 sugar (saccharide) units. **Complex carbohydrates,** or polysaccharides, are long chains of sugar units. Starch is a type of complex carbohydrate that is a major source of energy from foods of plant origin. Fiber, another type of complex carbohydrate, is discussed in the next section.

Carbohydrates used for immediate fuel are converted to glucose, a simple sugar that cells use for energy. An excess of carbohydrates is either stored in the liver and muscle cells as glycogen (long chains of glucose units—the animal equivalent of starch) or converted into and stored as fat. After the body's carbohydrate reserves are depleted, it starts burning fat.

Healthful, nutritive sources of carbohydrates include fruits and vegetables, pasta, cereal, and potatoes (Figure 31-3). The American Dietetic Association suggests natural sources of carbohydrates with an emphasis on complex carbohydrates, such as vegetables, legumes, and whole grain breads and cereals. Sugary foods, such as sweet desserts, candy, and soft drinks, also contain carbohydrates, but they are high in calories and low in nutritional value.

Fiber

Fiber is in a separate category, although it is a type of complex carbohydrate. Fiber does not supply energy or heat to the body. It is the tough, stringy part of vegetables and grains. Fiber is not absorbed by the body, but it serves these important digestive functions:

- Increasing and softening the bulk of the stool, thus promoting normal defecation
- Absorbing organic wastes and toxins in the body so that they can be expelled
- Decreasing the rate of carbohydrate breakdown and absorption

Therapeutically, fiber can help treat and prevent constipation, hemorrhoids, diverticular disease, and irritable bowel syndrome. It is linked to reduced blood cholesterol levels, reduction of gallstone formation, control of diabetes, and reduction in the risk of certain types of cancer and other diseases. Too little fiber can result in an increased risk of colon cancer, hypercholesterolemia (high blood cholesterol), and increased blood glucose levels after eating. Too much fiber can cause constipation, diarrhea, and other gastrointestinal disorders and can impair mineral absorption.

The recommended amount of fiber for adults is 20 to 35 grams a day. Because fiber works in conjunction with other substances and nutrients, it is advisable to get dietary fiber from a variety of food sources (Figure 31-4). Adequate water intake is especially important for fiber to work properly.

Fiber can be classified as soluble or insoluble. Soluble fiber, found in foods such as oats, dry beans, barley, and some fruits and vegetables, is the type that tends to absorb fluid and swell when eaten. It slows the absorption of food from the digestive tract, helps control the blood sugar level of diabetics, lowers blood cholesterol levels, and softens and increases the bulk of stools. Insoluble fiber, found in the bran in whole wheat bread and brown rice, for example, promotes regular bowel movements by contributing to stool bulk.

Lipids

Lipids in the diet include dietary fats and fat-related substances. Fats are a concentrated source of energy that the body can store in large amounts. Each gram of fat contains 9 calories (more than twice the calorie content of proteins and carbohydrates). About 95% of the lipids from plant and animal sources of food are fats. These simple lipids, or **triglycerides,** consist of glycerol (an alcohol) and three fatty

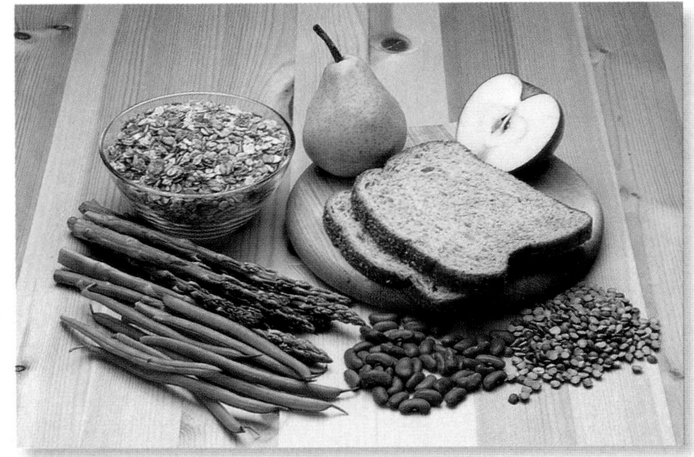

Figure 31-4. Dietary fiber serves many functions in the human body and is considered a basic food component.

acids. Chemical qualities of the fatty acids in a triglyceride determine the fat's characteristic flavor and texture. About 5% of dietary lipids are compound lipids such as cholesterol. Compound lipids are fat-related substances that are important components of cell membranes, nervous tissue, and some hormones. Compound lipids are vital to the transport of all fatlike substances within the body.

Lipids assist with important body functions and are essential to growth and metabolism. Among this nutrient's jobs are the following:

- Providing a concentrated source of heat and energy
- Transporting fat-soluble vitamins
- Storing energy in the form of body fat, which insulates and protects the organs
- Providing a feeling of satiety, or fullness, because it is digested more slowly than other nutrients

A lipid deficiency can interfere with the body's absorption and utilization of vitamins and can cause fatigue and dry skin. An excess of lipids, particularly some dietary fats, however, can lead to increased levels of triglycerides and cholesterol in the blood and an increased risk of heart and artery disease and other diseases. It is recommended that adults obtain no more than 30% of their daily calories from fat sources. Cholesterol intake should be limited to 300 milligrams per day. People with heart disease and certain other diseases or risks may benefit from even lower levels of lipid intake.

Saturated and Unsaturated Fats. The fats in food can be classified as either saturated fats or unsaturated fats (Figure 31-5). **Saturated fats** are derived primarily from animal sources and are usually solid at room temperature. They are found in meats and animal products such as butter, egg yolks, and whole milk. Coconut oil and palm oil are also saturated fats. Consumption of saturated fats should be restricted because these fats tend to raise blood cholesterol levels.

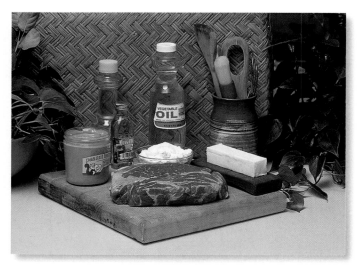

Figure 31-5. Foods that contain saturated fats include meat and butter. Most vegetable oils contain unsaturated fats.

Unsaturated fats are usually liquid at room temperature. They include most vegetable oils. Unsaturated fats can be divided into two classes:

1. Polyunsaturated fats, such as corn, soya, safflower, and sunflower oils
2. Monounsaturated fats, such as peanut, canola, and olive oils

Unsaturated fats can also be hydrogenated (have hydrogen added to their structures) so that they become solid at room temperature, as with margarine. Unsaturated fats tend to lower blood cholesterol.

The body needs essential fatty acids (primarily linoleic acid) for building and maintaining tissues. Because the body cannot produce these fatty acids, they must be supplied by food. Saturated fats in butter, egg yolks, and milk and unsaturated fats in corn, canola, sunflower, and safflower oils are good sources of essential fatty acids.

Cholesterol. **Cholesterol** is a fat-related substance produced by the liver that can also be obtained through dietary sources. Only animal-based foods contain cholesterol. It is essential to health because it:

- Serves as an integral part of cell membranes
- Provides the structural basis for all steroid hormones and vitamin D
- Serves as a constituent of bile, which aids in digestion

Lipid Levels in the Blood. Lipids, like other nutrients, are carried throughout the body in the bloodstream. When blood lipid levels become excessive, however, they pose certain risks. Doctors often order blood tests to determine the level of triglycerides and cholesterol in their patients' blood as a measure of overall health. High levels of cholesterol, especially if accompanied by high levels of triglycerides, may indicate an increased risk of heart disease, stroke, and peripheral vascular disease.

Lipids are not soluble in water; fats (or oil) and water do not mix. Because the fluid portion of blood is 90% water, lipids are encased in large molecules that are fat-soluble on the inside and water-soluble on the outside. These large molecules, called **lipoproteins,** carry lipids such as cholesterol and triglycerides through the bloodstream. Low-density lipoproteins (LDLs) and high-density lipoproteins (HDLs) are the two main types of lipoproteins. Cholesterol in blood is identified as HDL or LDL, depending on which type of lipoprotein carries it. High levels of LDL cholesterol in blood are a primary risk factor for heart attacks. High levels of LDL cholesterol most commonly occur in people whose diets are high in saturated fats. HDL cholesterol, commonly referred to as good cholesterol, carries excess cholesterol away from arteries and back to the liver for breakdown and elimination.

Patients can often reduce elevated cholesterol levels by increasing exercise and intake of soluble fiber and decreasing the dietary intake of saturated fats. (Table 31-2 lists the

TABLE 31-2 Saturated Fat and Cholesterol Contents of Various Foods

Food	Saturated Fat (g)	Cholesterol (mg)
Cheddar cheese (1 oz)	6.0	30
Mozzarella, part skim (1 oz)	3.1	15
Whole milk (1 c)	5.1	33
Skim milk (1 c)	0.3	4
Butter (1 tbsp)	7.1	31
Mayonnaise (1 tbsp)	1.7	8
Tuna in oil (3 oz)	1.4	55
Tuna in water (3 oz)	0.3	48
Lean ground beef, broiled (3 oz)	6.2	74
Leg of lamb, roasted (3 oz)	5.6	78
Bacon (3 slices)	3.3	16
Chicken breast, roasted (3 oz)	0.9	73

Source: U.S. Department of Agriculture.

saturated fat and cholesterol contents of various foods.) These measures tend to elevate the level of HDL cholesterol in the bloodstream and reduce the level of LDL cholesterol.

Vitamins

Vitamins are organic substances that are essential for normal body growth and maintenance and resistance to infection. Vitamins also help the body use other nutrients and assist in various body processes.

Most vitamins are absorbed directly through the digestive tract. They can be either water-soluble or fat-soluble. Water-soluble vitamins, such as vitamin C and the B vitamins, are not stored by the body and therefore must be replaced every day. Fat-soluble vitamins, such as vitamins A, D, E, and K, are stored for longer periods.

The amounts of vitamins the body needs are relatively small; however, a vitamin deficiency through lack of ingestion or absorption can lead to disease. Some vitamins can also cause health problems if taken in excess. Toxic levels of vitamin A, for example, can produce effects ranging from headache to liver damage. Because the level of vitamin intake is so essential to health, the Food and Nutrition Board of the National Research Council has established recommended dietary allowances (RDAs) for vitamins. For detailed information on specific vitamins, see Table 31-3.

Eating a well-balanced, nutritious diet minimizes the likelihood of vitamin deficiency. Many manufactured foods are also vitamin-fortified. Even so, some people choose to augment their diets with vitamin supplements (Figure 31-6). A physician or other member of the medical team may, in some instances, prescribe vitamin supplements for patients.

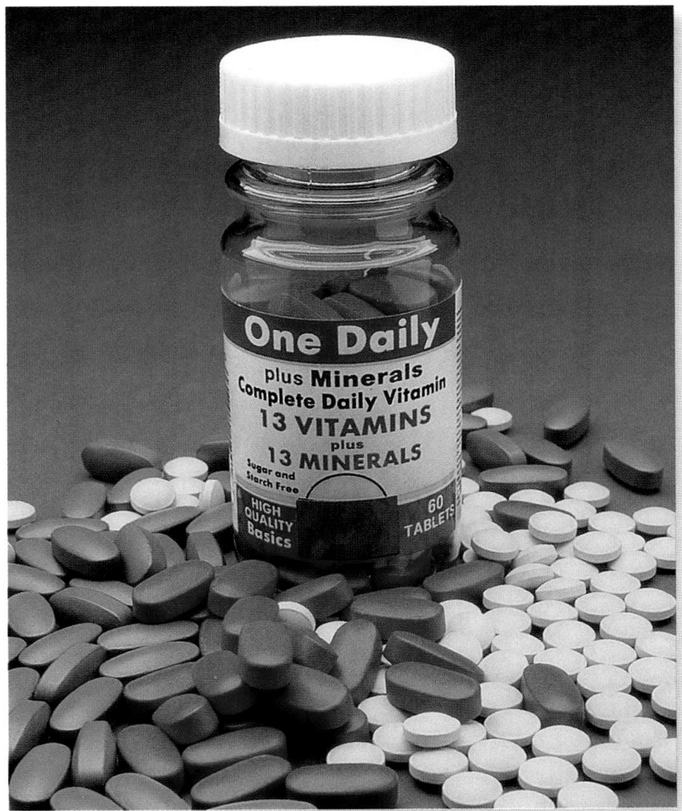

Figure 31-6. Some people use supplements to augment their dietary intake of vitamins.

Minerals

Minerals are natural, inorganic substances the body needs to help build and maintain body tissues and carry on life

TABLE 31-3 Vitamins				
Vitamin	**Functions**	**Adult RDA***	**Food Sources**	**Deficiencies and/ or Toxicities**
Vitamin A (retinol, provitamin, carotene)	Aids in night vision; cell growth and maintenance; normal reproductive function; health of skin, mucous membranes, and internal tracts	Males: 1000 μg retinol equivalents Females: 800 μg retinol equivalents	Milk fat; butter; egg yolks; meat; fish liver oil; liver; green, yellow, and orange leafy vegetables; yellow and orange fruits	Deficiency: night blindness; dry, rough skin; risk of internal infection Toxicity: headache, vomiting, joint pain, hair loss, jaundice, liver damage
Vitamin B_1 (thiamine)	Aids enzymes in breaking down and using carbohydrates; helps the nerves, muscles, and heart function efficiently	Males: 1.5 mg Females: 1.1 mg	Whole grains, brewer's yeast, organ meats, lean pork, beef, liver, legumes, seeds, nuts	Deficiency: beriberi with appetite loss, digestive problems, muscle weakness and deterioration, nervous disorders, heart failure
Vitamin B_2 (riboflavin)	Aids enzymes in metabolism of fats and proteins	Males: 1.2–1.5 mg Females: 1.0–1.1 mg	Dairy products, organ meats, green leafy vegetables, enriched and fortified grain products	Deficiency: cracks at lip corners, irritations at nasal angles, inflammation of the tongue, seborrheic dermatitis, anemia
Vitamin B_3 (niacin)	Aids enzymes in metabolism of carbohydrates and fats	Males: 15–19 mg Females: 13–15 mg	Meat, fish, poultry, enriched and fortified grain products	Deficiency: pellagra with dermatitis, diarrhea, inflammation of mucous membranes, dementia Toxicity: dilation of blood vessels; if sustained, abnormal liver function
Vitamin B_6 (pyridoxine)	Aids enzymes in synthesis of amino acids	Males: 2.0 mg Females: 1.6 mg	Chicken, fish, pork, liver, kidney, some vegetables, grains, nuts, legumes	Deficiency: convulsions, dermatitis, anemia Toxicity: loss of muscle coordination, severe sensory neuropathy
Folate (compounds)	Works with cobalamins in nucleic acid synthesis and metabolism of amino acids; maintains red blood cells	Males: 200 μg Females: 180 μg	Liver, yeast, legumes, green leafy vegetables, some fruits	Deficiency: glossitis, diarrhea, anemia, lethargy

continued ⟶

TABLE 31-3 Vitamins *(continued)*

Vitamin	Functions	Adult RDA*	Food Sources	Deficiencies and/ or Toxicities
Vitamin B_{12} (cobalamins)	Works with folate in nucleic acid synthesis and metabolism of amino acids; coenzyme in metabolism of fatty acids	2.0 μg	Seafood, meat, milk, eggs, cheese, brewer's yeast, blackstrap molasses	Deficiency: pernicious anemia, irreversible liver damage
Vitamin C (ascorbic acid)	Coenzyme involved in collagen production, capillary integrity, use of iron in hemoglobin, and synthesis of many hormones; improves absorption of iron; is an antioxidant	60 mg	Citrus fruits, mangoes, strawberries, green peppers, broccoli, potatoes, green leafy vegetables	Deficiency: scurvy with hemorrhages, loose teeth, poor wound healing Toxicity: stomachache, diarrhea
Vitamin D (calciferol)	Builds bones and teeth; helps maintain calcium-phosphorus balance in blood	5–10 μg	Egg yolks; butter; liver; fortified milk, margarine, and prepared cereals	Deficiency: rickets in children, osteomalacia in adults Toxicity: excess blood calcium and phosphorus, calcium deposits in soft tissue, bone pain, irreversible kidney and cardiovascular damage
Vitamin E (group)	Is an intracellular antioxidant; maintains cell structure; aids in formation of red blood cells	Males: 10 mg Females: 8 mg	Vegetable oils, margarine, shortening, wheat germ, nuts, green leafy vegetables	Deficiency: damage to cells, hemolytic anemia
Vitamin K (compounds)	Aids in blood clotting and bone growth	Males: 70–80 μg Females: 60–65 μg	Green leafy vegetables, milk, dairy products, meat, eggs, cereals, fruits, vegetables	Deficiency: slow blood clotting; hemorrhagic disease in newborns

Source: National Research Council, *Recommended Dietary Allowances,* 10th ed. (Washington, DC: National Academy Press, 1989).

*RDAs may vary for different age groups.

functions. Depending on the relative amounts the body requires, minerals fall into two categories:

1. Major minerals that the body needs in fairly large quantities, including calcium, magnesium, and phosphorus
2. Trace minerals that the body needs in tiny amounts, including iron, iodine, zinc, selenium, copper, fluoride, chromium, manganese, and molybdenum

Minerals essential to good health include calcium, iron, iodine, zinc, copper, magnesium, phosphorus, fluoride, manganese, chromium, molybdenum, and selenium. Calcium, iron, and iodine are the minerals in which people are most often deficient. Most minerals are absorbed in the intestines, and any excess is eliminated.

Minerals With Recommended Dietary Allowances. There are several minerals for which RDAs have been established. These minerals are calcium, iron, iodine, zinc, magnesium, phosphorus, and selenium.

Calcium. Calcium builds healthy bones and teeth, aids in blood clotting, and helps nerves and muscles function properly. It is found in dairy products, green leafy vegetables, broccoli, legumes, and the soft bones of sardines and salmon (Figure 31-7).

Calcium deficiency can cause poor bone growth and tooth development in children, osteoporosis in adults, and poor blood clotting. The normal requirement is 800 to 1200 milligrams per day.

Iron. Iron, one of the most important nutrients, is essential for the production of red blood cells, which transport oxygen throughout the body. It is also a component of enzymes needed for energy production. Although iron is found in a wide variety of foods, it is the most frequently deficient nutrient in people's diets. Liver, meat, poultry, fish, egg yolks, fortified breads and cereals, dark green vegetables, and dried fruits are good dietary sources of iron (Figure 31-8), although less than 20% of it is usually absorbed.

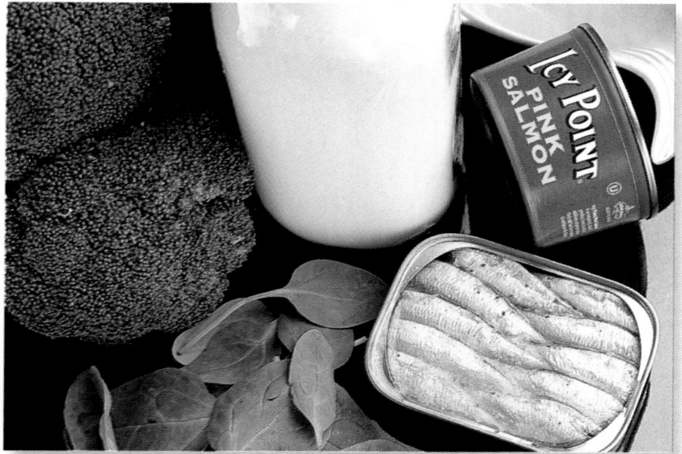

Figure 31-7. These foods are excellent sources of calcium, a mineral that is necessary for strong bones and teeth.

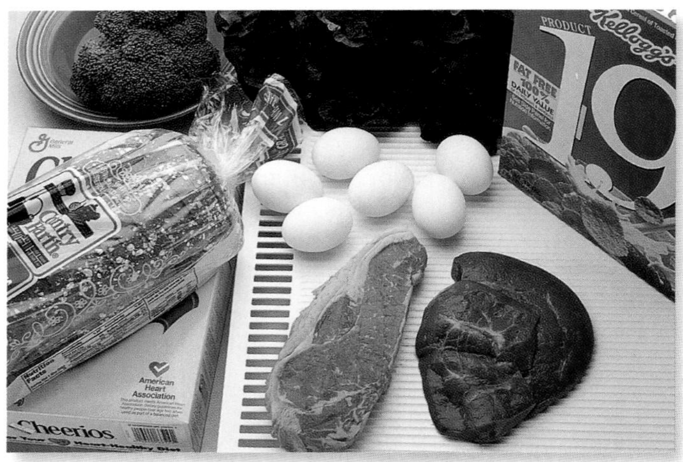

Figure 31-8. Iron, a mineral that is needed in small amounts, is found in a wide variety of foods.

Iron deficiency can cause anemia, a blood disorder that results in fatigue, weakness, and impaired mental abilities. At toxic levels iron may increase the risk of coronary heart disease. The daily requirement is 10 to 15 milligrams.

Iodine. Iodine plays a vital role in the activities of the thyroid hormones, which are involved in reproduction, growth, nerve and muscle function, and the production of new blood cells. Deficiency can cause an enlarged thyroid gland, known as goiter. Iodine can be obtained in seafood, iodized salt, and seaweed products. The daily requirement is 150 micrograms.

Zinc. Zinc promotes normal growth and wound healing and participates in many cell activities that involve proteins, enzymes, and hormones. It is found in liver, lamb, beef, eggs, oysters, and whole grain breads and cereals, although it is not always easily absorbed. Deficiency can result in growth retardation, impaired taste and smell, and reduced immune function. The daily requirement is 12 to 15 milligrams.

Magnesium. Magnesium activates cell enzymes, helps metabolize proteins and carbohydrates, maintains the structural integrity of the heart and other muscles, and aids in muscle contraction. Good sources include green leafy vegetables, nuts, legumes, bananas, and whole grain products. A deficiency may result from persistent vomiting or diarrhea, kidney disease, general malnutrition, alcoholism, and the use of certain medications. The daily requirement is 280 milligrams for women and 350 milligrams for men.

Phosphorus. Phosphorus is involved in bone and tooth formation, chemical reactions in the body, and energy production. It is found in dairy foods, animal foods, fish, cereals, nuts, and legumes. A deficiency of phosphorus can cause gastrointestinal, blood cell, and other disorders. Toxicity is harmful as well. The daily requirement is 800 milligrams for adults 25 and over.

Selenium. Selenium works with vitamin E to aid metabolism, growth, and fertility. It is found in seafood, kidney, liver, meats, grain products, and seeds. A daily dietary intake of 55 micrograms for women and 70 micrograms for men is recommended.

Minerals With Estimated Safe and Adequate Dietary Intakes. When data were sufficient to estimate a range of requirements—but insufficient for developing an RDA—the Food and Nutrition Board established a category of safe and adequate intakes for essential nutrients. The minerals in this category are copper, fluoride, chromium, manganese, and molybdenum.

Copper. Copper interacts with iron to form hemoglobin and red blood cells. It can be obtained through a wide variety of foods, such as liver, seafood, nuts and seeds, and whole grain products. Copper deficiency can cause anemia and central nervous system problems. The safe and adequate range of dietary copper for adults is 1.5 to 3.0 milligrams per day.

Fluoride. Fluoride is another contributor to bone and tooth formation, and it protects against tooth decay. Many municipal water supplies are fluoridated, and the mineral is also contained in saltwater fish, tea, and fluoridated toothpaste. Fluoride deficiency may predispose people to cavities and osteoporosis. Excess fluoride can cause discoloration and pitting of the teeth as well as other conditions. The range of safe and adequate intakes for adults is 1.5 to 4.0 milligrams per day.

Chromium. Chromium is essential for the body to use glucose, the primary food of cells. Foods containing chromium include calf's liver, American cheese, and wheat germ. A range of intakes between 50 and 200 micrograms per day is considered safe and adequate for adults.

Manganese. Manganese is part of several cell enzymes. It is also essential for bone formation and maintenance, insulin production, and nutrient metabolism. It is found in whole grain products, fruits, vegetables, and tea. A daily dietary intake of 2 to 5 milligrams for adults is recommended.

Molybdenum. Molybdenum helps in the metabolism of the mineral sulfur and the production of uric acid. The best sources are legumes, whole grains, milk, and organ meats such as liver and kidneys. The recommended range for dietary intake is 75 to 250 micrograms per day for adults.

Water

Water has no caloric value, but it contributes about 65% of body weight and is essential to the body's normal functioning. In general, water helps provide the body with other nutrients it needs and helps rid the body of what it does not need. Water has many functions, including these:

- Helping to maintain the balance of all the fluids in the body
- Lubricating the body's moving parts
- Dissolving chemicals and nutrients
- Aiding in digestion
- Helping to transport nutrients and secretions throughout the body
- Flushing out wastes
- Regulating body temperature through perspiration

The amount of water in the body directly affects the concentration and distribution of body fluids and all the functions related to them. The body maintains a careful balance between water consumed (in foods and beverages) and water lost (through urination, perspiration, and respiration). In a healthy fluid balance, water input equals water output. Measuring an ill person's level of water intake and output can help determine the best fluid replacement regimen to use.

People obtain most of their water from beverages such as tap water, milk, and fruit juices as well as coffee, tea, and soft drinks. On average, a person needs to drink six to eight glasses of water a day to maintain a healthy water balance. The daily need for water varies with size and age, the temperatures to which someone is exposed, the degree of physical exertion, and the water content of the foods one eats. Someone who is eating mostly foods with a high water content, such as fruits and vegetables, can drink a little less water than someone who is eating mostly foods with a low water content.

If people get too little water or lose too much water through vomiting, diarrhea, burns, or perspiration, they become dehydrated. Signs and symptoms of dehydration include dry lips and mucous membranes, weakness, lethargy, decreased urine output, and increased thirst. Severe dehydration can lead to hypovolemia, a reduction in the volume of blood in the body. Severe hypovolemia can result in inadequate blood pressure that affects the functioning of the heart, central nervous system, and various organs—a condition known as hypovolemic shock. If dehydration progresses so that water is lost from body cells, death usually occurs within a few days.

Procedure 31-1 explains how to educate patients to drink the right amount of water each day to prevent dehydration. Make sure patients know whether they are to drink extra fluids to replace fluids lost in an illness or to help rid the body of waste.

Principal Electrolytes and Other Nutrients of Special Interest

The principal electrolytes are essential to normal body functioning. Other nutrients, such as antioxidants, also merit special mention.

Principal Electrolytes. Although the principal electrolytes in the body—sodium, potassium, and chloride—are often excluded from lists of nutrients, they are essential dietary components. Electrolytes play an important role in maintaining body functions, such as normal heart rhythm.

PROCEDURE 31.1

Educating Adult Patients About Daily Water Requirements

Objective: To teach patients how much water their bodies need to maintain health

OSHA Guidelines: This procedure does not involve exposure to blood, body fluids, or tissues.

Materials: Patient education literature, patient's chart, pen

Method

1. Explain to patients how important water is to the body. Point out the water content of the body and the many functions of water in the body: maintaining the body's fluid balance, lubricating the body's moving parts, transporting nutrients and secretions.
2. Add any comments applicable to an individual patient's health status—for example, issues related to medication use, physical activity, pregnancy, and so on. Be aware that some elderly patients purposely limit their fluid intake because of incontinence or physical limitations that make getting to a bathroom difficult.
3. Explain that people obtain water by drinking water and other fluids and by eating water-containing foods. On average, a person should drink six to eight glasses of water a day to maintain a healthy water balance in which intake equals excretion. People's daily need for water varies with size and age, the temperatures to which they are exposed, degree of physical exertion, and the water content of foods eaten. Make sure you reinforce the physician's or dietitian's recommendations for a particular patient's water needs.

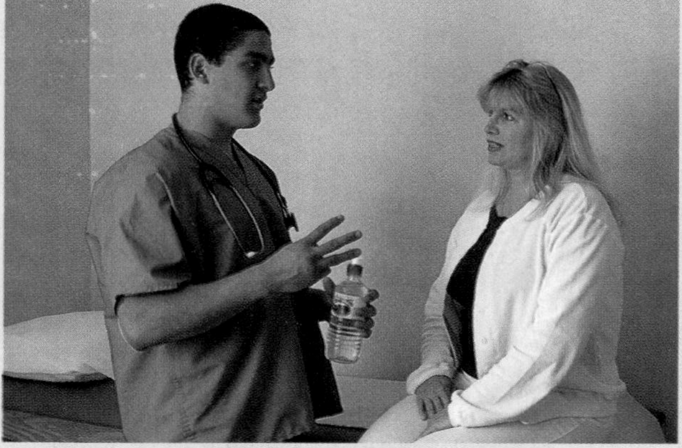

Figure 31-9. Using a personal water bottle that holds 16 ounces, the patient can make a point of drinking three to four full bottles daily.

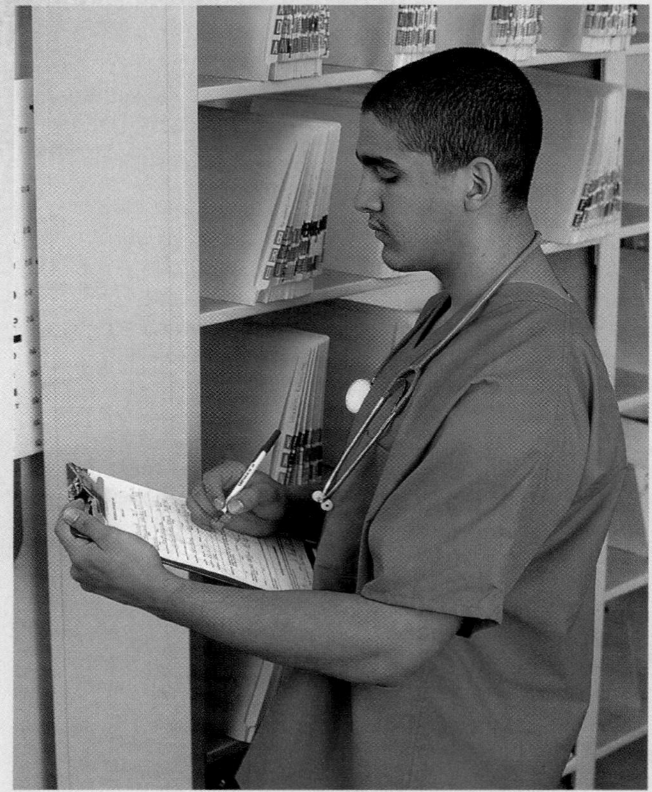

Figure 31-10. Always document patient education sessions in the patient's chart.

4. Caution patients that soft drinks, coffee, and tea are not good substitutes for water and that it would be wise to filter out any harmful chemicals contained in the local tap water or to drink bottled water, if possible.
5. Provide patients with tips about reminders to drink the requisite amount of water. Some patients may benefit from using a water bottle of a particular size, so they know they have to drink, say, three full bottles of water each day (Figure 31-9). Another helpful tip is to make a habit of drinking a glass of water at certain points in the daily routine, such as first thing in the morning and before lunch.
6. Remind patients that you and the physician are available to discuss any problems or questions.
7. Document any formal patient education sessions or significant exchanges with a patient in the patient's chart, noting whether the patient understood the information presented. Then initial the entry (Figure 31-10).

Sodium (Na) maintains fluid and acid-base balances, assists in the transport of glucose, and maintains normal conditions inside and outside cells. Salt is the main dietary source of sodium, and high salt intakes are normally associated with a diet high in processed foods. Too much sodium can be associated with high blood pressure in salt-sensitive individuals. Although many Americans consume far more, it is recommended that daily sodium intake be limited to 2.4 grams or less.

Potassium (K) is a crucial element in the maintenance of muscle contraction and fluid and electrolyte balance. It contributes to acid-base balance and the transmission of nerve impulses. Its role in fluid balance helps regulate blood pressure. Potassium occurs in unprocessed foods, particularly in fruits such as bananas, raisins, and oranges; many vegetables; and fresh meats (Figure 31-11). The minimum requirement is 1600 to 2000 milligrams per day.

Chloride (Cl) is essential in maintaining fluid and electrolyte balance, and it is a necessary component of hydrochloric acid, secreted into the stomach during digestion of food. Because dietary chloride comes almost entirely from sodium chloride, sources are essentially the same as those of sodium.

Antioxidants. **Antioxidants** are chemical agents that fight certain cell-destroying chemical substances called free radicals. In fact, antioxidants may help ward off cancer and heart disease by neutralizing free radicals, by-products of normal metabolism that may also form as a result of exposure to various damaging factors such as cigarette smoke, alcohol, or x-rays. Antioxidants may be added to foods and cosmetics as preservatives. The nutrients beta-carotene, vitamin C, vitamin E, and selenium (Figure 31-12) are natural antioxidants.

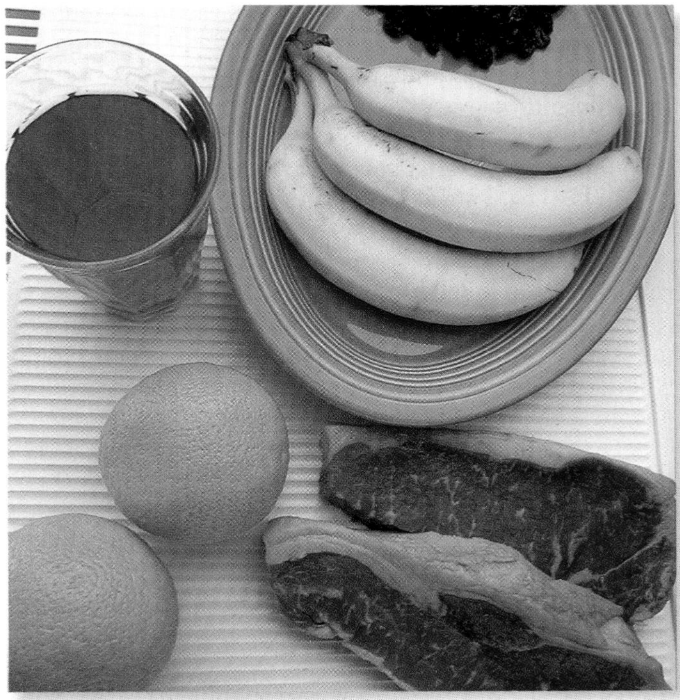

Figure 31-11. These foods are good sources of potassium.

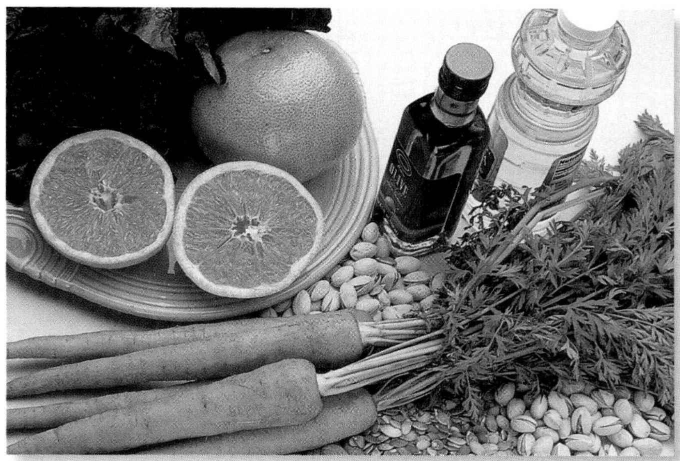

Figure 31-12. Antioxidants are substances in food that may offer protection against certain chronic diseases. Foods rich in beta-carotene, vitamin C, vitamin E, and selenium contain antioxidants.

Dietary Guidelines

A variety of dietary guidelines exist to help people get proper nutrition, reduce the occurrence of disease, and control their weight. These recommendations, which are issued by governmental agencies or private associations, are designed to encourage healthy eating habits.

Dietary guidelines suggest the types and quantities of food that people should eat each day. They may also contain recommendations about which types of foods to limit and which types of foods to increase.

Dietary Guidelines for Americans

The U.S. Department of Agriculture and the U.S. Department of Health and Human Services updated their Dietary Guidelines for Americans in 2000. These guidelines encourage people to eat a balanced diet and to limit consumption of less nutritious foods. Here are their recommendations.

- Eat a variety of foods to get the energy, protein, vitamins, minerals, and fiber you need for good health
- Balance the food you eat with physical activity—maintain or improve your weight to help reduce your chances of high blood pressure, heart disease, stroke, some types of cancer, and diabetes
- Choose a diet with plenty of grain products, vegetables, and fruits, which provide needed vitamins, minerals, fiber, and complex carbohydrates and can help you lower your intake of fat
- Choose a diet low in fat, saturated fat, and cholesterol to reduce your risk of heart attack and certain types of cancer

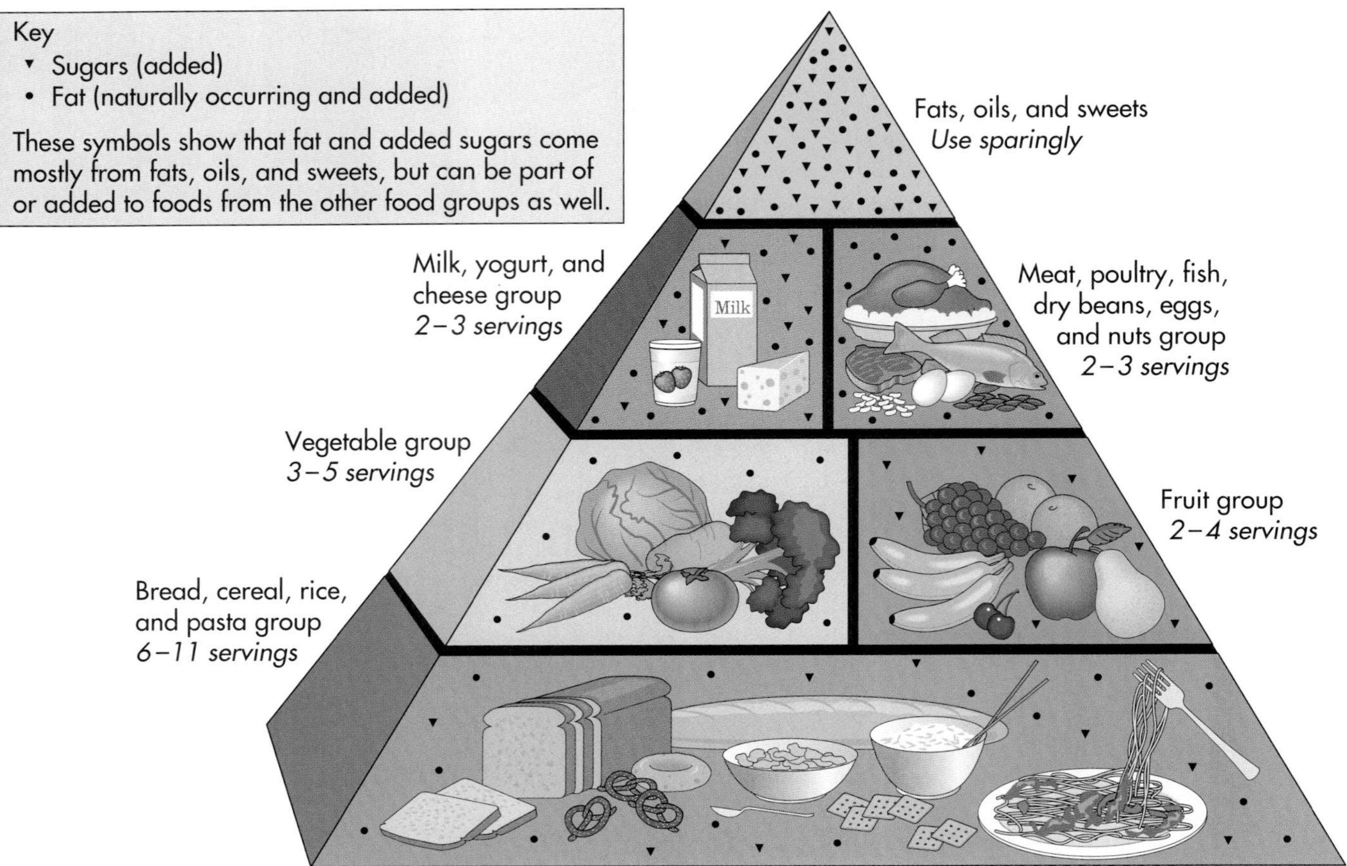

Figure 31-13. The U.S. Department of Agriculture's Food Guide Pyramid can be used to plan a nutritious, well-balanced diet.

- Choose a diet moderate in sugars—a diet with lots of sugars has too many calories and too few nutrients and can contribute to tooth decay
- Choose a diet moderate in salt and sodium to help reduce your risk of high blood pressure
- If you drink alcoholic beverages, do so in moderation—alcoholic beverages supply calories, but few or no nutrients

Food Guide Pyramid

In 1992 the U.S. Department of Agriculture introduced a new food pyramid, which serves as a nutritional guideline to replace previous pyramids, food wheels, and food groups. The pyramid is divided into six parts to show the quantities of food people should consume daily from each of five basic food groups (Figure 31-13). The sixth, and smallest, part of the pyramid represents fats, oils, and sweets, which should be eaten sparingly. The Food Guide Pyramid shows how the proportions of each basic food group contribute to a balanced diet.

Two symbols, a circle and a triangle, are used on the pyramid. The circle indicates fat that occurs naturally or is added, and the triangle indicates sugar that is added. These symbols show how fat and sugar—although they come mainly from fats, oils, and sweets—can occur naturally or be added to foods in the five basic food groups.

You can use the Food Guide Pyramid to explain nutritional guidelines to patients. If you post a colorful copy of it in your office—perhaps near the scale or on the wall of the examination room—you can use it as a visual aid when helping patients plan a balanced diet.

To help patients plan a balanced diet, you will need to know how much of a food equals a serving. For example, one serving of fruit equals one medium apple or orange, ½ cup canned fruit, or ¾ cup (6 ounces) fruit juice. You should refer to a chart similar to Table 31-4, which lists serving sizes for foods in each of the basic food groups. Serving sizes for young children are smaller; for example, serving sizes for toddlers and preschoolers are about half the sizes listed in the table.

The Food Guide Pyramid is a general guideline. It does not provide exact information about what to eat. Nutritional needs vary from person to person, depending on age, gender, and activity level (see Table 31-5). That is why the pyramid lists ranges of servings.

Some patients may have special dietary preferences or choices. Vegetarians do not eat meat, poultry, and fish. In order to provide vegetarians with guidelines for healthful eating, the American Dietetic Association has developed a Food Guide Pyramid specifically for these individuals (Figure 31-14).

TABLE 31-4 What Counts as a Serving?	
Food Group	**Food and Quantity**
Bread, cereal, rice, and pasta	1 slice bread 1 oz ready-to-eat cereal ½ c cooked cereal, rice, or pasta
Vegetable	1 c raw leafy vegetables ½ c other vegetables, cooked or raw ¾ c vegetable juice
Fruit	1 medium apple, banana, or orange ½ c chopped, cooked, or canned fruit ¾ c fruit juice
Milk, yogurt, and cheese	1 c milk or yogurt 1½ oz natural cheese 2 oz process cheese
Meat, poultry, fish, dry beans, eggs, and nuts	2–3 oz cooked lean meat, poultry, or fish ½ c cooked dry beans or 1 egg counts as 1 oz lean meat 2 tbsp peanut butter or ⅓ c nuts counts as 1 oz meat

Source: Nutrition and Your Health: *Dietary Guidelines for Americans,* 5th ed. (Washington, DC: U.S. Department of Agriculture and U.S. Department of Health and Human Services, 2000).

TABLE 31-5 Number of Servings Required for Different Calorie Levels			
Calorie Level (Common Individuals in Group)	**About 1600 (Many Women, Older Adults)**	**About 2200 (Children, Teen Girls, Most Men, Active Women)**	**About 2800 (Teen Boys, Active Men)**
Grain Products Group Servings	6	9	11
Vegetable Group Servings	3	4	5
Fruit Group Servings	2	3	4
Milk Group Servings	2–3*	2–3*	2–3*
Meat and Beans Group Servings	2 (5 oz total)	2 (6 oz total)	3 (7 oz total)
Total Fat (g)	53	73	93

Source: *Nutrition and Your Health: Dietary Guidelines for Americans,* 5th ed. (Washington, DC: U.S. Department of Agriculture and U.S. Department of Health and Human Services, 2000).

*Women who are pregnant or breast-feeding, teenagers, and young adults to age 24 need 3 servings.

American Cancer Society Guidelines

The American Cancer Society has set forth the following guidelines to aid in the prevention of cancer.

- Eat more high-fiber foods such as fruits, vegetables, and whole grain cereals
- Eat plenty of dark green and deep yellow fruits and vegetables rich in vitamins A and C
- Eat plenty of broccoli, cabbage, brussels sprouts, kohlrabi, and cauliflower
- Be moderate in consumption of salt-cured, smoked, and nitrite-cured foods, such as bacon and smoked sausage
- Cut down on total fat intake from animal sources and fats and oils
- Avoid obesity
- Be moderate in consumption of alcoholic beverages

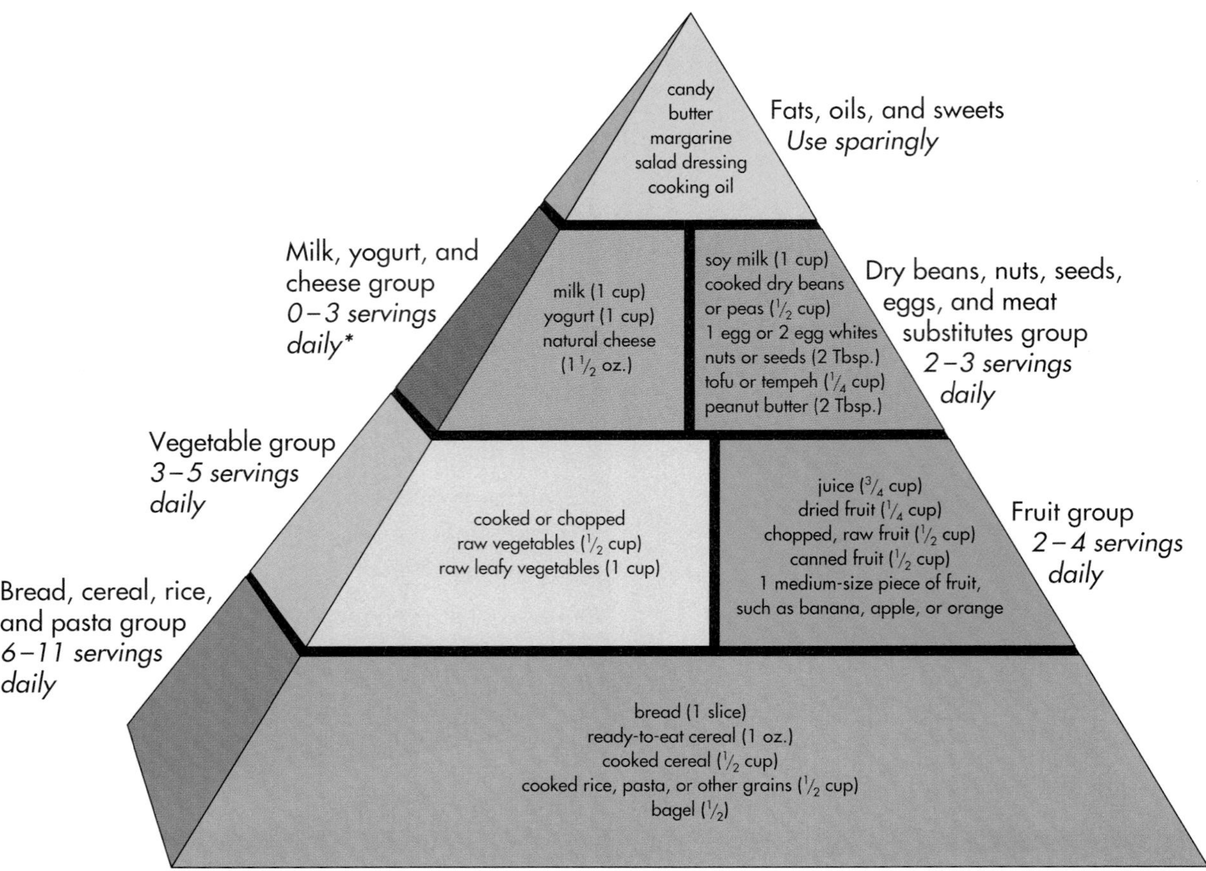

*Vegetarians who choose not to use milk, yogurt, or cheese need to select other food sources rich in calcium.

Figure 31-14. The American Dietetic Association's Food Guide Pyramid for Vegetarian Meal Planning can provide vegetarians with suggestions for healthy, balanced nutrition.

The American Cancer Society also advises that

> high-fat diets may contribute to the development of cancers of the breast, colon, and prostate. High-fiber foods might help reduce risk of colon cancer. A varied diet containing plenty of vegetables and fruits rich in vitamins A and C may reduce risk for a wide range of cancers. Salt-cured, smoked, and nitrite-cured foods have been linked to esophagus and stomach cancer.

Assessing Nutritional Levels

Doctors assess a patient's nutritional status by analyzing age, health status, height, weight, type of body frame, body circumference, percentage of body fat, nutritional and exercise patterns, and energy needs. They accomplish this assessment through direct measurement as well as through questionnaires and interviews. During the analysis, doctors take into account individual factors such as culture, beliefs, lifestyle, and education.

To measure fat as a percentage of body weight, doctors may perform a **skinfold test,** measuring the thickness of a fold of skin with a caliper (Figure 31-15). This measurement is often made on the triceps, midway between the shoulder and elbow. The test indicates the total percentage of fat, because about 50% of body fat is just below the skin and the volume of fat below the skin is related to the volume of inner fat. A trained individual must perform this test, which must be precise to be reliable.

The optimal percentage of body fat differs between men and women. For males younger than age 50, it is 10% to 14%; older than 50, 12% to 19%. In females younger than age 50, it is 14% to 23%; older than 50, 16% to 25%. Aging usually changes the ratio a bit because some muscle tissue is replaced by fat, even if weight remains constant.

Modifying Diets

A person's diet has a significant effect on health, appearance, and recovery from disease. After a physician or dietitian has established a patient's nutritional status, any necessary or beneficial dietary adjustments can be instituted. Dietary modification may be used alone or in combination with other therapies to prevent or treat illness. Factors affecting people's specific dietary needs may

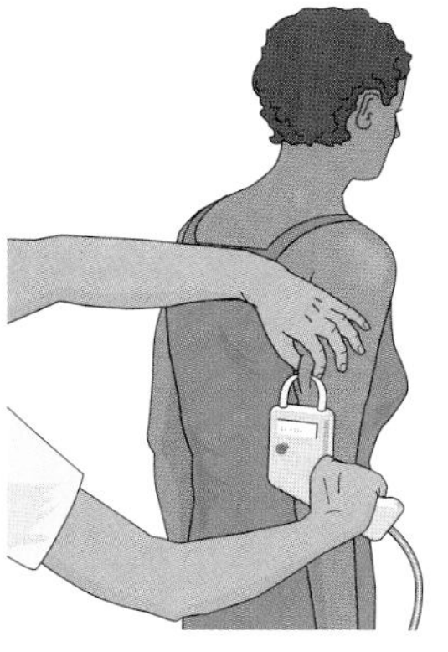

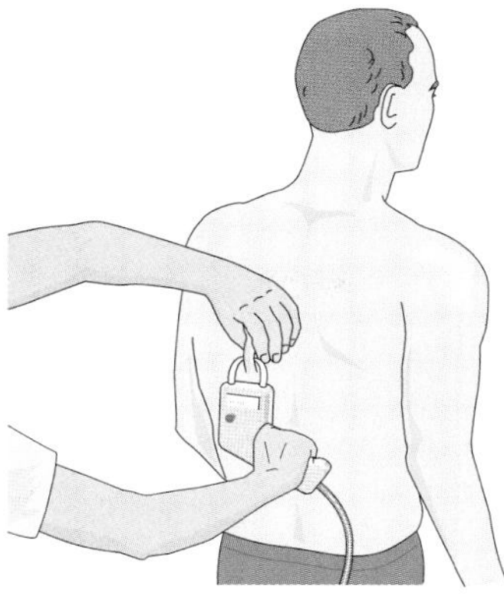

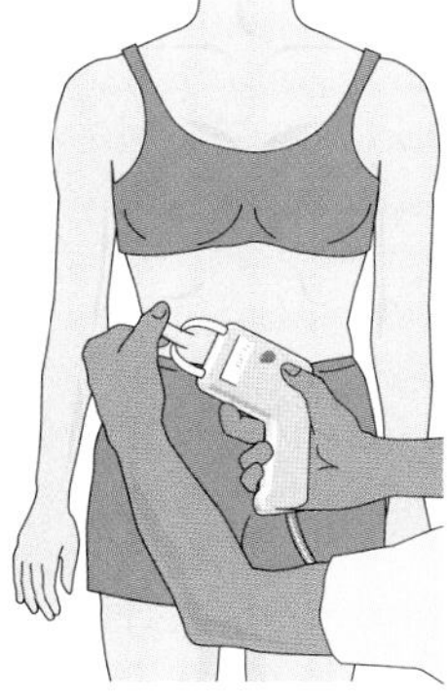

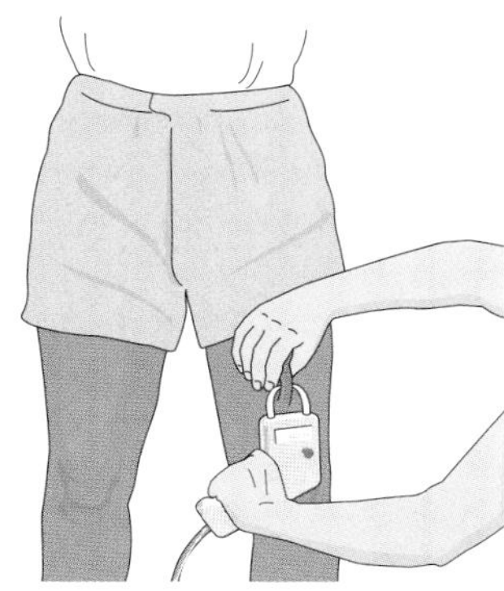

Figure 31-15. To estimate an individual's body fat percentage, a professional uses a tool called a caliper to measure the thickness of a fold of skin at one or more points on the body.

include pregnancy, injury, disease, vegetarianism, aging, genetic disorders, and substance abuse.

Adjustments in diet may involve any of the following:

- Restricting certain foods
- Emphasizing particular foods
- Changing daily caloric intake
- Changing the amount of a specific nutrient
- Changing textures of foods
- Altering the number of daily meals
- Changing variables such as bulk or spiciness

Physicians work with dietitians to determine the best diet therapy to initiate for individual patients. Diet therapy is based on many factors, including particular foods and nutrients associated with different diseases or body states.

Patients With Specific Nutritional Needs

Patients may have a variety of conditions that require special diets. In situations such as those that follow, you may need to educate patients about their diets and answer their questions. You may need to provide encouragement and emotional support and teach patients' caregivers how to perform physical tasks, such as holding utensils for patients during meals.

Patients With Allergies. Some patients have food allergies. Allergic reactions to food can range from sneezing or a rash to the potentially fatal state of anaphylaxis, described in Chapter 26. The scratch test described in Chapter 23 is used to determine which foods cause an allergic reaction.

Usually specific foods must be eliminated from or restricted in an allergic patient's diet. Procedure 31-2 provides information on discussing with the patient potential dangers of common foods and reactions to those foods.

Some of the most common food allergens are wheat, milk, eggs, and chocolate. The doctor may confirm an allergy by eliminating and then reintroducing the patient's suspect foods one by one. The patient's allergy may decrease over time through systematic desensitization by means of allergy shots and other regimens.

If a food that is being eliminated or restricted was a primary source of nutrients for the patient, then the doctor must adjust the diet to include another source of those nutrients. For example, if a baby is allergic to milk, the doctor recommends a milk-substitute formula.

Patients With Anemia. Iron deficiency anemia, the most common type of anemia, is usually caused by chronic blood loss, a lack of iron in the diet, impaired intestinal absorption of iron, or an increased need for iron, as in pregnancy. A patient may need to take iron supplements and ingest more dietary iron as part of the treatment for this disorder. Foods high in iron include liver, egg yolks, dark green vegetables, beans, some dried fruits, and fortified breads and cereals.

Patients With Cancer. Most patients being treated for cancer undergo weight loss resulting both from the cancer and from treatments involving radiation or chemotherapy. To help their bodies fight off the cancer, these patients must increase their caloric intake. It is especially important that they get enough protein, because protein is needed to regenerate cells to replace the cells destroyed by the cancer and cancer treatments. These patients may also need to increase their intake of B vitamins and vitamins A, C, D, and E to support tissue growth and repair and promote efficient metabolism and use of all nutrients in the diet.

Encourage patients with cancer to follow the diet the physician sets for them. Patients may find this difficult, because cancer often produces loss of appetite. They may also experience nausea and vomiting. Educate patients about ways to make food more appealing and easier to digest. Consuming small meals at frequent intervals may help. Patients may also follow a liquid diet. Bringing food to room temperature or chilling it slightly may reduce food odors that can trigger nausea.

PROCEDURE 31.2

Alerting Patients With Food Allergies to the Dangers of Common Foods

Objective: To explain how patients can eliminate allergy-causing foods from their diets

OSHA Guidelines: This procedure does not involve exposure to blood, body fluids, or tissues.

Materials: Results of the patient's allergy tests, patient's chart, pen, patient education materials

Method

1. Identify the patient and introduce yourself.
2. Discuss the results of the patient's allergy tests (if available), reinforcing the physician's instructions. List the foods the patient has been found to be allergic to. Provide the patient with a checklist of those foods.
3. Discuss with the patient the possible allergic reactions those foods can cause.
4. Talk about how the patient can avoid or eliminate those foods from the diet. Point out that the patient needs to be alert to avoid the allergy-causing foods not only in their basic forms but also as ingredients in prepared dishes and packaged foods. (Patients allergic to peanuts, for example, should avoid products containing peanut oil as well as peanuts.) Tell the patient to read labels carefully and to inquire at restaurants about the use of those ingredients in dishes listed on the menu.
5. With the physician's or dietitian's consent, talk with the patient about the possibility of finding adequate substitutes for the foods if they are among the patient's favorites. Also discuss, if necessary, how the patient can obtain the nutrients in those foods from other sources (for example, the need for extra calcium sources if the patient is allergic to dairy products). Provide these explanations to the patient in writing, if appropriate, along with supplementary materials such as recipe pamphlets, a list of resources for obtaining food substitutes, and so on.
6. Discuss with the patient the procedures to follow if the allergy-causing foods are accidentally ingested.
7. Answer the patient's questions and remind the patient that you and the rest of the medical team are available if any questions or problems arise later on.
8. Document the patient education session or interchange in the patient's chart, indicate the patient's understanding, and initial the entry.

Patients With Diabetes. A special diet is one of the foundations of treatment for diabetes. Dietary guidelines for patients with diabetes must not only provide them with adequate nutrition but also keep their blood sugar level under control and interact appropriately with medication. Patient education is especially important, because patients with diabetes must comfortably maintain the dietary modifications over a lifetime.

The diet a physician or dietitian prescribes for someone with diabetes includes a specific number of calories, meals per day, amount of carbohydrates, and amounts of other nutrients. As a way to simplify the diet, a system of **food exchanges** is used. All food exchanges in a particular food category provide the same amounts of protein, fat, and carbohydrates. Food exchange lists can be obtained from a registered dietitian or the American Diabetes Association.

The list of exchanges is divided into six categories—vegetables, fruits, breads, meats, fats, and milk—and indicates how large a portion of each food in a category is equal to one "exchange" of food in that category. This information tells patients what portions of specific foods are interchangeable and whether they are eating the correct amounts of those foods. The list includes a variety of foods from which patients make their selections. It is important that patients with diabetes not skip a meal, because skipping meals disturbs the balance of blood sugar and metabolism.

Patients with diabetes who are dependent on insulin should eat regular meals at consistent times. Skipping or delaying meals can result in hypoglycemia or an insulin reaction. Patients should work with a registered dietitian and their physician to create a meal plan that keeps blood glucose levels as close to normal as possible. The medical team specifies the proportion of carbohydrates and calories in meals, depending on the type of insulin patients use and the timing of injections.

Fiber is also important for patients who have diabetes. Fiber can sometimes prevent a sharp rise in blood glucose after a meal and may reduce the amount of insulin needed. It is therefore recommended that people with diabetes gradually increase their fiber intake until it is at about 45 grams per day.

Patients Who Are Elderly. Universal nutritional guidelines for aging patients have not been developed. It is known, however, that energy and metabolic requirements usually decline with age, which calls for some dietary modification. The Food and Nutrition Board of the National Academy of Science recommends a 10% decrease in caloric intake for people over age 50 compared with that of young adults. Men and women above age 75 should decrease their intake another 10% to 15%. The exact adjustment, however, depends on the individual patient's condition and needs.

Because protein requirements do not change, elderly patients should select foods that provide ample protein in a smaller quantity of food. To achieve daily nutritional goals, patients may require supplements for iron, calcium, and other minerals, such as phosphorus and magnesium.

Because aging is often accompanied by decreased gastrointestinal muscle tone, elderly patients should increase their intake of high-fiber foods and drink plenty of water. Although all people need a certain amount of fat in their diet to help the body absorb vitamins, too much may lead to atherosclerosis. Elderly individuals should therefore keep fat intake to 20% of their total calories.

Certain factors can impair or impede eating in this age group and may even lead to malnutrition. If you recognize any of these factors, discuss them with the patient's doctor:

- Physical factors, such as chewing difficulty caused by tooth loss or poorly fitting dentures, swallowing difficulty, and lack of appetite caused by altered taste, smell, or sight
- Medications, which may adversely affect food intake or nutrient use
- Social factors, including apathy toward food caused by depression, grief, or loneliness
- Economic factors, including homelessness or lack of money for food or transportation

Patients With Heart Disease. Coronary heart disease is caused by atherosclerosis, which usually results from hyperlipidemia, or an excess of lipids in the bloodstream. Left untreated, this condition can lead to angina, heart attack, or stroke.

Patients can significantly lower their risk by reducing their blood cholesterol levels and losing weight if they are overweight. Patients who have coronary heart disease usually must reduce their consumption of fats to a level that provides less than 30% of their total caloric intake. Saturated fats should provide less than 10% of caloric intake. Patients who have had a heart attack or are at increased risk for a heart attack are also encouraged to increase their consumption of soluble fiber.

As a medical assistant, your role with these patients is to encourage them to follow the nutritional regimen prescribed by the doctor. Do not recommend other dietary changes. Instead, educate patients about ways to reduce the amount of fat in their diets, such as by substituting skim milk for whole milk.

Patients With Hypertension. Hypertension (high blood pressure) is a condition that affects more than 20% of American adults. Nutritional therapy for patients with hypertension involves the following:

- Restricting sodium intake to 2 to 3 grams per day, especially in salt-sensitive individuals
- Increasing potassium intake through consumption of fresh fruits and vegetables
- Ensuring adequate calcium intake to meet an RDA of 800 milligrams
- Eliminating or reducing alcohol use
- Decreasing total fat intake and obtaining no more than 10% of calories from saturated fats

Patients With Lactose Sensitivity. Lactose is the sugar contained in human and animal milk. It must be broken down in the body by the enzyme lactase to enable the body to digest dairy products. In people from some parts of the world, lactase is present in the body until age 3 or 4, after which it all but disappears. As a result, after early childhood many people have trouble digesting foods that contain lactose and eliminate these foods from their diets. People who are especially sensitive to dietary lactose are often referred to as being lactose intolerant.

Chemical preparations can help a person digest lactose. Those preparations may be added to certain foods, such as ice cream, for lactose-sensitive people. If people with a lactose sensitivity choose to avoid dairy products, they need to be sure to obtain protein and calcium from other sources.

Patients Who Are Overweight. Overweight is a common problem: more than one-third of American adults are overweight. Overweight patients weigh 10% to 20% more than is recommended for their height and gender. Patients who are more than 20% overweight are considered obese. Obesity can lead to medical complications such as elevated blood cholesterol levels, hypertension, diabetes, joint problems, respiratory problems, and heart disease.

Approaches to Weight Loss. Overweight may be approached with dietary modification alone, but an exercise program is usually included. Behavior modification is also a common element of weight-loss programs. In a weight-loss program, foods should be proportioned in accordance with the Food Guide Pyramid, and the diet should be appealing and enjoyable. The goal is to have the patient decrease daily caloric intake and increase physical activity at an appropriate rate while remaining comfortable and healthy.

Weight loss will not occur unless patients expend more energy than they consume. A physician or dietitian can calculate each person's daily caloric needs and determine how many calories must be cut from the diet and how much activity must be increased to result in weight loss. Foods that are high in nutrients but low in calories are desirable.

The **behavior modification** facet of weight loss includes such methods as keeping a food diary to pinpoint overeating patterns, controlling the stimuli associated with overeating, and providing rewards for successful behavior.

You can help overweight patients in their weight-loss efforts by teaching them to:

- Eat slowly, because the message that the stomach is full takes 20 minutes to register with the brain
- Eat five or six small meals daily
- Be patient—reliable weight loss occurs over time, not immediately

Motivation and Education. Because patients who are trying to lose weight may have trouble with motivation, they need as much support as possible. You can provide encouragement and education. You may be able to introduce the patient to low-calorie or low-fat recipes, for instance, and positively reinforce the patient's efforts by complimenting small, gradual successes.

You will no doubt need to explain that fad diets and diet drugs are seldom successful. Fad weight-loss methods can lead to vitamin, mineral, and protein deficiency; serious medical disorders; and even death. Tell patients to use the following criteria to identify fad diets:

- They promise ease and comfort in weight loss
- They promise extremely quick weight loss
- They include only a few foods, such as grapefruit or low-protein foods
- They require the purchase of some secret ingredient or pill
- They are often published in a book or magazine

Truly effective weight-loss regimens usually possess the following qualities:

- They include a variety of foods that contain adequate nutrients
- They include an activity component
- They may be safely followed over a long period of time

An effective program should be one in which the patient is able to lose weight (including fat) gradually and constantly, with some plateaus, and then maintain the loss indefinitely afterward. You can help patients with the challenge of maintaining their weight loss by recommending a reputable weight-loss group or a support group that will help them make the necessary lifestyle changes and remain motivated.

Pediatric Patients. During the first year of life, an infant experiences the most rapid period of growth and development that occurs during the life span. Breast milk and commercially prepared formula contain the balance of nutrients that infants' bodies need during that period. Cow's milk does not meet these standards.

The pace of growth is steadier and slower during childhood, with growth spurts throughout. Nutritional needs change to reflect growth, maturation, and increasing activity levels. Vitamin D and calcium are critical to tooth and bone formation, and fluoride strengthens teeth. Hunger regulates food intake in young children, but forcing children to eat can promote eating habits that lead to obesity.

Patients Who Are Pregnant or Lactating. Nutrition is especially important during pregnancy, when it provides for normal growth and health of the baby as well as the health of the pregnant woman. Doctors recommend that pregnant women gain a certain amount of weight during each trimester of pregnancy, with a total weight gain of about 25 to 35 pounds. The rate of weight gain should be 2 to 5 pounds in the first trimester and about 1 pound per week after that. Gaining too little or too much weight during pregnancy can result in serious complications.

Here are some nutritional suggestions for pregnant women:

- An additional 10 to 15 grams of protein a day in the form of meat, poultry, fish, eggs, and dairy products
- 1200 milligrams of calcium a day, preferably in the form of low-fat dairy products such as skim milk
- 30 milligrams of iron a day through meat, liver, egg yolks, grains, leafy vegetables, nuts, dried fruits, legumes, and supplements (it is difficult to meet the daily need with food alone)
- Folic acid intake of 400 micrograms a day through leafy vegetables, yeast, and liver as well as supplements
- Adequate fiber intake to prevent the constipation that often accompanies pregnancy
- Recommendations consistent with the Food Guide Pyramid and normal sodium and water intake

Breast-feeding has specific nutritional and dietary requirements as well, because breast milk is nutrient-rich and the body requires considerable energy and nutrients to produce it. The infant depends on this milk for the extensive growth that takes place during the first months of life. Lactating women need to consume an additional 500 calories and an additional 12 to 19 grams of protein per day as well as 260 to 280 micrograms of folic acid and 1200 milligrams of calcium.

Specific Modified Diets

Physicians may modify a patient's diet to treat or prevent certain conditions. Specific types of modified diets include changes in texture, nutrient level, frequency and timing of meals, and exclusions.

Texture. A patient may need changes in food consistency as a result of swallowing, chewing, or other gastrointestinal problems or to fulfill short-term needs that result from such events as laboratory tests or surgical procedures. The following special diets are based on texture.

- A clear-liquid diet consists solely of foods such as tea, broth, noncitrus juices, carbonated beverages, popsicles, and gelatin. A full-liquid diet is less restrictive and includes strained cooked cereals, plain ice cream, sherbet, pudding, and strained soups.
- A soft diet includes foods that are easy to chew, swallow, and digest. Foods that patients cannot tolerate and those high in fiber are eliminated from this diet.

- All foods in a pureed diet are put through a strainer so that they are in the form of a semisolid. Pureed foods are easy to chew and swallow.
- A high-fiber diet contains large amounts of fiber (greater than 40 grams) from sources such as fresh fruits, vegetables, and bran cereal. Physicians may prescribe this diet for patients with conditions such as diverticulosis and constipation. The diet increases the bulk of fecal matter and stimulates peristalsis (waves of alternating contraction and relaxation of the intestine that move contents through the intestine).

Nutrient Level. Doctors may make nutrient-level modifications in patients' diets before or after surgical or medical procedures or for patients who have specific conditions. The following special diets are based on nutrient levels.

- Doctors may prescribe low-sodium diets for patients who suffer from disease conditions affecting the cardiovascular system, liver, pancreas, and gallbladder, including edema and hypertension. The typical American diet contains 2 to 5 grams of sodium daily. For mild sodium restriction, daily intake is limited to 2 to 3 grams; the patient reduces salt in cooking, adds no salt at the table, and avoids processed foods. Moderate sodium restriction allows 1 gram per day; the patient adds no salt in cooking or at the table and limits high-sodium vegetables, meat, and milk. Severe restriction allows 500 milligrams per day and greatly limits high-sodium vegetables, meat, milk, and eggs.
- Doctors recommend low-cholesterol diets for patients with high blood cholesterol levels. Such diets involve replacing saturated fats with unsaturated fats, using low-fat or nonfat cooking methods, and restricting fatty foods.
- Doctors may prescribe reduced-calorie diets to promote weight loss in patients who are overweight.
- Doctors may recommend low-tyramine diets for patients who have migraine headaches and patients who are taking certain antidepressant drugs. The compound tyramine is found in aged cheeses, red wine, beer, cream, chocolate, and yeast.
- Doctors may order high-calorie, high-protein diets for patients who have infections, are recovering from burns or surgery, or have had weight loss caused by a severe illness. Food intake is increased to provide 3000 to 5000 calories per day. Protein usually accounts for the greatest caloric increase in these diets.
- Doctors may prescribe high-carbohydrate diets for patients with kidney diseases and some cardiac conditions.

You can help patients who need to make nutrient-level modifications by teaching them how to read food labels. All packaged foods carry a Nutrition Facts label that contains information on the ingredients, major nutrients, and recommended amounts of key nutrients in daily diets. Procedure 31-3 explains how to educate patients about reading food labels.

PROCEDURE 31.3

Teaching Patients How to Read Food Labels

Objective: To explain how patients can use food labels to plan or follow a diet

OSHA Guidelines: This procedure does not involve exposure to blood, body fluids, or tissues.

Materials: Food labels from products

Method

1. Identify the patient and introduce yourself.
2. Explain that food labels can be used as a valuable source of information when planning or implementing a prescribed diet.
3. Using a label from a food package, such as the ice-cream label shown in Figure 31-16, point out the Nutrition Facts section.
4. Describe the various elements on the label—in this case the ice-cream label.
   - Serving size is the basis for the nutrition information provided. One serving of the ice cream is ½ cup. There are 16 servings in the package of ice cream.
   - Calories and calories from fat show the proportion of fat calories in the product. One serving of the ice cream contains 170 calories; more than 45% of the calories come from fat.
   - The % Daily Value section shows how many grams (g) or milligrams (mg) of a variety of nutrients are contained in one serving. Then the label shows the percentage (%) of the recommended daily intake of each given nutrient (assuming a diet of 2000 calories a day). The ice cream contains 24% of a person's recommended daily saturated fat intake but only 3% of dietary fiber.
   - Recommendations for total amounts of various nutrients for both a 2000-calorie and a 2500-calorie diet are shown in chart form near the bottom of the label. These numbers

continued →

PROCEDURE 31.3

Teaching Patients How to Read Food Labels *(continued)*

© 2003 EDY'S GRAND ICE CREAM

Double Fudge Brownie

INGREDIENTS: CREAM, MILK, SUGAR, FUDGE SWIRL (SUGAR, CORN SYRUP, SKIM MILK, CREAM, COCOA PROCESSED WITH ALKALI, BITTER CHOCOLATE, MODIFIED FOOD STARCH, NATURAL FLAVOR, SODIUM ALGINATE, SALT), SKIM MILK, CHOCOLATE BROWNIE PIECES (SUGAR, FLOUR, SOYBEAN OIL, EGGS, COCOA PROCESSED WITH ALKALI, CORN SYRUP, WATER, NATURAL FLAVOR, SALT, LECITHIN, XANTHAN GUM), CORN SYRUP, COCOA PROCESSED WITH ALKALI, CELLULOSE GUM, MONO AND DIGLYCERIDES, GUAR GUM, CARRAGEENAN, DEXTROSE.

Nutrition Facts

Serving Size: 1/2 cup (65g)
Servings Per Container: 16

Amount Per Serving	
Calories 170 Calories From Fat 80	
	% Daily Value*
Total Fat 9g	14%
Saturated Fat 5g	24%
Cholesterol 25mg	9%
Sodium 40mg	2%
Total Carbohydrate 19g	6%
Dietary Fiber 1g	3%
Sugars 14g	
Protein 2g	
Vitamin A 6% • Vitamin C 0%	
Calcium 6% • Iron 2%	

*Percent Daily Values are based on a 2000-calorie diet. Your daily values may be higher or lower depending on your calorie needs.

	Calories	2000	2500
Total Fat	Less than	65g	80g
Sat Fat	Less than	20g	25g
Cholesterol	Less than	300mg	300mg
Sodium	Less than	2400mg	2400mg
Total Carbohydrate		300g	375g
Dietary Fiber		25g	30g

QUALITY GUARANTEED! If you are not completely satisfied with this product, please send us the numbers printed on the bottom of this carton and we will replace your purchase.

MANUFACTURED BY
EDY'S GRAND ICE CREAM
HOME OFFICE: 5929 COLLEGE AVE.
OAKLAND, CA 94618
MFG. PLT. NO. ON BOTTOM

Figure 31-16. Food labels are a source of nutrition information. This label provides facts on the nutrients and ingredients contained in this product.

© 2003 EDY'S GRAND ICE CREAM

No Sugar Added Butter Pecan

INGREDIENTS: MILK, SKIM MILK, SORBITOL, POLYDEXTROSE, MALTODEXTRIN, CREAM, ROASTED PECANS (PECANS, COCONUT OIL, BUTTER, SALT), WATER, BUTTER, NATURAL FLAVOR, CARAMEL COLOR, MONO AND DIGLYCERIDES, CELLULOSE GUM, XANTHAN GUM, CELLULOSE GEL, TURMERIC AND ANNATTO COLOR, SUNETT® ACESULFAME POTASSIUM, CARRAGEENAN, ASPARTAME.
SUNETT® IS A REGISTERED TRADEMARK OF HOECHST AG.
PHENYLKETONURICS: CONTAINS PHENYLALANINE.

Nutrition Facts

Serving Size: 1/2 cup (62g)
Servings Per Container: 16

Amount Per Serving	
Calories 110 Calories From Fat 45	
	% Daily Value*
Total Fat 5.0g	7%
Saturated Fat 2.0g	9%
Cholesterol 10mg	3%
Sodium 55mg	9%
Total Carbohydrate 12g	4%
Dietary Fiber 0g	0%
Sugars 3g	
Sugar Alcohols 4g	
Protein 3g	
Vitamin A 4% • Vitamin C 0%	
Calcium 8% • Iron 0%	

*Percent Daily Values are based on a 2000-calorie diet. Your daily values may be higher or lower depending on your calorie needs.

	Calories	2,000	2,500
Total Fat	Less than	65g	80g
Sat Fat	Less than	20g	24g
Cholesterol	Less than	300mg	300mg
Sodium	Less than	2400mg	2400mg
Total Carbohydrate		300g	375g
Dietary Fiber		25g	30g

QUALITY GUARANTEED! If you are not completely satisfied with this product, please send us the numbers printed on the bottom of this carton and we will replace your purchase.

MANUFACTURED BY
EDY'S GRAND ICE CREAM
HOME OFFICE: 5929 COLLEGE AVE.
OAKLAND, CA 94618
MFG. PLT. NO. ON BOTTOM

Figure 31-17. By reading this label, a patient would learn that this ice cream contains less fat and fewer calories than regular ice cream.

provide the basis for the daily value percentages.

- Ingredients are listed in order from largest quantity to smallest quantity. In this half-gallon of ice cream, cream, milk, and sugar are the most abundant ingredients.

5. Inform the patient that a variety of similar products with significantly different nutritional values are often available. Explain that patients can use nutrition labels, such as those shown in Figures 31-16 and 31-17, to evaluate and compare such similar products. Patients must consider what a product contributes to their diets, not simply what it lacks. To do this, patients must read the entire label. Compared with the regular ice cream, the "no sugar added" ice cream contains less fat, fewer carbohydrates, and an extra gram of protein, but it contributes an additional 15 milligrams of sodium and lacks fiber. It also uses an artificial sweetener that contains phenylalanine.

6. Ask the patient to compare two other similar products and determine which would fit in better as part of a healthy, nutritious diet that meets that patient's individual needs.

7. Document the patient education session in the patient's chart, indicate the patient's understanding, and initial the entry.

TABLE 31-6 Food Label Terms and Definitions

Term	Definition
Low calorie	Less than or equal to 40 calories per serving
Reduced calorie	At least 25% fewer calories per serving than the food it replaces
Cholesterol free	Less than or equal to 2 mg cholesterol per serving
Low cholesterol	Less than or equal to 20 mg cholesterol per serving
Reduced cholesterol	At least 25% less cholesterol per serving than the food it replaces
Low fat	Less than or equal to 3 g fat per serving
Reduced fat	At least 25% less fat per serving than the food it replaces
Sodium free	Less than or equal to 5 mg sodium per serving
Very low sodium	Less than or equal to 35 mg sodium per serving
Low sodium	Less than or equal to 140 mg sodium per serving
Reduced sodium	At least 25% less sodium per serving than the food it replaces

Source: U.S. Department of Health and Human Services, Food and Drug Administration.

You can also teach patients how to interpret the terms on food labels (Table 31-6). Understanding marketing terms simplifies the process of buying the right foods to meet special dietary needs.

Frequency and Timing of Meals. A patient's diet may also be modified by adjusting the standard three-meal pattern. The goal may be to eat six small meals rather than three large meals to minimize stress on organs affected by disease conditions—as in patients with an ulcer or hiatal hernia. In other cases meals may simply be timed to follow tests or therapeutic procedures.

Exclusion of Certain Foods. Physicians may order that specific foods be omitted from patients' diets for health reasons.

- In a bland diet, specific foods that cause irritation are eliminated, along with caffeine, alcohol, nicotine, aspirin, and some spices. A typical bland diet includes easily digested foods, such as mashed potatoes and gelatins. Raw fruits and vegetables, whole grain foods, and very hot or cold items are among foods to avoid. A physician may prescribe this type of diet for a patient with a peptic ulcer, for example.
- Exclusion diets are prescribed for patients who have food intolerances. These diets must eliminate foods that contain the offending substances but still provide the nutrients needed for good health. Intolerance to lactose, the sugar in milk, is fairly common. Intolerance to the amino acid phenylalanine—a condition present at birth—is fairly rare but very serious. Infants born in hospitals in the United States are tested for this intolerance because if these infants were to receive a standard diet, they would develop severe mental retardation. People with this condition, known as phenylketonuria (PKU), must be vigilant about checking labels on prepared foods as well as knowledgeable about the phenylalanine content of fresh foods.

Using Supplements and Parenteral Nutrition

When a patient has a loss or lack of appetite or cannot tolerate a normal meal, the doctor may prescribe a specially formulated food supplement that provides protein, carbohydrates, fat, vitamins, and minerals. A patient who is chronically ill, underweight, or anemic or who has just undergone surgery may take supplements orally or through a tube to the stomach or small intestine. If the supplement is being taken orally, encourage the patient to follow the prescribed directions.

When patients cannot tolerate receiving supplements enterally (by way of the digestive tract), they may be fed parenterally. **Parenteral nutrition** is provided to patients as specially prepared nutrients injected directly into their veins rather than given by mouth. Because a parenteral feeding bypasses the digestive system, the nutrients it contains must already be in a form the body can use as they enter the blood.

Patients Undergoing Drug Therapy

Drugs may change a patient's nutritional status and needs. Long-term drug therapy and multiple prescriptions make close nutritional monitoring a high priority.

Drug therapy can cause a change in food intake, a change in the body's absorption of a nutrient, or both. Likewise, foods can interfere with the metabolism and action of a drug. For example, laxatives and certain other types of drugs may suppress the appetite. Antihistamines, alcohol, insulin, thyroid hormones, and some other drugs can stimulate appetite. Anesthetics can interfere with taste. Calcium in milk can diminish the absorption of some antibiotics. Be sure to discuss any possible interactions with the physician or dietitian before discussing diet and drug regimens with a patient.

Eating Disorders

Eating disorders, characterized by extremely harmful eating behavior, can lead to health problems. These disorders can damage the body and even cause death. They are most common in adolescent girls and young women, although 10% to 15% of patients with eating disorders are male. Figure 31-18 lists signs and symptoms of common types of eating disorders.

Anorexia Nervosa

Anorexia nervosa is an eating disorder in which people starve themselves. They fear that if they lose control of eating, they will become grossly overweight. They lose an excessive amount of weight and become malnourished, and women often stop menstruating. The typical patient with anorexia nervosa is a high-achieving, white female in her teens or early 20s. The numbers of children and middle-aged women who suffer from the disorder, however, have been increasing.

The cause of anorexia remains unknown, but risk factors include the following:

- Coming from a family that has problems with alcoholism
- Suffering a childhood trauma, such as sexual abuse (20% to 50% of patients were sexually abused)
- Having a high stress level
- Suffering from depression
- Suffering from shame and low self-esteem
- Having an extreme need to be in control

It has also been noted that anorexia tends to run in families. The victim of anorexia often uses food as a way to deal with the psychological effects of trauma by numbing the emotions or as a means of getting some measure of control in life. Anorexia can be precipitated by any major life change.

Signs and Symptoms of Common Eating Disorders

Anorexia Nervosa

- Unexplained weight loss of at least 15%
- Self-starvation
- Excessive fear of gaining weight
- Malnourishment
- Cessation of menstruation in women
- Drastic reduction in food consumption
- Denial of feeling hungry
- Ritualistic eating habits
- Overexercising
- Unrealistic self-image as being obese
- Extremely controlled behavior

Bulimia

- Eating large quantities of food in a short period, followed by purging
- Pretexts for going to the bathroom after meals
- Using laxatives or diuretics to control weight
- Buying and consuming large quantities of food
- Feeling out of control while eating
- Maintaining a constant weight while eating a large amount of fattening foods
- Mood swings
- Awareness of having a disorder, but fear of not being able to stop
- Depression, self-deprecation, and guilt following the episodes

Binge Eating

- Bingeing on food, not followed by purging
- Weight gain

Figure 31-18. Be alert for these signs and symptoms of eating disorders when you work with patients.

This disorder can be fatal. The first stage of treatment is to restore normal nutrition. Patients may need to be hospitalized and fed intravenously or by nasogastric tube, which enters through the nose and delivers food into the stomach. Hospitalization may be necessary, because patients with excessive weight loss may develop cardiac and other medical disorders. These patients may also be at risk for suicide. The hospital stay may eventually provide patients with the structure and support they need to establish healthy eating patterns.

Psychotherapy is a cornerstone of treatment protocol. Therapy usually involves a combination of one-on-one and group therapy. Therapy groups that are single-sex rather than coed are preferable because of the different gender and peer group issues men and women face. Doctors may prescribe medication for depression and anxiety. The later stages of treatment include teaching patients and their families about nutrition concepts.

Bulimia

Bulimia is an eating disorder in which people eat a large quantity of food in a short time (bingeing) and then attempt to counter the effects of bingeing by self-induced vomiting, use of laxatives or diuretics, and/or excessive exercise. People with bulimia may use such behavior to try to gain control of their lives and weight.

Bulimia can be triggered when a slightly overweight person diets but fails to achieve the goal. Episodes are usually frequent, rapid, and uncontrollable. The behavior may occur only during periods of stress.

People with bulimia often diet when not bingeing. Psychologically, they believe their worth depends on being thin. Behind their cheerful exterior, they usually feel depressed, lonely, ashamed, and empty.

Most bulimics who seek help are in their early 20s and report that they have been bulimic for 4 to 6 years. Because they are more likely to want and seek help, they are slightly easier to treat than anorexics are.

Bulimia is usually not life-threatening, but it can cause the following serious health problems:

- Erosion of tooth enamel
- Enlarged salivary glands
- Lesions in the esophagus
- Stomach spasms
- Chemical and hormonal imbalances

As with anorexia, treatment for bulemia involves a combination of psychotherapy and medication. Dental work, medication for depression and anxiety, nutritional counseling, and support groups may be used. The goal is to establish a healthy weight and good eating patterns as well as to resolve the psychosocial triggers.

Getting Help

Studies show an unsatisfactory rate of recovery from eating disorders; only about half of anorexic patients fully recover. The disorders can become chronic, with periods of remission and relapse. Chronic anorexia can be fatal, and many people who do recover from eating disorders remain preoccupied with food.

If you suspect that a patient has an eating disorder, be alert for the following eating or activity patterns that the patient might mention in conversation:

- Skipping two or more meals a day or limiting caloric intake to 500 or fewer calories a day
- Eating a very large amount of food in an uncontrollable manner over the course of 2 hours
- Eating large quantities of food without being hungry
- Using laxatives, excessive exercise, vomiting, diuretics, or other purges for weight control
- Avoiding social situations because they may interfere with a diet or exercise
- Feeling disgust, depression, and guilt after a binge
- Feeling that food controls life

Patient Education

Whenever you teach patients about nutrition and diet, you help them take steps to improve their health. In most instances a physician or dietitian gives the patient instructions, which you then reinforce. Patients may feel more comfortable asking you questions about their diet than asking other members of the medical team. They may think their concerns are too trivial or simple for the physician or dietitian.

Because of your frequent contact with patients, you can play a major role in education. You can teach patients about the role of nutrition in helping to prevent specific medical conditions. You can also teach patients how to be wise consumers when they shop by reading food package labels. You will be better equipped to educate patients and answer their questions if you have a solid knowledge of diet and nutrition and if you stay current with recent research findings. See the Educating the Patient section for information on the relevance of such research. Before discussing a diet with any patient, be sure you understand the regimen the physician or dietitian is recommending as well as how to implement it.

If you are unsure of answers to any patient's questions, always ask the physician. Refer patients who have questions about meal patterns and food selections to the registered dietitian, if one is available.

Your Role in Patient Education

When discussing dietary requirements with a patient, keep in mind that the patient is always the focus of nutritional care. Specific factors to take into account include the following:

- Any psychological or lifestyle factors that affect food choices and behaviors. Learn about the patient's dietary likes and dislikes, as well as religious or cultural restrictions, before you suggest the use of specific foods in meeting dietary requirements.
- The patient's age and family circumstances. For example, parents need to know the specifics about an infant's or a child's diet. An elderly person's diet needs to be physically and economically manageable as well as nutritious.
- Diseases and disorders. For example, if the patient has chewing or breathing problems or is nauseous, the doctor will have to prescribe treatments or medications to address those problems.
- The patient's psychological condition. You can learn a great deal about psychological status through discussion and nonverbal cues. For instance, you might look for signs that the patient is frustrated with the dietary

Educating the Patient

Changes in Nutritional Recommendations

In the field of nutrition—as in other scientific fields—research continues to provide people with additional information. How that information is used and the speed with which it is communicated often depend on public service agencies and federal agencies responsible for nutritional guidance.

You can help answer patients' questions about the potential usefulness of new information by understanding the difference between initial research findings and those evaluated and endorsed by the government. In many cases information is not officially released or endorsed until the government has studied the facts and determined that they are accurate and concrete enough for public consideration. For example, initial findings have suggested the following information.

- Beta-carotene supplements may provide no benefit and may even be harmful.
- Certain fruit-derived flavenoids—pigmented antioxidants—may help halt the growth of cancer cells.
- Vitamin E may be effective in slowing the accumulation of artery-clogging plaque.
- Dark beer may reduce the risk of coronary artery disease.

Patients may read about research studies and ask whether they should make whatever dietary changes the findings suggest. You need to explain that such findings are preliminary and not formally approved by a government agency. Although the approval process is lengthy—requiring a significant amount of data and test results—it provides a system for protecting consumers from false nutritional claims.

Tell patients that once the government determines that a nutritional recommendation is warranted, it often acts on it. One example is the case of folate. Since the 1960s a number of studies have been conducted on the importance of folate in the diet. Over the years, those studies have yielded the following results.

- Folate offers protection from neural tube defects in unborn babies.
- Folate can reverse certain anemias.
- Folate may reduce the risk of cervical dysplasia.
- Folate appears to lower the likelihood of heart attacks.

As a result of these studies, the Department of Health and Human Services' Food and Drug Administration considered folate to be so important to all people that it approved the addition of folate to flour. Several nutrients have long been added to certain products to improve the products' nutritional value and to increase people's intake of important nutrients lacking in the general diet:

- Vitamin A and vitamin D, added to dairy products
- Iodine, added to salt
- Niacin, added to milled grain products
- Various vitamins and minerals, added to processed cereals

Explain to patients that nutritional recommendations change as scientists learn more about the ways various foods affect the human body and the exact amount of nutrients the body requires. Keep up to date on nutrition research so you can provide patients with the latest information and help them steer clear of unsubstantiated claims.

changes or is in denial about a problem. The greater the rapport you develop with a patient, the more you will be able to help.

Remind patients that eating healthfully will help them feel and look better and help their bodies work better. When the doctor prescribes therapeutic diets, be sure patients are fully aware of the reasons they must follow the diets. Help patients set realistic goals, and praise them for even the smallest accomplishments. Offer positive reinforcement for current and new good food habits.

As with all patient education, teaching methods such as role playing, repetition of concepts, and the use of literature and other media reinforce your discussion. Use printed and audiovisual materials such as those shown in Figure 31-19 (available from health agencies and other sources) to illustrate your points.

Patient education sessions can be formal or informal and can take place at any appropriate time and place, such as in the office, over the telephone, or during a treatment or procedure. If possible, let patients decide which arrangements they prefer, or let them know the schedule in advance.

Patients need your support and empathy in working toward diet and nutrition goals, whether preventive or therapeutic. Follow these guidelines for best results when discussing diets with patients.

- Treat each patient as an individual with unique eating habits, knowledge of nutrition, and ability to learn

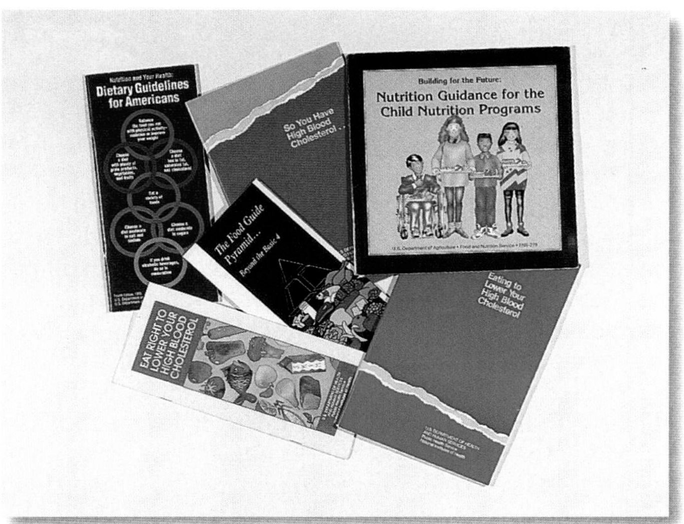

Figure 31-19. A variety of materials are available to help you teach patients about diet and nutrition.

- Teach a small amount of material at a time; 15- to 30-minute sessions are better than hour-long ones
- Keep explanations at the level of the patient's understanding and vocabulary
- Emphasize the patient's good eating behavior to reinforce it
- Let the patient play an active role in the learning process—for example, by helping to plan the diet
- Give the patient a written diet plan to take home as well as any other helpful materials you have to offer
- Suggest that the patient contact local support groups for people who are trying to maintain the same kind of diet

Keep in mind that patient education has become increasingly important for patients receiving managed care. Managed care providers want to see documentation of preventive care in patients' charts. Failure to provide documentation can jeopardize a patient's insurance coverage.

TABLE 31-7 Sources of Information About Specific Diet and Nutrition Issues

Organization	Address/Telephone Number
American Cancer Society	1599 Clifton Road NE Atlanta, GA 30329 (800) ACS-2345
American Diabetes Association	National Center 1211 Connecticut Avenue NW Washington, DC 20036 (202) 331-8303 (800) DIABETES
American Dietetic Association	120 S. Riverside Plaza Suite 2000 Chicago, IL 60606-6995 (800) 877-1600 (800) 366-1655
American Heart Association	7320 Greenville Avenue Dallas, TX 75231 (214) 373-6300
Anorexia Nervosa and Related Eating Disorders	P.O. Box 5102 Eugene, OR 97405 (541) 344-1144
National Association of Anorexia Nervosa and Associated Disorders	Box 7 Highland Park, IL 60035 (847) 831-3438
National Eating Disorders Association	603 Stewart Street Suite 803 Seattle, WA 98101 (206) 382-3587
Overeaters Anonymous (OA)	P.O. Box 44020 Rio Rancho, NM 87174 (505) 891-2664

Cultural Considerations

Eating is a personal and social activity, and cultural issues play an especially important part in diet and nutrition. A person's cultural heritage, religious background, family traditions, socioeconomic status, and personal beliefs help determine eating habits and preferences. Culture and lifestyle also help shape food purchasing and serving habits, likes and dislikes, meal timing and frequency, attitude toward food supplements, and tendency to snack.

Dietitians and nutritionists who design diets and recipes for patients know that to design successful diets, they must take into account cultural and lifestyle factors. You can increase the effectiveness of your patient education if you become familiar with the food habits and beliefs common to your patients' cultural backgrounds. Learn to recognize the eating patterns belonging to different cultures, and make a special effort to familiarize yourself with the food preferences of the ethnic groups most commonly represented among the patients in the practice where you work.

Outside Resources for Patient Education

Many community health agencies and organizations offer patient education materials and information about specific diet and nutrition issues. Some of them are listed in Table 31-7. Investigate your own community to find others, and keep the information on file.

Summary

Nutrition is a complex, highly technical topic that touches people's daily lives. It is part of your job to make good nutrition understandable and achievable for patients. You will play a major role in educating patients about special diets and in helping them implement dietary changes as instructed by physicians and dietitians. Your knowledge of basic nutritional principles and current nutritional findings will help you perform these tasks with confidence and competence.

You will need a basic understanding of metabolism and the role of calories in the diet. You must also be familiar with the body's daily requirements for protein, carbohydrates, fiber, fat, vitamins, minerals, and water and which foods can fulfill these requirements. The more you learn about foods and their nutritional value, the better able you will be to educate patients about meeting their particular nutritional needs.

Whenever you work with patients, be alert for body weights significantly above or below the ideal. It is also important to recognize indications of eating patterns that may lead to health problems such as obesity, anorexia nervosa, and bulimia.

Your knowledge about nutrition will help you teach patients a major means of supporting and improving their overall health. In some cases your work in this area will help patients avoid or recover from life-threatening medical conditions.

REVIEW

CHAPTER 31

CASE STUDY QUESTIONS

Now that you have completed this chapter, review the case study at the beginning of the chapter and answer the following questions:

1. What is the patient's probable diagnosis?
2. Do you think that the patient's attention to calorie intake is simply, as she says, preparation for the cheerleading competition?
3. Why is this patient experiencing muscle weakness?

Discussion Questions

1. Name four indications of anorexia nervosa that can be noted during a routine history and physical by a medical assistant.
2. An adult patient reads you his food journal for the previous week. His average daily intake of calcium is 540 milligrams. Is he getting enough calcium to supply his body's needs?
3. Using a normal clinical range of 90 to 171 for LDL cholesterol and a normal clinical range of 31 to 59 for HDL cholesterol, should you tell your patient that he is effectively controlling his cholesterol levels if he has readings of LDL 99 and HDL 56?

Critical Thinking Questions

1. A 16-year-old male has been diagnosed with mononucleosis. The doctor has asked you to explain changes within his diet that will speed up his recovery. His symptoms are fever, fatigue, and sore throat. What will you tell his mother about his new dietary needs?
2. A diabetic patient works as an office manager. She usually works through lunch and grabs fast food on the way home because she is too hungry to wait to cook a full meal. What can you tell her about her dietary habits? What can she do to ensure that her blood sugar levels are more stable?
3. A 63-year-old male goes to his doctor for a checkup. His patient history reveals that he has been obese for 8 years. At his last visit four months earlier, his blood pressure was 150/100. He is a heavy smoker with a desk job. His only hobby is watching sports on television. He admits that he is not following the diet you gave him four months ago. His only complaint is that he is tired a lot. His blood pressure is 160/110 today. What chronic disease is suggested by your intake information? What dietary and lifestyle habits does he need to change to lower his blood pressure?

Application Activities

1. Plan a well-balanced, health-promoting diet for one day for a 45-year-old man recently diagnosed with cardiovascular disease; do the same for a pregnant patient who is a lacto-ovo-vegetarian.
2. Have each member of the class report on the typical diet of a particular culture—Mexican, Asian, Mediterranean, Saudi, and so on. How does the diet satisfy nutritional requirements? In what areas is it outstanding or inadequate? How does the diet differ from a typical American diet?
3. Investigate and report on nutrient supplements that are not yet mainstream or are relatively new, such as 5-HTP, glucosamine, chondroitin, and lutein. What is the nutritional composition of each? What are people trying to use them for? Why? Do most physicians agree that these supplements are beneficial or harmless? Do you agree with these physicians' assessments? Why or why not?

Internet Activity

1. Find an Overeaters Anonymous (OA) meeting in your area. List the day, time, and location. Use the Web site **www.oa.org**.
2. What percentage of children are considered to be obese? Use the Web site **www.obesity.org.** Use the Web site noted in question 1 to name three health effects that have been observed in overweight children.
3. On average, what is the daily caloric goal for teenage boys and active men? Use the dietary guidelines listed at **www.mayoclinic.com**.

CHAPTER 32

Principles of Pharmacology

KEY TERMS

absorption
administer
controlled substance
dispense
distribution
dosage
dose
efficacy
excretion
generic name
indication
labeling
narcotic
opioid
pharmaceutical
pharmacodynamics
pharmacognosy
pharmacokinetics
pharmacology
pharmacotherapeutics
prescribe
prescription
prescription drug
toxicology
trade name
vaccine

AREAS OF COMPETENCE

2003 Role Delineation Study

CLINICAL

Patient Care

- Adhere to established patient screening procedures
- Prepare and administer medications and immunizations
- Maintain medication and immunization records
- Recognize and respond to emergencies
- Initiate IV and administer IV medications with appropriate training and as permitted by state law

GENERAL

Professionalism

- Display a professional manner and image
- Demonstrate initiative and responsibility

Legal Concepts

- Perform within legal and ethical boundaries
- Document accurately
- Follow employer's established policies dealing with the health-care contract
- Implement and maintain federal and state health-care legislation and regulations
- Comply with established risk management and safety procedures

Instruction

- Explain office policies and procedures

Operational Functions

- Perform inventory of office supplies and equipment

CHAPTER OUTLINE

- The Medical Assistant's Role in Pharmacology
- Drugs and Pharmacology
- Sources of Drugs
- The Food and Drug Administration (FDA)
- Pharmacodynamics
- Pharmacokinetics
- Pharmacotherapeutics
- Toxicology
- Sources of Drug Information
- Regulatory Function of the FDA
- Vaccines
- Patient Education About Drugs

OBJECTIVES

After completing Chapter 32, you will be able to:

32.1 Describe the five categories of pharmacology.

32.2 Differentiate between chemical, generic, and trade names for drugs.

32.3 Describe the major drug categories.

32.4 List the main sources of drug information.

32.5 Contrast over-the-counter and prescription drugs.

32.6 Compare the five schedules of controlled substances.

32.7 Describe how to register a physician with the Drug Enforcement Administration (DEA) for permission to administer, dispense, and prescribe controlled drugs.

32.8 Describe how vaccines work in the immune system.

32.9 Identify patient education topics related to the use of nonprescription and prescription drugs.

Introduction

Pharmacology, which is the science of drugs, is a great responsibility to any allied health professional. Medication mistakes made can injure or even cause the death of a patient. It is important to begin with a good working knowledge of the foundations of pharmacology. This chapter provides an overview of the role of drugs in ambulatory medical facilities.

CASE STUDY

You are a medical assistant working in a busy family practice office. You have been employed by this office for only one month. Your office manager tells you that because your performance to date has been excellent, you are being given the responsibility of maintaining the sample drug inventory and the office medications. The office has a space that is dedicated to the samples and office medications, but the area is very disorganized and your first task is to organize and implement an inventory system for the drugs.

As you read through this chapter, think about the steps you will take to design and implement an inventory system for your office's medications.

The Medical Assistant's Role in Pharmacology

You will be expected to have a basic knowledge of medications. There are increasing numbers of over-the-counter (OTC) drugs that were formerly available only with a **prescription,** a physician's written order to authorize the dispensing (and sometimes, administering) of drugs to a patient. The newly approved OTC drugs have been added to an array of drugs, many of which are available at supermarkets, that people purchase to treat themselves for ailments ranging from arthritis to colds to stomach ulcers.

As a medical assistant, you will need to be attentive to ensure that the physician is aware of all medications, both prescription and OTC, that a patient is taking. You also need to ask each patient about use of alcohol and recreational drugs (both past and present) as well as herbal remedies. You will need to educate the patient about the purpose of a drug and how to take the drug for maximum effectiveness and minimum adverse effects. As your state permits, you may also be asked to give drugs to a patient. Safe and effective drug therapy requires more of you than simply giving a drug or a prescription to a patient, however. Advanced skills that you will want to attain are described in the Tips for the Office section.

To handle these important functions, you must understand pharmacologic principles, be able to translate prescriptions, and be prepared to answer basic patient questions (Figure 32-2). You must also adhere to legal requirements and keep accurate records.

Drugs and Pharmacology

A drug is a chemical compound used to prevent, diagnose, or treat a disease or other abnormal condition. The study of drugs is called **pharmacology.** A specialist in pharmacology is called a pharmacologist. Included in pharmacology are **pharmacognosy** (the study of characteristics of

Tips for the Office

Expanding Your Knowledge of Medications

In the area of patient care, the 2003 AAMA Role Delineation Chart lists drug preparation and administration as a basic skill for medical assistants. Before you can administer medications safely, you must have a full knowledge of pharmacologic principles. You must also be able to read and understand all

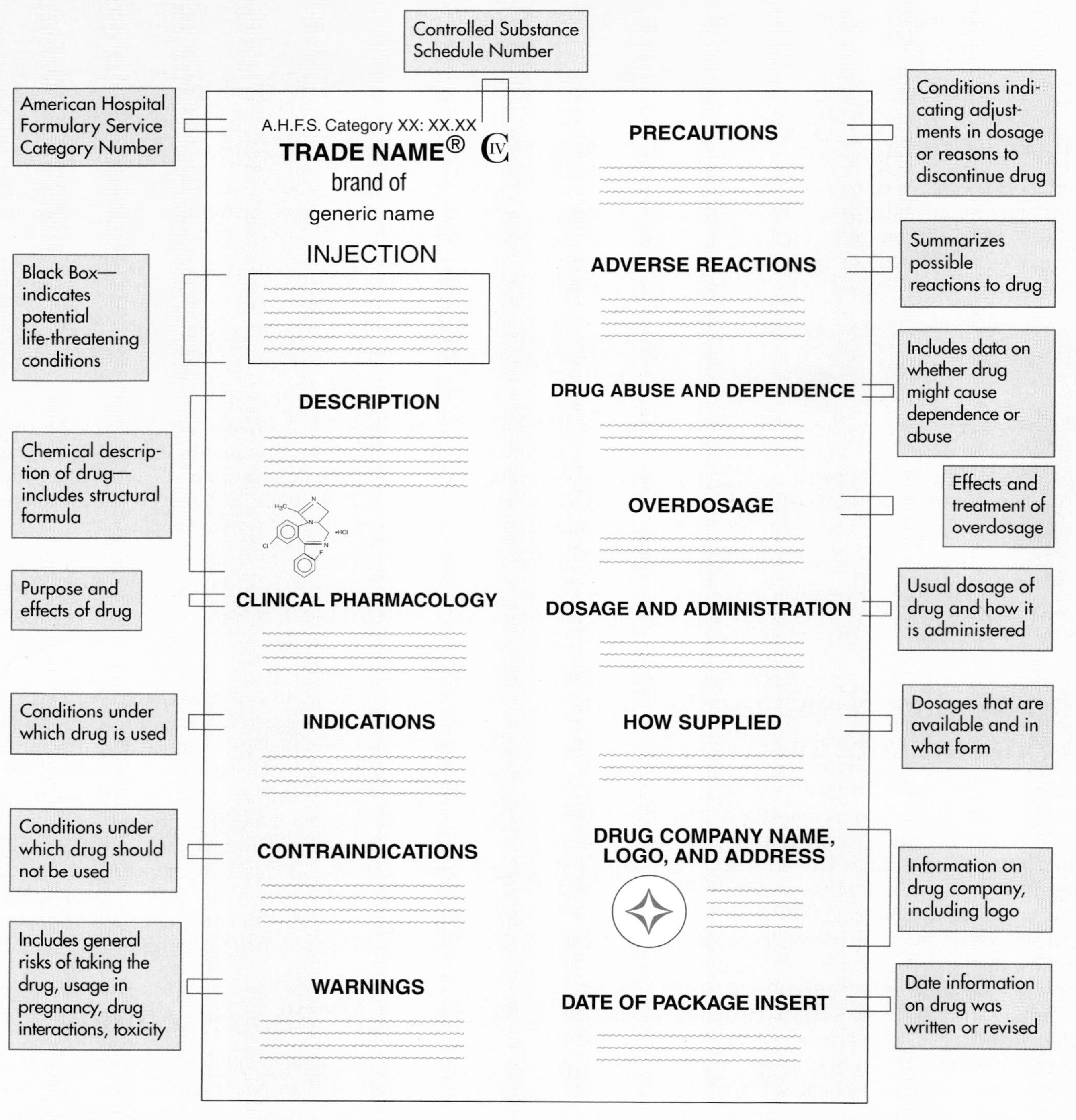

Figure 32-1. Use the package insert to become familiar with a drug's indications, contraindications, dosage, and adverse effects. Here is a representation of a package insert for an injectable drug.

continued →

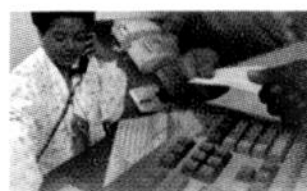

Tips for the Office

Expanding Your Knowledge of Medications *(continued)*

medical terms and abbreviations that appear on a prescription.

The Role Delineation Chart also includes the maintenance of medication records among the basic skills. You will need to use this skill whenever you record a patient's immunizations or transcribe prescription information.

Because controlled drugs are subject to many laws, you will be legally responsible for adhering to all related regulations. Laws require such activities as physician registration with the DEA, tight inventory control for drugs, and proper disposal of controlled drugs. These laws make it necessary for you to apply legal concepts to the practice on a daily basis.

Whenever a patient takes a nonprescription or prescription drug, your ability to provide helpful instructions will be vital. By educating the patient about how to use a drug properly, you will not only help the patient improve medically but also increase the probability of patient safety and compliance.

The most efficient way to prepare for all these responsibilities is to read the package inserts (Figure 32-1) and drug labels that accompany all medications, whether they are drugs from drug company representatives (the samples given to the practice to acquaint physicians with new drugs) or drugs ordered by the practice. Another excellent source of information is the *Physicians' Desk Reference,* or *PDR,* which most practices receive free of charge. To learn more about how drugs act in the body, you may want to read articles in professional journals. The Internet is also a valuable resource.

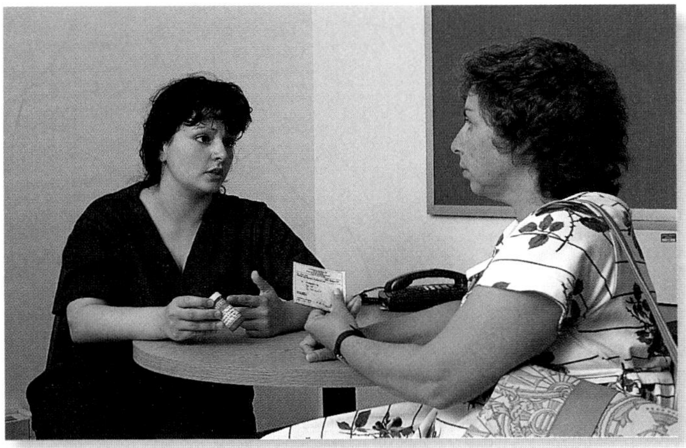

Figure 32-2. A medical assistant must be prepared to answer the patient's questions about a drug the doctor is prescribing.

natural drugs and their sources), **pharmacodynamics** (the study of what drugs do to the body), **pharmacokinetics** (the study of what the body does to drugs), **pharmacotherapeutics** (the study of how drugs are used to treat disease), and **toxicology** (the study of poisons or poisonous effects of drugs).

According to the Department of Justice's Drug Enforcement Administration (DEA) guidelines, a doctor **prescribes** a drug when he gives a patient a prescription to be filled by a pharmacy. To **administer** a drug is to give it directly by injection, by mouth, or by any other route that introduces the drug into a patient's body. A health-care professional **dispenses** a drug by distributing it, in a properly labeled container, to a patient who is to use it.

Sources of Drugs

Many drugs originate as natural products. Many other drugs originate in the chemical laboratory, as chemists seek to improve existing drugs.

Natural Products

Most often, drugs originate as substances from natural products, such as plants, animals, minerals, bacteria, or fungi. Figure 32-3 shows examples of natural sources of drugs. A pharmacognosist is a pharmacologist who specializes in the study of the characteristics of these drugs and their sources.

Plants. Perhaps the oldest source of drugs is plants. For hundreds of years, drugs have been made from seeds, bulbs, roots, stems, buds, leaves, or other parts of plants. Two examples of plant-derived drugs are digitoxin, which comes from the foxglove plant, and quinine, which comes from cinchona tree bark. There are countless others, and new drugs are developed from plants almost daily.

Animals. Animals are also used as a source of drugs. Certain animal substances have been shown to be compatible with human physiology. The following are examples of animal substances used as drugs:

- Glandular substances, such as insulin and thyroid hormones
- Fats and oils, such as cod-liver oil
- Enzymes, such as pancreatin and pepsin
- Antiserums and antitoxins for vaccines

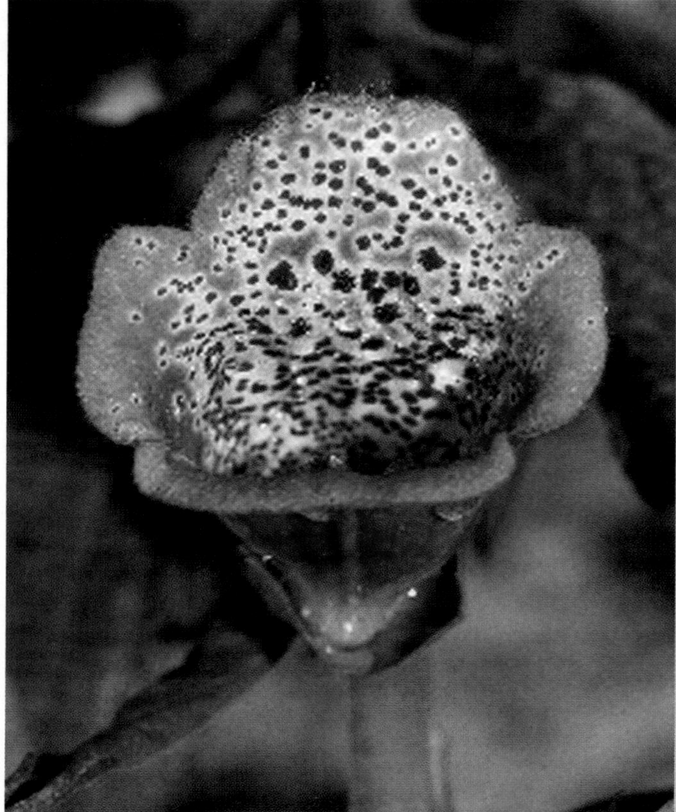

A

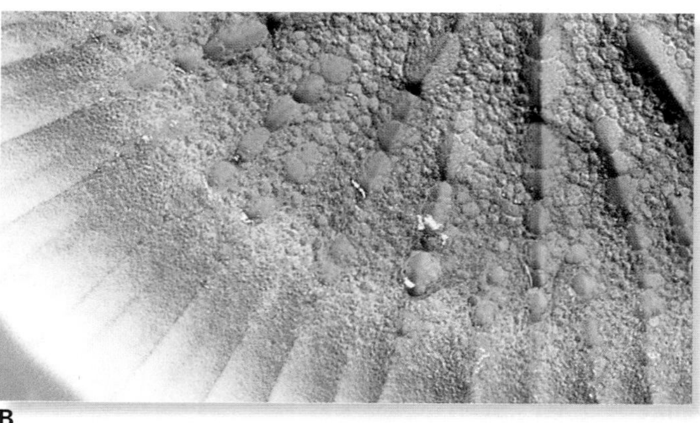

B

Figure 32-3. Many drugs originate as natural products. (a) The foxglove plant is the source of digitoxin. (b) Bacteria and yeasts are sources of many antibiotics.

Minerals. Mineral sources yield various substances that can be used as they occur naturally or can be mixed with other substances. Two drugs derived from mineral sources are potassium chloride and mineral oil.

Bacteria and Fungi. Simple organisms, such as bacteria and fungi, produce substances that are used to make certain antibiotics. Cephalosporins and penicillins are examples.

Chemical Development of Natural Products

After a pharmacognosist has identified the chemical properties of a natural product, a chemist conducts investigations that lead to the synthesis (chemical duplication) of one or more drugs, based on the pharmacognosist's findings. Some drugs are synthesized by strictly chemical methods. Others are duplicated by manipulating genetic information in a host organism. These types of manipulations can cause a host organism to produce a biologic product ordinarily produced only in another organism. For example, human insulin is produced by these means, also known as recombinant DNA techniques.

The Food and Drug Administration (FDA)

When chemists believe they have a drug that will be useful, they approach a drug company for further research and development, which is controlled by the Food and Drug Administration (FDA). The FDA is an agency of the Department of Health and Human Services. It regulates the manufacture and distribution of every drug used in the United States. By this point in the development process, the chemical formula has been identified, and a chemical name has been given to the drug.

The FDA requires that drug manufacturers perform clinical tests on new drugs before the drugs are used by humans. These tests include toxicity tests in laboratory animals, followed by clinical studies (frequently called clinical trials) in controlled groups of volunteers, such as the one shown in Figure 32-4. Some volunteers are patients; others are healthy subjects.

Clinical tests are designed to consider the ratio of benefits to the risk of adverse side effects. If the clinical tests prove that the drug is safe and effective, the FDA approves

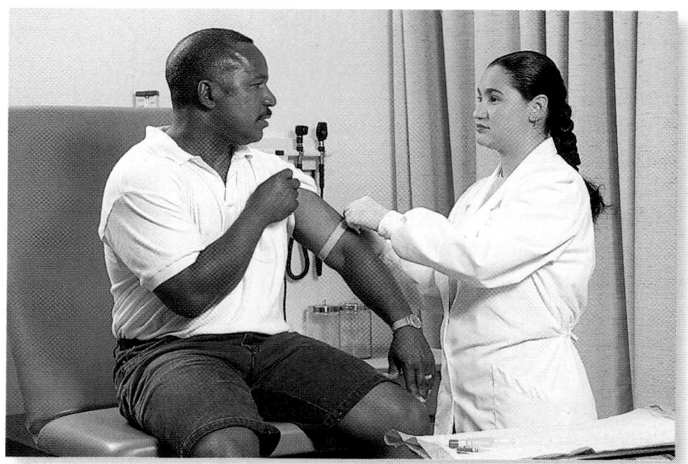

Figure 32-4. Tests such as blood tests provide baseline data on volunteers at the start of clinical trials.

it for marketing. The manufacturer must continue to demonstrate the drug's safety and **efficacy** (therapeutic value) and must submit reports whenever it discovers unexpected adverse reactions. The FDA can withdraw a drug from the market at any time if evidence suggests that it is no longer safe or effective.

During the clinical trials the **pharmaceutical** (drug) company studies all aspects of the pharmacology of the new drug. When the company seeks approval from the FDA, it must document the pharmacodynamics, pharmacokinetics, safety (how many and what kind of adverse effects), and efficacy of the drug. In addition, it must present data regarding the **dose,** the amount of drug given at one time.

Pharmacodynamics

Pharmacodynamics is the study of what a drug does to the body, that is, the mechanism of action or how the drug works to produce a therapeutic effect. Pharmacodynamics includes the interaction between the drug and target cells or tissues and the body's response to that interaction.

For example, when a patient with diabetes takes insulin, the drug acts by allowing the movement of glucose across cell membranes. This movement makes the glucose available to cells to use as an energy source. The end effect is a decrease in the blood glucose level.

Pharmacokinetics

Pharmacokinetics is what the body does to a drug, that is, how the body absorbs, metabolizes, distributes, and excretes the drug. It is important to understand these processes so that you will be able to explain to patients the reasons for taking a particular drug with food or for drinking plenty of water while taking a drug.

Absorption

Absorption is the process of converting a drug from its dose form, such as a tablet or capsule, into a form the body can use. For example, tablets or capsules are absorbed through the stomach or intestines into the bloodstream. Water, food, or a particular food may either hinder or assist the absorption of a specific drug through the stomach or intestines. Some drugs may irritate the digestive organs if they are taken without food or water. Because of such possible reactions, patients must precisely follow instructions for taking a drug with plenty of water, with food, or without food.

Injected drugs are absorbed through the skin (intradermally), through the tissue just beneath the skin (subcutaneously), or through muscle (intramuscularly), depending on the type of injection. Absorption allows the drug to enter the bloodstream and pass into tissues. Drugs that are administered intravenously are directly available to target cells from the bloodstream.

The extent and rate of drug absorption depend on several factors. One factor is the route of administration (see Chapter 33). When the drug is administered by mouth, for example, coatings on tablets or capsules and the amount and type of food consumed with the drug may affect absorption. Other factors involve the characteristics of the drug itself. For example, insulin products vary in rate of absorption, depending on their mode of preparation.

Metabolism

Drug metabolism is the process by which drug molecules are transformed into simpler products called metabolites. This transformation usually occurs in the liver, where enzymes break down the drug. Some drugs, however, are metabolized in the kidneys. Metabolism can be affected by disease, a patient's age or genetic makeup, characteristics of the drug, or other factors.

When drugs metabolized in the liver are prescribed for either children or the elderly, the dose is likely to be lower than that prescribed for young adults. Metabolism in children and the elderly is different from metabolism in other patients; the drugs may remain in the body longer and possibly reach harmful levels. The same concern holds true for any patient with impaired liver or kidney function if prescribed drugs are metabolized in the affected organ.

Distribution

Distribution is the process of transporting a drug from its administration site, such as the muscle of an injection site, to its site of action. Distribution also pertains to the length of time a drug takes to achieve maximum or peak plasma levels, that is, the length of time between dosing and availability in the bloodstream.

Excretion

Excretion describes the manner in which a drug is eliminated from the body. Most drugs are eliminated in urine. Drugs may also be excreted in feces, perspiration, saliva, bile, exhaled air, and breast milk.

Pharmacotherapeutics

Pharmacotherapeutics is the study of how drugs are used to treat disease. This area of pharmacology is sometimes called clinical pharmacology.

Drug Names

One drug may have several different names, including the drug's official name (also known as the **generic name**), international nonproprietary name, chemical name, and **trade name** (brand or proprietary name). To demonstrate, the trade-name antibacterial drug prescribed by physicians as Keflex or Biocef is also identified by the following names:

- Cephalexin (generic name)
- Cefalexin (international nonproprietary name)

- 7-(D-α-amino-α-phenylacetomido)-3-methyl-3-cephem-4-carboxylic acid, monohydrate (chemical name)

As a medical assistant, you will probably need to use only generic or trade names. In general, think of the generic name of a drug as a simple form of its chemical name. For each new drug marketed by a drug manufacturer, the United States Adopted Names (USAN) Council selects a generic name. This name is nonproprietary; that is, it does not belong to any one manufacturer. A generic name is also considered a drug's official name, which is listed in the *United States Pharmacopeia/National Formulary.* The 50 drugs most commonly dispensed in 2002 are listed in Table 32-1 by generic name, trade name, and category of pharmacologic activity. Notice that a drug may appear in the table more than once if its dispensing record was high for multiple trade names or for generic and trade names.

A drug's trade name is selected by its manufacturer. It is protected by copyright and is the property of the manufacturer. When a new drug enters the market, its manufacturer has a patent on that drug, which means that no other manufacturer can make or sell the drug for 17 years. When the patent runs out, any manufacturer can sell the drug under the generic name or a different trade name. The original manufacturer, however, is the only one allowed to use the drug's original trade name. For example, the antibiotic cephalexin has two trade names, Keflex and Biocef. These names are owned by different manufacturers.

A physician may prescribe a drug by its generic or trade name. Because generic drugs are usually less expensive, most physicians try to prescribe them if possible. Many states allow pharmacists to substitute a generic drug for a trade-name drug unless the physician specifies otherwise. In fact, most health insurance prescription plans now require the substitution of generic drugs for trade-name drugs (unless otherwise specified by a physician). Frequently, they also require the pharmacy to charge a higher copay amount for trade-name drugs than for generic drugs. Some prescription plans now offer a mail-in pharmacy through which a patient can obtain generic drugs with a reduced copayment or without any copayment.

Drug Categories

Drugs are categorized by their action on the body, general therapeutic effect, or the body system affected. Table 32-2 lists a variety of drug categories.

TABLE 32-1 The 50 Drugs Most Commonly Dispensed in U.S. Community Pharmacies in 2002

Category of Pharmacologic Activity	Trade Name	Generic Name
Analgesic	Hydrocodone w/APAP	Hydrocodone w/APAP
Analgesic, central acting	Ultram	Tramadol
Antianginal, antihypertensive	Norvasc	Amlodipine
Antianxiety	Ativan	Lorazepam
Antibiotic	Biaxin XL	Clarithromycin
	Cipro	Ciprofloxacin
	Levaquin	Levofloxacin
	Zithromax	Azithromycin
Anticoagulant	Coumadin	Warfarin
	Dilantin	Phenytoin
Anticonvulsant	Neurontin	Gabapentin
Anticonvulsant/miscellaneous	Depakote	Divalproex
Antidepressant	Lexapro	Escitalopram oxalate
	Paxil	Paroxetine
	Wellbutrin SR	Bupropion HCL
Antidiabetic	Glucophage XR	Metformin
	Glucotrol XL	Glipizide

continued →

TABLE 32-1 The 50 Drugs Most Commonly Dispensed in U.S. Community Pharmacies in 2002 *(continued)*

Category of Pharmacologic Activity	Trade Name	Generic Name
Antifungal	Diflucan	Fluconazole
	Nystatin	Nystatin
Antihistimine	Allegra	Fexofenadine
	Zyrtec	Cetirizine
Antihyperlipidemic	Lipitor	Atorvastatin
	Tricor	Fenofibrate
Antihypertensive	Prinivil	Lisinopril
	Toprol-XL	Metoprolol
Antihypertensive, ace inhibitor	Accupril	Quinapril
	Lotensin	Benazepril hydrochloride
	Monopril	Fosinopril sodium
Antiplatelet	Plavix	Clopidogrel bisulfate
Antiviral	Valtrex	Valacyclovir
Bronchodilator	Proventil	Albuterol
Calcium channel blocker, antihypertensive	Cartia XT	Diltiazem hydrochloride
Cardiac glycoside	Lanoxin	Digoxin
Cholinergic blocker, sympathomimetic	Combivent	Ipratropium/Albuterol
Conjugated estrogens	Premarin	Conjugated estrogens
Contraceptive	Ortho Tri-Cyclen	Norestimate/Ethinyl estradiol
CNS stimulant	Concerta	Methylphenidate XR
Diuretic	Lasix	Furosemide
Erectile dysfunction inhibitor	Viagra	Sildenafil citrate
Estrogen receptor modulator	Evista	Raloxifene
Gastric acid secretory depressant	Prevacid	Lansoprazole
GERD	Nexium	Esomeprazole
Glucocorticoid	Flonase	Fluticasone
	Nasonex	Mometasone
Hypnotic	Ambien	Zolpidem
Narcotic analgesic	Oxycontin	Oxycodone
NSAID	Bextra	Valdecoxib
	Celebrex	Celecoxib
	Vioxx	Rofecoxib
Osteoclast-mediated inhibitor	Fosamax	Alendronate
Sympathomimetic	Serevent	Salmeterol/Xinafoate
Thyroid hormone	Synthroid	Levothyroxine

Source: Adapted from "The Top 200 Prescriptions for 2002 by Number of US Prescriptions Dispensed," Rx List: The Internet Drug Index, www.rxlist.com.

TABLE 32-2 Selected Drug Categories

Drug Category	Examples Generic Name (Trade Name)	Action of Drug
Analgesic	Acetaminophen (Tylenol) Acetylsalicylic acid, or aspirin Morphine sulfate (MS Contin) Oxycodone HCl (Percocet)	Relieves mild to severe pain
Anesthetic	Lidocaine HCl (Xylocaine) Tetracaine HCl (Pontocaine) Thiopental sodium (Pentothal Sodium)	Prevents sensation of pain (generally, locally, or topically)
Antacid	Aluminum hydroxide (Basaljel) Calcium carbonate (Tums) Esomeprazole (Nexium) Lansoprazole (Prevacid)	Neutralizes stomach acid
Anthelmintic	Mebendazole (Vermox) Pyrantel pamoate (Combantrin, Antiminth)	Kills, paralyzes, or inhibits the growth of parasitic worms
Antiarrhythmic	Disopyramide phosphate (Norpace) Propafenone hydrochloride (Rythmol) Propranolol HCl (Inderal)	Normalizes heartbeat in cases of certain cardiac arrhythmias
Antibiotic	Amoxicillin (Amoxil) Azithromycin (Zithromax) Cefaclor (Ceclor) Ciprofloxacin (Cipro) Clarithromycin (Biaxin XL) Levofloxacin (Levaquin)	Kills microorganisms or inhibits or prevents their growth
Anticholinergic	Atropine sulfate (Isopto Atropine) Diclomine HCl (Bentyl) Scopolamine (Transderm-Scōp)	Blocks parasympathetic nerve impulses
Anticoagulant	Enoxaparin sodium (Lovenox) Heparin sodium (Hep-Lock) Warfarin sodium (Coumadin)	Prevents blood from clotting
Anticonvulsant	Clonazepam (Klonopin) Divalproex (Depakote) Phenobarbital sodium (Luminol Sodium) Phenytoin (Dilantin)	Relieves or controls seizures (convulsions)
Antidepressant (three types)		Relieves depression
Tricyclic	Amitriptyline HCl (Elavil) Doxepin HCl (Sinequan)	
Monoamine oxidase (MAO) inhibitors	Phenelzine sulfate (Nardil) Tranylcypromine sulfate (Parnate)	
Selective serotonin reuptake inhibitors (SSRIs)	Escitalopram (Lexapro) Fluoxetine HCl (Prozac) Paroxetine (Paxil) Sertraline HCl (Zoloft)	

continued ⟶

TABLE 32-2 Selected Drug Categories *(continued)*		
Drug Category	**Examples** **Generic Name (Trade Name)**	**Action of Drug**
Antidiarrheal	Bismuth subsalicylate (Pepto-Bismol) Kaolin and pectin mixtures (Kaopectate) Loperamide HCl (Imodium)	Relieves diarrhea
Antidote	Acetylcysteine (Mucosil) for acetaminophen (Tylenol) Flumazenil (Romazicon) for benzodiazepines, such as diazepam (Valium) or alprazolam (Xanax) Naloxone HCl (Narcan) for narcotics, such as morphine	Counteracts action of specific drug class
Antiemetic	Prochlorperazine (Compazine) Promethazine (Phenergan) Trimethobenzamide HCl (Tigan)	Prevents or relieves nausea and vomiting
Antifungal	Amphotericin B (Fungizone) Fluconazole (Diflucan) Nystatin (Mycostatin) Terbinafine (Lamisil)	Kills or inhibits growth of fungi
Antihistamine	Cetirizine HCl (Zyrtec) Diphenhydramine HCl (Benadryl) Fexofenadine (Allegra) Loratadine (Claritin)	Counteracts effects of histamine and relieves allergic symptoms
Antihypertensive	Amlodipine (Norvasc) Diltiazem hydrochloride (Cartia XL) Quinapril (Prinivil)	Reduces blood pressure
Anti-inflammatory (two types)		Reduces inflammation
Nonsteroidal (NSAIDs)	Celecoxib (Celebrex) Ibuprofen (Advil) Rofecoxib (Vioxx) Valdecoxib (Bextra)	
Steroids	Dexamethasone (Decadron) Methylprednisolone (Medrol) Prednisone (Deltasone) Triamcinoline (Kenalog)	
Antineoplastic	Bleomycin sulfate (Blenoxane) Dactinomycin (Cosmegen) Paclitaxel (Taxol) Tamoxifen citrate (Nolvadex)	Poisons cancerous cells
Antipsychotic	Chlorpromazine HCl (Thorazine) Clozapine (Clozaril) Haloperidol (Haldol) Risperidone (Risperdal) Thioridazine HCl (Mellaril)	Controls psychotic symptoms

continued ⟶

TABLE 32-2 Selected Drug Categories *(continued)*		
Drug Category	**Examples** **Generic Name (Trade Name)**	**Action of Drug**
Antipyretic	Acetaminophen (Tylenol) Acetylsalicylic acid, or aspirin	Reduces fever
Antiseptic	Isopropyl alcohol, 70% Povidone-iodine (Betadine)	Inhibits growth of microorganisms
Antitussive	Codeine Dextromethorphan hydrobromide (component of Robitussin DM)	Inhibits cough reflex
Bronchodilator	Albuterol (Proventil) Epinephrine (Epinephrine Mist) Salmeterol (Severent)	Dilates bronchi (airways in the lungs)
Cathartic (laxative)	Bisacodyl (Dulcolax) Casanthranol (Peri-Colace) Magnesium hydroxide (Milk of Magnesia)	Induces defecation, alleviates constipation
Contraceptive	Ethinyl estradiol and norgestimate (Ortho Cyclen) Norethindrone and ethinyl estradiol (Ortho-Novum) Norgestrel (Ovrette)	Reduces risk of pregnancy
Decongestant	Oxymetazoline HCl (Afrin) Phenylephrine HCl (Neo-Synephrine) Pseudoephedrine HCl (Sudafed)	Relieves nasal swelling and congestion
Diuretic	Bumetanide (Bumex) Furosemide (Lasix) Hydrochlorothiazide (Hydrodiuril) Mannitol	Increases urine output, reduces blood pressure and cardiac output
Expectorant	Guaifenesin (component of Robitussin)	Liquefies mucus in bronchi; allows expectoration of sputum, mucus, and phlegm
Hemostatic	Aminocaproic acid (Amicar) Phytonadione or vitamin K_1 (Mephyton) Thrombin (Thrombogen)	Controls or stops bleeding by promoting coagulation
Hormone replacement	Hydrocortisone (Hydrocortone Acetate) for adrenocortical deficiency Insulin (Humulin) for pancreatic deficiency Levothyroxine sodium (Synthroid) for thyroid deficiency	Replaces or resolves hormone deficiency
Hypnotic (sleep-inducing) or sedative	Chloral hydrate (Noctec) Ethchlorvynol (Placidyl) Secobarbital sodium (Seconal Sodium)	Induces sleep or relaxation (depending on drug potency and dosage)

continued →

TABLE 32-2 Selected Drug Categories *(continued)*

Drug Category	Examples Generic Name (Trade Name)	Action of Drug
Muscle relaxant	Carisoprodol (Rela or Soma) Cyclobenzaprine HCl (Flexeril)	Relaxes skeletal muscles
Mydriatic	Atropine sulfate (Allergan) for ophthalmic use Phenylephrine HCl (Alcon Efrin) for ophthalmic use or (Neo-Synephrine HCl) for nasal use	Constricts vessels of eye or nasal passage, raises blood pressure, dilates pupil of eye in ophthalmic preparations
Stimulant	Amphetamine sulfate (Benzadrine) for central nervous system Caffeine (No-Doz) for central nervous system; also component of many analgesic formulations and coffee	Increases activity of brain and other organs, decreases appetite
Vasoconstrictor	Dopamine HCl (Intropin) Norepinephrine bitartrate (Levophed)	Constricts blood vessels, increases blood pressure
Vasodilator	Enalopril (Vasotec) Lisinopril (Prinivil) Nitroglycerin (Nitrostat)	Dilates blood vessels, decreases blood pressure

Sources: *Physicians' Desk Reference; U.S. Pharmacopeia Dictionary.*

Note: Some drugs have a secondary category. When in doubt, check the *Physicians' Desk Reference* or *U.S. Pharmacopeia Dictionary.*

Indications and Labeling

An **indication** is the purpose or reason for using a drug. FDA-approved indications are part of a drug's **labeling.** Labeling also includes the form of the drug, such as tablet or liquid.

Regardless of category, some drugs may be used to treat several different conditions. Multiple uses are possible if the drug affects several body systems at once or if the drug's primary effect produces significant secondary effects in other body systems.

When a drug is used for multiple indications, one or more indications may not be in its labeling. Out-of-label prescribing is legal. Doctors who do it usually know from continuing education (seminars or journal articles) that such uses are generally accepted. For example, Benadryl (diphenhydramine) is an antihistamine used to treat allergic symptoms in both children and adults. Because it tends to make a patient sleepy but is safe for children, a pediatrician may use a low dose of Benadryl as a temporary sedative for a young child. Its use as a sedative, however, is not part of the labeling for Benadryl.

Another example of a drug with multiple uses is minoxidil. As a trade-name tablet, it is known as the antihypertensive Loniten; as a trade-name topical solution, it is known as the hair-growth stimulant Rogaine. In the case of minoxidil, both indications are approved, but the tablet labeling is for hypertension and the topical solution labeling is for hair growth.

It is important to be aware of these labeling considerations when dealing with questions from patients. Never assume that a drug is appropriate for only one use or that it is administered in only one form. Always consult the doctor or other sources of drug information before answering a patient's question.

Safety

The safety of a drug is determined by how many and what kinds of adverse effects are associated with it. An adverse effect may require immediate attention. It is not uncommon for a patient to call the physician's office with complaints of new symptoms soon after beginning therapy with a drug. Be alert for such complaints, because they could be signs of an adverse reaction to the drug or an interaction with another medication. These calls should be brought to the physician's attention. Some adverse effects are common whereas others are rare.

Efficacy

A patient may complain that a newly prescribed drug is not doing what the doctor said it would. There are a variety of explanations for such a complaint, including the following:

- The drug is working adequately, but the patient does not understand how it works
- The **dosage** (size, frequency, and number of doses) needs to be adjusted

- The drug has not yet reached a therapeutic level in the bloodstream
- The wrong drug was prescribed, or the wrong drug was dispensed by the pharmacy (this is rare, but possible)
- Some drugs work better in some patients than in others; not every drug is for everyone (this is particularly true of antihistamines)
- Some forms of a drug work better than others, such as tablets versus injection
- The generic drug does not work, but the trade-name drug does

Kinds of Therapy

There are several descriptive terms for drug therapy. Depending on a patient's condition, the physician may use drugs for any of the following kinds of therapy:

- Acute: Drug is prescribed to improve a life-threatening or serious condition, such as epinephrine for severe allergic reaction
- Empiric: Drug is prescribed according to experience or observation until blood or other tests prove another therapy to be appropriate, such as penicillin for suspected strep throat
- Maintenance: Drug is prescribed to maintain a condition of health, especially in chronic disease, such as insulin for diabetes mellitus
- Palliative: Drug is prescribed to reduce the severity of a condition or its accompanying pain, such as morphine for cancer
- Prophylactic: Drug is prescribed to prevent a disease or condition, such as immunizations or birth control drugs
- Replacement: Drug is prescribed to provide chemicals otherwise missing in a patient, such as hormone replacement therapy for a woman in menopause
- Supportive: Drug is prescribed for a condition other than the primary disease until that disease resolves, such as a corticosteroid for severe allergic reactions.
- Supplemental: Drug or nutrients are prescribed to avoid deficiency, such as iron for a woman who is pregnant

Toxicology

Toxicology is the study of the poisonous effects, or toxicity, of drugs, including adverse effects and drug interactions. Because you are likely to see evidence of immediate toxic effects only when administering a drug, this topic will be discussed in more detail in Chapter 33. You must be aware, however, of some possible toxic effects that may not be apparent right away:

- An adverse effect on a fetus when the drug crosses the placenta
- An adverse effect on infants when the drug passes easily into breast milk
- Adverse reactions reported in clinical trials, such as headache, drowsiness, gastric upset, or other effects
- An adverse effect in immunocompromised patients who are unable to metabolize a drug normally
- An adverse effect in pediatric or elderly patients or in patients with hypertension, diabetes mellitus, or other serious chronic conditions
- An adverse drug interaction when the drug is taken with another drug that is incompatible
- A carcinogenic (cancer-causing) effect in some patients

Nearly always, an adverse effect has been encountered in the clinical trials of a drug, and there will be mention of the adverse effect under that heading in the package insert or in accepted drug reference works. In the reports of clinical trials, however, the drug company must report *all* adverse effects noted during testing. As a result, effects that, at least theoretically, could not be caused by the drug are included. In dealing with patients who are about to begin drug therapy, it is best to avoid mentioning specific adverse effects associated with drugs. To do so could cause undue alarm, prompt patients to imagine they have the effects, or discourage patients from taking the needed medication. Always ask patients if they have any questions, and have the doctor answer patients' questions if they are drug related. Because patients will receive lists of adverse effects from the pharmacist, encourage them to discuss concerns with the pharmacist or to call the doctor's office. Also encourage patients to inform the doctor of adverse effects they experience after beginning drug therapy.

Sources of Drug Information

It is important to keep several up-to-date sources of drug information in the office for when you or the doctor need detailed information about a specific drug. Sources to refer to include the *Physicians' Desk Reference* (Figure 32-5),

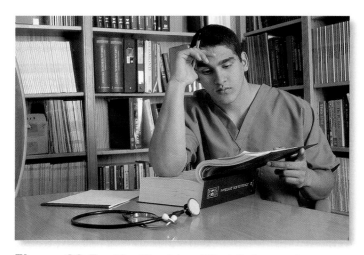

Figure 32-5. The *Physicians' Desk Reference* is one of several publications in which you can find current information on specific drugs.

Drug Evaluations, United States Pharmacopeia/National Formulary, and *American Hospital Formulary Service.*

Physicians' Desk Reference (PDR)

Medical Economics of Oradell, New Jersey, publishes the *Physicians' Desk Reference,* or *PDR,* annually, along with supplements twice a year. It sends the book free to doctors' offices and sells it through bookstores. The company also publishes separate editions for generic, nonprescription, and ophthalmologic drugs as well as a guide to drug interactions, adverse effects, and indications.

The *PDR* presents information provided by pharmaceutical companies about more than 2500 prescription drugs. The *PDR* has color-coded directories of drug categories, generic names, and trade names. It also lists each pharmaceutical company's name, address, emergency telephone number, and available products.

The drug information section is divided according to manufacturer, and the drugs are then grouped alphabetically within each manufacturer's subsection. The information closely resembles that on drug package inserts, which are illustrated in the Tips for the Office section. The package insert for each drug describes the drug, its purpose and effects (clinical pharmacology), indications, contraindications (conditions under which the drug should not be administered), warnings, precautions, adverse reactions, drug abuse and dependence, overdosage, dosage and administration, and how the drug is supplied (for example, tablets in different doses, liquid). Also included in this section are diagnostic compounds made by the drug companies.

A separate section of the *PDR* is devoted to color photographs of common drugs in various forms, also grouped by manufacturer. Other sections on poison control centers, controlled substances, and the system for reporting adverse reactions to vaccines could be important resources for you.

Drug Evaluations

Drug Evaluations is published once a year by the American Medical Association. It contains detailed information on more than 1000 drugs, including their names, efficacy, adverse reactions, and precautions.

United States Pharmacopeia/ National Formulary

The *United States Pharmacopeia/National Formulary,* or *USP/NF,* is the official source of drug standards in the United States and is published about every 5 years. By law, every drug sold under a name listed in the *USP/NF* must meet the strict standards of the *USP/NF.*

The *USP/NF* describes each drug approved by the federal government and lists its standards for purity, composition, and strength as well as its uses, dosages, and storage. The *NF* portion of the book provides the chemical formulas of the drugs.

American Hospital Formulary Service (AHFS)

The American Society of Hospital Pharmacists in Bethesda, Maryland, publishes the *American Hospital Formulary Service,* or *AHFS.* It sells the two-volume set by subscription and provides four to six supplements each year. The *AHFS* lists generic names and is divided into sections based on drug actions.

Regulatory Function of the FDA

After the FDA approves a drug, it continues its regulatory function to protect patients and consumers. The FDA reviews new-indication proposals (applications from companies for new indications for a drug), OTC proposals (applications for OTC status of a prescription drug), and further clinical trial results. If an adverse effect appears many times, for example, the FDA may withdraw the causative drug from the market.

Drug Manufacturing

The FDA also regulates drug manufacturing. It ensures that drugs shipped between states have the proper identity, strength, purity, and quality. Each manufacturer must consistently identify each drug by a particular color, form, shape, size, and label. It must produce every dose at the same tested strength, using the exact formula approved by the FDA. The manufacturer must also use high-quality, contaminant-free ingredients.

Nonprescription, or Over-the-Counter, Drugs

A nonprescription, or OTC, drug is one that the FDA has approved for use without the supervision of a licensed health-care practitioner. The consumer must follow the manufacturer's directions to use the drug safely. Some drugs, such as aspirin and vitamin supplements, have been OTC drugs for many years. The number of prescription drugs that have been granted OTC status is increasing. Although OTC drugs are safe when used as directed on the package, patient education contributes significantly to their safe use.

Prescription Drugs

A **prescription drug** is one that can be used only by order of a physician and must be dispensed by a licensed health-care professional, such as a pharmacist, physician, podiatrist, or licensed midwife. Some prescription drugs are dispensed as over-the-counter medications at much lower dosages.

Controlled Substances

A **controlled substance** is a drug or drug product that is categorized as potentially dangerous and addictive. The

TABLE 32-3 Schedules of Controlled Substances

Schedule	Abuse Potential	Examples
I	High	Heroin, LSD, methaqualone
II	High	Amphetamines, codeine, meperidine, morphine, secobarbital
III	Lower than Schedule II	Benzphetamine, butabarbital, methyltestosterone, talbutal
IV	Lower than Schedule III	Some benzodiazepines, chloral hydrate, fenfluramine, pentazocine
V	Lower than Schedule IV	Antitussives or antidiarrheals that combine small amounts of opioids (narcotics), such as codeine, dihydrocodeine, or diphenoxylate, with other drugs

Source: U.S. Department of Justice, *Physician's Manual,* March 1990.

greater the potential, the more severe the limitations on prescribing it. Use of these controlled drugs is strictly regulated by federal laws. States, municipalities, and institutions must adhere to these laws but may also impose their own regulations.

Comprehensive Drug Abuse Prevention and Control Act. The Comprehensive Drug Abuse Prevention and Control Act, also known as the Controlled Substances Act (CSA) of 1970, is the federal law that created the Drug Enforcement Administration (DEA) and strengthened drug enforcement authority. The CSA designates five schedules, according to degree of potential for a substance to be abused or used for a nontherapeutic effect. The five schedules and examples of substances in each are outlined in Table 32-3.

Drugs that are Schedule I substances have a high abuse potential or pose unacceptable dangers. In the United States these drugs are legal only for research. Doctors are not allowed to prescribe these drugs, which include heroin, LSD, marijuana, and peyote.

Drugs that are Schedule II substances have a high potential for abuse and may cause physical or psychological dependence. They do have therapeutic uses, however, for which they require written prescriptions. Prescriptions for these drugs may not be renewed. Examples of these drugs include dextroamphetamines (Dexedrine), secobarbital (Seconal), and opioids. **Opioids** are natural or synthetic drugs that produce opium-like effects, such as codeine, morphine, and meperidine (Demerol). Government agencies use the popular term **narcotics** for opioids.

Drugs that are Schedule III substances have a lower abuse potential than do drugs that are Schedule I or II substances and may cause moderate-to-low physical or psychological dependence. Prescriptions for these drugs may be given orally or in writing. Prescriptions may include refills, but refills are limited to five refills within 6 months of the original prescription. Benzphetamine (Didrex), butabarbital (Butisol), and methyltestosterone (Virilon) are examples of Schedule III drugs. Some drugs can belong to both Schedules II and III, depending on strength per tablet or capsule.

Drugs that are Schedule IV substances have a lower abuse potential than do drugs that are Schedule III substances and have various therapeutic uses. Prescriptions may include refills, but refills are limited to five refills within 6 months of the original prescription. These drugs include pentazocine (Talwin), fenfluramine, and diazepam (Valium).

Drugs that are Schedule V substances have a lower abuse potential than do drugs that are Schedule IV substances and have varied therapeutic uses. Most Schedule V drugs are dispensed like other nonopioid prescription drugs, but some may be dispensed without a prescription, depending on state regulations. Most of these drugs are antidiarrheals or antitussives that contain small amounts of opioids, such as codeine, dihydrocodeine, or diphenoxylate.

Sometimes the DEA reclassifies drugs. For example, a Schedule III drug may eventually be found to be less addictive than originally determined and therefore reclassified as a Schedule IV drug.

Controlled Substance Labeling. The Controlled Substances Act also set up a labeling system to identify controlled substances. An example of this label is shown in Figure 32-6. The large C means that the drug is a controlled substance, and the Roman numeral inside the C corresponds to the DEA schedule to which the drug belongs.

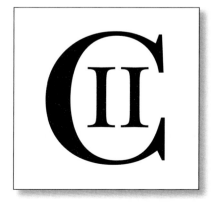

Figure 32-6. This symbol indicates that the drug is a Schedule II controlled substance.

Doctor Registration. Under the CSA, doctors who administer, dispense, or prescribe any controlled substance must register with the DEA and must have a current state license to practice medicine and, if required, a state controlled substance license. They must also comply with all aspects of the CSA, as outlined in Procedure 32-1.

To register the doctor with the DEA, submit DEA Form 224 (Figure 32-7), called the Application for Registration Under Controlled Substances Act of 1970. Send the form and the appropriate fee to the Drug Enforcement Administration, Registration Unit, Central Station, P.O. Box 28083, Washington, DC 20038-8083, or the nearest regional office. This registration must be renewed every 3 years with DEA Form 224a. The renewal steps are outlined in Procedure 32-2. The DEA should automatically send this form to the doctor's office at least 45 days before the renewal is due.

Doctors who administer or dispense drugs at more than one office must register at each location. Each registration is assigned a unique number, which identifies to suppliers and pharmacies that the doctor is properly authorized.

Ordering Drugs That Are Controlled Substances. A doctor who needs Schedule II drugs for the practice must order them by using the U.S. Official Order Forms—Schedules I & II (DEA Form 222), which you can obtain from the DEA (Figure 32-8). (DEA Form 222 is also used by research facilities such as pharmaceutical laboratories to order Schedule I drugs for research purposes; medicinal uses are not approved for Schedule I drugs.) One copy of the form goes to the DEA for overall surveillance of drug distribution. In most states this form can be used to obtain Schedule II drugs from the normal drug supplier.

When Schedule II drugs are ordered from an out-of-state company, some states require the doctor to send a copy of the purchase agreement (not the DEA Form 222) to the state attorney general's office within 24 hours of placing the order.

Schedules III through V drugs require less complicated ordering. They require only the doctor's DEA registration number.

Drug Security. Always store drugs that are controlled substances in a locked cabinet or safe. If required by state law, use double locks for opioids. The doctor should keep the key(s) at all times, except when asking you to add to or take from the stock (if this is a task medical assistants are permitted to perform in your state). If controlled drugs are stolen from the doctor's office, call the regional DEA office at once. Also notify the state bureau of narcotic enforcement and the local police. File all reports required by the DEA and other agencies as a follow-up.

Record Keeping. A doctor who administers or dispenses (as opposed to prescribing) controlled drugs to patients must maintain two types of records: dispensing records and inventory records. Note that these requirements

PROCEDURE 32.1

Helping the Physician Comply With the Controlled Substances Act of 1970

Objective: To comply with the Controlled Substances Act of 1970

OSHA Guidelines: This procedure does not involve exposure to blood, body fluids, or tissues.

Materials: DEA Form 224, DEA Form 222, DEA Form 41, pen

Method

1. Use DEA Form 224 (shown in Figure 32-7) to register the physician with the Drug Enforcement Administration. Be sure to register each office location at which the physician administers or dispenses drugs covered under Schedules II through V. Renew all registrations every 3 years using DEA Form 224a.
2. Order Schedule II drugs using DEA Form 222, shown in Figure 32-8, as instructed by the physician. (Stocks of these drugs should be kept to a minimum.)
3. Include the physician's DEA registration number on every prescription for a drug in Schedules II through V.
4. Complete an inventory of all drugs in Schedules II through V every 2 years (as permitted in your state; this task may be reserved to other health-care professionals).
5. Store all drugs in Schedules II through V in a secure, locked safe or cabinet (as permitted in your state).
6. Keep accurate dispensing and inventory records for at least 2 years.
7. Dispose of expired or unused drugs according to the DEA regulations. Always complete DEA Form 41 (shown in Figure 32-9) when disposing of controlled drugs.

continued ⟶

DEA Form – 224 (Aug 1994) OMB No. 1117-0014

APPLICATION FOR REGISTRATION
UNDER
CONTROLLED SUBSTANCES ACT OF 1970

Please **PRINT** or **TYPE** all entries.

No registration may be issued unless a completed application form has been received (21 CFR 1301.32).

Name (Last, First, Middle)

Proposed Business Address

City State Zip Code

DRUG ENFORCEMENT ADMINISTRATION
CENTRAL STATION
P.O. BOX 28083
WASHINGTON, D.C. 20038 – 8083
For **INFORMATION**, Call: **(202) 307 – 7255**

See "Privacy Act" information on reverse.

THIS BLOCK FOR DEA USE ONLY

REGISTRATION CLASSIFICATION: Submit Check or Money Order Payable to the **Drug Enforcement Administration** in amount indicated on enclosed fee schedule (3 year registration period).

• FEE MUST ACCOMPANY APPLICATION

1. BUSINESS ACTIVITY: (Check one box only)
   A ☐ Retail Pharmacy B ☐ Hospital/Clinic C ☐ Practitioner ________ *(Specify Medical Degree, e.g., DDS, DO, DVM, MD, NP, PA, etc.)* D ☐ Teaching Institution (Instructional purposes only)

2. SCHEDULES: (Check all applicable schedules in which you intend to handle controlled substances. See Schedules on Reverse of Instruction Sheet.)
   Schedule II ☐ Narcotic Schedule II ☐ Nonnarcotic Schedule III ☐ Narcotic Schedule III ☐ Nonnarcotic Schedule IV ☐ Schedule V ☐

3. ☐ CHECK HERE IF YOU REQUIRE ORDER FORMS.

4. **ALL APPLICANTS MUST ANSWER THE FOLLOWING:**
   (a) Are you currently authorized to prescribe, distribute, dispense, conduct research, or otherwise handle the controlled substances in the schedules for which you are applying, under the laws of the State or jurisdiction in which you are operating or propose to operate?
   ☐ YES – State License No. ________ ☐ NOT APPLICABLE ☐ PENDING
   ☐ YES – State Controlled Substance No. ________ ☐ NOT APPLICABLE ☐ PENDING
   (b) Has the applicant ever been convicted of a crime in connection with controlled substances under State or Federal law?
   ☐ YES ☐ NO
   (c) Has the applicant ever surrendered or had a Federal controlled substance registration revoked, suspended, restricted, or denied?
   ☐ YES ☐ NO
   (d) Has the applicant ever had a State professional license or controlled substance registration revoked, suspended, denied, restricted, or placed on probation?
   ☐ YES ☐ NO
   (e) If the applicant is a corporation (other than a corporation whose stock is owned and traded by the public), association, partnership, or pharmacy, has any officer, partner, stockholder or proprietor been convicted of a crime in connection with controlled substances under State or Federal law, or ever surrendered or had a Federal controlled substance registration revoked, suspended, restricted or denied, or ever had a State professional license or controlled substance registration revoked, suspended, denied, restricted, or placed on probation?
   ☐ YES ☐ NO ☐ NOT APPLICABLE

IF THE ANSWER TO QUESTION(S) (b), (c), (d), or (e) is YES, include a statement using the space provided on the REVERSE of this part.

Print or Type Name Here – Sign Below Applicant's Business Phone No.

SIGN HERE ➤ Signature of applicant or authorized individual Date

Title (If the applicant is a corporation, institution, or other entity, enter the TITLE of the person signing on behalf of the applicant (e.g., President, Dean, Procurement Officer, etc.…))

5. CERTIFICATION FOR FEE EXEMPTION

☐ CHECK THIS BLOCK IF APPLICANT HEREON IS A FEDERAL, STATE, OR LOCAL GOVERNMENT OPERATED HOSPITAL OR INSTITUTION.

Practitioners cannot be exempted from payment of the fee. The undersigned hereby certifies that the applicant named hereon is a Federal, state, or local government operated hospital or institution, and is exempt from the payment of the application fee.

Signature of Certifying Official Date

Print or Type Name

Print or Type Title

WARNING: **Section 843(a)(4) of Title 21, United States Code, states that any person who knowingly or intentionally furnishes false or fraudulent information in this application is subject to imprisonment for not more than four years, a fine of not more than $30,000.00 or both.**

Mail the Original and 1 copy with FEE to the above address. Retain 3rd copy for your records. **FEES ARE NOT REFUNDABLE.**

VOID

Figure 32-7. DEA Form 224 must be completed to register the physician with the Drug Enforcement Administration.

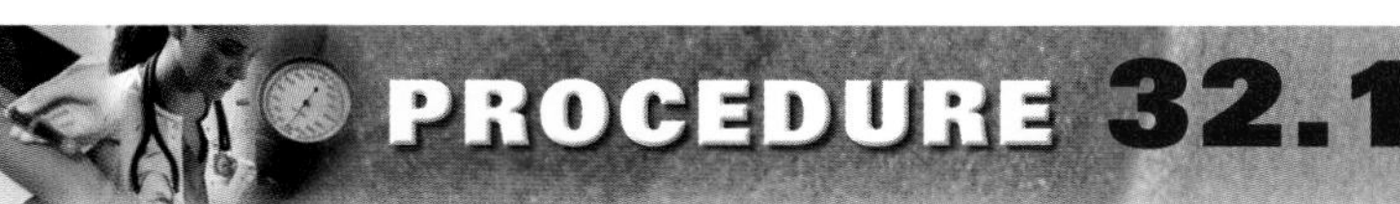

PROCEDURE 32.1

Helping the Physician Comply With the Controlled Substances Act of 1970 *(continued)*

See Reverse of PURCHASER'S Copy for Instructions

No order form may be issued for Schedule I and II substances unless a completed application form has been received. (21 CFR 1305.04).

OMB APPROVAL No. 1117-0010

TO: *(Name of Supplier)* | STREET ADDRESS

CITY and STATE | DATE

TO BE FILLED IN BY SUPPLIER

SUPPLIERS DEA REGISTRATION No.

TO BE FILLED IN BY PURCHASER

LINE No.	No. of Packages	Size of package	Name of Item	National Drug Code	Packages Shipped	Date Shipped
1						
2						
3						
4						
5						
6						
7						
8						
9						
10						

◄ LAST LINE COMPLETED *(MUST BE 10 OR LESS)* SIGNATURE OF PURCHASER OR ATTORNEY OR AGENT

Date Issued | DEA Registration No. | Name and Address of Registrant

Schedules

Registered as a | No. of this Order Form

DEA Form -222 (Oct. 1992)

U.S. OFFICIAL ORDER FORMS - SCHEDULES I & II
DRUG ENFORCEMENT ADMINISTRATION
SUPPLIER'S Copy 1

VOID

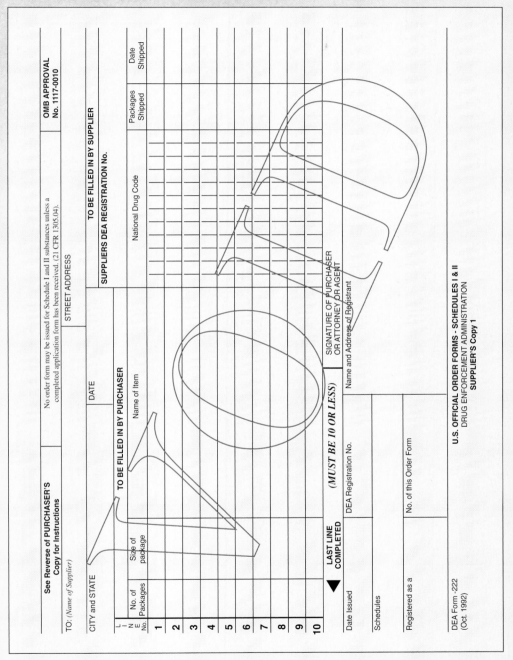

Figure 32-8. Use DEA Form 222 to order Schedule II drugs.

continued →

PROCEDURE 32.1

Helping the Physician Comply With the Controlled Substances Act of 1970 *(continued)*

OMB Approval No. 1117-0007	DEPARTMENT OF JUSTICE/DRUG ENFORCEMENT ADMINISTRATION REGISTRANTS INVENTORY OF DRUGS SURRENDERED	PACKAGE No.

The following schedule is an inventory of controlled substances which is hereby surrendered to you for proper disposition.

FROM: *(Include Name, Street, City, State and ZIP Code in space provided below).*

Signature of applicant or authorized agent

Registrant's DEA Number

Registrant's Telephone Number

NOTE: CERTIFIED MAIL (Return Receipt Requested) IS REQUIRED FOR SHIPMENTS OF DRUGS VIA U.S. POSTAL SERVICE: See instructions on reverse of form.

NAME OF DRUG OF PREPARATION Registrants will fill in Columns 1, 2, 3, and 4 Only.	Number of Containers	CONTENTS *(Number of grams, tablets, ounces or other units per container)*	Controlled Substance Content *(Each Unit)*	FOR DEA USE ONLY		
				DISPOSITION	QUANTITY	
					GMS.	MGS.
1	*2*	*3*	*4*	*5*	*6*	*7*
1						
2						

The controlled substances surrendered in accordance with Title 21 of the Code of Federal Regulations, Section 1307.21, have been received in _______packages purporting to contain the drugs listed on this inventory and have been: **(1) Forwarded tape-sealed without opening; (2) Destroyed as indicated and the remainder forwarded tape-sealed after verifying contents; (3) Forwarded tape-sealed after verifying

DATE: ________________ 19 ____ **DESTROYED BY:** ________________________________

••Strike out lines not applicable **WITNESSED BY:** ________________________________

INSTRUCTIONS

1. List the name of the drug in column 1, the number of containers in column 2, the size of each container in column 3, and in column 4 the controlled substance content of each unit described in column 3; e.g., morphine sulfate tabs., 3 pkgs., 100 tabs., 1/4 gr. (16 mg.) or morphine sulfate tabs., 1 pkg., 83 tabs., 1/2 gr. (32 mg.), etc.
2. All packages included on a single line should be identical in name, content and controlled substance strength.
3. Prepare this form in quadruplicate. Mail two (2) copies of this form to the Special Agent in Charge, under separate cover. Enclose one additional copy in the shipment with the drugs. Retain one copy for your records. One copy will be returned to you as a receipt. No further receipt will be furnished to you unless specifically requested. Any further inquiries concerning these drugs should be addressed to the DEA District Office which serves your area.
4. There is no provision for payment for drugs surrendered. This is merely a service rendered to registrants enabling them to clear their stocks and records of unwanted items.
5. Drugs should be shipped tape-sealed via prepaid express or certified mail (return reciept requested) to Special Agent in Charge, Drug Enforcement Administration, of the DEA District Office which serves your area.

PRIVACY ACT INFORMATION

AUTHORITY: Section 307 of the Controlled Substances Act of 1970 (P.L. 91-513).
PURPOSE: To document the surrender of controlled substances which have been forwarded by registrants to DEA for disposal.
ROUTINE USES: This form is required by Federal Regulations for the surrender of unwanted Controlled Substances. Disclosures of information from this system are made to the following categories of users for the purposes stated.
A. Other Federal law enforcement and regulatory agencies for law enforcement and regulatory purposes.
B. State and local law enforcement and regulatory agencies for law enforcement and regulatory purposes.
EFFECT: Failure to document the surrender of unwanted Controlled Substances may result in prosecution for violation of the Controlled Substances Act.

Public reporting burden for this collection of information is estimated to average 30 minutes per response, including the time for reviewing instructions, searching existing data sources, gathering and maintaining the data needed, and completing and reviewing the collection of information. Send comments regarding this burden estimate or any other aspect of this collection of information, including suggestions for reducing this burden, to the Drug Enforcement Administration, Records Management Section, Washington, D.C. 20537; and to the Office of Management and Budget, Paperwork Reduction Project No. 1117-0007, Washington, D.C. 20503.

DEA Form – 41
(Jun. 1986)

Figure 32-9. Use DEA Form 41 to report disposal of controlled drugs.

PROCEDURE 32.2

Renewing the Physician's DEA Registration

Objective: To accurately complete DEA Form 224a to renew the physician's DEA registration on time

OSHA Guidelines: This procedure does not involve exposure to blood, body fluids, or tissues.

Materials: Calendar, tickler file (optional), DEA Form 224a, pen

Method

1. Calculate a period of 3 years from the date of the original registration or the most recent renewal. Note that date as the expiration date of the physician's DEA registration.
2. Subtract 45 days from the expiration date, and mark this date on the calendar as a reminder to submit renewal forms. You might also put a reminder to submit renewal forms in the physician's tickler file for that date.
3. If you receive registration renewal paperwork (DEA Form 224a) from the DEA well before the submission date, put it in a safe place until you can complete it and have the physician sign it.
4. If you do not receive renewal paperwork by the submission date, call your regional DEA office to request DEA Form 224a or send written notice that no form was received and a request for the renewal form to:

   Drug Enforcement Administration
   Registration Unit
   Central Station
   P.O. Box 28083
   Washington, DC 20038-8083
5. Before the expiration deadline, complete DEA Form 224a as instructed on the form, and have the physician sign it. Prepare or request a check for the fee.
6. Submit the original and one copy of the completed form with the appropriate fee to the DEA so that it will arrive before the deadline. Keep one copy for the office records.

do not apply to doctors who prescribe but neither administer nor dispense controlled drugs.

Dispensing Records. The dispensing record for Schedule II drugs must be kept separate from the patient's regular medical record. Each time a drug is administered or dispensed, the doctor must note the date, the patient's name and address, the drug, and the quantity dispensed.

The dispensing record for Schedules III through V drugs must include the same information. The record for these drugs may be kept in the patient's medical record unless the doctor charges for the drugs dispensed. All dispensing records must be kept for 2 years and are subject to inspection by the DEA.

Inventory Records. A doctor who regularly dispenses controlled drugs must also keep inventory records of all stock on hand. This regulation applies to all scheduled drugs. To take an inventory, count the amount of each drug on hand. Compare this amount with the amount of the drug ordered and the amount dispensed to patients.

The controlled drug inventory must be repeated every 2 years. You must include copies of invoices from drug suppliers in the inventory record. All inventories and records of Schedule II drugs must be kept separate from other records. Inventories and records of other controlled drugs must be separate or easily retrievable from ordinary business and professional records. All records on controlled drugs must be retained for 2 years and made available for inspection and copying by DEA officials if requested.

Disposing of Drugs. If the doctor asks you to dispose of any outdated, noncontrolled drugs, you may flush them down the toilet or put them in the trash, depending on state law. Incineration may be required for large amounts of injectable and topical drugs. In some instances the doctor may hire an outside company to incinerate the drugs. If not, you may ask the local hospital to incinerate them for you if this is permitted by state law.

If the doctor needs to dispose of controlled drugs, such as expired samples, obtain DEA Form 41 (Figure 32-9), called Registrants Inventory of Drugs Surrendered, which is available from the nearest DEA office. Complete the form, have the doctor sign it, and call the DEA to obtain instructions for disposal of the drugs. If you must ship them, use registered mail. After the drugs have been destroyed, the DEA will issue the doctor a receipt, which you should keep in a safe place.

If doctors terminate their medical practice, they must return their DEA registration certificate and any unused copies of DEA Form 222 to the nearest DEA office. To prevent unauthorized use, write the word *VOID* across the front of these forms. Regional DEA offices will tell doctors how to dispose of any remaining controlled drugs.

Common Abbreviations Used in Prescriptions

Abbreviation	Meaning
ṫ	one
ṫṫ	two
ṫṫṫ	three
a	before
$\overline{AA}$, $\overline{aa}$	of each
a.c., ac	before meals
ad lib	as desired
amt	amount
aq.	aqueous
b.i.d., BID, bid	twice a day
$\bar{c}$	with
cap, caps	capsules
cc	cubic centimeter
d	day
D/C, d/c	discontinue
Dil, dil	dilute
dr	dram
Dr	doctor
D/W	dextrose in water
Dx, dx	diagnosis
Fl, fl, fld	fluid
gal	gallon
gm, Gm, g	gram
gr	grain
gt, gtt	drop(s)
H, hr, h	hour
HS, h.s., hs	hour of sleep or at bedtime
IM	intramuscular
IU	international unit
IV	intravenous
kg	kilogram
L, l	liter
liq	liquid
m, min	minim
mcg, μg	microgram
mEq	milliequivalent
mEq/L	milliequivalents per liter
mg	milligram
mL, ml	milliliter
mm	millimeter
noc, noct	night
npo, NPO	nothing by mouth
NS	normal saline
o.d.	once a day
O.D., OD	right eye
oint	ointment
O.S., OS	left eye
O.U., OU	both eyes
oz	ounce
$\bar{p}$	after, past
p.c., pc	after meals
per	by or with
po, per os	by mouth
PRN, p.r.n., prn	whenever necessary
pt	pint
Pt	patient
pulv	powder
q.	every
q.a.m., qam	every morning
q.d., qd	every day
q.h., qh	every hour
q2h, q2	every 2 hours
qhs	every night
q.i.d., qid	four times a day
qns, QNS	quantity not sufficient
qod	every other day
qs	quantity sufficient
℞, Rx	prescription, take
$\bar{s}$	without
SC, s.c., SQ, subq, SubQ	subcutaneous
Sig	directions
sol	solution
ss	one-half
stat, STAT	immediately
subling, SL	sublingual
S/W	saline in water
tab	tablet
Tbsp, tbsp	tablespoon
t.i.d., tid	three times a day
tinc, tr, tinct	tincture
top	topically
tsp	teaspoon
ung, ungt	ointment
U	unit
wt	weight

Figure 32-10. Physicians use many abbreviations when they write prescriptions.

Writing Prescriptions

Any drug that is not available over the counter requires a prescription. According to the Controlled Substances Act, doctors may issue prescriptions for controlled drugs only in the schedules for which they are registered with the DEA.

You must be familiar with the terms and abbreviations used in prescriptions (Figure 32-10), and you must become familiar with the doctor's style of writing. With this knowledge, you will be able to administer the prescribed drugs accurately (if allowed in your state) and to discuss the prescription accurately with a patient or pharmacist.

Every prescription has four basic parts: the superscription, inscription, subscription, and signature.

1. The superscription includes the date, the patient's full name and address, and the symbol ℞, which means "take thou" in Latin.
2. The inscription is the name of the drug (either generic or trade name) and the amount. It usually specifies the amount of drug in each dose of capsules, tablets, or suppositories in milligrams, such as "Banthine 50 mg." The inscription for oral liquid drugs typically uses milligrams per milliliter, such as "codeine sulfate 15 mg/ 5 mL." The inscription usually gives the amount for creams, ointments, and topical liquids as a percentage, such as "Spectazole 1% cream."
3. The subscription contains the directions to the pharmacist. It includes the size of each dose, the total number or amount of the drug to be dispensed for this prescription, and the form of the drug, such as tablets.
4. The signature, or transcription, refers to patient instructions. These are nearly always written using the abbreviations shown in Figure 32-10. Instructions generally follow the abbreviation Sig, which means "mark" in Latin. Many of these instructions appear in Latin, which the pharmacist must translate. The pharmacist includes the translated patient instructions on the prescription drug label.

A prescription also includes these items:

- Doctor's name, office address and telephone number, and DEA registration number
- Doctor's signature
- Number of times the prescription can be refilled
- Indication of whether the pharmacist may substitute a generic version of a trade-name drug at the patient's request

Prescriptions may be typed or handwritten in ink or indelible pencil on a prescription blank. Prescriptions for multiple medications may be written on a different form than that used for a single medication (Figure 32-11). In some states a prescription for Schedule II drugs must be prepared in triplicate on an official Department of Justice prescription form. When this form is required, the doctor keeps one copy, and the pharmacist keeps the original and sends the endorsed second copy to the Department of Justice.

The doctor may have you prepare prescriptions for signing. Because the doctor is responsible for the accuracy of prescriptions, you must be sure to write them clearly and correctly.

Prescription Blanks. Prescription blanks make prescription writing convenient and efficient. They are usually preprinted with the doctor's name, address, telephone number, state license number, and DEA registration number. Most blanks also provide space for writing the patient's name and address, the date, and other information. Some blanks are printed on colored paper or have a background design to minimize the risk of alteration,

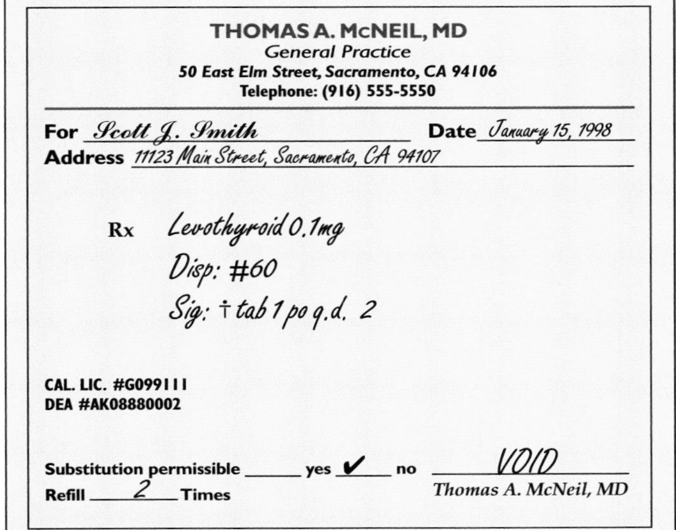

THOMAS A. McNEIL, MD
General Practice
50 East Elm Street, Sacramento, CA 94106
Telephone: (916) 555-5550

For *Scott J. Smith* **Date** *January 15, 1998*
Address *11123 Main Street, Sacramento, CA 94107*

Rx *Levothyroid 0.1mg*
Disp: #60
Sig: † tab 1 po q.d. 2

CAL. LIC. #G099111
DEA #AK08880002

Substitution permissible ____ **yes** ✔ **no** *VOID*
Refill *2* **Times** *Thomas A. McNeil, MD*

THOMAS A. McNEIL, MD
General Practice
CAL. LIC. #G099111 **50 East Elm Street, Sacramento, CA 94106**
DEA #AK08880002 **Telephone: (916) 555-5550**

For *Marjorie Smith* **Date** *January 7, 1998*
Address *11123 Main Street, Sacramento, CA 94107*

SIG:	LABEL MEDICATION	MG/CC	QUANTITY	REFILLS
Rx 1.	*Cyclobenzaprine*	*† tab 10mg po t.i.d.*	*90*	*∅*
Rx 2.	*Voltaren*	*† tab 50mg po b.i.d.*	*100*	*2*
Rx 3.	*Hydrocodone c̄ APAP*	*† tab 5/500mg po q4h prn pain*	*30*	*∅*
Rx 4.				
Rx 5.				

Substitution Permissible ____ **yes** ✔ **no** *VOID*
Thomas A. McNeil, MD

Figure 32-11. The physician may order drugs on a prescription blank (left) for a single medication or (right) for multiple medications.

CAUTION *Handle With Care*

Secure Handling of Prescription Pads

Because prescription pads are small, substance abusers can easily steal a single prescription sheet or an entire pad and use it to obtain controlled substances. To keep prescription pads secure, handle them with caution and follow these tips.

Storage and Use

- Keep all prescription pads, except the pad the physician is currently using, in a locked cabinet or a locked drawer in the physician's desk.
- Remind the physician to carry the current pad at all times or to keep it out of sight but easily accessible for writing prescriptions.
- Never ask the physician to sign prescription blanks in advance.
- Never use prescription blanks as notepaper.
- Suggest that the physician write prescribed amounts of medication in numerals and words—for example, "25 (twenty-five) capsules."

Printing and Preparation

- Order printing in colored ink that is not reproducible.
- Order prescription blanks with attached no-carbon-required duplicates to provide a permanent record of all prescriptions written. Keep the duplicate in the patient's record.
- Order tinted prescription blanks to allow easy detection of erasures or correction fluid.
- See to it that the phrase "℞ not valid for narcotics, barbiturates, or amphetamines" or "Not valid for Schedule II or III drugs" is preprinted in the center of each prescription blank. Use higher security and separate prescription blanks for these drugs.
- Do *not* allow the physician's DEA registration number to be preprinted on separate prescription blanks for Schedule II or III drugs.
- Have a sequencing number preprinted on all prescription blanks so that a missing blank will be noticed quickly.

counterfeiting, or loss. To prevent unauthorized use of prescription blanks, never leave them unattended. For tips on secure handling of prescription blanks, read the Caution: Handle With Care section.

If something about a prescription arouses suspicion, the pharmacist who receives it may call the doctor's office to verify it. You should be able to check the patient's records and tell the pharmacist whether the doctor wrote a prescription for that patient. If the prescription is a forgery, notify the doctor and, if she gives you authorization, notify the DEA.

The doctor should not use a prescription to obtain drugs for office stock. When the office needs drugs (other than Schedule II drugs), they should be obtained from a pharmacy with an order form. When the drugs are delivered, you should receive an invoice from the pharmacist.

Telephone Prescriptions. If requested by the doctor, you may telephone a new or renewal prescription to the patient's pharmacy. To do this, provide the pharmacist with the same information that would appear in a written prescription. You may not, however, telephone a prescription for a Schedule II drug. In an emergency situation, when a patient needs a drug immediately and no alternative is available, the doctor may telephone a prescription for a Schedule II drug. The amount must be limited to the period of emergency, and a written prescription must be sent to the pharmacist within 72 hours. The pharmacist must notify the DEA if a written prescription does not arrive within the specified time.

Telephone prescription renewals are called in on a daily basis from patients and pharmacies. The renewal requests may be called into the receptionist or left on a designated phone mail system. It is the medical assistant's responsibility to handle the prescription renewals in an appropriate manner. Here are some guidelines for handling office prescription renewal requests:

- Proper messages must be taken from the call or from the message system. The patient's name, phone number, pharmacy phone number, medication, dosage, and amount must be recorded and verified from the patient's medical chart.
- The patient's chart must be obtained for verification and for the physician. Do not give a prescription request to the physician without the chart.
- The physician must authorize the prescription renewal.
- The prescription renewal must be documented in the chart after the medication is called into the pharmacy.

An example of charting is as follows:

11/24/03 RX: Zyrtec 10mg, one tablet QD HS, # 30, 6 refills.______________________st

Note: Every conversation you have with patients regarding medications must be written into the medical chart.

- Prescriptions must be called in to the pharmacy the day they are requested. It is good customer service to call the patient after you have called the prescription into the pharmacy.

Vaccines

A **vaccine** is a special preparation made from microorganisms and administered to a person to produce reduced sensitivity to, or increased immunity to, an infectious disease. Vaccines are stored with the office supply of drugs and require similar handling. If you work in a pediatrician's office, you will handle the vaccines for childhood diseases. In an adult practice you can expect to see influenza vaccines and vaccines for diseases to which patients might be exposed in foreign travel.

It is important to know how vaccines work in the immune system. Immunity is discussed in detail in Chapter 1. Immunizations, particularly those for children, are discussed in Chapter 2. Adverse reactions to medications and vaccines are discussed in Chapter 33.

Through the action of the immune system, a patient can be protected from—or made not susceptible to—a disease. This immunity results from the formation of antibodies that destroy or alter disease-causing agents.

Antibody Formation

The human body creates antibodies in response to an invasion by an antigen (foreign substance). When an antigen enters the body, specialized white blood cells (lymphocytes) produce antibodies, which in turn combine with the antigens to neutralize them. This action arrests or prevents the reaction or disease that the antigen otherwise would cause. Specific antibodies always fight specific antigens.

Antigens can be bacteria, viruses, or other organisms that enter the body in spite of its natural defenses. Toxins, pollens, and drugs can also be antigens if the body reacts to them by forming antibodies. (Allergens are antigens that induce an allergic reaction.)

Vaccines contain organisms that have been killed or attenuated (weakened) in a laboratory. Because the organisms have been weakened, they stimulate antibody formation but do not overpower the body and cause disease. They may, however, still be strong enough to cause slight inflammation at the injection site and a fever. Some vaccines, such as those for the influenza viruses, may even produce some of the lesser effects of the disease against which they provide protection.

Immunizations made from organisms are called vaccines. Those made from the toxins of organisms are called toxoids. Some immunizations, such as polio vaccine, last a lifetime. Others, such as tetanus toxoid, do not. In the latter case booster immunizations must be used to stimulate the lymphocytes to produce antibodies again.

Timing of Immunizations

The Advisory Committee on Immunization Practices, the American Academy of Pediatrics, and the American Academy of Family Physicians jointly publish a schedule for immunizations (discussed in Chapter 2). This schedule covers children from infancy through 16 years of age. Just as children receive immunizations before exposure to disease, adults may receive immunizations for influenza or other diseases, including those to which an adult could be exposed during travel.

Patients are sometimes immunized after exposure. For example, if patients have been exposed to a serious disease and there is too little time for them to produce antibodies, they may receive an antiserum that contains antibodies to the disease-carrying organism. These immunizations are made from human or animal serum. If bacterial toxins (rather than bacteria) cause the disease, the patient may receive an antitoxin.

Antiserums and antitoxins must be used cautiously. They are usually reserved for life-threatening infectious diseases. Because patients can be allergic to substances in animal antiserums and antitoxins, human serums are usually preferred.

An example of a postexposure immunization is one given to a patient who has been exposed to hepatitis B virus (HBV). This patient should be given the antiserum hepatitis B immune globulin (HBV-Ig) within 7 days after exposure and again 28 to 30 days later. Because HBV-Ig is made from human serum, it causes relatively few adverse reactions. Another example involves a patient who may have been exposed to tetanus (lockjaw) organisms as the result of an injury such as a puncture wound. This patient may receive tetanus immune globulin (T-Ig, a human product) or tetanus antitoxin. Because tetanus antitoxin is made from horse serum, it may cause serious reactions in patients who are allergic to horses or horsehair.

For every vaccine in your medical office, you must be familiar with the indications, contraindications, dosages, administration routes, potential adverse effects, and methods of storage and handling. You must carefully read the package insert provided with each vaccine and, when necessary, consult drug reference books for further information.

Patient Education About Drugs

Your role as teacher cannot be underestimated with regard to drugs. In addition to providing specific instructions about different categories of drugs, you need to give your attention to all the drugs a patient is taking, whether prescription or over-the-counter.

Over-the-Counter Drugs

Even though patients can obtain OTC drugs without a prescription, they need to know several important facts to use them safely. That is why you should plan an education session with any patient whose medical history reveals use of OTC drugs or for whom a doctor has suggested an OTC drug.

In your patient education sessions, caution patients not to treat themselves with OTC drugs as a way to avoid medical care. For example, OTC drugs are available to treat recurrent yeast infections. Nonetheless, a patient should consult a doctor the first time she develops an infection.

Also inform patients that OTC drugs, which provide safe dosages for self-care only when used as directed, may not produce enough therapeutic benefit in some cases. In other cases they may mask symptoms or aggravate the problem.

Inform patients that many OTC drugs contain more than one active ingredient. These extra ingredients, such as aspirin or caffeine, can cause allergic or other undesirable effects.

It is important to advise patients that interactions can occur when a person takes more than one OTC drug at a time or takes an OTC and a prescription drug together. These interactions can lead to adverse reactions. For example, a patient who takes the prescription blood thinner warfarin (Coumadin) to prevent blood clots must avoid taking aspirin for pain relief. Taking these drugs together increases the risk of uncontrolled bleeding.

Prescription Drugs

Before patients begin drug therapy, you must inform them of certain considerations (such as when to take the drug) and drug safety precautions. As part of your patient education, provide instructions orally and, if possible, in writing. For commonly prescribed drugs, you may use preprinted information sheets published by the American Medical Association. Some pharmacies now routinely provide an information sheet with each dispensed drug. Figure 32-12 shows a sample of a drug information sheet.

Encouraging the Complete Medication List. Advise patients to inform the doctor of all drugs—prescription and OTC—they use regularly or periodically. Also advise patients to include past and present use of alcohol and recreational drugs as well as herbal remedies. When patients have more than one doctor, tell them to inform each doctor about all medications they are taking. Encourage them to keep up-to-date medication lists with dosages (some patients keep this information on their home computers). This information can help patients and health-care professionals prevent and monitor for drug interactions.

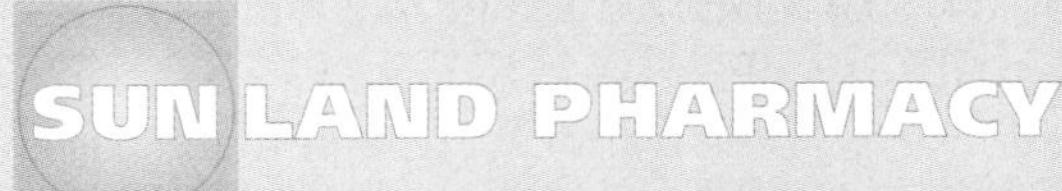

Patient Name: Jean Cranston
RX#: 711428172
Drug: Albuterol Inhalation Aerosol

COMMON USES:
To treat asthma, bronchitis, and other lung diseases.

HOW SHOULD I USE IT?
Follow your doctor's and/or the package instructions. Shake well before each use. Rinse mouth after each inhalation to avoid dryness. If breathing has not improved in 20 minutes, call doctor.

ARE THERE ANY SIDE EFFECTS?
Very unlikely, but report: Flushing, trembling, headache, nausea, vomiting, rapid heartbeat, chest pain, weakness, dizziness.

HOW DO I STORE THIS?
Store at room temperature away from moisture and sunlight. Do not puncture. Do not store in the bathroom. Rinse and clean inhaler regularly as described in package instructions.

Figure 32-12. Many pharmacies provide consumers with drug information sheets that accompany their prescriptions.

Encouraging the Complete Adverse Reaction List. Tell patients to inform each of their doctors of any adverse reactions (including allergic reactions) they have had to drugs. Previous adverse reactions may prompt a doctor to adjust a dosage or select a different drug. A history of drug allergies may contraindicate the use of a particular drug.

Educating for Patient Compliance. To help ensure that patients comply with instructions, confirm that they completely understand the name, dosage, and purpose of each drug prescribed for them. If patients must take more than one drug at a time, be sure they know the correct and relevant information for each one. Also teach patients to inform other health-care providers whenever there is a change in their medication regimen. In addition, cover each of the following points when educating patients about drugs.

- Explain how and when to take each drug to ensure its safety and effectiveness. Some drugs should be taken with food to minimize gastrointestinal irritation. Others should be taken on an empty stomach for proper absorption and metabolism. Some drugs must be taken once a day in the morning; others should be taken three or four times a day. If patients' medication schedules are complex, suggest that they create a chart, calendar, or diary to remind them of what drug to take and when, or create a schedule for them.
- Tell patients how long to take each drug. In the case of antibiotics, advise them to take all of the drug as scheduled, even if they feel better before finishing it. In the case of medicines prescribed for chronic disease, advise patients that they will need to continue taking the medication unless the doctor tells them to stop. Be aware that some drugs, such as prednisone, must be tapered off slowly to prevent adverse reactions.
- Explain how to identify possible adverse effects of each drug and safety measures related to adverse effects. For example, instruct patients to avoid certain activities, such as driving or operating machinery, while taking a drug that causes drowsiness. Also tell them to call the doctor if they experience adverse effects or any unusual reactions. If appropriate, inform patients that misuse of the drug may lead to dependence, and mention the dangers of drug dependence.
- Tell patients not to save old medications or share them with anyone else. Old medications and those taken by people other than the patient for whom they were prescribed can cause severe, unexpected adverse effects. Advise patients to check the expiration date on all drugs and to flush expired ones down the toilet.
- Suggest that patients avoid alcohol when taking a drug unless the doctor or pharmacist indicates otherwise. Alcohol interacts with some drugs, causing adverse effects such as lethargy, confusion, or coma.
- Tell patients to ask their pharmacists where to store each medication. Some drugs must be refrigerated. Others should be kept in a dry, cool area. Drugs should not usually be kept in a hot, damp place, such as a bathroom. They must always be kept out of the reach of children.
- Tell patients to take their drugs in a well-lit area so they can read each drug label carefully before taking each dose. They should never assume that they are taking the right medication without reading the label on the container. If patients have poor vision, print the name of the drug and the dosage schedule clearly on a separate piece of paper or card to attach to the medication container.
- Instruct patients to call the doctor if they have any questions about their drug therapy.

Summary

Pharmacology is the study of drugs, or pharmaceuticals. The pharmacologist studies pharmacognosy, pharmacokinetics, pharmacodynamics, pharmacotherapeutics, and toxicology. Pharmacognosy is the study of the characteristics of natural drugs and their sources. Pharmacokinetics pertains to how the body absorbs, metabolizes, distributes, and excretes a drug. Pharmacodynamics relates to a drug's mechanism of action, or how it affects the body. Pharmacotherapeutics addresses the use of drugs to prevent or treat disease. Toxicology is the study of poisons and the toxic effects of drugs, including adverse effects or drug interactions.

Every drug has several names, including chemical, generic, and trade names. Based on its action, a drug can belong to one of many classifications. These data can be found in the *Physicians' Desk Reference* and other sources of drug information.

Patients can obtain nonprescription (over-the-counter) drugs without a physician's order. For prescription drugs, patients must have a physician's written (or oral) order. For drugs that have been classified as controlled substances because they are potentially dangerous and addictive, extensive regulations apply. The physician must be registered with the Drug Enforcement Administration and follow the legal requirements of the Controlled Substances Act of 1970 to administer, dispense, and prescribe these drugs.

Immunizations usually contain killed or weakened organisms. They are used to provide immunity against specific diseases. Childhood immunizations should follow a recommended schedule. Other immunizations should be given as the need arises.

No matter what type of drug a patient must take, your role as an educator is an important one. You need to teach patients about specific drugs and required safety precautions. When you educate a patient carefully and thoroughly about a drug, you enhance the likelihood of patient compliance and safety.

REVIEW

CHAPTER 32

CASE STUDY QUESTIONS

Now that you have completed this chapter, review the case study at the beginning of the chapter and detail the steps you will take to design and implement an inventory system for your office's medications.

Discussion Questions

1. What do you think is most important about the foundations of pharmacology in direct patient care? How can you expand your knowledge of medications?
2. Distinguish between the chemical, generic, and trade names of a drug.
3. What is the protocol for prescription renewal for controlled substances?

Critical Thinking Questions

1. Why should children be immunized against diseases such as diphtheria and hepatitis B?
2. Why is patient education especially important for a patient who is receiving drug therapy?

Application Activities

1. Using the abbreviations in Figure 32-10, translate the following prescriptions:
   - triamterene 100 mg po b.i.d. p.c.
   - Benadryl 25–50 mg po hs prn insomnia
   - Rocephin 250 mg IM STAT
2. Using the *Physicians' Desk Reference,* find the information on indications, contraindications, warnings, drug abuse and dependence, and overdosage for each of the following drugs: Clinoril, fenfluramine hydrochloride, mirtazapine, Lipitor, Zocor, Lorazepam, Darvocet, and Serevent.
3. With your instructor, examine the required forms and discuss the prescribing requirements for controlled drugs in your state.

CHAPTER 33

Drug Administration

AREAS OF COMPETENCE

2003 Role Delineation Study

CLINICAL

Fundamental Principles

- Apply principles of aseptic technique and infection control
- Comply with quality assurance practices
- Screen and follow up patient test results

PATIENT CARE

- Prepare and administer medications and immunizations
- Maintain medication and immunization records
- Initiate IV and administer IV medications with appropriate training and as permitted by state law

GENERAL

Professionalism

- Display a professional manner and image
- Work as a member of the health-care team
- Treat all patients with compassion and empathy

Communication Skills

- Recognize and respect cultural diversity
- Adapt communications to individual's ability to understand
- Recognize and respond effectively to verbal, nonverbal, and written communications

Legal Concepts

- Perform within legal and ethical boundaries
- Document accurately
- Comply with established risk management and safety procedures

Instruction

- Explain office policies and procedures
- Teach methods of health promotion and disease prevention

* *Develop educational materials*

*Denotes advanced skills.

KEY TERMS

buccal
diluent
douche
infusion
intradermal (ID)
intramuscular (IM)
intravenous (IV)
ointment
route
solution
sublingual
transdermal
volume
Z-track method

CHAPTER OUTLINE

- Drug Administration and Scope of Practice
- Dosage Calculations
- Preparing to Administer a Drug

CHAPTER OUTLINE *(Continued)*

- Techniques of Administering Drugs
- Educating the Patient About Drug Administration
- Special Considerations
- Charting Medications
- Nonpharmacologic Pain Management

OBJECTIVES

After completing Chapter 33, you will be able to:

33.1 Discuss your responsibilities regarding drug administration.
33.2 Perform dosage calculations accurately.
33.3 Describe how to assess the patient before administering any drug.
33.4 Identify the seven rights of drug administration.
33.5 Describe the various techniques of drug administration you may be asked to perform.
33.6 Compare different types of needles and syringes.
33.7 Explain how to administer an intradermal, subcutaneous, or intramuscular injection.
33.8 Explain what information you need to teach the patient about drug use, interactions, and adverse effects.
33.9 Describe special considerations related to drug administration.
33.10 Describe nonpharmacologic ways to manage pain.

Introduction

Drug administration is one of the most important and most dangerous duties for a medical assistant. By following the procedures for proper drug administration, you can help restore patients to health. If you calculate dosages inaccurately, measure drugs incorrectly, or administer drugs improperly, patients' medications may have no therapeutic effect, may worsen their disease or abnormal condition, or may cause them to die.

To administer drugs safely and effectively to all patient groups, including pediatric, pregnant, and elderly patients, you must know and understand the principles of pharmacology as presented in Chapter 32. Chapter 33 prepares you to understand the fundamentals of drug administration, including the following:

- Routes of medication administration
- Dosage calculations
- Techniques involved with various types of parenteral injections
- Seven rights of drug administration
- Patient education

Because drug administration is a vital and common aspect of your job, you must familiarize yourself with the uses, contraindications, interactions, and adverse effects of common drugs. You should be familiar with the medications frequently prescribed in your practice. Furthermore, to be able to assume your role as educator, you must be comfortable with all aspects of drug administration so that you can instruct patients about the drugs prescribed to them.

Your responsibility in drug administration is great. Your critical thinking skills are important when performing this function. Self-directed lifelong learning is a key concept in direct patient care and drug administration.

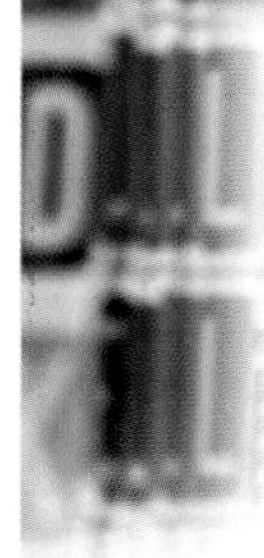

CASE STUDY

Jennifer has been a medical assistant for a year. She works with one physician in a busy multispecialty medical facility. She is very competent in her job and has a good working relationship with her physician based on mutual respect.

On one busy Monday morning, the physician orders injections and various procedures in three different exam rooms. Injections were ordered for two of the three patients. Jennifer is uncomfortable because she is unsure of what injections were ordered for each patient.

As you read through this chapter, think about what the medical assistant should do next and why.

Drug Administration and Scope of Practice

Many states have medical practice acts that define medical assistants' exact duties in drug administration. For example, an act may specify which drugs you are allowed to administer and by which **routes.** Because state laws vary, you need to research the scope of practice for medical assistants in the state where you will work.

Dosage Calculations

Before you can administer a drug, you may need to calculate the dose prescribed by the physician. To do so, you must understand various systems of measurement and ways to convert from one system to another.

Measurement Systems

In the United States three systems of measurement are used in pharmacology and drug administration. You must be able to use all three of these systems:

1. Metric
2. Apothecaries'
3. Household

Although most drug manufacturers and doctors use the metric system, some doctors still use the older apothecaries' system. You must also be familiar with the household system, because most patients use household measures when taking medicines at home.

To understand drug measurement, focus primarily on remembering the basic unit of volume and weight for each system, as shown in Table 33-1. **Volume** refers to the amount of space a drug occupies. Weight refers to its heaviness.

Metric System. The basic units of volume and weight in the decimal-based metric system are liters (L) to measure volume and grams (g) to measure weight. Prefixes are added to these basic units of measurement to indicate multiples—such as dekaliter or kilogram—or fractions—such as milliliter or microgram. Common metric equivalents are presented in Table 33-2. Note that a cubic centimeter (cc) is the amount of space occupied by 1 mL. Therefore, cc and mL are used interchangeably in prescriptions.

Apothecaries' System. The apothecaries' system uses minims, fluidrams, fluidounces, pints, quarts, and gallons to measure volume. It measures weight by grains, scruples, drams, ounces, and pounds. Common apothecaries' equivalents are outlined in Table 33-3. The apothecaries' system also uses Roman numerals to indicate the

TABLE 33-1 Comparing Selected Metric and Apothecaries' Measures (Approximate Values)

Measures of Volume	Measures of Weight
Metric vs. Apothecaries'	Metric vs. Apothecaries'
1 milliliter (mL) = 15–16 minims (min, ♏)	0.06 gram (g) or 60 milligrams (mg) = 1 grain (gr)
4 mL = 1 fluidram (fl dr, fʒ)	0.5 g or 500 mg = 7¾ gr
30 mL = 1 fluidounce (fl oz, f℥)	1 g or 1000 mg = 15 gr
500 mL = 1 pint (pt)	4 g = 1 dram (dr, ʒ)
1000 mL or 1 liter (L) = 1 quart (qt)	30 g = 1 ounce (oz, ℥)

TABLE 33-2 Common Metric Equivalents

Measures of Volume	Measures of Weight
0.001 liter (L) = 1 milliliter (mL) or 1 cubic centimeter (cc)	0.001 gram (g) or 1000 micrograms (μg) = 1 milligram (mg)
0.01 L = 1 centiliter (cL)	0.01 g = 1 centigram (cg)
0.1 L = 1 deciliter (dL)	0.1 g = 1 decigram (dg)
1 L = 1000 mL	1 g = 1000 mg or 0.001 kilogram (kg)
10 L = 1 dekaliter (daL)	10 g = 1 dekagram (dag)
100 L = 1 hectoliter (hL)	100 g = 1 hectogram (hg)
1000 L = 1 kiloliter (kL)	1000 g = 1 kg

TABLE 33-3 Common Apothecaries' Equivalents

Measures of Volume	Measures of Weight
60 minims (min, ♏) = 1 fluidram (fl dr, fʒ)	20 grains (gr) = 1 scruple (scr, ℈)
8 fl dr = 1 fluidounce (fl oz, f℥)	60 gr or 3 scr = 1 dram (dr, ʒ)
16 fl oz = 1 pint (pt)	8 dr = 1 ounce (oz, ℥)
2 pt = 1 quart (qt)	12 oz = 1 pound (℔)
4 qt = 1 gallon (gal)	

TABLE 33-4 Common Household Measurements

Measures of Volume
60 drops (gtt) = 1 teaspoon (tsp)
3 tsp = 1 tablespoon (tbsp)
6 tsp = 1 ounce (oz) or 2 tbsp
8 oz = 1 cup (c)
2 c = 1 pint (pt)
4 c = 1 quart (qt) or 2 pt

amount of the drug. For example, ASA gr X means "10 grains of acetylsalicylic acid (aspirin)." Note that in the metric system, the amount precedes the unit, whereas in the apothecaries' system, the amount follows the unit. Although this system is less popular than it once was, some doctors still use it.

Household System. The only household units of measurement that are used to measure drugs are units of volume. These include drops, teaspoons, tablespoons, ounces, cups, pints, quarts, and gallons. Common household equivalents are shown in Table 33-4.

Conversions Between Measurement Systems

At times you may need to convert from one measurement system to another. Because of the difference in basic units of measure, you must remember that conversions between systems are only approximate equivalents. If you use a conversion chart, read it carefully before administering a drug. Check it several times, and place a ruler under the line you are reading to be absolutely sure you are reading the chart properly. When you must calculate conversions instead of using a conversion chart, use either the ratio or the fraction method.

Basic Calculations. In some instances, you can use a basic formula to calculate drugs that have the same labels—such as milligrams and milligrams—and therefore do not require a conversion. The basic calculation that you would use looks like this:

$$\frac{\text{desired dose}}{\text{dose on hand}} \times \text{quantity of dose on hand}$$

Suppose that the physician orders aspirin, 10 grains. However, all that the office has on hand are 5-grain aspirins. Follow these steps to perform the basic calculation:

1. Verify that no conversion is necessary. In this example, because both measures are in grains, you do not need to convert the measurement.
2. Use the following formula and label all the parts:

$$\frac{\text{desired dose}}{\text{dose on hand}} \times \text{quantity of dose on hand}$$

$$\frac{10\,\cancel{\text{gr}}}{5\,\cancel{\text{gr}}} \times 1\text{ Tablet} = \frac{10}{5} = 2\text{ tablets}$$

Ratio Method. Suppose the doctor orders ASA gr X. Although this translates to 10 grains of aspirin in the apothecaries' system, the available tablets come in milligrams, a metric measurement. To convert from apothecaries' to metric measure, you must set up a ratio to solve for x, the unknown dose in milligrams. Follow these steps to convert the measurement.

1. Set up the first ratio:

$$x : 10\text{ gr}$$

2. Next set up the second ratio with the standard equivalent between the available and ordered measurements:

$$60\text{ mg} : 1\text{ gr}$$

3. Then use both ratios in a proportional equation that reads, x is to 10 gr as 60 mg is to 1 gr. Mathematically, this is written:

$$x : 10\text{ gr} :: 60\text{ mg} : 1\text{ gr}$$

4. Multiply the outer and then the inner parts of the proportion:

$$x \times 1\text{ gr} = 10\text{ gr} \times 60\text{ mg}$$

5. To solve for x, divide both sides of the equation by 1 gr, then do the arithmetic, canceling out like terms in

each numerator (top of the fraction) and denominator (bottom of the fraction):

$$\frac{x \times \cancel{1\,\text{gr}}}{\cancel{1\,\text{gr}}} = \frac{10\,\cancel{\text{gr}} \times 60\,\text{mg}}{1\,\cancel{\text{gr}}}$$

$$x = \frac{10 \times 60\,\text{mg}}{1}$$

$$x = \frac{600\ \text{mg}}{1}$$

$$x = 600\,\text{mg}$$

Fraction Method. Suppose the physician orders 300 mg of aspirin in the metric system. The tablets, however, are labeled in grains, an apothecaries' measure. To make this conversion, follow these steps.

1. Set up a fraction with the ordered dose on the top and the unknown amount on the bottom:

$$\frac{300\,\text{mg}}{x}$$

2. Next set up a fraction with the standard equivalent. Make sure that for this fraction you use units of measure on the top and the bottom that match the units of measure on the top and the bottom of the first fraction:

$$\frac{60\,\text{mg}}{1\ \text{gr}}$$

3. Then set up a proportion with both fractions:

$$\frac{300\,\text{mg}}{x} = \frac{60\,\text{mg}}{1\,\text{gr}}$$

4. Now cross multiply. Multiply the bottom left number by the top right number, and multiply the top left number by the bottom right number:

$$x \times 60\,\text{mg} = 300\,\text{mg} \times 1\,\text{gr}$$

5. To solve for x, divide both sides of the equation by 60, then do the arithmetic, canceling out like terms in the top and bottom of each fraction:

$$\frac{x \times \cancel{60\,\text{mg}}}{\cancel{60\,\text{mg}}} = \frac{300\,\cancel{\text{mg}} = 1\,\text{gr}}{60\,\cancel{\text{mg}}}$$

$$x = \frac{300 \times 1\,\text{gr}}{60}$$

$$x = \frac{300\,\text{gr}}{60}$$

$$x = 5\,\text{gr}$$

Calculations and Drug Doses

You may occasionally need to do some calculations to provide a prescribed drug dose. You can use the ratio method or the fraction method to calculate the dose. Because a patient's health or life can depend on your calculations, take the time to check and recheck your arithmetic. If you need extra practice in calculations, consider buying and using a dosage calculation workbook.

Ratio Method. Suppose the doctor orders 500 mg of ampicillin, but each tablet contains only 250 mg. To calculate how to provide this dose, follow these steps.

1. Set up a ratio with the unknown number of tablets and the amount of the drug ordered:

$$x : 500\ \text{mg}$$

2. Next set up a ratio with a single tablet and the amount of drug in a single tablet:

$$1\ \text{tab} : 250\ \text{mg}$$

3. Now put both of these ratios in a proportion:

$$x : 500\ \text{mg} :: 1\ \text{tab} : 250\ \text{mg}$$

4. Multiply the outer and then the inner parts of the proportion:

$$x \times 250\,\text{mg} = 500\,\text{mg} \times 1\,\text{tab}$$

5. To solve for x, divide both sides of the equation by 250 mg, then do the arithmetic, canceling out like terms in the top and bottom of each fraction:

$$\frac{x \times \cancel{250\,\text{mg}}}{\cancel{250\,\text{mg}}} = \frac{500\,\cancel{\text{mg}} \times 1\,\text{tab}}{250\,\cancel{\text{mg}}}$$

$$x = \frac{500\,\text{tabs}}{250}$$

$$x = 2\,\text{tabs}$$

As another example, the doctor orders 30 mg of Adalat, but each capsule contains only 10 mg. To calculate the prescribed drug dose using the ratio method, you would set up these equations:

$$x : 30\ \text{mg}$$

$$1\ \text{cap} : 10\ \text{mg}$$

$$x : 30\ \text{mg} :: 1\ \text{cap} : 10\ \text{mg}$$

$$x \times 10\ \text{mg} = 30\ \text{mg} \times 1\ \text{cap}$$

$$\frac{x \times \cancel{10\,\text{mg}}}{\cancel{10\,\text{mg}}} = \frac{30\,\cancel{\text{mg}} \times 1\,\text{cap}}{10\,\cancel{\text{mg}}}$$

$$x = \frac{30\,\text{caps}}{10}$$

$$x = 3\,\text{caps}$$

Fraction Method. For the same problem, you could use the fraction method to calculate how to provide the prescribed dose. Follow these steps for the fraction method.

1. Set up the first fraction with the dose ordered and the unknown number of capsules:

$$\frac{30\,\text{mg}}{x}$$

2. Set up the second fraction with the amount of drug in a capsule and a single capsule:

$$\frac{10\text{ mg}}{1\text{ cap}}$$

3. Then use both fractions in a proportion:

$$\frac{30\text{ mg}}{x} = \frac{10\text{ mg}}{1\text{ cap}}$$

4. Cross multiply. Remember to multiply the bottom left number by the top right number and multiply the top left number by the bottom right number:

$$x \times 10\text{ mg} = 30\text{ mg} \times 1\text{ cap}$$

5. To solve for x, divide both sides of the equation by 10 mg, then do the arithmetic, canceling out like terms in the top and bottom of each fraction:

$$\frac{x \times \cancel{10\text{ mg}}}{\cancel{10\text{ mg}}} = \frac{30\cancel{\text{ mg}} \times 1\text{ cap}}{10\cancel{\text{ mg}}}$$

$$x = \frac{30\text{ caps}}{10}$$

$$x = 3\text{ caps}$$

As another example, the doctor orders 120 mg of Armour thyroid but each tablet contains only 30 mg. To calculate the prescribed drug dose using the fraction method, you would set up these equations:

$$\frac{120\text{ mg}}{x}$$

$$\frac{30\text{ mg}}{1\text{ tab}}$$

$$\frac{120\text{ mg}}{x} = \frac{30\text{ mg}}{1\text{ tab}}$$

$$x \times 30\text{ mg} = 120\text{ mg} \times 1\text{ tab}$$

$$\frac{x \times \cancel{30\text{ mg}}}{\cancel{30\text{ mg}}} = \frac{120\cancel{\text{ mg}} \times 1\text{ tab}}{30\cancel{\text{ mg}}}$$

$$x = \frac{120\text{ tabs}}{30}$$

$$x = 4\text{ tabs}$$

Pediatric Dosage Calculations

Most pediatric dosage calculations are based on the child's age or body weight. The common formulas used for pediatric dosage calculations are Clark's rule and Fried's rule.

Clark's Rule

$$\frac{\text{weight of child}}{150\text{ lbs}} \times \text{adult dose} = \text{child's dose}$$

Fried's Rule

$$\frac{\text{age of child in months}}{150\text{ lbs}} \times \text{average adult dose}$$

$$= \text{child's dose}$$

Example. Katie has just turned 3 years old and weighs 30 pounds. Her mother wants to know how much cough syrup to give Katie. The directions have worn off the bottle and she can only make out the dosage for adults: 2 teaspoons every 4 hours. How much cough syrup should Katie receive?

The calculation based on Clark's rule would look like this:

$$\frac{30}{150} \times 10\text{ ml} = \text{Katie's dose}$$

$$\frac{1}{5} \times 10\text{ ml} = 2\text{ ml}$$

The calculation based on Fried's rule would look like this:

$$\frac{36}{150} \times 10\text{ ml} = \text{Katie's dose}$$

$$0.24 \times 10\text{ ml} = 2.4\text{ ml}$$

Preparing to Administer a Drug

Drugs may be administered for either local or systemic effects. Generally, drugs that have local effects are applied directly to the skin, tissues, or mucous membranes. Drugs that produce systemic effects are administered by routes that allow the drug to be absorbed and distributed in the bloodstream throughout the body. The importance of extreme care with drug dose and route is described in the Caution: Handle With Care section.

Before prescribing the route of administration for a drug, the doctor considers the drug's mechanism of action (described in the section on pharmacodynamics in Chapter 32); the drug's characteristics, cost, and availability; and the patient's physical and emotional state. The different routes of administration are described in Table 33-5 and discussed later in this chapter.

Assessment

Although the doctor gives the order to administer a drug, much of the responsibility is yours. Because you will often interview the patient, you must be alert to—and inform the doctor of—any change in the patient's condition that could affect drug therapy.

Injection Site. Part of your assessment is to locate and inspect the injection site. Find the injection site by using anatomical landmarks. Inspect the skin by checking for the following conditions:

- Moles
- Birthmarks
- Traumatic injury
- Redness
- Rash
- Edema
- Cyanosis

CAUTION *Handle With Care*

Dose and Route in Drug Administration

In the 2003 AAMA Role Delineation Chart, drug preparation and administration are included among the basic clinical skills for patient care. They require close attention to detail, strong patient assessment skills, and expert technique.

You must give close attention to both dose and route of administration, especially when one depends on the other. Not only must you give extreme care to dose and route, but frequently you must also check and recheck the ordered form of the drug (for example, tablet or extended release capsule). In the following examples, this crucial relationship is illustrated.

1. Prochlorperazine (Compazine) is an antiemetic drug for acute nausea and vomiting. It is given to both children and adults. When the vomiting is so severe that a tablet or capsule cannot be swallowed, the drug is administered in injectable or suppository form. This drug is available in the following forms:
   - 10 mL multidose vials with 5 mg of drug per mL, written as 5 mg/mL
   - 2 mL single-dose vials 5 mg/mL
   - 4 fl oz bottles of syrup 5 mg/5 mL (5 mg/1 tsp)
   - 5 mg tablets
   - 10 mg tablets
   - 2 mL prefilled disposable syringes 5 mg/mL
   - 2½ mg suppositories
   - 5 mg suppositories
   - 25 mg suppositories
   - 10 mg extended release capsules
   - 15 mg extended release capsules

   Because so many forms of this drug are available, there is a high risk of error in choosing the correct form. In addition, the route of administration can determine how much drug is delivered in one dose. For example, note that suppositories are available in 2½-mg, 5-mg, and 25-mg forms. If the 2½-mg dose were written as 2.5 mg, there might be confusion with the 25-mg dose suppository. Thus the 2½-mg suppository is always written this way, even in the PDR. This clarification helps prevent a child's receiving the adult dose of 25 mg, which could result in serious complications to the central nervous system. This possible confusion is a good example of how much difference a decimal point can make.

   Note also that in the syrup there is a 5-mg dose of drug per 5 mL (1 tsp), whereas in the other liquid forms (vials and prefilled syringes), there is a 5-mg dose of drug per 1 mL. The injectable form is five times more concentrated than the syrup. Therefore, if you were to administer the same amount of injectable liquid as syrup to a patient, you would give the patient five times more drug than in the syrup. Just as a child could be endangered with the 25-mg suppository, an adult could be endangered with the wrong form of liquid. Because elderly patients often receive syrup forms of medication, this instruction could be particularly confusing.
2. Allergy shots must be administered subcutaneously rather than intramuscularly to allow slower absorption of the serum. Within 30 minutes, a wheal and redness will appear if the patient has an allergic reaction. In such a case the patient requires further close monitoring. If the serum were injected intramuscularly, this reaction would not only be hidden (because of the deeper administration), it would also occur more rapidly (because of the faster rate of absorption). In fact, the patient could go into anaphylaxis, or anaphylactic shock, without any warning.

Check and recheck every order and drug label to prevent confusion and incorrect administration. This procedure is always worth the time it takes.

- Burns
- Tattoos
- Side of a mastectomy
- Paralyzed areas
- Warts

If you are unsure about any of these conditions, inform the physician.

Drug Allergies. During the assessment, it is important to ask the patient about any drug allergies. Even though you may see a patient on a regular basis, be in the habit of asking about drug allergies at every patient visit. Patients often see other physicians or specialists, who may have prescribed different medications. A patient could have had a drug reaction by a medication that has been prescribed by another physician. If applicable,

TABLE 33-5 Routes and Methods of Drug Administration

Route and Drug Forms	Method
Buccal route Tablets	Place drug between patient's gum and cheek. To ensure absorption, tell patient to leave tablet there until it dissolves and not to chew or swallow it. Tell the patient not to eat, drink, or smoke until tablet is completely dissolved.
Intradermal route Solutions Powders for reconstitution	Administer drug by injection into upper layers of patient's skin.
Intramuscular route Solutions Powders for reconstitution	Administer drug by injection into muscle.
Intravenous route Solutions (often in bags of 250, 500, or 1000 mL) Powders for reconstitution Blood and blood products	Administer drug by injection or infusion into vein.
Inhalation therapy (nasal or oral) Aerosols Sprays Mists or steam	Administer drug by inhalation to reach respiratory tract.
Oral route Tablets Capsules Liquids Lozenges	Give drug to patient to swallow.
Ophthalmic (eye) or otic (ear) route Solutions Ointments	Apply drug, usually as drops, in patient's eye or ear.
Rectal route Suppositories Solutions	Insert suppository into rectum. Administer solution as enema, using tube and nozzle.
Subcutaneous route Solutions Powders for reconstitution	Administer drug by injection into subcutaneous layer of skin.
Sublingual route Tablets Sprays	Place drug under patient's tongue. To ensure absorption, tell patient to leave tablet there until it dissolves and not to chew or swallow it. Tell the patient not to eat, drink, or smoke until tablet is completely dissolved.
Topical route Ointments Lotions Creams Tinctures Powders Sprays Solutions	Apply drug to patient's skin or rub into skin.

continued →

TABLE 33-5 Routes and Methods of Drug Administration *(continued)*	
Route and Drug Forms	**Method**
Transdermal route Patches	Apply drug to clean, dry, nonhairy area of skin.
Urethral route Solutions	Administer drug by instilling in bladder, using catheter.
Vaginal route Solutions Suppositories Ointments Foams Creams	Administer solution as douche, using tube and nozzle. Administer any other form by inserting into vagina with applicator.

document in the patient chart "NKDA" or "no known drug allergies."

Patient Condition. Before administering a drug, assess the patient's overall condition. For example, does the patient have a viral infection? Vaccines are not recommended if the patient has a viral infection such as a common cold. In addition, review the patient's drug list to ensure that any medications already being taken will not interfere with the ordered drug or route of administration. Also verify again that the ordered dose is appropriate for the patient's age and weight.

Patient Consent Form. Many physicians require that a patient sign a consent form before receiving an injection. This form provides general information regarding the medication or vaccine and lists the possible side effects or adverse reactions. If your physician requires a consent form, make sure that the patient signs the form and that you have answered any questions prior to giving the injection.

General Rules for Drug Administration

No matter what drug or administration route is ordered, follow these general rules when administering drugs.

- Give only the drugs the physician has ordered. Written orders are preferable, but oral orders are appropriate for emergencies. If you are unfamiliar with any aspect of a drug the physician orders, consult a drug reference work.
- Wash your hands before handling the drug. Prepare the drug in a well-lit area, away from distractions. Focus only on the task at hand.
- Calculate the dose if necessary. If you are unsure of your computation, ask another medical assistant, a nurse, or the physician to check it.
- Avoid leaving a prepared drug unattended, and never administer a drug that someone else has prepared.
- Ask the patient to state his name to ensure correct identification. Also ask the patient to tell you about any possible drug allergies. Do not rely on documentation in his chart; he may have developed a new allergy that has not yet been added to the record. Then verify any drug allergies in the chart.
- Be sure the physician is in the office when you administer a drug or vaccine. If the patient develops an anaphylactic reaction (sudden, severe allergic reaction) to the drug or vaccine, the physician must administer epinephrine. Some patients need to know how to administer this drug themselves. For information about epinephrine, see the Educating the Patient section.
- After administering the drug, ask the patient to remain in the facility for 10 to 20 minutes so that you can observe the patient for any unexpected effects. Give the patient specific instructions about the effects of the drug as well as general information about drug use.
- If the patient refuses to take the drug, flush it down the toilet. Do *not* return it to the original container. Be sure to document the refusal in the patient's record and tell the physician.
- If you make an error in drug administration, tell the physician immediately.
- Document immediately the drug and dose administered; never document administration before giving medicine.

To master your administration techniques, practice with classmates. When on the job, ask a coworker, perhaps a nurse or a more experienced medical assistant, to critique your technique.

Seven Rights of Drug Administration

When administering any drug, whether medication or vaccine, observe the seven "rights" of drug administration.

Educating the Patient

Using an Epinephrine Autoinjector

If you are working in a medical office that treats people with allergies, you must be familiar with epinephrine so that you can teach patients how to self-administer the drug. Epinephrine is a drug used to treat allergies so severe that exposure to the allergen may be life-threatening. The following reactions indicate the possibility of anaphylaxis, or anaphylactic shock, a severe allergic reaction:

- Flushing
- Sharp drop in blood pressure
- Hives
- Difficulty breathing
- Difficulty swallowing
- Convulsions
- Vomiting
- Diarrhea and abdominal cramps

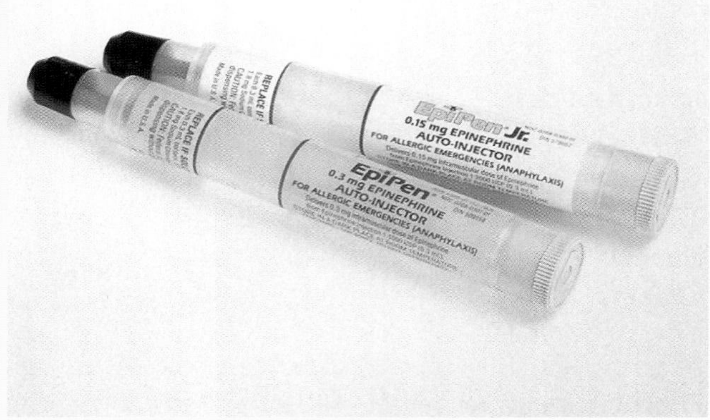

Figure 33-1. Epinephrine autoinjectors come prepackaged, containing the correct amount of the drug for an adult or a child (the junior unit).

If a patient with a severe allergy experiences any or all of these symptoms, the reaction can be fatal unless emergency treatment is given immediately. Therefore, patients who cannot always control their exposure to an allergen—for example, bee or wasp venom—must have access to an epinephrine autoinjector for emergency intramuscular use.

These injectors, which are prepackaged (Figure 33-1), deliver either 0.3 mg of epinephrine—a single dose for an adult—or 0.15 mg of epinephrine—a single dose for a child. A patient who is exposed to the allergen should use the injector if the allergy is confirmed or if the allergy is suspected and signs of anaphylaxis appear.

Teach the patient to follow these steps when using an autoinjector.

1. Remove the autoinjector from the packaging (box and/or plastic tube).
2. Pull back the gray cap.
3. Place the black tip of the injector on the outside of the upper thigh. (The injector can go through clothing.)
4. Press firmly into the thigh and hold for 10 seconds.
5. Remove the autoinjector and massage the injection site for a few minutes.
6. Call your physician or go to the emergency room of a nearby hospital. An autoinjector is designed as emergency supportive therapy only. It is not a replacement or substitute for immediate medical or hospital care.

Make sure the patient is thoroughly familiar with the parts of the autoinjector, how to activate it, how to use it, and what to do next. Ask the patient to explain the use of the autoinjector to you, as if you had never seen one. This approach not only reinforces the patient's understanding of the process but also improves the patient's self-confidence and points out any possible misconceptions. If the patient is very young or otherwise unable to use the autoinjector reliably, teach a family member or companion how to perform the process.

Never deviate from these seven steps. Adhering to these rights helps ensure that you administer the drug correctly. The seven rights refer to the following:

1. Right patient
2. Right drug
3. Right dose
4. Right time
5. Right route
6. Right technique
7. Right documentation

Right Patient. Always check the name on the order for a drug or vaccine in the patient's chart; then ask the patient to tell you her name. Be especially careful with a forgetful or confused patient, because she might answer to any name. Have a confused patient state her name, or check her name with an attending family member.

Right Drug. Carefully compare the name of the prescribed drug or vaccine in the patient's chart with the label on the drug container. As you check the drug name on the label, look at the expiration date. Never use a drug that has passed this date.

If you are unfamiliar with the drug, look it up in the *PDR* or other drug reference. Also, never prepare a drug from a container with a damaged or handwritten label. To ensure accuracy, read the label three times:

1. When you obtain the drug container from the cabinet
2. When you pour or prepare the drug from the container
3. When you put the container back in the cabinet (before leaving the medication room)

Right Dose. Compare the dose on the order in the patient's chart with the dose you prepare. To obtain the right dose, read the label closely. Do not confuse the dose contained in one tablet with the number of tablets in the container.

Right Time. Be sure to give the drug at the right time. If it must be given after meals, make sure the patient has eaten recently. For certain drugs, you must ensure that it is the correct time of day and the correct time in a series of doses. Timing is crucial with allergy shots because of possible reactions.

Right Route. Double-check to make sure the administration route you are preparing to use matches the route the doctor ordered. Check that the patient can receive the drug by this route and that the route seems appropriate. For example, if the patient has an injury at the specified injection site, consult the doctor for a possible alternative site or a different route.

Right Technique. Always use the proper administration technique. If you have not given a drug or vaccine by the ordered route recently, review the technique before administering the drug.

Right Documentation. Document the procedure immediately after administering the drug or vaccine to the patient. Do not wait until later, and do not document before administration. Be sure to include the date, time, drug or vaccine name, dose, administration route, patient reaction, patient education about the drug, and your initials. If the drug is a controlled substance, also document it on the controlled substance inventory record. Remember that correct documentation demands neat handwriting that others who care for the patient can read easily.

Techniques of Administering Drugs

The doctor may ask you to administer drugs by one of the routes outlined in Table 33-5. Because most patients take a prescription to a pharmacy to be filled and then take oral drugs at home, you rarely need to administer these drugs in the office. You are likely, however, to be asked to do the following.

- Place drugs in the patient's mouth between the cheek and gum or under the tongue
- Administer a drug by any means other than by mouth (if permitted in your state)
- Demonstrate how to use an inhaler
- Apply topical drugs (those applied to the skin)
- Administer or assist in administering drugs into the urethra, vagina, or rectum
- Administer medications to the eye or ear

These duties require you to master a variety of techniques to give drugs safely by any route.

Oral Administration

Drugs for oral administration include tablets, capsules, lozenges, and liquids. These drugs are absorbed relatively slowly as they travel along the gastrointestinal (GI) tract.

Oral administration is contraindicated in patients who have severe nausea, are comatose, or cannot swallow. Certain drugs are ineffective when administered orally, because the digestive process changes them chemically to an ineffective form or does not deliver them to the bloodstream quickly enough.

Many drugs, however, are most effective when given orally. These include antibiotics, vitamins, throat lozenges, and cough syrups. Although these drugs are familiar to most people, as a medical assistant, you must follow certain steps to ensure that the patient understands the drug and that the drug is administered safely and effectively. The steps for oral administration are outlined in Procedure 33-1.

Buccal and Sublingual Administration

Although buccal and sublingual drugs are placed in the mouth, they do not continue along the GI tract. Instead, they dissolve and are absorbed in the **buccal** area (between the cheek and gum) or the **sublingual** area (under the tongue), where they are placed. The medication is absorbed through tissue that is rich in capillaries, and the drug enters the bloodstream directly. Because the drug does not pass into the stomach or intestines before absorption, it produces a therapeutic effect more quickly than do oral drugs.

Specially formulated tablets may be given by the buccal or sublingual routes. Except for the point at which you give the tablet to the patient, the steps for administering buccal and sublingual drugs are the same as those for drugs administered orally (as outlined in Procedure 33-1). When you administer buccal or sublingual medications, your role usually involves teaching the patient how to administer these medications at home.

For both buccal and sublingual administration, tell the patient not to chew or swallow the tablet. Tell the patient

PROCEDURE 33.1

Administering Oral Drugs

Objective: To safely administer an oral drug to a patient

OSHA Guidelines: This procedure does not involve exposure to blood, body fluids, or tissues.

Materials: Drug order (in patient chart), container of oral drug, small paper cup (for tablets, capsules, or caplets) or plastic calibrated medicine cup (for liquids), glass of water or juice, straw (optional), package insert or drug information sheet

Method

1. Identify the patient and wash your hands.
2. Select the ordered drug (tablet, capsule, or liquid).
3. Check the seven rights, comparing information against the drug order.
4. If you are unfamiliar with the drug, check the PDR or other drug reference, read the package insert, or speak with the physician. Determine whether the drug may be taken with or followed by water or juice.
5. Ask the patient about any drug or food allergies. If the patient is not allergic to the ordered drug or other ingredients used to prepare it, proceed.
6. Perform any calculations needed to provide the prescribed dose. If you are unsure of your calculations, check them with a coworker or the physician.

If You Are Giving Tablets or Capsules

7. Open the container and tap the correct number into the cap (Figure 33-2). Do not touch the inside of the cap because it is sterile. If you pour out too many tablets or capsules and you have not touched them, tap the excess back into the container.
8. Tap the tablets or capsules from the cap into the paper cup.
9. Recap the container.
10. Give the patient the cup along with a glass of water or juice. If the patient finds it easier to drink with a straw, unwrap the straw and place it in the fluid. If patients have difficulty swallowing pills, have them drink some water or juice before putting the pills in the mouth. This additional fluid makes the pills float and allows patients to swallow quickly.

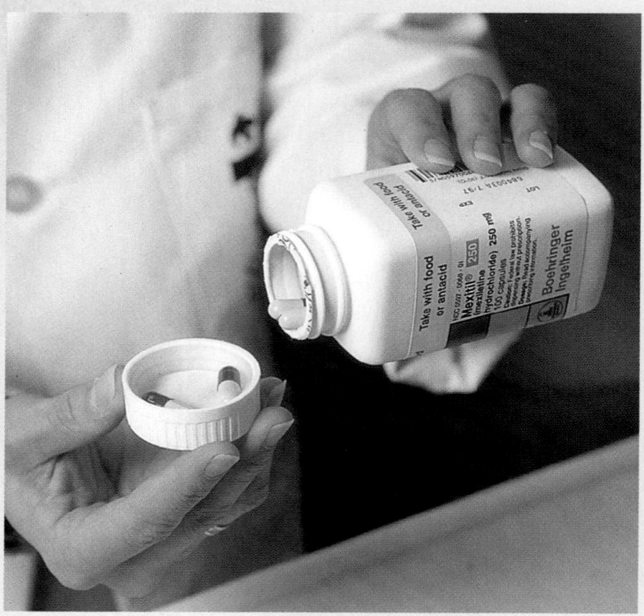

Figure 33-2. Tap tablets gently into the cap.

If You Are Giving a Liquid Drug

7. If the liquid is a suspension, shake it well.
8. Locate the mark on the medicine cup for the prescribed dose. Keeping your thumbnail on the mark, hold the cup at eye level and pour the correct amount of the drug. To prevent liquid drips from obscuring the label, keep the label side of the bottle on top as you pour (Figure 33-3), or put your palm over it.
9. After pouring the drug, place the cup on a flat surface, and check the drug level again. At eye level the base of the meniscus (the crescent-shaped form at the top of the liquid) should align with the mark that indicates the prescribed dose (Figure 33-4). If you poured out too much, discard it. Do not return it to the container because medicine cups are not sterile.
10. Give the medicine cup to the patient with instructions to drink the liquid. If appropriate, offer a glass of water or juice to wash down the drug.

continued ⟶

PROCEDURE 33.1

Administering Oral Drugs *(continued)*

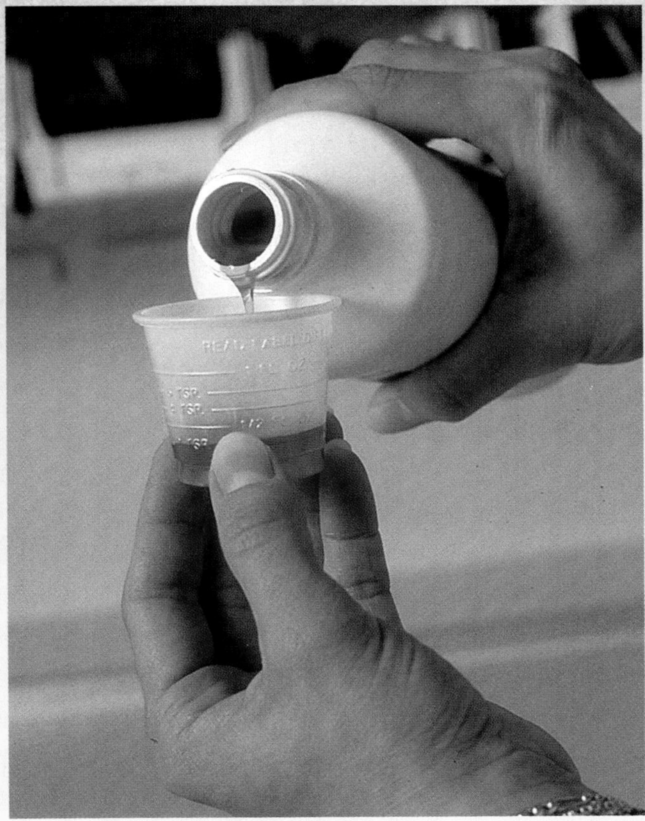

Figure 33-3. Pour a liquid drug into a calibrated medication cup.

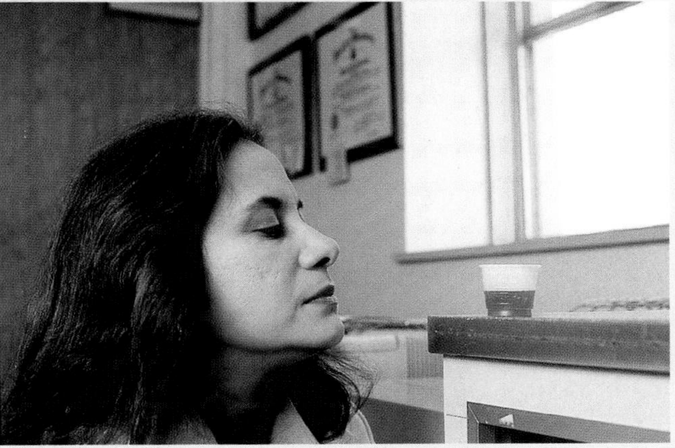

Figure 33-4. Read the measurement at eye level.

After You Have Given an Oral Drug

11. Wash your hands.

12. Give the patient an information sheet about the drug. Discuss the information with the patient and answer any questions she may have. If the patient has questions you cannot answer, refer her to the physician.

13. Document the drug administration with the date, time, drug name, dosage, expiration date, lot number, manufacturer, route, site, and significant patient reactions in the patient's chart. Also document patient education about the drug.

to place a buccal drug, such as hyoscyamine sulfate, between the cheek and gum until it dissolves, as shown in Figure 33-5. Explain that this area has a rich blood supply that promotes rapid drug absorption.

Tell the patient to place a sublingual drug, such as nitroglycerin, under the tongue until it dissolves, as shown in Figure 33-6. Explain that the capillaries in this area promote rapid drug absorption.

Instruct patients not to eat, drink, or smoke until after the tablet completely dissolves. Food and fluids wash the drug into the GI tract, slowing absorption or allowing gastric juices to destroy it. Smoking increases salivation, causing impaired absorption of the drug.

Remain with patients until their tablet dissolves to monitor for possible adverse reaction and to ensure that patients have allowed the tablet to dissolve in the mouth instead of chewing or swallowing it. Give patients an information sheet about the drug. Discuss it with them, and answer their questions. If they have questions you cannot answer, refer them to the doctor.

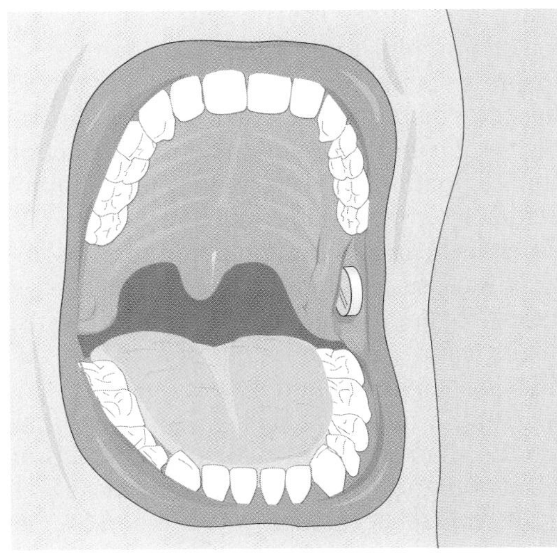

Figure 33-5. Place a buccal drug between the cheek and gum.

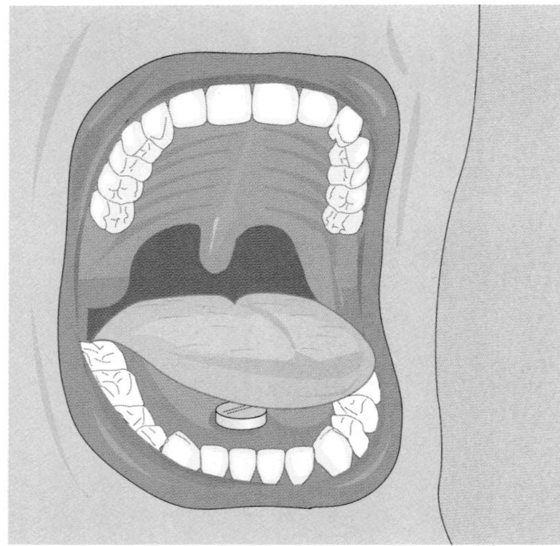

Figure 33-6. Place a sublingual drug under the tongue.

As always, immediately document the drug administration with the date, time, drug name, dose, route, site, and any significant patient reactions. Also document patient education about the drug.

Parenteral Administration

Parenteral administration is the administration of a substance such as a drug by muscle, vein, or any means other than through the GI tract (substances administered through the GI tract are usually given by mouth). It generally applies to giving drugs by injection. Although the parenteral route offers the advantage of rapid drug action, it has several potential drawbacks.

Parenteral administration poses more safety risks for the patient than administration by other routes. The reason is that after the drug has been injected, it cannot be retrieved. To reduce the risks, you must administer the drug expertly and observe the seven rights meticulously.

Parenteral administration increases your risk of potential exposure to blood-borne pathogens when performing injections and disposing of used needles. To minimize risks, follow Universal Precautions during injections. Also adhere to Occupational Safety and Health Administration (OSHA) and Environmental Protection Agency (EPA) regulations for disposing of contaminated needles and sharp items, as discussed in Chapter 1. Most offices provide a rigid, puncture-proof container for collecting disposable sharp instruments. This container should be self-sealing and have a lock-tight cap and a safety neck.

After using a needle, lancet, or syringe, immediately place it in the sharps container. To avoid puncturing yourself, do not force the needle, lancet, or syringe into the container. If you do accidentally stick yourself, notify the physician at once so you can be treated. OSHA requires medical follow-up for all workers who have been accidentally punctured.

Never let a sharps container become full. When the container is two-thirds full, seal it and follow your office procedure for container disposal.

Needles. When you administer a parenteral drug, you must select the appropriate needle, syringe, and drug form to use on the basis of the type of injection. The following are methods of injection:

- **Intradermal (ID),** or within the upper layers of the skin
- **Subcutaneous (SC),** or beneath the skin
- **Intramuscular (IM),** or within a muscle
- **Intravenous (IV),** or directly into a vein

Needles consist of a hub, hilt, shaft, lumen, point, and bevel (Figure 33-7). The hub of the needle fits onto the syringe. The needle tip is beveled (sloped at the opening). The bevel helps the needle cut through the skin with minimum trauma.

Needles are available in various gauges (inside diameters) and lengths (Figure 33-8). A needle's gauge is expressed with numbers. The smaller the number, the larger

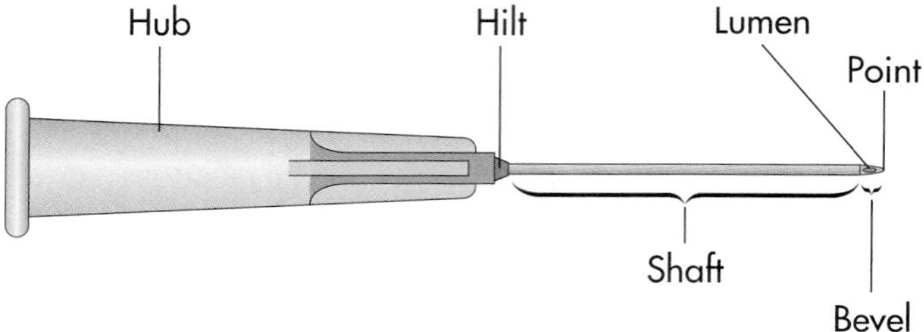

Figure 33-7. Understanding the parts of a needle will help you use it correctly.

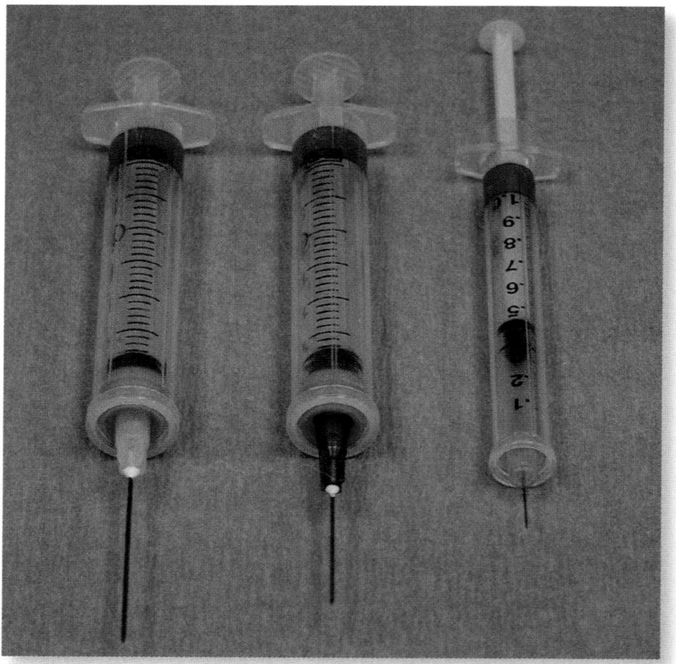

Figure 33-8. Choose a needle with a length, gauge, and bevel appropriate to the type of injection, the drug being injected, and the patient receiving the injection.

TABLE 33-6 Choosing a Needle		
Type of Injection	**Gauge of Needle**	**Length of Needle**
Intradermal	25–26 gauge	⅜–½ inch
Subcutaneous	23–27 gauge	½–¾ inch
Intramuscular	18–23 gauge	1–3 inches

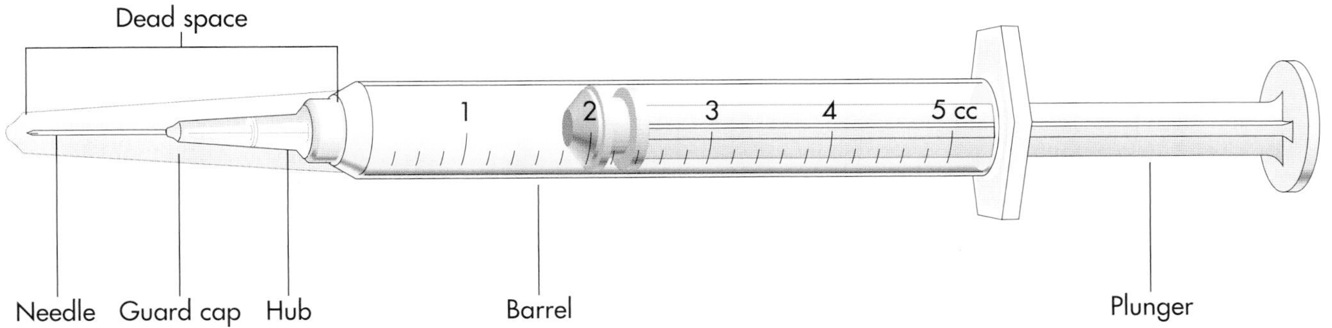

Figure 33-9. Know the parts of a standard syringe.

the gauge. For example, a 25-gauge needle is smaller than an 18-gauge needle. Use the right gauge for the type of injection and the viscosity (thickness) of the drug to be administered. For example, use a large-gauge needle for a highly viscous drug.

When selecting a needle, also consider its length. It must be long enough to penetrate the appropriate layers of tissue but not so long as to go too deep. Choose the correct needle length on the basis of the type of injection as well as the patient's size, amount of fatty tissue, and injection site. Table 33-6 lists the ranges of needle gauge and length typically used for intradermal, subcutaneous, and intramuscular injections.

Syringes. Syringes have two basic parts: a barrel and a plunger. The barrel is the calibrated cylinder that holds the drug. The plunger forces the drug through the barrel and out the needle, as shown in Figure 33-9. The syringe may be packaged with the needle attached and a guard cap over the needle, or the syringe and needle may be packaged separately.

Syringes come in many sizes and are calibrated according to how the syringe will be used. For example, the common 3-mL syringe is divided into tenths of a milliliter on one side and minims on the other. It is used to measure most drugs. A tuberculin (TB) syringe holds 1 mL and is calibrated in hundredths of a milliliter on one side and minims on the other for small doses of drugs (Figure 33-10). Insulin syringes are calibrated in units (U), commonly either 50 U or 100 U (Figure 33-10). Unlike other syringes, insulin syringes have permanently attached needles and no dead space (fluid remaining in the needle or syringe after the plunger is depressed fully). These differences help the patient self-administer the correct amount of insulin.

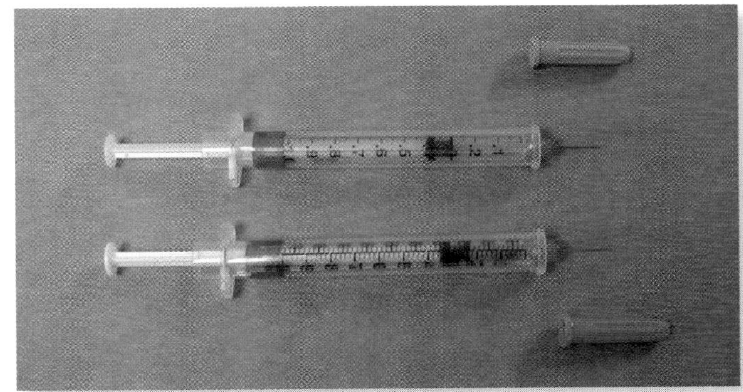

Figure 33-10. You may use the tuberculin syringe (top) to deliver small doses (up to 1.0 mL) of drugs. This insulin syringe (bottom) delivers precisely 100 U of insulin when filled with insulin of the proper concentration (100 U per mL).

Forms of Packaging for Parenteral Drugs. Parenteral drugs are supplied in the forms shown in Figure 33-11. They are ampules, cartridges, and vials.

- An ampule is a small glass or plastic container that is sealed to keep its contents sterile. It must be opened and used with care, as described in Procedure 33-2.
- A cartridge is a small barrel prefilled with a sterile drug. It slips into a special, reusable syringe assembly.
- A vial is a small bottle with a rubber diaphragm that can be punctured by needle. A vial contains a liquid or powder, which must first be reconstituted with a **diluent** (liquid used to dissolve and dilute a drug), as described in Procedure 33-3. It may contain a single or multiple dose. This procedure requires two needle and

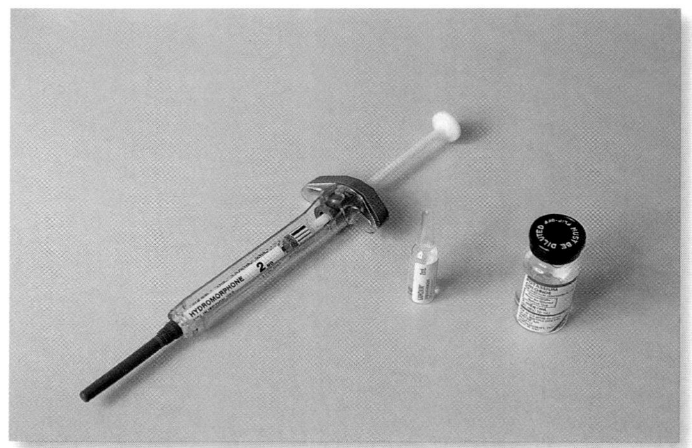

Figure 33-11. Injectable drugs may come in a cartridge (left), an ampule (center), or a vial (right).

syringe sets—one for inserting the diluent into the vial and another to draw and administer the reconstituted drug—to avoid using a contaminated needle. The first needle is considered contaminated when you set it down to mix the diluent and the drug.

Methods of Injection. Injections are the most common method of drug administration in a medical office. You need to be knowledgeable about all injection methods: intradermal, subcutaneous, intramuscular, and intravenous. You must also become proficient in administering intradermal, subcutaneous, and intramuscular injections, as permitted in your state.

Intradermal. An intradermal injection is administered into the upper layer of skin at an angle almost parallel to the skin, as described in Procedure 33-4. Common sites for intradermal injections are the forearm and back. Intradermal

PROCEDURE 33.2

Drawing a Drug From an Ampule

Objective: To safely open an ampule and draw a drug, using sterile technique

OSHA Guidelines

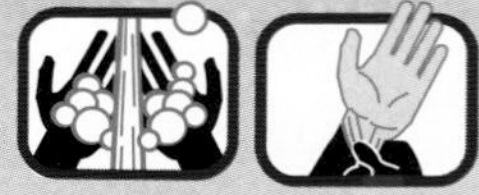

Materials: Ampule of drug, alcohol swab, 2-by-2-inch gauze square, small file (provided by the drug manufacturer), needle and syringe of the appropriate size

Method

1. Identify the patient. Wash your hands and put on examination gloves.
2. Gently tap the top of the ampule with your forefinger to settle the liquid to the bottom of the ampule.
3. Wipe the ampule's neck with an alcohol swab.
4. Wrap the 2-by-2-inch gauze square around the ampule's neck. Then snap the neck away from you (Figure 33-12). If it does not snap easily, score the neck with the small file and snap it again.
5. Insert the needle into the ampule without touching the side of the ampule.
6. Pull back on the plunger to aspirate (remove by vacuum or suction) the liquid. The drug is now ready for injection.

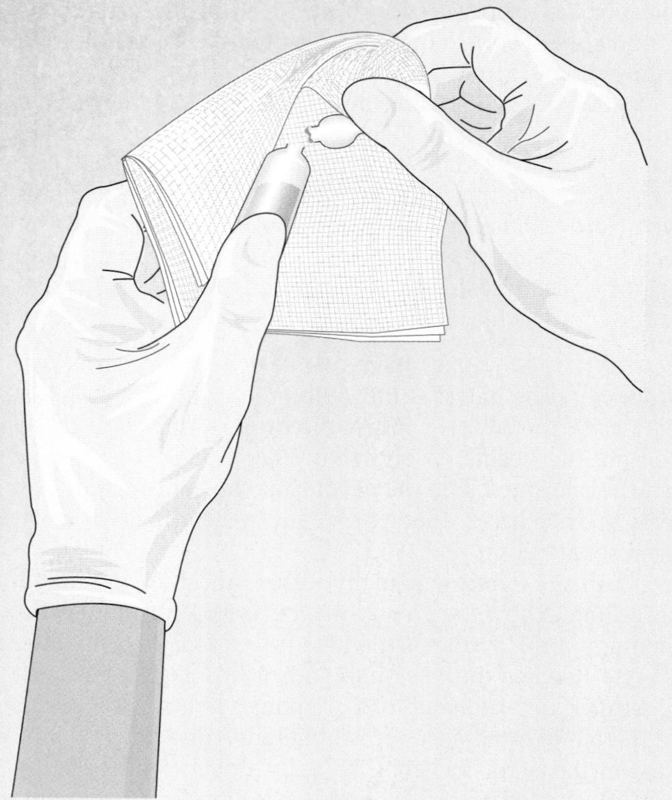

Figure 33-12. You must snap the neck of the ampule before inserting the needle.

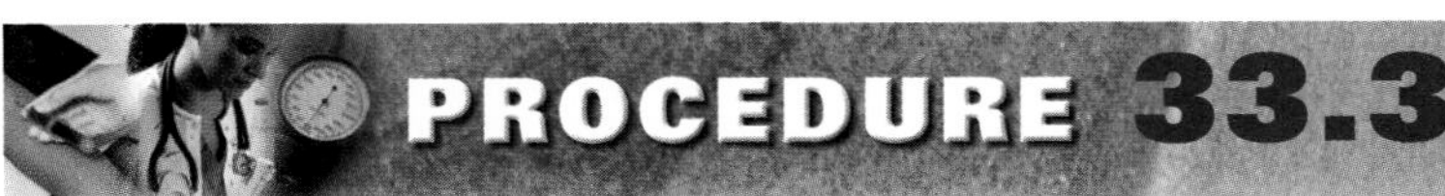

PROCEDURE 33.3

Reconstituting and Drawing a Drug for Injection

Objective: To reconstitute and draw a drug for injection, using sterile technique

OSHA Guidelines

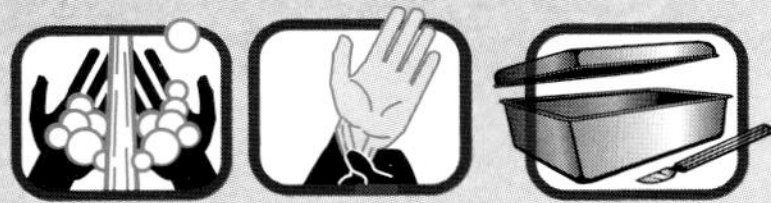

Materials: Vial of drug, vial of diluent, alcohol swabs, two disposable sterile needle and syringe sets of appropriate size, sharps container

Method

1. Identify the patient. Wash your hands and put on examination gloves.
2. Place the drug vial and diluent vial on the countertop. Wipe the rubber diaphragm of each with an alcohol swab.
3. Remove the cap from the needle and the guard from the syringe. Pull the plunger back to the mark that equals the amount of diluent needed to reconstitute the drug ordered. (This action aspirates air into the syringe.)
4. Puncture the diaphragm of the vial of diluent with the needle, and inject the air into the diluent. This action creates positive pressure that lets you draw the diluent easily (Figure 33-13). (If you do not add air, a vacuum forms, making it difficult to draw the diluent.)
5. Invert the vial and aspirate the diluent.
6. Remove the needle from the diluent vial, inject the diluent into the drug vial, and withdraw the needle. Properly dispose of this needle and syringe.
7. Roll the vial between your hands to mix the drug and diluent thoroughly. Do not shake the vial unless so directed on the drug label. When completely mixed, the solution in the vial should have no flakes. The solution will be clear or cloudy when completely mixed (depending on the drug).
8. Remove the cap and guard from the second needle and syringe.
9. Pull back the plunger to the mark that reflects the amount of drug ordered. Inject the air into the drug vial.
10. Invert the vial and aspirate the proper amount of the drug into the syringe (Figure 33-14). The drug is now ready for injection.

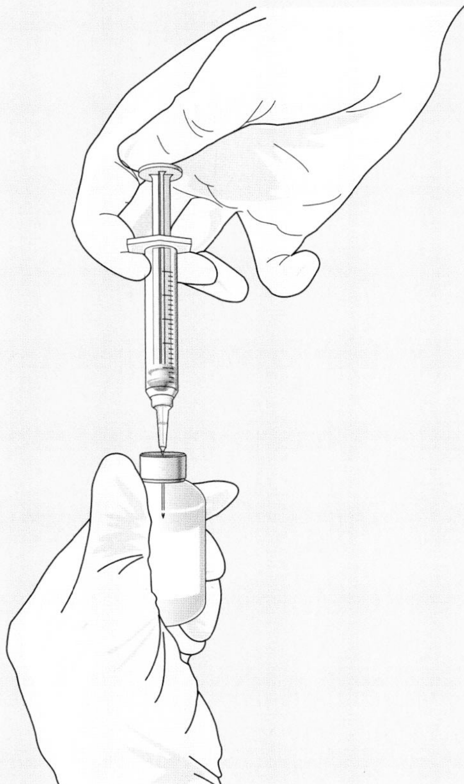

Figure 33-13. Injecting air into the diluent makes it easier to draw.

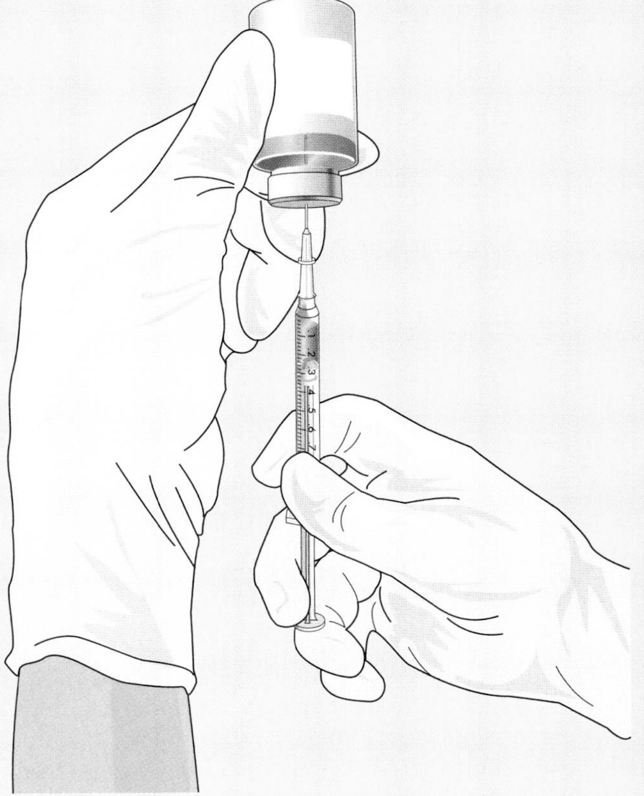

Figure 33-14. Invert the vial and draw the reconstituted drug.

PROCEDURE 33.4

Giving an Intradermal Injection

Objective: To administer an intradermal injection safely and effectively, using sterile technique

OSHA Guidelines

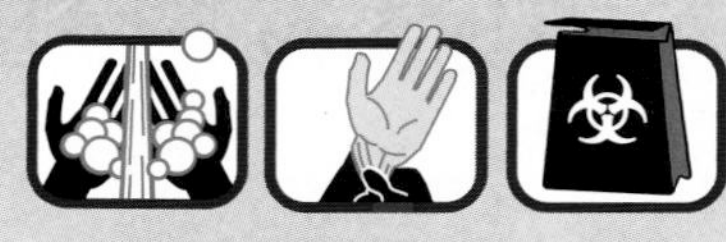

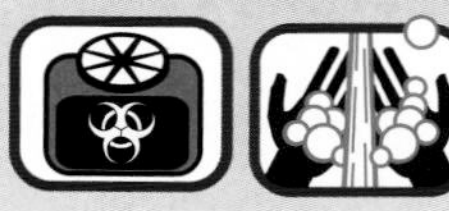

Materials: Drug order (in patient's chart), alcohol swab, disposable needle and syringe of the appropriate size filled with the ordered dose of drug, sharps container

Method

1. Identify the patient. Wash your hands and put on examination gloves.
2. Check the seven rights, comparing information against the drug order.
3. Identify the injection site on the patient's forearm. To do so, rest the patient's arm on a table with the palm up. Measure 2 to 3 finger-widths below the antecubital space and a hand-width above the wrist. The space between is available for the injection (Figure 33-15).
4. Prepare the skin with the alcohol swab, moving in a circle from the center out.
5. Let the skin dry before giving the injection. Otherwise, you could introduce antiseptic under the skin, which could cause irritation and falsify intradermal test results.
6. Hold the patient's forearm, and stretch the skin taut with one hand.
7. With the other hand, place the needle—bevel up—almost flat against the patient's skin. Press the needle against the skin and insert it.
8. Inject the drug slowly and gently. You should see the needle through the skin and feel resistance. As the drug enters the upper layer of skin, a wheal (raised area of the skin) will form (Figure 33-16).
9. After the full dose of the drug has been injected, withdraw the needle. Properly dispose of used materials and the needle and syringe immediately.
10. Remove the gloves and wash your hands.
11. Stay with the patient to monitor for unexpected reactions.
12. Document the injection with the date, time, drug name, dosage, expiration date, lot number, manufacturer, route, site, and significant patient reactions in the patient's chart. Also document patient education about the drug.

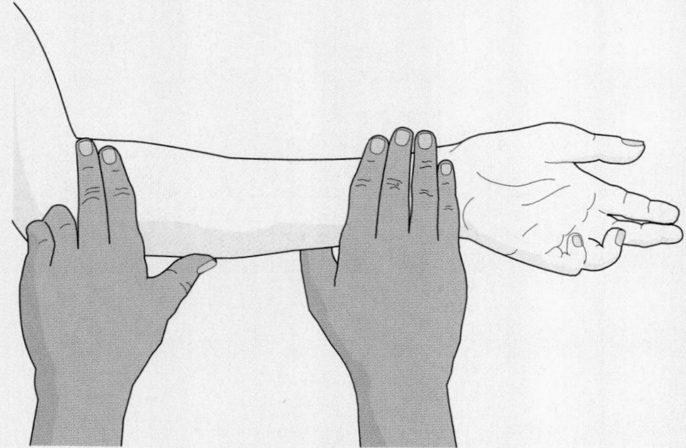

Figure 33-15. This space is available for intradermal injection sites.

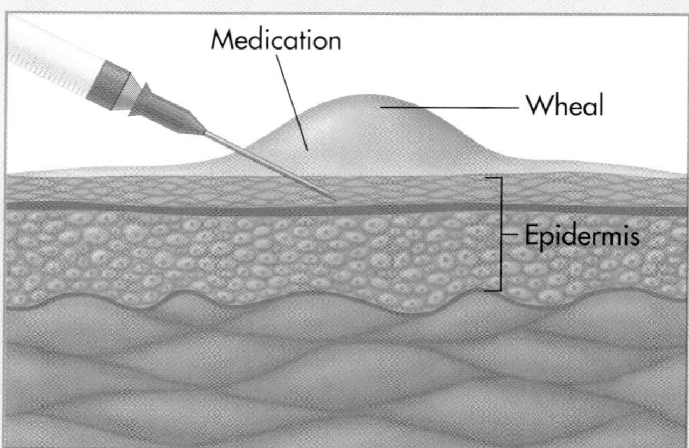

Figure 33-16. Medication collects under the skin, forming a wheal during an intradermal injection.

injections are usually used to administer a skin test, such as an allergy test or a TB test. When choosing an injection site on patients, avoid scarred, blemished, or hairy areas, because those features interfere with your ability to interpret test results on the skin.

The drug is injected under the top skin layer, and a little bubble or wheal is raised. If the body reacts to the drug, erythema (redness) and induration (hardening) occur. This reaction generally takes place 15 to 20 minutes after an allergy test and from 48 to 72 hours after a TB test.

Subcutaneous. Orally referred to as sub Q by most health-care professionals, a subcutaneous injection provides a slow, sustained release of a drug and a relatively long duration of action. Generally, 1 mL or less of a drug can be delivered by SC injection (Procedure 33-5). Various drugs, such as insulin and heparin, are commonly administered by SC injection.

Common subcutaneous injection sites include an area on the back between the shoulder blades, the outer sides of the upper arms and thighs, and the abdomen (except for a 2-inch area around the umbilicus). To prepare for an SC injection, select a site away from bones and blood vessels. Do not use an area that is edematous (swollen), scarred, or hardened or one that has a large amount of fat, because

PROCEDURE 33.5

Giving a Subcutaneous Injection

Objective: To administer a subcutaneous injection safely and effectively, using sterile technique

OSHA Guidelines

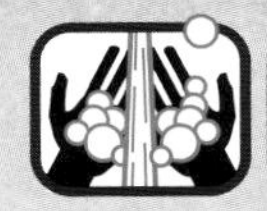
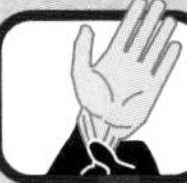

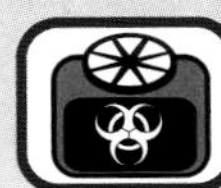
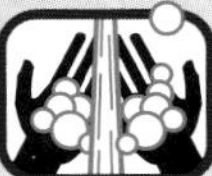

Materials: Drug order (in patient's chart), alcohol swabs, container of the ordered drug, disposable needle and syringe of the appropriate size, sharps container

Method

1. Identify the patient. Wash your hands and put on examination gloves.
2. Check the seven rights, comparing information against the drug order.
3. Prepare the drug and draw it up to the mark on the syringe that matches the ordered dose. Then pull the plunger back an additional 0.2 to 0.3 mL to create an air bubble. When you inject the drug, the air bubble helps seal the subcutaneous tissue (Figure 33-17).
4. Choose a site (Figure 33-18) and clean it with an alcohol swab, moving in a circle from the center out. Let the area dry.
5. Pinch the skin firmly to lift the subcutaneous tissue.
6. Position the needle—bevel up—at a 45° angle to the skin.
7. Insert the needle in one quick motion. Then release the skin, and aspirate by pulling back slightly on the plunger to check the needle placement (do not pull back if you are administering insulin or heparin). If pulling back on the plunger produces blood, placement is incorrect and you must begin again with a fresh needle and syringe. If pulling back on the plunger produces no blood, placement is correct. Inject the drug slowly (Figure 33-19).
8. After the full dose of the drug has been injected, place an alcohol swab over the site, and withdraw the needle at the same angle you inserted it.
9. Apply pressure at the puncture site with the alcohol swab.

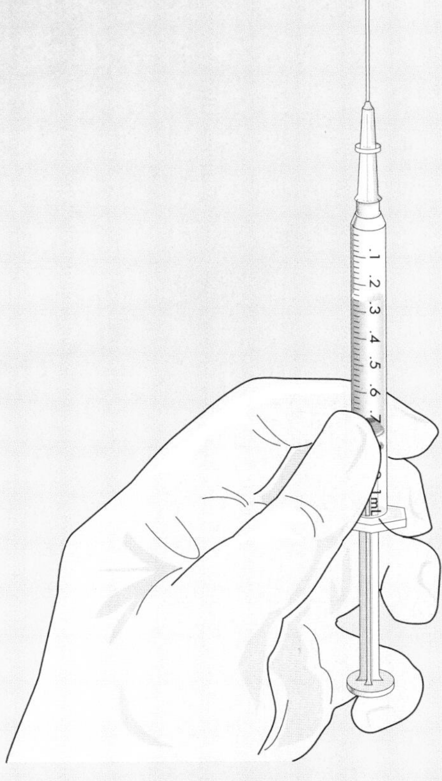

Figure 33-17. Pull back the plunger to create an air bubble in the syringe used in subcutaneous injection.

continued ⟶

PROCEDURE 33.5

Giving a Subcutaneous Injection *(continued)*

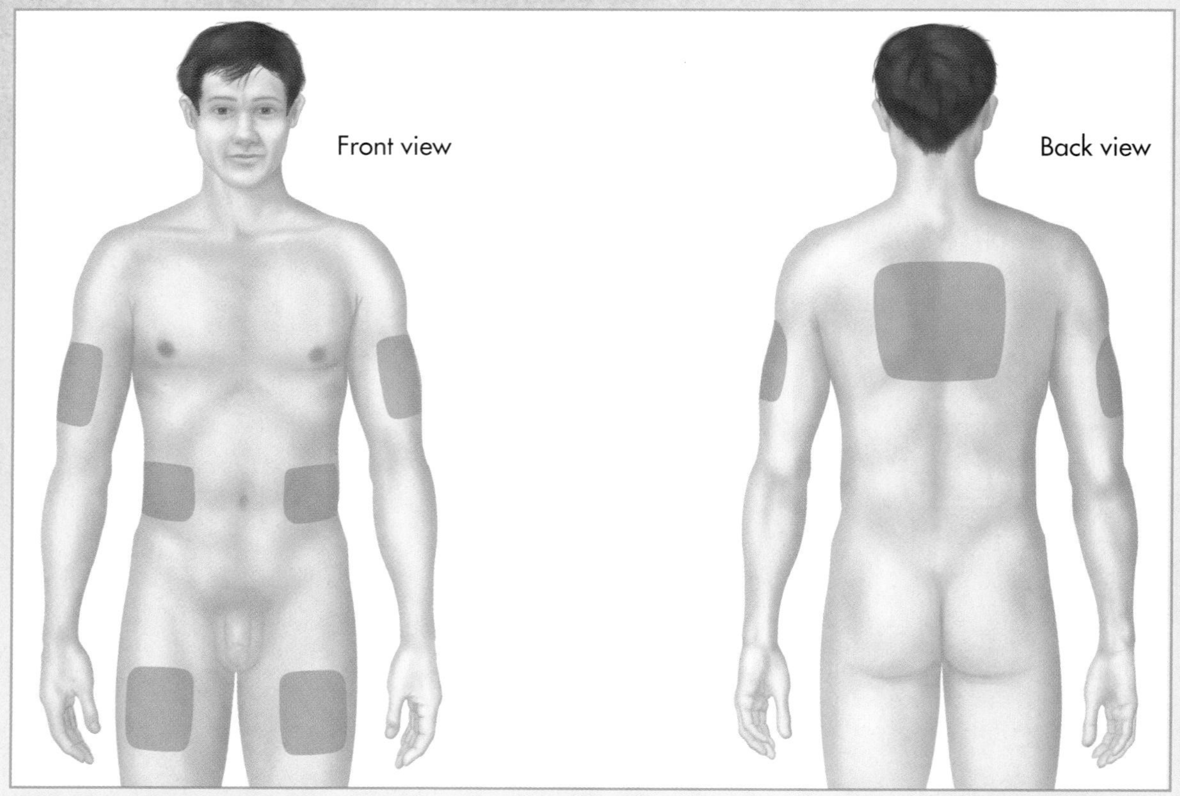

Figure 33-18. Many sites are available for subcutaneous injection.

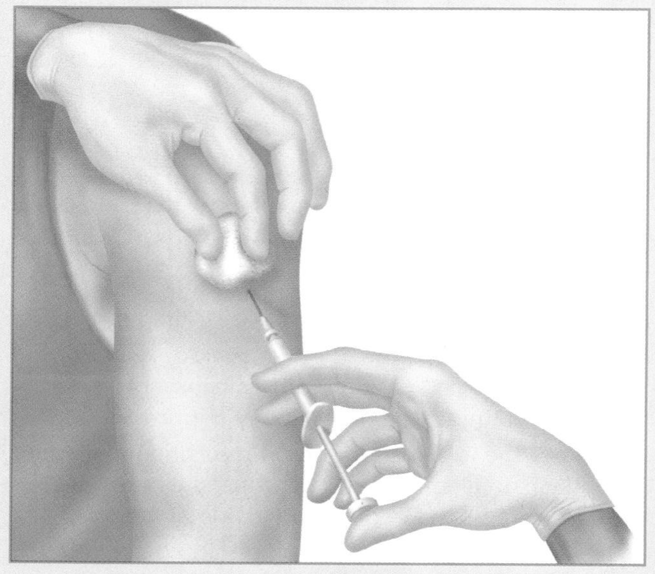

Figure 33-19. Perform a subcutaneous injection.

10. Massage the site gently to help distribute the drug, if indicated.
11. Properly dispose of the used materials and the needle and syringe.
12. Remove the gloves and wash your hands.
13. Stay with the patient to monitor for unexpected reactions.
14. Document the injection with the date, time, drug name, dosage, expiration date, lot number, manufacturer, route, site, and significant patient reactions in the patient's chart. Also document patient education about the drug.

these areas may not have the capillary network needed for absorption. When patients need regular SC injections, remember to rotate injection sites systematically. Begin the rotation pattern by giving injections in rows in the same area of the body (such as the abdomen). After all those sites have been used once, proceed to the next area on the body (such as the right leg), and follow a similar pattern there. Rotating sites promotes drug absorption and prevents hard subcutaneous lumps from forming.

At the injection site, ensure that you can pinch at least a 1-inch skin fold for the injection. If a patient is frail, dehydrated, or thin, you may need to use a site other than the back or abdomen to provide the necessary fold of skin.

Intramuscular. When a patient requires rapid drug absorption, you may be asked to administer an intramuscular injection, as described in Procedure 33-6. An IM injection usually irritates a patient's tissues less than an SC injection and allows administration of a larger amount of drug, usually 3 to 5 mL in an adult.

Common IM injection sites include the dorsogluteal, ventrogluteal, vastus lateralis, and deltoid muscles, illustrated in Figure 33-20. Before giving an IM injection, identify the site carefully to prevent injury to blood vessels and nerves in the area. As with SC injections, rotate sites if the patient must receive regular or multiple IM injections.

Take into consideration the patient's layer of fat when choosing an IM injection site. You want the injection to penetrate beyond the fat layer to muscle. If, for example, a patient is heavy in the buttocks and thighs, the deltoid may be the best site for administering an IM injection.

When giving an IM injection to a pediatric patient, use the smallest gauge needle, usually 22 to 25 gauge. Also use the shortest length needle that will allow you to reach muscle, usually 1 inch.

PROCEDURE 33.6

Giving an Intramuscular Injection

Objective: To administer an intramuscular injection safely and effectively, using sterile technique

OSHA Guidelines

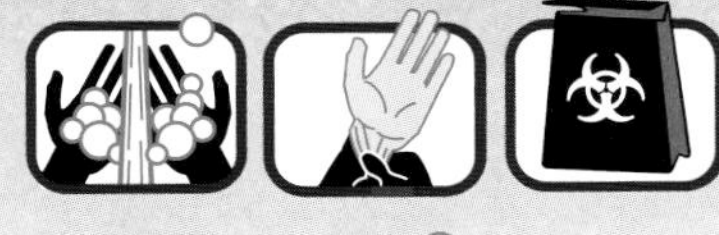

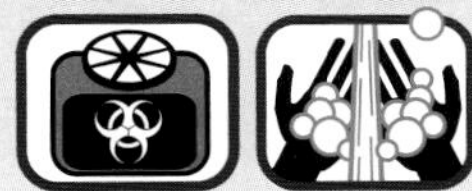

Materials: Drug order (in patient's chart), alcohol swabs, container of the ordered drug, disposable needle and syringe of the appropriate size, sharps container

Method

1. Identify the patient. Wash your hands and put on examination gloves.
2. Check the seven rights, comparing information against the drug order.
3. Prepare the drug and draw it up to the mark on the syringe that matches the ordered dose. Then pull the plunger back another 0.2 to 0.3 mL to add air. This air clears the drug from the needle and prevents drug seepage.
4. Choose a site (Figure 33-20) and gently tap it. Tapping stimulates the nerve endings and reduces pain caused by the needle insertion.
5. Clean the site with an alcohol swab, moving in a circle from the center out. Let the site dry.
6. Stretch the skin taut over the injection site.
7. Hold the needle and syringe at a 90° angle to the skin. Then insert the needle with a quick, dartlike thrust.
8. Release the skin and aspirate by pulling back slightly on the plunger to check the needle placement. If pulling back on the plunger produces blood, placement is incorrect and you must begin again with a fresh needle and syringe. If pulling back on the plunger produces no blood, placement is correct. Inject the drug slowly.
9. After the full dose of the drug has been injected, place an alcohol swab over the site. Then quickly remove the needle at a 90° angle.
10. Use the alcohol swab to apply pressure to the site and massage it, if indicated.
11. Properly dispose of used materials and the needle and syringe.
12. Remove the gloves and wash your hands.
13. Stay with the patient to monitor for unexpected reactions.
14. Document the injection with the date, time, drug name, dosage, expiration date, lot number, manufacturer, route, site, and significant patient reactions in the patient's chart. Also document patient education about the drug.

continued →

PROCEDURE 33.6

Giving an Intramuscular Injection *(continued)*

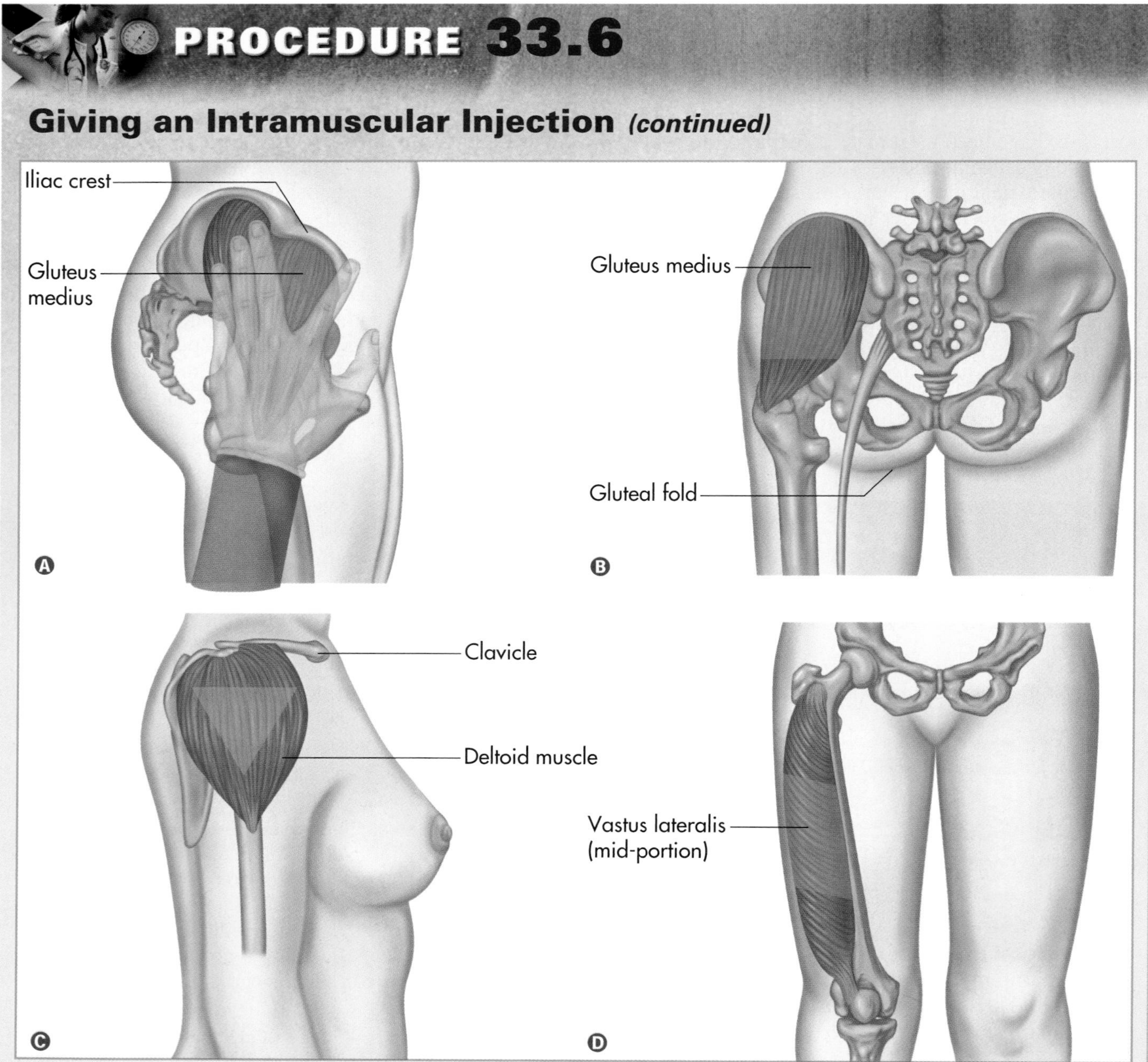

Figure 33-20. For intramuscular injection in an adult, use (a) the ventrogluteal site, (b) the dorsogluteal site, (c) the deltoid site, or (d) the vastus lateralis site.

Injection sites vary with age. For an infant or toddler, use the vastus lateralis muscle. For a child who has been walking for about a year, use the ventrogluteal or dorsogluteal site. For an older, well-developed child, use any adult site.

When injecting an IM drug that can irritate subcutaneous tissues, such as iron dextran (Imferon), use the **Z-track method,** illustrated in Figure 33-21. To do this, pull the skin and subcutaneous tissue to the side before inserting the needle at the site. After the drug is injected, release the tissue. This technique creates a zigzag path in the tissue layers, which prevents the drug from leaking into the subcutaneous tissue and causing irritation.

Intravenous. Although intravenous injections are not commonly performed in a medical office or by medical assistants, certain drugs may be administered this way. Drugs may also be mixed and dissolved into a **solution** (a homogeneous mixture of a solid, liquid, or gaseous substance in a liquid) and given by IV **infusion** (slow drip)

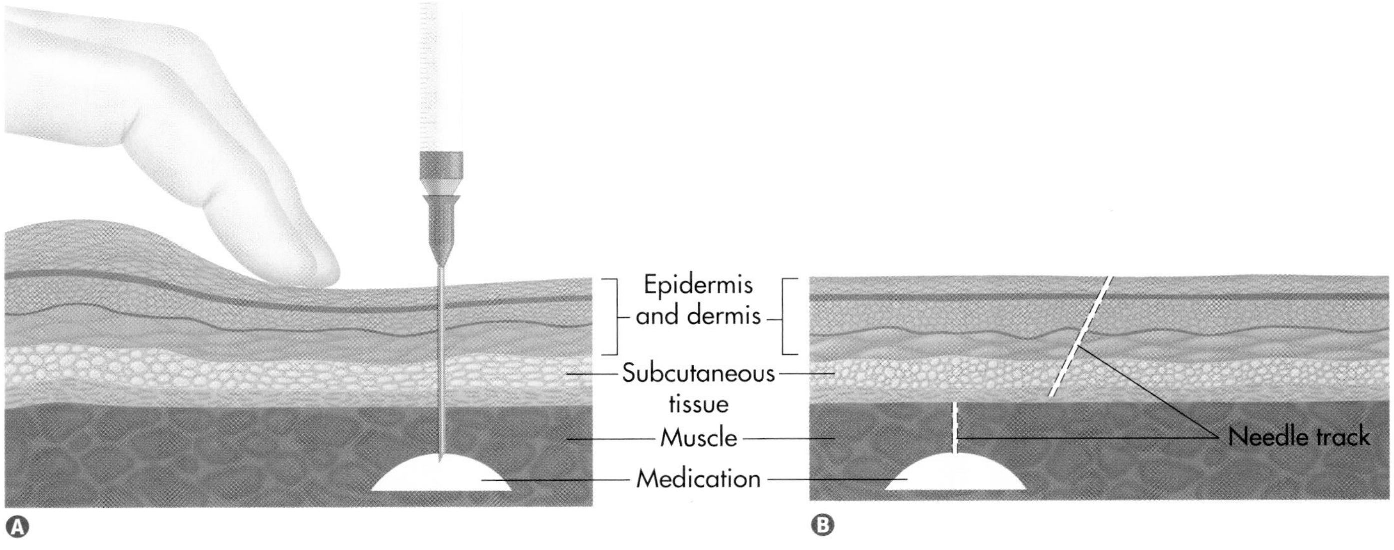

Figure 33-21. Use the Z-track method for IM injection of irritating solutions. (a) Pull the skin to one side before inserting the needle. (b) After injecting the drug, release the skin to seal off the needle track.

into a vein. Examples of IV drugs include powerful antibiotics, chemotherapeutic drugs, emergency drugs, and electrolytes. Because these drugs are introduced directly into the bloodstream, they produce an almost immediate effect. They also can cause sudden adverse reactions.

Although a doctor or nurse must administer an IV drug, you may assist by laying out supplies and equipment. When assisting with a venipuncture, gather the ordered drug and a tourniquet, bedsaver pad, gloves, iodine and alcohol swabs, venipuncture device, tape, and gauze pad, as ordered. Obtain other supplies and equipment, depending on the specific type of infusion or injection being administered.

Inhalation Therapy

Inhalation therapy can be administered through the mouth or nose. There are a number of disorders for which the physician may order an inhaler or aerosol form of medication. For example, an oral inhaler is frequently used by patients with asthma, whereas a nasal inhaler is frequently used for local treatment of nasal congestion. Nasal inhalers are also used to administer medicines for systemic effect, such as a vasopressin derivative for nocturnal bed-wetting.

Package inserts for inhaled drugs provide detailed descriptions of the correct procedure. If directed by the physician, however, you must teach the patient how to use an inhaler safely and correctly.

As with all drug administrations, check the seven rights, comparing information against the drug order. Ensure that you have the correct patient, the correct drug, and the correct form (oral or nasal) of inhaler. As you teach the patient, refer to the package insert, and show the patient where to find each step on the instruction sheet, so that he will be familiar with the steps when administering the inhaler at home.

Check the label of the inhaler to determine whether the inhaler must be shaken thoroughly before administration. If shaking the inhaler is indicated, stress this point with the patient. Otherwise, the drug will not be evenly distributed in the inhaler, and its effectiveness will be jeopardized. If indicated, a nasal inhaler must be shaken before administration to each nostril.

Tell patients to follow these steps when administering a nasal inhaler.

1. Wash hands and blow the nose to clear the nostrils as much as possible before using the inhaler.
2. Tilt the head back, and with one hand, place the inhaler tip about ½ inch into the nostril.
3. Point the tip straight up toward the inner corner of the eye. Angling the inhaler downward makes the drug run down the back of the throat, causing a burning sensation.
4. Use the opposite hand to block the other nostril.
5. Inhale gently while quickly and firmly squeezing the inhaler.
6. Remove the inhaler tip and exhale through the mouth.
7. Shake the inhaler and repeat the process in the other nostril.

If indicated in the package insert, instruct patients to keep the head tilted back and not to blow their nose for several minutes. They can then wash their hands while you immediately document the inhaler administration with date, time, drug, dose, route, and any significant patient reactions. Also record your patient education about inhaler use.

Topical Application

Topical application is the direct application of a drug on the skin. Topical drugs can take the form of creams, lotions, **ointments** (salves), tinctures, powders, sprays, and solutions, which are used for their local effects. They include antibacterial and antifungal drugs as well as corticosteroids.

To apply a cream, lotion, or ointment, use long, even strokes with a cotton-tipped applicator when rubbing it into the skin. Follow the direction of the hair growth to avoid irritating the hair follicles and skin. To apply a powder, shake it on but do not rub it in.

A specialized type of topical administration that produces a systemic effect is the **transdermal** system (or patch). A drug administered through the transdermal patch is absorbed through the skin directly into the bloodstream. The patch slowly and evenly releases a systemic drug, such as scopolamine, nitroglycerin, estrogen, or fentanyl, through the skin. The patient receives a timed-release dose, usually over a day or several days.

Because the release of a drug from a transdermal patch is often crucial to a patient's health, the package inserts with transdermal medications are extremely detailed. You must instruct the patient to follow the instructions precisely and to be sure to change the patch on the prescribed schedule.

If the doctor directs you to provide some education, your goal is to teach the patient how to apply and remove a transdermal drug unit safely and effectively. Refer to the package insert as you teach, and show the patient where each step is located on the instruction sheet. This identification gives the patient the reference needed for changing the patch at home.

Before showing and administering the patch, check the seven rights, comparing information against the drug order. Wash your hands and instruct the patient to do the same when preparing for transdermal system application.

Some patches come sealed in a protective pouch. The plastic backing is easily peeled off once the patch is removed from the pouch. The plastic backing on patches without a protective pouch must be manipulated carefully to allow its removal. Show the patient how to bend the sides of the latter type of transdermal unit back and forth until the clear plastic backing snaps down the middle.

For either type of patch, demonstrate how to peel off the clear plastic backing to expose the sticky side of the patch. Then show the patient how to apply the patch to a reasonably hair-free site, such as the abdomen. Figure 33-22 shows how to apply both types of patches. Advise the patient to avoid using the extremities below the knee or elbow, skin folds, scar tissue, or burned or irritated areas. Estrogen patches are usually placed on the hip. Wash your hands and instruct the patient to do the same after applying a transdermal system at home.

To remove the patch, instruct the patient to gently lift and slowly peel it back from the skin. Then wash the skin with soap and water, dry the area with a towel, and wash the hands. Explain that the skin may appear red and warm, which is normal. Reassure the patient that the redness will disappear. Instruct the patient to notify the doctor if the redness does not disappear in several days or if a rash develops.

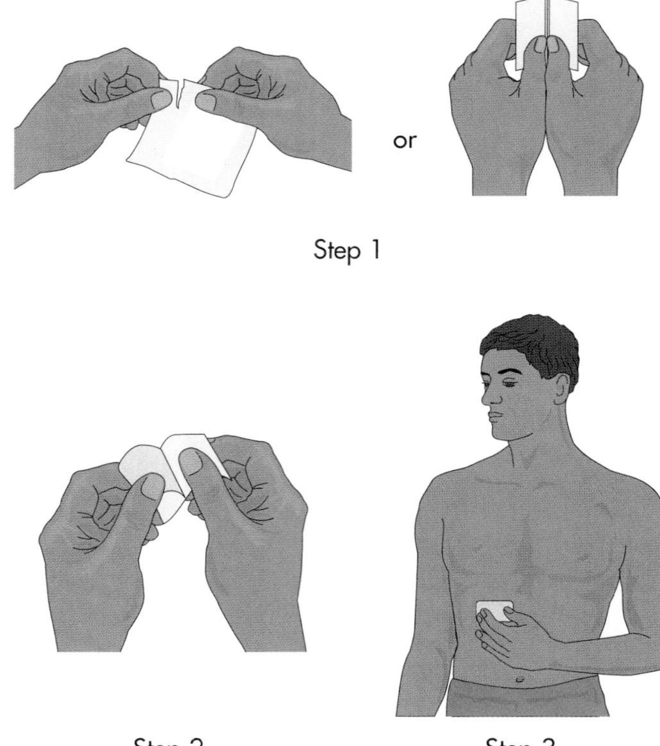

Figure 33-22. To apply a transdermal patch, first either (1) remove it from the pouch, or bend the sides back and forth until the backing snaps; then (2) peel the backing off the patch; and (3) apply the patch, sticky side down, to a clean, relatively hairless site.

Tell the patient never to apply a new patch to the site just used. It is best to allow each site to rest between applications. Some transdermal systems call for waiting 7 days before using a site again. Be sure to check the package directions regarding site rotation.

Patients frequently ask whether they can apply lotion or talc to the area after removing the patch. Tell them they may do so if the skin is dry. After answering any other questions, immediately document the drug application with date, time, drug, dose, route, and any significant patient reactions. Also record your patient education about transdermal system application and removal.

If the physician order calls for you to apply a transdermal patch, it is important that you wear gloves during this procedure. Even though the procedure is not invasive, the medication can absorb into your skin. Wash your hands thoroughly after you apply the transdermal patch.

Urethral Administration

The urethral route is used when antibiotic and antifungal drugs are needed locally—that is, at the site of infection—for some urinary tract infections. Depending on the nature of the infection and the duration of drug action, the physician or a nurse may instill liquid drugs only one time or several times a day for a week. Urethral administration is used in both men and women.

Urethral drug administration requires passing a small-diameter urinary catheter into the bladder, instilling a drug through it, and clamping the catheter to let the drug bathe the urinary bladder walls. The materials needed for catheterization are included in a urinary catheter kit.

When the physician or nurse administers a urethral drug, you may assist with the following steps as directed.

1. Use sterile technique. Wash your hands and gather the necessary supplies. Depending on the amount of drug to be administered, you will need either a syringe without a needle or tubing and a bag. You will also need a urinary catheter kit, sterile gloves, the prescribed drug, a drape, and a bedsaver pad.
2. Check the seven rights, comparing information against the drug order, and explain the procedure and the drug order to the patient.
3. Assist the patient into the lithotomy position, and drape her to preserve her modesty while exposing the vulva.
4. Place a bedsaver pad under the buttocks.
5. Open the catheter kit.
6. Put on sterile gloves.
7. Cleanse the vulva as you would to perform catheterization, using the materials in the kit. As you sweep down with the antiseptic swab, watch for the urethral opening to "wink," which helps you locate it accurately.
8. The physician or nurse will insert the lubricated catheter. Tell the patient that she should feel pressure, not pain, and that the physician or nurse is going to attach the syringe to the catheter and insert the drug (or attach the tubing and bag to the catheter and let the drug run in by gravity).
9. After instilling the drug, the physician or nurse will clamp the catheter and leave the drug in place for the ordered amount of time.
10. Stay with the patient not only to ensure that she remains still but also to reassure her that the full feeling in the bladder is normal. She may also say she feels the need to urinate. Advise her that this feeling, too, is normal and is caused by the catheter.
11. When the time is up, unclamp the catheter, gently remove it, and allow the patient to urinate. Assist the patient as needed.
12. While the patient is dressing, immediately document the drug instillation with date, time, drug, dose, route, and any significant patient reactions.

Vaginal Administration

Physicians usually prescribe vaginal drugs to treat local fungal infections. The drugs may also be used for local bacterial infections. They are usually packaged as suppositories (the most common form), solutions, creams, ointments, and foams. Patients frequently ask about administering vaginal medications, and they usually administer such medications at home. Therefore, you must be prepared to provide detailed patient education for this route of administration. The physician may ask you to administer the first dose as a means of teaching a patient the method to use at home, or you may be asked to administer a one-time-only dose.

To administer a vaginal suppository, follow these steps.

1. Wash your hands and gather the following materials: the prescription or drug order in the patient's chart, a cloth or paper drape, a bedsaver pad, gloves, cotton balls, water-soluble lubricant, and the prescribed drug.
2. Check the seven rights, comparing information against the drug order, and explain the procedure and the drug order to the patient.
3. Give the patient the opportunity to empty her bladder before beginning.
4. Assist the patient into the lithotomy position, and drape her to preserve her modesty while exposing the vulva.
5. Place a bedsaver pad under the buttocks.
6. Put on sterile gloves.
7. Cleanse the perineum with soap and water, using one cotton ball per stroke, and cleanse the center last, while spreading the labia.
8. Lubricate the vaginal suppository applicator in lubricant spread on a paper towel.
9. While spreading the labia with one hand, insert the applicator with the other (the applicator should be about 2 inches into the vagina and angled toward the sacrum).
10. Release the labia and push the applicator's plunger to release the suppository into the vagina.
11. Remove the applicator, and wipe any excess lubricant off the patient.
12. Help her to a sitting position, and assist with dressing if needed.
13. Document the administration with date, time, drug, dose, route, and any significant patient reactions.

Follow the same steps, using an appropriate applicator, for vaginal drugs in the forms of creams, ointments, gels, and tablets. The liquid form of vaginal medication is administered by performing a **douche** (vaginal irrigation). This process is similar to giving a urethral drug, but it requires a special irrigating nozzle.

Rectal Administration

Certain medications, such as drugs used to treat constipation, nausea, and vomiting, may be administered by the rectal route. These medications may be given in the form of suppositories or enemas and may produce local or systemic effects.

Rectal Suppository. Administering rectal suppositories is rarely done in a doctor's office except on a pediatric patient. The doctor may, however, ask you to give a first suppository to an adult as a means of patient education. To do so, follow these steps.

1. Check the seven rights, comparing information against the drug order.
2. Explain the procedure and the drug order to the patient.
3. Give the patient the opportunity to empty the bladder before beginning.
4. Help the patient into Sims' position (shown in Chapter 20, Figure 20-1).
5. Lift the patient's gown to expose the anus.
6. Put on gloves and remove the wrapper from the suppository.
7. Lubricate the tapered end of the suppository with about 1 tsp of lubricant.
8. While spreading the patient's buttocks with one hand, insert the suppository—tapered end first—into the anus with the other hand.
9. Gently advance the suppository past the sphincter with your index finger. Before it passes the sphincter, the suppository may feel as if it is being pushed back out the anus. When it passes the sphincter, it seems to disappear.
10. Use tissues to remove excess lubricant from the area.
11. Remove your gloves and ask the patient to lie quietly and retain the suppository for at least 20 minutes.
12. When the treatment is completed, help the patient to a sitting, then standing, position.
13. Wash your hands and immediately document the drug administration with date, time, drug, dose, route, and any significant patient reactions.

Retention Enema. Retention enemas are usually not administered in a physician's office. You may, however, be asked to perform this procedure in an unusual circumstance, such as for a frail, elderly patient with fecal impaction. The steps for administering a retention enema are as follows.

1. Check the seven rights, comparing information against the drug order.
2. Help the patient lie on the left side and bend the right knee.
3. Put a bedsaver pad under the patient's left hip.
4. Place the tip of a syringe into a rectal tube. Let a little rectal solution flow through the syringe and tube. While holding the tip up, clamp the tubing.
5. Lubricate the end of the tube.
6. Spread the patient's buttocks, and slide the tube into the rectum about 4 inches.
7. After the tube is in place, slowly pour the rectal solution into the syringe, release the clamp, and let gravity move the solution into the patient.
8. When you have administered the ordered amount of solution, clamp the tube, then remove it.
9. Using tissues, apply pressure over the anus for 20 seconds to stifle the patient's urge to defecate.
10. Wipe any excess lubricant or solution from the area, and encourage the patient to retain the enema for the time ordered.
11. When the time has passed, help the patient use a bedpan or direct the patient to a toilet to expel the solution.
12. Wash your hands and immediately document the drug administration with date, time, drug, dose, route, and any significant patient reactions.

Administering Medications to the Eye or Ear

Doctors commonly administer eye medications to assist patients in eye tests, reduce pressure in the eyes, relieve eye pain, and treat eye infections and inflammation. Refer to Procedure 21-2 in Chapter 21 for instructions on how to administer eye medications. Although most eye medications are administered for local effect, some contain drugs that are absorbed systemically. To prevent systemic absorption, the doctor may request that you apply pressure with one finger just below the inner corner of each eye after instilling medications. Continue applying pressure for 2 to 3 minutes, as directed.

Doctors often administer eardrops to treat patients' ear infections or inflammation, relieve ear pain, or loosen earwax. Like eye medications, eardrops are ordered primarily for their local effects. They are not usually absorbed systemically, nor do they cause systemic effects. Procedure 21-5 in Chapter 21 describes how to administer eardrops.

Educating the Patient About Drug Administration

Educating patients about what drugs do to the body and what the body does to drugs is discussed in detail in Chapter 50. You need to provide additional patient education, however, with regard to routes of administration. This education is extremely important; a patient who does not administer a drug correctly or safely may put health or life at risk.

Reading the Drug Package Label

You must check the *PDR* for information about any drug with which you are not familiar. Likewise, before you teach a patient how to administer a drug, you must review the specific administration instructions for the drug in the *PDR*. An important aspect of this kind of information is teaching the patient how to read a prescription drug label. Instruct the patient to be particularly alert for special instructions and warning labels, such as those shown in Figure 33-23.

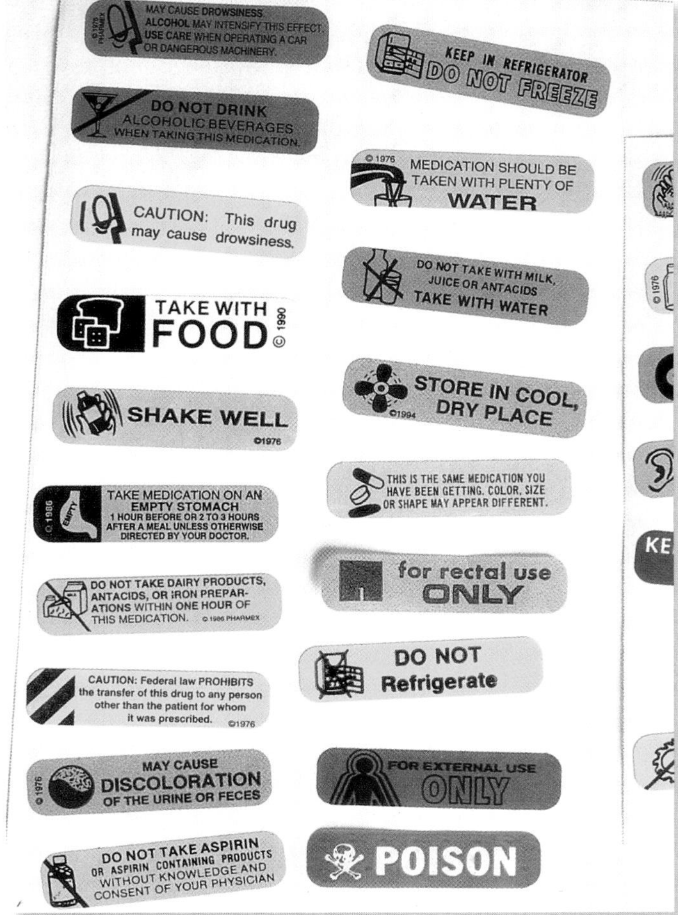
MAY CAUSE DROWSINESS. ALCOHOL MAY INTENSIFY THIS EFFECT. USE CARE WHEN OPERATING A CAR OR DANGEROUS MACHINERY.
KEEP IN REFRIGERATOR
DO NOT FREEZE
DO NOT DRINK ALCOHOLIC BEVERAGES WHEN TAKING THIS MEDICATION.
MEDICATION SHOULD BE TAKEN WITH PLENTY OF WATER
CAUTION: This drug may cause drowsiness.
DO NOT TAKE WITH MILK, JUICE OR ANTACIDS
TAKE WITH WATER
TAKE WITH FOOD
STORE IN COOL, DRY PLACE
SHAKE WELL
THIS IS THE SAME MEDICATION YOU HAVE BEEN GETTING. COLOR, SIZE OR SHAPE MAY APPEAR DIFFERENT.
TAKE MEDICATION ON AN EMPTY STOMACH 1 HOUR BEFORE OR 2 TO 3 HOURS AFTER A MEAL UNLESS OTHERWISE DIRECTED BY YOUR DOCTOR.
for rectal use ONLY
DO NOT TAKE DAIRY PRODUCTS, ANTACIDS, OR IRON PREPARATIONS WITHIN ONE HOUR OF THIS MEDICATION.
DO NOT Refrigerate
CAUTION: Federal law PROHIBITS the transfer of this drug to any person other than the patient for whom it was prescribed.
MAY CAUSE DISCOLORATION OF THE URINE OR FECES
FOR EXTERNAL USE ONLY
DO NOT TAKE ASPIRIN OR ASPIRIN CONTAINING PRODUCTS WITHOUT KNOWLEDGE AND CONSENT OF YOUR PHYSICIAN
POISON

Figure 33-23. Teach the patient to heed warning labels and instructions on drug bottles.

Interactions

Drug interactions should not be confused with adverse effects of drugs, discussed in Chapter 32. Patient education with regard to interactions is important. Interactions may occur between two prescription or nonprescription drugs or between a drug and food and may cause serious effects. Explain that the greater the number of drugs the patient takes, the greater the chance of a drug interaction.

Drug-Drug Interactions. Most drug interactions affect the absorption, distribution, metabolism, or excretion of the drugs. In some cases drug-drug interactions can affect the results of laboratory tests. When two drugs are taken at the same time, there are several possible interactions.

- The effects of both drugs are increased, causing either a toxic or beneficial effect. For example, when alcohol is combined with diazepam (Valium), there is the potential toxic effect of severe central nervous system depression, because one drug intensifies the effect of the other. An example of a beneficial effect is the combination of acetaminophen and codeine, which increases the activity of both drugs, allowing the physician to prescribe a lower dose of each. In fact, this combination of drugs is available in one tablet (Tylenol with codeine).
- The effects of both drugs are decreased, or one drug cancels out the effect of the other. For example, combining propanolol (Inderal) with albuterol (Proventil) causes each drug to lose its effectiveness.
- The effect of one of the drugs is increased by the other. For example, the effect of digoxin (Lanoxin) is increased by the presence of furosemide (Lasix), but the furosemide still works at the same degree of effectiveness as when administered alone.

To help prevent unintentional drug interactions, thoroughly assess the patient's medication use. Be sure to ask about medications prescribed by specialists as well as over-the-counter (OTC) drugs. Question the patient about past and present use of alcohol and recreational drugs as well as herbal remedies. Update the chart as needed. If you detect a potential for drug interactions, notify the physician.

Also teach patients about possible drug interactions and how to avoid or minimize them. For example, patients may need to take certain drugs at least 2 hours apart. Instruct patients to call the office if they think their drugs are interacting adversely.

Drug-Food Interactions. Interactions between a drug and food can alter a drug's therapeutic effect. For example, taking tetracycline with milk can reduce the drug's effectiveness because of decreased absorption from the GI tract. The drug-food interaction between a monoamine oxidase (MAO) inhibitor (such as Parnate, an antidepressant drug) and aged cheese or meat or other foods containing high levels of tyramine can produce a toxic effect. This interaction can cause a dangerous hypertensive crisis in which the patient's blood pressure rises quickly to dangerous levels, possibly leading to stroke and death.

Some drug-food interactions can affect the body's use of nutrients. For example, the cholesterol-lowering drugs cholestyramine resin and colestipol HCl may reduce the body's absorption of fat-soluble vitamins (A, D, E, and K) from food.

When teaching a patient about drug-food interactions, specify exactly which foods to avoid and when. For example, a patient may drink milk or eat food several hours before or after taking tetracycline, whereas a patient taking an MAO inhibitor must avoid foods that contain high levels of tyramine at all times. Explain what to expect if an interaction occurs, and describe how to deal with it.

Adverse Effects

Adverse effects or reactions associated with a drug and reported in the *PDR* are discussed briefly in the section on toxicology in Chapter 32. These responses are somewhat predictable and range from mild adverse reactions, such as stomach upset, to severe or life-threatening allergic responses. Unpredictable adverse effects can also occur; they are unique to each patient. Always advise the patient to report any change in overall health, because that change could be drug-related.

Elderly patients and patients with liver or kidney disease are more susceptible than others to adverse effects because these conditions affect drug metabolism and excretion. When drugs are not metabolized properly or excreted from the body quickly enough, drugs can reach toxic levels, even with normal doses.

To help prevent adverse effects, teach the patient to take the drug at the right time, in the right amount, and under the right circumstances. For example, the patient may need to take a cephalosporin with food to avoid nausea and diarrhea. Also teach the patient to recognize significant adverse effects and to call the office if any of them occur.

Special Considerations

Pediatric, pregnant, breast-feeding, or elderly patients or patients from different cultures require special considerations. When giving a drug to these patients, you must adjust patient care as needed.

Pediatric Patients

Children pose special challenges in drug administration and use. Their physiology and immature body systems may make drug effects less predictable because drugs are absorbed, distributed, metabolized, and excreted differently in children than in adults. Therefore, plan to observe a pediatric patient closely for adverse effects and interactions.

A child's small size may also increase the risk of overdose and toxicity. These factors may require dosage adjustments and careful measurement of small doses. To help administer drugs safely to pediatric patients, always check your calculations for providing a prescribed dose, and then ask a nurse or the doctor to double-check them.

Remember that administration sites and techniques for a child may differ from those for an adult. For example, fewer IM injection sites can be used for a young child. Also, the technique for eardrop administration varies slightly.

When dealing with an infant or young child, teach the parents—not the patient—about the drug. With an older child, include parents and patient in the teaching session. Be sure to use age-appropriate language when speaking to children.

It is important to use your therapeutic communication skills when working with pediatric patients. Pediatric patients are not like adults—they often have difficulty adjusting to medical procedures or illnesses. Children who do not understand what is happening to them can become problematic; some may see a physician visit as a punishment. It is important for you to be sensitive to the needs and reactions of pediatric patients. The first memorable exposure to an office visit will often determine how the child will react to physician visits for years to come.

Patience is important when working with pediatric patients. Infants and children can sense when you are irritated or annoyed. Pay close attention to your nonverbal communication as well as your verbal communication. New mothers are often apprehensive about invasive procedures when it concerns their children. Empathy and compassion are needed to ensure that the office visit is a pleasant one.

Administering medications to a pediatric patient may become a challenge if the child is not cooperative. It is important to ensure that the child receives the full dose as ordered.

Oral Medications. When administering oral medications to children, follow these guidelines:

- Use a calibrated dropper or spoon device to measure the ordered dose.
- Administer the medication to the side of the tongue; this method prevents the child from spitting out the medication.
- Hold the child until you are sure the medication is swallowed.
- If a small amount dribbles from the mouth, do not attempt to give more medication to the child.
- If the child vomits within 5 minutes and you can see the medication in the vomitus, you should readminister the medication after the child is calm. If you are unsure of readministering medication, consult with the physician.
- If the medication only comes in tablet form and the child is unable to swallow a tablet or capsule, verify in a drug reference to see if the medication can be crushed and given with food, such as applesauce.

Injections. Stress and anxiety will differ from child to child. When giving injections to pediatric patients, the following steps will help to ensure a smooth procedure:

- Distract the patient. Talk to the child while giving the injection. Often the injection is performed and over before the child realizes it.
- Praise the child. Say things that promote maturity and self-esteem.
- Use an anesthetic topical agent prior to the injection. This can be applied in the office or at home before the patient arrives in the office.
- Be swift. Do not allow a lot of time to pass before giving the injection. The faster the better.
- Try not to allow the child to see the syringe before giving the injection.

Pediatric Injection Sites. Pediatric patients have less muscle development than adults do, which limits the sites for intramuscular injections. The deltoid muscle is not developed enough for an injection and can be painful for the child. The sciatic nerve is larger in children; dorsogluteal injections are therefore not recommended because of the danger of hitting the sciatic nerve.

TABLE 33-7	Pregnancy Drug Risk Categories
Category	**Meaning**
A	Controlled studies in pregnant women have failed to demonstrate risk to the fetus.
B	There is no evidence of risk in humans, either because human findings show no risk or because there are no human findings but animal findings are negative.
C	Human studies are lacking, and animal findings are either positive for fetal risk or lacking as well. However, potential benefits may justify the potential risk.
D	There is positive evidence of risk. Nevertheless, potential benefits may outweigh the potential risk.
X	Fetal risk clearly outweighs any possible benefit to the patient.
NR	No rating is available.

Source: *2004* Physicians' Desk Reference, Thompson Healthcare.

The vastus lateralis and ventrogluteal sites are recommended for infants and children. The vastus lateralis site is good because it is a large and thick muscle that is developed before the child begins to walk. It is also the most desirable site for infants and children because it is not near major nerves and blood vessels. The vastus lateralis site is an easier site if you need to incorporate restraining methods.

The most common injections given to pediatric patients are vaccines. Most vaccines are given intramuscularly with a 25-gauge, ⅝-inch needle. Use your critical thinking and best judgment when selecting a needle.

Restraining Methods. Sometimes a pediatric patient will need to be restrained in order for you to administer an injection. Two medical assistants may be needed to safely restrain a child while giving an injection. Common restraining methods include the following:

- Have the child "hug the mother." The mother holds the child in front of her, with the child's thighs extended on either side of her torso. As the mother is talking to her child, make the injection in the vastus lateralis.
- Weight-bearing restraining is better than muscular control. Have the child sit on the edge of the exam table and use your weight to immobilize the child's legs against the table.

Pregnant Patients

When dealing with pregnant patients, remember that you are caring for two patients at once: the mother and her fetus. When you give the mother a drug, you may also be giving it to the fetus.

In addition, pregnancy-related changes in the mother's body can affect drug absorption, distribution, metabolism, and excretion. It is extremely important to double-check the drug in the *PDR* for toxicology or pregnancy warnings and to assess the patient carefully for therapeutic and adverse effects of the drug.

Some drugs can cause physical defects in the fetus if the mother takes them during pregnancy (especially in the first trimester). For this reason, you must be aware of the pregnancy drug risk categories (Table 33-7). These categories, established by the Food and Drug Administration (FDA), are based on the degree to which available information has ruled out risk to the fetus balanced against the drug's potential benefits to the patient. If the physician orders a high-risk drug for a pregnant patient, double-check the order with the physician before administering the drug.

Patients Who Are Breast-Feeding

Some drugs are excreted in breast milk and can thus be ingested by a breast-feeding infant. This ingestion can be dangerous because infants have immature body systems and cannot metabolize and excrete drugs that are safe for the mother. Some drugs, such as sedatives, diuretics, and hormones, can reduce the mother's flow of breast milk.

Whenever a drug is ordered for a patient who is breast-feeding, check a drug reference to see whether the drug is contraindicated during lactation. If so, consult the doctor. If not, teach the mother to recognize signs of adverse drug effects in her infant. If a mother must take a drug that affects lactation, advise her to supplement breast-feedings with infant formula.

Elderly Patients

Age-related changes in the body can affect drug absorption, metabolism, distribution, and excretion. These normal changes can be exaggerated by various diseases or disorders. Therefore, as people age, they have an increased risk of drug toxicity, adverse effects, or lack of therapeutic effects. Because of this risk, be especially alert when assessing an elderly patient who is on drug therapy.

Many elderly patients have complex, chronic diseases with unusual symptoms. This situation can make it difficult to tell whether a problem is caused by a drug. Listen closely to elderly patients and their family members; they are more likely to notice subtle changes than you are.

Patient *and family* education is important with elderly patients, particularly if they engage in polypharmacy (take several medications concurrently). Polypharmacy is common in elderly patients, and possible drug-drug interactions can be severe, as described in the Caution: Handle With Care section.

If an elderly patient is forgetful or confused, talk to the doctor about simplifying the medication schedule to reduce the risk of drug administration errors or omissions. Suggest the use of pill-organizing devices to help prevent forgotten doses or overdoses. If the patient has vision problems, provide drug instruction sheets in large type. To do this, either type instructions on a word processor in a large type size, enlarge the instructions on a photocopier, or clearly handwrite the instructions in large block letters. You might also contact a local association for the blind or visually impaired for devices and tips.

Patients From Different Cultures

Although cultural background is not likely to affect a drug's action in the body, it can affect a patient's understanding of drug therapy and compliance with it. For example, a patient who speaks little or no English cannot benefit from instructions given in English. To remedy this problem, obtain drug information sheets in the languages that are commonly spoken by patients of the practice. Use simple gestures and drawings to clarify difficult words or concepts. Also try to find a family member of the patient who speaks English.

To improve compliance, ask about the patient's feelings regarding medications and home remedies. Depending on cultural background, the patient may be more likely to use teas, poultices, and other home remedies than prescription or nonprescription drugs. If it appears that home remedies are not likely to affect the prescribed medication, tell the patient that it is all right to continue using the home remedies. Suggest adding the drug to the patient's usual routine to help it work better. Your cultural sensitivity may greatly increase the patient's compliance.

Charting Medications

Whenever a patient receives some form of treatment, such as medication, a record is kept of that treatment. Special problems or circumstances are also recorded, such as new symptoms, the patient's own statements, and how the patient tolerated the medications or treatment.

Most charting in the physician's office is documented on a progress note. A progress note is a document that is organized in a chronological sequence by date. The progress note is important because it serves as a communication tool that is utilized by all allied health-care members who are connected to that patient. The medical record is considered a legal document and is taken as proof that care was administered to the patient. All chart entries must be factual, accurate, complete, current, organized,

CAUTION *Handle With Care*

Avoiding Unsafe Polypharmacy

Before administering any drug by any route, you must know every drug, both prescription and nonprescription, that the patient is taking. Many patients, especially elderly ones, visit several doctors. It is entirely possible that each doctor may prescribe one or more drugs without being aware of other drugs the patient is taking. This practice can result in polypharmacy, which means taking several drugs at once. Polypharmacy can be safe, but if the doctor is unaware of the total drug profile, serious drug interactions can result.

When asking patients to identify *all* other drugs they are taking, including OTC drugs, keep in mind that patients may forget to mention all their medicines or OTC drugs to the doctor. Drugs that patients often forget to mention include antacids (such as Tums or Rolaids), birth control pills (some women do not think of these as medication), and medicines that are used only as needed, such as medicine for migraine headaches.

To help prompt patients about drugs they may have forgotten, ask patients who have seen an orthopedist or cardiologist whether pain medication has been prescribed. Ask women who have seen a gynecologist if they are using a patch or other form of hormone replacement therapy. Ask women of an appropriate age whether there is any chance they are pregnant. Ask a pregnant woman whether she is taking prenatal vitamin and mineral supplements. If a patient has been referred to any other doctor for any reason, ask whether that doctor prescribed medication.

After determining the total drug profile, you should:

- Update the patient's record.
- Consider possible drug interactions, consulting the *PDR* or other drug reference if needed.
- Inform the doctor of your findings.

and confidential. Avoid using words or statements that can be interpreted as your opinion. For example, if a patient gags and spits up cough syrup that you just administered, you would not write that the patient did not like the taste of the medication; you would simply state, "patient experienced difficulty in swallowing medication and expelled medication." Avoid terms like "appear" or "seems," which can lead you to draw assumptions without objective data to support them. Use abbreviations when appropriate because they allow you to say a great deal in a small space. Learn them well and use them carefully so that others can understand your notes. It is also useful and professional to learn the proper medical terms for symptoms and body functions.

Charting is not difficult, but it requires some practice. Review your office's charts to keep consistent with the charting methods used in them. Your own charting will be appropriate if you follow a few simple rules:

- Before you begin, make sure you have the right chart.
- Chart medications directly from the physician order.
- Be specific. Do not write "Gave Demerol for pain in the evening." Instead, write "(Date), Demerol 100 mg given IM in right upper outer quadrant of gluteus maximus for c/o sharp pain in left arm, lot number, expiration date, initials."
- Do not leave gaps or skip lines. If an entry does not fill a complete line, draw a straight line to fill the gap. Put your signature or initials at the right side directly after the note.
- If you make an error, do not erase it. Draw a line through the mistake. It should still be visible, so do not black it out. Initial it and write the word "error" on the line, then rechart the information correctly.
- Never use ditto marks.
- Write only in blue ink, never in pencil or another color ink.
- Write neatly in longhand.
- Spelling must be accurate.
- Use abbreviations and correct symbols.
- When you are unsure about charting, ask the physician.

Here is an example of a charted medication on a progress note:

When documenting an injection, you must include the following information:

- Date
- Name of patient
- Medication given
- Dose
- Route
- Location
- Lot number and expiration date
- Manufacturer
- Patient instructions and any other circumstances
- Initials

Nonpharmacologic Pain Management

Because of drug interactions, adverse effects, or the risk of dependence, many patients prefer not to take drugs to relieve chronic pain. To meet their needs, some practices now offer nonpharmacologic methods for managing pain, such as biofeedback, guided imagery, and relaxation exercises, in addition to traditional drug therapy. (For other alternative treatments, see Chapter 25.)

Biofeedback requires equipment that measures physical indicators of stress and relaxation, such as the galvanic skin response or pulse rate. This equipment provides feedback to help the patient recognize stress and relaxation responses and, ultimately, to control them. Biofeedback can help a patient learn to evoke relaxation, which helps block pain perception.

Guided imagery helps patients relax by teaching them to envision themselves in a calm, nurturing, wonderful place. Some cancer patients are taught to envision the cancer cells being eaten by healthy cells. Audiotapes and videotapes are available to help lead patients through these mental exercises.

Relaxation exercises involve learning special breathing techniques. Patients also learn how to relax different muscle groups.

Date	Patient Name: Jane Doe DOB 12/12/63 Progress Note
11/29/03	PPD, .1cc given ID, Rt. Forearm, Lot # 222-01, Exp. Date 12/05, ABC Pharmaceutical Co. Pt to return to office in 48–72 hours for screening results Patient tolerated well--ST/RMA

Summary

As a medical assistant, you must be prepared to administer drugs safely and effectively. Before you can do so, however, you must be familiar with the metric, apothecaries', and household systems of measurement. You must also be able to convert measures from one system to another and perform calculations to provide a prescribed dose. For both of these skills, you can use the ratio or fraction method.

When preparing to administer a drug, assess the patient for contraindications, and observe the general rules and seven rights of drug administration. Depending on the prescription, the drug may be administered by the oral, buccal, sublingual, intradermal, subcutaneous, intramuscular, nasal, topical, transdermal, vaginal, or rectal routes or as eyedrops or eardrops. If directed, assist the physician or nurse with urethral administration and IV drug injection or infusion.

Patient education is an important responsibility related to drug administration. You may need to instruct patients in the proper use of a prescribed drug. In addition, you may have to teach them to prevent or to recognize and report drug interactions and adverse effects.

Some patients require special consideration when receiving drugs. These include pediatric, pregnant, breastfeeding, and elderly patients as well as patients from different cultures.

Nonpharmacologic methods for managing chronic pain are gaining acceptance. Patients who are interested in learning about such methods should ask the physician for further information.

REVIEW

CHAPTER 33

CASE STUDY QUESTIONS

Now that you have completed this chapter, review the case study at the beginning of the chapter. Detail what you think the medical assistant should do next and why.

Discussion Questions

1. What effects may drug interactions produce?
2. Why should you observe the seven rights every time you prepare and administer a drug?
3. Compare subcutaneous and intramuscular drug administration in terms of technique and possible dosage levels.
4. Why is proper needle selection important when administering an injection?

Critical Thinking Questions

1. A foreign patient is in the office, and the physician has ordered a PPD. You ask the patient if he has had a reaction to a TB screen before, and the patient responds by telling you he has had the BCG vaccination as a child. What is BCG? What should you do? What can happen if you administer the PPD?
2. A patient in her first trimester of pregnancy calls the office saying she has acid indigestion. She says that before her pregnancy, she used to take Tagamet for acid indigestion and wants to know if it is safe to take it now. How can you find this information, and what should you do once you find it?
3. Mr. Lance, age 29, visits the office for his regular IM injection. As you are making a routine assessment, he tells you that the last time the drug was administered, he had a bad reaction to it. What should you do?

Application Activities

1. Perform the necessary calculations for the following conversions. Use a table of equivalents, if needed.
   - **a.** 350 mL = ____ L
   - **b.** 0.17 g = ____ mg
   - **c.** 3 tbsp = ____ tsp
   - **d.** ½ tsp = ____ gtt
   - **e.** 2 fl dr = ____ mL
2. Using the ratio or fraction method, calculate the following to provide a prescribed drug dose.
   - **a.** The doctor orders 60 mg of acetaminophen with codeine, but each tablet contains only 15 mg. How many tablets should the patient take?
   - **b.** The doctor orders 300 mg of theophylline anhydrous, but each tablet contains only 100 mg. How many tablets should the patient take?
   - **c.** The doctor orders 5 mg of glyburide, but each tablet contains only 1.25 mg. How many tablets should the patient take?
3. Using the basic formula of dose desired/dose on hand × quantity = dose, calculate the following to provide a prescribed drug dose.
   - **a.** The doctor orders 250 mg of a drug. You have 100-mg scored tablets on hand. How many tablets will you give the patient?
   - **b.** An injectable antibiotic is packaged as 100,000 units per cc. The doctor orders 400,000 units. How many packages will you administer parenterally to the patient?

CHAPTER 34

Electrocardiography and Pulmonary Function Testing

KEY TERMS

calibration syringe
cardiac cycle
deflection
depolarization
electrocardiogram (ECG)
electrocardiograph
electrocardiography
electrode
forced vital capacity (FVC)
Holter monitor
lead
polarity
pulmonary function test
spirometer
spirometry
stylus

AREAS OF COMPETENCE

2003 Role Delineation Study

CLINICAL

Fundamental Principles

- Apply principles of aseptic technique and infection control

Diagnostic Orders

- Perform diagnostic tests

Patient Care

- Prepare patient for examinations, procedures, and treatments

CHAPTER OUTLINE

- The Medical Assistant's Role in Electrocardiography and Pulmonary Function Testing
- Anatomy and Physiology of the Heart
- The Conduction System of the Heart
- The Electrocardiograph
- Preparing to Administer an ECG
- Applying the Electrodes and the Connecting Wires
- Operating the Electrocardiograph
- Troubleshooting: Artifacts and Other Problems
- Completing the Procedure
- Interpreting the ECG
- Exercise Electrocardiography (Stress Testing)
- Ambulatory Electrocardiography (Holter Monitoring)
- Anatomy and Physiology of the Respiratory System
- Pulmonary Function Testing
- Spirometry
- Performing Spirometry

OBJECTIVES

After completing Chapter 34, you will be able to:

34.1 Describe the anatomy and physiology of the heart.
34.2 Explain the conduction system of the heart.
34.3 Describe the basic patterns of an electrocardiogram (ECG).
34.4 Identify the components of an electrocardiograph and what each does.
34.5 Explain how to position the limb and precordial electrodes correctly.
34.6 Describe in detail how to obtain an ECG.

OBJECTIVES *(Continued)*

34.7 Identify the various types of artifacts and potential equipment problems and how to correct them.

34.8 Discuss how the ECG is interpreted.

34.9 Define exercise electrocardiography.

34.10 Explain the procedure of Holter monitoring.

34.11 Describe the anatomy and physiology of the lungs.

34.12 Describe various types of spirometers.

34.13 Describe the procedure of performing spirometry.

Introduction

It is not uncommon for patients to have cardiovascular or respiratory problems when they consult physicians. As a medical assistant, you may be responsible for performing screening and/or diagnostic testing in the physician's office. To correctly perform testing on the cardiac or respiratory system, you need to review the anatomy and physiology of the heart and the respiratory system. This chapter introduces you to the electrocardiograph instrument and how to administer an electrocardiogram. You will also learn how to apply electrocardiograph electrodes and wires, operate the instrument, and troubleshoot problems that can occur while recording the heart's electrical activity. Because many physicians perform more complex cardiac diagnostic testing, you will also learn about Holter monitors and stress testing. Pulmonary function testing is more commonplace now in physician's offices, and this chapter introduces you to the basics of performing a spirometry.

CASE STUDY

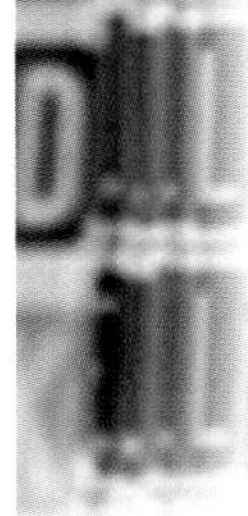

A 57-year-old woman has been having chest pain, discomfort in the chest, and a slight shortness of breath since the previous morning. She chose to come to the office where you are employed rather than the emergency room because she didn't think her symptoms were too severe. The physician orders an ECG and spirometry after reviewing the patient's history. The ECG reveals nonspecific wave changes, and the spirometry shows that the FVC is slightly decreased. The physician then orders a Holter monitor to be placed on the patient and requests that she be scheduled for an exercise electrocardiography.

As you read this chapter, consider the following questions:

1. What does the abbreviation ECG stand for? What is the diagnostic value of the ECG?
2. What is another name for a spirometry? What does FVC designate?
3. Why were the Holter monitor and stress tests ordered for this patient?

The Medical Assistant's Role in Electrocardiography and Pulmonary Function Testing

Electrocardiography and pulmonary function testing are two procedures you may be required to perform in a medical office. **Electrocardiography** is the process by which a graphic pattern is created from the electrical impulses generated within the heart as it pumps. It is often performed to evaluate symptoms of heart disease, to detect abnormal heart rhythms, to evaluate a patient's progress after a heart attack, or to check the effectiveness or side effects of certain medications. Electrocardiography is sometimes performed as part of a general examination.

Pulmonary function tests (PFTs) measure and evaluate a patient's lung capacity and volume. Such tests are commonly performed when a person suffers from shortness of breath, but they may also be performed as part of a general examination. Pulmonary function tests can help detect and diagnose pulmonary problems. They are also used to monitor certain respiratory disorders and to evaluate the effectiveness of treatment.

Anatomy and Physiology of the Heart

A description of the anatomy and physiology of the heart will help you better understand electrocardiography. It will also help you make sense of the electrical activity that electrocardiography records.

Anatomy of the Heart

The heart is a muscular pump that circulates blood throughout the body, carrying oxygen and nutrients to the tissues and removing waste products. The pumping action begins in the muscle tissue of the heart, called the myocardium.

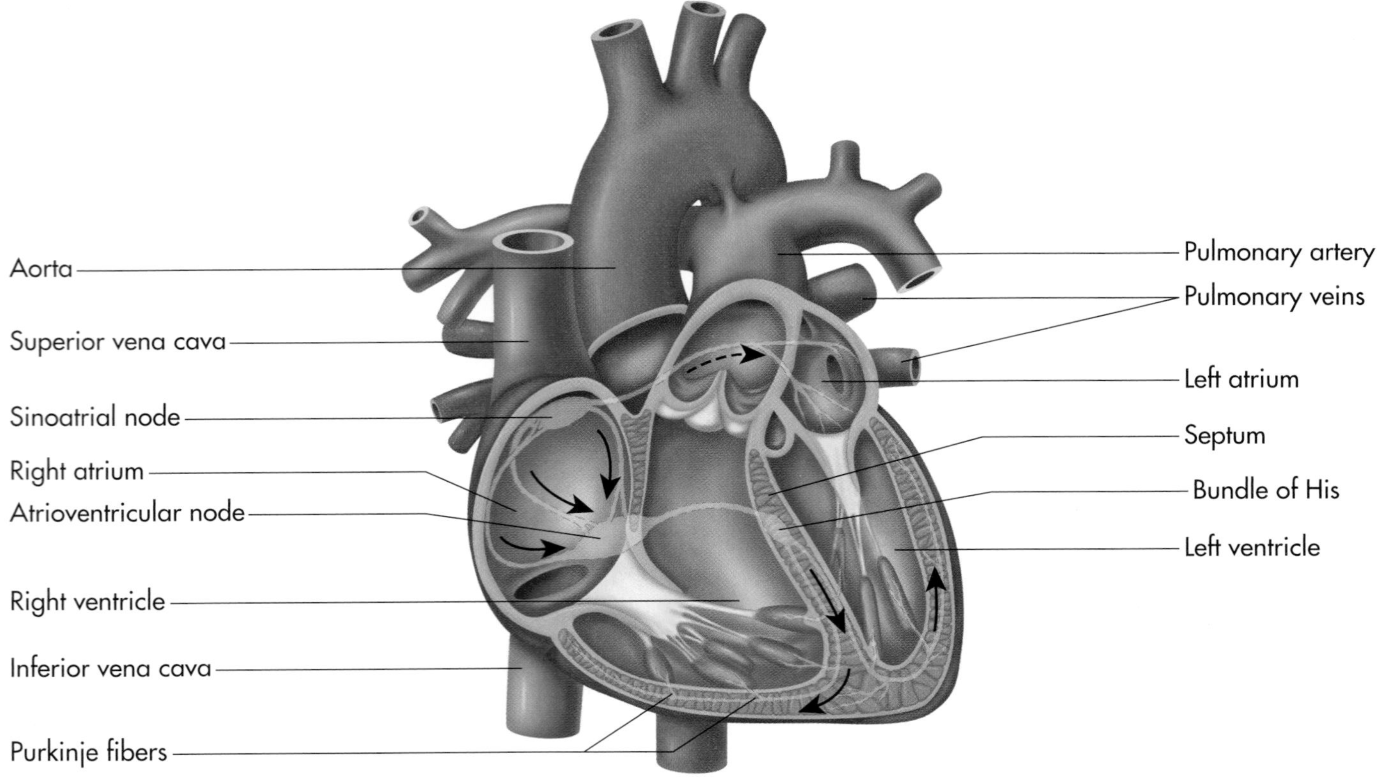

Figure 34-1. Electrical impulses control the cardiac conduction system. Each impulse begins in the sinoatrial node, progresses to the atrioventricular node, and then travels through the bundle of His, the right and left bundle branches, and the Purkinje fibers.

The heart is actually a double pump. The right side of the heart receives blood from the body by way of the superior vena cava and the inferior vena cava. From there, the pulmonary arteries deliver blood to the lungs, where the blood exchanges carbon dioxide for oxygen. Oxygenated blood flows into the left side of the heart through the pulmonary veins. Once in the heart, blood is pumped into the aorta, which pumps oxygenated blood to all parts of the body.

The heart has four sections, or chambers: two upper receiving chambers, the atria (singular, atrium), and two lower pumping chambers, the ventricles (Figure 34-1). Valves between each atrium and ventricle prevent blood from regurgitating (backing up) into the atrium while the ventricle contracts. Similar valves between the ventricles and the arteries into which they pump (the aorta and the pulmonary arteries) prevent blood from regurgitating into the ventricles when they relax. A partition, the septum, divides the heart into right and left sides.

Physiology of the Heart

The heart is divided into separate chambers that work as a single unit. Contraction of the atria, followed by contraction of the ventricles, moves the blood. This contraction phase is called systole. Systole is followed by a relaxation phase, called diastole. When you take someone's blood pressure, you are measuring the pressure during the contraction (systolic) and relaxation (diastolic) phases. This sequence of contraction and relaxation makes up a complete heartbeat, known as the **cardiac cycle.** Each cycle lasts an average of 0.8 second.

All the fibers in the cardiac muscle are interconnected and act as one muscle. Consequently, when one fiber is stimulated to contract, the entire group of fibers contracts. This property plays an important role in the conduction system of the heart.

The Conduction System of the Heart

The cardiac cycle is regulated by specialized tissues in the heart wall, shown in Figure 34-1, that transmit electrical impulses. These electrical impulses cause the heart muscle to contract and relax.

Transmission of electrical impulses in the heart begins in the sinoatrial (SA) node, also called the sinus node or the pacemaker of the heart. The sinoatrial node is a small bundle of heart muscle tissue in the superior wall of the right atrium that specializes in producing electrical impulses. The sinoatrial node sets the rhythm (or pattern) of the heart's contractions.

When the electrical impulse for muscle contraction is generated, it travels throughout the muscle of each atrium, causing atrial contraction. The impulse then travels to the atrioventricular (AV) node, another mass of specialized conducting cells, similar to those of the SA node. The AV node is located at the bottom of the right atrium, near the junction of the ventricles (the septum), where transmission of the impulse is slightly delayed. This delay gives the atria time to completely contract and fill the ventricles with blood.

The atrioventricular node then passes the impulse to the bundle of His (named after the Swiss physician Wilhelm His Jr. [1863–1934]), located in the septum between the ventricles. The bundle of His acts as a relay station, sending the impulse through a series of bundle branches to a network of cardiac conducting muscle fibers. These specialized muscle fibers, called Purkinje fibers (named after the Czech physiologist Jan Evangelista Purkinje [1787–1869]), are located in the ventricle walls. When the impulse reaches the Purkinje fibers, the ventricles contract.

Conduction and Electrocardiography

Electrocardiography records the transmission, magnitude, and duration of the various electrical impulses of the heart. Before you can understand how electrocardiography works, you must understand **polarity,** the condition of having two separate poles, one of which is positive and the other negative. A resting cardiac cell is polarized; that is, there is a negative charge inside and a positive charge outside. When the cardiac cell loses its polarity (a natural occurrence), depolarization occurs. **Depolarization** is the electrical impulse that initiates a chain reaction resulting in contraction. This wave of depolarization flows from the SA node to the ventricles and can be detected by **electrodes,** or electrical impulse sensors, that are placed on specific areas on the surface of the body. During electrocardiography, electrodes detect and record the electrical activity of the heart, including disturbances or disruptions in its rhythm.

Depolarization is always followed by a period of electrical recovery called **repolarization,** when polarity is restored. Following repolarization, the heart returns to a resting, polarized state. The electrical cycle is then repeated, leading to another cardiac cycle.

The Basic Pattern of the Electrocardiogram

The waves of electrical impulses responsible for the cardiac cycle produce a series of waves and lines on an **electrocardiogram** (abbreviated **ECG** or EKG), which is the tracing made by an **electrocardiograph,** an instrument that measures and displays these impulses (Figure 34-2). These peaks and valleys, called waves or **deflections,** are labeled with the letters P, Q, R, S, T, and U. Each letter represents a specific part of the pattern, as explained in Table 34-1. The recognition of abnormalities in the size of the waves or the various time intervals can aid in the diagnosis of certain types of heart problems.

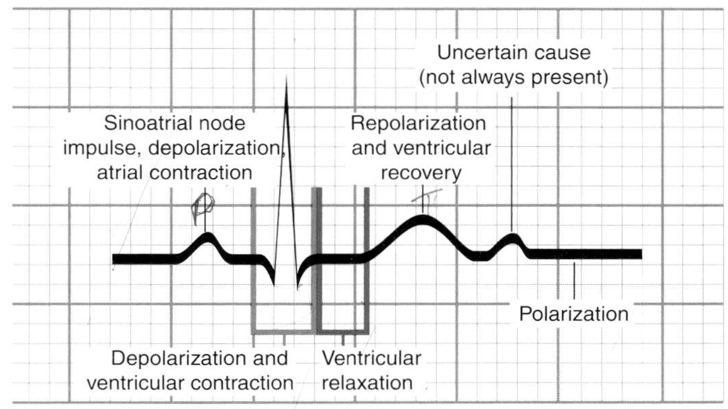

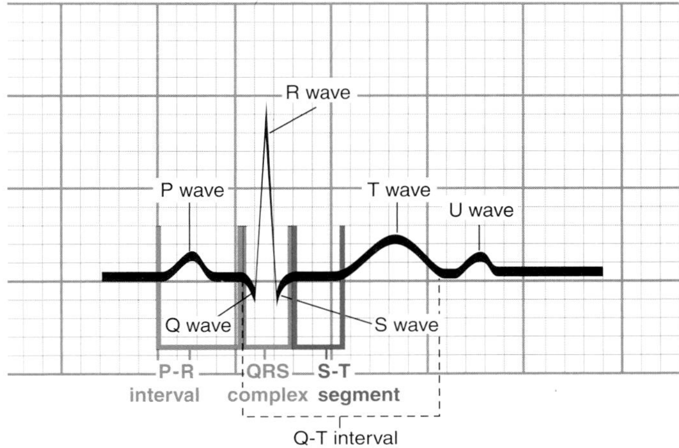

Figure 34-2. This ECG tracing shows the pattern of one cardiac cycle in a normal heart. These specific electrical impulses (top) represent the cycle of cardiac contraction and relaxation. The waves and lines (bottom) represent specific parts of the pattern.

The Electrocardiograph

Each type of electrocardiograph works in the same way. The electrical impulses produced by the heart can be detected through the skin; these impulses are measured, amplified, and recorded on the ECG. Detection begins with electrodes that conduct and transmit the electrical impulses to the electrocardiograph through insulated wires. An amplifier increases the signal, making the heartbeat visible. The **stylus,** a penlike instrument, records this movement on the ECG paper. The impulses received through various combinations of electrodes constitute different **leads,** or views of the electrical activity of the heart, that are recorded on the ECG.

Types of Electrocardiographs

Several different types of electrocardiographs are in use today. Two types are shown in Figure 34-3. The standard machine is a 12-lead electrocardiograph, which records the electrical activity of the heart simultaneously from 12 different views. A single-channel electrocardiograph records the electrical activity of one lead, and consequently, one

TABLE 34-1 Parts of the ECG

Name	Appearance	Represents
P wave	Small upward curve	Sinoatrial node impulse, wave of depolarization through atria, and resultant contraction
QRS complex	Includes Q, R, and S waves	Contraction (following depolarization) of ventricles; QRS complex is larger than P wave because ventricles are larger than atria
Q wave	Downward deflection	Impulse traveling down septum toward Purkinje fibers
R wave	Large upward spike	Impulse going through left ventricle
S wave	Downward deflection	Impulse going through both ventricles
T wave	Upward curve	Recovery (repolarization) of ventricles; repolarization of atria is not obvious because it occurs while ventricles are contracting and producing QRS complex
U wave	Small upward curve sometimes found after T wave	May be seen in normal individuals, in patients who experience slow recovery of Purkinje fibers, or in patients who have low potassium levels or other metabolic disturbances
P–R interval	Includes P wave and straight line connecting it to QRS complex	Time it takes for electrical impulse to travel from SA node to AV node
Q–T interval	Includes QRS complex, S–T segment, and T wave	Time it takes for ventricles to contract and recover, or repolarize
S–T segment	Connects end of QRS complex with beginning of T wave	Time between contraction of ventricles and recovery

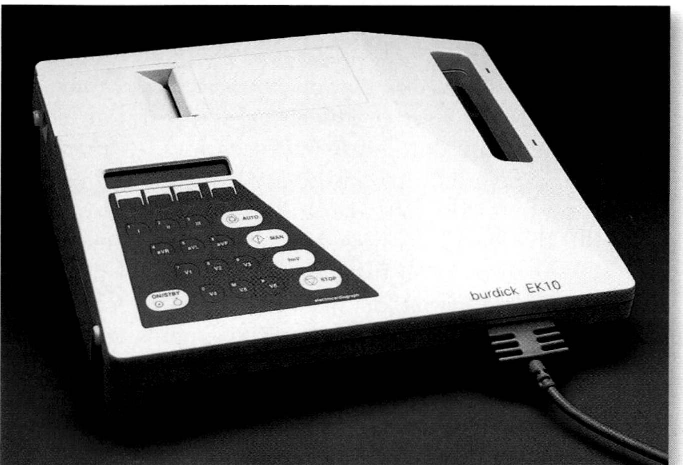

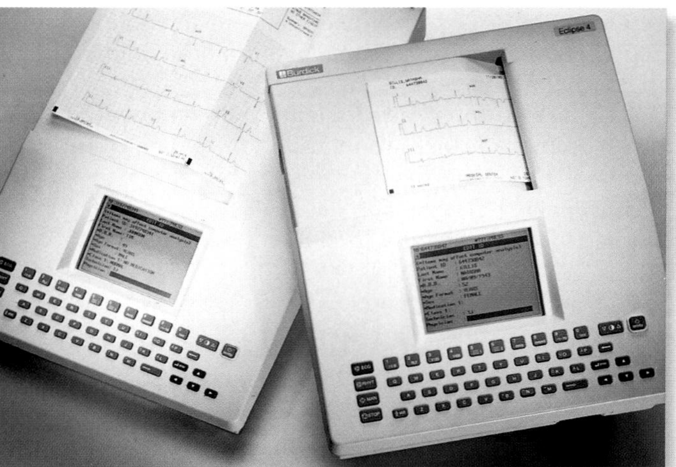

Figure 34-3. Single-channel (left) and multichannel (right) electrocardiographs are used to obtain an ECG.

view of the heart's electrical activity at a time. The record is printed on a long, thin strip of ECG paper. The most common single-channel units allow you to attach all electrodes at the same time and obtain a manual or automatic printout of individual leads. Some older units use fewer electrodes, requiring you to systematically attach, remove, and reposition the electrodes to obtain recordings from different leads.

The newer multichannel units record more than one lead at a time. These machines use wider paper and more than one stylus to record the leads.

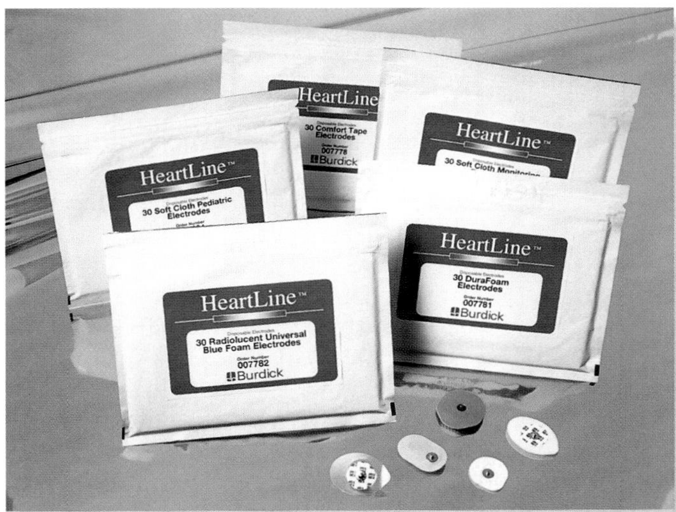

Figure 34-4. Disposable electrodes are available in several varieties.

Electrodes and Electrolyte Products

Electrodes are attached to the patient's skin during electrocardiography. There are several types of electrodes, including metal plate, suction bulb, and disposable electrodes. Disposable electrodes (Figure 34-4) are the most widely used.

The skin does not conduct electricity well. Consequently, an electrolyte (a substance that enhances transmission of electric current) is needed with each electrode. Disposable electrodes come with an electrolyte preparation in place, but you must apply an electrolyte to reusable electrodes. Electrolytes are available in the form of gels, lotions, and solutions and disposable pads impregnated with electrolyte (Figure 34-5).

When performing routine electrocardiography, you place electrodes on ten areas of the body: one each on the right arm (RA), left arm (LA), right leg (RL), and left leg (LL) and six on specific locations on the chest wall. The right leg is designated as the ground. You will move the fifth electrode to six different positions on the chest for successive readings. Evaluating different leads, that is, the electrical activity measured through various combinations of electrodes, enables the physician to pinpoint the origin of certain problems.

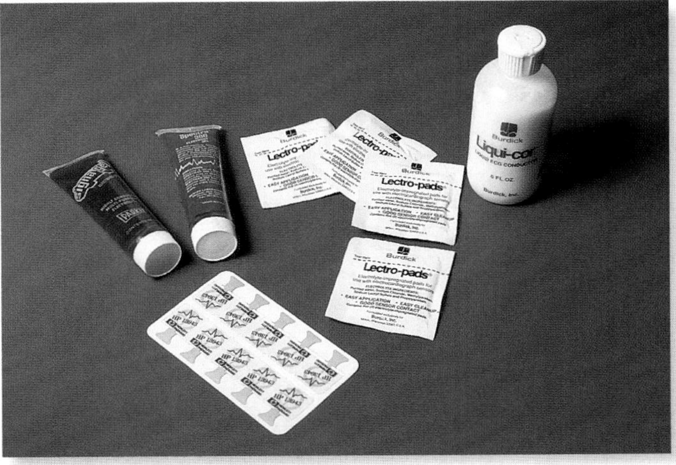

Figure 34-5. An electrolyte (in the form of gel, lotion, solution, or impregnated pad) must be applied to each electrode.

Leads

Each lead provides an image of the electrical activity of the heart from a different angle. Together, the images give the doctor a full picture of electrical activity moving up and down, left and right, and forward and backward through the heart. Monitoring the electrodes on the arms and legs in two different ways produces six leads that record electrical impulses that move up and down and left and right. The electrodes that are placed on the chest provide six more leads, showing electrical activity moving forward and backward (from the front of the body toward the back and vice versa).

Each lead is given a specific designation and code. The 12 leads are usually marked automatically on the ECG.

Limb Leads. Of the six leads that directly monitor electrodes on the arms and legs, three are standard leads and three are augmented leads. The standard leads each monitor two limb electrodes, recording electrical activity between them. These leads are also called bipolar leads, because they monitor two electrodes. The augmented leads monitor one limb electrode and a point midway between two other limb electrodes, recording electrical activity between the monitored electrode and the midway point. Because they directly monitor only one electrode, augmented leads are also called unipolar leads. The electrical activity recorded by these leads is very slight, requiring the machine to augment (amplify) the tracings to produce readable waves and lines on the ECG paper.

Precordial Leads. The six precordial, or chest, leads are unipolar leads. The electrodes are placed across the chest in a specific pattern (Figure 34-6). Each precordial lead monitors one electrode and a point within the heart. The precordial leads are each designated by a letter and a number. The designations for the 12 leads of a routine ECG are shown in Table 34-2. The table also indicates which electrodes and points are monitored by each lead. A common system of marking codes completes the information in the table. Other coding systems are in use; be sure to follow office policy or the doctor's preference when you code an ECG.

ECG Paper

ECG paper is provided in a long, continuous roll. If the paper is designed for use with a single-channel electrocardiograph, it is just wide enough for a single trace. Other ECG papers can accommodate several traces at once; these papers are used with multichannel electrocardiography. ECG paper consists of two layers and is both heat- and pressure-sensitive. The

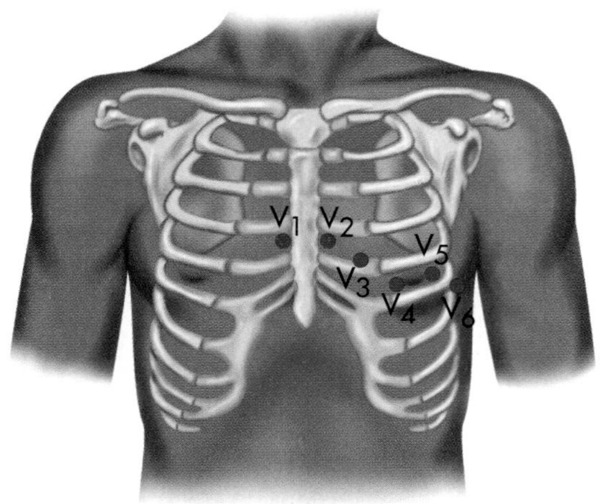

V_1 Fourth intercostal space (between the ribs), to the right of the sternum (breastbone)
V_2 Fourth intercostal space, to the left of the sternum
V_4 Fifth intercostal space, on the left midclavicular line
V_3 Fifth intercostal space, midway between V_2 and V_4
V_6 Fifth intercostal space, on the left midaxillary line
V_5 Fifth intercostal space, midway between V_4 and V_6

Figure 34-6. Six precordial electrodes are arranged in specific positions on the chest. Notice that electrode V_4 must be positioned before V_3 and V_6 before V_5.

heated stylus on the electrocardiograph serves as a "pen" that records the ECG pattern on the paper.

ECG paper (Figure 34-7) is marked with light and dark lines or with dots and lines. The pattern is standardized to permit uniform interpretation by any physician. Each small square, or square area delineated by dots, measures 1 mm by 1 mm. Each large square measures 5 mm by 5 mm.

The vertical, or short, axis of the paper records the voltage, or strength of the impulse; the horizontal axis measures time. Normally the paper moves through the machine at a speed of 25 mm per second. This means that the distance across 1 small square represents 0.04 second. The distance across 1 large square represents 0.2 second. The distance across 5 large squares represents 1.0 second. In 1 minute (60 seconds), the paper advances 300 large squares, or 1500 mm (150 cm).

Each electrocardiograph is standardized before use so that one small square represents 0.1 millivolt (mV). One large square represents 0.5 mV, and two large squares represent 1.0 mV.

Electrocardiograph Controls

The location of certain knobs and buttons on an electrocardiograph may vary from model to model. Certain features, however, are common to most machines. These include the standardization control, speed selector, sensitivity control, lead selector, centering control, stylus temperature control, marker control, and on/off switch.

Standardization Control. Before you obtain an ECG, you must correctly standardize the machine. The standardization control uses a 1-mV impulse to produce a standardization mark on the ECG paper. When you press the standardization control, the stylus should move up ten small squares, or 10 mm (1 cm) and remain there for

TABLE 34-2 ECG Lead Designations and Marking Codes

Lead	Electrodes and Points Monitored	Marking Codes
Standard limb		
I	RA and LA	•
II	RA and LL	••
III	LA and LL	•••
Augmented limb		
aVR	RA and (LA-LL)	-
aVL	LA and (RA-LL)	--
aVF	LL and (RA-LA)	---
Precordial		
V_1	V_1 and (LA-RA-LL)*	-•
V_2	V_2 and (LA-RA-LL)*	-••
V_3	V_3 and (LA-RA-LL)*	-•••
V_4	V_4 and (LA-RA-LL)*	-••••
V_5	V_5 and (LA-RA-LL)*	-•••••
V_6	V_6 and (LA-RA-LL)*	-••••••

*The point within the heart is identified by averaging the readings from the electrodes.

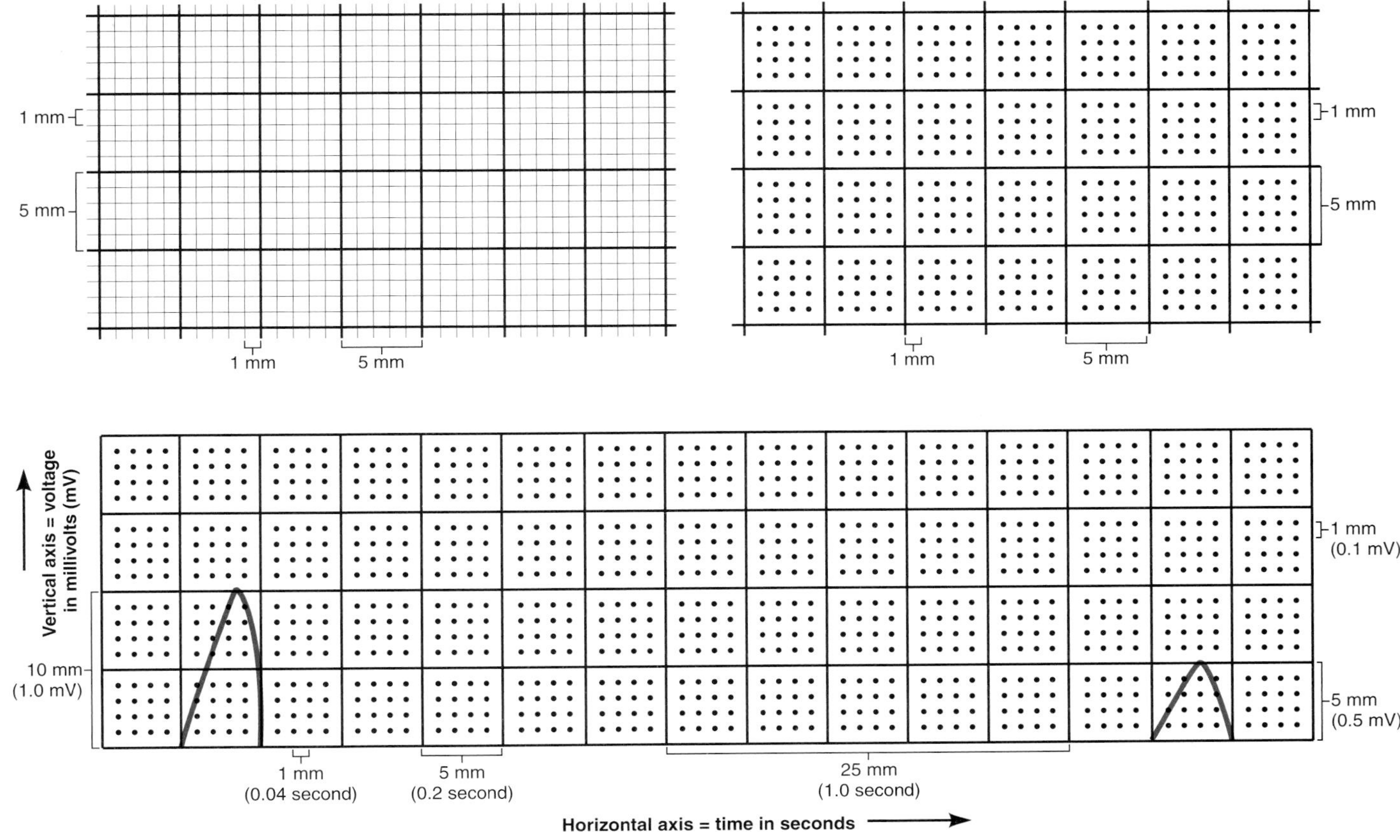

Figure 34-7. The pattern and spacing of lines or lines and dots on ECG paper are standardized and represent specific units of voltage and time.

0.08 second (two small squares, or 2 mm). If it does not, the instrument must be adjusted before you use it.

Speed Selector. The paper is normally set to run at 25 mm per second for adults. When you run an ECG on infants and children or on adults with a rapid heartbeat, the deflections may appear too close together. In these cases you may need to adjust the speed to 50 mm per second to separate the peaks and create a tracing that is easier to read. If you must set the speed at 50 mm per second, note it on the strip. Otherwise, a speed of 25 mm per second is assumed. In any case do not change the speed selection unless the doctor directs you to do so.

Sensitivity Control. The sensitivity control adjusts the height of the standardization mark and the tracing. It is normally set on 1. When the height of an ECG tracing is too high to fit completely on the paper, however, adjust this control to ½ to reduce the size of both the standardization mark and the tracing by one-half. For tracings that have very low peaks, set this control on 2 to double the standardization mark and the height of the tracing. Note this change on the strip.

Lead Selector. Most newer electrocardiographs have a setting that enables a standard 12-lead tracing to run automatically. All machines, however, have a lead selector that allows you to run each lead individually, in case you need to repeat a strip containing artifacts (erroneous marks or defects) during a run.

Centering Control. The centering control allows you to adjust the position of the stylus, which must be centered on the paper. (Centering the stylus simplifies the process of measuring wave heights for the person who interprets the ECG.)

Stylus Temperature Control. Another control allows you to adjust the temperature of the stylus. A higher temperature results in a heavier line, whereas a lower temperature results in a lighter, thinner line. The line should be clear without being so dark that it bleeds or smears on the ECG paper.

Marker Control. Most older machines have a marker control that allows you to place marking codes (Table 34-2) on the ECG paper to identify the lead during each run. Many newer machines do this automatically.

On/Off Switch. The on/off switch turns the machine on and off. Most machines have an indicator light that signals when the power is on.

Preparing to Administer an ECG

You must obtain a good-quality tracing when performing electrocardiography. To do so, you must be able to recognize an artifact or a generally defective ECG tracing when you see one. Proper technique is also essential to help you obtain the best-quality tracing. The following sections guide you through the process. The steps in obtaining a standard 12-lead ECG using a single-channel electrocardiograph are listed in Procedure 34-1.

Preparing the Room and Equipment

Be sure the room and equipment are properly set up before you begin to administer electrocardiography. The accuracy of an ECG can sometimes be affected by electric currents emitted from nearby machines. Although some electrocardiographs have filters to minimize outside electrical interference, it is always a good idea to perform electrocardiography in a room where all other electrical equipment is turned off. This equipment includes air conditioners, refrigerators, and fans as well as laboratory and diagnostic equipment.

The room should be in a quiet location, protected from interruptions. Because the patient must partially disrobe, adjust the room temperature to a comfortable level.

The examining table should be sturdy and comfortable. If the table is made of metal, it must be padded so the patient does not come in contact with any metal parts during the procedure.

Before using the electrocardiograph, check the date of its last inspection. Each machine should be periodically inspected and certified safe to use for a specific period of time. Using a machine only within this time period helps ensure your safety and that of the patient. Be sure to turn the machine on ahead of time to allow the stylus to warm up.

Preparing the Patient

Introduce yourself to the patient, explain the procedure, and answer any questions the patient has. Follow the steps described in Procedure 34-1 as you prepare the patient for

PROCEDURE 34.1

Obtaining an ECG

Objective: To obtain a graphic representation of the electrical activity of a patient's heart

OSHA Guidelines

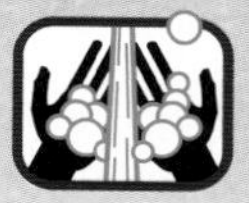
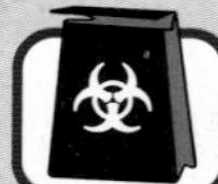

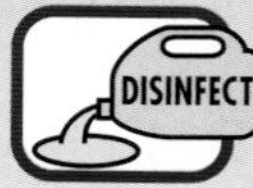

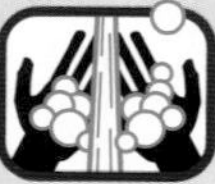

Materials: Electrocardiograph, ECG paper, electrodes, electrolyte preparation, wires, patient gown, drape, blanket, pillows, gauze pads, alcohol, moist towel, disposable shaving supplies (if needed)

Method

1. Turn on the electrocardiograph and, if necessary, allow the stylus to heat up.
2. Identify the patient, introduce yourself, and explain the procedure.
3. Wash your hands.
4. Ask the patient to disrobe from the waist up and remove jewelry, socks or stockings, and shoes. If the electrodes will be placed on the patient's legs, have the patient roll up his or her pant legs. Sometimes the electrodes are placed on the sides of the lower abdomen—check the manufacturer's instructions. Provide a gown if the patient is female, and instruct her to wear the gown with the opening in front.
5. Assist the patient onto the table and into a supine position. Cover the patient with a drape (and a blanket if the room is cool). If the patient experiences difficulty breathing or cannot tolerate lying flat, use a Fowler's or semi-Fowler's position, adjusting with pillows under the head and knees for comfort if needed.
6. Tell the patient to rest quietly and breathe normally. Explain the importance of lying still to prevent false readings.
7. Wash the patient's skin, using gauze pads moistened with alcohol. Then rub it vigorously with dry gauze pads to promote better contact of the electrodes.
8. If the patient's leg or chest hair is dense, put on examination gloves, and shave the areas where

continued ⟶

PROCEDURE 34.1

Obtaining an ECG *(continued)*

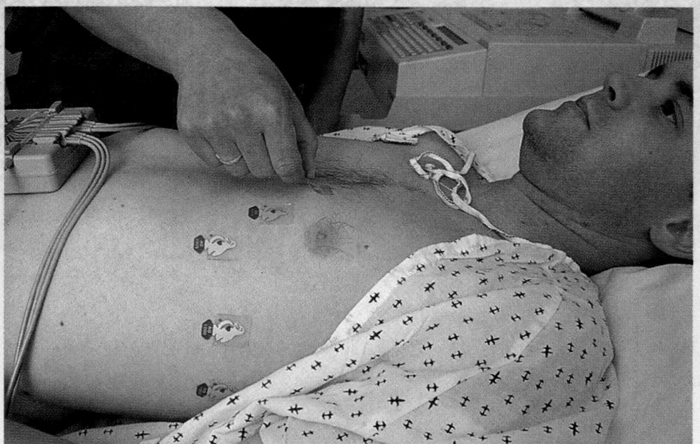

Figure 34-8. Place electrodes at the specified locations on the chest, arms, and legs.

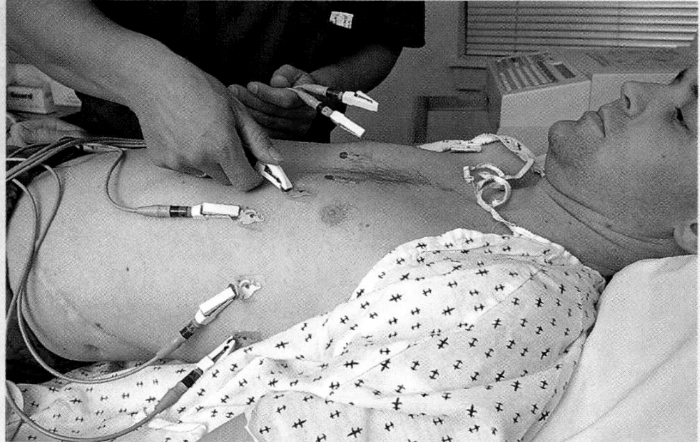

Figure 34-9. Attach wires and cables, draping wires over the patient to avoid tension that can result in artifacts.

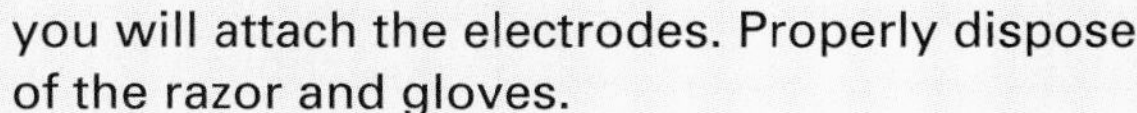

you will attach the electrodes. Properly dispose of the razor and gloves.

9. Apply electrodes to fleshy portions of the limbs, making sure that the electrodes on one arm and leg are placed similarly to those on the other arm and leg (Figure 34-8). The direction that the tabs (where the wires are fastened) are facing will vary. For disposable electrodes, peel off the backings, and press them into place. Reusable electrodes are rarely used.
10. Apply the precordial electrodes at specified locations on the chest.
11. Attach wires and cables, making sure all wire tips follow the patient's body contours.
12. Check all electrodes and wires for proper placement and connection; drape wires over the patient to avoid creating tension on the electrodes that could result in artifacts (Figure 34-9).
13. Enter the patient data into the electrocardiograph. Press the on, run, or record button. Older machines may require the following steps:
    - **a.** Set the paper speed to 25 mm per second or as instructed.
    - **b.** Set the sensitivity setting to 1 or as instructed.
    - **c.** Turn the lead selector to standardization mode.
    - **d.** Adjust the stylus so the baseline is centered.
    - **e.** Press the standardization button. The stylus should move upward above the baseline 10 mm (two large squares).
14. Run the strip.
    - **a.** If the machine has an automatic feature, set the lead selector to automatic.
    - **b.** For manual tracings, turn the lead selector to standby mode. Select the first lead (I), and record the tracing. Switch the machine to standby, and then repeat the procedure for all 12 leads.
15. Check tracings for artifacts.
16. Correct problems and repeat any tracings that are not clear.
17. Disconnect the patient from the machine.
18. Remove the tracing from the machine, and label it with the patient's name, the date, and your initials.
19. Disconnect the wires from the electrodes, and remove the electrodes from the patient.
20. Clean the patient's skin with a moist towel.
21. Assist the patient into a sitting position.
22. Allow a moment for rest, and then assist the patient from the table.
23. Assist the patient in dressing if necessary, or allow the patient privacy to dress.
24. Wash your hands.
25. Record the procedure in the patient's chart.
26. Properly dispose of used materials and disposable electrodes. Clean reusable electrodes, if used.
27. Clean and disinfect the equipment and the room according to OSHA guidelines.

CAUTION *Handle With Care*

Allaying Patient Anxiety About Having Electrocardiography

The most common reason for a patient's anxiety is not knowing what to expect from electrocardiography. The patient may be fearful of being hooked up to an electrical device and worried about receiving an electric shock.

Calmly and simply explain the procedure in detail, both before you begin and while you prepare the patient for the test. Assure her that it is a safe procedure that will last about 10 to 15 minutes. Explain that the machine measures the electrical activity of the heart and that no outside electricity will pass through the body. It is also helpful to explain why the doctor has ordered the procedure, without giving any diagnosis or prognosis.

Above all, talk to and listen to the patient. Encourage her to express her concerns and ask questions. Respond to the patient's concerns and questions calmly, fully, and respectfully.

Ensuring Patient Comfort

Ensuring that the patient is comfortable will help her feel more at ease. It will also result in less body movement and a more accurate ECG.

Each patient is an individual. You will need to find out from the patient what is and is not comfortable for her. First make sure the room temperature is right for the patient. If she says the room feels too cool, provide an extra blanket to prevent chills. Being chilly can make a patient shiver and increase her anxiety. If the patient says she feels too warm, do not provide a blanket.

Next ensure that the patient is comfortable on the examining table. Placing a small pillow under the head can help. Make sure, however, that the pillow does not touch the shoulders or raise them off the table. For most patients, placing a pillow under the knees helps relax the abdomen and lower extremities and prevents lower-back pain. Try this arrangement and let the patient decide whether it contributes to or detracts from her comfort. If the patient has trouble breathing, shift her into a Fowler's or semi-Fowler's position. Ask the patient which position is more comfortable, and use the position she chooses. If the patient chooses a position other than supine, be sure to note the position in her chart.

electrocardiography. Keep in mind that some patients are apprehensive about undergoing electrocardiography. Anxiety often stems from the fear of receiving an electric shock from the machine. See the Caution: Handle With Care section for ways to allay a patient's anxiety about having an ECG.

Applying the Electrodes and the Connecting Wires

You must prepare the patient's skin before applying the electrodes. Proper contact between an electrode and the skin allows for proper conduction of the impulses. Follow the steps described in Procedure 34-1 as you prepare the patient's skin. Depending on your office policy, you may be required to shave chest or leg hair if it is dense to ensure proper contact. Because you may be exposed to blood or broken skin when shaving a patient, observe Universal Precautions and wear gloves to prevent contact with potentially contaminated body fluids.

Electrodes

Disposable electrodes are the most commonly used type of electrode. Disposable electrodes come with the electrolyte product already applied. Simply remove the adhesive backing and press the electrode firmly into place on the skin. This type of electrode has largely replaced the metal plate and suction bulb electrodes from previous models. Because the electrolyte gel is prepackaged and measured, artifacts occurring from the placement of unequal amounts of electrolyte have been minimized.

Positioning the Electrodes

You must position electrodes at ten locations on the body (Figure 34-10). Remember, if the electrocardiograph has only five electrodes, you will need to move the fifth electrode to six different positions on the patient's chest to obtain the necessary tracings.

Limb Electrodes. Placement of limb electrodes need not be exact. Limb electrodes are most commonly placed on the inside of the fleshy part of the calf muscle and on the outside of the upper arm, but they are sometimes placed on the thigh and above the wrist. It is generally better to place arm electrodes on the upper arm because this reduces the amount of artifact caused by arm movement. Attach the electrodes to a smooth and fleshy part of each limb to ensure optimal conduction of impulses. Limb electrodes must always be placed at the same level on both arms and on both legs. If a patient has had a leg amputated, both leg electrodes should be placed on the thighs.

Precordial Electrodes. Unlike the limb electrodes, the precordial electrodes must be placed at specific locations

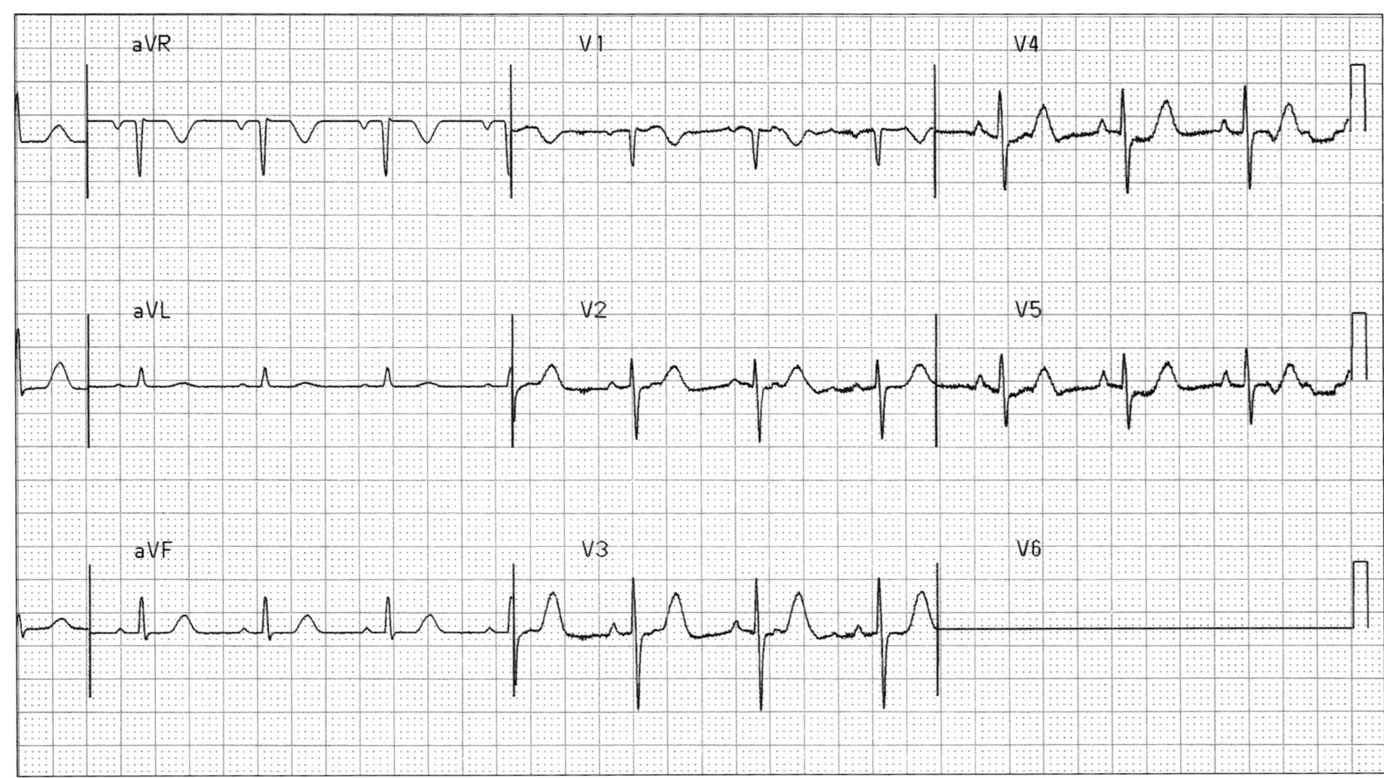

Figure 34-14. A flat line on one of the leads is caused by a loose or disconnected wire. (Courtesy of Burdick, Inc.)

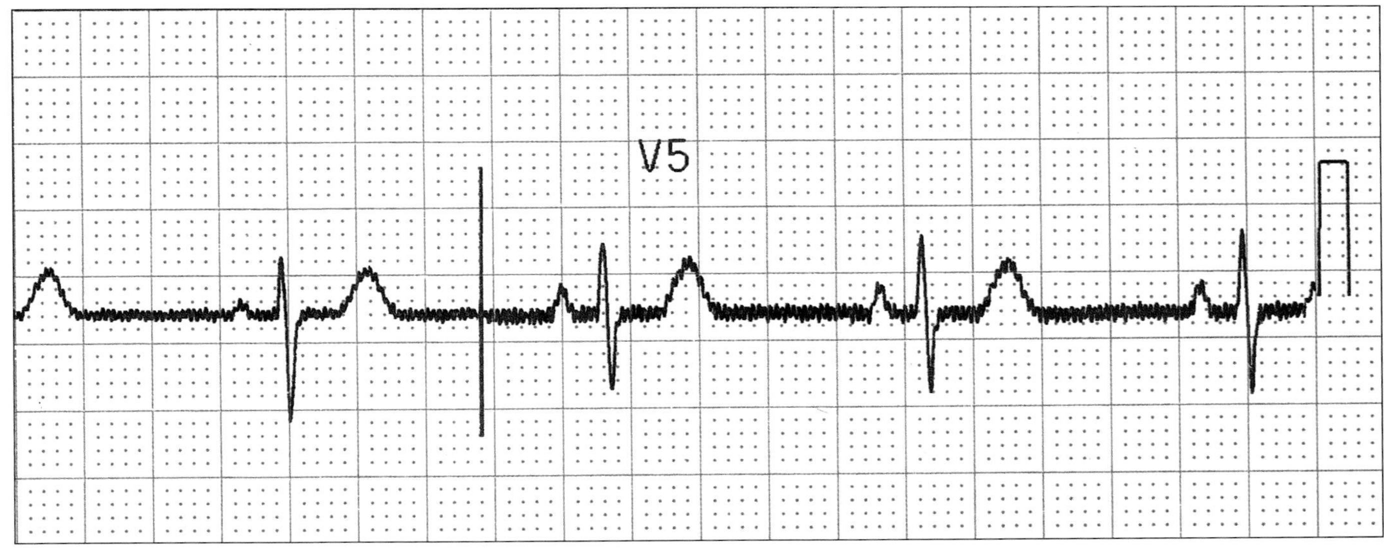

Figure 34-15. This type of artifact is caused by AC interference. (Courtesy of Burdick, Inc.)

small amount of electric current given off by another piece of electrical equipment. The line of the tracing will be jagged, consisting of a series of uniform, small spikes (Figure 34-15). Many of the newer electrocardiographs have filters to reduce or eliminate most of this interference.

AC interference can often be eliminated by turning off or unplugging other appliances in the room. It is also helpful to keep the examining table away from the wall, because wiring in the wall can contribute to AC interference. If these remedies do not work, check to see whether the electrodes are dirty or attached improperly or whether the machine is incorrectly grounded.

Somatic Interference. Somatic interference is caused by muscle movement. Tensing of voluntary muscles, shifting of body position, tremors, or even talking requires muscular contractions that generate electrical impulses.

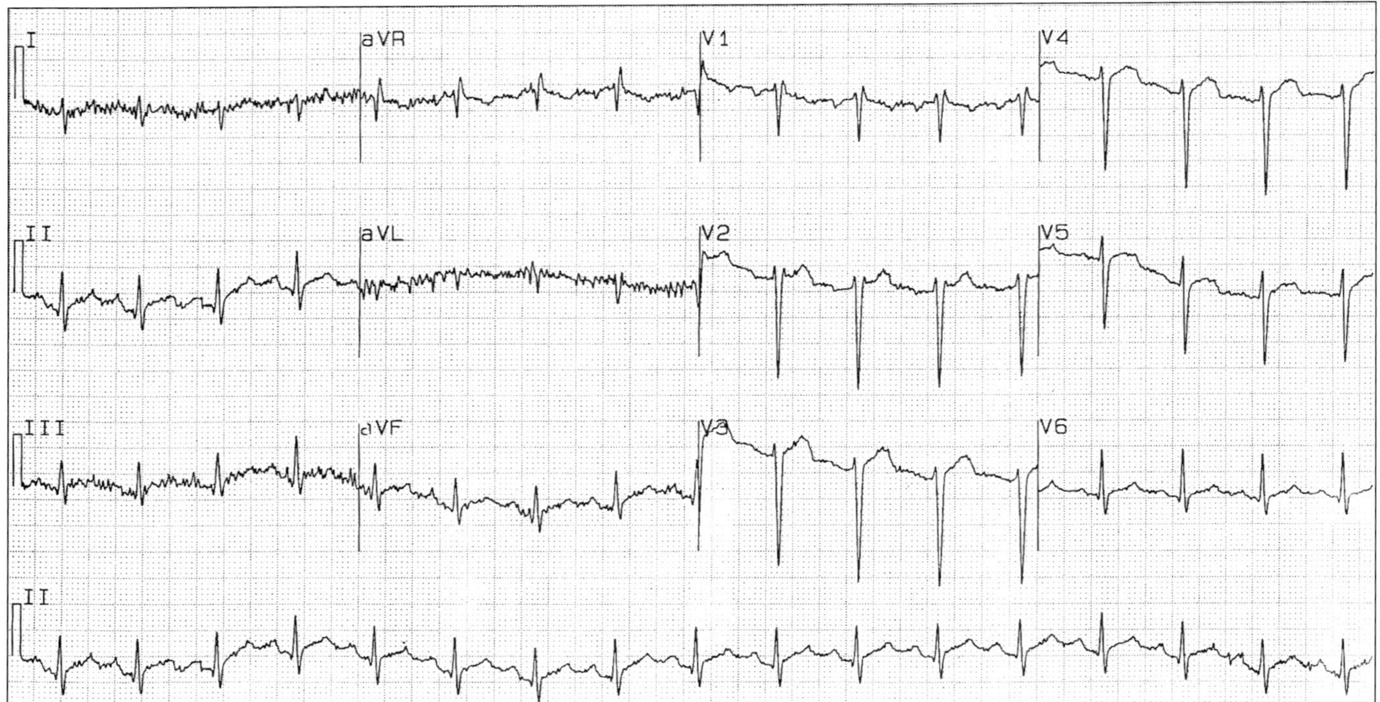

Figure 34-16. The somatic interference in this ECG was caused by patient tremors. (Courtesy of Burdick, Inc.)

A sensitive electrocardiograph detects these impulses. The result is erratic movement of the stylus during the tracing, leading to large, erratic spikes and a shifting baseline (Figure 34-16).

Eliminate this type of interference by reminding the patient to remain still and to refrain from talking. To reduce the chance of shivering, be sure the room temperature is comfortable. Make the patient comfortable to reduce shifting and moving.

Placing the limb electrodes closer to the trunk of the body—on the upper arms, close to the shoulder, and on the upper thighs—can reduce interference. Reducing patient anxiety by explaining the procedure can also help reduce somatic interference.

Certain nervous system disorders, such as Parkinson's disease, cause patients to experience involuntary movements that can cause interference. Placing the limb electrodes closer to the trunk of the body is often helpful; however, it may be necessary to interrupt the tracing until the tremors subside.

Identifying the Source of Interference

The source of interference on an ECG can often be identified by checking the tracings obtained on leads I, II, and III. If there is a problem with a particular limb electrode, the interference will be prominent in two leads. For prominent interference in the following pairs of leads, check the limb electrode indicated:

- Leads I and II, right arm electrode
- Leads I and III, left arm electrode
- Leads II and III, left leg electrode

If the cause of the artifact or the source of interference cannot be determined, stop the machine and notify your supervisor or the physician of the problem. Do not disconnect the patient from the electrocardiograph.

Completing the Procedure

When you are sure the quality of all ECG tracings is acceptable, disconnect the patient from the machine. First remove the tracing from the machine, and label it with the patient's name, the date, and your initials. Loosely roll long tapes from single-channel machines with the printed side facing in, and secure them with a rubber band. Do not use paper clips because they can cause extraneous marks on the tracing.

Next, disconnect the wires from the electrodes, and remove the electrodes from the patient. Wipe excess electrolyte from the patient's skin with a moist towel. Assist the patient to a sitting position, allowing a moment's rest before assisting the patient from the table. Help the patient dress if necessary, or allow the patient privacy to dress. Remove disposable paper covers from the table and pillows, clean surfaces according to OSHA guidelines, and discard all disposable materials in a biohazardous waste container.

Equipment Maintenance

If your machine has reusable electrodes, wipe off the electrolyte product, and wash the electrodes and rubber straps with a mild detergent. Metal plate electrodes must be polished with a fine grade of scouring powder. Do not use steel wool or metal-base polish because they will cause artifacts. Rinse the electrodes well, and dry them thoroughly before storing.

Mounting the Tracing

There are many types of ECG mounts or holders for single-channel ECG tracings. These mounts form a permanent record of the ECG and allow the doctor to read tracings from all 12 leads at once. Mounts are not typically necessary for multiple-channel ECG tracings because these are compact records of several leads. Several types of mounts are available, including slotted folders and folders with self-adhesive surfaces.

Interpreting the ECG

As a medical assistant, you are not responsible for interpreting an ECG. Knowing something about how ECGs are interpreted, however, may allow you to recognize a problem that requires immediate attention. Some of the features that are assessed by means of an ECG include heart rhythm, heart rate, the length and position of intervals and segments, and wave changes. A series of ECGs are often taken before a physician makes a diagnosis. The tracings are compared for changes in a patient's condition, progress, or response to a specific medication.

Heart Rhythm

The ECG is the best way to assess heart rhythm—the regularity of the heartbeat. A normal heart rhythm is indicated on the ECG by regularly spaced complexes. In a regularly spaced complex, the distance between one P wave and the next P wave—or one R wave and the next R wave—is consistent. The physician assesses the patient's rhythm by viewing the rhythm strip you obtain from lead II.

Irregularities in heart rhythm are called **arrhythmias.** Some arrhythmias do not cause problems, but many of them can be dangerous. It is important, therefore, to detect these irregularities with an ECG.

Heart Rate

The heart rate can easily be determined by counting the number of QRS complexes in a 6-second strip of the tracing (30 large squares at 25 mm per second) and multiplying by 10. Irregularities in heart rate may result from conduction abnormalities or reactions to certain drugs.

Intervals and Segments

Variations in the length and position of the intervals and segments can indicate many heart conditions, including conduction disturbances and **myocardial infarction,** or heart attack. For example, following a heart attack, the S–T segment will be elevated in the tracing for a period of time. Thus, the ECG can be used to determine not only the occurrence of a heart attack but also the approximate time it occurred. Electrolyte disturbances in the blood and drug reactions can also affect intervals and segments.

Wave Changes

The direction of certain waves may vary, depending on which lead is being viewed. Normally each wave should have a similar appearance in each of the leads. Changes in the height, width, or direction of a wave may indicate a problem. During the early stages of a heart attack, for example, the T wave forms a large peak. Not long afterward the T wave inverts and appears below the baseline.

Exercise Electrocardiography (Stress Testing)

The resting ECG does not always provide a doctor with enough information to diagnose a problem. Exercise electrocardiography, more commonly known as a stress test, assesses the heart's conduction system during exercise, when the demand for oxygen increases. This test measures a patient's response to a constant or increasing workload.

A stress test may be performed on a patient who has had surgery or a heart attack to determine how the heart is functioning. It is sometimes used to screen a patient for heart disease and to determine a patient's ability to undertake an exercise program.

During the procedure the patient is required to walk on a treadmill, pedal a stationary bicycle, or walk on a stair-stepping ergonometer while ECG readings are taken (Figure 34-17). An ergonometer measures work performed. You are responsible for preparing the patient for electrocardiography and monitoring blood pressure throughout the procedure. The test continues until the patient reaches a target heart rate, experiences chest pain or fatigue, or develops complications, such as tachycardia or dysrhythmia.

A patient who undergoes stress testing is often suspected of having a heart problem or is recovering from a heart attack or surgery. Consequently, there may be a risk of cardiac distress, heart attack, or cardiac arrest during testing. Because of the risks, the patient must be monitored by a physician throughout the test. Emergency medication and equipment, such as a defibrillator, must always be present in the room. The patient must sign an informed consent form before the procedure.

Because of the potential risk, patients may be apprehensive about the test. As a medical assistant, you can be instrumental in helping them feel comfortable about undergoing the procedure and in making the procedure as

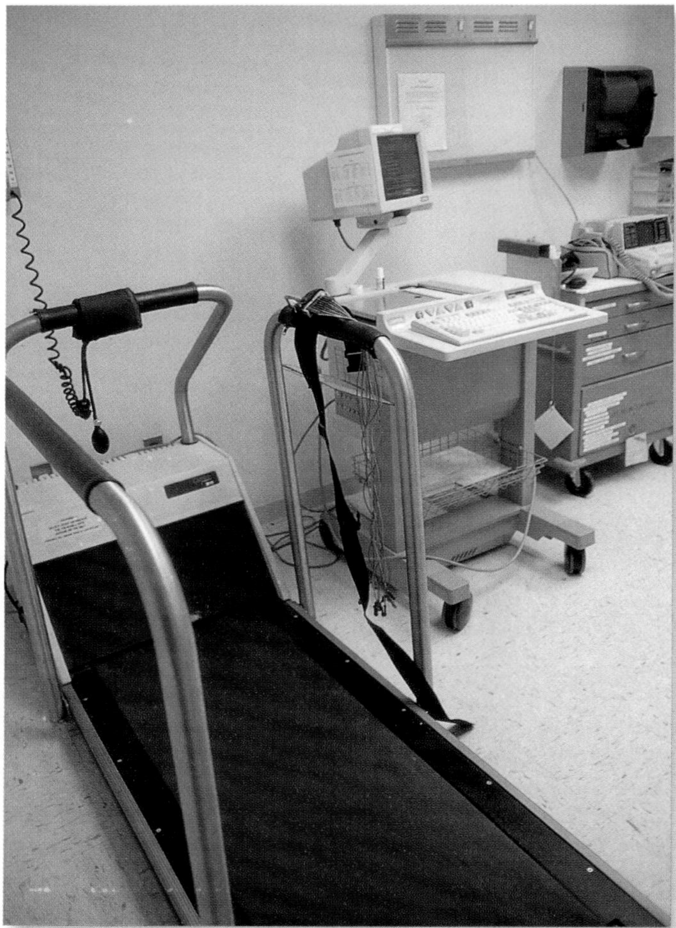

Figure 34-17. During a stress test, the patient exercises on special equipment to see how well the heart handles increased physical demands.

safe as possible for them. See the Caution: Handle With Care section for ways to help a patient safely undergo stress testing.

Ambulatory Electrocardiography (Holter Monitoring)

Patients who experience intermittent chest pain or discomfort may have a normal resting ECG and a normal stress test. When this is the case, the electrical activity of the patient's heart can be monitored over a 24-hour period of normal activity to help diagnose the problem. A special monitor, the Holter monitor, is used for this purpose.

Function of the Holter Monitor

The **Holter monitor** is an electrocardiography device that includes a small cassette recorder worn around a patient's waist or on a shoulder strap to record the heart's electrical activity. The monitor is connected to electrodes on the

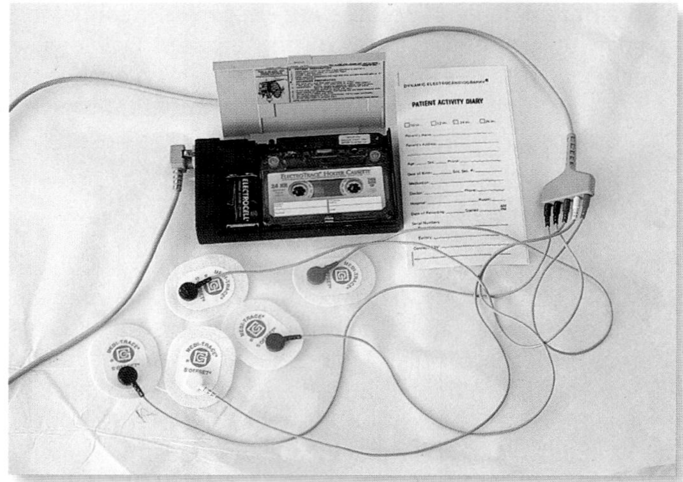

Figure 34-18. The Holter monitor is used to determine electrical activity of a patient's heart over a 24-hour period.

patient's chest (Figure 34-18). During the testing period, the patient is asked to perform usual daily activities and to keep a written log of activities undertaken and of stress or symptoms experienced. To aid in the diagnosis, some monitors allow patients to press an event button to mark the area on the recording whenever symptoms appear.

The patient returns to the office at the end of the 24-hour test period to have the monitor and electrodes removed. The tape is analyzed by a microcomputer in the office or at a reference laboratory, and a printout of the results is prepared. When the tracing has been evaluated, the doctor can correlate cardiac irregularities, such as arrhythmias or S–T segment changes, with the activities and symptoms listed in the patient's diary.

In addition to its role as a diagnostic tool, Holter monitoring can be used to evaluate the status of a patient who is recovering from a heart attack. It can indicate progress or the need to change therapy or modify the rehabilitation plan.

Patient Education

It is absolutely essential that the patient continue normal activities during Holter monitoring. Give the patient the following additional instructions.

- Record all activities, emotional upsets, physical symptoms, and medications taken.
- Wear loose-fitting clothing that opens in the front while wearing the monitor.
- Avoid going near magnets, metal detectors, and high-voltage areas, and avoid using electric blankets during the monitoring period. These devices and areas can interfere with the recording.
- Avoid getting the monitor wet. Do not take a bath or shower. A sponge bath is permissible.

Show the patient how to check the monitor to make sure it is working properly. This step is particularly important if

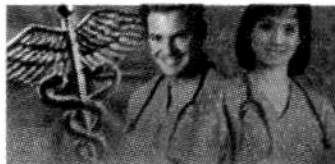

Career Opportunities

Respiratory Therapist *(continued)*

The respiratory therapist is also often responsible for testing equipment to make sure it is operating effectively. He may make minor repairs to faulty respiratory equipment or arrange for major repair work.

Workplace Settings

Most respiratory therapists work in hospitals. Sometimes, in emergency situations, they also work in ambulances. Increasing numbers of respiratory therapists, however, work in locations outside the hospital. These locations include nursing homes, physicians' offices, home health-care agencies, rehabilitation centers, clinics, medical equipment supply companies, and patients' homes.

Education

Approximately 400 colleges and universities in the United States offer respiratory care programs. To qualify for a program, you must be a high school graduate with a background in math and science.

The National Board for Respiratory Therapists has established two levels of respiratory care practitioners. A Certified Respiratory Therapy Technician (CRTT) has graduated from an approved program (usually 12 to 18 months), has 1 year of work experience, and has passed a voluntary written examination. A Registered Respiratory Therapist (RRT) has completed either a 2-year or 4-year approved program, has 1 year of work experience, and has passed a written and practical examination.

Where to Go for More Information

American Association for Respiratory Care
11030 Ables Lane
Dallas, TX 73429
(214) 243-2272

American Lung Association
1740 Broadway
New York, NY 10019
(212) 315-8700

Spirometry

Spirometry is a test used to measure breathing capacity. An instrument called a **spirometer** measures the air taken in by and expelled from the lungs. Several different measurements related to lung volume and capacity can be made with a spirometer (Table 34-4). Some of these measurements are made directly by the spirometer; others are calculated.

Forced Vital Capacity

Many measurements can be obtained during one particular maneuver—obtaining the **forced vital capacity (FVC)**, the greatest volume of air that can be expelled when a person performs rapid, forced expiration. To obtain the FVC, ask the patient to take as deep a breath as possible and to exhale into the spirometer as quickly and completely as possible. You can determine the lung's ability to function by taking into account the volume of air expelled and the time it takes to perform this maneuver.

Types of Spirometers

Many types of spirometers are used in physicians' offices. Each consists of a mouthpiece or a mouthpiece and a tube to carry air to the machine, a mechanism to measure the volume or flow of air, and a means of calculating and printing the results.

Computerized spirometers are available that can measure air volume and airflow, perform various calculations, and print a graphic representation of the information. Figure 34-24 shows a computerized spirometer.

Mechanical spirometers directly measure either the air volume displaced or airflow. Spirometers that directly measure airflow calculate air volume using flow rate and time values. The flow-sensing spirometer illustrated in Figure 34-25 calculates airflow by counting the rotations of a turbine.

Performing Spirometry

The technique for performing pulmonary function testing is similar for all types of spirometers. Successful spirometry depends on proper patient preparation and consistent technique in performing the procedure and analyzing the results. The steps involved in measuring forced vital capacity using a spirometer are described in detail here and outlined in Procedure 34-3.

Patient Preparation

When patients are scheduled for pulmonary function tests, inform them that the following conditions and activities may affect the test's accuracy:

- Viral infection or acute illness within the previous 2 to 3 weeks
- Serious medical condition, such as a recent heart attack
- Recent use of a prescribed medication if test order calls for spirometry before and after prescribed medication

TABLE 34-4 Pulmonary Function Tests	
Lung Capacity Tests	**Definition**
Vital capacity (VC)	Total volume of air that can be exhaled after maximum inspiration
Inspiratory capacity (IC)	Amount of air that can be inhaled after normal expiration
Functional residual capacity (FRC)	Amount of air remaining in lungs after normal expiration
Total lung capacity (TLC)	Total volume of lungs when maximally inflated
Forced vital capacity (FVC)	Greatest volume of air that can be expelled when person performs rapid, forced expiratory maneuver
Forced expiratory volume (FEV)	Volume of air expelled in first, second, or third second of FVC maneuver
Peak expiratory flow rate (PEFR)	Greatest rate of flow during forced expiration
Forced expiratory flow (FEF)	Average rate of flow during middle half of FVC
Maximal voluntary ventilation (MVV)	Greatest volume of air breathed per unit of time
Tidal volume (T_V)	Amount of air inhaled or exhaled during normal breathing
Minute volume (MV)	Total amount of air expired per minute
Inspiratory reserve volume (IRV)	Amount of air inspired over above-normal inspiration
Expiratory reserve volume (ERV)	Amount of air exhaled after normal expiration
Residual volume (RV)	Amount of air remaining in lungs after forced expiration

Adapted from *Illustrated Guide to Diagnostic Tests* (Springhouse, PA: Springhouse, 1998).

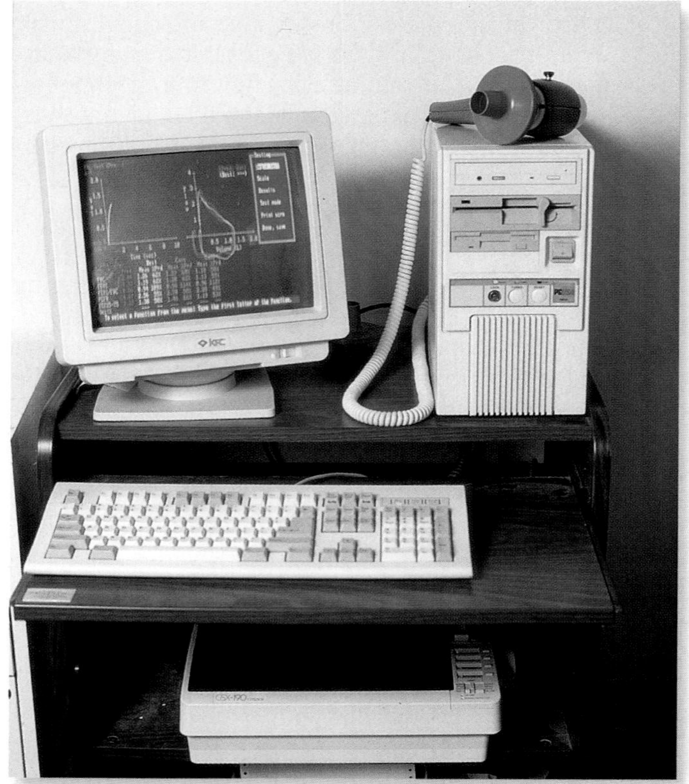

Figure 34-24. This computerized spirometer measures air volume and airflow.

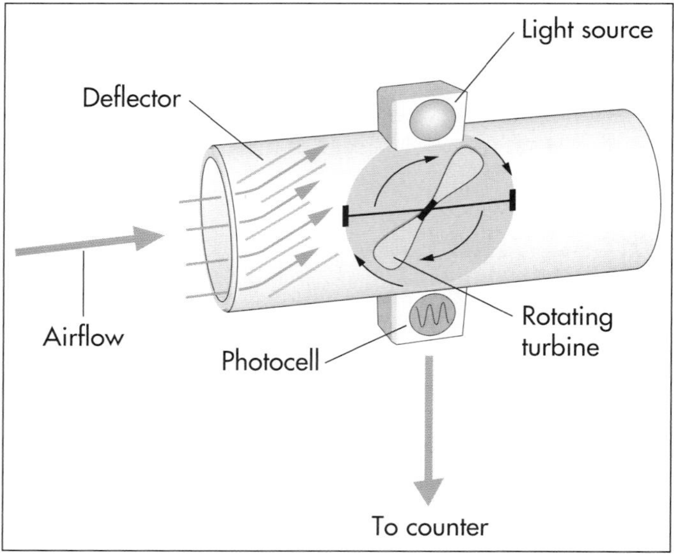

Figure 34-25. One type of flow-sensing spirometer uses a turbine to measure airflow directly from the lungs.

- Use of a sedative or opioid substance before the test
- Smoking or eating a heavy meal within 1 hour of taking the test

Review the conditions and activities with patients again on the day of the test to ensure that none apply. If

PROCEDURE 34.3

Measuring Forced Vital Capacity Using Spirometry

Objective: To determine a patient's forced vital capacity using a volume-displacing spirometer

OSHA Guidelines

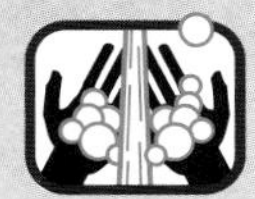
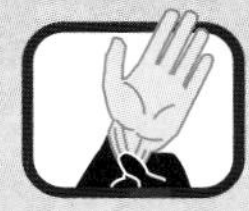
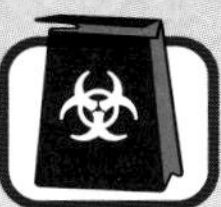
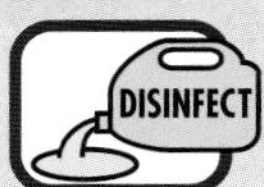

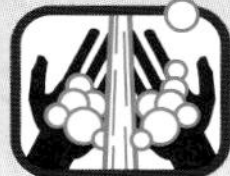

Materials: Adult scale with height bar, spirometer, patient tubing (tubing that runs from the mouthpiece to the machine), mouthpiece, nose clip, disinfectant

Method

1. Prepare the equipment. Ensure that the paper supply in the machine is adequate.
2. Calibrate the machine as necessary.
3. Identify the patient and introduce yourself.
4. Check the patient's chart to see whether there are special instructions to follow.
5. Ask whether the patient has followed instructions.
6. Wash your hands and put on examination gloves.
7. Measure and record the patient's height and weight.
8. Explain the proper positioning.
9. Explain the procedure.
10. Demonstrate the procedure.
11. Turn on the spirometer, and enter applicable patient data and the number of tests to be performed.
12. Ensure that the patient has loosened any tight clothing, is comfortable, and is in the proper position. Apply the nose clip.
13. Have the patient perform the first maneuver, coaching when necessary.
14. Determine whether the maneuver is acceptable.
15. Offer feedback to the patient and recommendations for improvement if necessary.
16. Have the patient perform additional maneuvers until three acceptable maneuvers are obtained.
17. Record the procedure in the patient's chart, and place the chart and the test results on the physician's desk for interpretation.
18. Ask the patient to remain until the physician reviews the results.
19. Properly dispose of used materials and disposable instruments.
20. Sanitize and disinfect patient tubing and reusable mouthpiece and nose clip.
21. Clean and disinfect the equipment and room according to OSHA guidelines.

there are no contraindications, weigh and measure patients. Use simple terms to explain the procedure and its purpose. Have them loosen tight clothing so they will be comfortable and their breathing will not be restricted in any way. The procedure is performed with patients sitting down. Make sure their legs are not crossed and that both feet are flat on the floor.

Explain that they need to wear a nose clip or hold the nose tightly closed to be sure that they will inhale and exhale through the mouth. The mouthpiece of the unit may be a disposable cardboard tube or a reusable rubber one that can be disinfected after use. If disposable mouthpieces are used, instruct patients to avoid biting down on them, because that will obstruct the flow of air. Be sure patients form a tight seal around the mouthpiece with their lips. Dentures normally help maintain a tight seal; however, they should be removed if they hinder the process.

Proper Positioning. Instruct patients to keep their chin and neck in the correct position during the procedure. The chin should be slightly elevated and the neck slightly extended. Bending the chin to the chest tends to restrict the flow of air and should be avoided (Figure 34-26). Some bending at the waist is acceptable.

Explaining and Demonstrating the Procedure. Tell patients to take the deepest breath possible, insert the mouthpiece into the mouth, form a tight seal, and then blow into the mouthpiece as hard and as fast as possible to completely exhale. Tell them to exhale as long as they can to force air from the lungs. Remind them that the initial force of their exhalation must be strong to get a valid reading. Demonstrate the procedure to show how the test is done correctly.

Performing the Maneuver

You can improve patients' performance during the maneuver by actively and forcefully coaching them. Urge patients to blow hard and to continue blowing. After a maneuver, give them feedback on their performance, and indicate corrective actions they can take to improve the next maneuver.

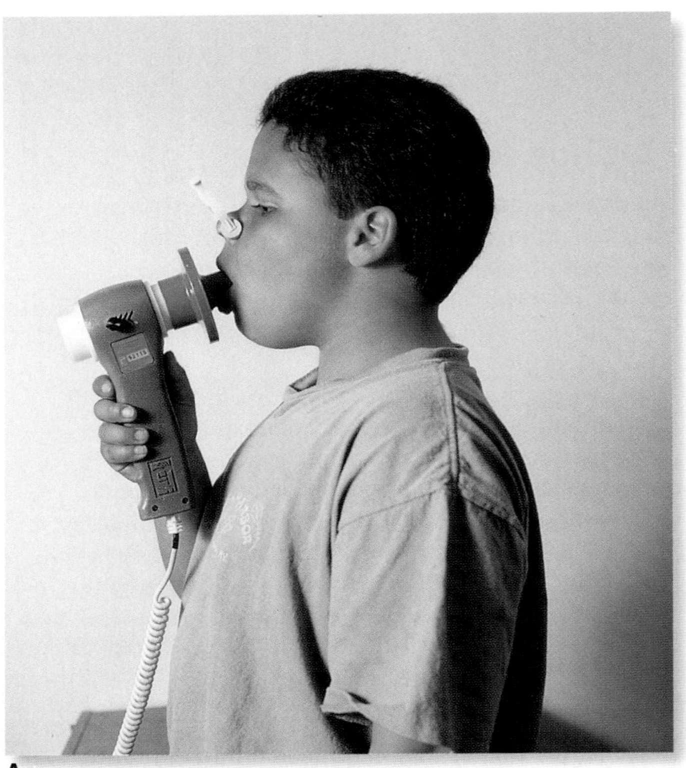

A

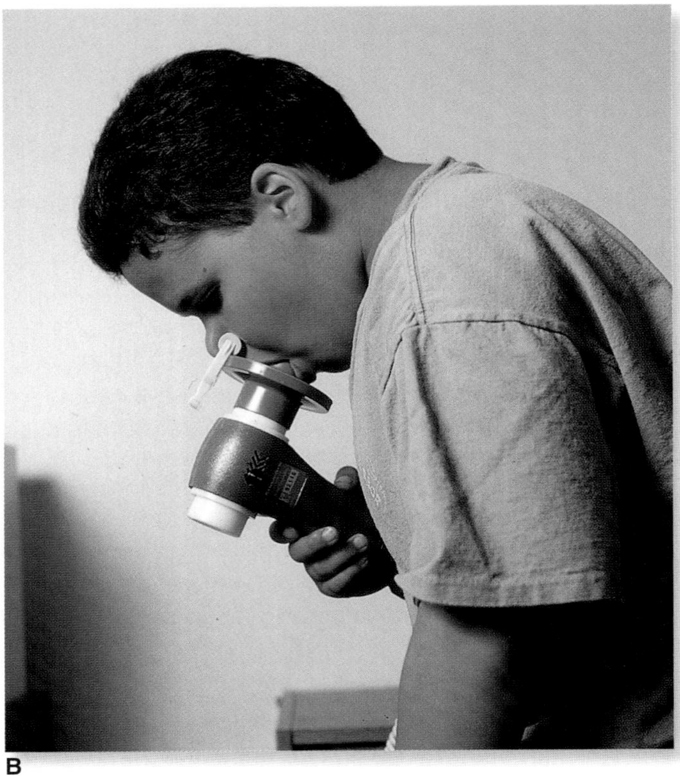

B

Figure 34-26. The patient must maintain the proper position during a pulmonary function test. (a) The chin should be slightly elevated and the neck slightly extended. (b) The neck should not approach the chest.

Some spirometers indicate whether a particular maneuver was of adequate force and duration to be measured. Adequate force does not, however, indicate that the maneuver was acceptable. An acceptable maneuver must have the following five features:

1. No coughing, particularly during the first second
2. A quick and forceful start
3. An adequate length of time (a minimum of 6 seconds)
4. A consistent and fast flow with no variability
5. Consistency with other maneuvers

Spirometry tracings plot volume and time. You will need to obtain three acceptable maneuvers, which may require more than three attempts. Observe the patient for signs of breathing difficulty, dizziness, light-headedness, or changes in pulse and blood pressure. If necessary, allow the patient to rest briefly before continuing. Notify the physician immediately if symptoms are severe.

Determining the Effectiveness of Medication. Spirometry is often used to determine the effectiveness of certain medications that a patient is taking. You will perform two sets of maneuvers if this determination is required. Instruct the patient to refrain from taking the prescribed medication on the day of the test. Before performing the test, confirm that the patient has followed this instruction. Conduct the first set of maneuvers, ensuring that they are acceptable. After obtaining the results, instruct the patient to take the prescribed medication. Allow the medication to take effect, and then perform a second set of maneuvers. Comparing the two sets of readings shows whether the medication has effectively improved the patient's lung function. Some computerized spirometers can graph both sets of readings together to simplify the comparison (Figure 34-27).

Special Considerations. On occasion you may have to deal with an uncooperative patient, one who cannot understand or follow directions, or one who cannot perform the procedure. In these situations patience and skill are essential to obtaining an acceptable spirometry tracing.

The doctor may be able to convince an uncooperative patient to perform the maneuver. You can help by taking a no-nonsense approach, perhaps stating that the doctor needs these test results to help the patient. Patients who cannot understand or follow directions—the very young, the very old, those who have limited proficiency in English, or those with a hearing impairment—may need extra attention and patience to obtain acceptable results. Explain the procedure in simple terms, and repeat instructions as necessary. If, after eight attempts, the patient is unable to perform the procedure, stop and report the situation to the doctor.

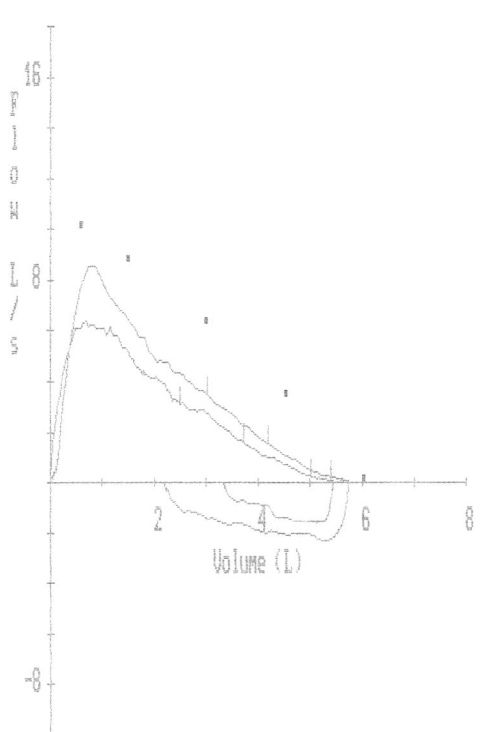

Figure 34-27. These spirometry tracings show air volume per second before and after use of a medication.

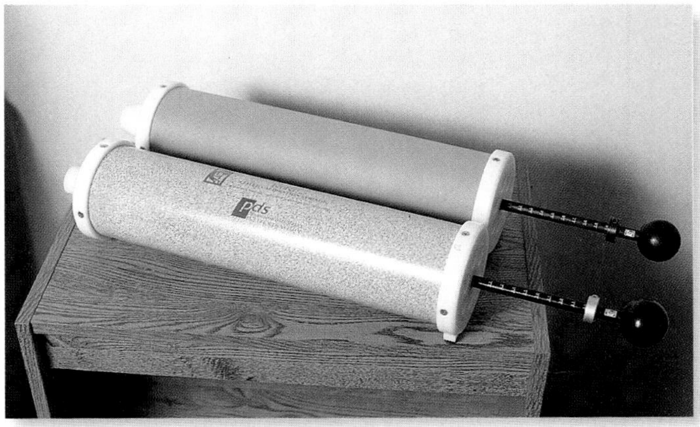

Figure 34-28. A calibration syringe delivers a fixed volume of air.

The Importance of Calibration

Spirometers should be calibrated each day they are used to ensure accurate readings. You may be required to perform this procedure. Calibration of a spirometer requires the use of a standardized measuring instrument called a **calibration syringe** (Figure 34-28). When the plunger is pulled back, this syringe contains a fixed volume of air. Connect the syringe to the patient tubing (the tubing that runs from the mouthpiece to the machine), and depress the plunger to inject the entire volume of air. The reading on the spirometer should be within ±3% of the stated volume. It is important to keep a calibration logbook for each spirometer.

While calibrating the spirometer, you can detect leaks by checking the volume/time graph. The volume should remain at a steady reading. If the volume declines with time, there is a leak somewhere in the system.

Infection Control

After a patient completes the pulmonary function test, you must clean the spirometer thoroughly to prevent transmission of microorganisms. If disposable mouthpieces and nose clips are used, discard them in a biohazardous waste container. If reusable mouthpieces and nose clips are used, clean and disinfect them between patients. Also change patient tubing between patients. Thoroughly clean and disinfect patient tubing before reusing it. Most important, wash your hands thoroughly before and after performing a pulmonary function test.

What the Results Reveal

Pulmonary function tests help the doctor evaluate ventilatory function of the lungs and chest wall. They are good screening tools for pulmonary disorders, such as pulmonary edema, chronic obstructive pulmonary disease, and asthma. These tests also help the doctor determine the nature of a patient's disorder, such as narrowing or obstruction of the airways. Pulmonary function tests can determine the severity of a patient's problem and response to therapy or medication.

Summary

Electrocardiography and pulmonary function testing play a vital role in the diagnosis and treatment of cardiac and pulmonary disease. As a medical assistant, you may be required to perform these procedures in the medical office.

To understand electrocardiography, you need to know the basics of the conduction system of the heart and the components of an electrocardiograph. To obtain accurate electrocardiogram readings, you must properly place the electrodes and be able to recognize artifacts and correct them.

Likewise, to provide accurate assessments of pulmonary function, you must use proper technique and recognize the acceptability of a spirometric maneuver. Because patient compliance is crucial for accurate results, effective patient education is vital to the process.

REVIEW

CHAPTER 34

CASE STUDY QUESTIONS

Now that you have completed this chapter, review the case study at the beginning of the chapter and answer the following questions:

1. What does the abbreviation ECG stand for? What is the diagnostic value of the ECG?
2. What is another name for a spirometry? What does FVC designate?
3. Why were the Holter monitor and stress tests ordered for this patient?

Discussion Questions

1. List the various types of control adjustments found on most electrocardiograph instruments.
2. For what reasons might a physician order an electrocardiogram?
3. Describe where to place the six precordial chest leads.

Critical Thinking Questions

1. For what reasons could a wandering ECG baseline occur? What are the solutions for these problems?
2. Stress testing is often ordered for patients suspected of having cardiac problems. Are there special precautions to consider for these patients, and if so, what are they?
3. What conditions or activities could affect the accuracy of a pulmonary function test?

Application Activities

1. Practice locating the areas for placement of precordial ECG electrodes on your chest.
2. Explain to another student how to use and care for a Holter monitor.
3. Practice explaining and demonstrating the procedure of obtaining a forced vital capacity to someone who is not familiar with the procedure.

CHAPTER 35

X-Rays and Diagnostic Radiology

AREAS OF COMPETENCE

2003 Role Delineation Study

CLINICAL

Patient Care

- Prepare patient for examinations, procedures, and treatments

GENERAL

Legal Concepts

- Prepare and maintain medical records
- Comply with established risk management and safety procedures

KEY TERMS

arthrography
barium enema
barium swallow
brachytherapy
cholangiography
contrast medium
diagnostic radiology
intravenous pyelography (IVP)
invasive
KUB radiography
mammography
MUGA scan
noninvasive
nuclear medicine
PET
radiation therapy
retrograde pyelography
SPECT
stereoscopy
teletherapy
thermography
ultrasound
xeroradiography

CHAPTER OUTLINE

- Brief History of the X-Ray
- Diagnostic Radiology
- The Medical Assistant's Role in Diagnostic Radiology
- Common Diagnostic Radiologic Tests
- Common Therapeutic Uses of Radiation
- Radiation Safety and Dose
- Storing and Filing X-Rays
- Electronic Medicine

OBJECTIVES

After completing Chapter 35, you will be able to:

35.1 Define x-rays and explain how they are used for diagnostic and therapeutic purposes.
35.2 Compare invasive and noninvasive diagnostic procedures.
35.3 Discuss the medical assistant's role in x-ray and diagnostic radiology testing.
35.4 Describe the imaging process and uses of the various types of x-rays.
35.5 Discuss the medical assistant's duties in preparing a patient for an x-ray.
35.6 Explain the risks and safety precautions associated with radiology work.
35.7 Describe proper procedures for filing and maintaining x-ray films and records.

Introduction

Diagnostic radiology has evolved immensely since the discovery of the simple x-ray beam. It has become a valuable screening and clinical diagnosis tool for physicians. In this chapter, you will learn the basics of noninvasive and invasive radiology as well as your role as a medical assistant in this testing. Safety issues for the administration of radiologic testing are discussed, as is the proper handling and storage of the actual films. In addition, you learn about preparing and instructing patients for the more common radiology procedures.

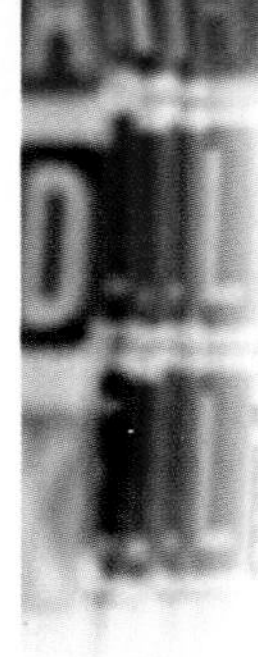

CASE STUDY

A 42-year-old woman has arrived at the office for her annual physical, part of which involves scheduling her to have a mammogram performed. The patient completes the procedure, which comes back revealing a small, abnormal density. The physician asks you to schedule the patient for a CT scan of the breast, which also reveals an abnormal mass. The patient decides that she wants to be more aggressive in determining if the small mass is cancerous, so you now schedule a mammotest, which is used to determine that the mass is benign with no evidence of cancer.

As you read this chapter, consider the following questions:

1. What special instructions should be given to the patient before her mammogram?
2. How is a CT scan performed?
3. When preparing a patient for a CT scan, what allergies should be disclosed during the patient interview?
4. Why was a mammotest requested by the physician?
5. What education requirements must you fulfill in order to work as a radiographer/sonographer?

Brief History of the X-Ray

In 1895 Wilhelm Konrad Roentgen (1845–1923) discovered the x-ray, or roentgen ray, a type of electromagnetic wave. It has a high energy level, traveling at the speed of light (186,000 miles per second), and an extremely short wavelength (one-billionth of an inch) that can penetrate solid objects. X-rays react with photographic film to produce a permanent record (x-ray, or radiograph). The x-ray image is lightest where the film is struck by the most x-ray energy. Differences in tissue densities produce the x-ray image, with the least dense being lightest and the most dense being darkest on the film.

Today there are both diagnostic and therapeutic uses for x-rays and radioactive substances. Radiologic technologists are trained medical personnel who are certified to perform certain radiologic procedures upon completion of a radiology curriculum lasting 2 to 4 years. Some radiologic technologists receive further training in radiology subspecialties, such as ultrasound, mammography, magnetic resonance imaging, and nuclear medicine. Radiographers, sonographers, radiation therapists, and nuclear medicine technologists are all radiologic technologists. Invasive radiologic procedures or procedures requiring a high degree of expertise are nearly always performed by a radiologist, a physician who specializes in radiology. A radiologist is also the physician who interprets the films for other physicians. Other specialists who perform radiologic procedures, either alone or with the assistance of a radiologist, include cardiologists, orthopedists, obstetricians, and oncologists.

Diagnostic Radiology

Diagnostic radiology is the use of x-ray technology for diagnostic purposes. Radiologic tests sometimes use contrast media as well as special techniques or instruments for viewing internal body structures and functions. A **contrast medium** is a substance that makes internal organs denser and blocks the passage of x-rays to the photographic film. Introducing contrast media into certain structures or areas of the body can provide a clearer image of organs and tissues and indications of how well they are functioning. Contrast media include gases (air, oxygen, or carbon dioxide), heavy metal salts (barium sulfate or bismuth carbonate), and iodine compounds. They can be administered orally, parenterally (for example, intravenously), or by routes that introduce them into an organ or body cavity (for example, by insertion). Types of diagnostic imaging include x-rays, computed tomography (CT), nuclear medicine, magnetic resonance imaging (MRI), and ultrasound.

Invasive Procedures

Diagnostic tests can be invasive or noninvasive. An **invasive** procedure (such as angiography) requires a radiologist to insert a catheter, wire, or other testing device into a patient's blood vessel or organ through the skin or a body orifice. All invasive tests require surgical aseptic technique. Some procedures, including angiography, are performed in a hospital or same-day surgical facility. The patient may need general anesthesia for some procedures. The anesthetist must closely monitor the patient who is under

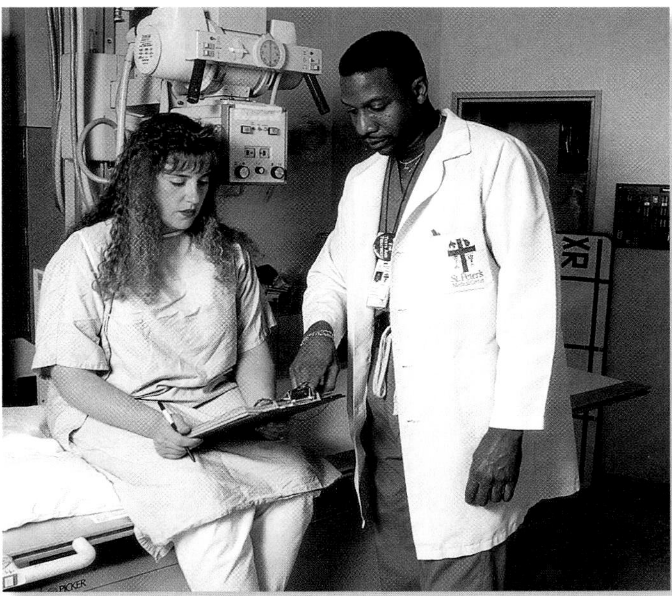

Figure 35-1. A standard x-ray is one of the most frequently performed radiologic tests.

anesthesia during and after the test for life-threatening complications, such as anaphylaxis.

Noninvasive Procedures

Noninvasive procedures, such as standard x-rays or ultrasound, use other technologies to view internal structures. They do not require inserting devices, breaking the skin, or the degree of monitoring needed with invasive procedures.

The most familiar equipment used for diagnostic imaging is the conventional x-ray machine, as shown in Figure 35-1. This machine consists of a table, an x-ray tube, a control panel, and a high-voltage generator. Other equipment used for diagnostic radiology includes instruments specifically designed for the test. Examples are a mammography unit, a scanner for CT, and a transducer for ultrasound.

The Medical Assistant's Role in Diagnostic Radiology

You may deal with diagnostic radiology in a radiology facility or in a medical office. Your duties in a radiology facility will include assisting a radiologic technologist or a radiologist in performing diagnostic radiologic procedures. Depending on the scope of practice in your state, you may be allowed to learn how to operate certain x-ray equipment. Even if you are not allowed to assist with an x-ray procedure or to operate x-ray equipment, you will probably provide preprocedure and postprocedure care of the patient.

Your duties in a medical facility, such as an orthopedic office, may include assisting a radiologic technologist in performing x-ray procedures. In an obstetric practice, you might assist a physician in performing an ultrasound examination of a pregnant woman. Even if you work in a medical office that does no radiologic testing, you must still provide a certain amount of preprocedure care. To properly explain a test to a patient and to assist a radiologic technologist or radiologist in performing a test, you must have a basic understanding of x-ray technology. You may also need in-service training to ensure accuracy and patient safety for some procedures.

Preprocedure Care

Preprocedure care varies somewhat, depending on the test. In general, however, you may do the following:

- Schedule the patient's appointment, if necessary. Inform the patient of the location, date, and time of the procedure.
- Provide preparation instructions. Advise the patient about diet restrictions or requirements (such as fasting or drinking liquids) as well as medication requirements (such as taking a laxative). Always check with the radiology facility for specific requirements, and be sure the patient receives this information.
- Explain the procedure to the patient briefly and clearly. Use proper terminology and nontechnical language, but do not talk down to the patient. Reinforce the doctor's reason for requesting the procedure, and provide any available written information about the test. Inform the patient about the length of the examination, about possible side effects or safety precautions and warnings, and about injections or uncomfortable steps.
- Ask pertinent questions. Obtain a medication history from the patient (current medications could interfere with some procedures). If the patient is a woman of childbearing age, ask whether she is pregnant or whether there is any chance she could be pregnant. Report the answers to the physician in a medical office or to the radiologic technologist in a radiology facility.

Care During and After the Procedure

If you work in a radiology facility, your responsibilities include preparing and guiding the patient through the procedure. You may also assist the radiologic technologist or the radiologist in performing the procedure by placing, removing, and developing film in the x-ray machine. Procedure 35-1 describes the general process of assisting with a radiologic procedure.

You may care for a patient and assist the radiologic technologist or radiologist during a wide variety of x-ray and other diagnostic imaging tests. Although requirements vary depending on the procedure, you will probably be

PROCEDURE 35.1

Assisting With an X-Ray Examination

Objective: To assist with a radiologic procedure under the supervision of a radiologic technologist

OSHA Guidelines: This procedure does not involve exposure to blood, body fluids, or tissue. You must wear a radiation exposure badge (dosimeter), however, and will be required to wear a garment containing a lead shield if you remain in the room during the operation of x-ray equipment

Materials: X-ray examination order, x-ray machine, x-ray film and holder, x-ray film developer, drape, patient shield

Method

1. Check the x-ray examination order and equipment needed.
2. Identify the patient and introduce yourself.
3. Determine whether the patient has complied with the preprocedure instructions.
4. Explain the procedure and the purpose of the examination to the patient.
5. Instruct the patient to remove clothing and all metals (including jewelry) as needed, according to body area to be examined, and to put on a gown. Explain that metals may interfere with the image. Ask whether the patient has any surgical metal or a pacemaker, and report this information to the radiologic technologist. Leave the room to ensure patient privacy.

Note: Steps 6 through 11 are nearly always performed by a radiologic technologist.

6. Position the patient according to the x-ray view ordered.
7. Drape the patient and place the patient shield appropriately.
8. Instruct the patient about the need to remain still and to hold the breath when requested.
9. Leave the room or stand behind a lead shield during the exposure.
10. Ask the patient to assume a comfortable position while the films are developed. Explain that x-rays sometimes must be repeated.
11. Develop the films.
12. If the x-ray films are satisfactory, instruct the patient to dress and tell the patient when to contact the physician's office for the results.
13. Label the dry, finished x-ray films, place them in a properly labeled envelope, and file them according to the policies of your office.
14. Record the x-ray examination, along with the final written findings, in the patient's chart.

asked to perform many of the duties described in Procedure 35-1. Although you are unlikely to position the patient, you should know that the position relative to the x-ray source determines the path of the x-rays and the sorts of images that result. Figure 35-2 illustrates common x-ray pathways and the images produced.

Common Diagnostic Radiologic Tests

A variety of radiologic imaging tests are available. Table 35-1 identifies some of the most frequently ordered tests and the disorders they are used to diagnose.

Contrast Media in Diagnostic Tests

Various procedures involve the use of contrast media to visualize body structures and observe their function. These procedures include angiography, arthrography, barium enema, barium swallow, cholangiography, cholecystography, fluoroscopy, intravenous pyelography, magnetic resonance imaging (sometimes), myelography, nuclear medicine studies, and retrograde pyelography.

As mentioned, contrast media can be administered by mouth, by needle or catheter into a blood vessel, or by a route that introduces the medium into an organ or body cavity (for example, into the colon). A contrast medium can cause adverse effects in some patients. Common adverse effects with oral agents include mild and transient abdominal cramping, constipation, nausea, vomiting, diarrhea, skin rashes, itching, heartburn, dizziness, and headache. Intravenous agents cause some of the same adverse effects as well as localized injection-site reactions and more serious reactions such as anaphylaxis. Because many contrast media contain iodine, a common allergen, patients should be questioned about known allergies to iodine or shellfish, which contain iodine, before procedures involving the use of contrast media. All patients should be observed during such procedures for signs of allergic reaction.

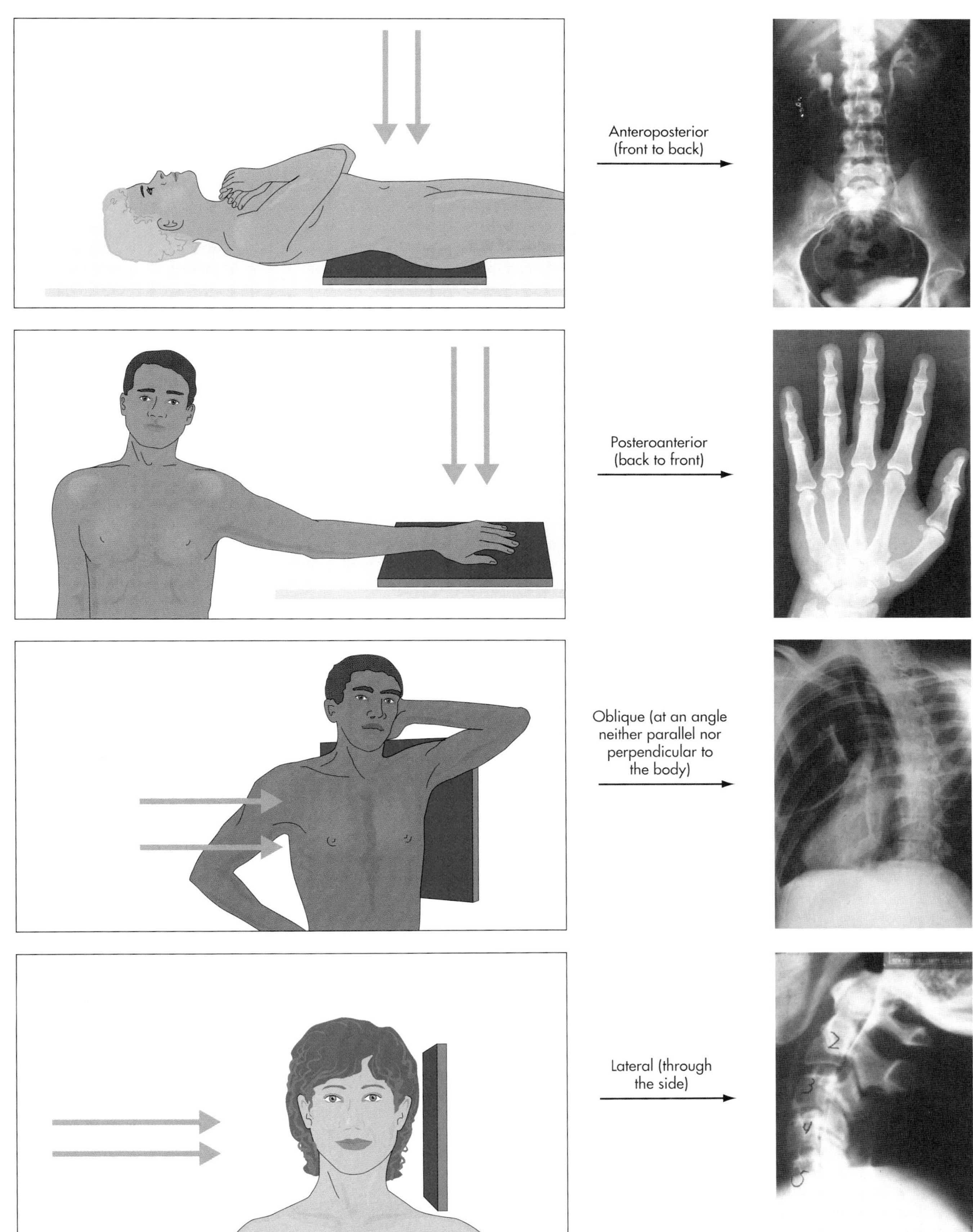

Figure 35-2. These are the x-ray pathways and resulting projections for the most common types of x-rays.

TABLE 35-1 Common Radiologic Tests and Disorders Diagnosed	
Test	**Disorders Diagnosed/Treated**
Angiography	
Cardiovascular	Status of blood flow, collateral circulation, malformed vessels, aneurysm, narrowing or blockages of vessels, presence of hemorrhage
Cerebral	Aneurysm, hemorrhage, evidence of cerebrovascular accident, arteriosclerosis
Gastrointestinal (GI)	Upper gastrointestinal bleeding
Pulmonary	Pulmonary emboli (especially when lung scan is inconclusive), evaluation of pulmonary circulation in some heart conditions before surgery
Renal	Abnormalities of blood vessels in urinary system
Arthrography	Joint conditions
Barium enema (lower GI series)	Obstructions, ulcers, polyps, diverticulosis, tumor, and motility problems of colon or rectum
Barium swallow (upper GI series)	Obstructions, ulcers, polyps, diverticulosis, tumor, and motility problems of esophagus, stomach, duodenum, and small intestine
Cholangiography, cholecystography	Gallstones, gallbladder or common bile duct stones or obstructions; ability of gallbladder to concentrate and store dye
Computed tomography (CT)	Aortic and heart aneurysms, disorders of liver and biliary systems, renal and pulmonary tumors, brain abnormalities (tumors, blood clots, evidence of cerebrovascular accident, outlines of brain ventricles), GI tract lesions, GI disorders (acute pseudocyst of pancreas, abdominal abscesses, biliary obstruction), breast diseases and disorders, spinal disorders; to guide biopsy procedures
Fluoroscopy	Structure, process, and function of organs in motion to detect abnormalities
Intravenous pyelography (IVP) (excretory urography)	Urinary system abnormalities, including renal pelvis, ureters, and bladder (for example, kidney stones); abnormal size, shape, or structure of kidneys, ureters, or bladder; space-occupying lesions; pyelonephrosis; hydronephrosis; trauma to the urinary system
KUB (kidneys, ureters, bladder) radiography	Size, shape, and position of urinary organs; urinary system diseases or disorders; kidney stones
Magnetic resonance imaging (MRI)	Cancerous tissue, atherosclerotic tissue, blood clots, tumors, and deformities, particularly of the heart valves, brain, spine, and joints
Mammography	Breast tumors and lesions
Myelography	Irregularities or compression of spinal cord
Nuclear medicine (radionuclide imaging)	Abnormal function (defects), lesions, or disorders of bone, brain, lungs, kidneys, liver, pancreas, thyroid, and spleen
Radiation therapy	Treatment of cancer
Retrograde pyelogram	Obstruction of ureters, bladder, or urethra (including tumors, stones, strictures, or blood clots); perinephritic abscess
Stereoscopy	Fractures, dense areas that indicate a tumor or increased pressure within the skull
Thermography	Breast tumors, breast abscesses, fibrocystic breast disease
Ultrasound	Abnormalities of gallbladder, liver, spleen, heart, kidneys, gonads, blood vessels, and lymph system; fetal conditions (including number of fetuses; age and sex of fetus; fetal development, position, and deformities)
Xeroradiography	Breast cancer, abscesses, lesions, calcifications

Fluoroscopy

X-rays can cause certain chemicals to fluoresce, or emit visible light. When x-rays penetrate a body structure and are directed onto a fluorescent screen, they produce an image the radiologist can view either directly or through special glasses. Usually, fluoroscopic procedures are performed by a radiologist rather than by a radiology technician or a medical assistant.

Many diagnostic procedures involve fluoroscopy, which allows viewing of internal organ movement or the movement of a contrast medium, such as barium sulfate, while the contrast medium travels through the alimentary canal. Fluoroscopy also guides the radiologist in locating a precise internal area that needs to be recorded on film.

Fluoroscopic images are sometimes photographed for further study. Photofluorography is a series of these photographs that records the body's internal movements over time. Cinefluorography is a motion picture of the images.

Angiography

Angiography requires a physician (usually a radiologist) to insert a catheter into the patient's vein (venography) or artery (arteriography). The test may be performed jointly by a radiologist and a vascular surgeon or other specialist. Typically, the femoral, brachial, or carotid artery is evaluated. The physician guides the catheter tip to the vessel being examined. Then the physician injects a contrast medium through the catheter and takes a series of x-rays to assess the vessel's blood flow and condition.

Because this procedure requires insertion of a catheter into a blood vessel and the use of local anesthesia, the patient is admitted to a hospital or same-day surgical facility. The physician who performs the examination provides the patient with instructions immediately before the procedure. You will, however, schedule the procedure, and you can encourage the patient to ask questions. Radiology facilities usually have information sheets for each procedure. If the patient has questions you cannot answer or if you have any doubt about preprocedure instructions, check with your supervisor.

Arthrography

Arthrography is performed by a radiologist, who uses a contrast medium and fluoroscopy to help diagnose abnormalities or injuries in the cartilage, tendons, or ligaments of the joints—usually the knee or shoulder. When preparing patients for arthrography or assisting with the procedure, follow these guidelines:

- Describe the procedure to patients, and inform them that the examination will take about 1 hour. Ask patients about possible allergies to contrast media, iodine, or shellfish. If they have any of these allergies, inform the radiologist immediately.
- Explain to patients that no special preprocedure preparations are necessary.
- Tell patients the doctor will first inject a local anesthetic to numb the area being examined. Then the doctor will inject the contrast medium (dye, air, or both) into the joint and will use a fluoroscope to evaluate the joint's function. Inform patients who are having a knee examined that the doctor may ask them to walk a few steps to spread the contrast medium.
- After the test is completed, advise patients that for 1 or 2 days they may experience some pain or swelling, particularly if the joint is exercised. Tell them to rest and avoid putting strain on the joint.

Barium Enema (Lower GI Series)

A **barium enema** is performed by a radiologist, who instills barium sulfate through the anus into the rectum and then into the colon, to help diagnose and evaluate obstructions, ulcers, polyps, diverticulosis, tumors, or motility problems of the colon or rectum. This procedure is called a lower GI (gastrointestinal) series, a series of x-rays of the colon and rectum. The two types of barium enema techniques are single-contrast, in which only barium is instilled into the colon, and double-contrast, in which air is forced into the colon to distend the tissue. The air may be added while the barium is present, after it has been expelled, or both. The double-contrast technique makes structures more visible by fluoroscopy and allows identification of small lesions. The digestive tract must be totally empty, requiring the patient to thoroughly cleanse the tract with a series of preparatory steps and to have nothing by mouth for 8 hours before the test, except for one cup of clear liquid on the morning of the test. In most facilities a nurse assists with a barium enema, but you may assist the patient before and after the procedure. If you do assist with a barium enema, you will have various responsibilities before, during, and after the procedure.

Before the Procedure. Include the following steps when you instruct a patient about the preparation for a barium enema:

- Schedule the patient's appointment in the morning so he can sleep through most of the period during which his digestive tract must be empty and thus avoid experiencing hunger unnecessarily.
- Describe the procedure to the patient, and tell him the examination will take 1 to 2 hours. Ask about possible allergies to contrast media, iodine, or shellfish, and report such allergies to the radiologist.
- Explain to the patient the importance of following the preparation instructions so the colon and rectum are free of residual material. (Residual material in the colon or rectum could cause blockages or shadows, resulting in an inaccurate test.) Preprocedure preparation on the day before the examination includes following an all-liquid diet beginning in the morning (coffee, tea, carbonated beverages, sherbet, clear gelatin, strained fruit juice, bouillon, clear broths, or

tomato juice; milk is not permitted) and taking prescribed amounts of electrolyte solution or other laxative preparations and fluids on a specified schedule. Tell the patient he may have one cup of coffee, tea, or water on the morning of the examination.

During the Procedure. Follow these steps when assisting during a barium enema:

- Have the patient undress and put on a gown.
- Tell the patient to expect some discomfort during the examination, as well as frequent side-to-side turning.
- Have the patient lie on his side. The radiologist inserts the enema tip, which is designed to help the patient hold the liquid, into the rectum and instills the barium sulfate into the colon. If the patient experiences cramping or the urge to defecate during instillation of the barium, instruct him to relax the abdominal muscles by breathing slowly and deeply through the mouth.
- Instruct the patient to remain still and hold his breath when x-rays are taken. Using a fluoroscope, the doctor observes the barium as it flows through the lower bowel and periodically takes x-rays while the patient is placed in various positions. You may be asked to assist with placing the patient in these positions.
- Tell the patient if a double-contrast study is being performed. Explain that air will be introduced into the colon to expand the colon tissue. Also tell the patient that the combination of air and barium provides a clearer view of structures than only one contrast medium would provide and allows possible identification of small lesions if they are present.
- Tell the patient that when the doctor has completed the barium portion of the examination, including x-rays with both barium and air, the patient should use the toilet and expel as much barium as possible. Explain that if enough barium is expelled, the doctor may take a final x-ray of the empty colon.
- Have the patient wait to dress until the doctor tells you that no additional x-rays are needed.

After the Procedure. After the radiologist has completed the barium enema, instruct the patient in postprocedure care. Tell the patient the following:

- He may now have a regular meal.
- The residual barium may make his stools appear whitish or lighter than usual, but this is normal.
- The barium may cause constipation, so he should drink extra water to help relieve constipation and to eliminate remaining barium sulfate. The physician may order a laxative to be taken if constipation is not relieved within 1 or 2 days.

Barium Swallow (Upper GI Series)

A **barium swallow** involves oral administration of a barium sulfate drink to help diagnose and evaluate obstructions, ulcers, polyps, diverticulosis, tumors, or motility problems of the esophagus, stomach, duodenum, and small intestine. This test is called an upper GI series. In preparation for this test, the patient can have nothing by mouth for at least 8 hours before the test. You will have various responsibilities before, during, and after the procedure.

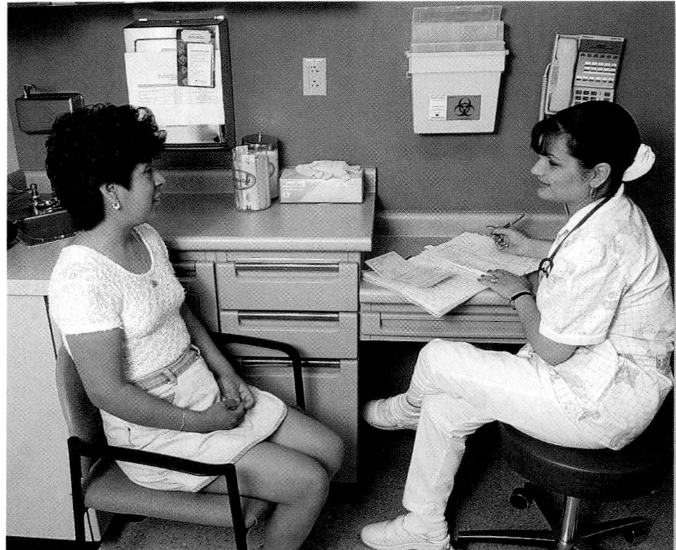

Figure 35-3. Preprocedure instruction is essential to a successful barium swallow procedure.

Before the Procedure. When instructing a patient about the preparation for an upper GI series (Figure 35-3), include the following steps:

- Schedule the patient's appointment in the morning so she can sleep through most of the period during which her digestive tract is empty and thus avoid experiencing hunger unnecessarily.
- Describe the procedure to the patient, and tell her the examination will take about 1 hour. If x-rays of the small bowel are needed, the test may take several hours. Ask about possible allergies to contrast media, iodine, or shellfish, and report such allergies to the radiologist.
- Explain to the patient the importance of following the preparation instructions so that the stomach is empty. Preprocedure requirements include having nothing by mouth (food or liquids) after midnight the night before the examination and no breakfast the morning of the examination. If the patient's small bowel is to be evaluated, also tell her to take the prescribed laxative preparation between 2:00 and 4:00 P.M. the day before the examination.
- Instruct the patient not to swallow water when brushing her teeth or rinsing her mouth and, if applicable, to stop smoking, because nicotine stimulates gastric secretions and can affect the test results.

Career Opportunities

Radiographer/Sonographer

To gain medical assistant credentials, you must fulfill the requirements of either the American Association of Medical Assistants (for a Certified Medical Assistant) or the American Medical Technologists (for a Registered Medical Assistant). After obtaining your medical assistant certification or registration, you may wish to acquire additional skills in specialty areas through course work or on-the-job training. Although this course work or training may not lead to an additional certification or degree, it will enable you to expand your role in the medical office and advance your career as the demand for skilled health professionals increases.

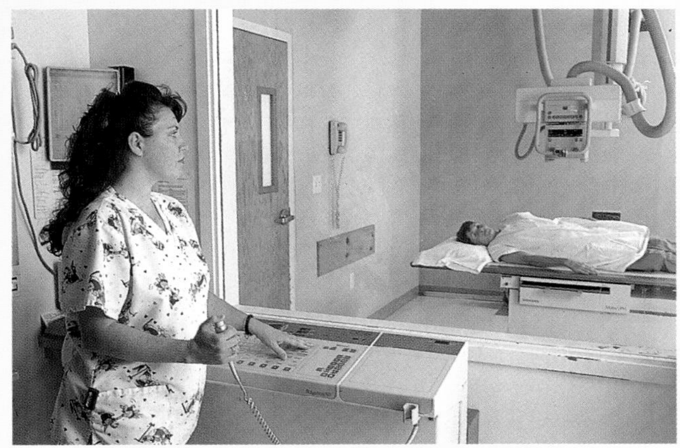

Skills and Duties

Radiographers and sonographers obtain images of internal organs, tissues, bones, and blood vessels. Physicians use these images to diagnose disease or to monitor health status.

A radiographer uses x-rays to produce the images. The radiographer positions the patient for imaging, covering parts of the body that are not to be x-rayed with a lead drape to protect them from the radiation. She then positions the x-ray machine, sets the controls, and makes the requested number of exposures.

The resulting black-and-white images can reveal whether a patient has a broken bone, tumor, ulcer, or other condition. Sometimes the radiographer or a physician administers a special material before the imaging process to make organs and blood vessels more visible on the x-ray film. The physician, usually a radiologist, examines the film and makes a diagnosis.

Sonographers use ultrasound machines that rely on sound waves rather than electromagnetic radiation to produce the images. The images are displayed on a television screen and can be videotaped or printed on film for further review by the physician.

The sonographer prepares the patient by applying a sound-enhancing gel. She then strokes the machine's handheld pad across the gel to create the image. She must be well-versed in anatomy to determine which parts of the image are important as she records measurements and data from the examination. Again, the physician uses the image to make a diagnosis and prescribe treatment if needed.

Sonographers can specialize in a variety of fields. Because sound waves are considered safe, sonography is frequently used in obstetrics and gynecology to take pictures of a fetus in the womb. Sonographers may also specialize in echocardiography, where they focus on heart problems.

Workplace Settings

Radiographers and sonographers most often work in hospitals. Some are employed in clinics, physicians' offices, and imaging centers. Radiographers may also work in dentists' offices, in mobile units, or in private industry. People in this field generally work 40-hour weeks, including some nights, weekends, and holidays.

Education

To become a radiographer or sonographer, you must complete an accredited 2- to 4-year program in radiography/sonography from an accredited vocational school, college, or university. (For those who are already employed in health care, a 1-year certificate program may be available.) Typically, such a program provides instruction in physics, biology, anatomy, medical terminology, radiation safety, and imaging techniques. The program may also include brief courses in nuclear medicine, computed tomography, magnetic resonance imaging, and radiation therapy—each of which can be further studied as a specialty.

After completing the program, you may take a national registry examination from the American Registry of Radiologic Technologists. The disciplines of sonography, nuclear medicine, and radiation therapy require a national registration examination for entry-level work. Radiographers must also have a license from the state to practice.

Where to Go for More Information

American Society of Radiologic Technologists
15000 Central Avenue SE
Albuquerque, NM 87123
(505) 298-4500

Society of Diagnostic Medical Sonographers
12770 Coit Road, Suite 508
Dallas, TX 75251
(214) 239-7367

During the Procedure. When assisting during an upper GI series, take the following steps:

- Have the patient undress and put on a gown.
- Explain to the patient that she will be drinking a barium sulfate drink that tastes chalky and resembles a milk shake.
- Have the patient stand and drink part of the barium. The radiologist will use a fluoroscope to observe the flow of the barium and to assess the functioning of the esophagus, stomach, duodenum, and small intestine as the barium passes through the structures. (The doctor will then direct the patient to drink additional barium and continue to observe the function of the various structures.)
- Place the patient on the x-ray table, and move her to different positions (if medical assistants are permitted to do so in your state) as instructed by the doctor, to allow x-rays to be taken of the upper digestive tract. Instruct the patient to remain still and hold her breath when x-rays are taken.

After the Procedure. After the physician completes the upper GI series, instruct the patient in postprocedure care. Give the patient the following information:

- She may now have a regular meal.
- Her stools may appear whitish or lighter than usual as the barium is eliminated, but this is normal.
- Sometimes another examination may be required after 24 hours to determine whether the barium has moved into the large intestine. If this test is indicated, tell the patient to follow a liquid diet (coffee, tea, carbonated beverages, sherbet, clear gelatin, strained fruit juices, bouillon, clear broths, or tomato juice; milk is not permitted) and to return in 24 hours.

Cholecystography and Cholangiography

Two similar tests performed by a radiologist are cholecystography and cholangiography. Both tests involve use of a contrast medium to view parts of the gallbladder.

Cholecystography. A radiologist uses cholecystography to detect gallstones and other abnormalities of the gallbladder. The doctor x-rays the patient's gallbladder after the patient has ingested an oral contrast medium. Cholecystography is usually used when ultrasound does not provide enough information for a diagnosis. You will be responsible for preparing the patient for the procedure and assisting during the procedure.

Before the Procedure. When instructing a patient about preparing for a cholecystography, follow these guidelines:

- Schedule the patient's appointment in the morning so he can sleep through most of the period during which his digestive tract is empty and thus avoid experiencing hunger unnecessarily.
- Describe the procedure to the patient, and explain that the examination will take about 1 to 2 hours. Ask the patient about possible allergies to contrast media, iodine, or shellfish, and report them to the radiologist.
- Explain to the patient the diet restrictions necessary to prepare for the test. Tell the patient to have a fat-free dinner (dry toast, tea, fruit, gelatin dessert) the evening before the examination. He should not smoke or have any food or liquids after midnight, and he should have no breakfast the morning of the examination.
- Instruct the patient to take the oral contrast medium (usually in tablet form) beginning about 2 hours after dinner or as prescribed by the doctor. The tablets should be taken one at a time, 5 minutes apart, with a small amount of water, until six tablets have been taken. Explain to the patient that the contrast agent may cause nausea or diarrhea but that nothing should be taken for these conditions. In the case of severe nausea, the doctor may prescribe an antiemetic; diarrhea is an expected result of the contrast medium used for this test.
- Some doctors also order a laxative for the patient to take the day before the examination.

During and After the Procedure. When assisting during a cholecystography, take the following steps:

- Have the patient undress and put on a gown.
- Have the patient lie on the x-ray table in the supine position (face up).
- Explain that the radiologist will take x-rays of the gallbladder, which will be filled with the contrast medium the patient took the night before. Then the radiologist will use a fluoroscope to study the gallbladder's function. A functioning gallbladder absorbs the contrast agent properly.
- Next give the patient a specially prepared fatty meal, which should stimulate the gallbladder to empty bile into the duodenum. After about 1 hour, the doctor takes more x-rays to study the gallbladder's function. A functioning gallbladder empties the contrast medium properly. A nonfunctioning gallbladder may indicate, for example, the presence of gallstones or obstruction of the bile ducts.
- After the examination advise the patient to return to a normal diet and to drink plenty of fluids to replace those lost with diarrhea.

Cholangiography. **Cholangiography** is similar to cholecystography and is performed by a radiologist to evaluate the function of the bile ducts. It involves injection of the contrast medium directly into the common bile duct (during gallbladder surgery) or through a T tube (after gallbladder surgery or during radiologic testing). X-rays are taken immediately after injection. Use the guidelines for cholecystography. In addition, follow these steps:

- Describe the procedure to the patient, and tell him the examination will take about 2 to 3 hours. Ask the patient about possible allergies to contrast media, iodine, or shellfish, and report them to the radiologist.
- Explain the preparation instructions to the patient. Tell the patient to eat a light evening meal the night before the examination, to take a laxative (as prescribed by the doctor), and to have no food or liquids after midnight. He should also have no solid food the morning of the examination.

Conventional Tomography and Computed Tomography

Conventional tomography produces tomograms, and computed tomography produces CT scans. These two techniques are frequently confused. Computers are involved in producing both kinds of images, but the computers are different and have different functions.

Conventional tomography uses a computerized x-ray camera that moves back and forth in an arc over the patient to produce a series of views of a body part. The computer sets the angle and layer for each arc; the camera produces one view per arc.

In CT scans produced by computed tomography, the x-ray camera rotates completely around the patient, and the computer compiles one cross-sectional view from each rotation of the camera. The patient is lying on a special table that gradually moves through the doughnut-shaped machine containing the rotating camera. Figure 35-4 compares the two kinds of images (tomogram and CT scan) with those produced by x-ray, magnetic resonance imaging (MRI), and myelography.

The preparation is essentially the same for the two procedures. Reassure the patient that he will not be inserted into an enclosed space, as is the case in magnetic resonance imaging. The patient will be able to see around the room during the test.

Tomograms and CT scans are used to diagnose abnormalities in almost all body structures, including the head, kidneys, heart, chest, liver, biliary tract, pancreas, GI tract, spine, pelvis, bones, and breast. When preparing the patient for a tomogram or a CT scan, use the following guidelines:

- Ask the patient about possible allergies to contrast media, iodine, or shellfish, and report them to the radiologist.
- Tell the patient that he will be placed on a table that moves through the scanner for CT scans or on an x-ray table for tomograms.
- Inform the patient that the procedure will last about 45 to 90 minutes and that he must lie still while the scans are taken. The patient may breathe normally while the CT scans are taken but must hold his breath for each of the tomograms.
- If a contrast medium will be used, advise the patient that it will be injected into a vein in the arm or on the back of the hand (except with a CT scan of the spine) to enhance detail of the structure being evaluated.
- If the patient is having a CT scan of the head or chest, instruct him not to eat anything for 4 hours or drink any liquids for 2 hours before the examination. Explain that he may experience mild nausea after injection of the contrast medium if the stomach is too full.
- If the patient is having tomograms or a CT scan of the abdomen or pelvis, tell him to obtain a preparation kit from the office or hospital the day before the examination. This kit includes a special drink the patient must take the night before the examination that helps outline the intestines. Inform the patient that the drink should not produce a laxative effect or any discomfort.
- Tell the patient to remove metallic objects that could interfere with the path of the x-rays. Also, ask if the patient has skin staples or metallic prostheses that could interfere.
- Inform the patient that a written report of the results should be available within 24 hours of the test and that a report will be sent to his primary care physician (or the referring physician).

Heart X-Ray

An x-ray of the heart, using a contrast medium, may be necessary to show the configuration of the heart and to reveal cardiac enlargement and aortic dilation. Angiography of the heart is called angiocardiography, in which a contrast medium is injected into a major blood vessel. X-rays are taken while the medium flows through the heart, lungs, and major vessels. Coronary arteriography uses a dye inserted through a catheter that has been passed through an artery to the heart. Both procedures require hospital admission, usually in a day surgery or ambulatory surgery unit.

Intravenous Pyelography

Also known as excretory urography, **intravenous pyelography (IVP)** is performed by a radiologist who injects a contrast medium into a vein. The doctor then takes a series of x-rays as the contrast medium travels through the kidneys, ureters, and bladder. IVP is used to evaluate urinary system abnormalities or trauma to the urinary system. In most facilities a nurse assists with IVP, but you may assist the patient before the procedure. If you assist with IVP, you will have several responsibilities both before and during the procedure.

Before the Procedure. When instructing a patient about the preparation for an IVP, include the following steps:

- Schedule the patient's appointment in the morning so she can sleep through most of the period during which her digestive tract is empty and thus avoid experiencing hunger unnecessarily.

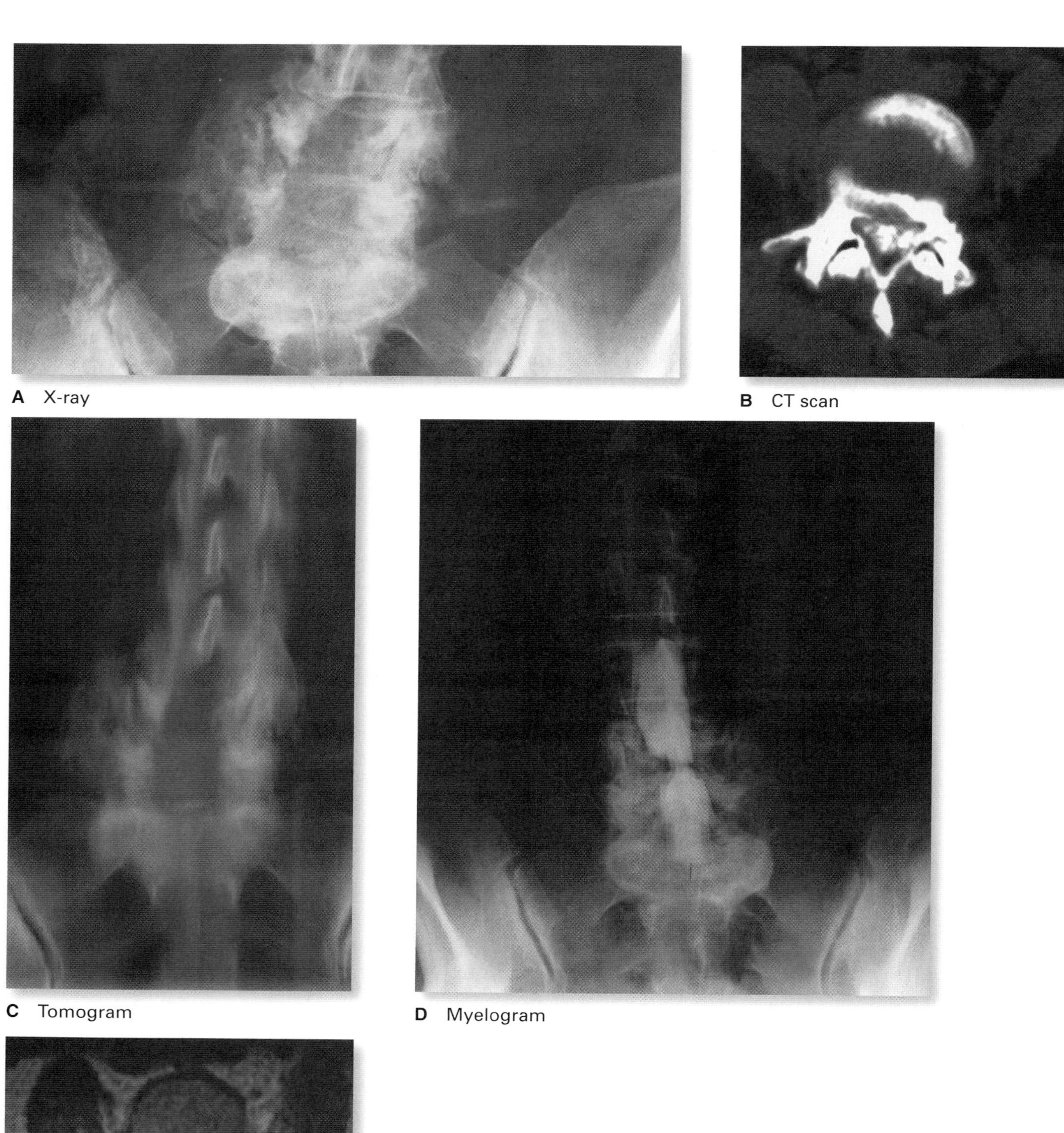

A X-ray

B CT scan

C Tomogram

D Myelogram

E MRI

Figure 35-4. These images of part of one patient's spine indicate scoliosis, degenerative disk disease, and osteoarthritis. Various techniques and x-ray pathways were involved: (a) x-ray, anteroposterior; (b) CT scan, full rotation; (c) tomogram, anteroposterior arc; (d) myelogram, posteroanterior; and (e) MRI, full rotation.

- Describe the procedure to the patient, and tell her that the examination will take about 1½ hours. Ask about possible allergies to contrast media, iodine, or shellfish, and report such allergies to the radiologist.
- Explain the importance of adhering to the preparation instructions, so that the bowel is free of any material that could obstruct the view of the urinary organs. Tell the patient to follow a liquid diet (coffee, tea, carbonated beverages, sherbet, clear gelatin, strained fruit juice, bouillon, clear broths, or tomato juice, but no milk) the day before the examination. The patient should take the prescribed amount of electrolyte solution or other laxative preparation as specified the night before the examination and have no food or liquids after midnight and no breakfast the morning of the examination. Some physicians also order an enema to be taken about 2 hours before the examination.

During and After the Procedure. When assisting during an IVP, you will generally proceed in this manner:

- Have the patient undress and put on a gown.
- Explain that a contrast medium will be injected into her vein (usually in the arm). Instruct her to inform the physician if she notices shortness of breath or itching after injection of the dye. This type of symptom can indicate an allergic reaction.
- Have the patient lie on the x-ray table, and move her to different positions as instructed by the physician, to allow x-rays to be taken of the urinary tract as the contrast medium is excreted. Instruct the patient to remain still and hold her breath when x-rays are taken.
- Note that some physicians place a compression device on the abdomen, which helps hold the contrast medium in the kidneys and ureters by exerting moderate pressure.
- After the physician takes the series of x-rays to evaluate urinary system function, ask the patient to urinate, and explain that a final x-ray will be taken.
- Inform the patient that she may resume a normal diet after the test and that the contrast medium will be eliminated in the urine.

Retrograde Pyelography

Retrograde pyelography is similar to the IVP, except that the doctor injects the contrast medium through a urethral catheter. This procedure, which evaluates function of the ureters, bladder, and urethra, is often used for patients with poor kidney function. Follow the same preparation and assistance instructions as for the IVP.

KUB (Kidneys, Ureters, and Bladder) Radiography

Also called a flat plate of the abdomen, **KUB radiography** is an x-ray of the abdomen used to assess the size, shape, and position of the urinary organs; to evaluate urinary system diseases or disorders; and to determine the presence of kidney stones. It can also be helpful in determining the position of an intrauterine device (IUD) or in locating foreign bodies in the digestive tract. No patient preparation is required. A KUB x-ray is taken by a radiologic technologist; thus, you follow the guidelines you would use for a patient having any type of standard, noninvasive x-ray.

Magnetic Resonance Imaging (MRI)

Nonionizing radiation and a strong magnetic field are combined in magnetic resonance imaging to allow the physician to examine internal structures and soft tissues of any area of the body. The combination of nonionizing radiation and magnetic field, which allows the MRI scanner to produce images based primarily on the water content of tissues, appears to have no harmful effects on the patient. The test may be performed with or without contrast. You will be responsible for preparing the patient for an MRI and assisting with the procedure.

Before the Procedure. When instructing a patient about preparing for an MRI, include the following steps:

- If a contrast medium is going to be used, ask the patient and inform the radiologist about possible allergies to contrast media, iodine, or shellfish.
- Screen the patient to determine whether any internal metallic materials are present. (This is especially important because a magnetic field is involved in creating the image.) Ask about a pacemaker, brain or aneurysm clips, brain or heart surgery, shunts and heart valves, other surgeries, and shrapnel or metal fragments (particularly in an eye).
- Ask the patient whether he is or has been a metalworker. If so, he may carry metal slivers, chips, or filings under his nails or skin.
- Describe the procedure to the patient, and explain that the examination will take between 45 minutes and 2 hours.
- Tell the patient he does not need to fast before the examination or follow any preprocedure diet, unless he is having an MRI of the pelvis. In that case instruct him to have no solid food for 6 hours and no liquids for 4 hours before the examination. Inform the patient that he may take prescription medications.
- Explain that he will not be required to drink an oral contrast preparation but that he should avoid caffeine for 4 hours before the examination. (Instruct women not to wear eye makeup the day of the examination, because eye makeup often contains metallic ingredients.)
- Tell the patient that he will probably have no side effects from the examination but that some nausea may occur as a result of the contrast medium.

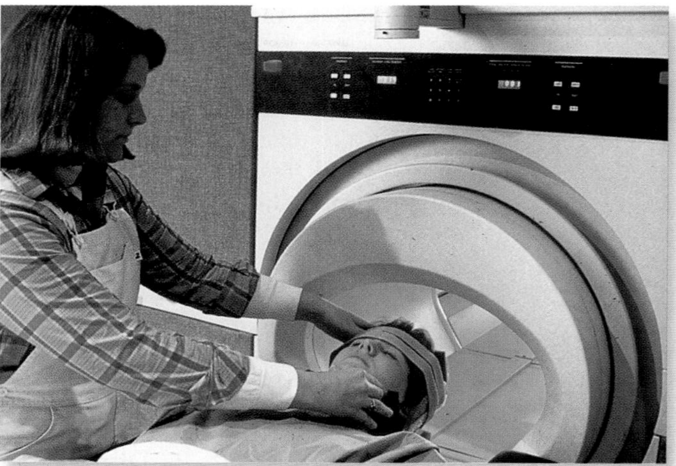

Figure 35-5. A patient who is claustrophobic or unable to lie still may require sedation during an MRI.

During and After the Procedure. When assisting during an MRI, you will need to follow these specific steps:

- Inform the patient that he may wear street clothing, unless it has metallic thread, metal stays or grippers, or thick elastic. Tell the patient that he will probably be asked to undress, however, and put on a gown.
- Have the patient lie on the padded table.
- Explain that the table will be placed inside a long, narrow tube about 22 inches in diameter and that he will hear a loud knocking noise as the machine scans. Warn the patient to remain still to avoid blurring the image and the consequent need for a retake. Note that physicians commonly order sedation for patients who are claustrophobic or cannot lie still for a long period (Figure 35-5).
- Advise the patient that although the technician will not be in the scanning room during the examination, she will maintain contact with a camera and a microphone. The patient may speak to the technician at any time in case of a problem, but he is encouraged to be still for each series.
- Inform the patient that his primary care physician or referring doctor should have a preliminary report of test results within about 24 hours.

Mammography

Mammography, the x-ray examination of the internal breast tissues, helps in diagnosing breast abnormalities (Figure 35-6). A specially trained radiologic technologist takes mammograms. Types of mammography include film-screen, thermography, diaphanography, and ultrasonography (ultrasound). Diaphanography is produced by directing a high-intensity light through the breast or soft tissue; images are then produced on a screen (a process called transillumination). Unlike other forms of mammography, diaphanography does not require ionizing radiation.

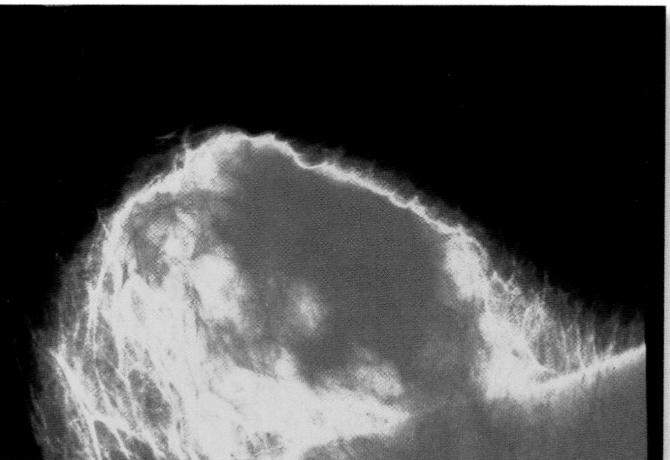

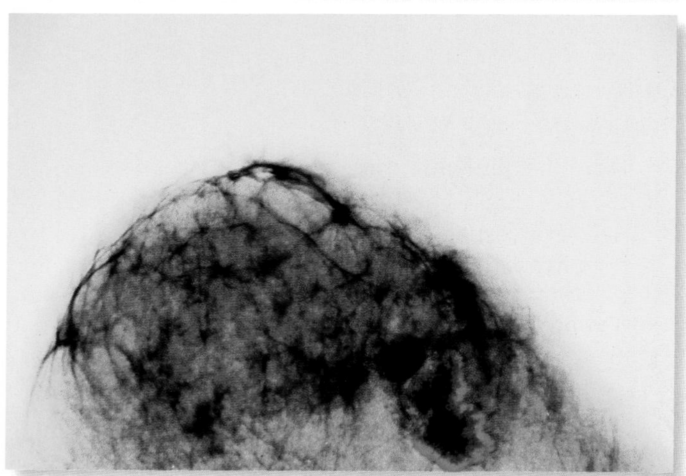

Figure 35-6. Mammograms can reveal the presence of tumors that are not detected by other means. The upper mammogram indicates normal breast tissue, whereas the lower suggests a malignancy.

You will have several responsibilities during both setup and patient care before and after mammography. A medical assistant does not assist during mammography in most states. Instead, you will prepare the patient for the procedure and ease her fears. The Educating the Patient section provides information on this topic.

Mammotest Biopsy Procedure

When a mammogram reveals an abnormality in the breast tissue, it is often treated in one of two ways—either the abnormality is followed for a period of time to see if there are any significant changes or a surgical excision biopsy is performed. Because so many abnormalities revealed by mammography are benign and present no health risk, physicians now perform stereotactic breast biopsies, which are less painful and less invasive than conventional excisional biopsies. The procedure is performed by a physician and a radiologic technologist and is similar to mammography except that the patient is lying face down rather than standing. The breast is compressed with a

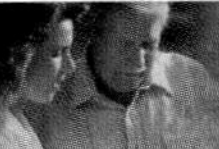

Educating the Patient

Preprocedure Care for Mammography

A patient who is scheduled for mammography must know the guidelines to follow before the examination. You can help educate the patient by instructing her in the following preprocedure care:

- The mammography should be scheduled for the first week after the patient's menstrual cycle. This timing helps minimize discomfort from compression of the breasts and ensures that the breasts are in their most normal state.
- No special preprocedure diet or medication requirements are necessary, but the patient should consider avoiding caffeine for 7 to 10 days before the examination (in some patients caffeine may cause swelling and soreness that would heighten discomfort during the procedure). Have the patient decrease caffeine intake gradually, however, to avoid getting headaches.
- The patient should shower or bathe as close as possible to the time of the mammography and wear loose clothing that is easy to remove. A blouse and pants or skirt work best to allow undressing only to the waist.
- The patient should not use deodorants, powders, or perfumes on the breasts or underarm areas before the examination, because these products could produce a false result on the x-ray.

In addition to providing these instructions, you may need to reassure a patient who is fearful about mammography. Explain that although mammography is uncomfortable, it is usually not painful. Describing how the procedure is performed may alleviate the patient's fears. Provide the patient with the following information:

- The procedure usually takes 15 to 20 minutes.
- A lead apron will be placed on the patient's abdominal area to protect her from unnecessary radiation exposure.
- The patient will be positioned in front of the machine. The technician will compress the left breast between the machine plates and take two x-rays—one horizontal view and one vertical view—of the left breast.
- The technician will then position and compress the right breast between the machine plates. Two x-rays will be taken of the right breast.
- If needed, the physician may order a mild pain reliever after the procedure to alleviate discomfort or aching.

compression paddle to confirm that the area of the breast with the lesion is correctly centered in the paddle window. A computer is used to help determine the exact positioning of the biopsy needle, and the physician takes a small sample of tissue to be examined by a pathologist for the presence of malignant cells. The attending physician later contacts the patient with the test results.

Myelography

Myelography is a kind of fluoroscopy of the spinal cord. The physician performs a lumbar puncture, removes some cerebrospinal fluid (CSF), and instills a contrast medium to evaluate spinal abnormalities, such as compression of the spinal cord. Sometimes the physician performs pneumoencephalography, which involves instilling air after removal of the CSF to allow visualization of the cerebral cavities.

The physician who performs myelography or pneumoencephalography must be skilled in performing lumbar puncture—most likely a radiologist, neurologist, neurosurgeon, or anesthetist. A radiologic technologist is typically the only other person present for the test. Although myelography is not used as frequently as it was before the invention of CT and MRI, it is still performed when these newer techniques do not provide enough information about the spinal canal. Myelography may be reserved for cases in which the clinical findings are unusual or the scanning results uncertain.

Nuclear Medicine

Also known as radionuclide imaging, **nuclear medicine** involves use of radionuclides, or radioisotopes (radioactive elements or their compounds). The radionuclides are administered orally, intravenously, or through routes that introduce them into organs or body cavities. The purpose is to evaluate the bone, brain, lungs, kidneys, liver, pancreas, thyroid, or spleen. Sometimes the entire body is scanned for "hot spots," or places where the radioisotope is concentrated.

For common nuclear medicine scans, the technician uses a scanner called a gamma camera. This scanner detects radiation from the radioisotope and converts it into an image (called a scintiscan or scintigram) to be photographed or displayed on a screen (see Figure 35-7). Some

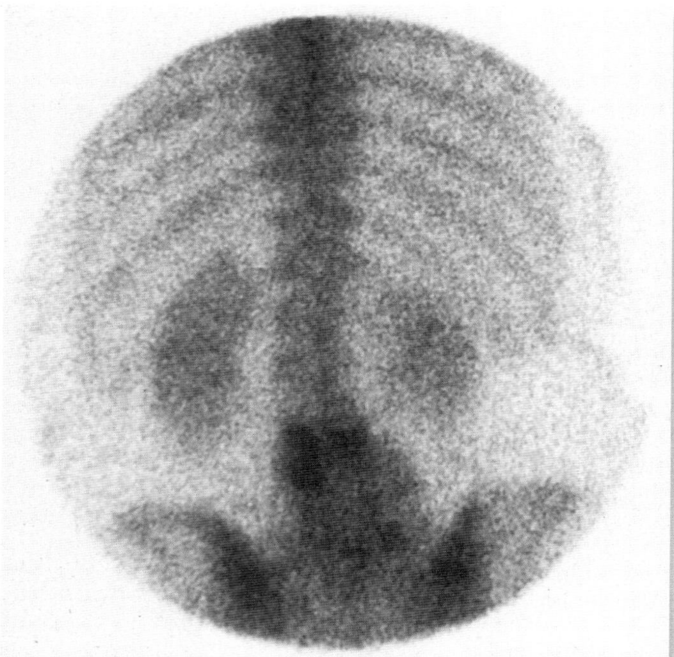

Figure 35-7. This bone scan of the spine (same patient as in Figure 35-4) shows the uptake of the radioactive contrast medium, which is darkest in the areas of inflammation.

images are produced immediately, whereas others may take up to several days. Radionuclide imaging exposes patients to lower doses of radiation than some radiologic techniques, because the amount of ionizing radiation in the isotope is less than that emitted from x-ray cameras.

Other nuclear medicine procedures include single photon emission computed tomography (SPECT), positron emission tomography (PET), and MUGA (multiple gated acquisition) scan.

- **SPECT** is often used to locate and determine the extent of brain damage from a stroke. The gamma camera detects signals induced by gamma radiation, and a computer converts these signals into either two- or three-dimensional images that are displayed on a screen.
- **PET** entails injecting isotopes combined with other substances involved in metabolic activity, such as glucose. These special isotopes emit positrons, which a computer processes and displays on a screen. PET is especially useful for diagnosing brain-related conditions, such as epilepsy, mental illnesses, and Parkinson's disease.
- The **MUGA scan** evaluates the condition of the heart's myocardium. It can be done while the patient is at rest or in stress (exercise) and involves the injection of radioisotopes that concentrate in the myocardium. The gamma camera allows the physician to measure ventricular contractions to evaluate the patient's heart wall.

When preparing a patient for a nuclear medicine procedure, describe the procedure and tell her how long the examination will take. Explain any preparation requirements and other special instructions, and tell the patient she will need to wait the required length of time for the uptake of the radioisotope. Length of examination and requirements for common scans are as follows:

- A bone scan lasts about 1 hour; it is done 2 to 3 hours after a 15-minute injection; the patient drinks 1 quart of liquid between the injection and the scan; a normal diet is permitted
- A liver/spleen or lung scan lasts approximately 1 hour; there are no diet restrictions
- A kidney scan lasts about 2 hours; there are no diet restrictions
- A thyroid uptake and scan test usually requires 2 days; the patient takes a capsule of contrast medium in the morning and has the scan on the first day; the patient returns 24 hours later for the second scan; there are no diet restrictions, except that the patient must have no fish because of its natural iodine content

Stereoscopy

Used primarily to study the skull, **stereoscopy** is an x-ray procedure that uses a specially designed microscope (stereoscopic, or Greenough, microscope) with double eyepieces and objectives to take films at different angles. Stereoscopy identifies fractures and dense areas to produce three-dimensional images. The images, which have depth as well as height and width, can indicate a tumor or increased pressure within the skull. No special preparation is required. Follow the guidelines you would use with any other noninvasive x-ray.

Thermography

Thermography is performed to diagnose breast tumors, breast abscesses, and fibrocystic breast disease. The procedure uses an infrared camera to take photographs that record variations in skin temperature as dark (cool areas), light (warm areas), or shades of gray (areas with temperatures between cool and warm). Tumors or inflammations produce more heat than healthy tissues and therefore show up lighter on these photographs; areas with lack of circulation are cooler than tissues with adequate circulation and show up as dark. Because no preparation requirements are necessary for this test, you need only to schedule the procedure and to assist as needed with reassurance during the examination.

Ultrasound

Ultrasound directs high-frequency sound waves through the skin over the area of the body being examined and produces an image based on the echoes. A radiologist or

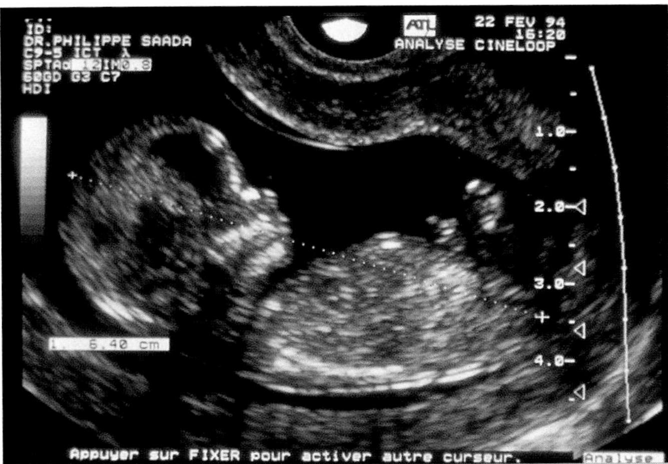

Figure 35-8. Ultrasound is commonly used to evaluate the health of a developing fetus.

an ultrasound radiologic technologist coats the body area with a special gel and passes a transducer (instrument similar to a microphone) over the area. As the transducer passes back and forth over the area, it picks up echoes from the sound waves, which a computer converts into an image on a screen. Ultrasound is used to detect abnormalities in the gallbladder, liver, spleen, heart, and kidneys. It is also safe to use in obstetrics to evaluate the developing fetus or to detect multiple fetuses, because it does not expose the patient (or the fetus) to radiation (Figure 35-8). In this case the obstetrician may perform the test in the office.

One form of ultrasound, called Doppler echocardiography, involves sound waves that echo against the flow of blood through vessels. Doppler echocardiography is usually performed by a cardiologist to determine whether blood flow is laminar (normal) or turbulent (disturbed).

When preparing the patient for an ultrasound or assisting with the examination, follow these guidelines:

- Describe the procedure to the patient and inform her that the examination will take about ½ to 2 hours, depending on the type of ultrasound. For example, a cardiac ultrasound takes about 1½ hours; pelvic, 1 to 2 hours; and abdominal, ½ to 1 hour.
- Explain the preparation requirements, which vary according to the type of ultrasound. Tell a patient who is having a gallbladder or liver ultrasound not to eat for several hours before the test. Tell a pregnant patient to drink the prescribed amount of water 1 hour before the examination and not to void. Advise a patient having a pelvic ultrasound to take the prescribed laxative (if indicated), drink three to four glasses of water within 1 hour, and not to void within 1 hour of the test. If the patient is having an abdominal ultrasound, instruct her to take a laxative the night before the examination and not to have any food or fluids for 8 hours before the test.
- Advise the patient to wear loose clothing that is easy to remove.

Xeroradiography

Xeroradiography is used to diagnose breast cancer, abscesses, lesions, and calcifications. The xeroradiographic x-rays are developed with a powder toner, similar to the toner in photocopiers, and the image is processed on specially treated xerographic paper. Xeroradiography uses lower exposure times and less radiation than standard x-rays.

Common Therapeutic Uses of Radiation

Used therapeutically, radiology is called **radiation therapy.** Radiation therapy is used to treat cancer by preventing cellular reproduction. The two types of radiation therapy are teletherapy and brachytherapy. **Teletherapy** allows deep penetration and is used primarily for deep tumors; it is done on an outpatient basis. The patient experiences minimal side effects, and superficial tissues are not damaged.

Localized cancers are treated with **brachytherapy.** In this technique the radiologist places temporary radioactive implants close to or directly into cancerous tissue. Both the staff and patient are subject to radiation exposure. Therefore, radiation safety precautions must be closely followed. When preparing the patient for radiation therapy, follow these guidelines:

- Describe the procedure to the patient, and explain how long the procedure will take, as determined by the radiologist and oncologist according to the diagnosis and the condition of the patient.
- Inform the patient that the radiologist or oncologist will explain the possible side effects of the treatment. Common side effects include nausea, vomiting, hair loss, ulceration of mucous membranes, weakness, and malaise. Other possible effects include localized burns on tissue and damage to organs in the path of treatment. Encourage the patient to discuss with the doctor (or the oncology nurse specialist) measures to relieve or minimize stress and discomfort.
- Advise the patient to immediately report any other symptoms to the doctor.

Radiation Safety and Dose

For many years after the discovery of the x-ray, the seriousness of radiation hazards was not addressed. In the 1920s the government of Great Britain took the first steps to limit x-ray exposure. Since World War II, studies have been performed, mostly on the effects of high-dose radiation.

Other studies on the effects of background radiation and nonradiologic versus radiologic (x-ray–related) risks have enabled scientists to assess the risks of diagnostic x-rays. Results from these studies show the risk of excess radiation from routine x-rays to be minimal.

Reducing Patient Exposure

Advances in diagnostic imaging technology, as well as limits to radiation exposure, have helped reduce the dose of radiation to which a patient is exposed during a diagnostic procedure. Another way to reduce the risk of excessive radiation exposure lies with the physician, who must assess the benefit-to-risk ratio when recommending a diagnostic radiology procedure. Because radiation has a cumulative effect, the physician must have valid medical reasons for ordering the test, particularly if the patient has recently had other x-rays. Some types of x-rays, such as mammograms, should be repeated regularly, however, because of their potential to prevent or promote treatment of life-threatening disorders.

According to a 1993 report by the National Council on Radiation Protection and Measurements (NCRP) titled *Limitation of Exposure to Ionizing Radiation,* one of the earliest pieces of legislation in the United States to limit occupational radiation exposure was enacted in the 1930s. The first legislation to limit public exposure, however, was not enacted until the 1950s. The NCRP report of 1993 set guidelines for protection from radiation in and out of the workplace. The two primary objectives outlined in the report are to prevent serious general tissue damage from radiation by limiting radiation dose to levels below known thresholds for such damage and to reduce the risk of cancer and genetic effects to a level that is balanced by potential benefits to the individual and society.

Because exposure to radiation always poses some degree of risk, the NCRP recommends that any activity involving radiation exposure be justified, or balanced against the expected benefits to society. Furthermore, the NCRP recommends that the cost, or detriment, to society from such activities be kept *a*s *l*ow *a*s *r*easonably *a*chievable (ALARA) and that individual dose limits be applied to ensure that justification and ALARA principles do not result in unacceptable levels of risk for individuals or groups.

The NCRP has developed detailed lists on radiation doses to achieve the primary objectives stated in the report. There are separate specific limits for occupational exposure and public exposure.

Safety Precautions

Understanding and following standard safety precautions are crucial for protection from radiation exposure. These precautions are essential to the health and safety of both medical personnel and patients.

Personnel Safety. If you work in a medical facility that performs radiologic tests, you are at risk for excessive radiation exposure. To protect yourself from radiation exposure, you must adhere to the following specific guidelines:

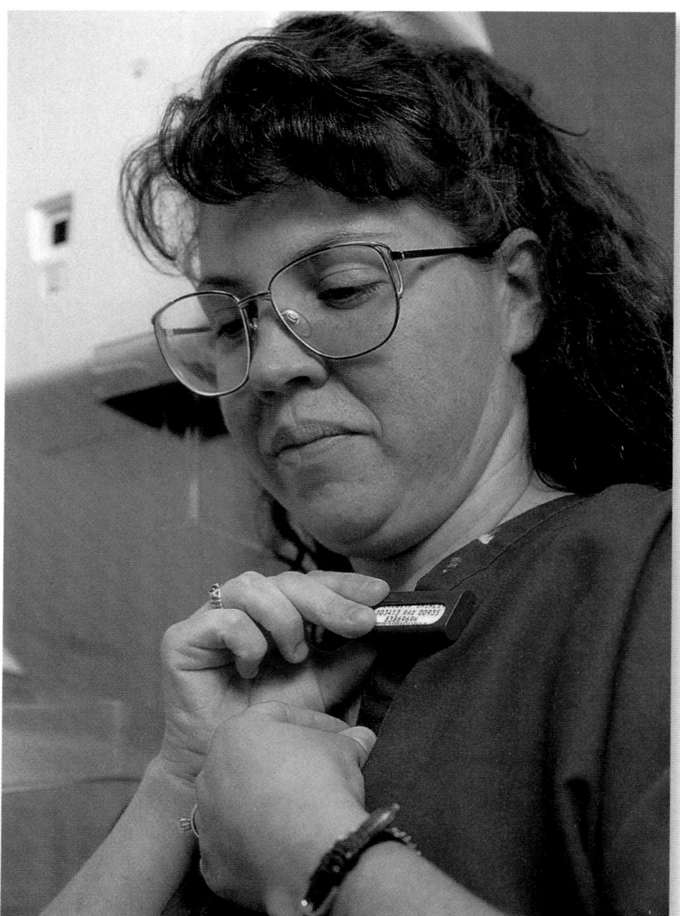

Figure 35-9. A radiation exposure badge contains a film that registers the levels of radiation to which a medical staff member is exposed at work.

- You (and other members of the medical staff) must always wear a radiation exposure badge, or dosimeter, which is a sensitized piece of film in a holder (Figure 35-9). You must have the badge checked regularly by specially qualified personnel, who measure the degree of radiation uptake on the film to determine the amount of radiation to which you have been exposed.
- Make sure that all equipment is in good working order and is checked routinely for radiation leakage and any other problems.
- Be aware that the technician and any other staff members present when equipment is operating should always wear a garment that contains a lead shield.

Patient Safety. You must follow all rules governing patient safety from radiation exposure. The Educating the Patient section explains safety measures and information that help protect a patient from exposure to unnecessary radiation.

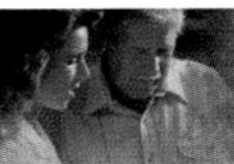

Educating the Patient

Safety With X-Rays

You are responsible for teaching the patient about x-ray safety. You will need to obtain pertinent patient history data, answer questions, and provide basic information on x-rays, possible side effects, and other important guidelines. Consider the following points when teaching the patient about x-ray safety.

Patient History

- Ask the patient about x-rays received in the past, including how many and what type, and about the possibility of exposure to radiation in the home, school, or workplace. Explain that the effects of radiation exposure are cumulative; that is, the effects are related to total exposure over the lifetime as well as to exposure from each procedure.
- Ask a female patient about the possibility of pregnancy. Use the 10-day rule—take an x-ray only within 10 days of the last menstrual period to avoid taking an x-ray of a patient who is unknowingly pregnant. If the patient knows that she is pregnant, do not schedule an x-ray unless approved by the radiologist.
- Inform the patient about possible side effects of radiation exposure. These effects include fetal abnormality or genetic mutation in a fetus (when a patient is pregnant) and the depression of bone marrow activity, which decreases the production of red blood cells and white blood cells.

Patient Questions

- Always answer questions in simple, easy-to-understand language; make explanations brief and clear. Do not use complex medical terms; however, do include proper terminology. Offer written information about the test, if available.
- Answer fully any questions about examinations, including descriptions of procedures; the doctor's reason for ordering them; their length, side effects, injections or other uncomfortable aspects; preprocedure requirements; cost and insurance issues; and availability of test results.
- Help the patient reduce fear or anxiety surrounding the scheduled test and feel comfortable and informed about the procedure.

General X-Ray Information

- Be aware of the most current guidelines established by the American College of Radiology. Always keep up with new studies on the risks of radiation exposure.
- Encourage the patient to ask questions about the need for x-rays ordered by the doctor and risks associated with those x-rays.
- If the patient's employer requires annual x-rays or a potential employer asks for preemployment x-rays, advise the patient to question the necessity of these tests. Suggest that the patient find out whether the doctor has x-rays on file that could be submitted.
- Advise the patient to discuss testing options with the doctor. For instance, if the doctor orders fluoroscopy, the patient might ask whether standard x-rays can be taken instead, because fluoroscopy often represents a higher risk for exposure to radiation than do standard x-rays. (Mobile x-ray examinations often pose a higher exposure risk as well.)
- Advise the patient to ask questions about x-ray safety standards in the office or hospital in which the tests are to take place.
- Tell the patient to avoid dental x-rays that are performed with wide-beamed plastic cones; narrow-beamed cones are more exact and less dangerous. In addition, educate the patient about the opinions of the American Dental Association and the National Conference of Dental Radiology, both of which believe that x-rays should not be performed solely for insurance claim purposes.
- Advise the patient to always ask for a lead apron over organs not being studied.
- Tell the patient to avoid retakes of x-rays because of blurriness or shadows (which are caused by movements or breathing) by remaining still when instructed to do so during x-ray examinations.
- Explain to the patient the importance of x-rays in proper diagnosis of disorders. Inform the patient about the constant improvements in equipment and x-ray procedures and the much lower doses of radiation now used in these procedures.
- Advise the patient to keep a family record of x-ray examinations.
- Educate a female patient without breast disease on the correct schedule for mammography examinations. The patient should have a baseline mammogram between ages 35 and 40; a mammogram every 1 to 2 years between ages 40 and 49; and an annual mammogram after age 50.
- Also tell the patient to see a doctor immediately if she notices a breast mass, lump, or nipple discharge.

Storing and Filing X-Rays

You will be responsible for storing x-ray films if you work in a radiology facility. Follow these guidelines for proper storage of x-rays:

- Keep fresh film on hand at all times.
- Maintain new and exposed films in as good a condition as possible by keeping them at a temperature between 50° and 70°F (between 10° and 20°C) and a relative humidity between 30% and 50%. Radiology facilities usually have one or more special rooms for films.
- Prevent pressure marks and keep expiration dates visible by storing packages on end; do not stack them on top of each other.
- Use a first-in, first-out method for using film (that is, use the oldest film first).
- Open film packages or boxes only in the darkroom.
- Do not store film near acid or ammonia vapors.

You will also be responsible for providing accurate record keeping of x-rays. See Procedure 35-2 for guidelines on documentation and filing techniques.

Remember that x-ray films are the property of the radiology facility or the doctor's office where they are taken. Although the films may be sent (or taken by the patient) to a hospital or another doctor for consultation, they should be returned to the original facility (for example, the radiologist's office). In some facilities, the images are stored on a specialized computer disk, and the patient receives a copy of films to take to another doctor or medical facility. The information, however, is the property of the patient. Thus, the patient need not return reports.

PROCEDURE 35.2

Documentation and Filing Techniques for X-Rays

Objective: To document x-ray information and file x-ray films properly

OSHA Guidelines: This procedure does not involve exposure to blood, body fluids, or tissues.

Materials: X-ray film(s), patient x-ray record card or book, label, film-filing envelopes, film-filing cabinet, inserts, marking pen

Method

1. Document the patient's x-ray information on the patient record card or in the record book (Figure 35-10). Include the patient's name, the date, the type of x-ray, and the number of x-rays taken.

X-RAY EXAMINATIONS RECORD

Patient	Date	Type X-Ray	No. Taken	Referring Doctor	Comments
Jill Cabot	2/16	Chest	4	Wapnir	
M. C. Gaines	2/16	Right knee	8	Wright	
J. Hale	2/19	Right wrist	6	McCarthy	
L. Becker	2/23	Left hip	4	Wright	
R. Bell	2/24	Chest	4	Wapnir	
Donna Lin	2/24	Sinuses	6	Harris	
Jon Carey	2/26	Right hand	2	Cohen	

Figure 35-10. Keeping accurate records of patient x-ray information is an important duty of the medical assistant.

continued ⟶

PROCEDURE 35.2

Documentation and Filing Techniques for X-Rays *(continued)*

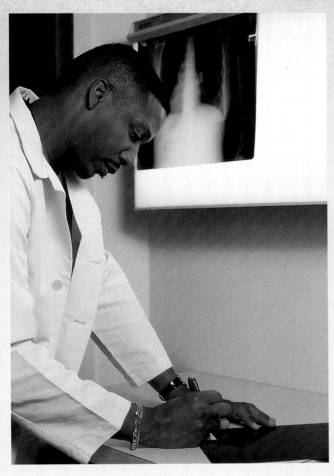

Figure 35-11. You may need to provide labeling information on an x-ray film before you file it.

2. Verify that the film is properly labeled with the referring doctor's name, the date, and the patient's name. To note corrections or unusual positions or to identify a film that does not include labeling, attach the appropriate label and complete the necessary information (Figure 35-11). Some facilities also record the name of the radiologist who interpreted the x-ray.
3. Place the processed film in a film-filing envelope. File the envelope alphabetically or chronologically (or according to your office's protocol) in the filing cabinet.
4. If you remove an envelope for any reason, put an insert or an "out card" in its place until it is returned to the cabinet.

Electronic Medicine

Recent major advances in telemedicine technology, including rapid video and computer-based communications of medical information, enable physicians to "examine" a patient in another city, view highly detailed medical images, consult with specialists in other cities, and supervise complex medical procedures. In addition, health-care personnel, including medical assistants, can participate in interactive teaching conferences by means of closed-circuit television.

In some cities emergency medical technicians (EMTs) are able to transmit an electrocardiogram (ECG) electronically to an emergency room physician to obtain lifesaving directives from the physician. These directives may involve administration of drugs or other measures the EMTs otherwise would not be permitted to perform without a physician's order. Similarly, some patients are monitored by cardiologists by the transmission of daily ECGs through telephone lines to the cardiologist's office.

Another new technology is stereotaxis, a magnetic neurosurgery procedure that allows surgeons to treat or remove brain tissue safely while being guided by a computer screen. Traditionally, neurosurgeons risked causing severe damage while gaining access to an affected area of a patient's brain. With stereotaxis, however, the computer screen shows a view of the brain containing a surgically implanted magnetic pellet in a safe area of the brain. The neurosurgeon then uses magnetic resonance imaging to guide the pellet, which is the size of a grain of rice, toward a critical area. Using this technique, the surgeon can avoid critical neurons and deliver treatment to the high-risk area. The pellet can be used to move a catheter, probe, or other implement into place to remove tissue or deliver a drug. Researchers hope to expand this technology to other parts of the body, such as the liver or blood vessels.

Summary

Diagnostic tests are an important part of medical care because they help doctors diagnose a variety of diseases and disorders. As a medical assistant, you will be asked to assist with patient care before, and sometimes during and after, diagnostic radiology procedures. Your responsibilities include providing instructions and explanations to patients, preparing patients for various tests, and assisting the doctor or technician with the procedures. Your duties may also include storing and filing x-rays.

Safety is a vital concern with radiologic tests. Understanding and following safety precautions will help you ensure your patients' health and well-being as well as your own.

CLINICAL SITE ASSESSMENT

NAME OF SITE ______________________________

ADDRESS ______________________________

SPECIALITY ______________________ SUPERVISOR ______________________

TELEPHONE # ______________________ FAX # ______________________

NUMBER OF STAFF ______________________

ADMINISTRATIVE/CLINICAL EXPERIENCE AVAILABLE TO STUDENTS
(*CHECK ALL THAT APPLY*)

____ FRONT OFFICE SKILLS

____ WORD PROCESSING SKILLS

____ MEASURE/RECORD VITAL SIGNS

____ BLOOD DRAWING (VENIPUNCTURE, FINGERSTICKS)

____ INJECTIONS

____ ELECTROCARDIOGRAMS

____ SPECIMEN COLLECTION/DIAGNOSTIC PROCEDURES
(urinalysis, blood sugar, cholesterol, etc.)

____ ASSISTING WITH MINOR SURGICAL PROCEDURES

I HAVE DETERMINED THAT THIS SITE MEETS THE NEED OF THE STUDENTS IN THE MEDICAL ASSISTING PROGRAM.

PRINT NAME OF UDS EVALUATOR ______________________________

SIGNATURE OF EVALUATOR ______________________________

DATE ______________________

Figure 36-1. A form such as this clinical site assessment is often used by the clinical coordinator to help determine if a clinical site will be appropriate for medical assisting externships.

- Providing professional liability insurance for the student, the educational institution, and the faculty
- Ensuring that the student is medically able to perform the assigned duties of the extern facility by providing proof of immunizations and health physicals

The clinical coordinator is the liaison between the externship site and the educational institution.

Screening. Students are placed in externship clinical sites by the clinical coordinator. It is not uncommon for the clinical site to screen students prior to their externship. This screening can include the following:

- Interviewing students prior to their externship.
- Asking students to provide a urine or hair sample for drug screening prior to the externship.
- Asking students to consent to a criminal background check prior to beginning their externship. Some medical facilities check only for felony convictions, whereas others check for misdemeanors and felonies. Honesty is the best policy for criminal background checks. Some institutions will waive some convictions as long as the student is honest and truthful about the conviction early in the process.
- Accepting students only if employment at the facility is the end result. The student may be asked to fill out an application and participate in a new employee orientation prior to beginning the externship.

Clinical Externship Timesheet
Medical Assistant Program

Instructions:
Students are expected to attend their clinical site for a minimum of 32 hours per week, and will not receive credit for more than ten hours per day. **For shifts greater than four hours, you must include a thirty-minute meal break.**

- Complete the log daily and fax the log each week to the school no later than 5 p.m. Friday.
- For each day attended, please include a brief description of the duties performed.
- The Timesheet must be signed and dated by both the student and the Clinical Site Supervisor.

Student Information

Name: ____________________

Program: ____________________

Home Phone: ____________________

Alt. Phone: ____________________

Clinical Site Information

Name: ____________________

Phone: ____________________

Rotation: ____________________

Assignment Dates: ____________________

Site Supervisor's Name: ____________________

	Date	Time In	Time Out	Total Hours	General Duties Performed *
Monday					
Tuesday					
Wednesday					
Thursday					
Friday					
Saturday					
TOTAL HOURS					

* Examples of General Duties include: Billing, Vital Signs, Lab Work, Filing, Charting, etc.

Student Signature: ____________________

Date: ____________________

Supervisor: ____________________

Supervisor Signature: ____________________

Date: ____________________

Figure 36-2. Students participating in an externship complete a weekly timesheet.

Time Sheets. Students are given time sheets to be completed on a daily basis and faxed to the educational facility at the end of every week. The clinical preceptor and the student both sign the time sheet (Figure 36-2). The student is monitored by the clinical coordinator and the program director for the duration of the externship. Weekly telephone calls and site visits are performed by the educational institution for each student. Some schools require weekly progress reports from each student. Figure 36-3 provides an example of this report. When students finish their externships, the preceptors will complete a final evaluation and the students will be graded on their externship performance (Figure 36-4).

Expectations of Externship Candidates

While in an externship, you are expected to be and look professional, report to the externship site as scheduled, and display initiative and a willingness to learn.

Professionalism. You are expected to conduct yourself in a professional manner at all times while attending your externship. You may feel that you are often criticized by the site preceptor. This normal part of learning is called **constructive criticism.** Constructive criticism is aimed at giving you feedback about your performance in order to

STUDENT WEEKLY PROGRESS REPORT

This form needs to be completed and signed each week. It must be faxed with the timesheet on Friday afternoon. It is designed to help you maximize your clinical externship experience. Having recognizable goals is the surest way to succeed!

Name: ____________________ Date: ____________________

Class Code: ____________________

Clinical Site: ____________________

Supervisor Signature: ____________________

Student Signature: ____________________

I. Goals for next week:

1. ____________________
2. ____________________
3. ____________________

II. Personal assessment of progress this week:

____

____

____

III. Supervisor's assessment of progress this week:

____

____

____

IV. Identify one task/item/event you are most proud of that occurred this week:

____

____

V. Did you meet your goals for this week? Why or why not?

____

____

Figure 36-3. A weekly progress report is a helpful way for students to track their externship goals and achievements.

MEDICAL ASSISTANT PROGRAM

EXTERNSHIP TRAINING PLAN

NAME:	INTERNSHIP PERIOD: / / TO / /
SITE NAME:	ADDRESS:
ON-SITE EMPLOYER REPRESENTATIVE:	PHONE #:

DIRECTIONS: THIS TRAINING PLAN WILL SERVICE TO SPECIFY THE APPLICATIONS AND EXPERIENCES THAT ARE TO BE SECURED DURING THEIR TRAINING. UPON COMPLETION OF THEIR TRAINING, PLEASE INDICATE YOUR APPRAISAL OF THE STUDENTS' PERFORMANCE BY DRAWING A CIRCLE AROUND THE NUMBER CORRESPONDING WITH THE ACHIEVEMENT LEVEL AS FOLLOWS:

1 = UNSATISFACTORY, 2 = FAIR, 3 = VERY GOOD, 4 = OUTSTANDING.

CIRCLE THE UA IF THE STUDENT WILL BE UNAVAILABLE TO DO THIS PROCEDURE, AND THE NA IF THIS IS NOT APPLICABLE TO THE STUDENTS' STUDIES.

EXTERNSHIP GOALS & OBJECTIVES/PERFORMANCE RATING SCALE

DURING THE EXTERNSHIP PERIOD, THE STUDENT WILL:

A.	DEVELOP EFFECTIVE "*FRONT OFFICE*" SKILLS INCLUSIVE OF SUCH ACTIVITIES AS; PATIENT COMMUNICATION, MEDICAL RECORDS, BILLING & COLLECTIONS, INSURANCE PROCESSING, AND COMPUTERIZED BUSINESS FUNCTIONS	1	2	3	4	UA	NA
B.	ACCURATELY MEASURE AND RECORD VITAL SIGNS, UTILIZING PROPER TECHNIQUE	1	2	3	4	UA	NA
C.	PERFORM STANDARD EKG RECORDING/ MOUNTING PER SITE PROTOCOL	1	2	3	4	UA	NA
D.	DEVELOP PROFICIENCY IN PARENTERAL MEDICATION ADMINISTRATION (INTRADERMAL, SUBQ, INTRAMUSCULAR)	1	2	3	4	UA	NA
E.	DEVELOP PROFICIENCY AND TECHNIQUE IN PERFORMING VENIPUNCTURE USING THE EVACUATED TUBE SYSTEM	1	2	3	4	UA	NA
F.	DEMONSTRATE EFFECTIVE SPECIMEN COLLECTION TECHNIQUE AND DIAGNOSTIC PROCEDURES (*i.e.*, URINALYSIS, BLOOD SUGAR, CHOLESTEROL, ETC.)	1	2	3	4	UA	NA

SIDE 1 OF 2

Figure 36-4. A form such as this one may be used by the clinical preceptor to evaluate a student's externship performance. (continued)

PROFESSIONAL ATTRIBUTES	PERFORMANCE RATING SCALE					
A. ORAL COMMUNICATIONS	1	2	3	4	UA	NA
B. ORGANIZATION & SAFETY	1	2	3	4	UA	NA
C. DEPENDABILITY & SELF-DIRECTION	1	2	3	4	UA	NA
D. COOPERATIVENESS	1	2	3	4	UA	NA
E. RECORDKEEPING	1	2	3	4	UA	NA
F. COLLABORATIVENESS/TEAMWORK	1	2	3	4	UA	NA
G. PATIENT RAPPORT/CONSIDERATION	1	2	3	4	UA	NA
H. ATTENDANCE/PUNCTUALITY	1	2	3	4	UA	NA

WHAT IS YOUR OVERALL OPINION OF THIS STUDENT'S PERFORMANCE?

( ) UNSATISFACTORY ( ) POOR ( ) FAIR ( ) GOOD ( ) VERY GOOD ( ) OUTSTANDING

THIS WILL CERTIFY THAT THE INTERN HAS COMPLETED ( ) HOURS AT THE SITE.

COMMENTS:

ON-SITE EVALUATOR'S SIGNATURE: ______________________________

DATE: ____________________

SIDE 2 OF 2

THIS PAGE IS STRICTLY FOR THE USE OF EDUCATION

TOTAL GOALS AND OBJECTIVE POINTS ________/________

\# OBJECTIVES EVALUATED = ________AVG POINTS

TOTAL ATTRIBUTE POINTS ________/________

\# ATTRIBUTES EVALUATED = ________AVG POINTS

AVERAGE OF TOTAL POINTS = ________________

GRADE POINT SCALE

A = 3.5–4.0

B = 2.5–3.4

C = 2.0–2.4

F = 1.9 OR LESS

FINAL GRADE = ________________

PROGRAM DIRECTOR SIGNATURE: ______________________________

DATE: ____________________

Figure 36-4. (continued)

improve that performance. You are not expected to know everything on your externship, but you are expected to be open to suggestions and ideas. It is not considered professional to question clinical preceptors during the learning experience. You may be exposed to some procedures that are not performed exactly as you were taught. Do not argue with preceptors about their skills. There is usually more than one way to get the desired result in patient care.

Your behavior is expected to be as professional as if you were an employee there. Foul language and inappropriate conversation is not tolerated in any workplace. You are expected to be professional with the patients under all circumstances. Medical facilities expect you to demonstrate empathy and compassion to every patient. Proper verbal skills and grammar are expected at all times. Do not use slang when communicating with office staff and patients. Personal phone calls should not be made during working hours; do not use the facility phone. Cell phones and pagers should be turned off during working hours.

Attendance. You are expected to report to your externship *every day* that you are assigned to a schedule. It is your responsibility to have several alternates to babysitting and transportation. Employers are seeking dependable and punctual medical staff and would not tolerate attendance problems with their own staff. In the event of an emergency, you are expected to report a call-off to the medical facility and the school two hours before the beginning of your shift, as would any other employee. Many medical facilities will not tolerate absenteeism or tardiness from an externship student, and they may ask the school to remove the student from the site.

Adhere to the facility's policy regarding breaks. Take breaks only when it is appropriate to do so. If you smoke, refrain from smoking during working hours and do not smoke in patient entrances. Lunch breaks are permitted under facility policies.

Professional Appearance. Medical facilities expect you to appear as a medical professional. Most require a uniform that consists of a scrub top and bottom and a lab jacket. Your scrubs should be clean, pressed, and well fitting. Shoes should be clean, white, and in good repair. Your name tag or badge should always be worn and visible to patients. Nails should be trimmed and polished in good taste in pale and neutral colors. Many medical facilities will not accept students with artificial nails, such as acrylics. Facial and tongue piercings are not acceptable when working with patients, and visible tattoos must be covered. Your hair should be a natural color and pulled back from your face and off your collar. Makeup should be conservative and in good taste. Perfumes and colognes should be avoided because patients with respiratory conditions or allergies may not be able to tolerate them.

Remember that you as a medical assisting student on an externship represent several things:

- The school you attend. It is important to maintain a good reputation in the medical community. You will depend on the reputation of the school to obtain a job.
- The profession of medical assisting. Participating in a medical assisting externship gives you an opportunity to represent the profession of medical assisting to patients and the community.
- Yourself. First impressions are lasting impressions. Make your first impression to the medical community an outstanding one.

Initiative and Willingness to Learn. During your externship, accept all assignments with enthusiasm and grace, no matter how mundane. These tasks are often a test on how well you accept orders and work within a medical team. Ask for additional work if you are idle, and look for tasks that need to be done. Keep a notebook and record the office policies and procedures. Be prepared to observe and participate in office procedures.

Preparing to Find a Position

The next phase of beginning your new career is seeking a position as a medical assistant. Most accredited schools have a career services department. Its primary focus is job placement after graduation. The department's counselors will assist you in writing your résumé, improving your interviewing skills, and learning about positions in your field. Many employers will contact a school's career services department to recruit medical personnel. It is important to work closely with the career services department in the beginning of your career to assist you in obtaining your first position.

Seeking Employment

In addition to working with a career services department, you can take advantage of a number of other resources in seeking employment within the field of medical assisting. These resources include classified ads, Internet sites, employment services, and networking with classmates and others.

Classified Ads and Internet Sites. Many prospective employers use classified advertisements in area newspapers to alert potential applicants to a career opportunity within their organization. The advertisement usually describes the duties and responsibilities of the position as well as the type of education and experience preferred.

When you are first beginning to seek a medical assisting position, don't become discouraged if you see advertisements asking for a specified amount of experience, such as 2 years. You must realize that employers place ads seeking an experienced candidate, but many will consider a new graduate because experienced candidates are not always available. Becoming credentialed will help you bridge the gap of experience. A local newspaper's classified advertisements are often a good place to start your search. There is usually a separate section listing health-related jobs.

It is important to explore all the possibilities when seeking employment opportunities. A medical assistant is qualified for a number of positions. New graduates can apply for the following positions:

- Unit secretary in hospitals
- Phlebotomist in labs
- Patient care associate or patient care technician in hospitals

- Entry-level medical coding and billing
- Customer service representative in medical-related companies
- Clinical or administrative position in physician offices

The Internet is another useful tool when seeking employment. Web sites often allow job seekers to post résumés online and to respond to advertisements that are posted by employers locally or statewide.

Employment Services. Employment and temporary agencies provide assistance in locating a specific job. Both types of agencies have a variety of job openings on file. Agencies also place classified ads. You should call to make an appointment with an employment counselor. Agencies usually require you to fill out an application, take a basic health-care test, and provide a résumé. If the agency has positions that match your skills, it contacts the employer. If the service has no appropriate listings, it will place your résumé on file.

Employment services are an excellent way to gain experience and select a position. You are given an opportunity to try out the office or facility at little commitment on your part. Many permanent opportunities can result from a temporary job assignment.

Networking. **Networking** involves making contacts with relatives, friends, and acquaintances who may have information about how to find a job in your field. People in your network may be able to give you job leads or tell you about openings. Word-of-mouth referrals—finding job information by talking with other people—can be very helpful. Other people may be able to introduce you to others who work in, or know people who work in, your field. Networking is a valuable tool. It can advance your career even while you are employed.

Joining a medical assisting organization and attending conferences are the easiest ways to network. Attend an organization's local chapter meetings and talk with as many people as possible. Remember to bring a pen and a notebook. Be prepared to exchange information with other attendees. Remember, networking is an exchange of information—it is not one-sided. What you learn through networking may enable you to provide others with information to help their job search or further their career.

Your classmates are often a good source of networking. It is important to build lasting friendships with your classmates and keep in touch after graduation. Oftentimes they will know of positions as they gain employment. Networking begins in the classroom.

Creating a Résumé

Your résumé is a vital part of the employment process. It provides potential employers with information about your educational and work history and other aspects of your background.

Components of a Résumé. In order to create a well-rounded, informative résumé, you need to include a wide variety of information about your background.

Personal Information. Include your name, address, telephone number, cell phone number, and e-mail address. Do not include your marital status or the number of children you have. You should not include your height, weight, interests, or hobbies unless you think they are relevant to the position.

Professional Objective. A professional objective is a brief, general statement that demonstrates a career goal. An example of an effective, professional objective is the following: "To work as a medical assistant, applying skills in patient relations and laboratory work while gaining increasing responsibility." If you want to list a specific career objective, such as applying your medical assisting skills in a pediatric medical facility, it would be best to mention it in the cover letter and not on your résumé.

Employment Experience. List the title of your most recent or last job first, the dates you were employed there, and a brief description of your duties. Choose jobs that have been the most beneficial to your working career. Do not clutter your résumé with needless details or irrelevant jobs. You can elaborate on specific duties in your cover letter and in the interview. Only include jobs you have held for a longer period of time, such as six months to a year.

Educational Background. In providing your educational history, list your highest degree first, the school attended, the dates, and the major field of study. Include educational experience that may be relevant to the job, such as certification, licensing, advanced training, and intensive seminars. Do not list individual classes on your résumé. If you have taken special classes that relate directly to the job you are seeking, list them in your cover letter.

Awards and Honors. List the awards and honors that are related to your career or that indicate excellence. Perfect attendance, academic honors, and student of the month are excellent traits that employers are seeking. Highlight this information prominently rather than writing it as an afterthought. You can make the most impact by displaying your best qualities at the beginning of this section.

Campus and Community Activities. List activities that show leadership abilities and a willingness to contribute. Include any volunteer work that you may have performed.

Professional Memberships and Activities. List any professional memberships that are related to your career. Student memberships are available through the American Medical Technologists (AMT) and the American Association of Medical Assistants (AAMA). You can contact the AMT and request a copy of the student by-laws and directions on how to form a student membership in your school. The AAMA provides continuing education through their local chapters. They sponsor local meetings periodically throughout the year. Employers like medical professionals who are involved in their disciplines. It demonstrates a commitment and dedication to their chosen field.

Summary of Skills. As you learn clinical and administrative skills, you will want to list them on your résumé. Under headings such as "Clinical Skills" or "Administrative Skills," list the skills you have acquired in school and on your externship. Some examples of clinical skills are the following:

- EKG
- Venipuncture
- Urinalysis
- Parenteral injections
- Aseptic technique
- Bandaging and first aid
- CPR
- Triage and vital statistics

Some examples of administrative skills are the following:

- ICD-9 and CPT coding
- Insurance claim form processing, HCFA
- Practice management software, Medisoft
- Pegboard accounting
- Typing, 45 wpm
- Microsoft Office software

References. Prior to the end of your externship, meet with your preceptor and ask for a **reference.** A reference is a recommendation for employment from the facility and the preceptor. A reference can be in the form of a letter from the facility, preceptor, or physician, or it can be a request to include these people on your reference list. It is professional to always ask before you list someone as a reference. References are important to career building because employers often like to inquire about a person prior to offering them employment. Your first references in medical assisting are your instructors and then the externship facility.

You will want three to five references, including employment, academic, and character references. Ask instructors for a general letter before you finish your program. Fellow members of professional associations or your classmates can provide character references, and your externship can provide an employment reference. Make certain that you ask your references for permission to use their names and phone numbers. Do not print your references on the bottom of your résumé. List them on a separate sheet of paper so that you can update the list as needed. On the bottom of your résumé, you should type "References available on request."

Choosing a Résumé Style. Three different résumé styles have been developed, each of which has specific advantages and disadvantages. You will want to choose a style or combination of styles that best describes your strengths and skills.

Functional Résumé. A **functional résumé** highlights specialty areas of your accomplishments and strengths. You can organize these in an order that supports your objective. Functional résumés are useful when you change careers, reenter the job market after an absence, or have had a variety of different, unconnected work experiences. Functional résumés are often not appropriate in highly traditional fields such as teaching, law, or health care, where the specific employers are the main interest. A sample of a functional résumé is shown in Figure 36-5.

Chronological Résumé. A **chronological résumé** is used by individuals who have job experience. List your most recent job first, and end with your first job. Chronological résumés are best when you stay in the same field as your prior jobs and when your employment history shows growth and development. Do not use a chronological résumé if you have gaps in your work history, if you have changed careers, if you have been in the same job for many years, or if you are looking for your first job. Figure 36-6 illustrates a chronological résumé.

Targeted Résumé. A **targeted résumé** is best if you are focused on a specific job target. The résumé should contain a clear, concise objective about what you are looking for. This résumé should list your skills, academic achievements, student honors, and other pertinent information that correlates with your objective. This type of information adds substance to your résumé when you have just graduated and do not have relevant job experience. Because the targeted résumé is an academic-type résumé, your skills, achievements, and community and volunteer work—your most significant assets—should be listed first. A sample of a targeted résumé is shown in Figure 36-7.

Résumé Writing Tips. Pay close attention to detail as you create your résumé. Here are some suggestions to help you:

- Organize your information by using a worksheet. List all the addresses, dates, phone numbers, and supervisors of previous positions that you have held. Write down brief descriptions of all the responsibilities and duties of your positions.
- List your educational institutions and their addresses, your dates of attendance, and the type of diploma or degree, including your major.
- Choose a résumé format that best describes your experience, education, and achievements.
- Use a computer and save your résumé on a disk.
- Proofread all spelling and grammar. Your completed résumé should be perfect. Do not rely on the spell-checking feature of your computer. Proofread your résumé line by line, and request that someone else also proofread your résumé.
- Select a high-quality résumé paper that is the standard size of 8½ by 11, with a weight between 16 and 25 pounds. Use an ivory or white paper with matching envelopes.

Donna Turner-Smith
18 Kingsley Road
Olmsted Falls, OH 44138
(440) 555-4279

PUBLIC HEALTH EDUCATION:

Instructed community groups on HIV awareness.
Instructed volunteers on how to set up community programs on domestic violence
Facilitated workshops for parents of teenagers
Provided in-services for public school teachers on signs and symptoms of substance abuse

COUNSELING:

Consulted with social workers on individual cases for suspected child abuse
Worked with parents from abused homes
Counseled individual abused children

ORGANIZATIONAL:

Grant writing for federal funds for HIV awareness programs
Served as a liaison for transitional shelters for victims of domestic violence
Served as a liaison between community health agencies and public schools

PROFESSIONAL WORK HISTORY:

1990–1997 Project SAFE, Plymouth, Michigan
HIV Public Health Instructor

1997–2004 Department of Child Health and Safety, Cleveland, Ohio
Public Health Educator

EDUCATION:

1990 B.S. Sociology, Eastern Michigan University, Ypsilanti, Michigan

References available upon request

Figure 36-5. A functional résumé is often used by people who are reentering the job market.

- Use clear and concise statements and sentences. Your writing should reflect a positive and confident tone. For example, if you are describing your duties as a server, use sentences that focus on customer service, cash management, and the training and development of new servers. Avoid using the word "I" because the reader already knows that the résumé is referring to you.
- Be truthful and honest about your strengths and abilities. Do not mislead or exaggerate any skills, talents, or experience.

Procedure 36-1 provides information on how to write a résumé.

Writing a Cover Letter

A cover letter is an introduction to your résumé. It is a tool that markets your résumé as well as your skills and abilities. Cover letters are just as important as your résumé in your job search. An effective cover letter motivates the employer to review the résumé and interview the candidate.

Your cover letter should be direct and to the point. It should be no longer than one page and is typed on paper that matches your résumé. If possible, your cover letter should be addressed to a specific person in the organization. You can call the hospital or facility and ask to whom you should address the letter. If a name is not available,

Anthony Dalton
1234 West 25th Street
Park Ridge, NJ 07656
(201) 555-8311

WORK EXPERIENCE:

September, 2000–Present NORTH BERGEN CLINIC FOUNDATION

Lead Medical Assistant for Cardiology practice
Patient preparation
EKG and Holter Monitor
Assist with Stress Testing
Patient follow-up

June, 1997–September, 2000 ST. JOSEPH HOSPITAL

Phlebotomist–inpatient and outpatient

March, 1997–June, 1997 ST. JOSEPH HOSPITAL

Medical Assisting Externship
Administrative and clinical responsibilities utilizing all medical assisting skills in the Emergency department.

- Patient Triage
- Foley catheters
- EKG
- Specimen collection
- Patient intake
- Insurance verification

EDUCATION AND CERTIFICATIONS:

Associate of Applied Science Degree, June 1997, Bergen Community College, Paramus, New Jersey, 07645

Certified Medical Assistant, August, 1997

References available upon request

Figure 36-6. A chronological résumé lists a person's job history in chronological order.

it is acceptable to address the letter to "Human Resource Manager" or "Recruitment Manager." Research the facility or hospital prior to writing the letter. This information can help you tailor your letter to show how your qualifications and interests directly relate to the needs of the company or medical facility. Make sure the description of your qualifications and interests reflects the words used by the company in the advertisement. Always be truthful about the information in the cover letter; employers often verify all facts presented in your résumé and cover letter. Check each cover letter for errors in spelling, grammar, and punctuation. An example of a cover letter is shown in Figure 36-8.

Sending a Résumé

When sending a résumé, make sure you have the correct name, address, and zip code of the facility. This information should be typed on a matching envelope. Many word-processing programs have an envelope template feature that allows you to print an envelope using the address in your cover letter. Do not hand-write envelopes; professionally

Kelly Adamson
220 Terrace Avenue
Mooresburg, TN 37811
(423) 555-2657

CAREER OBJECTIVE:
To obtain a challenging position as a medical assistant in a growth oriented ambulatory care facility

ACHIEVEMENTS:
Registered Medical Assistant
Certified Phlebotomy Technician
Registered Medical Office Specialist
Graduate of an Accredited Medical Assistant Program
OSHA Compliance Officer
American Heart BLS Instructor

SKILLS AND CAPABILITIES:
Front office and Clinical Medical Assistant Patient Triage
Specimen Collection Venipuncture
EKG and Holter Monitor Parenteral Injections
ICD-9 and CPT Coding Medical Billing

PROFESSIONAL EXPERIENCE:
September, 2000–Present Affiliated Physician Network, Mooresburg, Tennessee
Medical Assistant/Office Coordinator
June, 1996–September, 2000 Partners in Internal Medicine, Mooresburg, Tennessee
Medical Assistant

EDUCATION:
Sanford Brown Institute, Diploma, Medical Assisting 1996

AFFILIATIONS:
American Medical Technologists

References available upon request

Figure 36-7. A targeted résumé is often used by a person who is focusing on a specific job target.

appearing mail is often opened first. Make sure that you attach sufficient postage.

When you fax a résumé, verify the fax number and person or department you are faxing to. Make sure your name is on all the faxed pages. If your fax machine provides a fax completion printout, save it to verify that the fax was delivered.

Some classified ads request that you send your résumé via e-mail. In order to send your résumé in electronic form, you must first have an account with an Internet service provider (ISP). You will be asked by the ISP to select a log-in, or screen, name. Do not use a casual name for your log-in prospective employers will see your log-in name in their in-box. Instead, choose a name that is conservative and professional. Most e-mail programs have an attachment feature that will allow you to send a word-processing document via e-mail. Verify that your e-mail was sent by checking your sent items or your out-box.

PROCEDURE 36.1

Résumé Writing

Objective: To write a résumé that reflects a defined career objective and highlights your skills

Materials: Paper; pen; dictionary; thesaurus; computer or word processor

Method

1. Write your full name, address (temporary and permanent, if you have both), and telephone number (include the area code).
2. List your general career objective. You may also choose to summarize your skills. If you want to phrase your objective to fit a specific position, you should include that information in a cover letter to accompany the résumé.
3. List the highest level of education or the most recently obtained degree first. Include the school name, degree earned, and date of graduation. Be sure to list any special projects, courses, or participation in overseas study programs.
4. Summarize your work experience. List your most recent or most relevant employment first. Describe your responsibilities, and list job titles, company names, and dates of employment. Summer employment, volunteer work, and student externships may also be included. Use short sentences with strong action words such as *directed, designed, developed,* and *organized.* For example, condense a responsibility into "Handled insurance and billing" or "Drafted correspondence as requested."
5. List any memberships and affiliations with professional organizations. List them alphabetically or by order of importance.
6. Do not list references on the résumé; just state "References available on request."
7. Do not list the salary you wish to receive in a medical assisting position. Salary requirements should not be discussed until a job offer is received. If the ad you are answering requests that you include a required salary, it is best to state a range (no broader than $5,000 from lowest to highest point in the range for an annual salary).
8. Type your résumé on an 8½- by 11-inch sheet of high-quality white, off-white, or gray bond paper. Carefully check your résumé for spelling, punctuation, and grammatical errors.

Post your résumé and cover letter on the Internet by using a career job search Internet site. Most Internet job sites have local employers posting positions daily. A job search Internet site will provide clear directions on how to post your résumé and cover letter. Some school career services departments host online job fairs and will assist you in posting your résumé.

Preparing a Portfolio

Prior to the interviewing phase, you should organize all your employment documentation. A portfolio can help you. A **portfolio** is a collection of documents such as your résumé, cover letter, reference list or reference letters, awards for volunteer service in a health-related field, and student recognition certificates for student of the year or month, perfect attendance, or academic honors. Include a copy of your transcript, diploma or degree, and medical assisting credentials such as your CMA or RMA. You can also include any other certifications you hold, such as a CPR card. Some employers request proof of immunizations, so include that in your portfolio. Give your portfolio a professional presentation by printing your documents on a high-quality printer and organizing them in a nice binder. Look for a service that specializes in creating professional portfolios.

Interviewing

Preparation for your interview begins long before the interview itself. After you send your cover letters and résumés, you must make sure that prospective employers can reach you by telephone. You must practice how you are going to handle your interview, and you must plan what to wear and how to present yourself in the most professional way.

Before starting your job search, invest in an answering machine or voice mail to receive calls when you are not available. Be sure the outgoing message is clear, concise, and professional. Avoid cute messages or background music. An appropriate message would be "I'm unable to take your call at the moment, but your call is important to me. Please leave your name, number, the time you called, and a brief message after the tone, and I will call you back as soon as I can. Thank you." Also, make sure all household

Your Street Address
City, State, Zip Code

Date

Name of person to whom you are writing
Title
Company or Organization
Street Address
City, State, Zip Code

Dear Dr., Mr., Mrs., Miss, or Ms. ____________:

1st Paragraph: Tell why you are writing. Name the position or general area of work that interests you. Mention how you learned about the job opening. State why you are interested in the job.

2d Paragraph: Refer to the enclosed résumé and give some background information. Indicate why you should be considered as a candidate, focusing on how your skills can fulfill the needs of the company. Relate your experiences to their needs and mention results/achievements. Do not restate what is said on your résumé—you want to pull together all the information and tell how your background fits the position.

3d Paragraph: Close by making a specific request for an interview. Say that you will follow up with a phone call to arrange a mutually convenient interview time. Offer to provide any additional information that may be needed. Thank the employer for his/her time and consideration.

Sincerely,

(your handwritten signature)

Type your name

Enclosure

Figure 36-8. The object of a cover letter is to convince the recipient to read your résumé.

members who answer the phone (especially children) know proper phone etiquette and how to take a written message. When a prospective employer calls with an interview invitation, write down the interviewer's name, company or practice name, day, time, and location of the interview.

Interview Planning and Strategies

Just as the résumé is important for opening the door to opportunity, the job interview itself is critical for allowing you to present yourself professionally and to clearly articulate why you are the best person for the job. Being successful in a medical assisting career is centered on communication—both verbal and nonverbal. These communication skills will be assets during your job interviews. The following list provides some strategies that will help you improve your interviewing skills:

- Practice interviewing. Rehearse possible questions and be prepared to answer them directly. Have a friend or family member interview you as you sit in front of a mirror and observe your body language.
- Anticipate question types. Expect open-ended questions such as, What are your strengths? What are your weaknesses? Tell me about your best work experience. Can you give me an example how you have worked with others to solve a problem? Decide in advance what information and skills are pertinent to the position and reveal your strengths. For example, you could say, "While I was at school, I learned to get along with a diverse group of people."
- Learn about the company. Be prepared; research the company or medical facility. What is the type of specialty? How many physicians are there?
- Dress appropriately. Because much communication is nonverbal, dressing appropriately for the interview is important. In most situations, you will be safe if you wear clean, pressed, conservative business clothes in neutral colors. Do not wear current fashions or fad clothing to an interview. Pay special attention to grooming. Keep makeup light, and wear little jewelry. Make sure that your hair and nails are clean and styled conservatively. Do not carry a large purse, backpack, books, coat, or hat. Leave extra clothing in an outside office, and simply carry a pen, your portfolio with extra copies of your résumé, and a small pad for taking notes.
- Be punctual. A good first impression is important and can be lasting. If you arrive late for the interview, a prospective employer may conclude that you will be late in arriving to work. Make certain you know the location and the time of the interview. Allow time for traffic, parking, and other preliminaries.
- Be professional. Being too familiar in your manner can be a barrier to a professional interview. Never call anyone by his or her first name unless you are asked to. Know the interviewer's title and the pronunciation of his or her name. Do not sit down until the interviewer does.
- Exhibit appropriate interview behavior. Always greet the interviewer with a smile. The interview is an opportunity to sell yourself to the employer. Offer your hand for a firm, confident handshake, and be alert to the interviewer's body language. The flow of conversation during an interview should be natural. Maintain eye contact, pay attention to the interviewer, and show interest. Ask intelligent questions that you have prepared before the interview. Remember, the interview is an opportunity for both the prospective employer and the prospective employee to gather information and make a good impression. In addition to reviewing the experience listed on your résumé, the interviewer will evaluate your personality and behavior. At the same time, you will be observing the office and learning more about the position. Try to be aware of the office's atmosphere, its equipment and supplies, and the attitudes of the staff. Does it seem like a pleasant, professional place to work? Request a tour of the facility, and ask yourself if you would be happy in that work environment.
- Be poised and relaxed. Avoid nervous habits such as tapping your pencil, playing with your hair, or covering your mouth with your hand. Watch language such as "you know," "ah," "stuff like that." Use proper grammar and pronunciation as you talk with the interviewer—do not use slang. Do not smoke, chew gum, fidget, or bite your nails.
- Maintain comfortable eye contact. Look the interviewer in the eye and speak with confidence. Your eyes reveal much about you; use them to show interest, confidence, poise, and sincerity. Use other nonverbal techniques such as a firm handshake to reinforce your confidence.
- Relate your experience to the job. Use every question as an opportunity to show how your skills relate to the job. Use examples taken from school, previous jobs, your externship, volunteer work, leadership in student organizations, and personal experience to indicate that you have the personal qualities, aptitude, and skills needed for this job.
- Be honest. While it is important to be confident and stress your strengths, it is equally important to your sense of integrity to be honest. Dishonesty always catches up to you sooner or later. Someone will verify your background, so do not exaggerate your accomplishments, grade point average, or experience.
- Focus on how you can benefit the company. Don't ask about benefits, salary, or vacations until you are offered the job. During a first interview, try to show how you can contribute to the organization. Do not appear to be too eager to move up through the company or suggest that you are more interested in gaining experience than in contributing to the company.

PROCEDURE 36.2

Writing Thank-You Notes

Objective: To write an appropriate, professional thank-you note after an interview or externship

Materials: Paper; pen; dictionary; thesaurus; computer or word processor; #10 business envelope

Method

1. Write the letter within 2 days of the interview or completion of the externship. Begin by writing the date at the top of the letter.
2. Write the name of the person who interviewed you (or who was your mentor in the externship). Include credentials and title, such as Dr. or Director of Client Services. Write the complete address of the office or organization.
3. Start the letter with "Dear Dr., Mr., Mrs., Miss, or Ms. __________:"
4. In the first paragraph, thank the interviewer for his time and for granting the interview. Discuss some specific impressions, for example, "I found the interview and tour of the facilities an enjoyable experience. I would welcome the opportunity to work in such a state-of-the-art medical setting." If you are writing to thank your mentor for her time during your externship and for allowing you to perform your externship at her office, practice, or clinic, discuss the knowledge and experience you gained during the externship.
5. In the second paragraph, mention the aspects of the job or externship that you found most interesting or challenging. For a job interview thank-you note, state how your skills and qualifications will make you an asset to the staff. When preparing an externship thank-you letter, mention interest in any future positions.
6. In the last paragraph, thank the interviewer for considering you for the position. Ask to be contacted at his earliest convenience regarding his employment decision.
7. Close the letter with "Sincerely," and type your name. Leave enough space above your typewritten name to sign your name.
8. Type your return address in the upper left corner of the #10 business envelope. Then type the interviewer's name and address in the envelope's center, apply the proper postage, and mail the letter.

- Close the interview on a positive note. Thank the interviewer for his or her time, shake hands, and say that you are looking forward to hearing from him or her. On the way out of the office, thank the staff members involved in the interview. Ask for a business card from anyone whom you think you might want to send a thank-you note. After leaving the interview, write down any additional information you want to remember. Every interview provides you with information about the medical assisting profession. Even if an interview does not result in a job, you will have met new people, developed a larger network of professional contacts, and gained valuable interviewing experience.
- Follow up with a letter. After an interview, it is professional to send a thank-you letter to the person or persons from the company who conducted your interview. You should send this letter within two days of the interview. It may be brief, but it should express your appreciation for the opportunity to have met with the interviewer, reaffirm your interest in the organization, and state your desire to remain a part of the selection process. By sending a thank-you letter, you display common business courtesy, which can make a difference in the employer's hiring decision. Even if you are not interested in continuing the interview and selection process, you should thank the employer for holding the interview. Procedure 36-2 explains how to write and send a thank-you letter.
- Complete an application. Some employers ask you to complete an employment application at an interview even when you provide a résumé. You can use your résumé to help you complete the application. Fill out the application neatly. Spell all words correctly, and read and follow the instructions on the form carefully. Your application represents you; it must make a good first impression. Fill in all sections of the application—do not write "see résumé." An example of an application is shown in Figure 36-9.
- Comply with other aspects of the application process. As part of the application process, employers are required by federal law to request documents that prove your identity and eligibility to work in the United States. To maintain the safety and confidentiality of the medical office, hospital, or laboratory, employers may also check your police record, credit rating, and history of chemical or alcohol abuse. A drug screen

Date Called	Type of Work Applied For	Appointment Date	Appointment Time	Reschedule Date	Reschedule Time	Avail-ability	No Phone	GR	PC	Creden-tials	Pay Rate	Surplus Skill

Last Name	First	M.I.	Applicant Profile	Service Code	Pay Rate	Last Hiring Process Step

Address

City — State — Zip Code

Telephone No. — Social Security No. — Today's Date

Please print. Do not complete shaded areas.

EMPLOYMENT APPLICATION

EQUAL OPPORTUNITY EMPLOYER

KELLY Assisted Living®

FOR SUPERVISOR USE ONLY

Are you at least 18? ☐YES ☐NO

Are you familiar with the way a temporary help service works? *(Explain to applicant)* ☐YES ☐NO

Have you ever worked for a temporary help service? ☐YES ☐NO

Did you work for Kelly Assisted Living Services? ☐YES ☐NO

Where? ______

How long ago? ______

When could you start working for us? ______

How long do you plan to work on a temporary basis?

Can you work Monday through Friday? ☐YES ☐NO

Can you work Saturday? ☐YES ☐NO

Can you work Sunday? ☐YES ☐NO

Are you available ☐DAYS ☐EVENINGS ☐NIGHTS

Are you available as a Live-in? ☐YES ☐NO

What hours are you available? From______ To______

What form of transportation would you usually use to get to work? *(Car, Public transportation, Other)*

Did you bring your professional credentials with you today? ☐YES ☐NO ☐NONE REQUIRED

Check ☑ T if Trained; ☑ E if Experienced; ☑ T and E if Trained and Experienced.

T	E		T	E	
☐	☐	Home Health Aide	☐	☐	Other health-related positions
☐	☐	Homemaker			*Specify:* ______
☐	☐	Nurse Aide			______
☐	☐	Registered Nurse			______
☐	☐	Licensed Practical Nurse or Licensed Vocational Nurse			______

Do you have experience as a Live-in? ☐YES ☐NO

Check ☑ where work experience was obtained.

☐ Hospital ☐ Home ☐ Industry

☐ Nursing Home ☐ Clinic/Office ☐ Other ______

☐ Community Health

PRINTED IN U.S.A. 816 R9/90

Figure 36-9. Job applicants are often asked to fill out an application form like the one shown here. (Reprinted with permission from Kelly Assisted Living Services, Inc.)

may be requested. You may be asked to provide the needed documents or to give the employer authorization to obtain them.

Interview Questions

In order to prepare for your interview, you can anticipate that you may be asked any of the following questions:

- I see from your résumé that you graduated from ABC School. What did that school have to offer you that others did not?
- What is your five-year goal?
- Tell me about yourself.
- What do you consider to be your greatest strengths and weaknesses?
- How would your instructors describe you?
- What qualifications do you have that make you a good candidate for this position?
- How could you make a contribution to this facility?
- How well do you work with others?
- What is your concept of a team environment?
- How well do you work under pressure?
- Will you be able to work overtime?
- Do you have the flexibility to work various shifts?
- What has been your major accomplishment to date?
- Why did you choose medical assisting as your career?
- Do you have any questions that you would like to ask?

It is helpful to be prepared with any questions that you may have for the interviewer about the position or the facility. Questions about salary and benefits are not appropriate in a first interview.

An interviewer may ask you questions that you are not obligated to answer. These questions refer to age, race, sexual orientation, marital status, or number of children. Even if the questions sound harmless or the interviewer seems nonjudgmental, these questions have nothing to do with your skills or abilities. If the interviewer asks even one of these questions, you should reconsider whether you want to work for the organization.

If you are asked an inappropriate question during an interview, be polite and remain professional in declining to answer. You may simply state that you do not believe the requested information is necessary for the employer to evaluate your qualifications for the job. Try to move the discussion onto a more relevant topic.

Reasons for Not Being Hired

Employers in business were asked to list reasons for not hiring a job candidate. The 15 biggest complaints are the following:

1. Poor appearance, not being dressed properly, and being poorly groomed
2. Acting like a know-it-all
3. Not communicating clearly as well as poor voice, diction, and grammar
4. Lack of planning for the interview, with no purpose or goals communicated
5. Lack of confidence or poise
6. No interest in or enthusiasm for the job
7. Not being active in extracurricular school programs
8. Being interested only in the best salary offer
9. Poor school record, either in academics, attendance, or both
10. Unwillingness to begin in an entry-level position
11. Making excuses about an unfavorable record
12. No tact
13. No maturity
14. No curiosity about the job
15. Being critical of past employers

Salary Negotiations

Medical assisting salaries are varied and differ by geographic area. When you are a new graduate, you will begin your career as an entry-level medical assistant. As you gain experience, your compensation will reflect that. Salary ranges are determined by geographic location, medical specialty, years of experience, credentialing, and the job description.

The first step in determining your compensation needs is to know how much income is required to meet your living expenses. You will need to prepare a budget. Keep track of your overall expenditures and living expenses. Itemizing your basic living expenses can help you to prepare a budget. These living expenses can include:

- Rent
- Car payments or anticipated car payments
- Car insurance
- Food
- Utilities
- Student loans
- Credit cards
- Clothing
- Child care
- Other

Establishing a budget will give you an idea of the amount of income you may need. Once your budget is established, you have a negotiating benchmark. Employers will often ask you what you are looking for with regard to salary. If you answer directly, you may risk either quoting yourself out of a job or leaving money on the table. The best response to this question is to ask the employer the range of the position. Most positions have a low-to-high range. For example, the range for a specific position could be between $23,000 and $32,000 annually. Once you know the range, quote a little higher than what your budgetary amount is, which will give the employer room to negotiate down if necessary. Allow the employer to bring up salary first.

On the Job

Once you have a job, you must learn how to be an effective employee. There are many ways that your initiative enables the medical team in the office, hospital, clinic, or laboratory to function effectively. You must identify the important skills in your daily duties, stay competitive and marketable through continuing education, and integrate constructive criticism from your employee evaluations into your daily work and annual goals.

Employee Evaluations

Employee evaluations are usually held annually. An initial employment review generally occurs after a probationary period of 90 days. Evaluations describe an employee's performance. A completed evaluation is placed in an official record of employment. In most situations, the employee and the employer meet to discuss the employee's performance. The purpose of an annual evaluation should be to check the goals and values of both the employer and the employee to make sure they support each other.

An employee evaluation form typically outlines the most important qualities and abilities needed for the job. It evaluates the employee's strengths and weaknesses. This form may help determine whether an employee is worthy of a merit raise, which is a raise based on performance (as opposed to a cost-of-living raise). The quantity and quality of work are assessed on this form, as are initiative, judgment, and cooperation.

Continuing Education

After completing a medical assisting program, you should continue your education, setting specific educational advancement goals on a yearly basis. For example, you may decide to obtain further education to learn more about the medical specialty in which you work.

As medical research expands its discoveries and as new technologies emerge, the necessity for self-education increases. You must read to stay abreast of updates in medicine. The need for more highly specialized training presents you with an opportunity for growth in your education and career. Medical publications are the best source for the latest medical information (Figure 36-10). Local and state

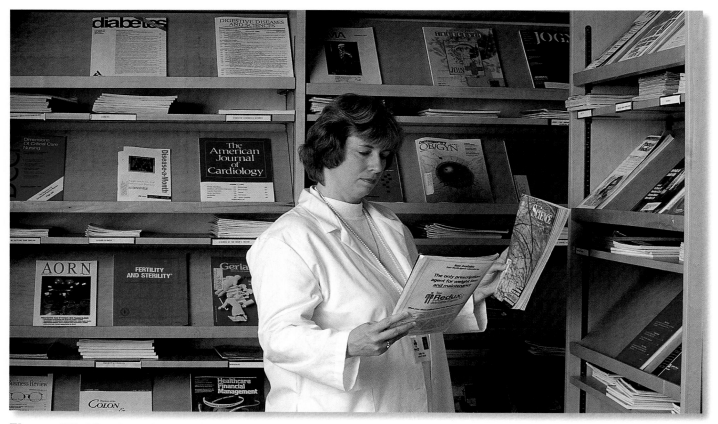

Figure 36-10. Part of self-education involves reading articles in professional and lay magazines about topics that relate to the medical practice in which you work.

medical assisting meetings also provide information about advances in the field. The Internet is a valuable source for staying current about today's technological advances.

Self-education is an important skill for the medical assistant. Stay up-to-date in topics about medicine, health care, wellness, insurance products, and pharmaceuticals. Patients may ask questions about information they have read or about the effectiveness of certain new treatments.

Summary

Medical assisting is an exciting field with many opportunities available to you. It is important to realize that the career phase begins with the externship and will continue for the duration of your career. Your résumé will be a lifelong document that summarizes your career endeavors. Your professionalism will become your reputation, and employment offers may cross your path even if you are not actively seeking them. Continuing education and credentialing will enhance your career, so you should make education and credentialing your short-term goal after completing your medical assisting program.

The profession of medical assisting allows you many directions to take your career and will enable you to make many career changes within this profession. For example, you may choose academics and teaching future medical assistants, or you may choose to pursue customer service or management positions in different areas within health care. Because medical assisting is one of the fastest-growing occupations, if you manage your career with professionalism and diligence and continue to learn, you will have many options for satisfying and successful employment.

REVIEW

CHAPTER 36

CASE STUDY QUESTIONS

Now that you have completed this chapter, review the case study at the beginning of the chapter and answer the following questions:

1. What should Sarah do about the ear irrigation?
2. How has she remembered all the previous procedures and not this one?
3. Will the clinical preceptor be disappointed or angry with her?

Discussion Questions

1. What specialty of medicine would provide an overall, well-rounded externship experience?
2. What accreditation does your school have, and how long is the externship requirement?
3. Describe constructive criticism.
4. List some ways in which you can become more confident in interviewing.

Critical Thinking Questions

1. Describe an effective medical assistant, and explain two ways that a new medical assistant can learn to be an efficient and effective employee.
2. What are among the most important skills a prospective employer seeks?
3. What is the best résumé type for a new graduate of a medical assisting program?

Application Activities

1. Bring in current classified advertisements from your local newspaper. Highlight all the positions that a medical assistant is qualified for. Discuss the different positions and describe how your qualifications would benefit the organization.
2. Stage mock interviews in your class in which the instructor interviews each student and the classmates critique the interview. Have students look for poise, confidence, and the ability to answer open-ended questions.
3. Invite a local recruiter to talk about interviewing skills. Stage an interview between the instructor and the recruiter. The instructor should behave in ways that are inappropriate for an interview. Write a paper describing what was wrong with the interview.
4. Practice answering interview questions in front of a mirror. Take a personal inventory of what you see. Write a one-page paper describing areas that need improvement as well as your best answers to interview questions.

APPENDIX I

Medical Assistant Role Delineation Chart

Administrative

Administrative Procedures

- Perform basic administrative medical assisting functions
- Schedule, coordinate, and monitor appointments
- Schedule inpatient/outpatient admissions and procedures
- Understand and apply third-party guidelines
- Obtain reimbursement through accurate claims submission
- Monitor third-party reimbursement
- Understand and adhere to managed care policies and procedures

* *Negotiate managed care contracts*

Practice Finances

- Perform procedural and diagnostic coding
- Apply bookkeeping principles
- Manage accounts receivable

* *Manage accounts payable*
* *Process payroll*
* *Document and maintain accounting and banking records*
* *Develop and maintain fee schedules*
* *Manage renewals of business and professional insurance policies*
* *Manage personnel benefits and maintain records*
* *Perform marketing, financial, and stragetic planning*

Clinical

Fundamental Principles

- Apply principles of aseptic technique and infection control
- Comply with quality assurance practices
- Screen and follow up patient test results

Diagnostic Orders

- Collect and process specimens
- Perform diagnostic tests

Patient Care

- Adhere to established patient screening procedures
- Obtain patient history and vital signs
- Prepare and maintain examination and treatment areas
- Prepare patient for examinations, procedures, and treatments
- Assist with examinations, procedures, and treatments
- Prepare and administer medications and immunizations
- Maintain medication and immunization records
- Recognize and respond to emergencies
- Coordinate patient care information with other health-care providers
- Initiate IV and administer IV medications with appropriate training and as permitted by state law

General

Professionalism

- Display a professional manner and image
- Demonstrate initiative and responsibility
- Work as a member of the health-care team
- Prioritize and perform multiple tasks
- Adapt to change
- Promote the CMA credential
- Enhance skills through continuing education
- Treat all patients with compassion and empathy
- Promote the practice through positive public relations

Communication Skills

- Recognize and respect cultural diversity
- Adapt communications to individual's ability to understand
- Use professional telephone technique
- Recognize and respond effectively to verbal, nonverbal, and written communications
- Use medical terminology appropriately
- Utilize electronic technology to receive, organize, prioritize, and transmit information
- Serve as liaison

Legal Concepts

- Perform within legal and ethical boundaries
- Prepare and maintain medical records
- Document accurately
- Follow employer's established policies dealing with the health-care contract
- Implement and maintain federal and state health-care legislation and regulations
- Comply with established risk management and safety procedures
- Recognize professional credentialing criteria
- * *Develop and maintain personnel, policy, and procedure manuals*

Instruction

- Instruct individuals according to their needs
- Explain office policies and procedures
- Teach methods of health promotion and disease prevention
- Locate community resources and disseminate information
- * *Develop educational materials*
- * *Conduct continuing education activities*

Operational Functions

- Perform inventory of supplies and equipment
- Perform routine maintenance of administrative and clinical equipment
- Apply computer techniques to support office operations
- * *Perform personnel management functions*
- * *Negotiate leases and prices for equipment and supply contracts*

* Denotes advanced skills

Source: This chart is part of the "AAMA Role Delineation Study: Occupational Analysis of the Medical Assisting Profession," released by the American Association of Medical Assistants in June 2003.

APPENDIX II

Prefixes and Suffixes Commonly Used in Medical Terms

a-, an- without, not
ab- from, away
ad-, -ad to, toward
adeno- gland, glandular
aero- air
-aesthesia sensation
-al characterized by
-algia pain
ambi-, amph-, amphi- both, on both sides, around
andr-, andro- man, male
angio- blood vessel
ano- anus
ante- before
antero- in front of
anti- against, opposing
arterio- artery
arthro- joint
-ase enzyme
-asthenia weakness
auto- self
bi- twice, double
bili- bile
bio- life
blasto-, -blast developing stage, bud
brachy- short
brady- slow
broncho- bronchial (windpipe)
cardio- heart
cata- down, lower, under
-cele swelling, tumor
-centesis puncture, tapping
centi- hundred
cephal-, cephalo- head
cerebr-, cerebro- brain
chol-, chole-, cholo- gall
chondro- cartilage
chromo- color
-cidal killing
-cide causing death
circum- around
-cise cut
co-, com-, con- together, with
-coele cavity
colo- colon
colp-, colpo- vagina
contra- against
cost-, costo- rib
crani-, cranio- skull
cryo- cold
cysto-, -cyst bladder, bag
-cyte, cyto- cell, cellular
dacry-, dacryo- tears, lacrimal apparatus
dactyl-, dactylo- finger, toe
de- down, from
deca- ten
deci- tenth
demi- half
dent-, denti-, dento- teeth
derma-, dermat-, dermato-, -derm skin
dextro- to the right
di- double, twice
dia- through, apart, between
dipla-, diplo- double, twin
dis- apart, away from
dorsi-, dorso- back
dynia- pain
dys- difficult, painful, bad, abnormal
e-, ec-, ecto- away, from, without, outside
-ectomy cutting out, surgical removal
em-, en- in, into, inside
-emesis vomiting
-emia blood
encephalo- brain
endo- within, inside
entero- intestine
ento- within, inner
epi- on, above
erythro- red
esthesio-, -esthesia sensation
eu- good, true, normal
ex-, exo- outside of, beyond, without
extra- outside of, beyond, in addition
fibro- connective tissue
fore- before, in front of
-form shape
-fuge driving away
galact-, galacto- milk
gastr-, gastro- stomach
-gene, -genic, -genetic, -genous arising from, origin, formation
glosso- tongue
gluco-, glyco- sugar, sweet
-gram recorded information
-graph instrument for recording
-graphy the process of recording
-gravida pregnant female
gyn-, gyno-, gyne-, gyneco- woman, female
haemo-, hemato-, hem-, hemo- blood
hemi- half
hepa-, hepar-, hepato- liver
herni- rupture
hetero- other, unlike
histo- tissue
homeo, homo- same, like
hydra-, hydro- water
hyper- above, over, increased, excessive
hypo- below, under, decreased
hyster-, hystero- uterus
-ia condition
-iasis condition of
-ic, -ical pertaining to
ictero- jaundice
idio- personal, self-produced
ileo- ileum
im-, in-, ir- not
in- in, into
infra- beneath
inter- between, among
intra-, intro- into, within, during
-ism condition, process, theory
-itis inflammation of
-ium membrane
-ize to cause to be, to become, to treat by special method
juxta- near, nearby
karyo- nucleus, nut
kata-, kath- down, lower, under
kera-, kerato- horn, hardness, cornea
kineto-, -kinesis, -kinetic motion
lact- milk
laparo- abdomen
latero- side
-lepsis, -lepsy seizure, convulsion
leuco-, leuko- white
levo- to the left
lipo- fat
lith-, -lith stone
-logy science of, study of
-lysis setting free, disintegration, decomposition
macro- large, long
mal- bad
-malacia abnormal softening
-mania insanity, abnormal desire
mast-, masto- breast
med-, medi- middle
mega-, megalo- large, great
meio- contraction
melan-, melano- black
meno- month
mes-, meso- middle
meta- beyond

-meter measure
metro-, metra- uterus
-metry process of measuring
micro- small
mio- smaller, less
mono- single, one
multi- many
my-, myo- muscle
myel-, myelo- marrow
narco- sleep
nas-, naso- nose
necro- dead
neo- new
nephr-, nephro- kidney
neu-, neuro- nerve
niter-, nitro- nitrogen
non-, not- no
nucleo- nucleus
-nuli none
ob- against
oculo- eye
odont- tooth
-odynia pain
-oid resembling
-ole small, little
olig-, oligo- few, less than normal
-oma tumor
onco- tumor
oo- ovum, egg
oophor- ovary
ophthalmo- eye
-opia vision
-opsy to view
orchid- testicle
ortho- straight
os- mouth, bone
-osis disease, condition of
oste-, osteo- bone
-ostomy to make a mouth, opening
oto- ear
-otomy incision, surgical cutting
-ous having
oxy- sharp, acid
pachy- thick
paedo, pedo- child
pan- all, every
par; para- alongside of, with; woman who has given birth
path-, patho-, -pathy disease, suffering
ped-, pedi-, pedo- foot
-penia too few, lack, decreased
per- through, excessive
peri- around
pes- foot
-pexy surgical fixation
phag-, phagia, phago-, -phage eating, consuming, swallowing
pharyng- throat, pharynx
phlebo- vein
-phobia fear, abnormal fear
-phylaxis protection
-plasia formation or development
-plastic molded
-plasty operation to reconstruct, surgical repair
-plegia paralysis
pleuro- side, rib
pluri- more, several
pneo-, -pnea breathing
pneumo- air, lungs
-pod foot
poly- many, much
post- after, behind
pre-, pro- before, in front of
presby-, presbyo- old age
primi- first
procto- rectum
proto- first
pseudo- false
psych- the mind
pulmon-, pulmono- lung
pyelo- pelvis (renal)
pyo- pus
pyro- fever, heat
quadri- four
re- back, again
reni-, reno- kidney
retro- backward, behind
rhino- nose
-rrhage, -rrhagia abnormal or excessive discharge, hemorrhage, flow
-rrhaphy suture of
-rrhea flow, discharge
sacchar- sugar
sacro- sacrum
salpingo- tube, fallopian tube
sarco- flesh
sclero- hard, sclera
-sclerosis hardening
-scopy examining
semi- half
septi-, septic-, septico- poison, infection
-spasm cramp or twitching
-stasis stoppage
steno- contracted, narrow
stereo- firm, solid, three-dimensional
stomato- mouth
-stomy opening
sub- under
super-, supra- above, upon, excess
sym-, syn- with, together
tachy- fast
tele- distant, far
teno-, tenoto- tendon
tetra- four
-therapy treatment
thermo-, -thermy heat
thio- sulfur
thoraco- chest
thrombo- blood clot
thyro- thyroid gland
-tome cutting instrument
tomo-, -tomy incision, section
trans- across
tri- three
-tripsy surgical crushing
tropho-, -trophy nutrition, growth
-tropy turning, tendency
ultra- beyond, excess
uni- one
-uria urine
urino-, uro- urine, urinary organs
utero- uterus, uterine
vaso- vessel
ventri-, ventro- abdomen
xanth- yellow

APPENDIX III

Latin and Greek Equivalents Commonly Used in Medical Terms

abdomen venter
adhesion adhaesio
and et
arm brachium; brachion (Gr*)
artery arteria
back dorsum
backbone spina
backward retro; opistho (Gr)
bend flexus
bile bilis; chole (Gr)
bladder vesica, cystus
blister vesicula
blood sanguis; haima (Gr)
body corpus; soma (Gr)
bone os, ossis; osteon (Gr)
brain encephalon
break ruptura
breast mamma; mastos (Gr)
buttock gloutos (Gr)
cartilage cartilago; chondros (Gr)
cavity cavum
chest pectoris, pectus; thorax (Gr)
child puer, puerilis
choke strangulo
corn clavus
cornea kerat (Gr)
cough tussis
deadly lethalis
death mors
dental dentalis
digestive pepticos
disease morbus
dislocation luxatio
doctor medicus
dose dosis (Gr)
ear auris; ous (Gr)
egg ovum
erotic erotikos (Gr)
exhalation exhalatio, expiro
external externus
extract extractum
eye oculus; ophthalmos (Gr)
eyelid palpebra
face facies
fat adeps; lipos (Gr)
female femella
fever febris
finger (or toe) digitus
flesh carnis, caro
foot pes
forehead frons
gum gingiva
hair capillus, pilus; thrix (Gr)
hand manus; cheir (Gr)
harelip labrum fissum; cheiloschisis (Gr)
head caput; kephale (Gr)
health sanitas
hear audire
heart cor; kardia (Gr)
heat calor; therme (Gr)
heel calx, talus
hysterics hysteria
infant infans
infectious contagiosus
injection injectio
intellect intellectus
internal internus
intestine intestinum; enteron (Gr)
itching pruritis
jawbone maxilla
joint vertebra; arthron (Gr)
kidney ren, renis; nephros (Gr)
knee genu
kneecap patella
lacerate lacerare
larynx guttur
lateral lateralis
limb membrum
lip labium, labrum; cheilos (Gr)
listen auscultare
liver jecur; hepar (Gr)
loin lapara
looseness laxativus
lung pulmo; pneumon (Gr)
male masculinus
malignant malignons
milk lac
moisture humiditas
month mensis
monthly menstruus
mouth oris, os; stoma, stomato (Gr)
nail unguis; onyx (Gr)
navel umbilicus; omphalos (Gr)
neck cervix; trachelos (Gr)
nerve nervus; neuron (Gr)
nipple papilla; thele (Gr)
no, none nullus
nose nasus; rhis (Gr)
nostril naris
nourishment alimentum
ointment unguentum
pain dolor; algia
patient patiens
pectoral pectoralis
pimple pustula
poison venenum
powder pulvis
pregnant praegnans, gravida
pubic bone os pubis
pupil pupilla
rash exanthema (Gr)
recover convalescere
redness rubor
rib costa
ringing tinnitus
scaly squamosus
sciatica sciaticus; ischiadikos (Gr)
seed semen
senile senilis
sheath vagina; theke (Gr)
short brevis; brachys (Gr)
shoulder omos (Gr)
shoulder blade scapula
side latus
skin cutis; derma (Gr)
skull cranium; kranion (Gr)
sleep somnus
solution solutio
spinal spinalis
stomach stomachus; gaster (Gr)
stone calculus
sugar saccharum
swallow glutio
tail cauda
taste gustatio
tear lacrima
testicle testis; orchis (Gr)
thigh femur
throat fauces; pharynx (Gr)
tongue lingua; glossa (Gr)
tooth dens; odontos (Gr)
touch tactus
tremor tremere
twin gemellus
ulcer ulcus
urine urina; ouran (Gr)
uterus hystera (Gr)
vagina vagina; kolpos (Gr)
vein vena; phlebos, phleps (Gr)
vertebra spondylos (Gr)
vessel vas
wash diluere
water aqua
wax cera
weak debilis
windpipe arteria aspera
wrist carpus; karpos (Gr)

* Parenthetical "Gr" means the preceding term is Greek. Other terms in the column are Latin.

APPENDIX IV
Abbreviations Commonly Used in Medical Notations

a before
a.c. before meals
AD right ear
ADD attention deficit disorder
ADL activities of daily living
ad lib as desired
ADT admission, discharge, transfer
AIDS acquired immunodeficiency syndrome
a.m.a. against medical advice
AMA American Medical Association
amp. ampule
amt amount
aq., AQ water; aqueous
AS left ear
ausc. auscultation
AU both ears
ax axis
Bib, bib drink
b.i.d., bid, BID twice a day
BM bowel movement
BP, B/P blood pressure
BPC blood pressure check
BPH benign prostatic hypertrophy
BSA body surface area
c., c̄ with
Ca calcium; cancer
cap, caps capsules
CBC complete blood (cell) count
cc cubic centimeter
C.C., CC chief complaint
CDC Centers for Disease Control and Prevention
CHF congestive heart failure
chr chronic
CNS central nervous system
Comp, comp compound
COPD chronic obstructive pulmonary disease
CP chest pain
CPE complete physical examination
CPR cardiopulmonary resuscitation
CSF cerebrospinal fluid
CT computed tomography
CV cardiovascular
d day
d/c, D/C discontinue, discharge
D & C dilation and curettage
DEA Drug Enforcement Administration
Dil, dil dilute
DM diabetes mellitus
DOB date of birth
DTP diptheria-tetanus-pertussis vaccine
Dr. doctor
DTs delirium tremens
D/W dextrose in water
Dx, dx diagnosis
ECG, EKG electrocardiogram
ED emergency department
EEG electroencephalogram
EENT eyes, ears, nose, and throat
EP established patient
ER emergency room
ESR erythrocyte sedimentation rate
FBS fasting blood sugar
FDA Food and Drug Administration
FH family history
Fl, fl, fld fluid
F/u follow-up
Fx fracture
GBS gallbladder series
GI gastrointestinal
Gm gram
gr grain
gt, gtt drops
GTT glucose tolerance test
GU genitourinary
GYN gynecology
HB, Hgb hemoglobin
HEENT head, ears, eyes, nose, throat
HIV human immunodeficiency virus
HO history of
h.s., hs, HS hour of sleep/at bedtime
Hx history
ICU intensive care unit
I & D incision and drainage
I & O intake and output
IM intramuscular
inf. infusion; inferior
inj injection
IT inhalation therapy
IUD intrauterine device
IV intravenous
KUB kidneys, ureters, bladder
L1, L2, etc. lumbar vertebrae
lab laboratory
liq liquid
LLL left lower lobe
LLQ left lower quadrant
LMP last menstrual period
LUQ left upper quadrant
MI myocardial infarction
MM mucous membrane
MRI magnetic resonance imaging
MS multiple sclerosis
NB newborn
NED no evidence of disease
no. number
noc, noct night
npo, NPO nothing by mouth
NPT new patient
NS normal saline
NSAID nonsteroidal anti-inflammatory drug
NTP normal temperature and pressure
N & V nausea and vomiting
NYD not yet diagnosed
OB obstetrics
OC oral contraceptive
o.d. once a day
OD overdose
O.D., OD right eye
oint ointment
OOB out of bed
OPD outpatient department
OPS outpatient services
OR operating room
O.S., OS left eye
OTC over-the-counter
O.U., OU both eyes
P & P Pap smear (Papanicolaou smear) and pelvic examination
PA posteroanterior
Pap Pap smear
Path pathology
p.c., pc after meals
PE physical examination
per by, with
PH past history
PID pelvic inflammatory disease
p/o postoperative
POMR problem-oriented medical record
PMFSH past medical, family, social history
PMS premenstrual syndrome
p.r.n., prn, PRN whenever necessary
Pt patient
PT physical therapy
PTA prior to admission
PVC premature ventricular contraction
pulv powder
q. every
q2, q2h every 2 hours
q.a.m., qam every morning

q.d., qd every day
q.h., qh every hour
qhs every night, at bedtime
q.i.d., QID four times a day
qns, QNS quantity not sufficient
qod every other day
qs, QS quantity sufficient
RA rheumatoid arthritis; right atrium
RBC red blood cells; red blood (cell) count
RDA recommended dietary allowance, recommended daily allowance
REM rapid eye movement
RF rheumatoid factor
RLL right lower lobe
RLQ right lower quadrant
R/O rule out
ROM range of motion
ROS/SR review of systems/systems review
RUQ right upper quadrant
RV right ventricle
Rx prescription, take
SAD seasonal affective disorder
s.c., SC, SQ, subq, SubQ subcutaneously
SIDS sudden infant death syndrome
Sig directions
sig sigmoidoscopy
SOAP subjective, objective, assessment, plan
SOB shortness of breath
sol solution
S/R suture removal
ss, $\overline{\text{ss}}$ one-half
Staph staphylococcus
stat, STAT immediately
STD sexually transmitted disease
Strep streptococcus
subling, SL sublingual
surg surgery
S/W saline in water
SX symptoms
T1, T2, etc. thoracic vertebrae
T & A tonsillectomy and adenoidectomy
tab tablet
TB tuberculosis
TBS, tbs. tablespoon
TIA transient ischemic attack
t.i.d., tid, TID three times a day
tinc, tinct, tr tincture
TMJ temporomandibular joint
top topically
TPR temperature, pulse, and respiration
tsp teaspoon
TSH thyroid stimulating hormone
Tx treatment
U unit
UA urinalysis
UCHD usual childhood diseases
UGI upper gastrointestinal
ung, ungt ointment
URI upper respiratory infection
US ultrasound
UTI urinary tract infection
VA visual acuity
VD venereal disease
Vf visual field
VS vital signs
WBC white blood cells; white blood (cell) count
WNL within normal limits
wt weight
y/o year old

APPENDIX V

Symbols Commonly Used in Medical Notations

Apothecaries' Weights and Measures

♏ minim
℈ scruple
ʒ dram
fʒ fluidram
℥ ounce
f℥ fluidounce
O pint
℔ pound

Other Weights and Measures

pounds
° degrees
′ foot; minute
″ inch; second
μm micrometer
μ micron (former term for micrometer)
mμ millimicron; nanometer
μg microgram
mEq milliequivalent
mL milliliter
dL deciliter
mg% milligrams percent; milligrams per 100 mL

Abbreviations

$\overline{aa}$, $\overline{AA}$ of each
$\bar{c}$ with
M mix (Latin *misce*)
m- meta-
o- ortho-
p- para-
$\bar{p}$ after
$\bar{s}$ without
ss, $\overline{ss}$ one-half (Latin *semis*)

Mathematical Functions and Terms

number
\+ plus; positive; acid reaction
− minus; negative; alkaline reaction
± plus or minus; either positive or negative; indefinite
× multiply; magnification; crossed with, hybrid
÷, / divided by
= equal to
≈ approximately equal to
> greater than; from which is derived
< less than; derived from
≮ not less than
≯ not greater than
≤ equal to or less than
≥ equal to or greater than
≠ not equal to
√ square root
$\sqrt[3]{}$ cube root
∞ infinity
: ratio; "is to"
∴ therefore
% percent
π pi (3.14159)—the ratio of circumference of a circle to its diameter

Chemical Notations

Δ change; heat
⇌ reversible reaction
↑ increase
↓ decrease

Warnings

Ⓒ Schedule I controlled substance
Ⓒ (II) Schedule II controlled substance
Ⓒ (III) Schedule III controlled substance
Ⓒ (IV) Schedule IV controlled substance
Ⓒ (V) Schedule V controlled substance
☠ poison
☢ radiation
☣ biohazard

Others

℞ prescription; take
□, ♂ male
○, ♀ female
ṫ one
ṫṫ two
ṫṫṫ three

APPENDIX VI

Professional Organizations and Agencies

American Academy of Dental Practice Administrators
1063 Whippoorwill Lane
Palatine, IL 60067
(312) 934-4404

American Academy of Medical Administrators
30555 Southfield Road, Suite 150
Southfield, MI 48076
(313) 540-4310

American Academy of Ophthalmology
655 Beach Street
San Francisco, CA 94109
(415) 561-8500

American Academy of Pediatrics
PO Box 927
Elk Grove, IL 60009-0927
(708) 228-5005

American Association for Medical Transcription
PO Box 576187
Modesto, CA 95355
(209) 527-9620

American Association for Respiratory Care
11030 Ables Lane
Dallas, TX 75229
(214) 243-2272

American Association of Medical Assistants
20 N. Wacker Drive, Suite 1575
Chicago, IL 60606
(312) 899-1500

American Cancer Society
777 Third Avenue
New York, NY 10017
(212) 586-8700

American College of Cardiology
9111 Old Georgetown Road
Bethesda, MD 20814
(301) 897-5400

American College of Physicians
2011 Pennsylvania Avenue, NW
Washington, DC 20006
(202) 261-4500

American Diabetes Association
Two Park Avenue
New York, NY 10016
(212) 683-7444

American Dietetic Association
216 West Jackson Boulevard, Suite 800
Chicago, IL 60606-6995
(800) 366-1655

American Health Information Management Association
(formerly the American Medical Record Association)
233 N. Michigan Avenue, Suite 2150
Chicago, IL 60601-5800
(312) 233-1100

American Heart Association
National Center
7272 Greenville Avenue
Dallas, TX 75231-4596
(800) 242-8721, or call your local center

American Hospital Association
One North Franklin, Suite 2706
Chicago, IL 60606
(312) 422-3000

American Lung Association
1740 Broadway
New York, NY 10019
(212) 315-8700

American Medical Association
Division of Allied Health Education and Accreditation
515 North State Street
Chicago, IL 60610
(312) 464-5000

American Medical Technologists
710 Higgins Road
Park Ridge, IL 60068
(847) 823-5169

American Occupational Therapy Association
4720 Montgomery Lane
PO Box 31220
Bethesda, MD 20824-1220
(301) 948-9626

American Pharmacists Association
2215 Constitution Avenue, NW
Washington, DC 20037-2985
(202) 628-4410

American Physical Therapy Association
1111 North Fairfax Street
Alexandria, VA 22314
(703) 684-2782

American Red Cross
17th and D Streets, NW
Washington, DC 20006
(202) 728-6400, or call your local chapter

American Red Cross
HIV/AIDS Education, Health and Safety Services
8111 Gatehouse Road, 6th Floor
Falls Church, VA 22042
(703) 206-7180

American Society for Cardiovascular Professionals
120 Falcon Drive, Unit 3
Fredericksburg, VA 22408
(540) 891-0079

American Society for Clinical Laboratory Science
7910 Woodmont Avenue, Suite 1301
Bethesda, MD 20814
(301) 657-2768

American Society of Clinical Pathologists
2100 West Harrison Street
Chicago, IL 60612
(312) 738-1336

American Society of Hand Therapists
401 North Michigan Avenue
Chicago, IL 60611
(312) 321-6866

American Society of Phlebotomy Technicians
PO Box 1831
Hickory, NC 28603
(704) 322-1334

American Society of Radiologic Technologists
15000 Central Avenue SE
Albuquerque, NM 87123
(505) 298-4500

The Arthritis Foundation
1314 Spring Street, NW
Atlanta, GA 30309
(404) 872-7100

Association of Surgical Technologists
7108-C South Alton Way
Englewood, CO 80112
(303) 694-9130

Association of Technical Personnel in Ophthalmology
50 Lee Road
Chestnut Hill, MA 02167
(617) 232-4433

Asthma and Allergy Foundation of America
1717 Massachusetts Avenue, Suite 305
Washington, DC 20036
(202) 265-0265

International Society for Clinical Laboratory Technology
818 Olive Street, Suite 918
St. Louis, MO 63101
(314) 241-1445

Joint Commission on Allied Health Personnel in Ophthalmology
2025 Woodlane Drive
St. Paul, MN 55125-2995
(800) 284-3937

Medical Group Management Association
104 Inverness Terrace East
Englewood Cliffs, CA 80112
(313) 799-1111

National Accrediting Agency for Clinical Laboratory Services
8410 West Bryn Mawr Avenue, Suite 670
Chicago, IL 60631
(312) 714-8880

National AIDS Hotline
215 Park Avenue South, Suite 714
New York, NY 10003
(800) 342-AIDS
(800) 344-SIDA (Spanish)

National Association of Medical Staff Services
PO Box 23590
Knoxville, TN 37933-1590
(615) 531-3571

National Cancer Institute
9000 Rockville Pike
Building 31, Room 10A18
Bethesda, MD 20205
(800) 4-CANCER

National Clearinghouse for Alcohol and Drug Information
PO Box 2345
Rockville, MD 20852
(301) 468-2600

National Health Council
1730 Street NW, Suite 500
Washington, DC 20036
(202) 785-3910

National Health Information Center
PO Box 1133
Washington, DC 20013-1133
(800) 336-4797

National Institute of Mental Health
Office of Communications
6001 Executive Boulevard, Room 8184, MSC 9663
Bethesda, MD 20892-9663
(301) 443-4513

National Institute on Aging
Building 31, Room 5C27
31 Center Drive, MSC 2292
Bethesda, MD 20892
(301) 496-1752

National Kidney Foundation
30 East 33rd Street
New York, NY 10016
(212) 889-2210

National Mental Health Association
2001 N. Beauregard Street, 12th Floor
Alexandria, VA 22311
(703) 684-7722

National Organization for Rare Disorders
100 Route 37, PO Box 8923
New Fairfield, CT 06812
(800) 999-NORD

National Phlebotomy Association
5615 Landover Road
Hyattsville, MD 20784
(301) 386-4200

National Rehabilitation Association
633 South Washington Street
Alexandria, VA 22314
(703) 836-0850

National Society for Histotechnology
4201 Northview Drive, Suite 502
Bowie, MD 20716-1073
(301) 262-6221

President's Council on Physical Fitness and Sports
Department of Health and Human Services
Washington, DC 20001
(202) 272-3421

Society of Diagnostic Medical Sonographers
12770 Coit Road, Suite 508
Dallas, TX 75251
(214) 239-7367

Glossary

Note: (†) Pronunciation from Stedman's Medical Dictionary 26th edition, all others from American Heritage 4th edition, in case you need to consult.

10× lens (tĕn) A magnifying lens in the ocular of a microscope that magnifies an image ten times. (27*)

24-hour urine specimen (twĕn′tē fôr our yŏŏr′ĭn spĕs′ə-mən) A urine specimen collected over a 24-hour period and used to complete a quantitative and qualitative analysis of one or more substances, such as sodium, chloride, and calcium. (29)

abduction (ab-dŭk′shŭn) (†) Movement away from the body. (8)

abscess (ăb′sĕs′) A collection of pus (white blood cells, bacteria, and dead skin cells) that forms as a result of infection. (24)

absorption (əb-sôrp′shən) The process by which one substance is absorbed, or taken in and incorporated, into another, as when the body converts food or drugs into a form it can use. (32)

accessibility (ăk-sĕs′ə-bĭl′ĭ-tē) The ease with which people can move into and out of a space. (2)

acetylcholine (as-e-til-kō′lēn) (†) A neurotransmitter released by the parasympathetic nerves onto organs and glands for resting and digesting. (8)

acetylcholinesterase (as′e-til-kō-lin-es′ter-ās) An enzyme within the nervous system that hydrolyzes acetylcholine to acetate and choline. (8)

acid-fast stain (ăs′ĭd făst stān) A staining procedure for identifying bacteria that have a waxy cell wall. (28)

acids (ăs′ĭds) Electrolytes that release hydrogen ions in water. (5)

acinar cells (as′i-nar sĕlz) (†) Cells in the pancreas that produce pancreatic juice. (13)

acquired immunodeficiency syndrome (AIDS) (ə-kwīrd im′yū-nō-dē-fish′en-sē sĭn′drōm′) (†) The most advanced stage of HIV infection; it severely weakens the body's immune system. (11)

acromegaly (ak-rō-meg′ă-lē) (†) A disorder in which too much growth hormone is produced in adults. (14)

acrosome (ak′rō-sōm) (†) An enzyme-filled sac covering the head of a sperm that aids in the penetration of the egg during fertilization. (17)

action potential (ăk′shən pə-tĕn′shəl) The flow of electrical current along the axon membrane. (9)

active transport (ak′-tiv trans-pórt) The movement of a substance across a cell membrane from an area of low concentration to an area of high concentration. (5)

acute (ə-kyōōt′) Having a rapid onset and progress, as acute appendicitis. (22)

addiction (ă-dĭk′shun) (†) A physical or psychological dependence on a substance, usually involving a pattern of behavior that includes obsessive or compulsive preoccupation with the substance and the security of its supply, as well as a high rate of relapse after withdrawal. (18)

adduction (ă-dŭk′shŭn) (†) Movement toward the body. (8)

adenoids (ăd′n-oidz′) See **pharyngeal tonsils.** (13)

administer (ăd-mĭn′ĭ-stər) To give a drug directly by injection, by mouth, or by any other route that introduces the drug into the body. (32)

adrenocorticotropic hormone (ă-drē′nō-kōr′ti-kō-trŏ′pik hōr′mōn) Hormone that stimulates the adrenal cortex to release its hormones. (14)

aerobes (âr′ōbs′) Bacteria that grow best in the presence of oxygen. (28)

aerobic respiration (â-rō′bĭk rĕs′pə-rā′shən) A process that requires large amounts of oxygen and uses glucose to make ATP. (8)

afebrile (ā-feb′ril) (†) Having a body temperature within one's normal range. (19)

afferent arterioles (ăf′ər-ənt ar-tēr′ē-ōlz) (†) Structures that deliver blood to the glomeruli of the kidneys. (16)

affiliation agreement (ə-fĭl′ē-ā′shən ə-grē′mənt) An agreement that externship participants must sign that states the expectations of the facility and the expectations of the student. (36)

agar (ā′gär′) A gelatinlike substance derived from seaweed that gives a culture medium its semisolid consistency. (28)

agglutination (ă-glū-ti-nā′shŭn) (†) The clumping of red blood cells following a blood transfusion. (10)

agranular leukocyte (ă-gran′-yu-lər lū′kō-sīt) (†) A type of leukocyte (white blood cell) with a solid nucleus and clear cytoplasm; includes lymphocytes and monocytes. (30)

agranulocyte (ă-gran′yū-lō-sīt) (†) See **agranular leukocyte.** (10)

albumins (ăl-byōō′mĭns) The smallest of the plasma proteins. Albumins are important for pulling water into the bloodstream to help maintain blood pressure. (10)

aldosterone (al-dos′ter-ōn) (†) A hormone produced in the adrenal glands that acts on the kidney. It causes the body to retain sodium and excrete potassium. Its role is to maintain blood volume and pressure. (14)

alimentary canal (ăl′ə-mĕn′tə-rē kə-năl′) The organs of the digestive system that extend from the mouth to the anus. (13)

allele (ə-lēl′) Any one of a pair or series of **genes** that occupy a specific position on a specific **chromosome.** (5)

allergen (ăl′ər-jən) An antigen that induces an allergic reaction. (11)

alopecia (ăl′ə-pē′shə) The clinical term for baldness. (6)

alveolar glands (al-vē′ō-lăr glăndz) (†) Glands that make milk under the influence of the hormone **prolactin.** (17)

alveoli (ăl-vē′ə-lī′) Clusters of air sacs in which the exchange of gases between air and blood takes place; located in the lungs. (12)

amblyopia (am-blē-ō′pē-ă) (†) Poor vision in one eye without a detectable cause. (15)

amino acids (ə-mē′nō ăs′ĭds) Natural organic compounds found in plant and animal foods and used by the body to create protein. (31)

amnion (ăm′nē-ən) The innermost membrane enveloping the embryo and containing amniotic fluid. (17)

anabolism (ə-năb′ə-lĭz′əm) The stage of metabolism in which substances such as nutrients are changed into more complex substances and used to build body tissues. (31)

* Parenthetical numbers indicate the chapter in which the entry is a key term or is first defined in context. Entries not followed by a chapter number are important terms related to material covered but not specifically defined in the text.

anaerobe (ăn′ə-rōb′) A bacterium that grows best in the absence of oxygen. (28)

anal canal (ā′nəl kə-năl′) The last few centimeters of the rectum. (13)

anaphylaxis (an′ă-fī-lak′sis) A severe allergic reaction with symptoms that include respiratory distress, difficulty in swallowing, pallor, and a drastic drop in blood pressure that can lead to circulatory collapse. (11)

anatomical position (ăn′ə-tŏm′ĭ-kəl pə-zĭsh′ən) When the body is standing upright and facing forward with the arms at the side and the palms of the hands facing forward. (5)

anatomy (ə-năt′ə-mē) The scientific term for the study of body structure. (5)

anemia (ə-nē′mē-ə) A condition characterized by low red blood cell count. This condition decreases the ability to transport oxygen throughout the body. (10)

anergic reaction (an-er′jik rē-ăk′shən) A lack of response to skin testing that indicates the body's inability to mount a normal response to invasion by a pathogen. (3)

anesthesia (ăn′ĭs-thē′zhə) A loss of sensation, particularly the feeling of pain. (24)

anesthetic (ăn′ĭs-thĕt′ik) A medication that causes anesthesia. (24)

aneurysm (ăn′yə-rĭz′əm) A serious and potentially life-threatening bulge in the wall of a blood vessel. (10)

angiography (an-jē-og′ră-fē) (†) An x-ray examination of a blood vessel, performed after the injection of a contrast medium, that evaluates the function and structure of one or more arteries or veins. (23)

angiotensin II (an-jē-ō-ten′sin to͞o) (†) A hormone that raises blood pressure and causes the secretion of another hormone called **aldosterone.** (16)

anorexia nervosa (ăn′ə-rĕk′sē-ə nûr-vō′sə) An eating disorder in which people starve themselves because they fear that if they lose control of eating they will become grossly overweight. (31)

antagonist (ăn-tăg′ə-nĭst) A muscle that produces the opposite movement of the **prime mover.** (8)

antecubital space (an-te-kyū′bi-tăl spās) The inner side or bend of the elbow; the site at which the brachial artery is felt or heard when a pulse or blood pressure is taken. (19)

anterior (ăn-tîr′ē-ər) Anatomical term meaning toward the front of the body; also called ventral. (5)

antibodies (ăn′tĭ-bod′ēs) Highly specific proteins that attach themselves to foreign substances in an initial step in destroying such substances, as part of the body's defenses. (1)

antidiuretic hormone (an′tē-dī-yū-ret′ik hôr′mōn′) (†) A hormone that increases water reabsorption, which decreases urine production and helps to maintain blood pressure. (14)

antigen (an′tĭ-jən) A foreign substance that stimulates white blood cells to create antibodies when it enters the body. (1)

antihistamines (ăn′tē-hĭs′tə-mēnz) Medications used to treat allergies. (11)

antimicrobial (an′tē-mī-krō′bē-ăl) (†) An agent that kills microorganisms or suppresses their growth. (28)

antioxidants (ăn′tē-ŏk′sĭ-dənt) Chemical agents that fight cell-destroying chemical substances called free radicals. (31)

antiseptic (ăn′tĭ-sĕp′tĭk) A cleaning product used on human tissue as an anti-infection agent. (2)

anuria (an-yū′rē-ă) (†) The absence of urine production. (29)

aortic valve (ā-ôr′tĭk vălv) Heart valve that is a semilunar valve and that is situated between the left ventricle and the aorta. (10)

apex (ā′pĕks) The left lower corner of the heart, where the strongest heart sounds can be heard. (19)

apical (ap′i-kăl) (†) Located at the **apex** of the heart. (19)

apocrine gland (ap′ō-krin glănd) (†) A type of sweat gland. It produces a thicker type of sweat than other sweat glands and contains more proteins. (6)

aponeurosis (ap′ō-nū-rō′sis) (†) A tough, sheet-like structure that is made of fibrous connective tissue. It typically attaches muscles to other muscles. (8)

appendicitis (ə-pĕn′dĭ-sī′tĭs) Inflammation of the appendix. (13)

appendicular (ap′en-dik′yū-lăr) The division of the skeletal system that consists of the bones of the arms, legs, pectoral girdle, and pelvic girdle. (7)

approximation (ə-prŏk′sə-mā′shən) The process of bringing the edges of a wound together, so the tissue surfaces are close, to protect the area from further contamination and to minimize scar and scab formation. (24)

aqueous humor (a′kwē-əs hyo͞o′mər) A liquid produced by the eye's ciliary body that fills the space between the cornea and the lens. (15)

areflexia (ā-rē-flek′sē-ă) (†) The absence of **reflexes.** (9)

areola (ă-rē′ō-lă) (†) The pigmented area that surrounds the nipple. (17)

arrector pili (ă-rek′tōr pī′lī) (†) Muscles attached to most hair follicles and found in the dermis. (6)

arrhythmia (ə-rĭth′mē-ə) Irregularity in heart rhythm. (10)

arterial blood gases (är-tîr′ē-əl blŭd găs′ses) A test that measures the amount of gases, such as oxygen and carbon dioxide, dissolved in arterial blood. (22)

arthrography (ar-throg′ră-fē) (†) A radiologic procedure performed by a radiologist, who uses a contrast medium and fluoroscopy to help diagnose abnormalities or injuries in the cartilage, tendons, or ligaments of the joints—usually the knee or shoulder. (35)

arthroscopy (är-thŏs′kə-pē) A procedure in which an orthopedist examines a joint, usually the knee or shoulder, with a tubular instrument called an arthroscope; also used to guide surgical procedures. (23)

articular cartilage (ar-tik′yu-lăr kär′tl-ĭj) (†) The cartilage that covers the **epiphysis** of long bones. (7)

artifact (är′tə-făkt′) Any irrelevant object or mark observed when examining specimens or graphic records that is not related to the object being examined; for example, a foreign object visible through a microscope or an erroneous mark on an ECG strip. (27)

ascending colon (ə-sĕnd′ĭng kō′lən) The segment of the large intestine that runs up the right side of the abdominal cavity. (13)

ascending tracts (ə-sĕnd′ĭng trăkts) The tracts of the spinal cord that carry sensory information to the brain. (9)

asepsis (ă-sep′sis) (†) The condition in which pathogens are absent or controlled. (1)

astigmatism (ə-stĭg′mə-tĭz′əm) A condition in which the cornea has an abnormal shape, which causes blurred images during near or distant vision. (15)

atherosclerosis (ăth′ə-rō-sklə-rō′sĭs) The accumulation of fatty deposits along the inner walls of arteries. (10)

atlas (ăt′ləs) The first cervical vertebra. (7)

atoms (ăt′əmz) The simplest units of all matter. (5)

atria (ā′trē-ă) (†) [*Singular:* **atrium**] Chambers of the heart that receive blood from the veins and circulate it to the ventricles. (10)

atrial natriuretic peptide (ā′trē-ăl nā′trē-yū-ret′ik pep′tīd) (†) A hormone secreted by the heart that regulates blood pressure. (14)

atrioventricular bundle (ā′trē-ō-ven-trik′yū-lar bŭn′dl) (†) A structure that is located between the ventricles of the heart and that sends the electrical impulse to the Purkinje fibers. (10)

atrioventricular node (ā′trē-ō-ven-trik′yū-lar nōd) A node that is located between the atria of the heart. After the electrical impulse reaches the atrioventricular node, the atria contract and the impulse is sent to the ventricles. (10)

audiologist (aw-dē-ol′ōjist) (†) A health-care specialist who focuses on evaluating and correcting hearing problems. (21)

audiometer (aw-dē-om′ĕ-ter) An electronic device that measures hearing acuity by producing sounds in specific frequencies and intensities. (21)

auditory tube (ô′dĭ-tôr′ē to͞ob) A structure that connects the middle ear to the throat. Also called the **eustachian tube.** (15)

auricle (ôr′ĭ-kəl) The outside part of the ear, made of cartilage and covered with skin. (15)

auscultated blood pressure (ô′skəl-tāt-ĕd blŭd prĕsh′ər) Blood pressure as measured by listening with a stethoscope. (19)

auscultation (ô′skəl-t ā′shən) The process of listening to body sounds. (20)

autoclave (aw′tō-klāv) (†) A device that uses pressurized steam to sterilize instruments and equipment. (2)

automated external defibrillator (AED) (ô′tə-mā′tĭd ĭk-stûr′nəl dē-fib′ri-lā-ter) A computerized defibrillator programmed to recognize lethal heart rhythms and deliver an electrical shock to restore a normal rhythm. (26)

autonomic (ô′tə-nŏm′ĭk) A division of the peripheral nervous system that connects the central nervous system to viscera such as the heart, stomach, intestines, glands, blood vessels, and bladder. (9)

autosome (ô′tə-sōm′) A chromosome that is not a sex chromosome. (5)

axial (ăk′sē-əl) The division of the skeletal system that consists of the skull, vertebral column, and rib cage. (7)

axilla (ăk-sĭl′ə) Armpit; one of the four locations for temperature readings. (19)

axis (ak′-səs) The second vertebra of the neck on which the head turns. (7)

axon (ăk′sŏn′) A type of nerve fiber that is typically long and branches far from the cell body. Its function is to send information away from the cell body. (9)

bacillus (ba-sil′ŭs) (†) A rod-shaped bacterium. (28)

bacterial spore (băk-tîr′ēăl spôr) A primitive, thick-walled reproductive body capable of developing into a new individual; resistant to killing through disinfection. (1)

barium enema (bâr′ē-əm ĕn′ə-mə) A radiologic procedure performed by a radiologist who administers barium sulfate through the anus, into the rectum, and then into the colon to help diagnose and evaluate obstructions, ulcers, polyps, diverticulosis, tumors, or motility problems of the colon or rectum; also called a lower GI (gastrointestinal) series. (35)

barium swallow (bâr′ē-əm swŏl′ō) A radiologic procedure that involves oral administration of a barium sulfate drink to help diagnose and evaluate obstructions, ulcers, polyps, diverticulosis, tumors, or motility problems of the esophagus, stomach, duodenum, and small intestine; also called an upper GI (gastrointestinal) series. (35)

baroreceptors (bar′ō-rē-sep′ters) (†) Structures, located in the aorta and carotid arteries, that help regulate blood pressure. (10)

bases (bā′sēz′) Electrolytes that release hydroxyl ions in water. (5)

basophil (bā-sō-fil) (†) A type of granular leukocyte that produces the chemical histamine, which aids the body in controlling allergic reactions and other exaggerated immunologic responses. (10)

behavior modification (bĭ-hāv′yər mŏd′ə-fĭ-kā-shən) The altering of personal habits to promote a healthier lifestyle. (31)

bicarbonate ions (bī-kar′bon-āt ī′onz) Elements formed when carbon dioxide gets into the bloodstream and reacts with water. In the alimentary canal, these ions neutralize acidic chyme arriving from the stomach. (12)

bicuspids (bī-kŭs′pĭds) Teeth with two cusps. There are two in front of each set of molars. (13)

bicuspid valve (bī-kŭs′pĭd vălv) Heart valve that has two cusps and that is located between the left atrium and the left ventricle. Also known as the mitral valve. (10)

bile (bīl) A substance created in the liver and stored in the gallbladder. Bile is a bitter yellow-green fluid that is used in the digestion of fats. (13)

bilirubin (bili-rū′bin) (†) A bile pigment formed by the breakdown of hemoglobin in the liver. (10)

bilirubinuria (bil′i-rū-bi-nū′rē-ă) (†) The presence of bilirubin in the urine; one of the first signs of liver disease or conditions that involve the liver. (29)

biliverdin (bil-i-ver′din) (†) A pigment released when a red blood cell is destroyed. (10)

biochemistry (bī′ō-kĕm′ĭ-strē) The study of matter and chemical reactions in the body. (5)

biohazard symbol (bī-ō-hăz′ərd sĭm′bəl) A symbol that must appear on all containers used to store waste products, blood, blood products, or other specimens that may be infectious. (27)

biohazardous materials (bī-ō-hăz′ərd-əs mə-tîr′ə-əls) Biological agents that can spread disease to living things. (1)

biohazardous waste container (bī-ō-hăz′ərd-əs wāst kən-tā′nər) A leakproof, puncture-resistant container, color-coded red or labeled with a special biohazard symbol, that is used to store and dispose of contaminated supplies and equipment. (1)

biopsy (bī′ŏp′sē) The process of removing and examining tissues and cells from the body. (11)

biopsy specimen (bī′ŏp′sē spĕs′ə-mən) A small amount of tissue removed from the body for examination under a microscope to diagnose an illness. (24)

bioterrorism (bī-ō′tĕr′ə-rĭz′əm) The intentional release of a biologic agent with the intent to harm individuals. (26)

blastocyst (blas′tō-sist) A **morula** that travels down the uterine tube to the uterus and is invaded with fluid. It then implants into the wall of the uterus. (17)

blood-borne pathogen (blŭd-bôrn păth′ə-jən) A disease-causing microorganism carried in a host's blood and transmitted through contact with infected blood, tissue, or body fluids. (3)

blood-brain barrier (blŭd brān băr′ē-ər) A structure that is formed from tight capillaries to protect the tissues of the central nervous system from certain substances. (9)

B lymphocyte (bē lĭm′fə-sīt′) A type of nongranular leukocyte that produces antibodies to combat specific pathogens. (30)

bone conduction (bōnkən-dŭk′shən) The process by which sound waves pass through the bones of the skull directly to the inner ear, bypassing the outer and middle ears. (21)

botulism (bŏch′ə-lĭz′əm) A life-threatening type of food poisoning that results from eating improperly canned or preserved foods that have been contaminated with the bacterium *Clostridium botulinum.* (8)

brachial artery (brā′kē-ăl är′tə-rē) An artery that provides a palpable pulse and audible vascular sounds in the antecubital space (the bend of the elbow). (19)

brachytherapy (brak-ē-thăr′ă-pe′)(†) A radiation therapy technique in which a radiologist places temporary radioactive implants close to or directly into cancerous tissue; used for treating localized cancers. (35)

brain stem (brān stēm) A structure that connects the cerebrum to the spinal cord. (9)

bronchi (brŏn-kī) The two branches of the trachea that enter the lungs. (12)

bronchial tree (brŏng′kē-al trē) A series of tubes that begins where the distal end of the trachea branches. (12)

bronchioles (brŏng′kē-ōlz) A part of the respiratory tract that branches from the tertiary bronchi. (12)

buccal (bŭk′ăl)(†) Between the cheek and gum. (33)

bulbourethral glands (bŭl′bō-yū-rē′thrăl glăndz)(†) Glands that lie beneath the prostate and empty their fluid into the urethra. Their fluid aids in sperm movement. (17)

buffy coat (buf′ē kōt) The layer between the packed red blood cells and plasma in a centrifuged blood sample; this layer contains the white blood cells and platelets. (30)

bulimia (bo͞o-lē′mē-ə) An eating disorder in which people eat a large quantity of food in a short period of time (bingeing) and then attempt to counter the effects of bingeing by self-induced vomiting, use of laxatives or diuretics, and/or excessive exercise. (31)

bursitis (bər-sī′tĭs) Inflammation of a bursa. (7)

calcaneus (kal-kā′nē-ŭs)(†) The largest tarsal bone; also called the heel bone. (7)

calcitonin (kal-si-tō′nin) A hormone produced by the thyroid gland that lowers blood calcium levels by activating osteoblasts. (14)

calibrate (kăl′ə-brāt) to determine the caliber of (19)

calibration syringe (kăl′ə-brā′shən sə-rĭnj′) A standardized measuring instrument used to check and adjust the volume indicator on a spirometer. (34)

calorie (kăl′ə-rē) A unit used to measure the amount of energy food produces; the amount of energy needed to raise the temperature of 1 kg of water by 1°C. (31)

calyces (kă′lĭ-sēz′) Small cavities of the renal pelvis of the kidney. (16)

canaliculi (kan-ă-lik′yū-lī) Tiny canals that connect lacunae to each other. (7)

capillary (kăp′ə-lĕr′ē) Branches of arterioles and the smallest type of blood vessel. (10)

capillary puncture (kăp′ə-lĕr′ē pŭngk′chər) A blood-drawing technique that requires a superficial puncture of the skin with a sharp point. (30)

carboxypeptidase (kar-bok-sē-pep′ti-dās) (†) A pancreatic enzyme that digests proteins. (13)

carcinogen (kär-sĭn′ə-jən) A factor that is known to cause the formation of cancer. (11)

cardiac catheterization (kär′dē-ăk′ kath′ē-ter-ī-zā′shun)(†) A diagnostic method in which a catheter is inserted into a vein or artery in the arm or leg and passed through blood vessels into the heart. (23)

cardiac cycle (kär′dē-ăk′ sī′kəl) The sequence of contraction and relaxation that makes up a complete heartbeat. (34)

carditis (kar-dī′tis)(†) Inflammation of the heart. (10)

carpal (kär′pəl) Bones of the wrist. (7)

carpal tunnel syndrome (kär′pəl tŭn′əl sĭn′drōm′) A painful disorder caused by compression of the median nerve in the carpal tunnel of the wrist. (7)

carrier (kăr′ē-ər) A reservoir host who is unaware of the presence of a pathogen and so spreads the disease while exhibiting no symptoms of infection. (1)

cast (kăst) A rigid, external dressing, usually made of plaster or fiberglass, that is molded to the contours of the body part to which it is applied; used to immobilize a fractured or dislocated bone. (26)
Cylinder-shaped elements with flat or rounded ends, differing in composition and size, that form when protein from the breakdown of cells accumulates and precipitates in the kidney tubules and is washed into the urine. (29)

catabolism (kə-tăb′ə-lĭz′əm) The stage of metabolism in which complex substances, including nutrients and body tissues, are broken down into simpler substances and converted into energy. (31)

cataracts (kăt′ə-răkts′) Cloudy areas that form in the lens of the eye that prevent light from reaching visual receptors. (15)

catheterization (kath′ē-ter-ī-ză′shun)(†) The procedure during which a catheter is inserted into a vessel, an organ, or a body cavity. (29)

caudal (kôd′l) See **inferior.** (5)

cecum (sē′kəm) The first section of the large intestine. (13)

cell body (sĕl bŏd′ē) The portion of the neuron that contains the nucleus and organelles. (9)

cell membrane (sĕl mĕm′brān′) The outer limit of a cell that is thin and selectively permeable. It controls the movement of substances into and out of the cell. (5)

cells (sĕlz) The smallest living units of structure and function. (5)

cellulitis (sel-yū-lī′tis) Inflammation of cellular or connective tissue. (6)

cellulose (sĕl′yə-lōs′) A type of carbohydrate that is found in vegetables and cannot be digested by humans; commonly called fiber. (13)

Celsius (centigrade) (sĕl′sē-əs) One of two common scales for measuring temperature; measured in degrees Celsius, or °C. (19)

central nervous system (CNS) (sĕn′trəl nûr′vəs sĭs′təm) A system that consists of the brain and the spinal cord. (9)

centrifuge (sĕn′trə-fyo͞oj′) A device used to spin a specimen at high speed until it separates into its component parts. (27)

cerebellum (sĕr′ə-bĕl′əm) An area of the brain inferior to the cerebrum that coordinates complex skeletal muscle coordination. (9)

cerebrospinal fluid (CSF) (ser′ē-brō-spī-năl flo͞o′ĭd) The fluid in the subarachnoid space of the meninges and the central canal of the spinal cord. (9)

cerebrum (sĕr´ə-brəm) The largest part of the brain; it mainly includes the cerebral hemispheres. (9)

Certificate of Waiver tests (sər-tĭf´ĭ-kĭt wā´vər tĕsts) Laboratory tests that pose an insignificant risk to the patient if they are performed or interpreted incorrectly, are simple and accurate to such a degree that the risk of obtaining incorrect results is minimal, and have been approved by the Food and Drug Administration for use by patients at home; laboratories performing only Certificate of Waiver tests must meet less stringent standards than laboratories that perform tests in other categories. (27)

cerumen (sə-rōō´mən) A waxlike substance produced by glands in the ear canal; also called earwax. (20)

cervical enlargement (sûr´vĭ-kəl in-lär´j-mənt) The thickening of the spinal cord in the neck region. (9)

cervical orifice (sûr´vĭ-kəl ôr´ə-fĭs) The opening of the uterus through the cervix into the vagina. (17)

cervicitis (ser-vi-sī´tis) Inflammation of the cervix. (17)

cervix (sûr´vĭks) The lowest portion of the uterus that extends into the vagina. (17)

chain of custody (chān kŭs´tə-dē) A procedure for ensuring that a specimen is obtained from a specified individual, is correctly identified, is under the uninterrupted control of authorized personnel, and has not been altered or replaced. (26)

chancre (shang´ker) (†) A painless ulcer that may appear on the tongue, the lips, the genitalia, the rectum, or elsewhere. (3)

chemistry (kĕm´ĭ-strē) The study of the composition of matter and how matter changes. (5)

chemoreceptor (kē´mō-rĭ-sĕp´tôr) Any cell that is activated by a change in chemical concentration and results in a nerve impulse. The olfactory or smell receptors in the nose are an example of a chemoreceptor. (15)

chief cells (chēf sĕlz) Cells in the lining of the stomach that secrete **pepsinogen**. (13)

chief complaint (chēf kəm-plān´t) The patient's main issue of pain or ailment. (18)

cholangiography (kō-lan-jē-og´ră-fē) (†) A test that evaluates the function of the bile ducts by injection of a contrast medium directly into the common bile duct (during gallbladder surgery) or through a T-tube (after gallbladder surgery or during radiologic testing) and taking an x-ray. (35)

cholecystography (kō-lē-sis-tog´ră-fē) (†) A gallbladder function test performed by x-ray after the patient ingests an oral contrast agent; used to detect gallstones and bile duct obstruction. (23)

cholesterol (kə-lĕs´tə-rôl) A fat-related substance that the body produces in the liver and obtains from dietary sources; needed in small amounts to carry out several vital functions. High levels of cholesterol in the blood increase the risk of heart and artery disease. (31)

chordae tendineae (kōr´dē ten-din´ā) (†) Cord-like structures that attach the cusps of the heart valves to the papillary muscles in the ventricles. (10)

choroid (kôr´oid´) The middle layer of the eye, which contains the iris, the ciliary body, and most of the eye's blood vessels. (15)

chromosome (krō´mə-sōm´) Thread-like structures comprised of DNA. (5)

chronic (krŏn´ĭk) Lasting a long time or recurring frequently, as in chronic osteoarthritis. (22)

chronic obstructive pulmonary disease (COPD) (krŏn´ĭk ob-strŭk´tĭv pŏŏl´mə-nĕr´ē dĭ-zēz´) A disease characterized by the presence of airflow obstruction due to chronic bronchitis or emphysema. It is typically progressive. Cigarette smoking is the leading cause. (13)

chronological résumé (krŏn´ə-lŏj´ĭ-kəl rĕz´ŏŏ-mā´) The type of résumé used by individuals who have job experience. Jobs are listed according to date, with the most recent being listed first. (36)

chylomicron (kī-lō-mi´kron) The least dense of the lipoproteins; it functions in lipid transportation. (10)

chyme (kīm) (†) The mixture of food and gastric juice. (13)

chymotrypsin (kī-mō-trip´sin) (†) A pancreatic enzyme that digests proteins. (13)

ciliary body (sĭl´ē-ĕr´ē bŏd´ē) A wedge-shaped thickening in the middle layer of the eyeball that contains the muscles that control the shape of the lens. (15)

circumduction (ser-kŭm-dŭk´shŭn) Moving a body part in a circle; for example, tracing a circle with your arm. (8)

cirrhosis (sĭ-rō´sĭs) A long-lasting liver disease in which normal liver tissue is replaced with nonfunctioning scar tissue. (13)

clavicle (klăv´ĭ-kəl) A slender, curved long bone that connects the sternum and the scapula; also called the collar bone. (7)

clean-catch midstream urine specimen (klēn-kăch mĭd´strēm yŏŏr´ĭn spĕs´ə-mən) A type of urine specimen that requires special cleansing of the external genitalia to avoid contamination by organisms residing near the external opening of the urethra and is used to identify the number and types of pathogens present in urine; sometimes referred to as midvoid. (29)

cleavage (klē´vĭj) The rapid rate of mitosis of a zygote immediately following fertilization. (17)

clinical coordinator (klĭn´ĭ-kəl kō-ôr´dn-ā´tor) The person associated with the medical assisting school that procures externship sites and qualifies them to ensure that they provide a thorough educational experience. (36)

clinical diagnosis (klĭn´ĭ-kəl dī´əg-nō´sĭs) A diagnosis based on the signs and symptoms of a disease or condition. (20)

clinical drug trial (klĭn´ĭ-kəl drŭg trī´əl) An internationally recognized research protocol designed to evaluate the efficacy or safety of drugs and to produce scientifically valid results. (3)

clitoris (klĭt´ər-ĭs) Located anterior to the urethral opening in females. It contains erectile tissue and is rich in sensory nerves. (17)

coagulation (kō-ăg´yə-lā´shən) The process by which a clot forms in blood. (10)

coccus (kŏk´əs) A spherical, round, or ovoid bacterium. (28)

coccyx (kŏk´sĭks) A small, triangular-shaped bone consisting of three to five fused vertebrae. (7)

cochlea (kŏk´lē-ăr) A spiral-shaped canal in the inner ear that contains the hearing receptors. (15)

colitis (kə-lī´tĭs) Inflammation of the colon. (13)

colonoscopy (kō-lon-os´ kŏ-pē) (†) A procedure used to determine the cause of diarrhea, constipation, bleeding, or lower abdominal pain by inserting a scope through the anus to provide direct visualization of the large intestine. (23)

colony (kŏl´ə-nē) A distinct group of microorganisms, visible with the naked eye, on the surface of a culture medium. (28)

colposcopy (kol-pos´kŏ-pē) (†) The examination of the vagina and cervix with an instrument called a colposcope to identify abnormal tissue, such as cancerous or precancerous cells. (22)

common bile duct (kŏm´ən bīl dŭkt) Duct that carries bile to the duodenum. It is formed from the merger of the cystic and hepatic ducts. (13)

complement (kŏm´plə-mənt) A protein present in serum that is involved in specific defenses. (11)

complete proteins (kəm-plēt´ prō´ten´) Proteins that contain all nine essential amino acids. (31)

complex carbohydrates (kəm-plĕks´ kär´bō-hī´drāt´s) Long chains of sugar units; also known as polysaccharides. (31)

complex inheritance (kəm-plĕks´ ĭn-hĕr´ĭ-təns) The inheritance of traits determined by multiple genes. (5)

compound (kŏm´pound´) A substance that is formed when two or more atoms of more than one element are chemically combined. (5)

compound microscope (kŏm´pound´ mī´krə-skōp´) A microscope that uses two lenses to magnify the image created by condensed light focused through the object being examined. (27)

computed tomography (kəm-pyōōt´ĕd tō-mogra-fē) (†) A radiographic examination that produces a three-dimensional, cross-sectional view of an area of the body; may be performed with or without a contrast medium. (23)

concussion (kən-kŭsh´ən) A jarring injury to the brain; the most common type of head injury. (26)

conductive hearing loss (kon-dŭk-tiv´ hēr´ing lôs) (†) A type of hearing loss that occurs when sound waves cannot be conducted through the ear. Most types are temporary. (15)

condyle (kon´dīl) (†) Rounded articular surface on a bone. (7)

cones (kōnz) Light-sensing nerve cells in the eye, at the posterior of the retina, that are sensitive to color, provide sharp images, and function only in bright light. (15)

conjunctiva (kŏn´jŭngk-tī´və) The protective membrane that lines the eyelid and covers the anterior of the sclera, or the white of the eye. (15)

conjunctivitis (kən-jŭngk´tə-vī´tĭs) A contagious infection of the conjunctiva caused by bacteria, viruses, and allergies. The symptoms may include discharge, red eyes, itching, and swollen eyelids; also commonly called pinkeye. (15)

connective (kə-nĕk´tĭv) A tissue type that is the framework of the body. (5)

consumable (kən-sōō´mə-bəl) Able to be emptied or used up, as with supplies. (4)

constructive criticism (kən-stre´k-tiv kr´i-tə-si-zəm) A type of critique that is aimed at giving an individual feedback about his or her performance in order to improve that performance. (36)

contraindication (kŏn´trə-ĭn´dĭ-kā´-shən) A symptom that renders use of a remedy or procedure inadvisable, usually because of risk. (2)

contrast medium (kŏn´trast´ mē´dē-əm) A substance that makes internal organs denser and blocks the passage of x-rays to photographic film. Introducing a contrast medium into certain structures or areas of the body can provide a clear image of organs and tissues and highlight indications of how well they are functioning. (35)

controlled substance (kən-trōld´ sŭb´stəns) A drug or drug product that is categorized as potentially dangerous and addictive and is strictly regulated by federal laws. (32)

control sample (kən-trōl´ săm´pəl) A specimen that has a known value; used as a comparison for test results on a patient sample. (27)

contusion (kon-tŭ´shŭn) (†) A closed wound, or bruise. (26)

convolutions (kŏn´və-lōō´shənz) The ridges of brain matter between the sulci; also called **gyri.** (9)

cornea (kôr´nē-ə) A transparent area on the front of the outer layer of the eye that acts as a window to let light into the eye. (15)

coronary sinus (kôr´ə-nĕr´ē sī´nəs) The large vein that receives oxygen-poor blood from the cardiac veins and empties it into the right atrium of the heart. (10)

corpus callosum (kôr´pəs ka-l´ō-səm) A thick bundle of nerve fibers that connects the cerebral hemispheres. (9)

corpus luteum (kôr´pŭs lū-tē´ŭm) (†) A ruptured follicle cell in the ovary following ovulation. (17)

cortex (kôr´təks´) The outermost layer of the cerebrum. (9)

cortisol (kōr´ti-sol) (†) A steroid hormone that is released when a person is stressed. It decreases protein synthesis. (14)

costal (kos´tăl) (†) Cartilage that attaches true ribs to the sternum. (7)

coxal (koks-al´) (†) Pertaining to the bones of the pelvic girdle. The coxa is composed of the ilium, ischium, and pubis. (7)

cranial (krā´-nē-ăl) (†) See **superior.** (5)

cranial nerves (krā´nē-ăl nûrvs) (†) Peripheral nerves that originate from the brain. (9)

crash cart (krăsh kärt) A rolling cart of emergency supplies and equipment. (26)

creatine phosphate (krē´ă-tēn fos´fāt) (†) A protein that stores extra phosphate groups. (8)

cricoid cartilage (krī´koyd kär´tl-ĭj) (†) A cartilage of the larynx that forms most of the posterior wall and a small part of the anterior wall. (12)

cryotherapy (krī´ō-thĕr´ə-pē) The application of cold to a patient's body for therapeutic reasons. (25)

cryosurgery (krī´ō-sûr´jə-rē) The use of extreme cold to destroy unwanted tissue, such as skin lesions. (24)

crystals (krĭs´təls) Naturally produced solids of definite form; commonly seen in urine specimens, especially those permitted to cool. (29)

culture (kŭl´chər) In the sociological sense, a pattern of assumptions, beliefs, and practices that shape the way people think and act. (20)
To place a sample of a specimen in or on a substance that allows microorganisms to grow in order to identify the microorganisms present. (28)

culture and sensitivity (C and S) (kŭl´chər sĕn´sĭ-tĭv´ə-tē) A procedure that involves culturing a specimen and then testing the isolated bacteria's susceptibility (sensitivity) to certain antibiotics to determine which antibiotics would be most effective in treating an infection. (28)

culture medium (kŭlchər mē´de-əm) A substance containing all the nutrients a particular type of microorganism needs to grow. (28)

Cushing's disease (kush´ingz dĭ-zēz´) A condition in which a person produces too much **cortisol** or has used too many steroid hormones. Some of the signs and symptoms include buffalo hump obesity, a moon face, and abdominal stretch marks; also called hypercortisolism. (14)

cuspids (kŭs′pĭdz) The sharpest teeth; they act to tear food. (13)

cyanosis (sī′ə-no′sĭs) A bluish color of skin that results when the supply of oxygen is low in the blood. (6)

cystic duct (sĭs′tĭk dŭkt) The duct from the gallbladder that merges with the hepatic duct to form the common bile duct. (13)

cystitis (sis-tī′tis) (†) Inflammation of the urinary bladder caused by infection. (16)

cytokines (sī′tō-kīnz) A chemical secreted by T lymphocytes in response to an antigen. Cytokines increase T and B cell production, kill cells that have antigens, and stimulate red bone marrow to produce more white blood cells. (11)

cytokinesis (sī′tō-ki-nē′sis) (†) Splitting of the cytoplasm during cell division. (5)

cytoplasm (sī′tə-plăz′əm) The watery intracellular substance that consists mostly of water, proteins, ions, and nutrients. (5)

debridement (dā-brēd-mont′) (†) The removal of debris or dead tissue from a wound to expose healthy tissue. (24)

decibel (dĕs′ə-bəl) A unit for measuring the relative intensity of sounds on a scale from 0 to 130. (21)

deep (dēp) Anatomical term meaning closer to the inside of the body. (5)

defecation reflex (def-ĕ-kā′shŭn rē′flĕks′) The relaxation of the anal sphincters so that feces can move through the anus in the process of elimination. (13)

deflection (dĭ-flĕk′shən) A peak or valley on an electrocardiogram. (34)

dehydration (dē-hī′drā′shən) The condition that results from a lack of adequate water in the body. (26)

dendrite (dĕn′drīt′) A type of nerve fiber that is short and branches near the cell body. Its function is to receive information from the neuron. (9)

deoxyhemoblobin (dē-oks-ē-hē-mō-glō′bin) (†) A type of hemoglobin that is not carrying oxygen. It is darker red in color than hemoglobin. (10)

depolarization (dē-pō′lăr-i-za-shŭn) (†) The loss of polarity, or opposite charges inside and outside; the electrical impulse that initiates a chain reaction resulting in contraction. (34)

depolarized (dē-pō′lăr-īzd) (†) A state in which sodium ions flow to the inside of the cell membrane, making the outside less positive. Depolarization occurs when a neuron responds to stimuli such as heat, pressure, or chemicals. (9)

depression (di′-pre-shan) The lowering of a body part. (8)

dermatitis (dûr′mə-tī′tĭs) Inflammation of the skin. (6)

dermis (dûr′mĭs) The middle layer of the skin, which contains connective tissue, nerve endings, hair follicles, sweat glands, and oil glands. (6)

descending colon (dĭ-sĕnd′ĭng kō′lən) The segment of the large intestine after the transverse colon that descends the left side of the abdominal cavity. (13)

descending tracts (dĭ-sĕnd′ĭng trăkts) Tracts of the spinal cord that carry motor information from the brain to muscles and glands. (9)

detrusor muscle (dē-trŭs′or mŭs′əl) A smooth muscle that contracts to push urine from the bladder into the urethra. (16)

diabetes mellitus (dī′ə-bē′tĭs mə-lī′təs) Any of several related endocrine disorders characterized by an elevated level of glucose in the blood, caused by a deficiency of insulin or insulin resistance at the cellular level. (14)

diagnostic radiology (dī′əg-nos′tik rā′dē-ŏl′ə-jē) The use of x-ray technology to determine the cause of a patient's symptoms. (35)

diapedesis (dī′ă-pĕ-dē′sis) (†) The squeezing of a cell through a blood vessel wall. (10)

diaphragm (dī′ə-frăm′) A muscle that separates the thoracic and abdominopelvic cavities. (5)

diaphysis (dī′-af′i-sis) The shaft of a long bone. (7)

diastolic pressure (dī′ə-stŏl′ĭk prĕsh′ər) The blood pressure measured when the heart relaxes. (10)

diathermy (dī′ə-thûr′mē) A type of heat therapy in which a machine produces high-frequency waves that achieve deep heat penetration in muscle tissue. (25)

diencephalon (dī-en-sef′ă-lon) (†) A structure that includes the thalamus and the hypothalamus. It is located between the cerebral hemispheres and is superior to the brain stem. (9)

differential diagnosis (dĭf′ə-rĕn′shəl dī′əg-nō′sĭs) The process of determining the correct diagnosis when two or more diagnoses are possible. (20)

diffusion (di-fyū′zhŭn) (†) The movement of a substance from an area of high concentration to an area of low concentration. (5)

digital examination (dĭj′ĭ-tl ĭg-zam′ə-nā′shən) Part of a physical examination in which the physician inserts one or two fingers of one hand into the opening of a body canal such as the vagina or the rectum; used to palpate canal and related structures. (20)

diluent (dĭl′yo͞o-ənt) A liquid used to dissolve and dilute another substance, such as a drug. (33)

disaccharide (dī-sak′ă-rīd) (†) A type of carbohydrate that is a simple sugar. (13)

disinfectant (dĭs′ĭn-fĕk′tănt) A cleaning product applied to instruments and equipment to reduce or eliminate infectious organisms; not used on human tissue. (2)

disinfection (dĭs′ĭn-fĕk′shən) The destruction of infectious agents on an object or surface by direct application of chemical or physical means. (1)

dislocation (dĭs′lō-kā′shən) The displacement of a bone end from a joint. (26)

dispense (dĭ-spĕns′) To distribute a drug, in a properly labeled container, to a patient who is to use it. (32)

distal (dĭs′təl) Anatomical term meaning farther away from a point of attachment or farther away from the trunk of the body. (5)

distal convoluted tubule (dĭs′təl kon′vō-lū-ted tū′byūl) The last twisted section of the renal tubule; it is located after the loop of Henle. Several of these tubules merge together to form collecting ducts. (16)

distribution (dĭs′trĭ-byo͞o′shən) The biochemical process of transporting a drug from its administration site in the body to its site of action. (32)

diverticulitis (dī′ver-tik-yū-lī′tis) (†) Inflammation of the diverticuli, which are abnormal dilations in the intestine. (13)

DNA (dē′ĕn-ā′) A nucleic acid that contains the genetic information of cells. (5)

dorsal (dôr′səl) See **posterior.** (5)

dorsal root (dôr′səl ro͞ot) A portion of a spinal nerve that contains axons of sensory neurons only. (9)

dorsiflexion (dōr-si-flek′shŭn) (†) Pointing the toes upward. (8)

dosage (dō′sāj) The size, frequency, and number of doses. (32)

dose (dōs) The amount of a drug given or taken at one time. (32)

douche (dōōsh) Vaginal irrigation, which can be used to administer vaginal medication in liquid form. (33)

drainage catheter (drā′nĭj kăth′ĭ-tər) A type of catheter used to withdraw fluids. (29)

dressings (drĕs′ĭngs) Sterile materials used to cover a surgical or other wound. (24)

ductus arteriosus (dŭk′tŭs ar-tēr′ē-ō′sus) (†) The connection in the fetus between the pulmonary trunk and the aorta. (17)

ductus venosus (duk′tŭs ven-ō′sus) (†) A blood vessel that allows most of the blood to bypass the liver in the fetus. (17)

duodenum (dōō′ə-dē′nəm) The first section of the small intestine. (13)

dwarfism (dwôrf′ĭzm) A condition in which too little growth hormone is produced, resulting in an abnormally small stature. (14)

dysmenorrhea (dis-men-ŏr-ē′ă) (†) Severe menstrual cramps that limit daily activity. (17)

dyspnea (disp-nē′ă) (†) Difficult or painful breathing. (19)

ear ossicles (îr os′i-kl) (†) Three tiny bones called the malleus, the incus, and the stapes located in the middle ear cavity. They are the smallest bones of the body. (15)

eccrine gland (ek′rin glănd) (†) The most numerous type of sweat gland. Eccrine sweat glands produce a watery type of sweat and are activated primarily by heat. (6)

echocardiography (ek′ō-kar-dē-og′ră-fē) (†) A procedure that tests the structure and function of the heart through the use of reflected sound waves, or echoes. (23)

ectoderm (ek′tō-derm) (†) The primary germ layer that gives rise to nervous tissue and some epithelial tissue. (17)

eczema (ĕk′sə-mə) Inflammatory condition of the skin. (6)

edema (ĭ-dē′mə) An excessive buildup of fluid in body tissue. (10)

effectors (ĭ-fĕk′tərs) Muscles and glands that are stimulated by motor neurons in the peripheral nervous system. (9)

efferent arterioles (ĕf′ər-ənt ar-tēr′ē-ōlz) (†) Structures that deliver blood to peritubular capillaries that are wrapped around the renal tubules of the nephron in the kidneys. (16)

efficacy (ĕf′ĭ-kə-sē) The therapeutic value of a procedure or therapy, such as a drug. (32)

electrocardiogram (ECG or EKG) (ĭ-lĕk′trō-kär′dē-ə-grăm′) The tracing made by an **electrocardiograph.** (34)

electrocardiograph (ĭ-lĕk′trō-kär′dē-ə-grăf′) An instrument that measures and displays the waves of electrical impulses responsible for the cardiac cycle. (34)

electrocardiography (ĭ-lĕk′trō-kär′dē-ŏg′rə-fē) The process by which a graphic pattern is created to reflect the electrical impulses generated by the heart as it pumps. (34)

electrocauterization (ĭ-lĕk′trō-kô′tər-ĭ-zā′shən) The use of a needle, probe, or loop heated by electric current to remove growths such as warts, to stop bleeding, and to control nosebleeds that either will not subside or continually recur. (24)

electrodes (ĭ-lĕk′trōds′) Sensors that detect electrical activity. (34)

electroencephalography (ĭ-lĕk′trō-ĕn-sĕf′ə-lŏ′grə-fē) A procedure that records the electrical activity of the brain as a tracing called an electroencephalogram, or EEG, on a strip of graph paper. (23)

electrolytes (ĭ-lĕk′trə-līts) Substances that carry electrical current through the movement of ions. (5)

electromyography (ĭ-lĕk′trō-mī-og′rə-fē) A procedure in which needle electrodes are inserted into some of the skeletal muscles and a monitor records the nerve impulses and measures conduction time; used to detect neuromuscular disorders or nerve damage. (23)

electron microscope (ĭ-lĕk′trŏn mī′krə-skōp′) A microscope that uses a beam of electrons instead of a beam of light; can magnify an image several million times. (27)

elevation (e-lə-vā′-shən) The raising of a body part. (8)

embolism (ĕm′bə-lĭz′əm) An obstruction in a blood vessel. (22)

embolus (ĕm′bə-ləs) A portion of a thrombus that breaks off and moves through the bloodstream. (10)

embryonic period (em-brē-on′ik pîr′ē-əd) (†) The second through eighth weeks of pregnancy. (17)

endocardium (en-dō-kar′dē-ŭm) (†) The innermost layer of the heart. (10)

endochondral (en-dō-kon′drăl) (†) A type of ossification in which bones start out as cartilage models. (7)

endocrine gland (ĕn′də-kra-n glănd) A gland that secretes its products directly into tissue, fluid, or blood. (5)

endoderm (ĕn′dō-derm) (†) The primary germ layer that gives rise to epithelial tissues only. (17)

endogenous infection (ĕn′-dŏj′ə-nəs ĭn-fĕk′shən) An infection in which an abnormality or malfunction in routine body processes causes normally beneficial or harmless microorganisms to become pathogenic. (1)

endolymph (ĕn′dō-limf) (†) A fluid in the inner ear. When this fluid moves, it activates hearing and equilibrium receptors. (15)

endometriosis (en′dō-mē-trē-ō′sis) (†) A condition in which tissues that make up the lining of the uterus grow outside the uterus. (17)

endometrium (en′dō-mē′trē-ŭm) (†) The innermost layer of the uterus. It undergoes significant changes during the menstrual cycle. (17)

endomysium (en′dō-miz′ē-ŭm) (†) A connective tissue covering that surrounds individual muscle cells. (8)

endoscopy (ĕn-dôs′kə-pē) Any procedure in which a scope is used to visually inspect a canal or cavity within the body. (23)

endosteum (en-dos′tē-ŭm) (†) A membrane that lines the medullary cavity and the holes of spongy bone. (7)

enzyme immunoassay (EIA) (ĕn′zīm im′yū-nō-as′ā) (†) The detection of substances by immunological methods. This method involves an antigen, an antibody specific for the antigen, and a second antibody conjugated to an enzyme. (29)

enzyme-linked immunosorbent assay (ELISA) test (ĕn′zīm-lĭngkt im′yū-nō-sōr′bent ăs′ā tĕst) (†) A blood test that confirms the presence of antibodies developed by the body's immune system in response to an initial HIV infection. (3)

eosinophil (ē-ō-sin′ō-fil) (†) A type of granular leukocyte that captures invading bacteria and antigen-antibody complexes through phagocytosis. (30)

epicardium (ep-i-kar′dē-ŭm) (†) The outermost layer of the wall of the heart. Also known as the **visceral pericardium.** (10)

epidermis (ĕp′ĭ-dûr′mĭs) The most superficial layer of the skin. (6)

epididymis (ep-i-did′i-mis) (†) An elongated structure attached to the back of the testes and in which sperm cells mature. (17)

epididymitis (ep-i-did-i-mī′tis) (†) Inflammation of an **epididymis.** Most cases result from infection. (17)

epiglottic cartilage (ep-i-glot′ik kär′tl-ĭj) (†) A cartilage of the larynx that forms the framework of the epiglottis. (12)

epiglottis (ep-i-glot-ĭ´tis) (†) The flap-like structure that closes off the larynx during swallowing. (12)

epilepsy (ĕp´ə-lĕp´sē) A condition that occurs when parts of the brain receive a burst of electrical signals that disrupt normal brain function; also called **seizures.** (9)

epimysium (ep-i-mis´ē-ŭm) (†) A thin covering that is just deep to the fascia of a muscle. It surrounds the entire muscle. (8)

epinephrine (ĕp´ə-nĕf´rĭn) An injectable medication used to treat anaphylaxis by causing vasoconstriction to increase blood pressure. (11) A hormone secreted from the adrenal glands. It increases heart rate, breathing rate, and blood pressure. (14)

epiphyseal disk (ep-i-fiz´ē-ăl dĭsk) (†) A plate of cartilage between the **epiphysis** and the **diaphysis.** (7)

epiphysis (e-pif´i-sis) (†) The expanded end of a long bone. (7)

epistaxis (ĕp´i-stak´sis) Nosebleed. (26)

epithelial tissue (ep-i-thē´lē-ĕl tĭsh´o͞o) (†) A tissue type that lines the tubes, hollow organs, and cavities of the body. (5)

erectile tissue (ĭ-rĕk´təl tĭsh´o͞o) A highly specialized tissue located in the shaft of the penis. It fills with blood to achieve an erection. (17)

erythema (er-i-thē´mă) Redness of the skin. (25)

erythroblastosis fetalis (ĕ-rith´rō-blas-tō´sis fe´tăl-is) (†) A serious anemia that develops in a fetus with Rh-positive blood as a result of antibodies in an Rh-negative mother's body. (10)

erythrocytes (ĭ-rĭth´rə-sīt´s) Red blood cells. (10)

erythrocyte sedimentation rate (ESR) (ĭ-rĭth´rə-sīt´ sĕd´ə-mən-tā´shən rāt) The rate at which red blood cells, the heaviest blood component, settle to the bottom of a blood sample. (30)

erythropoietin (ĕ-rith-rō-poy´ē-tin) (†) A hormone secreted by the kidney and is responsible for regulating the production of red blood cells. (10)

esophageal hiatus (ĭ-sŏf´ə-jē´əl) Hole in the diaphragm through which the esophagus passes. (13)

estrogen (ĕs´trə-jən) A female sex hormone; when produced during ovulation, estrogen causes a buildup of the lining of the uterus (womb) to prepare it for a possible pregnancy. (14)

ethmoid (ĕth´moyd) (†) Bones located between the sphenoid and nasal bone that form part of the floor of the cranium. (7)

etiologic agent (ē´tē-ə-lŏj´ĭk ā´jənt) A living microorganism or its toxin that may cause human disease. (28)

eustachian tube (yo͞o-stā´shən to͞ob) An opening in the middle ear, leading to the back of the throat, that helps equalize air pressure on both sides of the eardrum. (21)

eversion (ē-ver´zhŭn) (†) Turning the sole of the foot laterally. (8)

excretion (ĭk-skrē´shən) The elimination of waste by a discharge; in drug metabolism, the manner in which a drug is eliminated from the body. (32)

exocrine gland (ĕk´sə-krĭn glănd) A gland that secretes its product into a duct. (5)

exogenous infection (ĕk-sŏj´ə-nəs ĭn-fĕk´shən) An infection that is caused by the introduction of a pathogen from outside the body. (1)

expiration (ĕk´spə-rā´shən) The process of breathing out; also called exhalation. (12)

extension (ĭk-stĕn´shən) An unbending or straightening movement of the two elements of a jointed body part. (8)

external auditory canal (ĭk-stûr´nəl ô´dĭ-tôr´ē kə-năl´) Canal that carries sound waves to the tympanic membrane; commonly called the ear canal. (15)

extrinsic eye muscles (ĭk-strĭn´ sĭk ī mŭs´əlz) The skeletal muscles that move the eyeball. (15)

facultative (fak-ŭl-tā´tiv) (†) Able to adapt to different conditions; in microbiology, able to grow in environments either with or without oxygen. (28)

Fahrenheit (făr´ən-hīt) One of two common scales used for measuring temperature; measured in degrees Fahrenheit, or °F. (19)

fallopian tubes (fə-l´ō-pē-ən tübz) Tubes that extend from the uterus on each side and that open near an ovary. (17)

fascia (fash´e-ă) (†) A structure that covers entire skeletal muscles and separates them from each other. (8)

fascicle (făs´ĭ-kəl) Sections of a muscle divided by connective tissue called perimysium. (8)

febrile (fĕb´rəl) Having a body temperature above one's normal range. (19)

feces (fē´sēz) Material found in the large intestine and made from leftover chyme. Faces are eventually eliminated through the anus. (13)

femoral (fem´ō-răl) (†) Relating to the femur or thigh. (5)

femur (fē´mər) The bone in the upper leg; commonly called the thigh bone. (7)

fenestrated drape (fĕn´ĭ-strāt´ĕd drāp) A drape that has a round or slitlike opening that provides access to the surgical site. (20)

fertilization (fer´til-i-zā´shŭn) The process in which an egg unites with a sperm. (17)

fetal period (fēt´l pîr´ē-əd) A period that begins at week nine of pregnancy and continues through delivery of the offspring. (17)

fiber (fī´bər) The tough, stringy part of vegetables and grains, which is not absorbed by the body but aids in a variety of bodily functions. (31)

fibrinogen (fī-brin´ō-jen) (†) A protein found in plasma that is important for blood clotting. (10)

fibroid (fī´broid´) A benign tumor in the uterus composed of fibrous tissue. (17)

fibromyalgia (fī-brō-mī-al´jē-ă) (†) A condition that exhibits chronic pain primarily in joints, muscles, and tendons. (8)

fibula (fĭb´yə-lə) The lateral bone of the lower leg. (7)

filtration (fĭl-trā´shən) A process that separates substances into solutions by forcing them across a membrane. (5)

fimbriae (fi´m-brē-ə) Fringe-like structures that border the entrances of the **fallopian tubes.** (17)

first morning urine specimen (fûrst môr´nĭng yo͝or´ĭn spĕs´ə-mən) A urine specimen that is collected after a night's sleep; contains greater concentrations of substances that collect over time than specimens taken during the day. (29)

fixative (fĭk´sə-tĭv) A solution sprayed on a slide immediately after the specimen is applied. It is used to preserve and hold the cells in place until a microscopic examination is performed. (4)

flexion (flek´shŭn) (†) A bending movement of the two elements of a jointed body part. (8)

floater (flō´tər) A nonsterile assistant who is free to move about the room during surgery and attend to unsterile needs. (24)

fluidotherapy (flo͞o´ĭd-ōthĕr´ə-pē) A technique for stimulating healing, particularly in the hands and feet, by placing the affected body part in a container of glass beads that are heated and agitated with hot air. (25)

follicle (fŏl´ĭ-kəl) An accessory organ of the skin that is found in the dermis and the sites at which hairs emerge. (6)

follicle-stimulating hormone (FSH) (fŏl´ĭ-kəl stim´yū-lā-ting hôr´mōn´) A hormone that in females stimulates the production of estrogen by the ovaries; in males, it stimulates sperm production. (14)

follicular cells (fə-li´-kyə-lər selz) Small cells contained in the primordial follicle along with a large cell called a primary **oocyte.** (17)

folliculitis (fŏ-lik-yū-lī´tis) (†) Inflammation of the hair follicle. (6)

fomite (fō´mīt) (†) An inanimate object, such as clothing, body fluids, water, or food, that may be contaminated with infectious organisms and thus serve to transmit disease. (1)

fontanel (fän-tə-n´el) The soft spot in an infant's skull that consists of tough membranes that connect to incompletely developed bone. (7)

food exchange (fo͞od ĭks-chānj´) A unit of food in a particular food category that provides the same amounts of protein, fat, and carbohydrates as all other units of food in that category. (31)

foramen magnum (fə-rā´-mən mag-nəm) The large hole in the occipital bone that allows the brain to connect to the spinal cord. (7)

foramen ovale (fō-rā´men ō-va´lē) (†) A hole in the fetal heart between the right atrium and the left atrium. (17)

forced vital capacity (FVC) (fôrst vīt´l kə-păs´ĭ-tē) The greatest volume of air that a person is able to expel when performing rapid, forced expiration. (34)

formalin (fōr-mă-lin) (†) A dilute solution of formaldehyde used to preserve biological specimens. (24)

formed elements (fôrmd ĕl´ə-mənts) Red blood cells, white blood cells, and platelets; comprise 45% of blood volume. (30)

fracture (frăk´chər) Any break in a bone. (23)

frequency (frē´kwən-sē) The number of complete fluctuations of energy per second in the form of waves. (21)

frontal (frŭn´tl) Anatomical term that refers to the plane that divides the body into anterior and posterior portions. Also called coronal. (5)

functional re´sume´ (fŭngk´shə-nəl rĕz´o͞o-mā´) A re´sume´ that highlights specialty areas of a person's accomplishments and strengths. (36)

fungus (fŭng´gəs) A eukaryotic organism that has a rigid cell wall at some stage in the life cycle. (28)

gait (gāt) The way a person walks, consisting of two phases: stance and swing. (25)

ganglia (găng´glē-ə) Collections of neuron cell bodies outside the central nervous system. (9)

gastic juice (găs´trĭk jüs) Secretions from the stomach lining that begin the process of digesting protein. (13)

gastritis (gă-strī´tĭs) Inflammation of the stomach lining. (13)

gastroesophageal reflux disease (GERD) (gas´trō-ē-sof´ă-jē´ălrē´flĕks dĭ-zēz´) A condition that occurs when stomach acids are pushed into the esophagus and cause heartburn. (13)

gene (jēn) A segment of DNA that determines a body trait. (5)

general physical examination (jĕn´ər-əl fĭz´ĭ-kəl ĭg-zăm´ə-nā´shən) An examination performed by a physician to confirm a patient's health or to diagnose a medical problem. (4)

generic name (jə-nĕr´ĭk nām) A drug's official name. (32)

giantism (jī´an-tizm) (†) A condition in which too much growth hormone is produced in childhood, resulting in an abnormally increased stature. (14)

glans penis (glanz pē´nĭs) A cone-shaped structure at the end of the penis. (17)

glaucoma (glou-kō´mə) A condition in which too much pressure is created in the eye by excessive aqueous humor. This excess pressure can lead to permanent damage of the optic nerves, resulting in blindness. (15)

globulins (glob´yū-lin) (†) Plasma proteins that transport lipids and some vitamins. (10)

glomerular capsule (glō-măr´yū-lăr kăp´səl) (†) A capsule that surrounds the **glomerulus** of the kidney. (16)

glomerular filtrate (glō-măr´yū-lăr fĭl´trāt´) (†) The fluid remaining in the **glomerular capsule** after **glomerular filtration.** (16)

glomerular filtration (glō-măr´yū-lăr fĭl-trā´shən) (†) The process by which urine forms in the kidneys as blood moves through a tight ball of capillaries called the glomerulus. (16)

glomerulonephritis (glō-măr´yū-lō-nef-rī´tis) (†) An inflammation of the glomeruli of the kidney. (16)

glomerulus (glō-măr´yū-lŭs) (†) A group of capillaries in the renal corpuscle. (16)

glottis (glot´is) (†) The opening between the vocal cords. (12)

glucagon (glo͞o´kə-gŏn´) A hormone that increases glucose concentrations in the bloodstream and slows down protein synthesis. (14)

glycogen (glī´kə-jən) An excess of glucose that is stored in the liver and in skeletal muscle. (13)

glycosuria (glī-kō-sū´rē-ă) (†) The presence of significant levels of glucose in the urine. (29)

gonads (gō´nădz) The reproductive organs; namely, in women, the ovaries, and in men, the testes. (14)

gonadotropin-releasing hormone (GnRH) (gō´nad-ō-trō´pinrĭ-lēs´ĭng hôr´mōn´) Hormone that stimulates the anterior pituitary gland to release **follicle stimulating hormone (FSH).** (17)

goniometer (gō-nē-ä´-me-tər) A protractor device that measures range of motion. (25)

gout (gowt) (†) A medical condition characterized by an elevated uric acid level and recurrent acute arthritis. (7)

G-protein (jē-prō´tēn) (†) A substance that causes enzymes in the cell to activate following the activation of the hormone-receptor complex in the cell membrane. (14)

gram-negative (grăm´nĕg´ə-tĭv) Referring to bacteria that lose their purple color when a decolorizer has been added during a Gram's stain. (28)

gram-positive (grăm´pŏz´ĭ-tĭv) Referring to bacteria that retain their purple color after a decolorizer has been added during a Gram's stain. (28)

Gram's stain (grămz stān) A method of staining that differentiates bacteria according to the chemical composition of their cell walls. (28)

granular leukocyte (grăn´yə-lər lo͞o´kə-sīt´) A type of leukocyte (white blood cell) with a segmented nucleus and granulated cytoplasm; also known as a polymorphonuclear leukocyte. (30)

granulocyte (gran´yū-lō-sīt) (†) See **granular leukocyte.** (10)

Grave's disease (grāvz dĭ-zēz´) A disorder in which a person develops antibodies that attack the thyroid gland. (14)

gray matter (grā măt´ər) The inner tissue of the brain and the spinal cord that is darker in color than **white**

matter. It contains all the bodies and dendrites of nerve cells. (9)

growth hormone (GH) (grōth hôr′mōn′) A hormone that stimulates an increase in the size of the muscles and bones of the body. (14)

gustatory receptors (gə′s-tə-tör-ē ri-se′p-tər) Taste receptors that are found on taste buds. (15)

gyri (jī′rī) (†) The ridges of brain matter between the sulci; also called **convolutions.** (9)

hapten (hap′tĕn) (†) Foreign substances in the body too small to start an immune response by themselves. (11)

hairy leukoplakia (hâr′ē lū-kō-plā′kē-ă) (†) A white lesion on the tongue associated with AIDS. (3)

hazard label (hăz′ərd lā′bəl) A shortened version of the Material Safety Data Sheet; permanently affixed to a hazardous substance container. (27)

helper T-cells (hĕl′pər tē′sĕlz) White blood cells that are a key component of the body's immune system and that work in coordination with other white blood cells to combat infection. (3)

hematemesis (hē′-mă-tem′ĕ-sis) The vomiting of blood. (26)

hematocrit (hē′mă-tō-krit) (†) The percentage of the volume of a sample made up of red blood cells after the sample has been spun in a centrifuge. (30)

hematology (hēmə-tŏl′ə-jē) The study of blood. (30)

hematoma (hē′mə-tō′mə) A swelling caused by blood under the skin. (26)

hematuria (hē-mă-tu′rē-ă) (†) The presence of blood in the urine. (29)

hemocytoblast (hē′mă-tō-sī′tō-blast) (†) Cells of the red bone marrow that produce most red blood cells. (10)

hemoglobin (hē′mə-glō′bĭn) A protein that contains iron and bonds with and carries oxygen to cells; the main component of erythrocytes. (6)

hemoglobinuria (hē′mō-glō-bi-nū′rē-ă) (†) The presence of free **hemoglobin** in the urine; a rare condition caused by transfusion reactions, malaria, drug reactions, snake bites, or severe burns. (29)

hemolysis (hē-mol′ĭ-sis) (†) The rupturing of red blood cells, which releases hemoglobin. (30)

hemorrhoids (hĕm′ə-roidz′) Varicose veins of the rectum or anus. (13)

hemostasis (hē′mō-stā-sis) (†) The stoppage of bleeding. (10)

hepatic duct (hĭ-păt′ĭk dŭkt) A duct that leaves the liver carrying bile and merges with the cystic duct to form the common bile duct. (13)

hepatic lobule (he-păt′ĭk lob′yūl) (†) Smaller divisions within the lobes of the liver. (13)

hepatic portal system (he-pat′ik pôr′tl sĭs′təm) (†) The collection of veins carrying blood to the liver. (10)

hepatic portal vein (hĭ-păt′ĭk pôr′tl vān) A blood vessel that carries blood from the other digestive organs to the **hepatic lobules.** (13)

hepatitis (hĕp′ə-tī′tĭss) Inflammation of the liver usually caused by viruses or toxins. (13)

hepatocytes (hep′ă-tō-sītz) (†) The cells within the lobules of the liver. Hepatocytes process nutrients in the blood and make bile. (13)

hernia (hûr′nē-ə) The protrusion of an organ through the wall that usually contains it, such as a hiatal or inguinal hernia. (13)

herpes simplex (her′pēz sĭm′plĕks) (†) A medical condition characterized by an eruption of one or more groups of vesicles on the lips or genitalia. (6)

herpes zoster (her′pēz zos′ter) (†) A medical condition characterized by an eruption of a group of vesicles on one side of the body following a nerve root. (6)

hilum (hī′lŭm) (†) The indented side of a lymph node. (10) The entrance of the renal sinus that contains the renal artery, renal vein, and ureter. (16)

Holter monitor (hol′tər mŏn′ĭ-tər) An electrocardiography device that includes a small portable cassette recorder worn around a patient's waist or on a shoulder strap to record the heart's electrical activity. (34)

homologous chromosome (hŏ-mŏl′ō-gŭs krō′mə-sōm′) (†) Members in each pair of chromosomes. (5)

hormone (hôr′mōn′) A chemical secreted by a cell that affects the functions of other cells. (14)

human chorionic gonadotropin (HCG) (hyo͞o′mən kō-rē-on′ik gō′nad-ō-trō′pin) A hormone secreted by cells of the embryo after implantation. It maintains the corpus luteum in the ovary so it will continue to secrete estrogen and progesterone. (17)

human immunodeficiency virus (HIV) (hyo͞o′mən im′yū-nō-dē-fish′en-sē vī′rəs) A retrovirus that gradually destroys the body's immune system and causes AIDS. (11)

humerus (hyü′-mə-rəs) The bone of the upper arm. (7)

humors (hyo͞o′mərz) Fluids of the body. (11)

hydrotherapy (hī′drə-thĕr′ə-pē) The therapeutic use of water to treat physical problems. (25)

hyoid (hī′-ȯid) The bone that anchors the tongue. (7)

hyperextension (hī′per-eks-ten′shŭn) (†) Extension of a body part past the normal anatomical position. (8)

hyperglycemia (hī′pər-glī-sē′mē-ə) High blood sugar. (26)

hyperopia (hī-per-ō′pē-ă) A condition that occurs when light entering the eye is focused behind the retina; commonly called farsightedness. (15)

hyperpnea (hī-per-nē′ă) (†) Abnormally deep, rapid breathing. (19)

hyperreflexia (hī′per-rē-flek′sē-ă) Reflexes that are stronger than normal reflexes. (9)

hypertension (hī′pər-tĕn′shən) High blood pressure. (10)

hyperventilation (hī′pər-vĕn′tl-ā′shən) The condition of breathing rapidly and deeply. Hyperventilating decreases the amount of carbon dioxide in the blood. (12)

hypodermis (hī′pə-dûr′mĭs) The subcutaneous layer of the skin that is largely made of adipose tissue. (6)

hypoglycemia (hī′pō-glī-sē′mē-ə) Low blood sugar. (26)

hyporeflexia (hī′pō-rē-flek′sē-ă) (†) A condition of decreased reflexes. (9)

hypotension (hī′pō-tĕn′shən) Low blood pressure. (19)

hypothalamus (hī′pō-thăl′ə-məs) A region of the **diencephalon.** It maintains homeostasis by regulating many vital activities such as heart rate, blood pressure, and breathing rate. (9)

hypovolemic shock (hī′per-vō-lē′mē-ă shŏk) (†) A state of shock resulting from insufficient blood volume in the circulatory system. (26)

hysterectomy (hĭs′tə-rĕk′tə-mē) Surgical removal of the uterus. (17)

ileocecal sphincter A structure that controls the movement of **chime** from the **ileum** to the **cecum.** (13)

ileum (ĭl′ē-əm) The last portion of the small intestine. It is directly attached to the large intestine. (13)

ilium (ĭ′-lē-əm) The most superior part of the hip bone. It is broad and flaring. (7)

immunity (ĭ-myo͞on′ĭ-tē) The condition of being resistant or not susceptible to pathogens and the diseases they cause. (1)

immunization (im′yū-nī-zā-shən) The administration of a vaccine or toxoid to protect susceptible individuals from communicable diseases. (2)

immunocompromised (im′yū-nō-kom′pro-mīzd) (†) Having an impaired or weakened immune system. (3)

immunofluorescent antibody (IFA) test (im′yū-nō-flūr-es′ent ăn′tĭ-bŏd-ē tĕst) (†) A blood test used to confirm enzyme-linked immunosorbent assay (ELISA) test results for HIV infection. (3)

immunoglobulins (im′yū-nō-glob′yū-linz) (†) A class of structurally related proteins that include IgG, IgA, IgM, and IgE; also called **antibodies.** (11)

impetigo (im′pĭ-tī′gō) A contagious skin infection usually caused by germs commonly called staph and strep. (6)

impotence (ĭm′pŏ-tens) (†) A disorder in which a male cannot maintain an erect penis to complete sexual intercourse; also called erectile dysfunction. (17)

incision (ĭn-sĭzh′ən) A surgical wound made by cutting into body tissue. (24)

incisors (ĭn-sī′zərz) The most medial teeth. They act as chisels to bite off food. (13)

incomplete proteins (ĭn′kəm-plēt′ prō′tēnz′) Proteins that lack one or more of the essential amino acids. (31)

incontinence (in-kon′ti-nens) (†) The involuntary leakage of urine. (16)

incus (ĭng′kəs) A small bone in the middle ear, located between the malleus and the stapes; also called the anvil. (21)

indication (ĭn′dĭ-kā′shən) The purpose or reason for using a drug, as approved by the FDA. (32)

induration The process of hardening or of becomming hard. (2)

infection (ĭn-fĕk′shən) The presence of a pathogen in or on the body. (11)

inferior (ĭn-fîr′ē-ər) Anatomical term meaning below or closer to the feet; also called caudal. (5)

inflammation (ĭn′flə-mā′shən) The body's reaction when tissue becomes injured or infected. The four cardinal signs are redness, heat, pain, and swelling. (11)

infundibulum (in-fŭn-dib′yū-lŭm) (†) The funnel-like end of the uterine tube near an ovary. It catches the secondary oocyte as it leaves the ovary. (17)

infusion (in-fyū′zhŭn) (†) A slow drip, as of an intravenous solution into a vein. (33)

inner cell mass (ĭn′ər sĕl măs) A group of cells in a blastocyte that gives rise to an embryo. (17)

inorganic (ĭn′ôr-găn′ĭk) Matter that generally does not contain carbon and hydrogen. (5)

insertion (ĭn-sûr′shən) An attachment site of a skeletal muscle that moves when a muscle contracts. (8)

inspection (ĭn-spĕk′shən) The visual examination of the patient's entire body and overall appearance. (20)

inspiration (in(†)-spə-rā′-shən) The act of breathing in; also called inhalation. (12)

insulin (ĭn′sə-lĭn) A hormone that regulates the amount of sugar in the blood by facilitating its entry into the cells. (14)

intercalated disc (in-ter′kă-lā-ted disk) (†) A disk that connects groups of cardiac muscles. This disc allows the fibers in that group to contract and relax together. (8)

interferon (in-ter-fēr′on) (†) A protein that blocks viruses from infecting cells. (11)

interneuron (in′ter-nū′ron) (†) A structure found only in the central nervous system that functions to link sensory and motor neurons together. (9)

interphase (in′ter-fāz) (†) The state of a cell carrying out its normal daily functions and not dividing. (5)

interstitial cell (in-ter-stish′ăl sĕl) A cell located between the seminiferous tubules that is responsible for making testosterone. (17)

intestinal lipase (ĭn-tĕs′tĭ-n lip′ās) An enzyme that digests fat. (13)

intradermal (ID) (in′tră-der′măl) Within the upper layers of the skin. (33)

intradermal test (in′tră-der′măl tĕst) An allergy test in which dilute solutions of allergens are introduced into the skin of the inner forearm or upper back with a fine-gauge needle. (23)

intramembranous (in-trə-me′m-brə-nəs) A type of ossification in which bones begin as tough fibrous membranes. (7)

intramuscular (IM) (in′tră-mŭs′kyū-lăr) Within muscle; an IM injection allows administration of a larger amount of a drug than a subcutaneous injection allows. (33)

intraoperative (in′tră-ŏp′ər-ə-tĭv) Taking place during surgery. (24)

intravenous IV (ĭn′trə-vē′nəs) Injected directly into a vein. (33)

intravenous pyelography (IVP) (ĭn′trə-vē′nəs pī′ĕ-log′ră-fē) (†) A radiologic procedure in which the doctor injects a contrast medium into a vein and takes a series of x-rays of the kidneys, ureters, and bladder to evaluate urinary system abnormalities or trauma to the urinary system; also known as excretory urography. (35)

intrinsic factor (ĭn-trĭn′zĭk făk′tər) A substance secreted by **parietal cells** in the lining of the stomach. It is necessary for vitamin B_{12} absorption. (13)

invasive (ĭn-vā′sĭv) Referring to a procedure in which a catheter, wire, or other foreign object is introduced into a blood vessel or organ through the skin or a body orifice. Surgical asepsis is required during all invasive tests. (35)

inversion (ĭn-vûr′zhən) Turning the sole of the foot medially. (8)

ions (ī′ənz) Positively or negatively charged particles. (5)

iris (ī′rĭs) The colored part of the eye, made of muscular tissue that contracts and relaxes, altering the size of the pupil. (15)

ischium (is′-kē-əm) A structure that forms the lower part of the hip bone. (7)

islets of Langerhans (ī′lĭt lan′ger-hans) Structures in the pancreas that secrete insulin and glucagon into the bloodstream. (14)

jaundice (jôn′dĭs) A condition characterized by yellowness of the skin, eyes, mucous membranes, and excretions; occurs during the second stage of hepatitis infection. (3)

jejunum (jə-jo͞o′nəm) The mid-portion and the majority of the small intestine. (13)

juxtaglomerular apparatus (jŭks′tă-glŏ-mer′yū-lăr ăp′ə-răt′əs) (†) A structure contained in the nephron and made up of the macula densa and **juxtaglomerular cells.** (16)

juxtaglomerular cells (jŭks′tă-glŏ-mer′yū-lăr sĕlz) Enlarged smooth muscle cells in the walls of either the afferent or efferent arterioles. (16)

Kaposi's sarcoma (kap′ō-sēz sar-kō′mă) Abnormal tissue occurring in the skin, and sometimes in the lymph nodes and organs, manifested by reddish-purple to dark blue patches or spots on the skin. (3)

keratin (kĕr′ə-tĭn) A tough, hard protein contained in skin, hair, and nails. (6)

keratinocyte (kĕ-rat′i-nō-sīt) (†) The most common cell type in the epidermis of the skin. (6)

KOH mount (kā′ō-āch mount) A type of mount used when a physician suspects a patient has a fungal infection of the skin, nails, or hair and to which potassium hydroxide is added to dissolve the keratin in cell walls. (28)

Krebs cycle (krēbz sī′kəl) Also called the citric acid cycle. This cycle generates ATP for muscle cells. (8)

KUB radiography (kā′yōō-bē rā′dē-og′ră-fē) (†) The process of x-raying the abdomen to help assess the size, shape, and position of the urinary organs; evaluate urinary system diseases or disorders; or determine the presence of kidney stones. It can also be helpful in determining the position of an intrauterine device (IUD) or in locating foreign bodies in the digestive tract; also called a flat plate of the abdomen. (35)

kyphosis (kī-fō′sis) A deformity of the spine characterized by a bent-over position; more commonly called humpback. (20)

labeling (lā′bəl-ĭng) Information provided with a drug, including FDA-approved indications and the form of the drug. (32)

labia majora (lā′bē-ă mă′jôr-ă) The rounded folds of adipose tissue and skin that serve to protect the other female reproductive organs. (17)

labia minora (lā′bē-ă mī′nôr-ă) The folds of skin between the labia majora. (17)

labyrinth (lăb′ə-rĭnth′) The inner ear. (21)

laceration (lăs′ə-rā′shən) A jagged, open wound in the skin that can extend down into the underlying tissue. (24)

lacrimal apparatus (lăk′rə-məl ăp′ə-răt′əs) A structure that consists of the lacrimal glands and nasolacrimal ducts. (15)

lacrimal gland (lăk′rə-məl glănd) A gland in the eye that produces tears. (15)

lactase (lăk′tās) (†) An enzyme that digests sugars. (13)

lactic acid (lăk′tĭk ăs′ĭd) A waste product that must be released from the cell. It is produced when a cell is low on oxygen and converts pyruvic acid. (8)

lactogen (lak′tō-jen) Substance secreted by the placenta that stimulates the enlargement of the mammary glands. (17)

lacunae (lə-kü-na) Holes in the matrix of bone that hold osteocytes. (7)

lag phase (lăg fāz) The initial phase of wound healing, in which bleeding is reduced as blood vessels in the affected area constrict. (24)

lamella (lə-me′-lə) Layers of bone surrounding the canals of osteons. (7)

lancet (lăn′sĭt) A small, disposable instrument with a sharp point used to puncture the skin and make a shallow incision; used for capillary puncture. (30)

laryngopharynx (lă-ring′gō-far-ingks) (†) The portion of the pharynx behind the **larynx.** (13)

larynx (lăr′ĭngks) The part of the respiratory tract between the pharynx and the trachea that is responsible for voice production; also called the voice box. (12)

lateral (lăt′ər-əl) A directional term that means farther away from the midline of the body. (5)

lead (lēd) A view of a specific area of the heart on an electrocardiogram. (34)

lens (lēnz) A clear, circular disc located in the eye, just posterior to the iris, that can change shape to help the eye focus images of objects that are near or far away. (21)

leukemia (lōō-kē′mē-ə) A medical condition in which bone marrow produces a large number of white blood cells that are not normal. (10)

leukocytes (lōō-kə-sīt′s) White blood cells. (10)

leukocytosis (lū′kō-sī-tō′sis) (†) A white blood cell count that is above normal. (10)

leukopenia (lū′kō-pē′nē-ă) (†) A white blood cell count that is below normal. (10)

ligament (lĭg′ə-mənt) A tough, fibrous band of tissue that connects bone to bone. (7)

ligature (lĭg′ə-chŏŏr′) Suture material. (24)

lingual frenulum (ling′gwăl fren′yū-lŭm) (†) A flap of mucosa that holds the body of the tongue to the floor of the oral cavity. (13)

lingual tonsils (ling′gwăl ton′silz) (†) Two lumps of lymphatic tissue on the back of the tongue that act to destroy bacteria and viruses. (13)

linoleic acid (lin-ō-lē′ik as′id) (†) An essential fatty acid found in corn and sunflower oils. (13)

lipoproteins (lip-ō-prō′tēnz) Large molecules that are fat-soluble on the inside and water-soluble on the outside and carry lipids such as cholesterol and triglycerides through the bloodstream. (31)

lobe (lōb) The frontal, parietal, temporal, or occipital regions of the cerebral hemisphere. (9)

loop of Henle (lōōp hen′lē) The portion of the renal tubule that curves back toward the renal corpuscle and twists again to become the distal convoluted tubule. (16)

lumbar enlargement (lŭm′bər ĕn-lärj′mənt) The thickening of the spinal cord in the low back region. (9)

lunula (lū′nū-lă) The white half-moon–shaped area at the base of a nail. (6)

lupus erythematosis (lōō′pəs er-ə-the′-tō′-səs) An autoimmune disorder in which a person produces antibodies that target the person's own cells and tissues. (11)

luteinizing hormone (LH) (lū′tē-in-iz-ing hôr′mōn′) (†) Hormone that in females stimulates ovulation and the production of estrogen; in males, it stimulates the production of testosterone. (14)

lymph (lĭmf) A pale fluid found between cells that is collected by the lymphatic system and returned to the bloodstream. (10)

lymphedema (limf′e-dē′mă) The blockage of lymphatic vessels that results in the swelling of tissue from the accumulation of lymphatic fluid. (11)

lymphocyte (lĭm′fō-sīt) (†) An agranular leukocyte formed in lymphatic tissue. Lymphocytes are generally small. See **T lymphocyte** and **B lymphocyte.** (10)

lysozyme (lī′sō-zīm) (†) An enzyme in tears that destroys pathogens on the surface of the eye. (11)

macrophage (măk′rə-fāj′) A type of phagocytic cell found in the liver, spleen, lungs, bone marrow, and connective tissue. Macrophages play several roles in humoral and cell-mediated immunity, including presenting the antigens to the lymphocytes involved in these defenses; also known as monocytes while in the bloodstream. (1)

macula densa (mak′yū-lă den′sa) (†) An area of the distal convoluted tubule that touches afferent and efferent arterioles. (16)

macular degeneration (mak′yū-lăr dē-jen-er-ā′shŭn) (†) A progressive disease that usually affects people over the age of 50. It occurs when the retina no longer receives an adequate blood supply. (15)

magnetic resonance imaging (măg-nĕt′ĭk rĕz′ə-nəns ĭ-măj′ing) A viewing technique that uses a powerful magnetic field to produce an image of internal body structures. (23)

major histocompatibility complex (MHC) (mā′jər his′tō-kom-pat-i-bil′i-tē kəm-plĕks) A large protein complex that plays a role in T cell activation. (11)

malignant (mə-lĭg′nənt) A type of tumor or neoplasm that is invasive and destructive and that tends to metastasize; it is commonly known as cancerous. (11)

malleus (măl′ē-əs) A small bone in the middle ear that is attached to the eardrum; also called the hammer. (21)

maltase (mawl-tās) An enzyme that digests sugars. (13)

mammary glands (mam′ă-rē glăndz) Accessory organs of the female reproductive system that secrete milk after pregnancy. (17)

mammography (mă-mŏg′rə-fē) X-ray examination of the breasts. (35)

mandible (man′-də-bəl) A bone that forms the lower portion of the jaw. (7)

manipulation (mə-nĭp′yə-la′shən) The systematic movement of a patient's body parts. (20)

marrow (mer′-ō) A substance that is contained in the medullary cavity. In adults, it consists primarily of fat. (7)

mastoid process (mas′-tō′id pr′ä-ses) A large bump on each temporal bone just behind each ear. It resembles a nipple, hence the name mastoid. (7)

matrix (mā′trĭks) The material between the cells of connective tissue. (5)

matter (măt′er) Anything that takes up space and has weight. Liquids, solids, and gases are matter. (5)

maturation phase (măch′ə-rā′shən fāz) The third phase of wound healing, in which scar tissue forms. (24)

maxillae (mak-si′-lə) A bone that forms the upper portion of the jaw. (7)

Mayo stand (mā′ō stănd) A movable stainless steel instrument tray on a stand. (24)

medial (mē′dē-əl) A directional term that describes areas closer to the midline of the body. (5)

medical asepsis (mĕd′ĭ-kəl ə-sĕp′sĭs) Measures taken to reduce the number of microorganisms, such as hand washing and wearing examination gloves, that do not necessarily eliminate microorganisms; also called clean technique. (24)

medical practice act (mĕd′ĭ-kəl prăk′tĭs ăkt) A law that defines the exact duties that physicians and other health-care personnel may perform. (22)

medullary cavity (me′-de-ler-ē ka′-və-tē) The canal that runs through the center of the **diaphysis.** (7)

megakaryocytes (meg-ă-kar′ē-ō-sīts) (†) Cells within red blood marrow that give rise to platelets. (10)

meiosis (mī-ō′sis) (†) A type of cell division in which each new cell contains only one member of each chromosome pair. (5)

melanin (mĕl′ə-nĭn) A pigment that is deposited throughout the layers of the epidermis. (6)

melanocyte (mĕl′ă-nō-sīt) (†) A cell type within the epidermis that makes the pigment **melanin.** (6)

melatonin (mĕl′ə-tō′nĭn) A hormone that helps to regulate circadian rhythms. (14)

membrane potential (mĕm′brān′ pə-tĕn′shəl) The potential inside a cell relative to the fluid outside the cell. (9)

meninges (mĕ-nin′jēz) (†) Membranes that protect the brain and spinal cord. (9)

meningitis (mĕn′ĭn-jī′tĭs) An inflammation of the **meninges.** (9)

meniscus (mə-nĭs′kəs) The curve in the air-to-liquid surface of a liquid specimen in a container. (19)

menopause (mĕn′ə-pôz′) The termination of the menstrual cycle due to the normal aging of the ovaries. (17)

menses (mĕn′sēz) The clinical term for menstrual flow. (17)

menstral cycle (mĕn′stro͞o-əl sī′kəl) The female reproductive cycle. It consists of regular changes in the uterine lining that lead to monthly bleeding. (17)

mensuration (mĕn′sə-rā′-shən) The process of measuring. (20)

mesoderm (mez′ō-derm) (†) The primary germ layer that gives rise to connective tissue and some epithelial tissue. (17)

metabolism (mĭ-tăb′ə-lĭz′əm) The overall chemical functioning of the body, including all body processes that build small molecules into large ones (anabolism) and break down large molecules into small ones (catabolism). (5)

metacarpals (me-tə-k′är-pəl) The bones that form the palms of the hand. (7)

metastasis (mə-tăs′tə-sĭs) The transfer of abnormal cells to body sites far removed from the original tumor. (23)

metatarsals (mĕt′ə-tär′salz) The bones that form the front of the foot. (7)

microbiology (mī′krō-bī-ŏl′ə-jē) The study of microorganisms. (28)

microorganism (mī′krō-ôr′gə-nĭz′əm) A simple form of life, commonly made up of a single cell and so small that it can be seen only with a microscope. (1)

micropipette (mī′krō-pĭ-pet′) A small pipette that holds a small, precise volume of fluid; used to collect capillary blood. (30)

microvilli (mī′krō-vil′-ī) (†) Structures found in the lining of the small intestine. They greatly increase the surface area of the small intestine so it can absorb many nutrients. (13)

micturition (mik-chū-rish′ŭn) (†) The process of urination. (16)

midsagittal (mid′saj′i-tăl) (†) Anatomical term that refers to the plane that runs lengthwise down the midline of the body, dividing it into equal left and right halves. (5)

minerals (mĭn′ər-əlz) Natural, inorganic substances the body needs to help build and maintain body tissues and carry on life functions. (31)

mirroring (mĭr′ər-ĭng) Restating in your own words what a person is saying. (18)

mitosis (mī-tō′sĭs) A type of cell division that produces ordinary body, or somatic, cells; each new cell receives a complete set of paired chromosomes. (5)

mitral valve (mī′trăl vălv) (†) See **bicuspid valve.** (10)

mobility aids (mō′bəl-ə-tē ādz) Devices that improve one's ability to move from one place to another; also called mobility assistive devices. (25)

molars (mō′lərz) Back teeth that are flat and are designed to grind food. (13)

mold (mōld) Fungi that grow into large, fuzzy, multicelled organisms that produce spores. (28)

molecule (mŏl′ĭ-kyo͞ol′) The smallest unit into which an element can be divided and still retain its properties; it is formed when atoms bond together. (5)

monocytes (mŏn′ō-sīts) (†) A large white blood cell with an oval or horseshoe-shaped nucleus that defends the body by phagocytosis; develops into a macrophage when it moves from blood into other tissues. (10)

monosaccharide (mon-ō-sak′ă-rīd) (†) A type of carbohydrate that is a simple sugar. (13)

mons pubis (m′änz py′ü-bəs) A fatty area that overlies the public bone. (17)

mordant (môr´dnt) A substance, such as iodine, that can intensify or deepen the response a specimen has to a stain. (28)

morphology (môr-fŏl´ə-jē) The study of the shape or form of objects. (30)

morula (mōr´ū-lă) (†) A zygote that has undergone cleavage and results in a ball of cells. (17)

motor (mō´tər) Efferent neurons that carry information from the central nervous system to the effectors. (9)

mucocutaneous exposure (myü-kō-kyü´-tā-nē-əs ik-spō´-zhər) Exposure to a pathogen through mucous membranes. (3)

mucosa (myo͞o-kō´sə) The innermost layer of the wall of the alimentary canal. (13)

mucous cells (myo͞o´kəs sĕlz) Cells that are found in the salivary glands and the lining of the stomach and that secrete mucous. (13)

MUGA scan (mŭg´ə skăn) A radiologic procedure that evaluates the condition of the heart's myocardium; it involves injection of radioisotopes that concentrate in the myocardium, followed by the use of a gamma camera to measure ventricular contractions to evaluate the patient's heart wall. (35)

multi-unit smooth muscle (mŭl´tə-yo͞o´nĭt smo͞oth mŭs´əl) A type of smooth muscle that is found in the iris of the eye and in the walls of blood vessels. (8)

murmur (mûr´mər) An abnormal heart sound heard when the ventricles contract and blood leaks back into the atria. (10)

muscle tissue (mŭs´əl tĭsh´o͞o) A tissue type that is specialized to shorten and elongate. (5)

muscle fatigue (mŭs´əl fa-tēg´) A condition caused by a buildup of lactic acid. (8)

muscle fiber (mŭs´əl fī´bər) Muscle cells that are called fibers because of their long lengths. (8)

muscular dystrophy (mŭs´kyə-lər dis´trō-fē) (†) A group of inherited disorders characterized by a loss of muscle tissue and by muscle weakness. (8)

mutation (myo͞o-ta´shən) An error that sometimes occurs when DNA is duplicated. When it occurs, it is passed to descendent cells and may or may not affect them in harmful ways. (5)

myasthenia gravis (mī-as-thē´nē-ă grav´is) An autoimmune disorder that is characterized by muscle weakness. (8)

myelin (mī´ə-lĭn) A fatty substance that insulates the axon and allows it to send nerve impulses quickly. (9)

myelography (mī´ē-log´ră-fē) An x-ray visualization of the spinal cord after the injection of a radioactive contrast medium or air into the spinal subarachnoid space (between the second and innermost of three membranes that cover the spinal cord). This test can reveal tumors, cysts, spinal stenosis, or herniated disks. (23)

myocardial infarction (mī´ō-kär´dē-ăl ĭn-fark´shən) A heart attack that occurs when the blood flow to the heart is reduced as a result of blockage in the coronary arteries or their branches. (10)

myocardium (mī´ō-kär´dē-əm) The middle and thickest layer of the heart. It is made primarily of cardiac muscle. (10)

myofibrils (mī-ō-fī´brils) (†) Long structures that fill the sarcoplasm of a muscle fiber. (8)

myoglobin (mī-ō-glō´bin) (†) A pigment contained in muscle cells that stores extra oxygen. (8)

myoglobinuria (mī´ō-glō-bi-nūrē-ă) The presence of myoglobin in the urine; can be caused by injured or damaged muscle tissue. (29)

myometrium (mī´ō-mē´trē-ŭm) (†) The middle, thick muscular layer of the uterus. (17)

myopia (mī-ō´pē-ə) A condition that occurs when light entering the eye is focused in front of the retina; commonly called nearsightedness. (15)

myxedema (mik-se-dē´mă) (†) A severe type of hypothyroidism that is most common in women over the age of 50. (14)

nail bed (nāl bĕd) The layer beneath each nail. (6)

narcotic (när-kŏt´ĭk) A popular term for an opioid and term of choice in government agencies; see **opioid.** (32)

nasal (nā´zəl) Relating to the nose. The nasal bones fuse to form the bridge of the nose. (7)

nasal conchae (nā´zəl kon´kē) (†) Structures that extend from the lateral walls of the nasal cavity. (12)

nasal mucosa (nā´zəl myo͞o-kō´sə) The lining of the nose. (20)

nasal septum (nā´zəl sĕp´təm) A structure that divides the nasal cavity into a left and right portion. (12)

nasolacrimal duct (nā-zō-lăk´rə-məl dŭkt) A structure located on the medial aspect of each eyeball. These ducts drain tears into the nose. (15)

nasopharynx (nā´zō-far´ingks) (†) The portion of the pharynx behind the nasal cavity. (13)

natural killer (NK) cells (năch´ər-el kĭl´ər selz) Non-B and non-T lymphocytes. NK cells kill cancer cells and virus-infected cells without previous exposure to the antigen. (11)

needle biopsy (nēd´l bī´ŏp´sē) A procedure in which a needle and syringe are used to aspirate (withdraw by suction) fluid or tissue cells. (24)

neonatal period (nē-ō-nā´tăl pîr´ē-əd) (†) The first four weeks of the postnatal period of an offspring. (17)

neonate (nē´ə-nāt´) An infant during the first four weeks of life. (17)

nephrons (nef´ronz) (†) Microscopic structures in the kidneys that filter blood and form urine. (16)

nerve fiber (nûrv fī´bər) A structure that extends from the cell body. It consists of two types: axons and dendrites. (9)

nerve impulse (nûrv ĭm´pŭls´) Electrochemical messages transmitted from neurons to other neurons and effectors. (9)

nervous tissue (nûr´vəs tĭsh´o͞o) A tissue type located in the brain, spinal cord, and peripheral nerves. (5)

networking (nĕt´wûrk´ĭng) Making contacts with relatives, friends, and acquaintances that may have information about how to find a job in your field. (36)

neuralgia (no͝o-răl´jə) A medical condition characterized by severe pain along the distribution of a nerve. (9)

neuroglial cell (nū-rog´lē-ăl sĕl) (†) Non-neuronal type of nervous tissue that is smaller and more abundant than neurons. Neuroglial cells support neurons. (9)

neuron (no͝or´ŏn´) A nerve cell; it carries nerve impulses between the brain or spinal cord and other parts of the body. (5)

neurotransmitter (no͝or´ō-trăns´mĭt-ər) A chemical within the vesicles of the synaptic knob that is released into the postsynaptic structures when a nerve impulse reaches the synaptic knob. (9)

neutrophil (nū´trō-fil) (†) A type of granular leukocyte that aids in phagocytosis by attacking bacterial invaders; also responsible for the release of pyrogens. (10)

nocturia (nok-tū´rē-ă) (†) Excessive nighttime urination. (29)

noninvasive (non-in-vā´siv)(†) Referring to procedures that do not require inserting devices, breaking the skin, or monitoring to the degree needed with invasive procedures. (35)

nonsteroidal hormone (non-stĕr´oyd-al hôr´mōn´)(†) A type of hormone made of amino acids and proteins. (14)

norepinephrine (nōr´ep-i-nef´rin)(†) A neurotransmitter released by sympathetic neurons onto organs and glands for fight-or-flight (stressful) situations. (8)

normal flora (nôr´məl flō´ră) Beneficial bacteria found in the body that create a barrier against pathogens by producing substances that may harm invaders and using up the resources pathogens need to live. (1)

nosocomial infection (nos-ō-kō´mē-ăl ĭn-fĕk-shən) An infection contracted in a hospital. (2)

nuclear medicine (nōō´klē-ər mĕd´ĭ-sĭn) The use of radionuclides, or radioisotopes (radioactive elements or their compounds), to evaluate the bone, brain, lungs, kidneys, liver, pancreas, thyroid, and spleen; also known as radionuclide imaging. (35)

nucleases (nū´klē-ās-ez) Pancreatic enzymes that digest nucleic acids. (13)

nucleus (nōō´klē-əs)(†) The control center of a cell; contains the chromosomes that direct cellular processes. (5)

O and P specimen (ō ənd pē spĕs´ə-mən) An ova and parasites specimen, or a stool sample, that is examined for the presence of certain forms of protozoans or parasites, including their eggs (ova). (28)

objectives (ob-jek´tĭvs) The set of magnifying lenses contained in the nosepiece of a compound microscope. (27)

occipital (ŏk-sĭp´ĭ-tl) Relating to the back of the head. The occipital bone forms the back of the skull. (7)

occult blood (ə-kŭlt blŭd) Blood contained in some other substance, not visible to the naked eye. (4)

ocular (ŏk´yə-lər) An eyepiece of a microscope. (27)

oil-immersion objective (oilĭ-mûr´zhən əb-jĕk´tĭv) A microscope objective that is designed to be lowered into a drop of immersion oil placed directly above the prepared specimen under examination, eliminating the air space between the microscope slide and the objective and producing a much sharper, brighter image. (27)

ointment (oint´mənt) A form of topical drug; also known as a salve. (33)

olfactory (ŏl-făk´tə-rē) Relating to the sense of smell. (15)

oliguria Insufficient production (or volume) of urine. (29)

onychectomy (ŏn-i-kek´tō-mē) The removal of a fingernail or toenail. (24)

oocyte (ōō-sīt)(†) The immature egg. (17)

oogenesis (ō-ō-jen´ĕ-sis)(†) The process of egg cell formation. (17)

ophthalmologist (ŏf-thəl-mŏl´ə-jĭst) A medical doctor who is an eye specialist. (21)

ophthalmoscope (of-thal´mōskōp)(†) A hand-held instrument with a light; used to view inner eye structures. (23)

opioid (ō´-pē-ȯid) A natural or synthetic drug that produces opium-like effects. (32)

optic chiasm (ŏp´tĭk kī´azm)(†) A structure located at the base of the brain where parts of the optic nerves cross. It carries visual information to the brain. (14)

optical microscope (op´ti-kăl mī´krə-skōp´) A microscope that uses light, concentrated through a condenser and focused through the object being examined, to project an image. (27)

opportunistic infection (ŏp´ər-tōōnĭs´tĭk ĭn-fĕk-shən) Infection by microorganisms that can cause disease only when a host's resistance is low. (1)

optometrist (ŏp-tŏm´ĭ-trĭst) A trained and licensed vision specialist who is not a physician. (21)

orbicularis oculi (ōr-bik´yū-lā´ris ok´yū-lī) The muscle in the eyelid responsible for blinking. (15)

orbit (ôr´bĭt) The eye socket, which forms a protective shell around the eye. (21)

organ (ôr´gan) Structure formed by the organization of two or more different tissue types that carries out specific functions. (5)

organelle (ôr´gə-nəl´) A structure within a cell that performs a specific function. (5)

organic (ôr-găn´ĭk) Pertaining to matter that contains carbon and hydrogen. (5)

organism (ôr´gə-nĭz´əm) A whole living being that is formed from organ systems. (5)

organ system (ôr´gən sĭs´təm) A system that consists of organs that join together to carry out vital functions. (5)

origin (ôr´ə-jĭn) An attachment site of a skeletal muscle that does not move when a muscle contracts. (8)

oropharynx (ōr´ō-far´ingks)(†) The portion of the pharynx behind the oral cavity. (13)

osmosis (ŏz-mō´sĭs) The diffusion of water across a semipermeable membrane such as a cell membrane. (5)

ossification (ä-sə-fə-kā´-shən) The process of bone growth. (7)

osteoblast (os´tē-ō-blast)(†) Bone-forming cells that turn membrane into bone. They use excess blood calcium to build new bone. (7)

osteoclast (os´tē-ō-klast)(†) Bone-dissolving cells. When bone is dissolved, calcium is released into the bloodstream. (7)

osteocyte (äs´-tē-ə-sīt) A cell of osseous tissue; also called a bone cell. (7)

osteon (äs´-tē-ən) Elongated cylinders that run up and down the long axis of bone. (7)

osteoporosis (ôs´tē-ō-pə-rō´sĭs) An endocrine and metabolic disorder of the musculoskeletal system, more common in women than in men, characterized by hunched-over posture. (22)

osteosarcoma (os´tē-ō-sar-kō´mă) A type of bone cancer that originates from osteoblasts, the cells that make bony tissue. (7)

otologist (ō-tol´ō-jist)(†) A medical doctor who specializes in the health of the ear. (21)

oval window (ō´vəl wĭn´dō) The beginning of the inner ear. (15)

ovulation (ō´vyə-lā´shən) The process by which the ovaries release one ovum (egg) approximately every 28 days. (17)

oxygen debt (ŏk´sĭ-jən) A condition that develops when skeletal muscles are used strenuously for a minute or two. (8)

oxyhemoglobin (oks-ē-hē-mō-glō´bin) (†) Hemoglobin that is bound to oxygen. It is bright red in color. (10)

oxytocin OT (ok-sē-tō´sin)(†) A hormone that causes contraction of the uterus during childbirth and the ejection of milk from mammary glands during breast-feeding. (14)

packed red blood cells (păkt rĕd blud sĕlz) Red blood cells that collect at the bottom of a centrifuged blood sample. (30)

palate (pal´ăt)(†) The roof of the mouth. (13)

palatine (pa´-lə-tīn) Bones that form the anterior potion of the roof of the mouth and the **palate.** (7)

palatine tonsils (pal´ă-tīn tŏn´sils) (†) Two masses of lymphatic tissue located at the back of the throat. (13)

palpation (păl-pā´shən) A type of touch used by health-care providers to determine characteristics such as texture, temperature, shape, and the presence of movement. (20)

palpatory method (pal-pa´tôr´ē mĕth´əd) Systolic blood pressure measured by using the sense of touch. This measurement provides a necessary preliminary approximation of the systolic blood pressure to ensure an adequate level of inflation when the actual auscultatory measurement is made. (19)

palpitations (păl´pĭ-tā´shənz) Unusually rapid, strong, or irregular pulsations of the heart. (26)

pancreatic amylase (pan-krē-at´ik am´il-ās) (†) An enzyme that digests carbohydrates. (13)

pancreatic lipase (pan-krē-at´ik lip´ās) (†) An enzyme that digests lipids. (13)

papillae (pə-pĭl´ē) The "bumps" of the tongue in which the taste buds are found. (15)

paranasal sinuses (par-ă-nā´zəl sī´nŭs-ĕz) Air-filled spaces within skull bones that open into the nasal cavity. (12)

parasite (păr´ə-sīt´) An organism that lives on or in another organism and relies on it for nourishment or some other advantage to the detriment of the host organism. (28)

parasympathetic (păr´ə-sĭm´pə-thĕt´ĭk) (†) A division of the autonomic nervous system that prepares the body for rest and digestion. (9)

parathyroid hormone (par-ă-thī´royd hôr´mōn´) (†) A hormone that helps regulate calcium levels in the bloodstream. (17)

parenteral nutrition (pă-ren´ter-ăl nōō-trĭsh´ən) Nutrition obtained when specially prepared nutrients are injected directly into patients' veins rather than taken by mouth. (31)

paresthesias (par-es-thē´zē-ăs) (†) Abnormal sensations ranging from burning to tingling. (9)

parietal Bones that form most of the top and sides of the skull. (7)

parietal cells (pă-rī´ĕ-tăl sĕlz) Stomach cells that secrete hydrochloric acid, which is necessary to convert **pepsinogen** to **pepsin.** Parietal cells also secrete **intrinsic factor,** which is necessary for vitamin B_{12} absorption. (13)

parietal pericardium (pă-rī´ĕ-tăl per-i-kar´dē-ŭm) (†) The layer on top of the visceral pericardium. (10)

parotid glands (pă-rot´id glăndz) (†) The largest of the salivary glands. The parotid glands are located beneath the skin just in front of the ears. (13)

patch test (păch tĕst) An allergy test in which a gauze patch soaked with a suspected allergen is taped onto the skin with nonallergenic tape; used to discover the cause of contact dermatitis. (23)

patella (pə-té-lə) The bone commonly referred to as the kneecap. (7)

pathogen (păth´ə-jən) A microorganism capable of causing disease. (1)

patient compliance (pā´shənt kəm-plī´əns) Obedience in terms of following a physician's orders. (20)

pectoral girdle The structure that attaches the arms to the axial skeleton. (7)

pelvic girdle The structure that attaches the legs to the axial skeleton. (7)

pepsin (pep´sin) (†) An enzyme that allows the body to digest proteins. (13)

pepsinogen (pep-sin´ō-jen) (†) Substance that is secreted by the chief cells in the lining of the stomach and becomes **pepsin** in the presence of acid. (13)

peptidases (pep´ti-dās-ez) (†) Enzymes that digest proteins. (13)

percussion (pər-kŭsh´ən) Tapping or striking the body to hear sounds or feel vibration. (20)

percutaneous exposure (per-kyū-tā´nē-ŭs ĭk-spō´zhər) (†) Exposure to a pathogen through a puncture wound or needlestick. (3)

pericardium (per-i-kar´dē-ŭm) (†) A membrane that covers the heart and large blood vessels attached to it. (10)

perilymph (per´i-limf) (†) A fluid in the inner ear. When this fluid moves, it activates hearing and equilibrium receptors. (15)

perimetrium The thin layer that covers the myometrium of the uterus. (17)

perimysium (per-i-mis´ē-ŭm) (†) The connective tissue that divides a muscle into sections called fascicles. (8)

periosteum The membrane that surrounds the **diaphysis** of a bone. (7)

peripheral nervous system (pə-rĭf´ər-əl nûr´vəs sĭs´təm) A system that consists of nerves that branch off the central nervous system. (9)

peristalsis (pĕr´ĭ-stôl´sĭs) The rhythmic muscular contractions that move food through the digestive tract. (8)

phagocyte (făg´ə-sīt´) A specialized white blood cell that engulfs and digests pathogens. (1)

phagocytosis (fag´ō-sī-tō´sis) (†) The process by which white blood cells defend the body against infection by engulfing invading pathogens. (11)

phalanges The bones of the fingers. (7)

pharmaceutical (fär´mə-sōō´tĭ-kəl) Pertaining to medicinal drugs. (32)

pharmacodynamics (far´mă-kō-dī-nam´iks) (†) The study of what drugs do to the body: the mechanism of action, or how they work to produce a therapeutic effect. (32)

pharmacognosy (far-mă-kog´nō-sē) (†) The study of characteristics of natural drugs and their sources. (32)

pharmacokinetics (far´mă-kō-kinet´iks) (†) The study of what the body does to drugs: how the body absorbs, metabolizes, distributes, and excretes the drugs. (32)

pharmacology (fär´ma-kŏl´ə-jē) (†) The study of drugs. (32)

pharmacotherapeutics (far´mă-kō-thĕr´ə-pyōō´tĭks) The study of how drugs are used to treat disease; also called clinical **pharmacology.** (32)

pharyngeal tonsils (fă-rin´jē-ăl tŏn´səls) (†) Two masses of lymphatic tissue located above the palatine tonsils; also called adenoids. (13)

pharynx (făr´ĭngks) Structure below the mouth and nasal cavities that is an organ of the respiratory system as well as the digestive system. (12)

phenylketonuria (PKU) (fen´il-kē´tō-nū´rē-ă) (†) A genetically inherited disorder in which the body cannot properly metabolize the nutrient phenylalanine, resulting in the buildup of phenylketones in the blood and their presence in the urine. The accumulation of phenylketones results in mental retardation. (5)

phlebotomy (flĭ-bŏt´ə-mē) The insertion of a needle or cannula (small tube) into a vein for the purpose of withdrawing blood. (30)

photometer (fō-tŏm´ĭ-trē) An instrument that measures light intensity. (27)

physical therapy (fĭz´ĭ-kəl thĕr´ə-pē) A medical specialty that uses cold, heat, water, exercise, massage, traction, and other physical means to treat musculoskeletal, nervous, and cardiopulmonary disorders. (25)

physician's office laboratory (POL) (fĭ-zĭsh′ənz ô′fĭs lăb′rə-tôr′ē) A laboratory contained in a physician's office; processing tests in the POL produces quick turnaround and eliminates the need for patients to travel to other test locations. (27)

physiology (fĭz′ē-ŏl′ə-jē) The science of the study of the body's functions. (5)

pineal body (pin′ē-ăl bŏd′ē) A small gland located between the cerebral hemispheres that secretes melatonin. (14)

placenta (plə-sĕn′tə) An organ located between the mother and the fetus. It permits the absorption of nutrients and oxygen. In some cases, harmful substances such as viruses are absorbed through the placenta. (17)

plantar flexion (plan′tăr flek′shŭn) (†) Pointing the toes downward. (8)

plasma (plăz′mə) The fluid component of blood, in which formed elements are suspended; makes up 55% of blood volume. (30)

platelets (plāt′lĭts) Fragments of cytoplasm in the blood that are crucial to clot formation; also called thrombocytes. (30)

pleura (plūr′ă) (†) The membranes that surround the lungs. (12)

pleuritis A condition in which the **pleura** become inflamed, which causes them to stick together. It can also cause an excess amount of fluid to form between the membranes. (12)

plexus (plĕk′səs) A structure that is formed when spinal nerves fuse together. It includes the cervical, brachial, and lumbosacral nerves. (9)

pneumothorax (nū-mō-thōr′aks) (†) The presence of air or gas in the pleural cavity. The lung typically collapses with pneumothorax. (12)

polar body (pō′lər bŏd′ē) A nonfunctional cell that is one of two small cells formed during the division of an oocyte. (17)

polarity (pō-lăr′ĭ-tē) The condition of having two separate poles, one of which is positive and the other, negative. (34)

polarized (pō′lə-rīzd′) The state in which the outside of a cell membrane is positively charged and the inside is negatively charged. Polarization occurs when a neuron is at rest. (9)

polysaccharide (pol-ē-sak′ă-rīd) (†) A type of carbohydrate that is a starch. (13)

positron emission tomography A radiologic procedure that entails injecting isotopes combined with other substances involved in metabolic activity, such as glucose. These special isotopes emit positrons, which a computer processes and displays on a screen. (35)

posterior (pŏ-stîr′ē-ar) Anatomical term meaning toward the back of the body. Also called dorsal. (5)

postnatal period (pōst-nā′tăl pîr′ē-əd) (†) The period following childbirth. (17)

postoperative (pōst-ŏp′ər-ə-tĭv) Taking place after a surgical procedure. (24)

posture (pŏs′chər) Body position and alignment. (25)

premenstrual syndrome (PMS) (prē-me′n-strə-wal sin′-drōm) (†) A syndrome that is a collection of symptoms that occur just before the menstrual period. (17)

prenatal period (prē-nā′tăl pîr′ē-əd) (†) The period that includes the embryonic and fetal periods until the delivery of the offspring. (17)

preoperative (prē-ŏp′ər-ə-tĭv) Taking place prior to surgery. (24)

prepuce (prē′pūs) (†) A piece of skin in the uncircumcized male that covers the glans penis. (17)

presbyopia (prez-bē-ō′pē-ă) A common eye disorder that results in the loss of lens elasticity. Presbyopia develops with age and causes a person to have difficulty seeing objects close up. (15)

prescribe (prĭ-skrīb′) To give a patient a prescription to be filled by a pharmacy. (32)

prescription (prĭ-skrĭp′shən) A physician's written order for medication. (32)

prescription drug (prĭ-skrĭp′shən drŭg) A drug that can be legally used only by order of a physician and must be administered or dispensed by a licensed health-care professional. (32)

primary germ layer (prī′mĕr′ē jûrm lā′ər) An inner cell mass that organizes into layers: the ectoderm, mesoderm, and endoderm. (17)

prime mover (prīm mo͞o′vər) The muscle responsible for most of the movement when a body movement is produced by a group of muscles. (8)

primordial follicle (prī-mōr′dēl-ăl fŏl′ĭ-kəl) (†) A structure that develops in the ovarian cortex of a female infant before she is born. (17)

proctoscopy (prok-tos′kō-pē) An examination of the lower rectum and anal canal with a 3-inch instrument called a proctoscope to detect hemorrhoids, polyps, fissures, fistulas, and abscesses. (23)

proficiency testing program (prə-fĭ′shən-cē tĕst′ĭng prō′grăm′) A required set of tests for clinical laboratories; the tests measure the accuracy of the laboratory's test results and adherence to standard operating procedures. (27)

progesterone (prō-jĕs′tə-rōn′) A female steroid hormone primarily produced by the ovary. (14)

prognosis (prŏg-nō′sĭs) A prediction of the probable course of a disease in an individual and the chances of recovery. (20)

prolactin (PRL) (prō-lak′tin) (†) A hormone that stimulates milk production in the mammary glands. (14)

proliferation phase (prə-lĭf′ər-ā′shən fāz) The second phase of wound healing, in which new tissue forms, closing off the wound. (24)

pronation (prō-nā′shŭn) (†) Turning the palms of the hand downward. (8)

prostaglandin (pros-tă-glan′din) (†) A local hormone derived from lipid molecules. Prostaglandins typically do not travel in the bloodstream to find their target cells because their targets are close by. This hormone has numerous effects, including uterine stimulation during childbirth. (14)

prostate gland (prŏs′tāt′ glănd) A chestnut-shaped gland that surrounds the beginning of the urethra in the male. (17)

prostatitis (pros-tă-tī′tis) Inflammation of the prostate gland, which can be acute or chronic. (17)

proteinuria (prō-tē-nū′rē-ă) An excess of protein in the urine. (29)

protozoan (prō′-tə-zō′ən) A single-celled eukaryotic organism much larger than a bacterium; some protozoans can cause disease in humans. (28)

protraction (prō-trăk′shən) Moving a body part anteriorly. (8)

proximal (prok′si-măl) (†) Anatomical term meaning closer to a point of attachment or closer to the trunk of the body. (5)

proximal convoluted tubule (prok′si-măl kon′vō-lū-ted tū′byūl) (†) The portion of the renal tubule that is directly attached to the glomerular capsule and becomes the loop of Henle. (16)

psoriasis (sə-rī′ə-sĭs) A common skin condition characterized by reddish-silver scaly lesions most often found on the elbows, knees, scalp, and trunk. (6)

puberty (pyoo͞′bər-tē) The period of adolescence when a person begins to develop secondary sexual traits and reproductive functions. (22)

pulmonary circuit (po͞ol′mə-nĕr′ē sûr′kĭt) The route that blood takes from the heart to the lungs and back to the heart again. (10)

pulmonary trunk (po͞ol′mə-nĕr′ē trŭngk) A large artery that branches into the pulmonary arteries and carries blood to the lungs. (10)

pulmonary valve (po͞ol′mə-nĕr′ē vălv) A heart valve that is a semilunar valve. It is situated between the right ventricle and the pulmonary trunk. (10)

pubis (pyü′-bəs) The area that forms the front of a hip bone. (7)

pulmonary function test (po͝ol′mə-nĕr′ē fŭngk′shən tĕst) A test that evaluates a patient's lung volume and capacity; used to detect and diagnose pulmonary problems or to monitor certain respiratory disorders and evaluate the effectiveness of treatment. (34)

puncture wound (pŭngk′chər wound) A deep wound caused by a sharp, pointed object. (24)

pupil (pyo͞o′pəl) The opening at the center of the iris, which grows smaller or larger as the iris contracts or relaxes, respectively; it regulates the amount of light that enters the eye. (15)

Purkinje Fibers (per′kin-jē fī′bərz) Cardiac fibers that are located in the lateral walls of the ventricles. (10)

pyelonephritis (pī′ĕ-lō-ne-frī-tis) (†) A urinary tract infection that involves one or both of the kidneys. (16)

pyrogens (pī′ō-jenz) (†) Fever-producing substances released by neutrophils. (30)

quadrants (kwŏd′rəntz) Four equal sections, such as those into which the abdomen is figuratively divided during an examination. (20)

qualitative analysis (kwŏl′ĭ-tā′tĭv ə-năl′ĭ-sĭs) In microbiology, identification of bacteria present in a specimen by the appearance of colonies grown on a culture plate. (28)

qualitative test response (kwŏl′ĭ-tā′tĭv tĕst rĭ-spŏns′) A test result that indicates the substance tested for is either present or absent. (27)

quality assurance program (kwŏl′ĭ-tē ə-sho͝or′əns prō′gram′) A required program for clinical laboratories designed to monitor the quality of patient care, including quality control, instrument and equipment maintenance, proficiency testing, training and continuing education, and standard operating procedures documentation. (27)

quality control (QC) (kwŏl′ĭ-tē kən-trōl′) An ongoing system, required in every physican's office, to evaluate the quality of medical care provided. (28)

quality control program (kwŏl′ĭ-tē kən-trōl′ prō′grăm′) A component of a quality assurance program that focuses on ensuring accuracy in laboratory test results through careful monitoring of test procedures. (27)

quantitative analysis (kwŏn′tĭ-tā′tĭv ə-năl′ĭ-sĭs) In microbiology, a determination of the number of bacteria present in a specimen by direct count of colonies grown on a culture plate. (28)

quantitative test results (kwŏn′tĭ-tā′tĭv tĕst rĭ-zŭltz′) The concentration of a test substance in a specimen. (27)

radial artery (rā′dē-əl är′tə-rē) An artery located in the groove on the thumb side of the inner wrist, where the pulse is taken on adults. (19)

radiation therapy (rā′dē-ā′shən thĕr′ə-pē) The use of x-rays and radioactive substances to treat cancer. (35)

radius (rā-dā-əs) The lateral bone of the forearm. (7)

random urine specimen (răn′dəm yo͝or′ ĭn spĕs′ ə-mən) A single urine specimen taken at any time of the day; the most common type of sample collected. (29)

range of motion (ROM) (rānj mō′shən) The degree to which a joint is able to move. (25)

reagent (rē-ā′jənt) A chemical or chemically treated substance used in test procedures and formulated to react in specific ways when exposed under specific conditions. (27)

recovery position (rĭ-kŭv′ər-ē pə-zĭsh′ən) The position a person is placed in after receiving first aid for choking or cardiopulmonary resuscitation. (26)

rectum (rĕk′təm) The last section of the sigmoid colon that straightens out and becomes the anal canal. (13)

reference (rĕf′ər-əns) A recommendation for employment from a facility or a preceptor. (36)

reference laboratory (rĕf′ər-əns lăb′rə-tôr′ē) A laboratory owned and operated by an organization outside the physician's practice. (27)

reflex (rē′flĕks′) A predictable automatic response to stimuli. (9)

refraction examination (rĭ-frăk′shən ĭg-zăm′ə-nā′shən) An eye examination in which the patient looks through a succession of different lenses to find out which ones create the clearest image. (23)

refractometer (rē-frak-tom′ĕ-ter) (†) An optical instrument that measures the refraction, or bending, of light as it passes through a liquid. (29)

relaxin (rē-lak′sin) (†) A hormone that comes from the corpus luteum. It inhibits uterine contractions and relaxes the ligaments of the pelvis in preparation for childbirth. (17)

renal calculi (rē′nəl kăl′kyə-lī′) Kidney stones. (16)

renal column (rē′nəl kŏl′əm) The portion of the **renal cortex** between the **renal pyramids.** (16)

renal corpuscle (rē′nəl kôr′pə-səl) Corpuscle that is composed of the glomerulus and the glomerular capsule. The filtration of blood occurs here. (16)

renal cortex (rē′nəl kôr′tĕks′) The outermost layer of the kidney. (16)

renal medulla (rē′nəl mĭ-dŭl′ə) The middle portion of the kidney. (16)

renal pelvis (rē′nəl pĕl′vĭs) The internal structure of the kidney. Urine flows from the renal pelvis down the ureter. (16)

renal pyramids (rē′nəl pĭr′ə-mĭdz) Triangular-shaped areas in the medulla of the kidney. (16)

renal sinus (rē′nəl sī′nəs) The medial depression of a kidney. (16)

renal tubule (rē′nəl tū′byūl) Structure that extends from the glomerular capsule of a nephron and is comprised of the proximal convoluted tubule, the loop of Henle, and the distal convoluted tubule. (16)

renin (ren′in) (†) A hormone secreted by the kidney that helps to regulate blood pressure. (16)

repolarization (rē′pō-lăr-i-zā′shŭn) (†) The process of returning to the original polar (resting) state. (9)

reservoir host (rĕz′ər-vwär′ hōst) An animal, insect, or human whose body is susceptible to growth of a pathogen. (1)

respiratory volume (rĕs′pər-ə-tôr′ē vŏl′yo͞om) The different volumes of air that move in and out of the lungs during different intensities of breathing. These volumes can be measured to assess the healthiness of the respiratory system. (12)

retina (rĕt′n-ə) The inner layer of the eye; contains light-sensing nerve cells. (15)

retraction (rĭ-trăk′shən) Moving a body part posteriorly. (8)

retrograde pyelography (rĕt′rə-grăd′ pī′ĕ-log′ră-fē) (†) A radiologic procedure in which the doctor injects a contrast medium through a urethral catheter and takes a series of x-rays to evaluate function of the ureters, bladder, and urethra. (35)

retroperitoneal (re-trō-per-ə-ə-nē′-əl) An anatomical term that means behind the peritoneal cavity. It is where the kidneys lie. (16)

rhabdomyolysis (rab′dō-mī-ol′i-sis) (†) A condition in which the kidneys have been damaged due to toxins released from muscle cells. (8)

Rh antigen (ăr′ăch an′tĭ-jən) A protein first discovered on the red blood cells of rhesus monkeys, hence the name Rh. (10)

RhoGAM (rō′găm) A medication that prevents an Rh-negative mother from making antibodies against the Rh antigen. (10)

RNA (ăr′ĕn-ā′) A nucleic acid used to make protein. (5)

rods (rŏdz) Light-sensing nerve cells in the eye, at the posterior of the retina, that function in dim light but do not provide sharp images or detect color. (15)

rosacea (rō-ză′shē-ă) (†) A condition characterized by chronic redness and acne over the nose and cheeks. (6)

rotation (rō-tā′shən) Twisting a body part. (8)

route (ro͞ot) The way a drug is introduced into the body. (33)

sacrum (sa′-krəm) A triangular-shaped bone that consists of five fused vertebra. (7)

sagittal (saj′i-tăl) (†) An anatomical term that refers to the plane that divides the body into left and right portions. (5)

sanitization (săn′ĭ-tĭ-zā′shən) (†) A reduction of the number of microorganisms on an object or a surface to a fairly safe level. (1)

sarcolemma (sar′kō-lem′ă) The cell membrane of a muscle fiber. (8)

sarcoplasm The cytoplasm of a muscle fiber. (8)

sarcoplasmic reticulum (sar-kō-plaz′mik re-tik′yū-lŭm) The endoplasmic reticulum of a muscle fiber. (8)

SARS (severe acute respiratory syndrome) (särz) A severe and acute respiratory illness characterized by fever and a nonproductive cough that progresses to the point at which insufficient oxygen is present in the blood. (20)

saturated fat (săch′ə-rā′tĭd făt) Fats, derived primarily from animal sources, that are usually solid at room temperature and that tend to raise blood cholesterol levels. (31)

scabies (skā′bēz) Skin lesions that are very itchy and caused by a burrowing mite. Scabies is most commonly found between the fingers and on the genitalia. (6)

scapula (sk′a-pyə-la) Thin, triangular-shaped, flat bones located on the dorsal surface of the rib cage; also called shoulder blades. (7)

Schwann cell (shwahn sĕl) (†) A neuroglial cell whose cell membrane coats the axons. (9)

sciatica (sī-ăt′ĭ-kə) Pain in the low back and hip radiating down the back of the leg along the sciatic nerve. (9)

sclera (sklîr′ə) The tough, outermost layer, or "white," of the eye, through which light cannot pass; covers all except the front of the eye. (15)

scoliosis (skō′lē-ō′sĭs) A lateral curvature of the spine, which is normally straight when viewed from behind. (7)

scratch test (skrăch tĕst) An allergy test in which extracts of suspected allergens are applied to the patient's skin and the skin is then scratched to allow the extracts to penetrate. (23)

scrotum (skrō′təm) In a male, the sac of skin below the pelvic cavity that contains the testes. (17)

sebaceous (sĭ-bā′shəs) A type of oil gland found in the dermis. (6)

sebum (sē′bŭm) (†) An oily substance produced by sebaceous glands. (6)

seizure (sē′zhər) A series of violent and involuntary contractions of the muscles; also called a convulsion. (9)

sella turcica (sel′ă tŭr′sē-kă) (†) A deep depression in the sphenoid bone where the pituitary gland sits. (7)

semen (sē′mən) Sperm and the various substances that nourish and transport them. (17)

semicircular canals (sĕm′ē-sûr′kyə-lər kə-năl z′) Structures in the inner ear that help a person maintain balance; each of the three canals is positioned at right angles to the other two. (15)

seminal vesicles (sem′-năl ves′i-klz) (†) A pair of convoluted tubes that lie behind the bladder. These tubes secrete a fluid that provides nutrition for the sperm. (17)

seminiferous tubules (sem′i-nif′ér-ŭs tū′byūlz) (†) These tubes contain spermatogenic cells and are located in the lobules of the testes. (17)

sensorineural hearing loss (sen′sōr-i-nūr′ăl hîr′ĭng lôs) This type of hearing loss occurs when neural structures associated with the ear are damaged. Neural structures include hearing receptors and the auditory nerve. (15)

sensory (sĕn′sə-rē) Afferent neurons that carry sensory information from the periphery to the central nervous system. (9)

sensory adaptation (sĕn′sə-rē ăd′ăp-tā′shən) A process in which the same chemical can stimulate receptors only for a limited amount of time until the receptors eventually no longer respond to the chemical. (15)

septic shock (sĕp′tĭk shŏk) A state of shock resulting from massive, widespread infection that affects the blood vessels' ability to circulate blood. (26)

serosa (se-rō′să) (†) The outermost layer of the alimentary canal; also known as the visceral peritoneum. (13)

serous cells (sēr′ŭs sĕlz) (†) One of two types of cells that make up the salivary glands. These cells secrete a watery fluid that contains amylase. (13)

serum (sēr′ŭm) (†) The clear, yellow liquid that remains after a blood clot forms; it is separated from the clotted elements by centrifugation. (30)

sex chromosome (sĕks krō′mə-sōm′) Chromosome of the 23rd pair. (5)

sex-linked trait (sĕks lĭngk trāt) Traits that are carried on the sex chromosomes, or X and Y chromosomes. (5)

sigmoid colon (sig-moid ko-lən) An S-shaped tube that lies between the **descending colon** and the **rectum.** (13)

sigmoidoscopy (sig′moy-dos′kŏ-pē) A procedure in which the interior of the sigmoid area of the large intestine, between the descending colon and the rectum, is examined with a sigmoidoscope, a lighted instrument with a magnifying lens. (23)

sinoatrial node (sī′nō-ā′trē-ăl nōd) (†) A small bundle of heart muscle tissue in the superior wall of the right atrium that sets the rhythm (or pattern) of the heart's contractions; also called sinus node or pacemaker. (10)

sinusitis (sī′nə-sī′tĭs) Inflammation of the lining of a sinus. (12)

skinfold test (skĭn´ tĕst) A method of measuring fat as a percentage of body weight by measuring the thickness of a fold of skin with a caliper. (31)

slit lamp (slĭt lămp) An instrument composed of a magnifying lens combined with a light source; used to provide a minute examination of the eye's anatomy. (23)

smear (smîr) A specimen spread thinly and unevenly across a slide. (28)

solution (sə-lo͞o´shən) A homogeneous mixture of a solid, liquid, or gaseous substance in a liquid, such as a dissolved drug in liquid form. (33)

somatic (sō-măt´ĭk) A division of the peripheral nervous system that connects the central nervous system to skin and skeletal muscle. (9)

SPECT (spĕkt) Single photon emission computed tomography; a radiologic procedure in which a gamma camera detects signals induced by gamma radiation and a computer converts these signals into two- or three-dimensional images that are displayed on a screen. (35)

speculum (spĕk´yə-ləm) An instrument that expands the vaginal opening to permit viewing of the vagina and cervix. (22)

spermatids (sper´mă-tidz) (†) Immature sperm before they develop their flagella (tails). (17)

spermatocytes (sper´mă-tō-sīts) (†) The cells that result when **spermatogonia** undergo mitosis. (17)

spermatogenesis (sper´mă-tō-jen´ĕ-sis) (†) The process of sperm cell formation. (17)

spermatogenic cells (sper´mă-tō-jen´ik sĕlz) (†) The cells that give rise to sperm cells. (17)

spermatogonia (sper´mă-tō-gō´nē-ă) (†) The earliest cell in the process of **spermatogenesis.** (17)

sphenoid A bone that forms part of the floor of the cranium. (7)

sphincter (sfĭngk´tər) A valve-like structure formed from circular bands of muscle. Sphincters are located around various body openings and passages. (8)

sphygmomanometer (sfig´mō-mănom´ĕ-ter) (†) An instrument for measuring blood pressure; consists of an inflatable cuff, a pressure bulb used to inflate the cuff, and a device to read the pressure. (19)

spinal nerves (spī´năl nûrvs) (†) Peripheral nerves that originate from the spinal cord. (9)

spirillum (spī-ril´ŭm) (†) A spiral-shaped bacterium. (28)

spirometer (spī-rom´ĕ-ter) (†) An instrument that measures the air taken in and expelled from the lungs. (34)

spirometry (spī-rom´ĕ-trē) (†) A test used to measure breathing capacity. (34)

splint A device used to immobilize and protect a body part. (26)

splinting catheter (splĭnt´ĭng kăth´ĭ-tər) A type of catheter inserted after plastic repair of the ureter; it must remain in place for at least a week after surgery. (29)

sprain (sprān) An injury characterized by partial tearing of a ligament that supports a joint, such as the ankle. A sprain may also involve injuries to tendons, muscles, and local blood vessels and contusions of the surrounding soft tissue. (26)

stain (stān) In microbiology, a solution of a dye or group of dyes that impart a color to microorganisms. (28)

standard (stăn´dərd) A specimen for which test values are already known; used to calibrate test equipment. (27)

Standard Precautions (stăn´dərd prĭ-kô´shənz) A combination of Universal Precautions and Body Substance Isolation guidelines; used in hospitals for the care of all patients. (1)

stapes (stā´pēz) A small bone in the middle ear that is attached to the inner ear; also called the stirrup. (21)

stereoscopy (ster-ē-os´kŏ-pē) (†) An x-ray procedure that uses a specially designed microscope (stereoscopic, or Greenough, microscope) with double eyepieces and objectives to take films at different angles and produce three-dimensional images; used primarily to study the skull. (35)

sterile field (stĕr´əl fēld) An area free of microorganisms used as a work area during a surgical procedure. (24)

sterile scrub assistant (stĕr´əl skrŭb ə-sĭs´tənt) An assistant who handles sterile equipment during a surgical procedure. (24)

sterilization (stĕr´ə-lĭ-zā´shən) The destruction of all microorganisms, including bacterial spores, by specific means. (1)

sterilization indicator (stĕr´ə-lĭ-zā´shən ĭn´dĭ-kā´shən) A tag, insert, tape, tube, or strip that confirms that the items in an autoclave have been exposed to the correct volume of steam at the correct temperature for the correct amount of time. (2)

steroid hormone (stîr´oid´ hôr´mōn´) A hormone derived from steroids that are soluble in lipids and can cross cell membranes very easily. (14)

sternum (st´ər-nəm) A bone that forms the front and middle portion of the rib cage; also called the breastbone or breast plate. (7)

stethoscope (stĕth´ə-skōp´) An instrument that amplifies body sounds. (19)

strabismus (strə-bĭz´məs) A condition that results in a lack of parallel visual axes of the eyes; commonly called crossed eyes. (15)

strain (strān) A muscle injury that results from overexertion or overstretching. (26)

stratum basale (straťŭm bā-să´le) (†) The deepest layer of the epidermis of the skin. (6)

stratum corneum (straťŭm kōr´nē-ŭm) (†) The most superficial layer of the epidermis of the skin. (6)

stressor (stres´or) (†) Any stimulus that produces stress. (14)

stress test (strĕs tĕst) A procedure that involves recording an electrocardiogram while the patient is exercising on a stationary bicycle, treadmill, or stair-stepping ergometer, which measures work performed. (23)

striations (strī-ā´shŭns) (†) Bands produced from the arrangement of filaments in myofibrils in skeletal and cardiac muscle cells. (8)

stroke (strōk) A condition that occurs when the blood supply to the brain is impaired. It may cause temporary or permanent damage. (26)

stylus (stī´ləs) A penlike instrument that records electrical impulses on ECG paper. (34)

subarachnoid space (sŭb-ă-rak´noyd spās) (†) An area between the arachnoid mater and the pia mater. (9)

subclinical case (sŭb-klin´i-kăl kās) (†) An infection in which the host experiences only some of the symptoms of the infection or milder symptoms than in a full case. (1)

subcutaneous (SC) (sŭb´kyo͞o-tā´nē-əs) Under the skin. (6)

sublingual (sŭb-ling´gwăl) (†) Under the tongue. (33)

sublingual gland (sŭb-ling´gwăl glănd) (†) The smallest of the salivary glands. (13)

submandibular gland (sŭb-man-dib´yū-lăr glănd) (†) The gland that is located in the floor of the mouth. (13)

submucosa (sŭb-mū-kō´să) (†) The layer of the alimentary canal located between the mucosa and the muscular layer. (13)

substance abuse (sŭb′stəns ə-byōōz′) The use of a substance in a way that is not medically approved, such as using diet pills to stay awake or consuming large quantities of cough syrup that contains codeine. Substance abusers are not necessarily addicts. (18)

sucrose (sū′krōs) (†) An enzyme that digests sugars. (13)

sulci (sŭl′si) (†) The grooves on the surface of the cerebrum. (9)

superficial (sōō′pər-fĭsh′əl) Anatomical term meaning closer to the surface of the body. (5)

superior (sōō′-pîr′-ē-ər) Anatomical term meaning above or closer to the head; also called cranial. (5)

supernatant (sū-per-nā′tănt) (†) The liquid portion of a substance from which solids have settled to the bottom, as with a urine specimen after centrifugation. (29)

supination (sū′pi-nā′shŭn) (†) Turning the palm of the hand upward. (8)

surgical asepsis (sûr′jə-kəl ă-sep′sis) (†) The elimination of all microorganisms from objects or working areas; also called sterile technique. (24)

susceptible host (sə-sĕp′təbal hōst) An individual who has little or no immunity to infection by a particular organism. (1)

suture (sōō′chər) Fibrous joints in the skull. (7) A surgical stitch made to close a wound. (24)

symmetry (sĭm′ĭ-trē) The degree to which one side of the body is the same as the other. (20)

sympathetic (sĭm′pə-thĕt′ĭk) A division of the autonomic nervous system that prepares organs for fight-or-flight (stressful) situations. (9)

synaptic knob (si-nap′tik nŏb) (†) The end of the axon branch. (9)

synergist (sĭn′ər-jist′) Muscles that help the **prime mover** by stabilizing joints. (8)

synovial (sin-ō-vā-əl) A type of joint, such as the elbow or knee, that is freely moveable. (7)

systemic circuit (sĭ-stĕm′ĭk sûr′kĭt) The route that blood takes from the heart through the body and back to the heart. (10)

systolic pressure (sĭ-stŏl′ĭk prĕsh′ər) The blood pressure measured when the left ventricle of the heart contracts. (10)

tachycardia (tak′i-kar′dē-ă) (†) Rapid heart rate, generally in excess of 100 beats per minute. (26)

tachypnea Abnormally rapid breathing. (19)

targeted résumé (tär′gĭt-əd rĕz′ōō-mā′) A résumé that is focused on a specific job target. (36)

tarsals (tär′-səlz) Bones of the ankle. (7)

taste bud (tāst bŭd) A structure that is made of taste cells (a type of chemoreceptor) and supporting cells. (15)

teletherapy (tel-ĕ-thār′ăpē) (†) A radiation therapy technique that allows deeper penetration than brachytherapy; used primarily for deep tumors. (35)

temporal (tem′-p(a)-rəl) Bones that form the lower sides of the skull. (7)

tendon (tĕn′dən) A cordlike fibrous tissue that connects muscle to bone. (8)

terminal (tûr′mə-nəl) Fatal. (3)

testes (tĕs′tēz) The primary organs of the male reproductive system. Testes produce the hormone **testosterone.** (17)

testosterone (tĕs-tŏs′tə-rōn′) A hormone produced by the testes that maintains the male reproductive structures and male characteristics such as deep voice, body hair, and muscle mass. (14)

tetanus (tĕt′n-əs) A disease caused by *clostridium tetani* living in the soil and water; more commonly called lockjaw. (8)

thalamus (thăl′ə-məs) Structure that acts as a relay station for sensory information heading to the cerebral cortex for interpretation; a subdivision of the **diencephalon.** (9)

therapeutic team (thĕr′ə-pyōō′tĭk tēm) A group of physicians, nurses, medical assistants, and other specialists who work with patients dealing with chronic illness or recovery from major injuries. (25)

thermography (ther-mog′ră-fē) (†) A radiologic procedure in which an infrared camera is used to take photographs that record variations in skin temperature as dark (cool areas), light (warm areas), or shades of gray (areas with temperatures between cool and warm); used to diagnose breast tumors, breast abscesses, and fibrocystic breast disease. (35)

thermotherapy (ther′mō-thār′ă-pē) (†) The application of heat to the body to treat a disorder or injury. (25)

thrombocytes (throm′bō-sīts) See **platelets.** (30)

thrombophlebitis (thrŏm′bō-flĕ-bī′tis) (†) A medical condition that most commonly occurs in leg veins when a blood clot and inflammation develop. (10)

thrombus (thrŏm′bəs) A blood clot that forms on the inside of an injured blood vessel wall. (10)

thymosin (thī′mō-sin) (†) A hormone that promotes the production of certain lymphocytes. (14)

thymus gland (thī′məs glănd) A gland that lies between the lungs. It secretes a hormone called **thymosin.** (14)

thyroid cartilage (thī′roid′ kär′tl-ĭj) The largest cartilage in the larynx. It forms the anterior wall of the larynx. (12)

thyroid hormone (thī′roid′ hôr′mōn′) A hormone produced by the thyroid gland that increases energy production, stimulates protein synthesis, and speeds up the repair of damaged tissue. (14)

thyroid stimulating hormone (thī′roid′ stim′yū-lā-ting hôr′mōn′) A hormone that stimulates the thyroid gland to release its hormone. (14)

tibia (ti-bē-ə) The medial bone of the lower leg; commonly called the shin bone. (7)

timed urine specimen (tīmd yŏŏr′ĭn spĕs′ ə-mən) A specimen of a patient's urine collected over a specific time period. (29)

tinnitus (ti-nī′tus) (†) An abnormal ringing in the ear. (15)

tissue (tĭsh′ōō) A structure that is formed when cells of the same type organize together. (5)

T lymphocyte (tē lĭm′fə-sīt) A type of nongranular leukocyte that regulates immunologic response; includes helper T cells and suppressor T cells. (30)

topical (tŏp′ĭ-kəl) Applied to the skin. (24)

toxicology (tŏk′sĭ-kŏl′ə-jē) The study of poisons or poisonous effects of drugs. (32)

trachea (trā′kē-ə) The part of the respiratory tract between the larynx and the bronchial tree that is tubular and made of rings of cartilage and smooth muscle; also called the windpipe. (12)

traction (trăk′shən) The pulling or stretching of the musculoskeletal system to treat dislocated joints, joints afflicted by arthritis or other diseases, and fractured bones. (25)

trade name (trād nām) A drug's brand or proprietary name. (32)

transcutaneous absorption (trans-kyū-tā′nē-ŭs əb-sorp′shən) (†) Entry (as of a pathogen) through a cut or crack in the skin. (4)

transdermal (trans-der´mel) A type of topical drug administration that slowly and evenly releases a systemic drug through the skin directly into the bloodstream; a transdermal unit is also called a patch. (33)

transverse (trăns-vŭrs´) Anatomical term that refers to the plane that divides the body into superior and inferior portions. (5)

transverse colon (trăns-vûrs´ kō´lən) The segment of the large intestine that crosses the upper abdominal cavity between the ascending and descending colon. (13)

trichinosis (trik-i-nō´sis) (†) A disease caused by a worm that is usually ingested from undercooked meat. (8)

tricuspid valve (trī-kŭs´pid vălv) (†) A heart valve that has three cusps and is situated between the right atrium and the right ventricle. (10)

triglycerides (trī-glĭs´ə-rīd´z) Simple lipids consisting of glycerol (an alcohol) and three fatty acids. (31)

trigone (trī´gōn) (†) The triangle formed by the openings of the two ureters and the urethra in the internal floor of the bladder. (16)

trypsin (trip´sin) (†) A pancreatic enzyme that digests proteins. (13)

tubular reabsorption (tū´byū-lăr) (†) The second process of urine formation in which the glomerular filtrate flows into the proximal convoluted tubule. (16)

tubular secretion (tū´byū-lăr sĭ-krē´shən) (†) The third process of urine formation in which substances move out of the blood in the peritubular capillaries into renal tubules. (16)

tympanic membrane (tĭm-păn´ĭk mĕm´brān´) A fibrous partition located at the inner end of the ear canal and separating the outer ear from the middle ear; also called the eardrum. (15)

tympanic thermometer (tim-pan´ik ther-mom´ĕ-ter) A type of electronic thermometer that measures infrared energy emitted from the tympanic membrane. (19)

ulna (əl´-nə) The medial bone of the lower arm. (7)

ultrasonic cleaning (ŭl´trə-sŏn´ĭk klēn´ĭng) A method of sanitization that involves placing instruments in a cleaning solution in a special receptacle that generates sound waves through the cleaning solution, loosening contaminants. Ultrasonic cleaning is safe for even very fragile instruments. (2)

ultrasound The noninvasive theraputic or diagnostic use of ultrasound for examination of internal body structures. (35)

umbilical cord (ŭm-bĭl´ĭ-kəl kôrd) The rope-like connection between the fetus and the placenta. It contains the umbilical blood vessels. (17)

Universal Precautions (yōō´nə-vur´səl prĭ-kô´shənz) Specific precautions required by the Department of Health and Human Services' Centers for Disease Control and Prevention (CDC) to prevent health-care workers from exposing themselves and others to infection by blood-borne pathogens. (1)

unsaturated fats (ŭn-săch´ə-rā´tĭd făts) Fats, including most vegetable oils, that are usually liquid at room temperature and tend to lower blood cholesterol. (31)

urea (yŏŏ-rē´ə) Waste product formed by the breakdown of proteins and nucleic acids. (16)

ureters (yŏŏ-rē´tərz) Long, slender, muscular tubes that carry urine from the kidneys to the urinary bladder. (16)

urethra (yŏŏ-rē´thrə) The tube that conveys urine from the bladder during urination. (16)

uric acid (yŏŏr´ĭk as´id) Waste product formed by the breakdown of proteins and nucleic acids. (16)

urinalysis (yŏŏr´ə-năl´ĭ-sĭs) The physical, chemical, and microscopic evaluation of urine to obtain information about body health and disease. (29)

urinary catheter (yŏŏr´ə-nĕr´ē kăth´ĭ-tər) A sterile plastic tube inserted to provide urinary drainage. (29)

urinary pH (yŏŏr´ə-nĕr´ē pē´ăch) A measure of the degree of acidity or alkalinity of urine. (29)

urine specific gravity (yŏŏr´ĭn spĭ-sĭf´ĭk grăv´ĭ-tē) A measure of the concentration or amount (total weight) of substances dissolved in urine. (29)

urobilinogen (yūr-ō-bī-lin´ō-jen) (†) A colorless compound formed by the breakdown of hemoglobin in the intestines. Elevated levels in urine may indicate increased red blood cell destruction or liver disease, whereas lack of urobilinogen in the urine may suggest total bile duct obstruction. (29)

uterus (yōō´tər-əs) A hollow, muscular organ that functions to receive an embryo and sustain its development; also called the womb. (17)

uvula (yōō´vyə-lə) The part of the soft palate that hangs down in the back of the throat. (13)

vaccine (văk-sēn´) A special preparation made from microorganisms and administered to a person to produce reduced sensitivity to, or increased immunity to, an infectious disease. (32)

vagina (və-jī´nə) A tubular organ that extends from the uterus to the labia. (17)

vaginitis (vaj-i-nī´tis) (†) Inflammation of the vagina characterized by an abnormal vaginal discharge. (17)

varicose veins (văr´i-kōs vānz) (†) Distended veins that result when vein valves are destroyed and blood pools in the veins, causing these veins to dilate. (10)

vas deferens (văs´ dĕf´ər-ənz) A tube that connects the epididymis with the urethra and that carries sperm. (17)

vasectomy (və-sĕk´tə-mē) A male sterilization procedure in which a section of each vas deferens is removed. (23)

vasoconstriction (vā´sō-kon-strik´shŭn) (†) The constriction of the muscular wall of an artery to increase blood pressure. (10)

vasodilation (vā-sō-dī-lā´shŭn) (†) The widening of the muscular wall of an artery to decrease blood pressure. (10)

vector (vĕk´tər) A living organism, such as an insect, that carries microorganisms from an infected person to another person. (1)

venipuncture (ven´i-pŭnk-chŭr) (†) The puncture of a vein, usually with a needle, for the purpose of drawing blood. (30)

ventilation (vĕn´tə-lā´shən) Moving air in and out of the lungs; also called breathing. (12)

ventral (vĕn´trəl) See **anterior.** (5)

ventral root (vĕn´trəl rōōt) A portion of the spinal nerve that contains axons of motor neurons only. (9)

ventricle (vĕn´trĭ-kəl) Interconnected cavities in the brain filled with cerebrospinal fluid. (9)

ventricular fibrillation (ven-trik´yū-lăr fī-bri-lā´shŭn) An abnormal heart rhythm that is the most common cause of cardiac arrest. (26)

verbalizing (vûr´bə-līz´-ĭng) Stating what you believe the patient is suggesting or implying. (18)

vermiform appendix (uer′mi-fōrm ə-pĕn′dĭks)(†) A structure made mostly of lymphoid tissue and projecting off the cecum. It is commonly referred to as simply the appendix. (13)
vesicles (vĕs′ĭ-kəlz) Small sacs within the synaptic knobs that contain chemicals called neurotransmitters. (9)
vestibular glands (ves-tib′yū-lăr glăndz)(†) Glands that secrete mucus into the vestibule of the female during sexual excitement. (17)
vestibule (vĕs′tə-byo͞ol′) The area in the inner ear between the semicircular canals and the cochlea. (15)
vial (vī′əl) A small glass bottle with a self-sealing rubber stopper. (24)
vibrio (†)(vib′rē-ō) A comma-shaped bacterium. (28)
virulence (vîr′yə-ləns) A microorganism's disease-producing power. (1)
virus (vī′rəs) One of the smallest known infectious agents, consisting only of nucleic acid surrounded by a protein coat; can live and grow only within the living cells of other organisms. (28)
visceral pericardium (vis′er-ăl per-i-kar′dē-ŭm)(†) The innermost layer of the pericardium that lies directly on top of the heart; also known as the **epicardium.** (10)
visceral smooth muscle (vĭs′ər-əl smo͞oth mŭs′əl) A type of smooth muscle containing sheets of muscle that closely contact each other. It is found in the walls of hollow organs such as the stomach, intestines, bladder, and uterus. (8)
vitamins (vī′tə-mĭnz) Organic substances that are essential for normal body growth and maintenance and resistance to infection. (31)
vitreous humor (vĭt′rē-əs hyo͞o′mər) A jellylike substance that fills the part of the eye behind the lens and helps the eye keep its shape. (15)
volume (vŏl′yo͞om) The amount of space an object, such as a drug, occupies. (33)
vomer (vō′-mər) A thin bone that divides the nasal cavity. (7)
warts (wôrts) Flesh-colored skin lesions with distinct round borders that are raised and often have small fingerlike projections; also called verruca. (6)
Western blot test (wĕs′tərn blŏt tĕst) A blood test used to confirm enzyme-linked immunosorbent assay (ELISA) test results for HIV infection. (3)
wet mount (wĕt mount) A preparation of a specimen in a liquid that allows the organisms to remain alive and mobile while they are being identified. (28)
white matter (hwīt măt′ər) The outer tissue of the spinal cord that is lighter in color than **gray matter.** It contains myelinated axons. (9)
whole blood (hōl blŭd) The total volume of plasma and formed elements, or blood in which the elements have not been separated by coagulation or centrifugation. (30)
whole-body skin examination (hōl bŏd′ē skĭn ĭg-zăm′ə-nā′shən) An examination of the visible top layer of the entire surface of the skin, including the scalp, genital area, and areas between the toes, to look for lesions, especially suspicious moles or precancerous growths. (23)
Wood's light examination (wo͝odz līt ĭg-zăm′ə-nā′shən) A type of dermatologic examination in which a physician inspects the patient's skin under an ultraviolet lamp in a darkened room. (23)
xeroradiography (zē′rō-rā′dē-og′ră-fē)(†) A radiologic procedure in which x-rays are developed with a powder toner, similar to the toner in photocopiers, and the x-ray image is processed on specially treated xerographic paper; used to diagnose breast cancer, abscesses, lesions, or calcifications. (35)
xiphoid process (zif′oyd prŏs′ĕs)(†) The lower extension of the breastbone. (26)
yeast (yēst) A fungus that grows mainly as a single-celled organism and reproduces by budding. (28)
yolk sac (yōk săk) The sac that holds the materials for the nutrition of the embryo. (17)
zona pellucida (zō′nă pe-lū′sid-ă)(†) A layer that surrounds the cell membrane of an egg. (17)
zygomatic (zī-gə-m′a-tik) The bones that form the prominence of the cheeks. (7)
zygote (zī′gō) The cell that is formed from the union of the egg and sperm. (17)
Z-track method (zē′trăk mĕth′əd) A technique used when injecting an intramuscular (IM) drug that can irritate subcutaneous tissue; involves pulling the skin and subcutaneous tissue to the side before inserting the needle at the site, creating a zigzag path in the tissue layers that prevents the drug from leaking into the subcutaneous tissue and causing irritation. (33)

Photo Credits

CHAPTER 1 Fig. 1.1, Fig. 1.2: © Corbis-Bettmann; Fig. 1.4: © Biology Media/Photo Researchers, Inc.; Fig. 1.7: © Tony Freeman/PhotoEdit; Fig. 1.8: © Photo Researchers, Inc.; Fig. 1.9: © David Kelly Crow; Fig. 1.10, 1.11, Fig. 1.12: © Cliff Moore; Fig. 1.13: Courtesy Tyco Healthcare/Kendall; Fig. 1.14: © Cliff Moore; Fig. 1.16, Fig. 1.17: © David Kelly Crow; Fig. 1.18: Robert Matthews.

CHAPTER 2 Fig. 2.1, Fig. 2.2: © Cliff Moore; Fig. 2.3: © Barry Slaven/Medical Images, Inc.; Fig. 2.5: © Cliff Moore; Fig. 2.6: Courtesy Pelton and Crane Company; Fig. 2.7: Courtesy Pelton and Crane Company; Fig. 2.8: © Cliff Moore; Fig. 2.9: Courtesy Barnstead International.

CHAPTER 3 Page 53: © EP063 Eyewire/Getty; Fig. 3.2: © Gary Watson/SPL/Photo Researchers, Inc.; Fig. 3.4: © SIU/Photo Researchers, Inc.

CHAPTER 4 Fig. 4.1: © David Kelly Crow; Fig. 4.2, Fig. 4.3, Fig. 4.4: © Cliff Moore; Fig. 4.6, Fig. 4.7, Fig. 4.8, Fig. 4.9a–d: © David Kelly Crow.

CHAPTER 5 Fig. 5.10b, Fig. 5.11b, Fig. 5.12b, Fig. 5.13b: © Ed Reschke.

CHAPTER 6 Fig. 6.2a–c: © SPL/Photo Researchers, Inc.; Fig. 6.3: © Victor B. Eichler, Ph.D.; Fig. 6.6a: © SPL/Custom Medical Stock Photos; Fig. 6.6b: © John Radcliff/Photo Researchers, Inc.; Fig. 6.6c: © John Radcliff/Photo Researchers, Inc.

CHAPTER 7 Fig. 7.2: © Ed Reschke; Fig. 7.9b: © Martin M. Rotker.

CHAPTER 9 Fig. 9.1: © Ed Reschke.

CHAPTER 10 Fig. 10.7: © Carolina Biological/Visuals Unlimited; Fig. 10.9: © Don W. Fawcett, from Bloom, W. and Fawcett, D.W., Textbook of Histology, 10th edition. W.B. Saunders Co., 1975. Photo by T. Kuwabara; Fig. 10.14b: © Bill Longcore/Photo Researchers, Inc.; Fig. 10.15, Fig. 10.16, 10.17, Fig. 10.18, Fig. 10.19: © Ed Reschke; Fig. 10.22: © SPL/Photo Researchers, Inc.; Fig. 10.23c: © G.W. Willis/Visuals Unlimited; Fig. 10.23d: © George Wilder/Visuals Unlimited.

CHAPTER 12 Fig. 12.2: © CNRI/Phototake.

CHAPTER 18 Fig. 18.1, Fig. 18.2, Fig. 18.3: © David Kelly Crow.

CHAPTER 19 Fig. 19.2: Courtesy ALARIS Medical Systems, Inc.; Fig. 19.3: © David Kelly Crow; Fig. 19.6, Fig. 19.7, Fig. 19.9: Courtesy of Total Care Programming; Fig. 19.14, Fig. 19.15: Shirley Zeiberg.

CHAPTER 20 Fig. 20.2, Fig. 20.3, Fig. 20.4, Fig. 20.5, Fig. 20.6, Fig. 20.7: © Terry Wild Studio; Fig. 20.8, Fig. 20.12: Courtesy of Total Care Programming.

CHAPTER 21 Page 328: Ken Lax; Fig. 21.2: Sara Matthews; Fig. 21.3a–b, Fig. 21.4, Fig. 21.5: Courtesy Richmond Products, Inc.; Fig. 21.6: Stereo Optical Co., Inc., Chicago, IL. Copyright Vision Sciences Research Corporation, San Ramon, CA. Developed by Dr. Arthur P. Ginsburg; Fig. 21.7: Courtesy Richmond Products, Inc.; Fig. 21.8, Fig. 21.9, Fig. 21.10, Fig. 21.11, Fig. 21.12: Ken Lax; Fig. 21.14: © Bonnie Kamin/PhotoEdit; Fig. 21.15, Fig. 21.17, Fig. 21.18, Fig. 21.19: © Terry Wild Studio.

CHAPTER 22 Fig. 22.1: © David Kelly Crow; Fig. 22.3, Fig. 22.4: © C.C. Duncan/Medical Images, Inc.; Fig. 22.5: © David Kelly Crow; Fig. 22.7: Courtesy Scoliosis Association (UK); Fig. 22.8: Ken

Lax; Fig. 22.9: © David Kelly Crow; Fig. 22.10: Ken Lax; Fig. 22.13: © C.C. Duncan/Medical Images, Inc.

CHAPTER 23 Fig. 23.1: © John Radcliffe/SPL/Photo Researchers, Inc.; Fig. 23.3: © Cliff Moore; Fig. 23.5: Shirley Zeiberg; TA 23.2: page 385: © Blair Seitz/Photo Researchers, Inc.; Fig. 23.6: © Nicholas Thomas/Medical Images, Inc.; Fig. 23.7: © Martin M. Rotker; Fig. 23.8: © BioPhoto/Photo Researchers, Inc.; Fig. 23.9: © Tom Meyers/Photo Researchers, Inc.; Fig. 23.10: Ken Lax; Fig. 23.12: © CNRI/SPL/Photo Researchers, Inc.; Fig. 23.13: © C.C. Duncan/Medical Images, Inc.; Fig. 23.14: © Grant Pix/Photo Researchers, Inc.; Fig. 23.15: Ken Lax; Fig. 23.16a: © Terry Wild Studio; Fig. 23.16b, Fig. 23.17: Ken Lax; Fig. 23.18: © BioPhoto/Photo Researchers, Inc.; Fig. 23.20: © Herb Snitzer/Medical Images, Inc.

CHAPTER 24 Page 415: © Leslie O'Shaughnessy/Medical Images, Inc.; Fig. 24.1: © Barry Slaven/Medical Images, Inc.; Fig. 24.6, Fig. 24.7, Fig. 24.12: © David Kelly Crow; Fig. 24.13, Fig. 24.14, Fig. 24.15: © Cliff Moore; Fig. 24.16: Courtesy of Total Care Programming; Fig. 24.17, Fig. 24.18, Fig. 24.19, Fig. 24.21, Fig. 24.22, Fig. 24.23, Fig. 24.24: © Cliff Moore; 24.20: © The McGraw-Hill Companies, Inc./Joe DeGrandis.

CHAPTER 25 Fig. 25.4: Courtesy of Total Care Programming; Page 453: © C.C. Duncan/Medical Images, Inc.; Fig. 25.5a–d: © David Kelly Crow; Fig. 25.7: Courtesy of Total Care Programming.

CHAPTER 26 Fig. 26.10: © Cliff Moore; Page 479: © Michael Neuman/PhotoEdit; Fig. 26.15: Courtesy of Total Care Programming.

CHAPTER 27 Fig. 27.1: © David Kelly Crow; Page 508: Ken Lax; Fig. 27.3, Fig. 27.4, Fig. 27.5, Fig. 27.6, Fig. 27.7: © Cliff Moore; Fig. 27.8: © Larry Mulvehill/Photo Researchers, Inc.; Fig. 27.12: © Cliff Moore; Fig. 27.13: Courtesy Becton Dickinson; Fig. 27.15: Courtesy Lukens Medical Corp.

CHAPTER 28 Fig. 28.1a: © NIBSC/Photo Researchers, Inc.; Fig. 28.1b: © SPL/Photo Researchers, Inc.; Fig. 28.1c: © R.J. Erwin/Photo Researchers, Inc.; Fig. 28.2a–b: © Oliver Meckes/Photo Researchers, Inc.; Fig. 28.2c: © Volker Steger/Peter Arnold, Inc.; Fig. 28.2d, Fig. 28.3: © Morendum Animal Health, Ltd./SPL/Photo Researchers, Inc.; Fig. 28.4a–b: © David Scharf/Peter Arnold, Inc.; Fig. 28.5a: © J.H. Robinson/Photo Researchers, Inc.; Fig. 28.5b: © Dickson Despommier/Photo Researchers, Inc.; Fig. 28.5c: © Dr. Tony Brain/SPL/Photo Researchers, Inc.; Fig. 28.5d: © Scott Camazine/Photo Researchers, Inc.; Fig. 28.5e: © SIU/Peter Arnold, Inc.; Fig. 28.6a–f, Fig. 28.7, Fig. 28.8, Fig. 28.9, Fig. 28.13: © Cliff Moore; Fig. 28.15a–b: © Martin M. Rotker; Fig. 28.16: Courtesy Orion Diagnostica, OY, Finland/Life Sign, LLC; Fig. 28.18: © John Durham/SPL/Photo Researchers, Inc.; Fig. 28.20: © Dr. E. Buttane/Peter Arnold, Inc.; Fig. 28.21: Courtesy Becton Dickinson Diagnostic Systems; Fig. 28.22: © Cliff Moore.

CHAPTER 29 Fig. 29.5: © David Kelly Crow.

CHAPTER 30 Page 595: © Terry Wild Studio; Fig. 30.12: Courtesy Becton Dickinson; Fig. 30.13: Courtesy of Total Care Programming; Fig. 30.14, Fig. 30.15, Fig. 30.16: © Terry Wild Studio; Fig. 30.17: Courtesy Total Care Programming; Fig. 30.21: © Nicholas Thomas/Medical Image, Inc.; Fig. 30.28: © Terry Wild Studio; Fig. 30.29, Fig. 30.30, Fig. 30.31, Fig. 30.32: Courtesy Becton Dickinson.

CHAPTER 31 Fig. 31.1: © Spangler Studio/Merrill Property; Fig. 31.2, Fig. 31.3: Ken Lax; Fig. 31.4: © Tom Dunham; Fig. 31.5, Fig. 31.6: © Elaine Shay/Merrill Property; Fig. 31.7, Fig. 31.8: Ken Lax; Fig. 31.9, Fig. 31.10: © David Kelly Crow; Fig. 31.11, Fig. 31.12: Ken Lax; Fig. 31.19: Robert Matthews.

CHAPTER 32 Fig. 32.2: © David Kelly Crow; Fig. 32.3a: © R.J. Erwin/Photo Researchers, Inc.; Fig. 32.3b: © Andrew McClenaghan/SPL/Photo Researchers, Inc.; Fig. 32.4: © Terry Wild Studio; Fig. 32.5: © David Kelly Crow.

CHAPTER 33 Fig. 33.1: Center Laboratories; Fig. 33.2, Fig. 33.3, Fig. 33.4: © Cliff Moore; Fig. 33.8, Fig. 33.10: Courtesy of Total Care Programming; Fig. 33.11, Fig. 33.23: © Cliff Moore.

CHAPTER 34 Fig. 34.3a–b, Fig. 34.4: Courtesy Burdick, Inc.; Fig. 34.5: © Cliff Moore; Fig. 34.8, Fig. 34.9: © David Kelly Crow Fig. 34.17: © Cliff Moore; Fig. 34.18, 34.19, Fig. 34.20, Fig. 34.21, Fig. 34.22: © David Kelly Crow; Page 738: © Robert Crandall/Medical Images, Inc.; Fig. 34.24, Fig. 34.26a–b, Fig. 34.28: © Cliff Moore.

CHAPTER 35 Fig. 35.1: © Cliff Moore; Fig. 35.2a–d: © Martin M. Rotker; Fig. 35.3: © Cliff Moore; Page 753: © David Kelly Crow; Fig. 35.4a: Courtesy of Radiology Affiliates of Central NJ, PA; Mercerville, NJ; Fig. 35.4b: Courtesy of Virtual Healthscan; Fig. 35.4c: Courtesy of Mercer Medical Center, Dept. of Radiology, Trenton, NJ; Fig. 35.4d: Courtesy of Virtual Healthscan; Fig. 35.4e: Courtesy of MRI Center at Lawrenceville, NJ; Fig. 35.5: © NIH/Science Source/Photo Researchers, Inc.; Fig. 35.6a: © Stephen Gerard/Science Source/Photo Researchers, Inc.; Fig. 35.6b: © Scott Camazine/Photo Researchers, Inc.; Fig. 35.7: Courtesy of Mercer Medical Center, Dept. of Radiology, Trenton, NJ; Fig. 35.8: © P. Sadda/Eurelios/SPL/Photo Researchers, Inc.; Fig. 35.9, Fig. 35.11: © Cliff Moore.

CHAPTER 36 Fig. 36.10: © David Kelly Crow.

Text and Line Art Credits

CHAPTER 2 Fig. 2.12: Adult immunization, (National Coalition for Adult Immunization. Reprinted with permission.).

CHAPTER 3 Table 3.1: Source: Centers for Disease Control and Prevention; Table 3.2: Source: US Department of Health and Human Services; Food and Drug Administration and AIDSInfo; Table 3.3: Source: *"State Health Facts Online,"* The Henry J. Kaiser Family Foundation, www.kff.org. This information was reprinted with permission from the Henry J. Kaiser Family Foundation. The Kaiser Family Foundation, based in Menlo Park, California, is a nonprofit, independent national health care philanthropy and is not associated with Kaiser Permanente or Kaiser Industries.

CHAPTER 5 Fig. 5.2: Seeley-*Essentials of Anatomy and Physiology* 5th ed. McGraw-Hill © 2005; Fig. 5.6–5.13: Shier-*Hole's Essentials of Human Anatomy and Physiology* 8th ed. McGraw-Hill © 2003.

CHAPTER 6 Fig. 6.1, 6.4, 6.6: Shier-*Hole's Essentials of Human Anatomy and Physiology* 8th ed. McGraw-Hill © 2003; Fig. 6.5: Mader-*Understanding Human Anatomy and Physiology* 4th ed. McGraw-Hill © 2001.

CHAPTER 7 Fig. 7.1, 7.3, 7.4, 7.6–7.9, 7.12: Shier-*Hole's Essentials of Human Anatomy and Physiology* 8th ed. McGraw-Hill © 2003; Fig. 7.5: Mader-*Understanding Human Anatomy and Physiology* 4th ed. McGraw-Hill © 2001; Fig. 7.10, 7.11: Saladin-*Anatomy and Physiology: The Unity of Form and Function* 3rd ed. McGraw-Hill © 2004; Fig. 7.11: Saladin-*Anatomy and Physiology: The Unity of Form and Function* 3rd ed. McGraw-Hill © 2004.

CHAPTER 8 Fig. 8.1–8.9: Shier-*Hole's Essentials of Human Anatomy and Physiology* 8th ed. McGraw-Hill © 2003.

CHAPTER 9 Fig. 9.2–9.4, 9.7, 9.8: Shier-*Hole's Essentials of Human Anatomy and Physiology* 8th ed. McGraw-Hill © 2003; Fig. 9.5: Mader-*Understanding Human Anatomy and Physiology* 4th ed. McGraw-Hill © 2001; Fig. 9.6: Saladin-*Anatomy and Physiology: The Unity of Form and Function* 3rd ed. McGraw-Hill © 2004.

CHAPTER 10 Fig. 10.1–10.6, 10.8, 10.10–10.14, 10.20–10.21, 10.23–10.29: Shier-*Hole's Essentials of Human Anatomy and Physiology* 8th ed. McGraw-Hill © 2003.

CHAPTER 11 Fig. 11.1–11.2: Shier-*Hole's Essentials of Human Anatomy and Physiology* 8th ed. McGraw-Hill © 2003.

CHAPTER 12 Fig. 12.1–12.3: Mader-*Understanding Human Anatomy and Physiology* 4th ed. McGraw-Hill © 2001; Context (pg 202) Scale to determine the severity of snoring, adapted from The Mayo Clinic's Sleep Disorders Center.

CHAPTER 13 Fig. 13.1–13.12: Shier-*Hole's Essentials of Human Anatomy and Physiology* 8th ed. McGraw-Hill © 2003.

CHAPTER 14 Fig. 14.1–14.2: Shier-*Hole's Essentials of Human Anatomy and Physiology* 8th ed. McGraw-Hill © 2003.

CHAPTER 15 Fig. 15.1, 15.4, 15.5: Shier-*Hole's Essentials of Human Anatomy and Physiology* 8th ed. McGraw-Hill © 2003; Fig. 15.2–15.3: Mader-*Understanding Human Anatomy and Physiology* 4th ed. McGraw-Hill © 2001.

CHAPTER 16 Fig. 16.1–16.6: Shier-*Hole's Essentials of Human Anatomy and Physiology* 8th ed. McGraw-Hill © 2003.

CHAPTER 17 Fig. 17.1–17.11: Shier-*Hole's Essentials of Human Anatomy and Physiology* 8th ed. McGraw-Hill © 2003.

CHAPTER 19 Fig. 19.8: *Source:* Kathryn Booth, *Health Care Science Technology,* 1st ed. Peoria, IL: Glencoe/McGraw-Hill, 2004.

CHAPTER 20 Fig. 20.11: Adapted from The National Cancer Institute includes these instructions and illustrations in the brochure *Breast Exams: What You Should Know* (NIH Publications No. 90-2000).

CHAPTER 22 Fig. 22.2: From Corbin et. al., *Concepts of Physical Fitness* 11/e © 2003 The McGraw-Hill Companies. Reprinted by permission. All rights reserved; Fig. 22.14: From Seeley *Anatomy & Physiology* 6th ed. © 2003 The McGraw-Hill Companies. Reprinted by permission. All rights reserved.

CHAPTER 24 Fig. 24.20: *Source:* Keir, Wise, and Krebs, *Medical Assisting Administrative and Clinical Competencies,* 5th ed. 2003, p. 763.

CHAPTER 25 Fig. 25.6: *Source:* McGraw-Hill *Health Care Science Technology* by Booth, 2004; Fig. 25.8: teaching a patient to walk with crutches, borrowed from McGraw-Hill *Health Care Science Technology* by Booth, 2004.

CHAPTER 26 Fig. 26.20: *Source: Glencoe Health Care Science Technology,* Booth 2004, p. 98; Fig. 26.21: *Source: Glencoe Health Care Science Technology,* Booth 2004, p. 101, Fig. 4.8.

CHAPTER 27 Fig. 27.11: (Courtesy of Medical Chemical Corp.)

CHAPTER 28 Table 28.3: Source: Centers for Disease Control, Health Topics A to Z. Atlanta, Georgia, 2003 http://www.cdc.gov/health/default.htm.

CHAPTER 30 Fig. 30.3: Source: Adapted from Norbert W. Tietz, ed., *Clinical Guide to Laboratory Tests,* 3rd ed. (Philadelphia: W.B. Saunders, 1995.)

CHAPTER 31 Table 31.1: Adapted from Marvin R. Levy et. al., *Life & Health: Targeting Wellness* (New York: McGraw-Hill, 1992; Table 31.3: Reprinted with permission from (Recommended Dietary Allowances: 10th Edition) © (1989) by the National Academy of Sciences, courtesy of the National Academies Press, Washington, D.C.; Table 31.4–31.5: Source: Nutrition and Your Health: *Dietary Guidelines for Americans,* 5th ed. (Washington, DC: U.S. Department of Agriculture and U.S. Department of Health and Human Services, 2000.); Fig. 31.14: *Source:* 1998 American Dietetic Association. Reprinted with permission.

CHAPTER 32 Table 32.1: Adapted from "The Top 200 Prescriptions for 200 by Number of US Prescriptions Dispensed." RxList: The Internet Drug Index, www.rxlist.com.; Table 32.2: Sources: *Physicians' Desk Reference: U.S. Pharmacopeia Dictionary;* Table 32.3: Source: U.S. Department of Justice, *Physician's Manual,* March 1990.

CHAPTER 33 Table 33.7: Source: *2004 Physicians' Desk Reference,* Thompson Healthcare.

CHAPTER 34 Fig. 34.11: Courtesy of Burdick, Inc., Milton, Wisconsin; Fig. 34.12–34.16: Courtesy of Burdick, Inc; Table 34.4: Adapted from *Illustrated Guide to Diagnostic Tests* (Springhouse, PA: Springhouse, 1998).

CHAPTER 36 Fig. 36.9: (reprinted with permission from Kelly Assisted Living Services, Inc.) Context (pg. 786) *Source: Peak Performance: Success in College and Beyond,* 4th ed., Sharon K. Ferret, McGraw-Hill, 2003. Text (pg. 787) *Source:* Highline Community College, Counceling/Career Center, Des Moines, WA.

Index

Page numbers in **boldface** indicate figures. Page numbers followed by (b) indicate box features, (p) procedures, and (t) tables, respectively.